Clinical Guidelines
for Advanced Practice Nursing

■ ■ ■ ■ ■ ■ ■ ■ ■

An Interdisciplinary Approach

SECOND EDITION

Edited by

Geraldine M. Collins-Bride, RN, ANP-BC, MS

Health Sciences Clinical Professor
Adult Nurse Practitioner
University of California, San Francisco
School of Nursing
Department of Community Health Systems

JoAnne M. Saxe, RN, ANP-BC, MS, DNP

Health Sciences Clinical Professor
Adult Nurse Practitioner
University of California, San Francisco
School of Nursing
Department of Community Health Systems

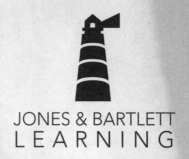

JONES & BARTLETT
LEARNING

World Headquarters
Jones & Bartlett Learning
5 Wall Street
Burlington, MA 01803
978-443-5000
info@jblearning.com
www.jblearning.com

Jones & Bartlett Learning books and products are available through most bookstores and online booksellers. To contact Jones & Bartlett Learning directly, call 800-832-0034, fax 978-443-8000, or visit our website, www.jblearning.com.

Substantial discounts on bulk quantities of Jones & Bartlett Learning publications are available to corporations, professional associations, and other qualified organizations. For details and specific discount information, contact the special sales department at Jones & Bartlett Learning via the above contact information or send an email to specialsales@jblearning.com.

The authors, editor, and publisher have made every effort to provide accurate information. However, they are not responsible for errors, omissions, or for any outcomes related to the use of the contents of this book and take no responsibility for the use of the products and procedures described. Treatments and side effects described in this book may not be applicable to all people; likewise, some people may require a dose or experience a side effect that is not described herein. Drugs and medical devices are discussed that may have limited availability controlled by the Food and Drug Administration (FDA) for use only in a research study or clinical trial. Research, clinical practice, and government regulations often change the accepted standard in this field. When consideration is being given to use of any drug in the clinical setting, the health care provider or reader is responsible for determining FDA status of the drug, reading the package insert, and reviewing prescribing information for the most up-to-date recommendations on dose, precautions, and contraindications, and determining the appropriate usage for the product. This is especially important in the case of drugs that are new or seldom used.

Production Credits

Publisher: Kevin Sullivan
Acquisitions Editor: Amanda Harvey
Editorial Assistant: Sara Bempkins
Associate Production Editor: Cindie Bryan
Marketing Manager: Elena McAnespie
V.P., Manufacturing and Inventory Control: Therese Connell
Compositor: Arlene Apone
Cover Design: Kristin E. Parker
Associate Photo Researcher: Lauren Miller
Cover Image: © Comstock/Thinkstock
Photo credit for Florence Nightingale Image: Courtesy of the National Library of Medicine
Printing and Binding: Courier Kendallville
Cover Printing: Courier Kendallville

Some images in this book feature models. These models do not necessarily endorse, represent, or participate in the activities represented in the images.

Library of Congress Cataloging-in-Publication Data
Clinical guidelines for advanced practice nursing : an interdisciplinary approach / [edited by] Geraldine M. Collins-Bride, JoAnne M. Saxe. – 2nd ed.
     p. ; cm.
  Rev. ed. of: Nurse practitioner/physician collaborative practice / edited by Geraldine M. Collins-Bride and JoAnne M. Saxe. San Francisco, Calif. : School of Nursing, University of California, UCSF Nursing Press, c1998.
  Includes bibliographical references and index.
  ISBN 978-0-7637-7414-1 (pbk.)
  1. Nurse practitioners. 2. Primary care (Medicine). 3. Nursing. I. Collins-Bride, Geraldine M. II. Saxe, JoAnne M. III. Nurse practitioner/physician collaborative practice.
  [DNLM: 1. Advanced Practice Nursing–Guideline. 2. Clinical Protocols–standards–Guideline. 3. Nursing Care–methods–Guideline. WY 128]
  RT82.8.C5553 2012
  610.73--dc23
                    2011019904

6048
Printed in the United States of America
15   10 9 8 7 6 5

DEDICATION

To our patients and students, we appreciate the many lessons that we have learned from you and the trust that you have given us over the years. We are privileged to have been your healthcare provider and/or mentor.

GCB and JMS

To my "boys" (Bob, Patrick, & Brendan) who are ecstatic that this book is finished! Thanks for putting up with my many late nights and missed dinners. And to my sister Tricia who loved the written word and was one of my biggest fans. Miss you Trish.

GCB

To my mother, Patricia, father, John, husband, Noel, daughters, Kelly, Jocelyn and Lydia, son-in-law, Benny, daughter-in-law, Marlene and all of my wonderful brothers and sisters for your years of support, love and laughter. Thank you for all that you are and do!

JMS

CONTENTS

Acknowledgments   xiii
Contributors   xv
Introduction   xxiii

 Legal Scope of Advanced Nursing Practice   1
Brian Budds and JoAnne M. Saxe
Introduction   1
Overview of Scope of Practice Legal Framework   1
Issues Related to Collaborative Practice
    and Documentation   4
Concluding Remarks   5

SECTION I   Pediatric Health Maintenance and Promotion   7

2   First Well-Baby Visit   9
Annette Carley
I.   Introduction and general background   9
II.   Database   9
III.   Assessment   11
IV.   Goals of first well-baby visit   11
V.   Plan   11
VI.   Resources and tools   12

3   Care of the Postneonatal Intensive Care Unit Graduate   13
Annette Carley
I.   Introduction and general background   13
II.   Database   15
III.   Assessment   16
IV.   Goals of clinical management   17
V.   Plan   17
VI.   Resources and tools   17

4   0 to 3 Years of Age Interval Visit   19
Ann Birenbaum Baker
I.   Introduction   19
II.   Database   19
III.   Assessment   21
IV.   Plan   21

5   3 to 6 Years of Age Interval Visit   25
Angel K. Chen
I.   Introduction and general background   25
II.   Database   25
III.   Assessment   26
IV.   Plan   27

6   6 to 11 Years of Age Interval Visit   29
*Bridget Ward Gramkowski and
Ann Birenbaum Baker*
I.   Definition   29
II.   Database   29
III.   Assessment   30
IV.   Plan   31

7   The Adolescent and Young Adult (12–21 Years of Age) Interval Visit   35
Erica Monasterio
I.   Introduction and general background   35
II.   Database   36
III.   Assessment   38
IV.   Plan   39
V.   Self management resources   40
Appendix 7-1: Childhood and Adolescent
    Immunization Schedules   43

8   Developmental Assessment: Screening for Developmental Delay and Autism   57
Abbey Alkon
I.   Introduction   57
II.   Developmental surveillance and
    screening algorithm   58
III.   Screening instruments   61
IV.   Psychometrics   61
V.   Conclusion   69
VI.   Clinician resources   69

SECTION II Common Pediatric Presentations 73

9 Atopic Dermatitis in Children 75
Karen G. Duderstadt and Nan Madden

I.   Introduction and general background   75
II. Database   75
III. Assessment   79
IV. Goals of clinical management   79
V.   Plan   80
VI. Self-management   83
VII. Psychosocial and emotional support   83

10 Attention-Deficit/Hyperactivity Disorder in Children and Adolescents 85
Naomi Schapiro

I.   Introduction   85
II. Overview   85
III. Database: history   86
IV. Database: physical examination   88
V.   Assessment   88
VI. Plan   89

11 Childhood Asthma 95
Andrea Crosby, Nan Madden, and Shannon Thyne

I.   Introduction and general background   95
II. Database   95
III. Assessment   96
IV. Goals of clinical management   96
V.   Plan   96

12 Childhood Depression 103
Damon Michael Williams

I.   Introduction   103
II. Database guidelines   104
III. Assessment   105
IV. Plan   106
V.   Self-management resources   109

13 Child Maltreatment 111
Naomi Schapiro

I.   Introduction   111
II. Database   113
III. Assessment   117
IV. Plan   118

14 Failure to Thrive During Infancy 121
Annette Carley

I.   Introduction and general background   121
II. Database   122
III. Assessment   123
IV. Goals of clinical management   123
V.   Plan   124
VI. Resources   125

15 Urinary Incontinence in Children 127
Angel K. Chen

I.   Introduction and general background   127
II. Database   129
III. Assessment   131
IV. Goals of clinical management   134
V.   Plan   134
VI. Self-management resources and tools   140

SECTION III Gynecology 143

16 Abnormal Uterine Bleeding 145
Kim K. O-Hair, Geraldine Collins-Bride, and Fran Dreier

I.   Introduction and general background   145
II. Database   148
III. Assessment   150
IV. Goals of clinical management   150
V.   Plan   150
VI. Self-management resources and tools   155

17 Amenorrhea and Polycystic Ovary Syndrome 157
Pilar Bernal de Pheils

I.   Introduction and general background   157
II. Database   159
III. Assessment   161
IV. Goals of clinical management   161
V.   Plan   161
VI. Self-management resources and tools   169

18 Cervical, Vaginal, and Vulvar Cancer Screening 171
Mary M. Rubin and Lynn Hanson

I.   Introduction and general background   171
II. Database   179
III. Assessment   179

IV. Goals of clinical management 180
V. Plan 180

19 Female and Male Sterilization 183
Janis Luft
I. Introduction and general background 183
II. Database 184
III. Assessment 184
IV. Plan 184
V. Self-management resources 185

20 Hormonal Contraception 187
Lynn Hanson
I. Introduction and general background 187
II. Database 195
III. Assessment 196
IV. Goals of clinical management 196
V. Plan 196
Appendix 20-1: Comparison of Oral
Contraceptives 200

21 Menopause Transition 209
Priscilla Abercrombie
I. Introduction and general background 209
II. Database 210
III. Assessment 211
IV. Goals of clinical management 212
V. Plan 212
VI. Self-management resources and tools 216
VII. Clinical practice guidelines 216

22 Nonhormonal Contraception 219
Kimberley Chastain
I. Introduction and general background 219
II. Database 223
III. Assessment 224
IV. Goals of clinical management 224
V. Plan 224
VI. Self-management resources and tools 225

23 Urinary Incontinence in Women 227
Janis Luft
I. Introduction and general background 227
II. Initial evaluation 228
III. Assessment 229
IV. Goals of clinical management 229
V. Plan 230
VI. Self-management resources and tools 233

SECTION IV Obstetric Health Maintenance and Promotion 235

24 The Initial Prenatal Visit 237
Rebekah Kaplan
I. Definition and background 237
II. Database 237
III. Assessment 239
IV. Plan 239
V. Internet resources 240

25 Prenatal Genetic Screening 245
Deborah Anderson and Amy J. Levi
I. Introduction and general background 245
II. Database 246
III. Assessment 247
IV. Plan 247

26 The Return Prenatal Visit 249
Rebekah Kaplan and Margaret Hutchison
I. Definition and background 249
II. Database 249
III. Assessment 251
IV. Plan 251

27 The Postpartum Visit 255
Jenna Shaw-Battista
I. Introduction and general background 255
II. Database 255
III. Assessment 256
IV. Plan 256

28 Guidelines for Medical Consultation and Referral During Pregnancy 259
Jenna Shaw-Battista

SECTION V Common Obstetric Presentations 261

29 Anemia in Pregnancy 263
Laurie Jurkiewicz
I. Introduction and general background 263
II. Database 264
III. Assessment 264
IV. Plan 264

30 **Birth Choices for Women with a Previous Cesarean Delivery 267**

Rebekah Kaplan

I.   Introduction and general background 267
II. Data collection 267
III. Risks and benefits of TOL versus repeat cesarean delivery 267
IV. Assessment 269
V.   Plan 269
VI. Internet resources for providers, patients, and families 269

31 **Common Discomforts of Pregnancy 273**

Cynthia Belew and Jamie Meyerhoff

I.   Introduction to common discomforts of pregnancy 273
II. Musculoskeletal 273
III. Gastrointestinal tract 276
IV. Heartburn 278

32 **Gestational Diabetes Mellitus: Early Detection and Management in Pregnancy 285**

Maribeth Inturrisi, Julio Diaz-Abarca, and JoAnne M. Saxe

I.   Introduction and general background 285
II. Database 286
III. Assessment 286
IV. Plan 288

33 **Preeclampsia 291**

Jenna Shaw-Battista

I.   Introduction and general background 291
II. Database 291
III. Assessment 292
IV. Plan 292

34 **Prenatal Genetic Diagnosis 295**

Deborah Anderson and Amy J. Levi

I.   Introduction and general background 295
II. Database 295
III. Assessment 296
IV. Plan 296

35 **Preterm Labor Management 297**

Mary Barger

I.   Introduction and general background 297
II. Database 297

III. Assessment 298
IV. Plan 298

36 **Urinary Tract Infection: Prevention and Management in Pregnancy 301**

Mary Barger

I.   Introduction and general background 301
II. Database 301
III. Assessment 302
IV. Plan 302

SECTION VI **Adult Health Maintenance and Promotion 305**

37 **Healthcare Maintenance of the Adult 307**

Hattie C. Grundland and JoAnne M. Saxe

I.   Introduction and general background 307
II. Database 307
III. Assessment 308
IV. Plan 309

38 **Healthcare Maintenance for Adults with Developmental Disabilities 319**

Geraldine Collins-Bride and Clarissa Kripke

I.   Introduction and general background 319
II. Database 322
III. Assessment 324
IV. Plan 325
V.   Self-management resources and tools 334

39 **Healthcare Maintenance for Transgendered Individuals 337**

Charles E. Williamson

I.   Introduction and general background 337
II. Database 337
III. Assessment 338
IV. Plan 338
V.   Self-management resources and tools 339

40 **Postexposure Prophylaxis for HIV Infection 343**

Barbara Newlin

I.   Definition and overview 343
II. Database 343

III. Assessment 348
IV. Plan 348
V. Clinician and patient resources 349

SECTION VII Common Adult Presentations 353

41 Abscess Assessment and Management 355

Rosalie D. Bravo

I. Introduction and general background 355
II. Database 355
III. Assessment 356
IV. Plan 356

42 Anemia 361

Michelle M. Marin

I. Introduction and general background 361
II. Database 365
III. Physical examination 367
IV. Assessment 367
V. Goals of clinical management 370
VI. Plan 370
VII. Self-management resources and tools 372

43 Anticoagulation Therapy (Oral) 373

Fran Dreier and Linda Ray

I. Introduction 373
II. Patient education and safety 378

44 Anxiety 387

Esker-D Ligon and Donald E. Tarver II

I. Introduction and general background 387
II. Database 388
III. Assessment 389
IV. Plan 390
V. Special populations 392
VI. Self-management resources and tools 393

45 Asthma in Adolescents and Adults 395

Susan L. Janson

I. Introduction and general background 395
II. Database 396
III. Assessment 397
IV. Goals of clinical management to control asthma 399
V. Plan 399

46 Benign Prostatic Hyperplasia 409

Jean N. Taylor-Woodbury

I. Introduction and general background 409
II. Database 410
III. Assessment 411
IV. Goals of clinical management 411
V. Plan 411
VI. Self-management resources and tools 414
Appendix 46-1: The American Urological Association (AUA) Symptom Index for Benign Prostatic Hyperplasia (BPH) and the Disease Specific Quality of Life Question 415
Appendix 46-2: Benign Prostatic Hyperplasia (BPH) Impact Index ("Bother" Score) 416

47 Chronic Obstructive Pulmonary Disease 417

Lynda A. Mackin

I. Introduction and general background 417
II. Database 417
III. Goals of clinical management 418
IV. Components of COPD management 419
V. Care from a population health perspective 422

48 Chronic Nonmalignant Pain Management 423

Kellie McNerney, JoAnne M. Saxe, and Kelly Pfeifer

I. Introduction and general background 423
II. Database 424
III. Assessment 425
IV. Goals of clinical management 425
V. Plan 425
VI. Patient education 435
VII. Chronic pain support resources and tools 435

49 Chronic Viral Hepatitis 437

Miranda Surjadi

I. Introduction and general background 437
II. Database 438
III. Assessment 441
IV. Goals of clinical management 441
V. Plan 442
VI. Self-management resources and tools 444

50 Congestive Heart Failure 445

Barbara Boland

I. Introduction and general background 445
II. Database 446

III. Assessment 447
IV. Goals of clinical management 447
V. Plan 447
VI. Self-management resources and tools 450

51 Dementia 451
Jennifer Merrilees
I. Introduction and general background 451
II. Database 452
III. Assessment 456
IV. Goals of clinical management 456
V. Plan 456
VI. Assessment and management of concomitant conditions 459
VII. Assessment of the status of the family and caregiver 459
VIII. General resources 459

52 Depression 461
Matt Tierney and Beth Phoenix
I. Introduction and general background 461
II. Database 463
III. Assessment 464
IV. Goals of clinical management 465
V. Plan 466
VI. Self-management resources and tools 466

53 Diabetes Mellitus 475
Barbara A. Boland
I. Introduction, general background, prevalence, and incidence 475
II. Database 475
III. Assessment 476
IV. Goals of clinical management 477
V. Plan 477
VI. Self-management resources and tools 482

54 Epilepsy 485
M. Robin Taylor and Paul Garcia
I. Definition and description 485
II. Database 485
III. Assessment 486
IV. Goals of clinical management 486
V. Plan 486
VI. Self-management resources 490

55 Low Back Pain 491
H. Kate Lawlor
I. Introduction and general background 491
II. Database 491
III. Assessment 496
IV. Plan 496
V. Self-management resources and tools 500

56 Gastroesophageal Reflux Disease 501
Karen C. Bagatelos, Geraldine Collins-Bride, and Fran Dreier
I. Definition and overview 501
II. Database 502
III. Assessment 503
IV. Goals of clinical management 503
V. Plan 503
VI. Self-management resources 506

57 Herpes Simplex Infections 509
Hattie C. Grundland and Geraldine Collins-Bride
I. Introduction and general background 509
II. Database 510
III. Assessment 511
IV. Goals of clinical management 511
V. Plan 512
VI. Self-management resources and tools 514

58 Hypertension 515
Judith Sweet
I. Introduction and definition 515
II. Database 515
III. Assessment 518
IV. Goals of clinical management 518
V. Plan and management 518

59 Intimate Partner Violence (Domestic Violence) 527
Cecily Cosby, JoAnne M. Saxe, and Janice Humphreys
I. Introduction 527
II. Database 528
III. Assessment 531
IV. Goals of clinical management 531
V. Plan 532
VI. Self-management resources and tools 533

Irritable Bowel Syndrome 537

Karen C. Bagatelos and Geraldine Collins-Bride

I. Definition and overview 537
II. Database 538
III. Assessment 538
IV. Goals of clinical management 539
V. Plan 539
VI. Self-management eResources 543

61 Neck Pain 545

Rossana Segovia-Bain

I. Introduction and general background 545
II. Database 547
III. Assessment 549
IV. Goals of clinical management 549
V. Plan 549
VI. Self-management resources and tools 552

62 Obesity 553

*Sherri Borden, David Besio,
and Geraldine Collins-Bride*

I. Introduction and general background 553
II. Database 555
III. Assessment 556
IV. Goals of clinical management 557
V. Plan 557
VI. Self-management resources 564

63 Osteoarthritis 567

Diane Putney and JoAnne M. Saxe

I. Introduction and general background 567
II. Database 568
III. Assessment 571
IV. Goals of clinical management 572
V. Plan 572
VI. Self-management resources and tools 579
VII. Acknowledgments 580

 Primary Care of HIV-Infected Adults 583

Suzan Stringari-Murray

I. Introduction 583
II. Database 586

III. Assessment 590
IV. Plan 590

65 Smoking Cessation 597

Kellie McNerney and Vicki Smith

I. Introduction and general background 597
II. Database 599
III. Assessment 600
IV. Plan 600
V. Self-management resources and support 602
VI. Consultation 602

66 Thyroid Disorders 605

JoAnne M. Saxe

I. Introduction and general background 605
II. Database 606
III. Assessment 607
IV. Goals of clinical management 610
V. Plan 610
VI. Self-management resources and tools 612

67 Upper Extremity Tendinopathy: Bicipital Tendinopathy, Lateral Epicondylitis, and DeQuervain's Tenosynovitis 615

Barbara J. Burgel

I. Introduction and general background 615
II. Database 616
III. Assessment 618
IV. Goals of clinical management 618
V. Plan 618
VI. Self-management resources and tools 620

68 Wound Care 623

Nancy A. Stotts

I. Introduction and general background 623
II. Database 623
III. Assessment 626
IV. Goals of clinical management 626
V. Plan 626
VI. Self-management resources and tools 628

Index 629

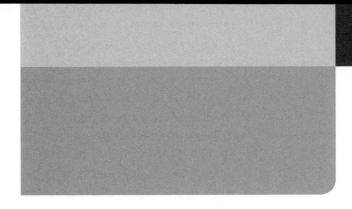

ACKNOWLEDGMENTS

The Editors would like to acknowledge the following individuals for their contributions to the publication of this book:

- Rocel Ryan, our wonderful editorial assistant for her editorial and organizational skills and emotional support during some difficult moments! We congratulate Rocel for joining the nursing profession this year as a new RN.

- Dr. Carmen Portillo, Chair of the Department of Community Health Systems in the School of Nursing at UCSF for her support and commitment to publishing.

- Faculty colleagues at UCSF in the Schools of Nursing, Medicine, Pharmacy, and Dentistry and the Department of Physical Therapy who contributed much time and expertise as authors and reviewers of this manuscript. We are grateful for having such an esteemed team.

CONTRIBUTORS

Editors and Authors

Geraldine M. Collins-Bride, RN, ANP-BC, MS
Clinical Professor & Vice Chair of Faculty Practice
Department of Community Health Systems

Director of Clinical Education & Training
Office of Developmental Primary Care
Department of Family and Community Medicine
University of California, San Francisco
San Francisco, CA

JoAnne M. Saxe, RN, ANP-BC, MS, DNP*
Clinical Professor
Associate Director, Adult Nurse Practitioner Masters
    Specialty Program
Department of Community Health Systems
University of California, San Francisco School of Nursing
San Francisco, CA

Adult Nurse Practitioner
Glide Health Services
San Francisco, CA

Authors

Priscilla Abercrombie, RN, NP, PhD, AHN-BC
Associate Clinical Professor
Department of Community Health Systems
Nurse Practitioner
San Francisco General Hospital, Women's Health Center
Osher Center for Integrative Medicine & Chronic Pelvic Pain Clinic
University of California, San Francisco
San Francisco, CA

Abbey Alkon, RN, PNP, PhD
Professor
Director, California Childcare Health Program
Department of Family Health Care Nursing
University of California, San Francisco
San Francisco, CA

Deborah Anderson, MS, CNM
Associate Clinical Professor
Department of Obstetrics, Gynecology & Reproductive Sciences
San Francisco General Hospital Division
University of California, San Francisco School of Nursing
San Francisco, CA

Karen C. Bagatelos, RN, MSN, FNP
Assistant Clinical Professor & Nurse Practitioner
Department of Community Health Systems
Department of Medicine, Division of Gastroenterology
University of California, San Francisco
San Francisco, CA

Mary Barger, RN, CNM, MPH, PhD
Assistant Professor
Department of Family Health Care Nursing
University of California, San Francisco
San Francisco, CA

Cynthia Belew, CNM, MS
Associate Clinical Professor
Department of Obstetrics, Gynecology & Reproductive Sciences
University of California, San Francisco School of Nursing
San Francisco General Hospital Division
San Francisco, CA

Pilar Bernal de Pheils, RN, MS, FNP-BC, CNM, FAAN*
Clinical Professor
Department of Family Health Care Nursing
University of California, San Francisco
San Francisco, CA

David Besio, MS, RD
Clinical Dietitian
UCSF Adult Weight Management Program
Nutrition and Food Services
University of California, San Francisco Medical Center
San Francisco, CA

Ann Birenbaum Baker, RN, MS, CPNP
Pediatric Nurse Practitioner
Well Baby Nursery
University of California, San Francisco
San Francisco, CA

Barbara A. Boland, RN, MS, ANP-BC, CDE
Edward S. Cooper Practice
University of Pennsylvania Health System
Philadelphia, PA

Sherri Borden, RN, ANP, CNS
Adult Nurse Practitioner & Psychiatric Clinical Nurse Specialist
    & Assistant Clinical Professor
Department of Community Health Systems
University of California, San Francisco School of Nursing
San Francisco, CA

Rosalie D. Bravo, RN, MS, ACNP-BC
Assistant Clinical Professor
Acute Care Nurse Practitioner Program
Department of Physiological Nursing
Acute Care Nurse Practitioner, Division of Emergency Medicine
University of California, San Francisco
San Francisco, CA

Brian Budds, RN, MS, JD
Adult Nurse Practitioner/Attorney at Law
Associate Clinical Professor
Department of Community Health Systems
University of California, San Francisco School of Nursing
San Francisco, CA

Adjunct Professor
University of San Francisco School of Law
San Francisco, CA

Barbara J. Burgel, RN, ANP-BC, PhD, FAAN
Clinical Professor & Certified Occupational Health
    Nurse Specialist
Department of Community Health Systems
University of California, San Francisco School of Nursing
San Francisco, CA

Annette Carley, RN, MS, NNP-BC, PNP-BC
Associate Clinical Professor
Clinical Coordinator, Advanced Practice Neonatal Nursing
    (APNN) Program
Department of Family Health Care Nursing
University of California, San Francisco
San Francisco, CA

Kimberley Chastain, RN, FNP-BC, MSN
Clinician III/Clinician Trainer
Planned Parenthood
San Francisco, CA

Angel K. Chen, RN, MSN, CPNP
Assistant Clinical Professor
Department of Family Health Care Nursing
University of California, San Francisco
San Francisco, CA

Cecily Cosby, RN, MSN, PhD, FNP-C, PA-C, DFAAPA
Professor
Interim Director, Doctor of Nursing Practice (DNP) Program
Samuel Merritt University
Oakland, CA

Lucy S. Crain, MD, MPH, FAAP*
Clinical Professor of Pediatrics Emerita
Consultant in Developmental Pediatrics, ML Johnson Child
    Developmental Unit
Lucile Packard Childrens Hospital, Stanford University
University of California, San Francisco
San Francisco, CA

Andrea Crosby, RN, FNP
Assistant Clinical Professor & Family Nurse Practitioner
Department of Family Health Care Nursing
Assistant Clinical Director, Pediatric Asthma Clinic
    (2007–2010)
Children's Health Center, San Francisco
    General Hospital
University of California, San Francisco
San Francisco, CA

Julio Diaz-Abarca, RN, MSN, CNM
Assistant Clinical Professor
Department of Obstetrics, Gynecology &
    Reproductive Sciences
University of California, San Francisco School of Nursing
San Francisco, CA

Fran Dreier, RN, MHS, FNP*
Associate Clinical Professor & Nurse Practitioner
Department of Community Health Systems
University of California, San Francisco School of Nursing
San Francisco, CA

Karen G. Duderstadt, PhD, RN, CPNP, PCNS
Clinical Professor
Department of Family Health Care Nursing
University of California, San Francisco
San Francisco, CA

Paul Garcia, MD
Professor of Clinical Neurology
Director of Clinical Epilepsy Services
University of California, San Francisco
San Francisco, CA

Bridget Ward Gramkowski, RN, MS, CPNP
Pediatric Nurse Practitioner
Pediatric Associates
San Jose, CA

Hattie C. Grundland, RN, MS, ANP-BC
Assistant Clinical Professor & Nurse Practitioner
Department of Community Health Systems
University of California, San Francisco School of Nursing
San Francisco, CA

Lynn Hanson, RN, MS, WHNP
Associate Clinical Professor & Nurse Practitioner
Department of Obstetrics, Gynecology Faculty Practice
University of California, San Francisco
San Francisco, CA

Janice Humphreys, PhD, RN, NP, FAAN*
Associate Professor & Vice-Chair for Academic Personnel
Department of Family Health Care Nursing
University of California, San Francisco
San Francisco, CA

Margaret Hutchison, RN, MS, CNM
Associate Clinical Professor
Director of Outpatient Services, Nurse-Midwives
    of San Francisco
San Francisco General Hospital
Department of Obstetrics, Gynecology
    & Reproductive Sciences
University of California, San Francisco
San Francisco, CA

Maribeth Inturrisi, RN, MS, CNS, CDE
Assistant Professor
Department of Family Health Care Nursing
Coordinator & Nurse Educator Consultant for the California
    Diabetes and Pregnancy Program
University of California, San Francisco
San Francisco, CA

Certified Diabetes Educator
Sweet Success Program
Sutter Pacific Physician Foundation
San Francisco, CA

Susan L. Janson, DNSc, RN, ANP-C, CNS, AE-C, FAAN
Professor of Nursing and Medicine
Mary Harms/Nursing Alumni Endowed Chair
Department of Community Health Systems
University of California, San Francisco

Laurie Jurkiewicz, RN, MS, CNM
Assistant Clinical Professor
Department of Obstetrics, Gynecology & Reproductive Sciences
University of California, San Francisco School of Nursing
San Francisco General Hospital Division
San Francisco, CA

Rebekah Kaplan, RN, MS, CNM
Associate Clinical Professor
Department of Obstetrics, Gynecology & Reproductive Sciences
University of California, San Francisco
San Francisco General Hospital Division
San Francisco, CA

Clarissa Kripke, MD, FAAFP
Associate Clinical Professor
Director, Office of Developmental Primary Care
Department of Family and Community Medicine
University of California, San Francisco
San Francisco, CA

H. Kate Lawlor, RN, MS, ANP
Associate Clinical Professor & Nurse Practitioner
Department of Community Health Systems, School of Nursing
Instructor, Foundations of Patient Care
School of Medicine
University of California, San Francisco
San Francisco, CA

Amy J. Levi, RN, PhD, CNM, FACNM
Clinical Professor & Certified Nurse–Midwife
Director, Interdepartmental Nurse–Midwifery Education Program
University of California, San Francisco
San Francisco, CA

Esker-D Ligon, RN, MSN, ANP-BC
Assistant Clinical Professor & Nurse Practitioner
Department of Community Health Systems
University of California, San Francisco School of Nursing
San Francisco, CA

Janis Luft, RN, MSN, NP
Associate Clinical Professor & Women's Health
    Nurse Practitioner
Department of Obstetrics, Gynecology & Reproductive Sciences
University of California, San Francisco
San Francisco, CA

Lynda A. Mackin, RN, PhD, GNP-BC, ANP-BC, CNS
Associate Clinical Professor
Department of Physiological Nursing
University of California, San Francisco
San Francisco, CA

Nan Madden, RN, MS, CNS, PNP
Associate Clinical Professor
Department of Family Health Care Nursing
University of California, San Francisco
San Francisco, CA

Clinical Director, Pediatric Asthma Clinic
Children's Health Center
San Francisco General Hospital
San Francisco, CA

Michelle M. Marin, RN, MS, ANP-BC
Assistant Clinical Professor & Nurse Practitioner
Department of Community Health Systems
University of California, San Francisco School of Nursing
San Francisco, CA

Kellie McNerney, RN, FNP, MS
Assistant Clinical Professor & Nurse Practitioner
Department of Community Health Systems
University of California, San Francisco School of Nursing
San Francisco, CA

Jennifer Merrilees, RN, MS, PhD(c)
Associate Professor & Clinical Nurse Specialist
Memory and Aging Center
University of California, San Francisco
San Francisco, CA

Jamie Meyerhoff, RN, CNM
Certified Nurse–Midwife
Midwifery & Women's Health Care at Geneva Woods
Anchorage, AK

Erica Monasterio, RN, MN, FNP-BC
Clinical Professor
Department of Family Health Care Nursing
Division of Adolescent Medicine, Department of Pediatrics
University of California, San Francisco
San Francisco, CA

Barbara Newlin, RN, MN, ANP-BC
Assistant Clinical Professor
Department of Community Health Systems
University of California, San Francisco School of Nursing
San Francisco, CA

Kim K. O'Hair, RN, MSN, NP
Assistant Clinical Professor & Nurse Practitioner
Department of Obstetrics, Gynecology Faculty Practice
University of California, San Francisco
San Francisco, CA

Kelly Pfeifer, MD
Family Physician
Medical Director, San Francisco Health Plan
San Francisco, CA

Beth Phoenix, RN, PhD, CNS
Associate Health Sciences Clinical Professor
Director, Psychiatric Mental Health Graduate Nursing Program
Department of Community Health Systems
University of California, San Francisco School of Nursing
San Francisco, CA

Diane C. Putney, MN, RN, FNP-BC
Department of Orthopedic Surgery
Kaiser Permanente
South San Francisco, CA

Linda Ray, RN, MSN, ANP-BC
Adult Nurse Practitioner
Anticoagulation Clinic, University of California San Francisco
    Medical Center
Assistant Clinical Professor, School of Pharmacy
University of California, San Francisco
San Francisco, CA

Mary Rubin, RN-C, PhD, CRNP, FAANP
Associate Clinical Professor
Department of Obstetrics, Gynecology & Reproductive Sciences
Gynecology, Oncology/Dysplasia Clinical Research
    Nurse Coordinator
Helen Diller Family Comprehensive Cancer Center
University of California, San Francisco
San Francisco, CA

Naomi A. Schapiro, RN, PhD(c), CPNP
Clinical Professor
Department of Family Health Care Nursing
University of California, San Francisco
San Francisco, CA

Rossana Segovia-Bain, RN, MS, ANP-BC, COHN-S*
Assistant Clinical Professor & Nurse Practitioner
Department of Community Health Systems
University of California, San Francisco School of Nursing
San Francisco, CA

Jenna Shaw-Battista, RN, PhD, NP, CNM
Assistant Clinical Professor
Department of Family Health Care Nursing
University of California, San Francisco
San Francisco, CA

Nancy A. Stotts, RN, EdD, FAAN
Professor Emeritus
Department of Physiological Nursing
University of California, San Francisco
San Francisco, CA

Suzan Stringari-Murray, RN, MS, ANP-BC
Clinical Professor
Director, Adult Nurse Practitioner Program
Department of Community Health Systems
University of California, San Francisco School of Nursing
San Francisco, CA

Miranda Surjadi, RN, MS, ANP-BC
Assistant Clinical Professor
Department of Community Health Systems
University of California, San Francisco School of Nursing
San Francisco, CA

Judith Sweet, RN, MS, FNP
Associate Clinical Professor & Nurse Practitioner
Division of General Internal Medicine
University of California, San Francisco
San Francisco, CA

Donald E. Tarver II, MD
Assistant Clinical Professor
Department of Community Health Systems
University of California, San Francisco School of Nursing
San Francisco, CA

Chief Consulting Psychiatrist
Glide Health Services
San Francisco, CA

M. Robin Taylor, MSN, FNP
Clinical Research Manager
Department of Neurology
University of California, San Francisco
San Francisco, CA

Jean N. Taylor-Woodbury, RN, MS, ANP-BC
Assistant Clinical Professor
Department of Community Health Systems
University of California, San Francisco School of Nursing
San Francisco, CA

Shannon Thyne, MD
Associate Professor of Clinical Pediatrics
University of California, San Francisco
San Francisco, CA

Medical Director, Pediatric Asthma Clinic
San Francisco General Hospital
San Francisco, CA

Matt Tierney, RN, NP, CNS
Director, OBIC & COPE Clinics
San Francisco General Hospital Division of Substance Abuse
    and Addiction Medicine
University of California, San Francisco
San Francisco, CA

Damon Michael Williams, RN, PMHNP-BC, MS
Family Psychiatric Nurse Practitioner
Portland, OR

Charles Williamson, RN, MS, ANP-BC

Reviewers

Brian Alldredge, PharmD
Professor of Clinical Pharmacy & Neurology
Associate Dean, Academic Affairs
University of California, San Francisco School of Pharmacy
San Francisco, CA

Amy (Meg) Autry, MD
Professor
Department of Obstetrics, Gynecology &
    Reproductive Sciences
University of California, San Francisco
San Francisco, CA

Peter Berman, MD, MPH
Assistant Clinical Professor
Department of Family and Community Medicine
University of California, San Francisco
San Francisco, CA

Lisa Benaron, MD
Medical Director, Far Northern Regional Center
CHCF Health Care Leadership Program Fellow
University of California, San Francisco Center for the
    Health Professions
San Francisco, CA

Judith Bishop, CNM, MPH
Clinical Professor
Department of Obstetrics, Gynecology &
    Reproductive Sciences
University of California, San Francisco School of Medicine
San Francisco, CA

Laura P. Breckenridge, RN, MSN, CPNP
Certified Pediatric Nurse Practitioner
Primary Care
San Mateo, CA

Allison Bryant, MD, MPH
Assistant Adjunct Professor
Division of Obstetrics & Gynecology, Perinatal Medicine
    & Genetics
University of California, San Francisco
San Francisco, CA

Virginia Carrieri-Kohlman, RN, DNSc, FAAN
Professor
Department of Physiological Nursing
University of California, San Francisco
San Francisco, CA

Aaron B. Caughey, MD, MPP, MPH, PhD
Professor and Chair
Department of Obstetrics & Gynecology
Julie Neupert Stott Director
Center for Women's Health
Oregon Health & Science University
Portland, OR

R. Krishna Chaganti, MD, MS
Assistant Clinical Professor
Division of Rheumatology
University of California, San Francisco
San Francisco, CA

Angelique Champeau, RN, MN, CPNP
Pediatric Nurse Practitioner
UCSF Children's Hospital
Division of Urology Faculty Practice
University of California, San Francisco
San Francisco, CA

Kanu Chatterjee, MD
Clinical Professor of Medicine
University of Iowa, Carver College of Medicine
Iowa City, IA

Emeritus Professor of Medicine
Division of Cardiology
University of California, San Francisco
San Francisco, CA

Hubert Chen, MD, MPH
Assistant Professor of Medicine
Division of Pulmonary and Critical Care
University of California, San Francisco
San Francisco, CA

Sharon Christian, JD
Center for the Health Professions
University of California, San Francisco
San Francisco, CA

Carole Deitrich, APRN, MS
Professor Emerita & Gerontological Nurse Practitioner
Department Physiological Nursing
University of California, San Francisco
San Francisco, CA

Dana Drew-Nord, PhD, APRN, BC
Assistant Adjunct Professor
Department of Community Health Systems
University of California, San Francisco School of Nursing
San Francisco, CA

Susannah Ewing, RN, NP
Nurse Practitioner
Department of Obstetrics, Gynecology Faculty Practice
University of California, San Francisco
San Francisco, CA

Katharine Fast, MD
Allergy & Immunology
San Francisco, CA

Rena K. Fox, MD
Associate Professor of Clinical Medicine
Division of General Internal Medicine
University of California, San Francisco
San Francisco, CA

Roxanne Garbez, RN, PhD, ACNP
Associate Clinical Professor
Director, Acute Care Nurse Practitioner Program
Department of Physiological Nursing
University of California, San Francisco
San Francisco, CA

Amy E. Gilliam, MD
Assistant Clinical Professor
Department of Dermatology
University of California, San Francisco
San Francisco, CA

Courtney Giraudo, RN, MS, CNS, CPNP
Pediatric Nurse Practitioner
Whitney NICU Follow-Up Clinic
California Pacific Medical Center
San Francisco, CA

Richard Goldwasser, MD
Private Practice (specializing in child, adolescent, and
  adult psychiatry)
Mill Valley, CA

Psychiatrist Consultant
Redwood Coast & North Bay Regional Centers

Josephina T. Gomez, MSN, FNP-BC
Nurse Practitioner
San Francisco Wound Care and Reconstructive Surgery Center
St. Mary's Medical Center
San Francisco, CA

Terri Hupfer, RN, MSN, NNP
Clinical Nurse Coordinator
Regional Spina Bifida Program
Kaiser Permanente
Oakland, CA

Kathryn Johnson, RN, MSN, Psych CNS, Adult PMHNP
Assistant Clinical Professor
Department Community Health Systems
University of California, San Francisco School of Nursing
San Francisco, CA

Henry J. Kahn, MD
Director, Student Health and Counseling Services
University of California, San Francisco
San Francisco, CA

James Kahn, MD
Professor of Medicine
UCSF HIV/AIDS Program at San Francisco General Hospital
San Francisco, CA

Cynthia Kane Hyman, RN, MS, CNS-BC
Clinical Nurse Specialist
Staff Development, Inpatient Mental Health Service
ABSMC Herrick Campus
Berkeley, California

Steven R. Kayser, PharmD
Professor Emeritus
Associate Dean for Global Affairs
Department of Clinical Pharmacy
University of California, San Francisco
San Francisco, CA

Victoria F. Keeton, RN, MS, CPNP, CNS
Assistant Clinical Professor
Department of Family Health Care Nursing
University of California, San Francisco
San Francisco, CA

Susan J. Kelley, RN, PhD, FAAN
Dean and Professor
College of Health and Human Sciences
Georgia State University
Atlanta, GA

Christine Kennedy, RN, PNP, PhD, FAAN
Professor
Jack & Elaine Koehn Endowed Chair in Pediatric Nursing
Department of Family Health Care Nursing
University of California, San Francisco
San Francisco, CA

Sharon Knight, MD
Associate Clinical Professor
Department of Obstetrics, Gynecology & Reproductive Sciences
University of California, San Francisco
San Francisco, CA

Sarah Malin-Roodman, RN, NP, MS
Nurse Practitioner
Lyon Martin Health Services
San Francisco, CA

Umesh Masharani, MD
Professor of Clinical Medicine
University of California, San Francisco
San Francisco, CA

Carol A. Miller, MD
Clinical Professor, Pediatrics
Medical Director, Well Newborn Nursery
University of California, San Francisco
San Francisco, CA

Gina Moreno-John, MD, MPH
Professor of Clinical Medicine
Attending Physician
Division of General Internal Medicine
University of California, San Francisco
San Francisco, CA

Rebecca S. Neuwirth, RN, MSN, NP-C, WHNP-BC
Adult Nurse Practitioner
Golden Gate Community Health
San Francisco, CA

Don C. Ng, MD
Clinical Professor of Medicine
Attending Physician
Division of General Internal Medicine
University of California, San Francisco
San Francisco, CA

Sarah B. Pawlowsky, PT, DPT, OCS
Assistant Clinical Professor
Faculty Practice, Department of Physical Therapy &
    Rehabilitation Science
University of California, San Francisco
    School of Medicine
San Francisco, CA

Laurence Peiperl, MD
Health Sciences Associate Clinical Professor
    of Medicine
University of California, San Francisco
San Francisco, CA

Chief Consulting Physician
Glide Health Services
San Francisco, CA

Michael S. Policar, MD, MPH
Clinical Professor
Department of Obstetrics, Gynecology
    & Reproductive Sciences
University of California, San Francisco
San Francisco, CA

Steven Protzel, PharmD
Community Pharmacist
Assistant Clinical Professor (Volunteer)
Department of Clinical Health Services
University of California, San Francisco
San Francisco, CA

Patricia Purcell, RN, FNP-BC, MS
Nurse Practitioner
Southeast Health Center
Department of Public Health
San Francisco, CA

Patricia A. Robertson, MD
Professor & Endowed Chair for Obstetric and
    Gynecologic Education
Director of Medical Student Education
Department of Obstetrics, Gynecology & Reproductive Sciences
University of California, San Francisco
San Francisco, CA

Ronald J. Ruggiero, PharmD
Pharmacist Specialist in Women's Health
Clinical Professor
Departments of Clinical Pharmacy and Obstetrics, Gynecology &
    Reproductive Sciences
University of California, San Francisco
San Francisco, CA

Ellen Scarr, APRN-BC, MS, FNP, WHNP
Clinical Professor
Department of Family Health Care Nursing
University of California, San Francisco
San Francisco, CA

Suzanne Seger, RN, CNM
Associate Clinical Professor
Division of Obstetrics & Gynecology, Perinatal Medicine & Genetics
University of California, San Francisco
San Francisco, CA

Brian Shaffer, MD
Assistant Professor
Division of Maternal-Fetal Medicine
University of California, San Francisco
San Francisco, CA

Renée Smith, MPH, CNM
Assistant Professor
Samuel Merritt University, School of Nursing
Oakland, CA

Vicki Smith, MS, RN, NP
Assistant Clinical Professor
Department of Community Health Systems
Institute on Health and Aging
University of California, San Francisco
San Francisco, CA

Nancy Stark, RN, MS, ANP, PMHCNS
Assistant Clinical Professor & Nurse Practitioner
Department of Community Health Systems
University of California, San Francisco School of Nursing
San Francisco, CA

Mary M. Sullivan RN, DNP, ANP-BC, CDE
Diabetes Clinical Nurse Specialist
University of California, San Francisco
San Francisco, CA

Mari-Paule Thiet, MD
Director, Division of Maternal-Fetal Medicine
Vice Chair of Patient Safety and Quality Assurance
Department of Obstetrics, Gynecology &
    Reproductive Sciences
University of California, San Francisco
San Francisco, CA

Dzung X. Vo, MD
Clinical Fellow, Adolescent Medicine
University of California, San Francisco
San Francisco, CA

Sharon Whittemore, BSN, MS, RN, ARNP-BC
Nurse Practitioner
Division of Orthosurgery-Spine
University of California, San Francisco
San Francisco, CA

Sharon Wiener, RN, CNM, MPH
Associate Clinical Professor
Department of Obstetrics, Gynecology & Reproductive Sciences
University of California, San Francisco
San Francisco, CA

Elisabeth Wilson, MD, MPH
Associate Professor
Department of Family and Community Medicine
University of California, San Francisco
San Francisco, CA

Allen Wong, DDS, EdD
Assistant Professor
Director, Hospital Dentistry Program
University of the Pacific, Arthur. A. Dugoni School of Dentistry
San Francisco, CA

* These individuals are authors and reviewers.

INTRODUCTION

Welcome to the second edition of our clinical guidelines text for advanced practice nurses and other clinicians in primary care. This new text, *Clinical Guidelines for Advanced Practice Nursing: An Interdisciplinary Approach, Second Edition,* builds upon the work of nurse practitioners, certified nurse–midwives and clinical nurse specialists which began over 30 years ago in the ambulatory care center at the University of California, San Francisco. It targeted across the life span health promotion and common problems seen in primary care settings.

In this edition, the editors and contributing authors have written evidenced-supported clinical guidelines on common, complex chronic health problems, and included new chapters on health promotion for select vulnerable populations (adults with developmental disabilities and transgendered individuals). We are excited about the addition of several new chapters that address several prevalent and often problematic chronic issues in primary care: childhood depression, childhood ADHD, developmental assessment/screening for developmental delay and autism, anticoagulation therapy, chronic pain, and dementia.

Our text strives to integrate an interdisciplinary approach to clinical decision making and thus is a collaborative effort with contributions from a variety of health disciplines: nursing, pharmacy, medicine, dentistry, nutrition, and physical therapy. This text includes:

- Sections on Pediatrics, Gynecology, Obstetrics, and Adult Medicine
- S-O-A-P (Subjective-Objective-Assessment-Plan) formatting for easy reference
- Client/patient educational resources to enhance self-management efforts
- Recommendations for situations when advanced practice nurses should consider physician or specialty consultation
- Access to online decision support and patient self-management resources and tools via the Jones & Bartlett Learning web-based library
- Section on legal scope of practice for advanced practice nurses

Our hope is that this text will provide a substantial and timely resource for a variety of busy clinicians. We also anticipate that this text will be an important addition to decision support toolkits that clinicians rely upon for providing individualized, patient-centered care.

Geraldine M. Collins-Bride, RN, ANP-BC, MS
JoAnne M. Saxe, RN, ANP-BC, MS, DNP

"Let us always be open to acknowledge, respect, and learn from great leaders in any field or discipline. Let us always be able to critique the work of any leader to move forward ideas and substantive knowledge for the betterment of humanity. For, indeed, great progress is largely contingent upon thoughtful reflections, critiques, and the creative use of worthwhile ideas."

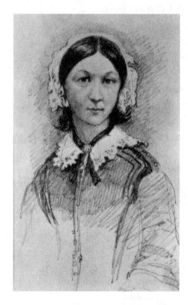

— Florence Nightingale

LEGAL SCOPE OF ADVANCED NURSING PRACTICE

Brian Budds and JoAnne M. Saxe

▌ Introduction

Nurses, like all healthcare professionals, must act within the scope of practice as outlined in statutes and regulations. Failure to comply with this by exceeding the permissible scope of practice could result in professional discipline or even criminal prosecution. Advanced practice nurses (e.g., clinical nurse specialists, nurse anesthetists, nurse midwives, or nurse practitioners) frequently encounter issues related to the scope of their practice.

These issues may arise as part of the individual nurse's ethical and professional concern or as a result of professional "friction" between nursing and other healthcare professions. This is especially so when the advanced practice nurse's scope overlaps with areas that have traditionally been viewed as the practice of medicine. Regardless of what may trigger such concerns, it is imperative that advanced practice nurses and practice managers know how to ascertain what is and is not part of their scope of practice and what actions they may need to take to be in compliance with the applicable law or regulation. Clear understanding of one's scope of practice can lead to enhanced collaboration among professionals, decreased professional tension, and more effective provision of health care in clinical settings.

Two key questions emerge when considering the issue of advanced practice nursing and scopes of practice. The first is the extent of what one, by virtue of being an advanced practice nurse, can do. Thus, the advanced practice nurse—or perhaps the clinical manager of a setting in which the advanced practice nurse is working or a collaborating physician—wants to know the duties an advanced practice nurse may legally perform. Second, one must understand what constitutes the outer boundaries of a clinician's scope of practice. For example, one must know if there needs to be a supervisory relationship and, if so, of what nature and how it should be documented.

Of course, it would be wonderful if those answers were always clear, concise, and readily available. Although that may occasionally be the case, it is not the rule. As such, this chapter outlines for advanced practice nurses and those responsible for the management of advanced nursing practice in the clinical setting how to approach these questions and where to begin to find that information necessary to properly understand the limits of one's scope of practice and what steps need to be taken to ensure that one's practice is consistent with the appropriate legal framework.

In a number of states (including the jurisdictions of Puerto Rico and Washington, DC), it is necessary for nurses to develop written documentation to support their expanded practice. Different states use different terms to describe these documents and require different specific elements be addressed. In most cases, the specific requirements for each state can be found in statutes or regulations, as discussed later. An explanation of practice guidelines, such as *Standardized Procedures* that are used in California, can be viewed at http://www.rn.ca.gov/pdfs/regulations/npr-b-20.pdf

▌ Overview of Scope of Practice Legal Framework

▌ State Regulation of Professional Practice

Control of the scope of practice of healthcare professionals rests at the level of state government. Although there are some areas of professional practice—including those relating to the advanced practice nursing roles—for which federal regulations have an impact, the basic definitions and limits of professional practice are determined at the state level.

This can sometimes lead to confusion. For example, some federal regulations dealing with reimbursement requirements for federally funded programs, such as Medicare and Medicaid, do address what can or should be done by advanced practice nurses. One such example is found in the Medicare Conditions of Participation for Rural Health Clinics (2010).[1] The regulations require that participating rural health clinic staff include one or more physician assistant or nurse practitioner. They further require that the physician assistant or nurse practitioner work with the physician on staff to develop and review clinic policies.

However, although compliance with these federal regulations is required for reimbursement for services, the individual healthcare

---

[1] 42 CFR 491 et seq (This citation is to the Code of Federal Regulations. This particular chapter of the code addresses the regulations applied to healthcare providers who participate in the Medicare Program. These regulations can be accessed from the website of the Centers for Medicare and Medicaid, found at: www.cms.hhs.gov)

practitioner's practice is directly regulated by the state in which she or he is licensed to practice. Thus, although the Medicare Conditions of Participation may not require that advanced practice nurses work with physicians in these settings, the rules governing who can become a nurse practitioner and what scope of practice the person has are set by the individual states and are subject to significant variation from state to state.

▌ Sources: Statutes

There are several sources of authority for the regulation of professional practice within states (and other jurisdictions within the United States). The most basic and important of these are statutes. Statutes are laws or acts passed by the legislative body of a particular jurisdiction. As such, statutes represent the voice of the people's elected representatives with regard to permissible activities.

Each state enacts a professional practice act addressing the specific health professions within the jurisdiction. In general, these statutes define the training requirements of healthcare professionals and what behaviors are allowed in the practice of the profession. For example, the State of California sets the basic legal framework for the practice of nursing in its Business and Professions Code (Nursing Practice Act, 2008). Similarly, the provisions for the practice of medicine, physical therapy, dentistry, and so forth are found in other sections of the Business and Professions Code.

Although not universally the case, most of these laws—known as practice acts—are relatively easy to locate. Most states have some board or agency charged with the regulation of each of the specific healthcare professions. Using California as an example, the statutes governing the practice of nursing authorize the Board of Registered Nursing to manage the practice of nursing within California. This state agency has a website (http://www.rn.ca.gov) on which it makes available links to the specific statutes relating to the practice of nursing within California (California Board of Registered Nursing, 2010c). An interactive list allowing one to link to boards of registered nursing throughout the country can be found at the website of the National Council of State Boards of Nursing (https://www.ncsbn.org/515.htm).

When looking at state statutes to understand issues relating to scope of practice it should be kept in mind that statutes may be written in fairly general and expansive language rather than in point-by-point specifics. One can think of the statutes as setting out the broad parameters of a professional practice without spelling out each particular specific aspect of the practice. Examples of the broad language include this excerpt from the Washington State statute defining advanced practice nursing:

> "Advanced registered nursing practice" means the performance of the acts of a registered nurse and the performance of an expanded role in providing healthcare services as recognized by the medical and nursing professions, the scope of which is defined by rule by the commission. Upon approval by the commission, an advanced registered nurse practitioner may prescribe legend drugs and controlled substances contained in

Schedule V of the Uniform Controlled Substances Act, chapter 69.50 RCW, and Schedules II through IV subject to RCW 18.79.240(1)(r) or (s).

Nothing in this section prohibits a person from practicing a profession for which a license has been issued under the laws of this state or specifically authorized by any other law of the state of Washington.

This section does not prohibit (1) the nursing care of the sick, without compensation, by an unlicensed person who does not hold himself or herself out to be an advanced registered nurse practitioner, or (2) the practice of registered nursing by a licensed registered nurse or the practice of licensed practical nursing by a licensed practical nurse (Revised Code of Washington, 2009).

▌ Sources: Regulations

Another authority for the control of advanced nursing practice can be found in regulations, which like statutes have the force of law. Regulations are not the result of the legislative process but, rather, rules or orders issued by an arm of government, such as a particular agency.

The process of developing regulations typically involves those who have particular expertise in an area drawing up specific rules, making them available for public comment, and then promulgating or issuing them publicly.

Because regulations are often developed by the agency or arm of government closest to the actual profession, they often are more detailed and specific than statutes. Regulations often spell out the details of how to implement the vision of the legislature as stated in the statutes.

State health boards often provide links to scope of practice regulations. However, it is easier to find these links in some states than in others. Should it be difficult to find a direct link to an individual state's law and regulations, the reader may choose to do an Internet search on such terms as "advanced practice nursing statutes" or "nursing regulations" and the particular state's name. Should this not help, one could always call the particular licensing agency and ask how to access the statutes and regulations governing nursing or the specific aspect of advanced practice nursing in which one is interested.

Like statutes, regulations are readily available to the public. For example, in California, regulations addressing the practice of nursing are found in the California Code of Regulations. Regulations in Title 16 address specifics relating to the practice of health professions, whereas those in Title 22 regulate how health care is provided in licensed institutions. Both require specific language. An example is the regulation describing what must appear in a "standardized procedure" document, required to allow registered nurses to practice beyond their usual scope of practice.

The website of a particular state's agency charged with the regulation of healthcare professionals often has links to the state regulations surrounding a particular profession available on that website.

For example, the Commonwealth of Massachusetts Board of Registration in Nursing has its website as part of the larger Health and Human Services Agency's section of the state government website (www.mass.gov). Under "Nursing," one can choose the link to "Statutes, Rules and Regulations" (Commonwealth of Massachusetts, 2010).

▍ *Sources: Statements of Regulatory Agencies*

Unfortunately, even a thorough reading and analysis of all pertinent statutes and regulations may not yield a definitive answer to all questions regarding one's scope of practice. The issue at question may be complex enough that a simple answer may not be available in the statutes and regulations. For example, it may not be precisely clear what an advanced practice nurse may do in a very specific clinical setting under specific circumstances.

When this is the case, the governing body (e.g., Board of Registered Nursing) may issue an advisory statement or some sort of information addressing the specific concern. These statements can be extremely helpful in allowing clinical practices and individual practitioners to understand what is permissible or required in a particular circumstance.

For example, the California Board of Registered Nursing makes multiple documents and sources of information about these issues available on its website (California Board of Registered Nursing, 2010b). Among the documents listed, the Board has made available a statement helping to explain the statutes and regulations in regard to the roles of nurse practitioners and certified nurse specialists working in long-term care settings (California Board of Registered Nursing, 2010a).

Although this kind of statement can be extremely helpful in understanding the complexities of the statutes and regulations, it does not of itself have the force of law. Even so, should a practice issue ever come to the point of being litigated, courts may be inclined to give deference to the statement of specific regulatory agencies.

▍ *Sources: Attorney General Opinions*

In some circumstances, issues are very complex and even contentious. Sometimes these situations result in an agency or some member of government seeking an official opinion from the State's Attorney General to clarify issues. This may often be the case when there has been substantial change in existing statutes and regulations that has led to confusion or even turf battles.

One example of this can be found in an opinion of the Michigan Attorney General (1980) about the ability of physicians to grant "unlimited authority" to advanced practice nurses to prescribe medications. One can see in reading this opinion the evolution of Michigan law that led to confusion about just how much authority may be delegated and under what circumstances.

In this example, a member of the State Legislature asked the Attorney General to issue an opinion. As is often the case, the opinion carefully lays out what the issues are and what the history

has been that has led to the question. Then, the Attorney General issues an opinion as to how she or he understands the law.

Like the statements of the regulatory agencies, an Attorney General's opinion does not carry the force of law. That is to say, such an opinion does not necessarily fully resolve the issue at controversy. However, courts routinely grant "great respect" or "great weight" to the opinions of attorneys general in cases that come before them. Thus, such opinions often have the power to effectively resolve a particular issue within a jurisdiction.

▍ *Sources: Statements of Professional Organizations*

Professional organizations that represent the interest of advanced practice nurses may issue statements or information about a particular topic related to scope of practice. As with the other opinions cited here, these opinions or statements, although often very helpful, do not carry the force of law. One thing to keep in mind is that often these statements may be issued by the organization in its role as an advocate for the particular profession or advanced practice role.

A particularly helpful service offered by many professional organizations is a regular legislative update. These updates often review legislation that has been passed or proposed within a year and that impacts the particular area of practice covered by the organization.

These updates, rather than clarify specific issues, are intended to inform readers of new laws and regulations and potential trends within the states. For example, a 2009 report in *Advance for Nurse Practitioners* reports on the failure of two bills introduced in Connecticut to remove a mandatory collaborative agreement and the pledge of a legislator to continue efforts toward that end in the future (Ford, 2009).

▍ *Other Sources*

There are other sources available to help understand scope of practice issues as they relate to advanced practice nursing. Two deserve at least a brief mention as part of this discussion.

The Center for the Health Professions is part of the University of California, San Francisco. The Center engages in numerous activities to improve health care through research and development projects. Among their efforts has been research into scope of practice of health professionals. Their publication of an "Overview of Nurse Practitioner Scopes of Practice in the United States—Discussion" is a very valuable tool for understanding the state of scope of practice regulation and for accessing particular information (Christian, Dower, & O'Neill, 2007).

Another valuable tool is a textbook devoted to issues relating to nurse practitioner practice and legal issues. Carolyn Buppert's (2008) *Nurse Practitioner's Business Practice and Legal Guide* addresses, among other topics, specifics about state regulation of nurse practitioner practice. It is hoped that this discussion orients advanced practice nurses to the resources for determining and understanding their particular scope of practice.

Issues Related to Collaborative Practice and Documentation

Once the advanced practice nurse has been able to identify the resources for understanding scope of practice it is imperative to determine the level of independence with which she or he can practice and the level of collaboration that is required by her or his jurisdiction. Furthermore, if there are requirements related to collaborative practice, one needs to be able to determine how to meet and appropriately document those requirements.

It has been widely noted that there is significant disparity in the terminology used to describe advanced practice nursing. For example, statutory language describing the nature of the required relationship between advanced practice nurses and physicians can include such terms as "supervise," "collaboration with," "delegate," and even "collegial working relationship" (Ritter & Hansen-Turton, 2008). Furthermore, we have already seen that the nature of this relationship can lead—as it did in Michigan—to repeated changes in legislation and regulation that, in the end, required an Attorney General Opinion to sort it out.

Although not a comprehensive list, the following issues are offered as a guide for understanding the possible requirements and methods of documenting compliance. The practitioner should consider each of these areas when attempting to set up practice or understand the extent of their scope of practice.

Fully Independent Practice

As of 2007, 11 states allowed nurse practitioners to practice independently of physicians. That is, in such states the nurse practitioner is permitted to diagnose, treat, and prescribe medications without supervision by or collaboration with a physician. Alaska, Oregon, and Washington are examples of states that have this kind of broad scope of practice.

Some Collaboration, Supervision, or Delegation Required

Most states require documentation of some sort of relationship with physician colleagues for the advanced practice nurse to practice within that scope of practice. The nature of the "collaboration," "supervision," or "delegation" may vary significantly from state to state.

Many states with this kind of requirement also require that there be a written agreement that sets forth the terms under which this relationship is defined. California's requirement of standardized procedures is an example of this need.

Collaborative or Supervisory Agreement Necessary for the Advanced Practice Nurse to Prescribe Medications In Most States

Apart from the other elements of advanced practice nursing, such as diagnosis, ordering of diagnostic tests, and ordering of treatments, the issue of prescribing medications can be particularly difficult. The history of political and legislative difficulties in approaching this issue has been well documented elsewhere. The key issue here is that the advanced practice nurse wishing to have prescribing as part of her or his practice needs to be sure that all particular scope of practice requirements are met.

In some states, advanced practice nurses must sign prescriptive agreements to prescribe, order, or furnish drugs. An example of this is found in the Minnesota legal framework, which allows for advanced practice without a written agreement but requires one for the advanced practice nurse to be able to prescribe (Public Health Occupations, 2006a and 2006b).

Precise Nature of the Supervision or Collaboration Required

In situations in which a supervisory or collaborative relationship is required, advanced practice nurses need to understand the precise nature of what is required. Furthermore, when that relationship requires documentation, as in a collaborative practice agreement or a standardized procedure, the nature of the relationship should be spelled out in the agreement.

State regulations may spell out what needs to be included in such an agreement and can be very helpful in drafting such an agreement. North Carolina's regulations are an example of how one can find excellent guidance in translating the statutes and the regulations into a workable document (North Carolina Board of Nursing, 2010). Issues that may arise or need to be documented properly include the following:

1. On-site supervision requirements: Only a few jurisdictions require that a physician supervisor be physically present. When practicing in those states, advanced practice nurses should be aware of and document regulations relating to:
   ► Length of time (i.e., percentage of working day) that the supervisor must be on-site
   ► What precisely constitutes "on-site" within that jurisdiction
   ► Whether there exists any exemption or modified requirements for working in a particular area, such as remote rural setting or medically underserved setting.
2. Chart review: A small number of jurisdictions require some level of advanced practice nurse chart review by collaborating physicians. In those states, attention should be paid to:
   ► The precise number or percentage of charts required to be reviewed in a specific period of time.
   ► What constitutes a need for review and how it is to be documented.
   ► Whether there is a particular type of chart (e.g., one involving an adverse outcome) that requires review.
3. Limitations on oversight for the collaborating physician.

In jurisdictions and settings that require some sort of physician oversight, the question necessarily arises as to how many practitioners may be supervised by a particular physician. These issues may arise in terms of the number of nurse practitioners with whom a physician may enter into a collaborative relationship, the number of individual practitioners that may be supervised at one time in an on-site situation, and other settings. For example, the question arises in those jurisdictions that require anesthesiologist supervision of certified nurse anesthetists.

Advanced practice nurses and those physicians with whom they enter into collaborative relationships should be clear about the specific limitations and requirements of the oversight required. In those jurisdictions and situations that require documentation of this relationship, it should be made clear in the practice agreement how many individuals are to be supervised and in what manner.

Concluding Remarks

From this discussion, the reader should appreciate three important themes about the legal scope of advanced nursing practice and clinical guidelines:

1. The advanced practice nurse must have a thorough understanding of the respective state's nurse practice act. There are several sources that provide context for one's professional scope of practice.
2. The advanced practice nurse must be able to clearly communicate with other registered nurses, physicians, healthcare administrators, and healthcare consumers their scope of nursing practice.
3. The advanced practice nurse must communicate, often in writing, the legal scope of their practice in a clear, concise, and flexible manner that is in keeping with regulatory law and community standards.

REFERENCES

Buppert, C. (2008). *Nurse practitioner's business practice and legal guide* (3rd ed.). Sudbury, MA: Jones and Bartlett.

California Board of Registered Nursing. (2010a). *Nurse practitioners and clinical nurse specialists in long-term care settings.* Retrieved from http://rn.ca.gov/pdfs/regulations/npr-b-22.pdf

California Board of Registered Nursing. (2010b). *Nurse practitioner information.* Retrieved from http://rn.ca.gov/regulations/np.shtml

California Board of Registered Nursing. (2010c). *Practice information.* Retrieved from http://www.rn.ca.gov/regulations/practice.shtml

Christian, S., Dower, C., & O'Neill, E. (2007). *Overview of nurse practitioner scopes of practice in the United States.* Retrieved from http://futurehealth.ucsf.edu/Public/Publications-and-Resources/Content.aspx?topic=Overview_of_Nurse_Practitioner_Scopes_of_Practice_in_the_United_States.

Commonwealth of Massachusetts, Nursing Licensing. (2010). Retrieved from http://www.mass.gov/?pageID=eohhs2subtopic&L=6&L0=Home&L1=Government&L2=Laws%2c+Regulations+and+Policies&L3=Department+of+Public+Health+Regulations+%26+Policies&L4=Regulations+and+Other+Publications+-+M+to+P&L5=Nursing+Licensing&sid=Eeohhs2

Ford, J. (2009). Annual legislative update: A state-by-state report on 2009. *Advance for Nurse Practitioners, 17*(12), 31.

Medicare Conditions of Participation, 42 C.F.R. §§491 et seq. (2010). Retrieved from http://www.cms.hhs.gov

North Carolina Board of Nursing. (2004). *Collaborative practice agreement—a guide for implementation.* Retrieved from http://ncbon.org/content.aspx?id=658

North Carolina Board of Nursing. (2010). Retrieved from http://ncbon.org

Nursing Practice Act, Cal. Bus. & Prof. Code §§2700 et seq. (2008). Retrieved from http://www.leginfo.ca.gov/calaw.html

Public Health Occupations. (2006a). Minn. Stat. Ann. §148.171.

Public Health Occupations. (2006b). Minn. Stat. Ann. §148.235.

Revised Code of Washington §18.79.050. (2009). Nursing care.

Ritter, A., & Hansen-Turton, T. (2008). The primary care paradigm shift: An overview of the state-level legal framework governing nurse practitioner practice. *The Health Lawyer, 20*(4), 21.

State of Michigan. Op. Att'y Gen. No. 5630 (Jan. 22, 1980). Retrieved from http://www.ag.state.mi.us/opinion/datafiles/1980s/op05630.htm

PEDIATRIC HEALTH MAINTENANCE AND PROMOTION

FIRST WELL-BABY VISIT

Annette Carley

I. Introduction and general background

The birth of a child creates new challenges for a family. The initial outpatient visit affords the provider an opportunity to establish an ongoing relationship with the infant and family, follow-up on residual issues from birth, and individualize and prioritize healthcare needs. For healthy infants, the American Academy of Pediatrics recommends that this initial visit occur within the first week after discharge, dependent on the duration of the initial hospitalization (Hagan, Shaw, & Duncan, 2008).

A. Follow-up of healthy infant after vaginal or cesarean delivery

1. For vaginal delivery, discharge typically at 48 hours; follow-up should occur within 48–72 hours of discharge.

2. For cesarean delivery, where discharge typically occurs at 96 hours, follow-up should occur within 1 week of discharge (Hagan et al., 2008).

B. Follow-up of infant after early discharge

1. Early discharge (i.e., hospital discharge between 24 and 48 hours) may be offered to healthy singleton infants, born at 37–41 weeks gestation, who are appropriately grown for gestational age, have no abnormal physical findings, and who were born vaginally after an uncomplicated prenatal course. Family, environmental, and social risks should be identified and addressed. Before discharge the infant must have completed a minimum of two successful feedings; had such issues as jaundice (if present) adequately addressed; and demonstrated adequate voiding and stooling (Committee on Fetus & Newborn, 2010). However, normal newborns may not void or stool within the first day of life. If discharge of the otherwise normal infant who has not voided or stooled is being considered, a documented plan for follow-up must be ensured and parents instructed about findings that warrant immediate follow-up (e.g., vomiting, inconsolability, or abdominal distention).

2. Plan for follow-up care should be confirmed and documented before discharge (Hagan et al., 2008).

C. Follow-up of premature and late premature infant after discharge

1. Premature infants less than 37 weeks gestational age are commonly discharged at or near their due date. At discharge they should demonstrate cardiorespiratory—hemodynamic—and—thermal stability, and adequate weight gain. Exact standards for discharge are lacking, but most centers consider discharge after completion of the 35th to 37th postconceptual week and stabilization of weight at 1,800–2,000 g.

   a. Those with a complicated clinical course or birth weight less than 1,500 g are typically also followed by a specialty clinic versed in premature infant care and outcome.

2. Late preterm (i.e., 34–37 weeks gestation), also known as "near term" infants, are frequently discharged using the same guidelines as term infants; however, this may underestimate some ongoing needs because of their immaturity or small size. Although no clear recommendations exist for timing of follow-up, the initial outpatient visit should occur no later than the first week following discharge.

3. Enhanced risks in this population that may complicate the early neonatal period or result in rehospitalization after discharge include hyperbilirubinemia, poor feeding, dehydration, and thermal instability (Raju, Higgins, Stark, & Leveno, 2006).

II. Database (may include but is not limited to)

A. Subjective

1. History and review of systems

   a. Parental concerns including feelings of readiness, stress, adequacy, and support

b. Birth and health history to date
   i. Maternal age, gravida, and parity
   ii. Pregnancy complications, including substance exposure, infections, hypertensive disorders, and poor prenatal care
   iii. Delivery method, complications, and use of anesthesia
   iv. Birth complications, including premature rupture of membranes, meconium, need for resuscitation, and low Apgar scores at birth
   v. Birth date
   vi. Gestational age
   vii. Birth weight
   viii. Discharge weight and age at discharge
   ix. Nursery complications, including jaundice
c. Family, social, and environmental history
   i. Mothers age, health, occupation, and level of education
   ii. Fathers age, health, occupation, and level of education
   iii. Siblings age and health
   iv. Family history including such conditions as asthma, allergies, chronic lung disease, diabetes, renal dysfunction, mental health disorders, heart disease, hematologic disorders, and tuberculosis
   v. Social or environmental concerns, such as unemployment, marital problems, physical abuse, substance exposure, and adjustment to newborn in home
   vi. Family source of support and religious affiliation
d. Nutrition history
   i. Bottle feeding infants: type, frequency, and volume of feedings; proper preparation of formula; strength of suck; burping
   ii. Breastfeeding infants: frequency; duration; perceived satiety; strength of suck; single versus two breasts used for feeding; maternal breast fullness before feeding and emptying after feeding; use of breast pump; use of other devices, such as breast shields or supplemental nursing systems
e. Review of systems and clinical findings

B. Objective

1. Physical examination findings
   a. Skin: turgor, color, perfusion; note presence of rashes, birthmarks, dermal breaks, skin tags or pits, or jaundice
   b. Head–eyes–ears–nose–throat
      i. Assess size, shape, symmetry of head and fontanels; note presence of cephalohematoma, caput, or cranial molding
      ii. Assess red reflex, ocular mobility, intactness of palate, and patency of nares; note presence of ocular opacification and dacryostenosis
   c. Chest and thorax
      i. Assess character of respirations; respiratory rate (normal 30–60 breaths per minute); shape and contour of thorax; breast size and shape; note presence of dyspnea; chest asymmetry; nipple discharge or tenderness
   d. Cardiovascular
      i. Assess heart rate (normal 100–180 beats per minute), rhythm, perfusion, quality of pulses; note presence of arrhythmias or murmurs
   e. Abdomen and rectum
      i. Assess symmetry, tone, presence of bowel sounds, anal patency, timing of first stool, stage of umbilical healing; note presence of distension and tenderness
   f. Genitourinary
      i. Assess appearance of external genitalia, timing of first void, voiding pattern, kidney size by palpation (normally 4–5 cm in size); note presence of ambiguous genitalia or abnormal kidney size
   g. Musculoskeletal
      i. Assess extremities, presence of digits, intactness of spine, movement of hips; note presence of deviation of gluteal cleft, hair tufts, or sacral dimple
   h. Neurobehavioral
      i. Assess activity, tone, state regulation, and symmetry of movements; note presence of clonus and irritability

   (Hagan et al., 2008; Hernandez & Glass, 2005).

2. Establish a growth trend, including comparative measurements of head circumference, weight and length from birth, and adjust for gestational age as indicated (Hagan et al., 2008).

3. Observe parent–child interactions, including holding, comforting, responsiveness, confidence, and mutual support

4. Review supportive data from relevant diagnostic tests including:
   a. Results of neonatal screen (Phenylketonuria (PKU), sickle cell, and congenital hypothyroidism mandated by all states)

i. PKU screening should occur after 24 hours of age, but less than the seventh postnatal day. If done before 24 hours of age, the infant must be rescreened to eliminate erroneous results.

ii. Sickle cell screening should occur before discharge, with confirmation of positive results before 2 months of age.

iii. Congenital hypothyroid screening is done at the second to fourth postnatal day, or immediately before discharge if discharge occurs before 48 hours of age (U.S. Preventive Health Services Task Force, 2007; U.S. Preventive Health Services Task Force, 2008a; U.S. Preventive Health Services Task Force, 2008b).

b. Hearing screen recommended, although not mandated, for all infants within the first month of age (U.S. Preventive Health Services Task Force, 2008c).

c. Immunizations deferred until 2 months postnatal age, except hepatitis B vaccine, which is recommended for all infants before 1 month. If immunization is received at birth, follow Centers for Disease Control and Prevention recommendations for subsequent dosing (CDC, 2008).

d. Refer to yearly Recommended Immunization Schedule at www.cdc.gov/vaccines or http://www.aap.org/pressroom/aappr-immunization-issuekit.htm (*Appendix 1*, Childhood and Adolescent Immunization schedules, 2010).

III. Assessment

A. Determine the diagnosis
Determine client's current health status, and identify general health risks based on gender, age, ethnicity, or other factors.

B. Motivation and ability
Determine caregiver and family willingness and ability to follow through with treatment plans.

IV. Goals of first well-baby visit

A. Screening or diagnosing
Choose a practical, cost-effective approach to screening and diagnosis, while abiding by mandated screening protocols.

B. Treatment
Select a treatment plan that achieves appropriate growth and development, is individualized for the caregiver and child, and maximizes caregiver compliance.

V. Plan

A. Screening
Elicit a thorough history and perform a thorough physical examination, with growth and development assessments at this and all well-child visits.

B. Diagnostic tests
1. Newborn screening as required by individual state, but must include assessment for congenital hypothyroidism, phenylketonuria, and sickle cell.

2. Hearing screen recommended.

C. Client education and anticipatory guidance (Hagan et al., 2008)
1. Nutrition
   a. Support the mother's nutritional needs for calories, liquids, and adequate rest and emotional and social support.
   b. Encourage breastfeeding or support bottle feeding as indicated.
   c. Milk intake considered adequate if baby has five to eight wet diapers and three to four stools per day, and is gaining weight appropriately. Initial stools with breastfeeding may be loose.
   d. Healthy infants should need no extra water, because both breast milk and formula provide adequate fluid for the newborn.
   e. Exclusive breastfeeding considered the ideal source of nutrition for the first 4–6 months; for formula feeders, always use iron-fortified formula, and provide 2 oz. every 2–3 hours; increase if infant seems hungry.
   f. Counsel about safety with milk preparation and storage.

2. Growth and development

3. Safety, including use of car seats; exposures, such as tobacco; back-to-sleep; cardiopulmonary resuscitation; when to call the provider; and illness prevention.

4. Referrals as indicated, including encouraging mother to seek appropriate postpartum follow-up

for herself. Women, Infant & Children referral should be initiated for eligible families.

5. Family transition to parenthood and well-being, including obtaining adequate rest, developing routines.

VI. Resources and tools

A. Patient and client education

1. The American Academy of Pediatrics website contains a variety of links of interest to parents, including a parenting corner. Visit: http://www .aap.org/

2. American Association of Family Practitioners sponsors a website called Family Doctor.org, which provides resources and links of interest to parents. Visit: www.familydoctor.org

REFERENCES

Arnold, S., & Bernstein, H. H. (2000). Newborn discharge: A time to be especially thoughtful. *Contemporary Pediatrics, 17*(10), 47–69.

Committee on Fetus & Newborn. (2010). Policy statement: Hospital stay for healthy term newborns. *Pediatrics, 125*(2), 405–409. Retrieved from http://aappolicy.aappublications.org/cgi/reprint /pediatrics;125/2/405.pdf

Deloian, B. J., & Berry, A. (2009). Developmental management of infants. In C. E. Burns, A. M. Dunn, M. A. Brady, N. B. Starr, & C. G. Blosser (Eds.), *Pediatric primary care* (4th ed., pp. 71–90). St. Louis, MO: Saunders.

Department of Health & Human Services. Centers for Disease Control and Prevention. (2008). *Recommended immunization schedule for persons aged 0 through 6 years.* Retrieved from http://www.cdc.gov/vaccines/recs/schedules/downloads/child /2009/09_0-6yrs_schedule_pr.pdf

Gaylord, N. M., & Yetman, R. J. (2009). Perinatal conditions. In C. E. Burns, A. M. Dunn, M. A. Brady, N. B. Starr, & C. G. Blosser (Eds.), *Pediatric primary care* (4th ed., pp. 1035–1079). St. Louis, MO: Saunders.

Hagan, J. F., Shaw, J. S., & Duncan, P. M. (2008). Supervision: First week visit. In J. F. Hagan, J. S. Shaw, & P. M. Duncan (Eds.), *Bright futures: Guidelines for health supervision of infants, children, and adolescents* (3rd ed., pp. 289–302.). Elk Grove Village, IL: American Academy of Pediatrics.

Hernandez, J. A., & Glass, S. M. (2005). Physical assessment of the newborn. In P. J. Thureen, J. Deacon, J. A. Hernandez, & D. M. Hall, *Assessment and care of the well newborn* (pp. 119–172). Philadelphia: W. B. Saunders.

Raju, T. N. K., Higgins, R. D., Stark, A. R., & Leveno, K. J. (2006). Optimizing care and outcome for late-preterm (near term) infants: A summary of the workshop sponsored by the National Institute of Child Health and Human Development. *Pediatrics, 118*(3), 1207–1214.

U.S. Preventive Health Services Task Force. (2007). *Screening for sickle cell disease in newborns.* Retrieved from http://www.ahrq.gov/clinic/uspstf07 /sicklecell/sicklers.htm

U.S. Preventive Health Services Task Force. (2008a). *Screening for congenital hypothyroidism.* Retrieved from http://www.ahrq.gov/clinic/uspstf /uspscghy.htm

U.S. Preventive Health Services Task Force. (2008b). *Screening for phenylketonuria.* Retrieved from http://www.ahrq.gov/clinic/uspstf08/pku /pkurs.htm

U.S. Preventive Health Services Task Force. (2008c). *Universal screening for hearing loss in newborns.* Retrieved from http://www.ahrq.gov/clinic /uspstf08/newbornhear/newbhearrs.htm

CARE OF THE POST-NEONATAL INTENSIVE CARE UNIT GRADUATE

Annette Carley

I. Introduction and general background

Greater numbers of recuperating infants, shorter hospital stays, and complex health demands have increased the need for comprehensive post–neonatal intensive care unit (NICU) care. Survival to discharge has improved across all gestational ages, although many survivors have residual disabilities requiring specialized care, expertise by providers versed in the needs of the fragile infant, and a provider who can intervene early (Carley, 2008; Kelly, 2006b). The American Academy of Pediatrics (AAP) has identified four categories of post-NICU patients who are considered high risk at discharge: (1) premature infants, (2) those with special health needs or who are dependent on technology, (3) those at risk because of social or family issues, and (4) those for whom early death is anticipated. Essential elements at discharge include physiologic stability, active caretaker involvement and preparation to assume care, and an integrated plan for follow-up care and management (Committee on Fetus & Newborn, 2008).

A. Common issues for the post-NICU population include

1. The infant who is premature at discharge

    Premature infants constitute over 12% of births, and late preterm infants (of gestational age 34–36 weeks) account for most of the recent increase in numbers of preterm infants. An analysis of data from 2002 suggested that infants completing the 34th, 35th, and 36th gestational week accounted

for 12.7%, 21.9%, and 40.1%, of the preterm population, respectively (Davidoff et al., 2006). With decreasing gestational age the incidence of neonatal complications increases; however, even late preterm infants are at risk for issues, such as impaired thermoregulation, poor feeding and nutrition, gastroesophageal reflux and other gastrointestine issues, late-onset sepsis, jaundice, or neurodevelopment impairment. Often managed as their term counterparts, these infants are at risk for rehospitalization after illness in the early postnatal period (Darcy, 2009; Doyle, Ford, & Davis, 2003).

2. Chronic lung disease (CLD)

    CLD is the leading cause of pediatric lung disease occurring secondary to pulmonary system immaturity or dysfunction and the additive effects of therapies, such as oxygen or mechanical ventilation support. Also referred to as "bronchopulmonary dysplasia," CLD commonly affects the premature infant, and despite overall improved survival and advances, such as exogenous surfactant therapy, it affects more than half of infants less than 1,000-g birth weight. Infants with CLD are at increased risk of pulmonary infections, long-term growth failure, and development delay (Verna, Sridhar, & Spitzer, 2003).

    a. Postdischarge therapies that may be used to optimize pulmonary function and growth include supplemental oxygen or ventilation, cardiorespiratory monitors, diuretics, and bronchodilators (Kelly, 2006b).

    b. Supplemental oxygen aims to optimize growth and stamina, and prevent development of cor pulmonale.

    c. Home mechanical ventilation, although rarely needed, may be used for those infants unable to wean from mechanical ventilation before hospital discharge (Committee on Fetus & Newborn, 2008).

3. Apnea

    Apnea is a serious condition for the neonate, and may result from pulmonary disorders; infection; brain injury; or metabolic derangements, such as hypoglycemia. Apnea is also a common complication in the preterm population, caused by immature central regulation of respiratory effort, and may be managed with oxygen or ventilator support, respiratory stimulants (e.g., methylxanthines), and cardiopulmonary monitoring. Although typically resolved by 42–44 weeks postconceptual age, apnea caused by immaturity in some infants (known as "apnea of prematurity") may persist until the time of discharge (Verna et al., 2003).

4. Gastroesophageal reflux disease (GERD)

   Infants born prematurely, those whose early course included structural or functional disorders of the gastrointestinal tract, those with pulmonary conditions requiring surgical intervention, and those with neurologic compromise are at risk for GERD. GERD may lead to erosive esophageal injury, and may be associated with serious conditions, such as apnea, bronchospasm, aspiration, or long-term growth failure (Verna et al., 2003).

   a. Physiologic reflux is common in infants; up to two-thirds of all infants less than 4 months of age exhibit regurgitation.

   b. Pathologic reflux, also known as GERD, is associated with complications including apnea, bronchospasm, esophagitis, esophageal strictures, and failure to thrive. It may be managed conservatively with small, frequent feedings; upright positioning; medications to optimize gastric emptying; or may necessitate surgical management for intractable cases (Verna et al., 2003). Some providers advocate use of thickened feedings; success of this strategy has shown variable results, although a recent meta-analysis of randomized clinical trials supported a moderate effect in healthy infants (Horvath, Dziechciarz, & Szajewska, 2008).

5. Postnatal growth restriction

   Premature infants are at increased risk for poor feeding and growth failure, and at discharge typically are below their healthy term counterparts in weight. Growth risks are compounded by the effects of chronic illness and genetic potential. Premature infants frequently need higher calories and nutrients than their healthy term counterparts. Diligently applied nutritional support plays a key role in supporting adequate long-term growth.

   a. Human milk is the ideal food for all infants regardless of gestational age; if human milk is not available, premature formula and postdischarge formula may be indicated to optimize catch-up growth (Greer, 2007).

   b. Premature infants may require additional supplementation to support nutrient requirements for protein; calcium; phosphorus; sodium; vitamins, such as B_{12}, B_6, D, E, and K; and trace minerals, such as zinc, copper, magnesium, selenium, and carnitine (Greer, 2007; Shah & Shah, 2009; Verna et al., 2003).

   c. Recuperating infants, especially preterm infants attempting to achieve adequate catch-up growth, may require up to 165 kcal/kg/d.

   Chronic health issues creating increased nutritional demands, such as CLD or growth failure, may warrant increased caloric goals (Verna et al., 2003).

   d. Structural or functional comorbidities, such as orofacial anomalies or altered tone, may complicate the nutritional plan (Kelly, 2006b).

6. Neurobehavioral and sensory deficits

   Infants recovering from the effects of initial illness or prematurity, and the NICU environment, may have residual neurobehavioral challenges including developmental delays, learning disabilities, hyperactivity, and cerebral palsy. Additionally, sensory deficits may include hearing or vision loss, auditory processing disorders, or language delay. Up to 50% of infants less than 1,000-g birth weight have some learning disability at school age (Verna et al., 2003).

   a. Hearing screening is recommended universally for all infants, and indicated for the NICU infant before discharge. Up to 50% of abnormal hearing screens occur in NICU graduates (Kelly, 2006b), and up to 10% of preterm infants may have severe sensorineural hearing loss (Verna et al., 2003). Exposure to ototoxic medications enhances this risk. Early intervention (i.e., at age < 6 months) enhances language development (Kelly, 2006a).

   b. Vision screening is recommended for preterm infants less than 1,500-g birth weight (or < 28 weeks gestation); those with a complicated medical course; and those exposed to supplemental oxygen. The first examination typically occurs at 31–33 weeks postconceptual age, with regular follow-up until vascular maturity is ensured at 3–6 months (Kelly, 2006b).

   c. Formal developmental assessment is indicated for all at-risk infants including those born preterm or with a complicated clinical course.

   d. Goals of developmental follow-up include optimizing growth and development to maximize long-term potential; integrating the infant into family and community; and providing early intervention to reduce medical, social, and emotional burden (Allen, 2005).

7. Dependence on technology

   Infants with unresolved cardiopulmonary issues, such as apnea, chronic hypoxia, or growth failure, may require technologic support in the home after discharge.

   a. Pulmonary support may be achieved with supplemental oxygen, cardiopulmonary monitoring, or the use of mechanical ventilation.

b. Weaning from ventilatory support is dictated by the infant demonstrating normal oxygen saturation, resolution of apnea or bradycardia, and showing appropriate growth.

c. Use of in-home technology requires vigilant attention to safety and hygiene, consistent education, and support of caretakers. Mechanical ventilation requires dedicated personnel and ongoing caretaker support including respite.

d. Nutritional support may be achieved with complementary enteral feedings or parenteral nutrition. In-home use of intermittent orogastric gavage or gastrostomy feedings requires vigilant attention to safety and hygiene, and education and support of caretakers. Efforts should concentrate on encouraging oral feeding skills.

e. Weaning from supplemental nutritional support can be considered when the infant demonstrates consistent appropriate growth, under the supervision of a nutrition specialist (Kelly, 2006b; Verna et al., 2003).

f. A plan for emergency management in the case of equipment malfunction must be in place (Committee on Fetus & Newborn, 2008).

8. Postnatal infection

Convalescing post-NICU patients, especially preterm infants, are at risk for complications related to infections, including respiratory syncytial virus (RSV) and influenza virus. Their increased vulnerability to infections may result in acute decompensation and the need for rehospitalization (Allen, 2005). At-risk infants discharged during peak RSV transmission seasons (i.e., October through March in the United States) should receive RSV prophylaxis in addition to routine immunizations given at recommended intervals (Department of Health & Human Services, Centers for Disease Control & Prevention, 2008; Kelly, 2006).

B. *Additional issues for the post-NICU population may include*

1. Social and environmental risks

The AAP identifies premature birth, need for hospitalization, presence of birth defects, and infant disability as risks for family dysfunction and child abuse. These risks are compounded by family and environmental risks, such as low socioeconomic status, lack of social supports, substance exposure, and lack of family involvement during the infant's hospitalization. Identifying strategies to enhance infant safety and family functioning before discharge is encouraged (Committee on Fetus & Newborn, 2008).

a. Vulnerable child syndrome is recognized as a potential outcome caused by the effects of protracted neonatal hospitalization, parental anxiety or depression, impact of the illness on the family, or lack of social supports. This has been associated with excess health care use and risk of impaired infant developmental outcome (Allen et al., 2004).

b. A posttraumatic stress disorder has been reported in parents of infants in the NICU, caused by ongoing stress of the hospitalization and uncertainty of neonatal outcome (Shaw et al., 2009).

2. Infant with anticipated early death

To enhance the quality of remaining life, infants with terminal disorders may be discharged to the home for hospice care. Discharge planning and follow-up care attends to family needs and concerns, and occurs with the involvement of home nursing. Necessary elements include creating a plan for management of infant pain and discomfort; securing arrangements for equipment or supplies; and providing ongoing support to parents, siblings, or extended family members (Committee on Fetus & Newborn, 2008).

II. **Database** (may include but is not limited to)

A. *Subjective database*

1. History and review of systems

a. Parental concerns including feelings of readiness, stress, adequacy, and support.

b. Birth and health history to date.

i. Birth history, including gravida and parity, pregnancy complications, delivery method and birth complications, Apgar scores

ii. Infant birth date, weight, and gestational age

iii. Neonatal course including complications

c. Family, social and environmental history.

i. Maternal age, health, occupation, and level of education

ii. Paternal age, health, occupation, and level of education

iii. Sibling ages, health, and history of prematurity

iv. Family history including chronic conditions

v. Parental head circumference and stature to compare with infant measurements

vi. Social or environmental concerns, such as unemployment, abuse, marital problems, and lack of support

d. Nutrition history.

i. Date feedings initiated, formula versus breast milk, nipple versus gavage, feeding tolerance, complications

ii. Parenteral nutrition support, use of hyperalimentation, peripheral versus central vascular access

e. Review of systems and clinical findings.

i. Dysmorphic features, which may suggest a genetic syndrome

ii. Skin, including rashes, birthmarks, scars, or jaundice

iii. Head, ears, eyes, nose, and throat including

   a. High arched palate caused by oral intubation

   b. Nostril distortion caused by feeding tube

   c. Head circumference: poor head growth in the premature infant strongly predictive of impaired cognitive function, academic performance, and behavioral issues

iv. Chest and thorax, including character of respirations, respiratory rate, and shape and contour of the thorax; findings may include

   a. Hyperexpansion caused by air trapping

   b. Tachypnea caused by chronic hypoxia

   c. Hypercarbia

v. Cardiovascular, including presence of murmurs, perfusion, and quality of pulses

vi. Abdomen and rectum, including stool pattern, distention, and inguinal or umbilical hernias

vii. Genitourinary, including voiding pattern

viii. Musculoskeletal, including symmetry of movements, strength, and tone

ix. Neurobehavioral, including activity, tone, state regulation, and tremulousness

x. Immune, including immunizations received before discharge

   a. Follow Centers for Disease Control and Prevention recommendations for dosing by chronologic age

(Department of Health & Human Services. Centers for Disease Control & Prevention, 2008). Refer to yearly Recommended Immunization Schedule at www.cdc.gov/vaccines or http://www.aap.org/pressroom /aappr-immunization-issuekit.htm (see *Appendix 1*, Childhood and Adolescent Immunization schedules, 2010)

xi. Supportive data from relevant diagnostic tests including

   a. Results of neonatal screen (phenylketonuria, sickle cell, and congenital hypothyroidism screening mandated in all states)

   b. Hearing screening

   c. Vision screening

   d. Developmental screening

   e. Laboratory studies including baseline blood gas, oxygen saturation, electrolytes

   f. Imaging studies including most recent chest radiograph, cranial ultrasound, or other cranial imaging study

B. Objective

1. Physical examination findings

   a. Establish a growth trend including comparative measurements of head circumference, weight, and length from birth. Plot, and adjust for gestational age.

   b. Thorough physical examination including vital signs and blood pressure.

   c. Essential to take into account size at birth (Table 3-1) and to use growth charts corrected for gestational age for accurate assessment of postnatal growth.

2. Observation of parent–child interactions, including holding, comforting, responsiveness, confidence, and mutual support.

3. Laboratory studies as clinically indicated, such as blood gas, electrolytes, or complete blood count.

4. Chest radiograph as clinically indicated.

III. Assessment

A. Determine the diagnosis

Determine client's current health status, and identify general health risks based on gender, age, ethnicity, and other factors.

TABLE 3-1 Birth Weight Classifications

Extremely Low Birth Weight	Very Low Birth Weight	Low Birth Weight
< 1,000 g at birth	< 1,500 g at birth	< 2,500 g at birth

Source: World Health Organization (2010). *Low birth weight (percentages).* Retrieved from http://www.who.int/whosis/indicators/2007LBW/en/index.html.

B. *Severity*

Assess the severity of illness, as indicated.

C. *Motivation and ability*

Determine family willingness to understand and comply with the treatment plan.

IV. Goals of clinical management

A. *Screening or diagnosing*

Choose a practical, cost-effective approach to screening and diagnosis, while abiding by mandated screening protocols. Post-NICU infants need careful, ongoing assessment related to neurobehavioral and growth risks, and individualized screening based on clinical findings.

B. *Treatment*

Select a treatment plan that optimizes growth and development, is individualized for the caregiver and child, and maximizes caregiver acceptance.

V. Plan

A. *Screening*

Elicit a thorough history and perform a thorough physical examination, including growth and developmental assessment at all visits.

B. *Diagnostic tests*

If not already performed before discharge, these should include

1. Newborn screen as required by individual state.

2. Hearing screen.

3. Vision screen.

4. Developmental assessment, often done by referral to a specified neonatal follow-up clinic facility. Premature and at-risk infants may be seen as frequently as four to five times in the first year of life, and are followed to school age (Leonard, 1988). However, there are no standardized guidelines for high-risk follow-up care (Committee on Fetus & Newborn, 2004).

C. *Management*

A primary provider should be identified and accept responsibility for orchestrating care. Post-NICU patients may be managed cooperatively with a variety of consultant and subspecialty services, including but not limited to nutrition services, dysmorphology and genetics, pulmonary, cardiology, gastroenterology, hematology, neurodevelopmental, and surgery. Specific intervals vary dependent on the complexity of the infant's history and current condition (Committee on Fetus & Newborn, 2008).

D. *Client education*

1. Concerns and feelings

Assist the family with expressing concerns and feelings about having a complex neonatal patient in the home, and coping with uncertainties related to the infant's health status or anticipated development.

2. Information

Provide verbal and written information related to
a. Health maintenance
b. Nutrition
c. Growth and development
d. Safety
e. Anticipated referrals and follow-up plans

VI. Resources and tools

A. *Parent–client–provider tools*

1. The AAP website contains resources for caregivers, including information about high-risk neonatal growth, development, and health needs (www.aap.org).

2. The March of Dimes provides multiple neonatal and perinatal resources for providers and parents (http://www.marchofdimes.com).

REFERENCES

Allen, E. C., Manuel, J. C., Legault, C., Naughton, M. J., Pivor, C., & O'Shea, T. M. (2004). Perception of child vulnerability among mothers of former premature infants. *Pediatrics, 113*(2), 267–273.

Allen, M. C. (2005). Risk assessment and neurodevelopmental outcomes. In H. W. Taeusch, R. A. Ballard, & C. A. Gleason, *Avery's diseases of the newborn* (8th ed., pp. 1026–1042). Philadelphia, PA: Elsevier.

Carley, A. (2008). *Beyond the NICU: Can at-risk infant patients be better served.* Retrieved from http://nursing.advanceweb.com/Article/Beyond-the-NICU-2.aspx

Committee on Fetus & Newborn. (2004). Follow-up care of high-risk infants. *Pediatrics, 114*(5), 1377–1397.

Committee on Fetus & Newborn. (2008). Hospital discharge of the high-risk neonate. *Pediatrics, 122*(5), 1119–1126.

Darcy, A. E. (2009). Complications of the late preterm infant. *Journal of Perinatal & Neonatal Nursing, 23*(1), 78–86.

Davidoff, M. J., Dias, T., Damus, K., Russell, R., Bettegowda, V. R., Dolan, S., et al. (2006). Changes in the gestational age distribution among U.S. singleton births: Impact on rates of late preterm birth, 1992 to 2002. *Seminars in Perinatology, 30*, 8–15.

Department of Health & Human Services. Centers for Disease Control & Prevention. (2008). *Recommended immunization schedule for persons aged 0-through 6 years.* Retrieved from http://www.cdc.gov/vaccines/recs/schedules/downloads/child/2009/09_0-6yrs_schedule_pr.pdf

Doyle, L. W., Ford, G., & Davis, N. (2003). Health and hospitalizations after discharge in extremely low birth weight infants. *Seminars in Neonatology, 8*(2), 137–145.

Dusick, A. M., Poindexter, B. B., Ehrehkranz, R. A., & Lemons, J. A. (2003). Growth failure in the preterm infant: Can we catch up? *Seminars in Perinatology, 27*(4), 302–310.

Greer, F. R. (2007). Post-discharge nutrition: What does the evidence support? *Seminars in Perinatology, 31*, 89–95.

Horvath, A., Dziechciarz, P., & Szajewska, H. (2008). The effect of thickened-feed interventions on gastroesophageal reflux in infants: Systematic review and meta-analysis of randomized, controlled trials. *Pediatrics, 122*(6), 1268–1277.

Kelly, M. M. (2006a). The medically complex premature infant in primary care. *Journal of Pediatric Health Care, 20*(6), 367–373.

Kelly, M. M. (2006b). Primary care issues for the healthy premature infant. *Journal of Pediatric Health Care, 20*(5), 293–299.

Leonard, C. H. (1988). High-risk infant follow-up programs. In R. A. Ballard, *Pediatric care of the ICN graduate* (pp. 17–23). Philadelphia, PA: W. B. Saunders.

Shah, M. D., & Shah, S. R. (2009). Nutrient deficiencies in the premature infant. *Pediatric Clinics of North America, 56*(5), 1069–1083.

Shaw, R. J., Bernard, R. S., Deblois, T., Ikuta, L. M., Ginzburg, K., & Koopman, C. (2009). The relationship between acute stress disorder and posttraumatic stress disorder in the neonatal intensive care unit. *Psychosomatics, 50*(2), 131–137.

Verna, R. P., Sridhar, S., & Spitzer, A. R. (2003). Continuing care of NICU graduates. *Clinical Pediatrics, 42*(4), 299–315.

World Health Organization. (2010). *Low birth weight (percentages).* Retrieved from http://www.who.int/whosis/indicators/2007LBW/en/index.html

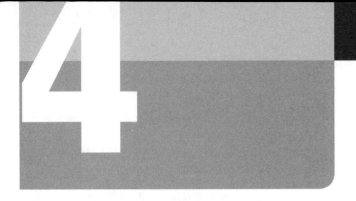

0 TO 3 YEARS OF AGE INTERVAL VISIT

Ann Birenbaum Baker

I. Introduction

The 0–3 years of age pediatric visit encompasses a wide range of physical and developmental growth. In infancy, babies go through dramatic physical growth while constantly developing gross and fine motor, language, and social skills that allow them to respond to their environment. As infants reach toddler age, their physical growth slows as they begin an intense exploration of their environment (Hockenberry, Wilson, Winkelstein, & Kline, 2003). This developmentally and physically diverse patient population requires additional consideration at each visit.

The physical examination of infants and toddlers aged 0–3 years may need a different approach than other age groups because they do not consistently respond to verbal instruction and developmentally may have stranger anxiety. Infants and toddlers may adjust to an examiner if they first watch the interaction between the examiner and their parent during the patient interview (Duderstadt, 2006). During this time, respecting a toddler's personal space and avoiding eye contact may help the toddler become comfortable before the examination. Instead of a head-to-toe examination, a more system-focused approach may be necessary with some patients. For example, auscultation can be completed first in infants before they become more active as the examination proceeds. Infants up to 6 months of age can usually be examined on the examining table, whereas infants older than 6 months and toddlers may feel more comfortable being examined in their parent's lap (Hockenberry & Barrera, 2007). In addition to assessing the child, it is also important to observe the parent–child interaction (Duderstadt, 2006). These interactions can give the provider clues to the parent–child dynamic, which is an important element of an overall assessment.

Health maintenance is a mutual goal for the patient and health provider and is aimed at potentiating the patient's state of well being. During periodic scheduled visits, a complete history is taken, an examination is performed, and potential health risks are identified. Counseling and guidance are provided in the areas of physical, behavioral, and emotional development. Cultural considerations, such as language barriers, cultural values, folk illnesses, recognizing one's own personal values, and working to eliminate health disparities related to race or ethnicity, are also important to incorporate into each visit (Duderstadt, 2006).

II. Database (may include, but is not limited to)

A. Subjective

1. Parental concerns

2. Interval history (if new patient include birth, patient and family medical history, and review of symptoms)
   a. Frequency and type of illness since last visit
   b. Medications
   c. Trauma or hospitalizations

3. Immunization status

4. Family and social history
   a. Changes from previous visit including new stressors
   b. Family planning
   c. Emotional support
   d. Means of financial support
   e. Child care arrangements
   f. Peer or social interactions including siblings, other children and adults, parents

5. Review of systems (Duderstadt, 2006)
   Maternal infections or drug use, prenatal history, history of preterm birth, birth history, neonatal history (including congenital anomalies and hospitalizations), and family medical history are important elements of the review of symptoms for this age group
   a. Skin: birth skin trauma, skin tags, dimples, cysts, extra digits, birth marks, hair, nails, diapering habits, clothing habits, behavioral history related to potential skin trauma
   b. Head: head growth, head trauma
   c. Eyes: focusing, eye discharge or swelling, infant history of being shaken, vision, abnormal head positioning

d. Ears: newborn hearing screening results, infant reaction to sound, infant vocalization, frequent colds, history of recurrent otitis

e. Nose, mouth, and throat: difficulty sucking or feeding, mouth sores or lesions, tooth eruption, breastfeeding, bottle use, mouthing habits, language acquisition, sucking on finger or pacifier, daycare, dental care

f. Respiratory: respiratory infections, reactive airway disease or asthma, eczema or skin allergies, daycare, immunization status, reflux or vomiting, breath holding, mouthing habits

g. Cardiovascular: heart murmur, cyanosis, failure to thrive

h. Gastrointestinal: stooling and voiding patterns, vomiting or reflux, weight gain and growth, constipation, toilet training, rectal bleeding, enuresis, urinary tract infections

i. Genitourinary: urinary stream, urinary tract infections, dysuria, hematuria, testes descended, vaginal discharge, enuresis

j. Skeletal: motor milestones, toe-walking, deformities, gait, bowing of legs, injuries

k. Neurologic: difficulty feeding, tongue thrust, developmental milestones, toe-walking, hand dominance, feeds self, poor coordination, seizures, staring spells, loss of consciousness, speech development, muscle tone

l. Lymph and endocrine: newborn screening results, weight gain, linear growth pattern, travel, lymphadenopathy

6. Review of behaviors

  a. Nutrition

    i. Milk

      a. Type: breast milk, formula, cow's milk

      b. Amount in 24 hours

      c. Method: breast, bottle (held or propped), cup

    ii. Type and amount of foods

    iii. Self-feeding: use of utensils

    iv. Meal routine: number of meals per day, where eaten and with whom

    v. Vitamins, fluoride, iron

  b. Oral health (American Academy of Pediatrics [AAP], 2003)

    i. Brushing teeth and wiping gums with moist rag

    ii. Parental oral health

    iii. Dental visit

    iv. Fluoride

c. Sleep patterns

  i. Daytime and nighttime sleeping: hours and routine

  ii. Where sleeping: co-sleeping, own room, crib, bed

  iii. Sleep positioning

  iv. Nightmares and night terrors

d. Elimination pattern and, if age appropriate, toilet training history

e. Developmental and behavioral appraisal (LaRosa & Glascoe, 2009)

  i. Periodically for early identification of developmental or behavioral disorders

  ii. 9 months: evaluate child's vision, hearing, motor skills, early communication skills, parent education

  iii. 18 months: evaluate motor, communication, and language skills plus autism screening

  iv. 24 or 30 months: evaluate motor, language, and cognitive skills plus autism screening

  v. Standardized developmental screening tools (see Chapter 8, Developmental Assessment: Screening for Developmental Delay and Autism)

f. Behavior

  i. Crying

  ii. Temper tantrums

  iii. Head banging

  iv. Body rocking

  v. Pacifier use

  vi. Thumb sucking

B. Objective

Physical examination (Duderstadt, 2006)

a. Height, weight, and head circumference through 36 months of age (Hockenberry & Barrera, 2007); refer to the following link for Centers for Disease Control and Prevention (CDC) growth charts: http://www.cdc.gov/growthcharts/charts.htm

b. Vital signs: heart rate, respirations, temperature, blood pressure (in children who are at risk or have chronic conditions), pain

c. General appearance: state of alertness, nutrition

d. Skin: hydration, rash, birthmark, scar

e. Head: anterior fontanel size, sutures, condition of hair and scalp, asymmetry

f. Eyes: eyelids, discharge, reactivity of pupils, corneal light reflex, red reflex, cover test, strabismus, nystagmus

g. Ears: external ear, external canal, tympanic membranes, pneumatic otoscopy

h. Nose: discharge, turbinates

i. Mouth and throat: presence of teeth, caries, occlusion status, tonsils

j. Neck: supple, rigid, palpable nodes

k. Chest: work of breathing, auscultation of lungs

l. Heart: rhythm, quality of heart sounds, presence of murmur, gallop or click, pulses, precordium, perfusion, color

m. Abdomen: umbilicus, liver, spleen, masses, bowel sounds

n. Genitalia
   i. Male: urethral meatus, foreskin, testes, inguinal canal, anus
   ii. Female: appearance of perineum, clitoris, vaginal introitus, hymen, discharge, anus

o. Musculoskeletal: muscle strength, range of motion, joints, extremities, spine, Ortolani and Barlow maneuvers for infants

p. Neurologic: motor function, symmetry, tone, gait, language, social development, primitive reflexes, and postural reflexes

III. Assessment

A. *Identify the child's general health risks based on age, gender, ethnicity, and specific health risks.*

B. *Determine the child's current health status.*

C. *Determine the motivation of the child's caregiver to change health-damaging behaviors or to promote and maintain health-promoting behaviors.*

D. *Delineate the child's ability to accomplish and master developmental milestones.*

IV. Plan

A. *Diagnostics (screening and secondary prevention tests)*
   A periodicity schedule for preventive pediatric health care is available through the AAP and Bright Futures at http://practice.aap.org/content.aspx?aid=1599 (AAP, 2007).

   1. Hearing risk assessment (Green & Palfrey, 2002; Harlor & Bower, 2009)
      a. Auditory skills monitoring
      b. Developmental surveillance

c. Assessment of parental concern

d. If risk factors are identified by review of symptoms or risk assessment children should have at least one diagnostic audiology assessment by 24–30 months of age

2. Vision screen (Green & Palfrey, 2002; Kelly, 2009)
   a. Detection of strabismus
   b. Vision
      i. Indirect assessment of vision for younger patients
      ii. Direct assessment of visual acuity in older patients able to comply with vision screening test
   c. Video that reviews practical techniques for children from birth to age 5 years can be found at www.aao.org/education/ped_vision/index.cfm

3. Iron deficiency (AAP, 2007; Kelly, 2009)
   a. Risk assessment screening at 4, 18, and 24 months of age; risk factors include history of prematurity, low birth weight, and diet
   b. Hemoglobin or hematocrit at 12 months of age

4. Lead poisoning (AAP, 2005; CDC, 2009; Kelly, 2009; Wengrovitz & Brown, 2009)
   a. Follow state screening plan available through the CDC (available at cdc.gov/nceh/lead/programs.htm)
   b. If no state screening plan in place, consider universal screening
      i. Blood lead level at 12 and 24 months of age
      ii. Universal screening also recommended for recent immigrants, foreign adoptees, and refugee children between ages 6 months and 16 years
   c. Targeted screening; see Figure 4-1 for suggested lead screening questions

5. Oral health screening (AAP, 2003; American Academy of Pediatric Dentistry [AAPD], 2009; Kelly, 2009)
   a. Risk assessment at 6, 9, 18, 24, and 30 months of age using a caries risk assessment tool (available through the AAPD)
   b. Dental referral at 12 months of age

6. Tuberculosis (AAP, 2007; Kelly, 2009)
   a. Risk assessment at 1 month of age
   b. Targeted screening

7. Lipid profile (Kelly, 2009)
   a. Risk assessment at age 2, 4, 6, 8, and 10 years

FIGURE 4-1 *Lead Screening Questionnaire*

PLEASE CIRCLE ONE: Male   Female   Age: _____ years

PLEASE CIRCLE ONE: 1. African American   3. Latino   5. White
                        2. Asian/Pacific Islander   4. Native American   6. Other

Address: _____

City _____

State _____   Zip code: _____

PLEASE CIRCLE YOUR ANSWERS TO THE FOLLOWING QUESTIONS:

1. Does your child live in or regularly visit a house, daycare center or a nursery school that was built before 1960?   Yes   No   I don't know

2. Is there any peeling, chipping, or powdery paint in the house, daycare center, or nursery school?   Yes   No   I don't know

3. Is the house, daycare center, or nursery school being remodeled or renovated?   Yes   No   I don't know

4. Does your child live within two to three blocks of a major highway or a heavily traveled road? (Give local examples)   Yes   No   I don't know

5. Does your child live near a battery manufacturing plant, construction area, or other industrial site?   Yes   No   I don't know

6. Is there anyone in the family who works with lead, for example, in the construction, welding, plumbing, painting, auto repair, pottery, ceramics or jewelry trades?   Yes   No   I don't know

7. Have any of your children, their playmates, or relatives been told that they have lead poisoning?   Yes   No   I don't know

8. Does your child eat, chew or put in his or her mouth nonfood items, such as painted surfaces, soil, or clay?   Yes   No   I don't know

9. Do you use ceramics or glazed pottery for storing or serving foods?   Yes   No   I don't know

10. Please circle any home remedies used by family or friends:

    • azarcon (rueda, coral, maria luisa, garcon, liga) or greta

    • pay-oo-lah (red powder for rash or fever) (frequently used by people of Hmong ethnicity)

    • alkohl (kohl, powder for skin infections, cosmetics (frequently used by people of Arab descent)

    • ghasard, bala goli or kandu (frequently used by people of Asian Indian descent)

Source: Collins-Bride, G., & Saxe, J. (Eds.). (1998). *Nurse Practitioner/Physician Collaborative Practice: Clinical Guidelines for Ambulatory Care.* San Francisco, CA: UCSF Nursing Press. Used with permission from the UCSF Nursing Press.

b. Risk factors
   i. Family history of dyslipidemia, premature cardiovascular disease, or diabetes
   ii. Disease states associated with cardiovascular disease
   iii. Body mass index greater than or equal to 85th percentile for age and gender, hypertension, insulin resistance
c. Hyperlipidemia screening if risk factors present

B. Treatment

Immunizations appropriate for age (refer to yearly Recommended Immunization Schedule at www.cdc.gov/vaccines or http://www.aap.org/pressroom/aappr-immunization-issuekit.htm; see *Appendix 1*, Childhood and Adolescent Immunization schedules 2010).

C. Patient and family education (Green & Palfrey, 2002)

Discussion of the following
a. Presenting concerns
b. Nutrition appropriate for age
c. Safety and accident prevention
d. Toilet training appropriate to age
e. Available community resources
f. Child-care arrangements and preschool plans
g. Growth and development appropriate for age with review of growth chart, physiologic development of lower extremities (bowed legs, knock knees)
h. Age-appropriate behavior of infant or toddler (including separation anxiety, fear of strangers, and sleep patterns)
i. Tantrums and limit setting
j. Possible reactions to indicated immunizations

D. Expected parent outcomes

Parents able to
a. Be reassured about their concerns
b. Verbalize knowledge of nutritional requirements appropriate for age: variable appetites; food fads, bottle habits (sleeping with bottle, juice in bottle, starting cup use); label reading
c. Verbalize safety precautions appropriate for age
d. Verbalize age-appropriate toilet training
e. Verbalize available community resources
f. Verbalize available child care arrangements and preschools and the appropriateness for their child
g. Verbalize understanding of age-appropriate growth and development including physiologic development of lower extremities

h. Verbalize understanding for age-appropriate behavior including sleep patterns and separation anxiety
i. Verbalize understanding of tantrums and limit setting in relation to development
j. Verbalize understanding of possible reactions to given immunizations including home treatment and temperature taking and grant informed consent before each immunization

REFERENCES

American Academy of Pediatric Dentistry. (2009). *Guideline on infant oral health care*. Retrieved from http://www.aapd.org/media/policies.asp

American Academy of Pediatrics. (2003). Oral health risk assessment timing and establishment of the dental home. *Pediatrics, 111*(5), 1113–1116.

American Academy of Pediatrics. (2005). Lead exposure in children: Prevention, detection, and management. *Pediatrics, 116*(4), 1035–1047.

American Academy of Pediatrics. (2007). *Recommendations for preventive pediatric health care (periodicity schedule)*. Retrieved from http://practice.aap.org/content.aspx?aid=1599

Centers for Disease Control and Prevention. (2009). *Lead poisoning prevention in newly arrived refugee children*. Retrieved from http://www.cdc.gov/nceh/lead/Publications/Refugeetoolkit/RTK_Resources.htm

Duderstadt, K. G. (Ed.). (2006). *Pediatric physical examination: An illustrated handbook*. San Francisco, CA: Mosby, Inc.

Green, M. D., & Palfrey, J. S. (2002). *Bright futures: Guidelines for health supervision of infants, children, and adolescents* (2nd ed.). Arlington, VA: National Center for Education in Maternal and Child Health.

Harlor, A. D., & Bower, C. (2009). Hearing assessment in infants and children: Recommendations beyond neonatal screening. *Pediatrics, 124*(4), 1252–1263.

Hockenberry, M. J., & Barrera, P. (2007). Communication and physical and developmental assessment of the child. In M. J. Hockenberry & D. Wilson, *Wong's nursing care of infants and children* (8th ed., pp. 141–204). St. Louis, MO: Mosby.

Hockenberry, M. J., Wilson, D. W., Winkelstein, M. L., & Kline, N. E. (2003). Communication and health assessment of the child and family. In M. J. Hockenberry & D. Wilson, *Wong's nursing care of infants and children* (7th ed., pp. 139–169). St. Louis, MO: Mosby.

Kelly, N. (2009, October 12). *Screening tests in children and adolescents*. UpToDate. Retrieved from http:www.uptodate.com/online/content/topic.do?topicKey=gen_pedi/6606&view=print

LaRosa, A., & Glascoe, F. P. (2009, September 30). *Developmental surveillance and screening in primary care*. UpToDate. Retrieved from http://www.uptodate.com/online/content/topic.do?topicKey=behavior/5562&view=print

Wengrovitz, A. M., & Brown, M. J. (2009). Recommendations for blood lead screening of Medicaid-eligible children aged 1–5 years: An updated approach to targeting a group at high risk. *MMWR: Recommendations and Reports, 58*, 1–11.

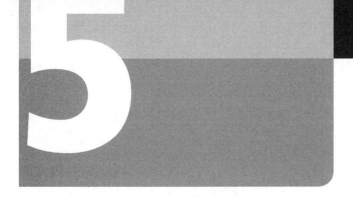

3 TO 6 YEARS OF AGE INTERVAL VISIT

Angel K. Chen

I. Introduction and general background

Health supervision and well-child visits are opportunities for the healthcare provider to assess a child's growth and development and to promote wellness in the child and family. In addition, the provider needs to address disease detection and prevention, and offer proper anticipatory guidance during the visit (Hagan, Shaw, & Duncan, 2008a).

Children between 3 and 6 years of age experience an explosion of language, mastery of physical skills, sense of self and peers, an increase in independence, and endless curiosity, all in preparation for a successful school entry milestone (Hagan, Shaw, & Duncan, 2008b). They cross from early childhood into the beginning stages of middle childhood.

The approach to preschoolers during their well-child visit is two-fold: although most of the history may still be provided by the parent or caretaker, children at this age may now participate in some of the interview and actively engage with the provider. Careful observation of their behavior in the examination room is also useful, including their interaction with the parent or caretaker, the environment, and the provider (Duderstadt, 2006). Healthcare maintenance visits in this age range include careful history; physical examination; screening studies (as appropriate); immunizations; anticipatory guidance; counseling at a yearly basis; and follow-up on an as-needed basis.

II. Database (may include but is not limited to)

A. Subjective

1. Parental and child concerns (chief complaint)
   a. History of present illness
2. Interval history
3. Past medical history
   a. Birth history
   b. Trauma, surgeries, or hospitalizations
   c. Dental home: date of last examination (if any); caries or dental work
4. Medication (include homeopathic or herbal supplements and vitamins)
5. Allergies (medication, environmental, and food)
6. Immunization status
7. Family history
8. Social history
   a. Daycare or preschool attendance; kindergarten
   b. Household members
   c. Means of financial support
9. Nutrition
   a. Iron-rich foods; intake of fruits, vegetables, and whole-grains; calcium sources (milk, cheese, and yogurt); and juice and water intake (source of water and fluoride)
   b. Eating habits and mealtime behavior
10. Elimination
    a. Potty training process and status; voiding habits
    b. Stooling patterns
11. Sleep (quality and quantity)
12. Developmental (see Chapter 8 on Developmental Assessment: Screening for Developmental Delay and Autism); evaluate overall school readiness
    a. Socioemotional: self-care skills, typical play, and description of self

    b. Language
        i. 3–4 year old: conversation and communication
        ii. 5–6 year old: articulation, full sentences, counts to 10, names four colors, tells simple story, and uses appropriate tenses and pronouns
    c. Cognitive
        i. 5–6 year old: comprehension, follows directions, and able to listen and attend
    d. Physical
        i. 3 year old: builds tower of cubes, throws ball, rides tricycle, walks up stairs, draws, and toilet training progress
        ii. 4 year old: hops on one foot; balances for 2 seconds; copies cross; dresses and undresses with minimal assistance; and pours, cuts, and mashes own food
        iii. 5–6 year old: balances on one foot, hops and skips, ties a knot, grasps a pencil, draws a person with six body parts, recognizes letters and numbers, copies squares and triangles, and dresses and undresses without assistance

13. Review of systems
    a. General
    b. Skin, hair, and nails: birthmarks, rashes
    c. Head–eyes–ears–nose–throat: headaches; ocular history (vision, eyes straight, eyelid droop, eye injury); hearing and history of otitis media; nasal congestion, allergies, and nosebleeds; oral health, dental brushing, and flossing; and sore throats and difficulty swallowing
    d. Chest and lungs: history of asthma or reactive airway disease, croup, bronchitis, or persistent cough
    e. Cardiac and heart: history of heart murmur, cyanosis, shortness of breath, and energy level
    f. Abdomen and gastrointestinal: appetite, diet, abdominal pain, vomiting, and diarrhea
    g. Genitourinary: incontinence, enuresis, urinary tract infections, dysuria, frequency, hematuria, vaginal discharge, and phimosis or balanitis
    h. Musculoskeletal: deformities, limb pains, injuries, and orthopedic appliances
    i. Neurologic: seizures, fainting spells, loss of consciousness, and gait
    j. Endocrine: recent weight gain or losses and linear growth patterns

B. Objective

1. Physical examination
    a. Weight, height, and body mass index
    b. Pulse, respiratory rate, and blood pressure
    c. General: state of alertness and orientation to space
    d. Skin, hair, and nails: hydration; rashes; birthmarks; scars; nail and hair health; and infestations (lice)
    e. Head–eyes–ears–nose–throat: symmetry of head; external inspection of eyes and lids, extraocular movement assessment, pupil examination, red reflex examination, cover and uncover examination, ophthalmoscopic examination of optic nerve and retinal vessels; tympanic membrane description and mobility; nasal discharge and turbinate status; dental condition, caries, gingival inflammation, and malocclusion; throat and tonsils; neck supple and palpable lymph nodes
    f. Chest and lungs: auscultation of lungs
    g. Cardiac and heart: rhythm, murmur, gallop, click, and pulses
    h. Abdomen: liver, spleen, masses, stool, and bowel sounds
    i. Genitourinary: external genitalia and rectal status; for males, circumcision or retractable foreskin, meatus, testes descended bilaterally; for females, perineum condition and hygiene, vaginal introitus, labial condition
    j. Musculoskeletal: muscle strength, range of motion, gait, and spine and back check
    k. Neurologic: CN II–XII; deep tendon reflexes; symmetry, tone, gait, strength; observe fine and gross motor skills; assess language acquisition, speech fluency, and clarity; and thought content and ability to understand abstract thinking

III. Assessment

A. Summary of health, growth, and development

1. Identify general health risks based on age, gender, past history, and ethnicity

2. Determine caregiver's motivation to change health-damaging behaviors and promote and maintain health-promoting behaviors

3. Identify ability to accomplish and master developmental milestones

IV. Plan

A. Screening (Hagan, Shaw, & Duncan, 2008c)

1. Vision screening

2. Audiometric screening

3. Lead screening and risk assessment (see resources and screening questions from http://www.brightfutures.org/healthcheck/labs/lead.html, and Chapter 4 for lead screening questionnaire)

4. Anemia screening and risk assessment (see resource and screening questions from http://www.brightfutures.org/healthcheck/labs/anemia)

5. Tuberculosis screening and risk assessment (see resources and screening questions from http://www.brightfutures.org/healthcheck/labs/tb.html)

6. Dyslipidemia screening and risk assessment (4 and 6 years; see resources and screening questions from http://www.brightfutures.org/healthcheck/labs/cholesterol.html)

7. Urinalysis (one time between 3 and 5 years of age)

B. Treatment

1. Immunizations (refer to yearly Recommended Immunization Schedule at www.cdc.gov/vaccines or http://www.aap.org/pressroom/aappr-immunization-issuekit.htm; see *Appendix 1*, Childhood and Adolescent Immunization schedules 2010)

2. Oral fluoride (if primary water source is deficient in fluoride)

C. Anticipatory guidance and family education (Hagan et al., 2008b)

1. Address child and parental–caregiver concerns

2. Family support and routine

   a. Family decisions, sibling rivalry, work balance, and discipline choices

   b. Temperament

3. Literacy

   a. Singing, talking, describing, observing, and reading

4. Peers

   a. Interactive games, play opportunities, social interactions, and taking turns

5. School readiness

   a. Preschool: structured learning experiences; friends; socialization; and able to express feelings of joy, anger, sadness, fear, and frustration

   b. Kindergarten and elementary school: establish routine, after-school care and activities, parent–teacher communication, friends, bullying, maturity, management of disappointments, and fears

6. Physical activity

   a. Limit screen time (television and computer) to 1–2 hours per day of appropriate programming; no television or DVD player in child's room

   b. Encourage 60 minutes of physical activity per day (5–6 year olds)

7. Healthy personal habits

   a. Daily routines including bedtime routine

   b. Oral health: daily brushing and flossing, adequate fluoride intake

   c. Discuss proper nutrition for age: well-balanced diet, breakfast everyday, five servings of fruits and vegetables per day, increased whole-grain consumption, two cups of milk or equivalent calcium intake per day, and limit high-fat and low-nutrient foods and drinks

8. Safety

   a. Car safety: seat or booster and safety helmets

   b. Pedestrian safety: falls from windows, outdoor safety, swimming safety, smoke detectors and carbon monoxide detectors, and guns and weapons in the home

   c. Stranger safety: reinforce rules about talking with and going with strangers if approached

   d. Sexual abuse prevention

D. Expected outcomes

1. Reassure child and parents about health concerns

2. Promote optimal health for children and their families

3. Promote family support and acceptable discipline approach

4. Promote social development

5. Encourage literacy activities

6. Empower parents to provide healthy eating habits and encourage physical activities; limit amount of television and computer time

7. Promote safety parameters at home, in the car, and in the neighborhood

8. Support school readiness

E. Consultation and referral

1. Dental home if not already established

2. Developmental testing if indicated

3. Subspecialty referral if indicated

F. Resources for families

1. Healthy Children (American Academy of Pediatrics): www.healthychidren.org; includes special section on preschoolers in "Ages and Stages"

2. Kids Health (Nemours Center for Child Health Media): www.Kidshealth.org

3. Bright Futures for Families: www.brightfuturesfor families.org

G. Resources for providers

1. National Association of Pediatric Nurse Practitioners: www.napnap.org

2. American Academy of Pediatrics: www.aap.org

3. Bright Futures: www.brightfutures.org

REFERENCES

Duderstadt, K. (2006). Approach to child & adolescent assessment. In K. Duderstadt (Ed.), *Pediatric physical examination: An illustrated handbook* (pp. 3–10). Philadelphia, PA: Mosby.

Hagan, J. F., Shaw, J. S., & Duncan, P. M. (Eds.). (2008a). Introduction to the bright futures visits. In American Academy of Pediatrics, *Bright futures: Guidelines for health supervision of infants, children, and adolescents* (3rd Ed., pp. 203–219). Elk Grove Village, IL: American Academy of Pediatrics.

Hagan, J. F., Shaw, J. S., & Duncan, P. M. (Eds.). (2008b). Rationale and evidence. In American Academy of Pediatrics, *Bright futures: Guidelines for health supervision of infants, children, and adolescents* (3rd ed., pp. 439–481). Elk Grove Village, IL: American Academy of Pediatrics.

Hagan, J. F., Shaw, J. S., & Duncan, P. M. (Eds.). (2008c). Rationale and evidence. In American Academy of Pediatrics, *Bright futures: Guidelines for health supervision of infants, children, and adolescents* (3rd ed., pp. 221–250). Elk Grove Village, IL: American Academy of Pediatrics.

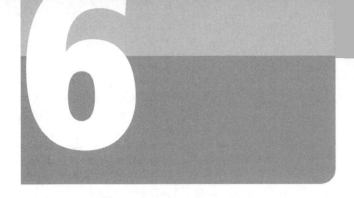

6 TO 11 YEARS OF AGE INTERVAL VISIT

Bridget Ward Gramkowski and Ann Birenbaum Baker

I. Definition

School-aged children spend less than half as much time with their parents than they did in their younger years (Hill & Stafford, 1980). Although parents are still the most important influence in their child's emotional and physical development, teachers and peers become increasingly important as the child approaches adolescence. Opportunities for mastery and early identification of learning issues are critical to promoting self-esteem and academic success (Santrock, 1999). The influence of media on this age group is also increasing, with "screen time" for children ages 6–11 years averaging more than 28 hours a week (Gold, 2009). The timing of puberty varies widely between ethnic groups and genders, and can start as early as 6 years in African American girls (Zuckerman, 2001). Early maturing girls are more likely to have internalizing behavior problems and more risk-taking behaviors (Obradović & Hipwell, 2010; Zuckerman, 2001).

Health maintenance is a mutual goal for the patient and healthcare provider and is aimed at promoting the patient's well-being. During periodic scheduled visits, a complete history is taken, an examination is performed, and potential health risks are identified. Counseling and guidance are provided to the patient and parent in the areas of physical, behavioral, and emotional development. Cultural considerations, such as language barriers, cultural values, folk illnesses, recognizing one's own personal values, and working to eliminate health disparities related to race or ethnicity, are also important to incorporate into each visit (Duderstadt, 2006).

II. Database (may include but is not limited to):

A. Subjective

1. Parent and child concerns

2. Interval history (American Academy of Pediatrics [AAP], 2000)

   a. Frequency and type of illness since last visit
   b. Chronic illnesses: current status and treatment plan
   c. Medications
   d. Trauma, hospitalizations, or emergency room visits
   e. Dental care status

3. Immunization status

4. Family and social history

   a. Changes from previous visit: emotional support, means of financial support, child welfare arrangements, and changes to family medical history
   b. Sibling rivalry, parental stress, living arrangements, and childcare
   c. Safety: screen for domestic violence, neighborhood, school or bullying, Internet, personal, and weapons
   d. Environmental risk factors: cigarette smoke, sun exposure, pollution, lead, and allergens

5. Developmental and behavioral history

   a. Problems or concerns
   b. Appraisal of coping styles: anxiety, anger, frustration, fear, and happiness
   c. Interaction with peers, teachers, adults, and family
   d. Amount and type of screen time per day and week, supervised versus alone
   e. Child's strengths and self-esteem
   f. Child's socialization skills and peer activities
   g. Parent's approach to sexuality and pubertal development
   h. Exposure to trauma, tobacco, alcohol, and drug use (Duderstadt & Schapiro, 2006; Santrock, 1999; Windom, 2006)

6. Review of daily habits

   a. Nutrition
      i. Calcium: type and amount in 24 hours
      ii. Type and amount of foods

     iii. Meal routine: 24-48 hour dietary recall, number of meals per day, at home and at school; frequency and type of snacks, family meal

     iv. Attitude toward food and body image

     v. Sweetened beverage intake

     vi. Fast food or junk food frequency and type

     vii. Physical activity: frequency, type, duration, and safety

     (American Heart Association [AHA] et al., 2006; Duderstadt & Schapiro, 2006)

  b. Sleep patterns

     i. Amount of sleep, scheduled bedtime, sleep hygiene (routines and sleep-promoting habits)

     ii. Sleepwalking

     iii. Teeth grinding, snoring, apnea, and daytime sleepiness

     iv. Nocturnal enuresis

     v. Nightmares

  c. School

     i. Name of school, location, and grade; new or continuing at previous year's school

     ii. Scholastic achievement or grades, other areas of achievement, and changes in performance

     iii. Attitude toward school, teachers, favorite subject, and future goals

     iv. Peer relationships

     v. School attendance and participation in activities

     vi. Reading, writing skills (have child demonstrate)

     vii. Learning differences, disabilities, and delays

7. Review of systems

  a. Skin: birthmarks, rashes, abrasions, and lesions

  b. Head–eyes–ears–nose–throat: headaches, head injuries, vision, corrective lenses or glasses, hearing, history of otitis, allergies, frequent colds, snoring, dental hygiene, dentist visit, difficulty swallowing, hoarseness, and sore throats

  c. Respiratory: reactive airway disease or asthma, croup, bronchitis, persistent cough, and cough at night or with exercise

  d. Cardiovascular: heart murmur, cyanosis, shortness of breath, energy level, and syncope

  e. Gastrointestinal: appetite, diet, abdominal pain, vomiting, diarrhea, and constipation

  f. Genitourinary: enuresis, urinary tract infection, dysuria, frequency, hematuria, vaginal discharge, Tanner stage, and menarche

  g. Skeletal: deformities, scoliosis, limb pains, injuries, orthopedic appliances, linear growth, and weight gain or loss

  h. Neurologic: seizures, fainting spells, loss of consciousness, gait, and cognitive disorders

  i. Lymph: lymphadenopathy, swollen tonsils, adenoids, and enlarged spleen

B. Objective

  a. Physical examination

     a. Height (plot on growth chart)

     b. Weight and body mass index (plot on growth chart)

     c. Blood pressure, pulse, and respiration

     d. Skin: hydration, lesions or rashes, scars, nevi, and birthmarks

     e. Head: hair growth and distribution, asymmetry

     f. Eyes: reactivity of pupils, red reflexes, fundus, extraocular movements, and cover–uncover test

     g. Ears: tympanic membrane description and mobility, cerumen, and external canal

     h. Nose: presence or absence of discharge, color of turbinates, and swelling

     i. Mouth: presence of teeth, caries, occlusion, braces, and lesions

     j. Neck: palpable nodes and presence of nuchal rigidity

     k. Chest: presence of ronchi; coarseness; wheeze or diminished breath sounds in lung fields; breast development (females); Tanner stage

     l. Cardiac: rhythm, presence of murmur, gallop, and click

     m. Abdomen: palpable organs, masses, tenderness, and guarding

     n. Genitalia: Tanner stage; circumcision and testes (males); general description of vaginal introitus, clitoris, labia (females)

     o. Musculoskeletal: muscle strength, range of motion, and scoliosis

     p. Neurologic: mental status examination; cerebellar testing; sensory, motor (fine and gross) status; deep tendon reflexes; and CN II–XII

III. Assessment

A. Determine the child's current health status

B. Identify the child's general health risks based on age, gender, and ethnicity, and specific health risks

C. *Determine the child's and caregiver's motivation to change health-damaging behaviors and promote and maintain health-promoting behaviors*

D. *Delineate the child's ability to accomplish and master developmental milestones*

IV. Plan

A. *Diagnostics (screening and secondary prevention tests)*

A periodicity schedule for preventive pediatric health care is available through the AAP and Bright Futures at http://practice.aap.org/content.aspx?aid=1599 (AAP, 2007).

1. Hearing risk assessment (Green & Palfrey, 2003; Harlor & Bower, 2009)

   Auditory skills monitoring annually or if indicated by parental or teacher concerns

2. Vision screen (Green & Palfrey, 2003; Kelly, 2009)

   Assess for defects in visual acuity annually and as needed using Snellen chart

3. Lead poisoning (AAP, 2005; CDC, 2009; Kelly, 2009) for recent immigrant, foreign adoptee, and refugee children between ages 6 months and 16 years

4. Oral health screening (AAP, 2003; American Academy of Pediatric Dentistry, 2009; Kelly, 2009)
   a. Assessment for caries, gingival health, and orthodontic needs
   b. Recommend routine dental visit every 6 months

5. Tuberculosis (TB) screening (AAP, 2007; Kelly, 2009)
   a. Targeted screening by purified protein derivative annually for children with the following
      i. Contacts of persons with active TB
      ii. Those who are foreign-born; those who travel to or have household visitors from a country with a high TB prevalence, such as Mexico, the Philippines, Vietnam, India, and China
      iii. Contacts with high-risk adults, including those who are homeless, incarcerated, infected with HIV, or intravenous drug users; and those with chronic conditions, such as diabetes mellitus, renal failure, malnutrition, or other immunodeficiencies

6. Dyslipidemia risk assessment (AAP, 2008; Kelly, 2009)
   a. Risk assessment at ages 2, 4, 6, 8, and 10 years
   b. Risk factors
      i. Family history of dyslipidemia, premature cardiovascular disease, or diabetes, or if family history is unknown
      ii. Children with disease states associated with cardiovascular disease
      iii. Body mass index $\geq$ 85th percentile for age and gender, hypertension, or insulin resistance
   c. If risk factors are present, test with fasting lipid profile; repeat testing in 3–5 years if results are within normal limits

B. *Treatment*

Immunizations appropriate for age (refer to yearly recommended immunization schedule at www.cdc.gov/vaccines or http://www.aap.org/pressroom/aappr-immunization-issuekit.htm. See *Appendix 1*, Childhood and Adolescent Immunization schedules 2010)

C. *Patient and family education (Figure 6-1)*

1. Discussion of parent and child concerns

2. Discussion of nutritional requirements, physical activities appropriate for age, and limitation of screen time to 1 hour per day

3. Child–parent discussion of safety: helmet use, car, sports, recreational activities, street, water, Internet, texting, and personal safety

4. Discussion of approaches to discipline within the family

5. Discussion of child's developmental need for peer interaction and socialization

6. Discussion of child–parent readiness for school and the adjustment if in school

7. Discussion of opportunities for mastery and self-esteem building

8. Ages 8–12 years: discussions of child's pubertal development and "body concerns"; discussion of child's relationship with peers, school, and family

9. Discussion of hygiene

D. *Expected child–parent outcomes*

1. Reassurance: in reference to the parent or child's concerns

2. Nutrition and physical activity: understands nutritional and physical activity recommendations appropriate for age

FIGURE 6-1   Safety, Nutrition, and Activity Guidelines for Your School-Aged Child

- *Recreational activities* should always be supervised and full appropriate safety gear worn. Helmets should be used with any wheeled devices. Traffic, street, and water safety are especially important areas to review.

- *Teach* your child to think carefully about his or her surroundings, particularly around new animals or people. Review the use of 911 and what to do if a child gets lost or separated. Model safe habits, such as seatbelt use, and instruct your child to wear his or her seatbelt appropriately for age and weight.

- *Prepare and Practice* for emergency situations in the home, such as fire or natural disaster. Make sure you have a planned reunification point (a school, firehouse, and so forth) in the event of a catastrophe. Have emergency supplies for at least 3 days. Have an emergency "go bag" with essential items if you are forced to leave home quickly. Include in the bag any medical needs, emergency instructions, and contact information. Instruct all your caregivers regarding the emergency plan and location of the go bag.

- *Computers* or any other device allowing on-line access should be closely monitored. Computers should be in public rooms of the home and parents should review Internet safety and use by setting clear limits and supervising closely.

NUTRITION TIPS (U.S. Department of Food And Agriculture, 2010):

- *Make half your grains whole:* whole-wheat bread, oatmeal, brown rice

- *Vary your veggies:* go dark green and orange with your vegetables

- *Focus on fruits:* fresh, frozen, canned, or dried, and go easy on the fruit juice

- *Get your calcium-rich foods:* low-fat and fat-free milk products several times a day

- *Go lean with protein:* eat lean or low-fat meat, chicken, turkey, fish, and dry beans

- *Change your oil:* fish, nuts, and liquid oils, such as corn, soybean, canola, and olive oil

- *Do not sugarcoat it:* try to avoid sweetened foods and beverages

ACTIVITY (Centers for Disease Control and Prevention, 2010):

- *60 minutes or more EVERY day!*

- *Limit* "screen time" (includes television, video games, and computer time) to 1 hour a day.

- *Vigorously exercise* at least 3 days a week. Some examples of vigorous activity include any games involving running and chasing; bicycle riding; jumping rope; martial arts; and sports, such as ice or field hockey, basketball, swimming, tennis, or gymnastics.

- *Strengthen muscles* by doing gymnastics, playing on a jungle gym, or climbing trees (www.treeclimbing.com for safety tips) at least 3 days a week.

- *Strengthen bones* with activities, such as jumping rope or running at least 3 days a week. Some examples of bone strengthening activities include such games as hop-scotch, hopping, skipping, jumping, jumping rope, and running, and such sports as gymnastics, basketball, volleyball, or tennis.

Adapted from: Centers for Disease Control and Prevention. (2010). *Physical activity for everyone.* Retrieved from http://www.cdc.gov/physicalactivity/everyone/guidelines/children.html and U.S. Department of Food and Agriculture, Food and Nutrition Service. (2010). *Team nutrition: My pyramid for kids.* Retrieved from http://www.fns.usda.gov/TN/kids-pyramid.html

3. Safety measures understood for helmet use, car boosters, sports, recreational activities, street, water, Internet, texting, and personal safety

4. Discipline and behavior: parents agree on an approach to discipline and implement it with consistency; no evidence of behavioral problems in the child

5. Developmental needs: parents understand the child's need for peer interaction, socialization, and opportunities for mastery

6. Education: parents assess school readiness and child's adjustment once in school

7. Sexuality: developmentally appropriate discussion and education (Santrock, 1999).

8. Ages 8–12 years: child able to freely verbalize "body concerns" and expectations of puberty; child able to freely verbalize relationships with peers, family, teachers, and participation in activities

9. Hygiene: parents and child understand recommended hygiene care

REFERENCES

American Academy of Pediatric Dentistry. (2009). *Guideline on infant oral health care.* Retrieved from http://www.aapd.org/media/policies.asp

American Academy of Pediatrics. (2003). Oral health risk assessment timing and establishment of the dental home. *Pediatrics, 111*(5), 1113–1116.

American Academy of Pediatrics. (2005). Lead exposure in children: Prevention, detection, and management. *Pediatrics, 116*(4), 1035–1047.

American Academy of Pediatrics. (2007). *Recommendations for preventive pediatric health care (periodicity schedule).* Retrieved from http://practice.aap.org/content.aspx?aid=1599

American Academy of Pediatrics. (2008). *Committee on nutrition policy statement: Cholesterol in childhood.* Retrieved from http://aappolicy.aappublications.org/cgi/content/full/pediatrics;101/1/141.

American Academy of Pediatrics. Committee on Practice and Ambulatory Medicine. (2000). Recommendations for preventive pediatric health care. *Pediatrics, 105*(3), 645–646.

American Heart Association, Gidding, S., Dennison, B., Birch, L., Daniels, S., Gilman, M., Lichtenstein, A., et. al. (2006). Dietary recommendations for children and adolescents: A guide for practitioners. *Pediatrics, 117*(2), 544–559.

Centers for Disease Control and Prevention. (2009). *Lead poisoning prevention in newly arrived refugee children.* Retrieved from http://www.cdc.gov/nceh/lead/Publications/Refugeetoolkit/RTK_Resources.htm

Duderstadt, K. G. (2006). Approach the child and adolescent assessment. In K. G. Duderstadt (Ed.), *Pediatric physical examination: An illustrated handbook* (pp. 3–10). San Francisco, CA: Mosby Inc.

Duderstadt, K. G., & Schapiro, N. (2006). Comprehensive information gathering. In K. G. Duderstadt (Ed.), *Pediatric physical examination: An illustrated handbook* (pp. 33–45). San Francisco, CA: Mosby Inc.

Gold, M. (2009, October 27). Kids watch more than a day of TV each week. *Los Angeles Times.* Retrieved from http://articles.latimes.com

Goldson, E., Hagerman, R., & Reynolds, A. (2003). Child development and behavior. In W. W. Green & J. S. Palfrey, *Bright futures: Guidelines for health supervision of infants, children, and adolescents* (2nd ed.). Arlington, VA: National Center for Education in Maternal and Child Health.

Green, W. W., & Palfrey, J. S. (2003). *Bright futures: Guidelines for health supervision of infants, children, and adolescents* (2nd ed.). Arlington, VA: National Center for Education in Maternal and Child Health.

Harlor, A. D., & Bower, C. (2009). Hearing assessment in infants and children: Recommendations beyond neonatal screening. *Pediatrics, 124*(4), 1252–1263.

Hill, C. R., & Stafford, F. P. (1980). Parental care of children: Time diary estimate of quantity, predictability, and variety. *Journal of Human Resources, 15,* 219–239.

Kelly, N. (2009, October 12). *Screening tests in children and adolescents.* UpToDate. Retrieved from http:www.uptodate.com/online/content/topic.do?topicKey=gen_pedi/6606&view=print

Obradovi, Ć. J., & Hipwell, A. (2010). Psychopathology and social competence during the transition to adolescence: The role of family adversity and pubertal development. *Developmental Psychopathology, 22*(3), 621–634.

Santrock, J. W. (1999). *Life-span development* (7th ed.). Dallas, TX: McGraw-Hill Companies.

Windom, A. (2006). Developmental parameters. In K. G. Duderstadt (ed.), *Pediatric physical examination: An illustrated handbook* (pp. 23–32). San Francisco, CA: Mosby Inc.

Zuckerman, D. (2001). *When little girls become women: Early onset of puberty in girls.* The Ribbon. Retrieved from http://www.center4research.org.

THE ADOLESCENT AND YOUNG ADULT (12–21 YEARS OF AGE) INTERVAL VISIT

Erica Monasterio

I. Introduction and general background

A. Developmental considerations

Adolescence, generally considered to encompass ages 12–21, is a time of enormous development and change in all domains of a young person's and a family's life. Bridging (and overlapping) childhood and young adulthood, adolescents experience the physical changes of growth and sexual maturation; continued developmental changes in both structure and function of their brains (a process not completed until the mid to late 20s); and cognitive, psychologic, and social changes related to both their physical changes and the roles and expectations of the culture and the society in which they live.

B. Adolescent consent and confidentiality

1. For the healthcare provider, the care of the adolescent may also be a time of transition, because it is the relationship that develops between the youth and the provider that becomes the key to the efficacy with which the provider can assess what services and interventions may be appropriate (Ford et al., 1997). The provider must develop an alliance with the youth, and addressing issues of confidentiality is the cornerstone of this alliance. Without assurances of confidentiality, the most vulnerable youth in need of attention and intervention, those who engage in behaviors that present a risk to their health, who are depressed or suicidal, and who report poor communication and lack of perceived support from their parents, may avoid health care altogether (Lehrer et al., 2007). For these reasons, it is recommended that providers seeing adolescents be prepared to spend time in the visit with both the parent and adolescent together, and with the adolescent alone, to get a full picture of the youth's strengths, risks, and overall physical and psychologic health status (Ford, English, & Sigman, 2004).

2. Although the involvement and participation of a caring adult in the care of adolescents is desirable, there are situations in which a young person may not feel able to involve their parent, or in which parental involvement could impair the youth's ability to seek or receive services. All states give adolescents some rights to both consent to and maintain privacy related to care for confidential issues (English, 2007). Laws vary significantly from state to state, and it is incumbent on the healthcare provider to be familiar with minor consent and confidentiality laws in their state of practice.

3. Effective communication with both youth and their caregivers about adolescent consent and confidentiality rights is essential to establishing rapport and eliciting pertinent information. A brief discussion of adolescent consent and confidentiality with the youth and parent, emphasizing the aspects of developing self-reliance and skills to manage their own health care, helps to set the stage. Assuring the parent that their presence and participation is valued, and that youth are always encouraged to communicate with their parents, reassures the parent that they are not being "shut out" of their child's care. Both parents and youth should be informed of the conditional nature of adolescent confidentiality rights because of obligations to protect the youth in the event that they are a danger to themselves or others or have been subjected to any reportable abuse. Once alone with the adolescent, it is helpful for the provider to elicit the youth's understanding of conditional confidentiality and provide a rationale for the personal nature of the questions that they will be asked.

C. Rationale for the psychosocial assessment

The leading causes of morbidity and mortality in adolescents (accidents, homicides, and suicides) are rooted in behavioral risk that the astute provider can identify and in which they can attempt to intervene (Heron & Tejada-Vera, 2009). For this reason, the major consensus guidelines focused on the care of adolescents (Guidelines for Adolescent Preventative Services from the American Medical Association and Bright Futures, from the Maternal-Child Health Bureau and the American Academy of Pediatrics) concur that a psychosocial assessment, focused to determine the strengths and risks of the youth and guide the physical and psychologic assessment and intervention process is recommended (Ford, Millstein, Halpern-Felsher, & Irwin, 1997; Hagen, Shaw, & Duncan, 2008).

D. Periodicity and focus of well adolescent care

1. Yearly well-adolescent visits are recommended, with an emphasis on prevention, education and counseling for both youth and their parents and guardians, screening for risk behaviors and their consequences, and counseling on healthy lifestyles (Rosen et al., 1997). Healthy People 2010 identified 21 critical objectives for youth, focusing on reducing deaths, unintentional injuries, violence, substance abuse, and mental health problems, and adverse reproductive health outcomes and reducing the proportion of adolescents who are overweight or obese, increasing the proportion who engage in vigorous physical activity that promotes cardiorespiratory fitness and reducing tobacco use by adolescents to reduce the early antecedents of chronic disease (U.S. Department of Health and Human Services, 2000).

2. According to Bright Futures, priority areas to address in the well-adolescent visit include the following:
   a. Physical growth and development (physical and oral health, body image, healthy eating, and physical activity).
   b. Social and academic competence (connectedness with family, peers, and community; interpersonal relationships; and school performance).
   c. Emotional well-being (coping, mood regulation and mental health, and sexuality).
   d. Risk reduction (tobacco, alcohol, or other drugs; pregnancy; and sexually transmitted infections [STIs]).
   e. Violence and injury prevention (safety belt and helmet use, driving [graduated license] and substance abuse, guns, interpersonal violence [dating violence], and bullying) (Hagen et al., 2008)

II. Database (may include but is not limited to)

A. *Subjective (to be obtained with both the youth and parent or caregiver present)*
   1. Client and parent or caregiver concerns
   2. History of any presenting concerns
   3. Past medical history
      a. Congenital or chronic conditions
      b. Surgery or hospitalizations
      c. Accidents or injuries, including injuries in sports activities that have required exclusion from play and head injuries resulting in loss of consciousness or memory loss
   4. Medications
      a. Drug, dose, prescriber, and medication adherence
      b. Revisit topic of medications once alone with the youth to determine if using any medications to treat or suppress STIs or to prevent pregnancy
   5. Dental
      a. Last dental visit
   6. Communicable diseases
      a. Varicella (documented disease)
      b. Hepatitis (birth in or travel to endemic areas, perinatal acquisition)
      c. Exposure to tuberculosis
   7. Immunizations
      a. Completion of childhood immunizations
      b. Initiation or completion of adolescent immunizations: refer to yearly Recommended Immunization Schedule at www.cdc.gov /vaccines or http://www.aap.org/pressroom /aappr-immunization-issuekit.htm

   See *Appendix 1*, Childhood and Adolescent Immunization schedules 2010.

   8. Allergies
      a. Seasonal allergies
      b. Food allergies or intolerances
      c. Drug reactions
   9. Family history
      a. First-degree relatives with a history of
         i. Hypertension
         ii. Hyperlipidemia
         iii. Cardiovascular disease
         iv. Sudden cardiac or unexplained death
         v. Cerebrovascular accidents

vi. Seizure disorder
vii. Diabetes
viii. Obesity
ix. Cancer
x. Mental health diagnoses
xi. Substance abuse
xii. Other medical or mental health problems

B. Subjective history (to be obtained only with the youth)

The psychosocial history, obtained after separating the youth and parent, must be adapted to the age, developmental stage, and interactive style of the adolescent. The mnemonic HEEADSSS (for *Home, Education/Employment, Eating, Activities, Drugs, Sexuality, Suicide/Depression/Self-image* and *Safety*) provides a flexible tool for guiding a discussion with an adolescent about the protective and risk factors in their lives (Goldenring & Rosen, 2004). A newer approach, SSHADESS (for *Strengths, School, Home, Activities, Drugs/substance use, Emotions/depression, Sexuality* and *Safety*) ensures that the provider starts with a focus on strengths that can then be built on in the context of the assessment and counseling (Ginsberg, 2007).

1. Home
   a. Who lives in the home
   b. How do family members get along
   c. Connectedness and engagement with and monitoring by parents

2. Education and employment
   a. School attendance
   b. School achievement (grades)
   c. School experience and connectedness to school
   d. Concerns about school
   e. Attitude toward school: good, poor, or indifferent
   f. Work: type and hours
   g. Goals: academic and career

3. Eating
   a. Body image
   b. Recent changes in weight
   c. Nutritional intake
   d. Eating patterns
   e. Family meals
   f. Dieting and weight control

4. Activities
   a. Peers: same gender, opposite gender, relationship quality (friends or romantic partners)
   b. Peer relationships: close friends or loner
   c. Outside interests: sports, music, dancing, hobbies, or organized activities
   d. Amount of daily screen time (television, computer and video games)

5. Drugs and alcohol
   a. Tobacco, alcohol and drug use (quantify frequency, intensity, patterns and context of use)
   b. Family substance use patterns

6. Sexuality
   a. Information appropriate for age
   b. Attracted to same, opposite, or both genders
   c. Sexually active
      i. Age of sexual debut
      ii. Number of partners
      iii. Gender of partners
      iv. Contraception type and frequency of use
      v. Type and frequency of protected or unprotected sex
      vi. Comfort or satisfaction with sexual activity
      vii. History of STIs

7. Suicide and depression
   a. Mood or energy level
   b. Depression
   c. Self-destructive behavior
   d. Suicidal thoughts or attempts

8. Safety
   a. Use of seatbelts
   b. Riding in or driving a car under the influence
   c. Use of protective equipment for leisure activities and sports
   d. Sense of safety or history of abuse in:
      i. Home
      ii. School
      iii. Relationships (peer and romantic)
      iv. Community

C. Review of systems

1. General health: fatigue, fever, weight change, appetite change, mood change, and sleep problems

2. Skin: lesions, rashes, and acne

3. Hematology: excessive bleeding, bruising, and lymphadenopathy

4. Head–eyes–ears–nose–throat: headaches, head injuries, vision problems, glasses, ear pain, decreased hearing, allergies, frequent colds, snoring, dental hygiene, last dentist visit, difficulty swallowing, hoarseness, and sore throats

5. Respiratory: asthma, frequent cough, wheezing, shortness of breath, and exercise-induced cough or wheezing

6. Cardiovascular: heart murmurs, chest pain, palpitations, syncope or near syncope, and shortness of breath on exertion

7. Gastrointestinal: abdominal pain, nausea, vomiting, diarrhea, constipation, and bloody stool

8. Genitourinary: enuresis, dysuria, frequency, hematuria, vaginal discharge, urethral discharge, testicular pain, vulvar lesions, and genital lesions

9. Skeletal: deformities or scoliosis, joint pain, joint swelling, injuries, and back pain

10. Neurologic: headache, seizures, syncope, dizziness, and numbness

11. Endocrine: polyuria and polydipsia

12. Female: menarche, last menstrual period, regularity and frequency, duration, dysmenorrhea, and premenstrual tension

13. Male: body hair and voice change

14. Psychologic and emotional: mood, stress, and mental health diagnoses and care source

D. Objective

1. Physical examination

   a. Height (measure and plot on growth chart if under 18)

   b. Weight (measure and plot on growth chart if under 18)

   c. Body mass index (BMI) (calculate and plot on BMI graph if under 18; overweight = age- and gender-specific BMI at ≥ 85th to 94th percentile; obesity = age- and gender-specific BMI at ≥ 95th percentile)

   d. Blood pressure, pulse, and respiration

   e. Vision (Snellen once in early, middle, and late adolescence; more frequently based on risk assessment)

   f. Hearing (audiometry only if positive responses to screening questions to determine risk for or evidence of hearing impairment)

   g. Mental status

   h. State of nutrition

   i. Skin: scars, tattoos, piercings, signs of self-injurious behavior, acne, and acanthosis nigricans

   j. Ears

   k. Eyes: include fundoscopic

   l. Nose: mucosa of septum

   m. Mouth: teeth (gums, caries, and occlusion)

   n. Pharynx

   o. Thyroid

   p. Lymph nodes
      i. Cervical
      ii. Axillary
      iii. Inguinal

   q. Breasts: inspect for sexual maturity rating (SMR), clinical breast examination after age 20 in females; gynecomastia in males

   r. Lungs: wheezing and adventitious sounds

   s. Heart: murmurs (upright and supine), rhythm, lower extremity pulses, and radio-femoral delay

   t. Abdomen: masses and hepatosplenomegaly

   u. Genitalia
      i. Males: inspect for SMR, signs of STIs, palpation of scrotum and testes for masses, and presence of hernia
      ii. Females: inspect for SMR, signs of STIs and dermatologic conditions of the vulva; use noninvasive (urine-based or high vaginal swab) screening tests for gonorrhea and *Chlamydia* when possible
      iii. Pelvic examination indicated at age 21 years to obtain first Pap smear or without a Pap smear if sexually active with signs and symptoms of STI, pregnancy, or pelvic infection, or to evaluate abnormal pubertal development, abnormal vaginal bleeding

   v. Musculoskeletal
      i. Back: range of motion and presence of scoliosis
      ii. Extremities: joint pain, swelling, and stability; range of motion
      iii. Twelve-point musculoskeletal screening (Kurowski & Chandran, 2000)

   w. Neurologic: strength, reflexes, coordination, and cranial nerves II–XII

III. Assessment

A. Identify the strengths and protective factors that will support the youth and family in successfully negotiating challenges in adolescence.

B. Identify the youth's specific health risks, based on family history, past medical history, and behavioral choices and activities in which the youth engages.

C. Determine the youth's current health status.

D. Determine the youth's motivation to modify

health-damaging behaviors and promote and maintain health-promoting behaviors.

E. *Determine the parent or caregiver's motivation to support the youth's behavior change plan as appropriate.*

IV. Plan

A. Screening

1. Psychosocial and behavioral assessment (annually) (Hagan et al., 2008).

2. Major depressive disorder screening when systems for diagnosis, treatment, and follow-up are in place, using such tools as the Patient Health Questionnaire for Adolescents or the Beck Depression Inventory–Primary Care Version (U.S. Preventive Services Task Force, 2009).

3. Alcohol and drug use risk assessment (annually), with follow-up in-depth assessment based on findings using a youth-specific alcohol and drug screening assessment tool, such as CRAFFT (Hagan et al., 2008).

4. Hemoglobin and hematocrit every 5–10 years starting in adolescence, more frequently if indicated based on risk (heavy or frequent menses, poor nutritional intake, limited dietary sources of iron, and history of iron-deficiency anemia) (Centers for Disease Control and Prevention, 1998).

5. Dyslipidemia screening (fasting total cholesterol, low-density lipoprotein, high-density lipoprotein, and triglycerides) at one late adolescent visit if no risk factors; initially at age 10 years and then every 2 years if BMI ≥ 85th percentile; add alanine aminotransferase, aspartate aminotransferase, and glucose if BMI is between 85th and 94th percentile and there are risk factors in the family history or physical examination or if BMI ≥ 95th percentile with or without risk factors (Barlow, 2007). Additionally, screen based on history of a parent with hyperlipidemia (cholesterol ≥ 240), first-degree relative with a history of premature (≤ 55 years old) atherosclerotic disease, myocardial infarction, or cerebrovascular accident (Daniels & Greer, 2008). These recommendations remain somewhat controversial, because there is insufficient evidence to support criteria to determine who should be included in targeted screening based on family history (Daniels & Greer).

6. Tuberculosis annually if HIV-positive or incarcerated, otherwise based on risk assessment (family member or household contact with tuberculosis or positive purified protein derivative, born in tuberculosis endemic country, travel with > 1 week residence in tuberculosis endemic country) (American Academy of Pediatrics, 2006).

7. Chlamydia screening annually for all sexually active females ≤ 25 years old; screening of high-risk young men is a clinical option (U.S. Preventive Services Task Force, 2001).

8. Gonorrhea screening annually for all sexually active young women and young men who have sex with men, and young men with multiple partners, and those seen in high-prevalence settings, such as adolescent clinics, correctional facilities, and STI clinics (Centers for Disease Control and Prevention, 2006a).

9. Syphilis screening for all pregnant women, young men who have sex with men and engage in high-risk sexual behaviors, commercial sex workers, youth who exchange sex for drugs, and youth in adult correctional facilities.

10. HIV screening once for all individuals between 13 and 64 years of age regardless of recognized risk factors (CDC, 2006b). Repeat HIV screening based on individual risk assessment.

11. Cervical cancer screening (Pap smear) for all women at age 21 regardless of sexual history, then every 2 years if benign (American Congress of Obstetricians and Gynecologists, 2009).

B. Immunization update

1. Because of the rapidly changing nature of immunization recommendations in terms of available immunizations and recommended schedule of administration, the reader is advised to consult the Centers for Disease Control and Prevention or the American Academy of Pediatrics websites for the current immunization schedule. Centers for Disease Control and Prevention National Immunization Program: http://www.cdc.gov/vaccines. American Academy of Pediatrics Red Book: http://www.aapredbook.org. See *Appendix 1*, Childhood and Adolescent Immunization schedules 2010.

2. Immunization lag: the following immunizations have commonly been missed in the adolescent

client and should be administered as "catch up" immunizations at the annual visit:

    a. Varicella #2

    b. Hepatitis A #2

    c. Tdap

    d. Meningococcal conjugate vaccine (MCV4)

    e. Human papilloma virus series

C. Anticipatory guidance

1. Normative development and developmental progression (discuss with youth and parent as appropriate)

    a. Adapt to youth's developmental stage and any concerns of youth or parent

    b. Include counseling regarding physical and psychosocial development

    c. Address levels of stress in youth and family and discuss healthy versus dysfunctional coping mechanisms

    d. Use an approach that is dynamic, interactive, and inclusive of the youth, prioritizing behaviors that the young person is interested in modifying and developing a change plan with rather than for the youth (Erickson, Gerstle, & Feldstein, 2005)

    e. Address parenting issues, emphasize continued importance of parental support and monitoring with consideration of age and developmental stage and gradual shift in locus of control from parent to youth

2. Nutrition and activity counseling (discuss with youth and parent as appropriate):

    a. Avoid skipping meals, particularly emphasize the importance of breakfast

    b. Drink adequate fluids, emphasize water and avoidance of high intake of soda, juice, sports drinks, and caffeinated drinks

    c. Increase intake of fruits and vegetables

    d. Avoid high caloric and low nutritional value snacks

    e. Build physical activity into everyday routine and limit "screen time"

    f. Refer overweight and obese patients to comprehensive moderate- to high-intensity programs that include dietary, physical activity, and behavioral counseling components (U.S. Preventive Services Task Force, 2010)

3. Safety, injury, and violence prevention counseling as appropriate to age and developmental stage and individual risk

    a. Use of protective gear for sports and leisure activities

    b. Automobile safety

       i. Seatbelt use

       ii. Counseling regarding alcohol and drug use and driving or riding with an impaired driver

    c. Nonviolent conflict resolution

    d. Dating and relationship safety and healthy relationships

4. Tobacco, alcohol, and other drug counseling as appropriate to age and developmental stage and individual risk (with youth alone, using a motivational counseling approach)

    a. Tobacco resistance and cessation

    b. Alcohol resistance and use modification

       i. Discuss binge drinking patterns, risks, and self-management

    c. Marijuana resistance and use modification

       i. Discuss impact of marijuana use on learning, school performance, goal setting, and decision-making

    d. Other substances of abuse related to individual risk, individual use, and community use patterns

5. Sexual health and risk reduction as appropriate to age and developmental stage and individual risk (with youth alone, using a motivational counseling approach)

    a. Relationship quality and sexual decision-making

    b. Encourage delaying onset of sexual activity with younger adolescents

    c. Contraception and pregnancy prevention

       i. Discuss access to emergency contraception with all youth regardless of current sexual activity

       ii. Counsel regarding contraceptive choice as appropriate to current and anticipated sexual activity

    d. STI and HIV risk reduction

       i. Discuss risk reduction approaches with all youth regardless of current sexual activity

V. Self management resources

A. For adolescents

1. http://www.teenhealthfx.com: Interactive website with a question and answer format by and for teenagers. The Adolescent/Young Adult Center for Health at the Goryeb Children's Hospital is

responsible for the content and operation of the site.

2. http://www.bam.gov: Centers for Disease Control and Prevention youth website with games and facts about health. Oriented towards middle school and early adolescents.

3. http://kidshealth.org/teen: Resources to increase teenagers' health awareness and empower young people to take an active role in their health. Operated by Nemours Children's Health Systems.

4. http://www.teengrowth.com: Interactive website specifically tailored toward health interests and general well-being of the teenage population. Information from a physician advisory board of experts on puberty, family, friends, sex, emotions, and nutrition. Includes links, crisis lines, and the opportunity to contact a doctor.

B. For parents or caregivers

5. http://www.4parents.gov: Resources for parents who wish to help their teenage children make healthy choices and avoid risk.

6. http://www.pamf.org/parents: Palo Alto Medical Foundation information for parents of teenagers and preteenagers about a variety of health and social issues.

7. http://www.parentingteensonline.com: On-line magazine with information about adolescent health in an "Ask the Expert" format. Content is focused on producing responsible and appropriate communications for parents and teenagers about important issues, such as health and wellness, relationships, technology and media, education, and finances.

8. http://www.talkingwithkids.org: Developed by Children Now and Kaiser Family Foundation. Basic information about talking with youth about challenging issues.

9. http://www.familiesaretalking.org: Developed by SIECUS with materials in English and Spanish for parents and youth with a focus on providing guidance and support for parents as the primary sexuality educators of their child.

C. For healthcare providers

10. http://www.ama-assn.org/ama/pub/physician-resources/public-health/promoting-healthy-lifestyles/adolescent-health.shtml: American Medical Association resources on promoting adolescent health including screening and periodicity recommendations.

11. http://www.ama-assn.org/ama/upload/mm/39/parentinfo.pdf: Parent information handouts on 15 adolescent topics ranging from vaccines to alcohol and drug use prevention.

12. http://www.brightfutures.org/bf2/pdf/pdf/AD.pdf: Bright Futures Guidelines for Health Supervision of Adolescents (2nd edition, revised). Developed by the American Academy of Pediatrics and the Maternal Child Health Bureau.

13. http://www.ahwg.net/knowledgebase/nodates.php?pid=79&tpid=2: Adolescent Health Working Group's "Adolescent Providers Toolkit Series" includes five Toolkit modules contain screening tools, brief office interventions and counseling guidelines, community resources and referrals, health education materials for teenagers and their parents or caregivers, literature reviews, and Internet resources.

REFERENCES

American Academy of Pediatrics. (2006). Tuberculosis. In L. Pickering, C. Baker, S. Long, & J. McMillan (Eds.), *Red book: 2006 report of the committee on infectious diseases* (27th ed., pp. 678–698). Elk Grove Village, IL: American Academy of Pediatrics.

American Congress of Obstetricians and Gynecologists. (2009). ACOG Practice Bulletin No. 109: Cervical Cytology Screening. *Obstetrics and Gynecology, 114*(6), 1409–1420.

Barlow, S. E. (2007). Expert committee recommendations regarding the prevention, assessment, and treatment of child and adolescent overweight and obesity: Summary report. *Pediatrics, 120*(Suppl. 4), S164–S192.

Centers for Disease Control and Prevention. (1998). Recommendations to prevent and control iron deficiency in the United States. *MMWR Recomm Rep, 47*(RR-3), 1–36.

Centers for Disease Control and Prevention. (2006a). *Sexually transmitted diseases treatment guidelines 2006. Special Populations.* Retrieved from http://www.cdc.gov/std/treatment/2006/specialpops.htm#specialpops2.

Centers for Disease Control and Prevention. (2006b). Revised recommendations for HIV testing of adults, adolescents, and pregnant women in health-care settings. *MMWR, 55*(RR-14), 1–17.

Daniels, S. R., & Greer, F. R. (2008). Lipid screening and cardiovascular health in childhood. *Pediatrics, 122*(1), 198–208.

English, A. (2007). Sexual and reproductive health care for adolescents: Legal rights and policy challenges. *Adolescent Medicine, 18*(3), 571–581.

English, A., & Ford, C. A. (2007). More evidence supports the need to protect confidentiality in adolescent health care. *Journal of Adolescent Health, 40*(3), 199–200.

English, A., Ford, C. A., & Santelli, J. S. (2009). Clinical preventive services for adolescents: Position paper of the society for adolescent medicine. *American Journal of Law and Medicine, 35*(2-3), 351–364.

Erickson, S. J., Gerstle, M., & Feldstein, S. W. (2005). Brief interventions and motivational interviewing with children, adolescents, and their parents in pediatric health care settings: A review. *Archives of Pediatrics & Adolescent Medicine, 159*(12), 1173–1180.

Ford, C., Millstein, S., Halpern-Felsher, B., & Irwin, C. (1997). Influence of physician confidentiality assurances on adolescents' willingness to disclose information and seek future health care. *Journal of the American Medical Association, 278*(12), 1029–1034.

Ford, C., English, A., & Sigman, G. (2004). Confidential health care for adolescents: Position paper for the society for adolescent medicine. *Journal of Adolescent Health, 35*(2), 160–167.

Ginsburg, K. R. (2007). Viewing our adolescent patients through a positive lens. *Contemporary Pediatrics, 24*, 6–76.

Goldenring, J. M., & Rosen, D. S. (2004). Getting into adolescent heads: An essential update. *Contemporary Pediatrics, 21*(1), 64–90.

Hagan, J. F., Shaw, J. S., & Duncan, P. M. (Eds.). (2008). *Bright futures: Guidelines for health supervision of infants, children, and adolescents* (3rd ed.). Elk Grove Village, IL: American Academy of Pediatrics.

Heron, M. P., & Tejada-Vera, B. (2009). Deaths: Leading causes for 2005. *National Vital Statistics Reports, 58*(8), 1–98.

Kurowski, K., & Chandran, S. (2000). The preparticipation athletic evaluation. *American Family Physician, 61*(9), 2683–2696.

Lehrer, J., Pantell, R., Tebb, K., & Shafer, M. (2007). Forgone health care among U.S. adolescents: Associations between risk characteristics and confidentiality concern. *Journal of Adolescent Health, 40*(3), 218–226.

Rosen, D. S., Elster, A., Hedberg, V., et al. (1997). Clinical preventive services for adolescents: Position paper of the society for adolescent medicine. *Journal of Adolescent Health, 21*(3), 203–214.

U.S. Department of Health and Human Services. (2000). *Healthy People 2010, volumes 1 and 2.* Washington, DC: U.S. Government Printing Office.

U.S. Preventive Services Task Force. (2001). *Screening for chlamydial infection: Recommendations and rationale.* Rockville, MD: Agency for Healthcare Research and Quality. Retrieved from: http://www.ahrq.gov/clinic/ajpmsuppl/chlarr.htm.

U.S. Preventive Services Task Force. (2004). *Screening for syphilis infection: Recommendation statement.* Agency for Healthcare Research and Quality, Rockville, MD. Retrieved from http://www.ahrq.gov/clinic/3rduspstf/syphilis/syphilrs.htm.

U.S. Preventive Services Task Force. (2009). Screening and treatment for major depressive disorder in children and adolescents: U.S. preventive services task force recommendation statement. *Pediatrics, 123*(4), 1223–1228.

U.S. Preventive Services Task Force. (2010). Screening for obesity in children and adolescents: U.S. preventive services task force recommendation statement. *Pediatrics, 125*(2), 361.

APPENDIX 7-1: CHILDHOOD AND ADOLESCENT IMMUNIZATION SCHEDULES

Lucy S. Crain

An Overview of Active and Passive Immunization: Introduction

Simply stated, vaccines prevent disease, with their ultimate goal being to eradicate or eliminate disease. Along with pure water and refrigeration, preventive vaccines are the most important public health development of the past century. United States public health history documents recorded nearly 48,164 annual cases of smallpox and 175,885 annual cases of diphtheria in 1900–1904, and no cases of these diseases in 2007. There were 16,000 cases of paralytic polio reported annually during 1951–1954, a period 4 years before vaccine licensure. Similarly, there were more than 503,000 cases of measles in 1958–1962, a period 5 years before the first measles vaccine was licensed. In the years before licensure of rubella vaccine in 1971, there were 40,000–50,000 cases of rubella annually in the United States, with hundreds of cases of congenital rubella syndrome. Although global eradication of smallpox was achieved in 1977, and poliomyelitis was eliminated from the Americas in 1991, prevention of other vaccine-preventable diseases, such as pertussis, diphtheria, rubella, mumps, measles, varicella, hepatitis A and B, and pneumococcal and meningococcal meningitis, depends on consistently high levels of immunization to ensure a protected or immune population. The *Red Book* report of the American Academy of Pediatrics Committee on Infectious Diseases is one of the most comprehensive compendia of vaccine information and discussions of infectious diseases, and in-depth discussion of various types of vaccines and their indications (American Academy of Pediatrics, 2009).

Epidemiologic studies confirm that population immunization rates of 90% or greater are desirable for adequate control and prevention of spread of most contagious infectious diseases. Although vaccines for smallpox, diphtheria, tetanus, and pertussis have been available for well over 60 years, the above data also note the significant number of vaccines that have been developed and licensed more recently. Well-child visits are scheduled to ensure timely administration of recommended vaccines at appropriate ages, according to immunization schedules published and updated regularly by the American Academy of Pediatrics in collaboration with the Centers for Disease Control and Prevention (CDC) and the U.S. Public Health Service. Childhood immunizations constitute the predominant basis for infectious disease prevention, assuming an immunized population of 90% or more adequately to protect against occasional exposures or possible epidemics.

Active and Passive Immunizations

The administration of all or part or modified form of a microorganism in order to produce the humoral or cellular responses in the recipient to the immunization agent constitutes active immunization. Modifications include purified antigens, genetically engineered antigens, or toxoids produced by those microorganisms. Active immunizations provoke an immune response that is similar to a natural infection, but without the risk of the actual infection. The result is the development of protective antibodies in the actively immunized child or adult. Such vaccines may include infectious agents that are attenuated (i.e., weakened or modified), live, genetically engineered, or killed units of infectious agents. The U.S. Food and Drug Administration maintains a website of such licensed vaccines and is an excellent reference (www.fda.gov/cber/vaccine/licvacc.htm).

The administration of an already formed antibody, such as immune globulin, constitutes passive immunization. Special circumstances indicate the need for passive immunization (i.e., when an individual is deficient in certain antibodies or the ability to produce antibodies, either from congenital or acquired immunodeficiencies or other lymphocyte defects). Another indication for passive immunization is its prophylactic use when a person is exposed to a high-risk disease and does not have time to produce adequate antibodies from active immunization. A third category is therapeutic indication, when a disease, such as botulism, tetanus, or other toxin-producing infection, is already present.

Current Concerns and Vaccination Rates

Immunizations have been so successful in the United States in preventing most of these diseases for more than a half century that many people, including parents, physicians, and nurses, have never seen a case of polio or possibly even measles, pertussis, or rubella. The unfortunate downside of such success is an increasing number of parents who choose to refuse immunizations for their children, assuming that their child will not be exposed, or assuming that he or she will be protected by the immune status of his or her schoolmates. Parental refusal can constitute religious exemptions and other formats, differing from state to state, to avoid mandatory compliance with adequate immunization status required for school entry at age 5. Parental refusal has resulted in communities and states where immunization rates have fallen to less than 50% (CDC, 2010b), which is far less than that required to have an immune "herd" or cohort of individuals to protect. This has led to several recent outbreaks of vaccine-preventable diseases, such as measles, mumps, and pertussis. The California Department of Health Services declared an epidemic of pertussis in July 2010 because of the excessively great and rapidly increasing number of cases reported. As of this time, several California infants have died of pertussis and others are hospitalized critically ill with the disease. The primary reservoir for community pertussis is the adult population, in which pertussis is a nagging 6-week illness marked by spasms of uncontrollable coughing, preceded by an upper respiratory prodrome. It is rarely recognized as a treatable and contagious infectious disease, increasing opportunities for affected adults to expose infants and children to pertussis. Infants are especially vulnerable to complications of pertussis, because the laryngospasm associated with the cough in unimmunized or incompletely immunized infants can be life-threatening. Also, infants can develop pneumonia as a complication of pertussis, and this also can be a cause of death. In addition, for young infants who survive pertussis, there are significant risks for brain damage, because of intracranial hemorrhages caused by the severity of their coughing spasms.

▌Vaccine Risk Versus Benefit Considerations

The morbidity and mortality associated with any of the vaccine-preventable diseases is significant and should be considered in any discussions of risk versus benefit of immunizations. Although immunizations may be momentarily painful at time of injection and associated local discomfort may ensue temporarily, complications include allergic reactions and, less commonly, syncope. More severe complications, including a shock-like reaction, are exceedingly rare. Vaccine package inserts are also a good source of information on potential complications, including data on incidence. For more detailed discussion of vaccine-associated safety issues, the CDC maintains an excellent website (http://www.cdc.gov/vaccinesafety/index.html).

Today's vaccines are remarkably safe and the benefits of prevention of life-threatening diseases are convincing to most healthcare providers and laypersons. However, the media and popular, nonscientifically or nonevidence based on-line and broadcast and print sources often sensationalize cases of untoward reactions to vaccines and the public has become skeptical and lacking in trust about vaccines. Many parents have accepted a popular misconception that vaccines contain harmful substances, such as mercury, and that these substances have been implicated in causing autism spectrum disorders. The basis for this incorrect information stems from an article by a British physician published in the *Lancet* in the 1990s, which has since been discredited and disproved by numerous studies, including an exhaustive review by the Institute of Medicine. There is no proven association with causation of autism and thimerosal, a mercurial preservative used in the past in vaccines. Thimerosal has not been included in vaccines in the United States (with the exception of multidose influenza vaccine for adult administration) for more than 10 years, and should not be a reason to avoid immunizations. It is important that parents be referred to reliable and scientifically accurate sources of information about vaccines so that they can choose to immunize and protect their child adequately against potentially life-threatening diseases. The CDC websites cited and the American Academy of Pediatrics *Red Book* are excellent sources of such information. Also, "parent friendly" information is found at the highly regarded Texas Children's Hospital website (www.vaccine.texaschildrenshospital.org), and the Every Child by Two sites (www.ecbt.org and www.vaccinateyourbaby.org). A myriad of frequently updated websites regarding vaccines are available on-line, and health professionals are advised to review such sources carefully before recommending them to their patients or to parents. Other important sources of information on vaccines include the Vaccine Adverse Event Reporting System, with information in reporting any adverse vaccine-related events experienced by children or adults (see http://vaers.hhs.gov and https://vaers.hhs.gov/esub/index).

Additional immunizations are recommended for adults, including the attenuated diphtheria–pertussis–tetanus combination, according to the U.S. Public Health Service Adult Preventive Health Care guidelines. For older adults and those with impaired immunity, zoster vaccine for prevention or amelioration of shingles and pneumococcal vaccine for prevention of pneumococcal pneumonia are recommended. Adults and children are advised to obtain hepatitis A immunization, especially if they live in or plan to travel in endemic areas. Immunization recommendations are frequently updated as new vaccines become available, and reference to current CDC guidelines is advised.

The appended immunization tables and recommended schedules attest to the ongoing development of safer, more effective vaccines through vigilant surveillance, quality control, and research and development. Additional immunization and epidemiologic data can be obtained online from http://www.cdc.gov and from www.cdc.gov/mmwr, the *Morbidity and Mortality Weekly Report*.

REFERENCES

American Academy of Pediatrics. (2009). *Red book: 2009 report of the committee on infectious diseases* (28th ed., pp. 1–2). Elk Grove Village, IL: American Academy of Pediatrics.

Centers for Disease Control and Prevention. (2010a). *Morbidity and mortality weekly report (MMWR)*. Retrieved from www.cdc.gov/mmwr.

Centers for Disease Control and Prevention. (2010b). *Vaccines & immunizations*. Retrieved from www.cdc.gov/vaccines.

Centers for Disease Control and Prevention. (2010c). *Vaccine safety*. Retrieved from http://www.cdc.gov/vaccinesafety/index.html.

Every Child by Two. (n.d.). Retrieved from www.ecbt.org.

Texas Children's Hospital. (n.d.). *The center for vaccine awareness and research*. Retrieved from www.vaccine.texaschildrenshospital.org.

U.S. Food and Drug Administration. (2010). *Complete list of vaccines licensed for immunization and distribution in the U.S.* Retrieved from www.fda.gov/cber/vaccine/licvacc.htm.

Vaccine Adverse Events Reporting System. (n.d.). Retrieved from http://vaers.hhs.gov.

Vaccine Adverse Events Reporting System. (n.d.). *Report an adverse event*. Retrieved from https://vaers.hhs.gov/esub/index.

Vaccinate Your Baby. (n.d.). Retrieved from www.vaccinateyourbaby.org.

RECOMMENDED ADULT IMMUNIZATION SCHEDULE
UNITED STATES—2010

Note: These recommendations *must* be read with the footnotes (on page 47) that follow containing number of doses, intervals between doses, and other important information.

FIGURE 1 Recommended Adult Immunization Schedule, by Vaccine and Age Group

Vaccine	19–26 Years	27–49 Years	50–59 Years	60–64 Years	≥ 65 years
Tetanus, diphtheria, pertussis (Td/Tdap)[1,*]	Substitute 1-time dose of Tdap for Td booster; then boost with Td every 10 yrs				Td booster every 10 yrs
Human papillomavirus (HPV)[2,*]	3 doses (females)				
Varicella[3*]	2 doses				
Zoster[4]				1 dose	
Measles, mumps, rubella (MMR)[5,*]	1 or 2 doses		1 dose		
Influenza[6,*]	1 dose annually				
Pneumococcal (polysaccharide)[7,8]	1 or 2 doses				1 dose
Hepatitis A[9,*]	2 doses				
Hepatitis B[10,*]	3 doses				
Meningococcal[11,*]	1 or more doses				

* Covered by the Vaccine Injury Compensation Program.

For all persons in this category who meet the age requirements and who lack evidence of immunity (e.g., lack documentation of vaccination or have no evidence of prior infection)

Recommended if some other risk factor is present (e.g., on the basis of medical, occupational, lifestyle, or other indications)

No recommendation

Report all clinically significant postvaccination reactions to the Vaccine Adverse Event Reporting System (VAERS). Reporting forms and instructions on filing a VAERS report are available at www.vaers.hhs.gov or by telephone, 800-822-7967.

Information on how to file a Vaccine Injury Compensation Program claim is available at www.hrsa.gov/vaccinecompensation or by telephone, 800-338-2382. To file a claim for vaccine injury, contact the U.S. Court of Federal Claims, 717 Madison Place, N.W., Washington, D.C. 2005; telephone, 202-357-6400.

Additional information about the vaccines in this schedule, extent of available data, and contraindications for vaccination is also available at www.cdc.gov/vaccine or from the CDC-INFO Contact Center at 800-CDC-INFO (800-232-4636) in English and Spanish, 24 hours a day, 7 days a week.

Use of trade names and commercial sources is for identification only and does not imply endorsement by the U.S. Department of Health and Human Services.

FIGURE 2 Vaccines That Might Be Indicated for Adults Based on Medical and Other Indications

Vaccine	Pregnancy	Immuno-compromising conditions (excluding human immunodeficiency virus [HIV])[3-5,13]	HIV infection[3-5,12,13] CD4+ T lymphocyte count <200 cells/μL	HIV infection ≥200 cells/μL	Diabetes, heart disease, chronic lung disease, chronic alcoholism	Asplenia[12] (including elective splenectomy and persistent complement component deficiencies)	Chronic liver disease	Kidney failure, end-stage renal disease, receipt of hemodialysis	Health-care personnel
Tetanus, diphtheria, pertussis (Td/Tdap)[1],*	Td	Substitute 1-time dose of Tdap for Td booster; then boost with Td every 10 yrs							
Human papillomavirus (HPV)[2],*			3 doses for females through age 26 yrs						
Varicella[3],*	Contraindicated	Contraindicated			2 doses				
Zoster[4]	Contraindicated	Contraindicated			1 dose				
Measles, mumps, rubella (MMR)[5],*	Contraindicated	Contraindicated			1 or 2 doses				
Influenza[6],*			1 dose TIV annually					1 dose TIV or LAIV annually	
Pneumococcal (polysaccharide)[7,8]					1 or 2 doses				
Hepatitis A[9],*					2 doses				
Hepatitis B[10],*					3 doses				
Meningococcal[11],*					1 or more doses				

*Covered by the Vaccine Injury Compensation Program.

For all persons in this category who meet the age requirements and who lack evidence of immunity (e.g., lack documentation of vaccination or have no evidence of prior infection)

Recommended if some other risk factor is present (e.g., on the basis of medical, occupations, lifestyle, or other indications)

No recommendation

These schedules indicate the recommended age groups and medical indications for which administration of currently licensed vaccines is commonly indicated for adults ages 19 years and older, as of January 1, 2010. Licensed combination vaccines may be used whenever any components of the combination are indicated and when the vaccine's other components are not contraindicated. For detailed recommendations on all vaccines, including those used primarily for travelers or that are issued during the years, consult the manufacturers' package inserts and the complete statements from the Advisory Committee on Immunization Practices (www.cdc.gov/vaccines/pubs/acip-list.htm).

The recommendations in this schedule were approved by the Centers for Disease Control and Prevention's (CDC) Advisory Committee on Immunization Practices (ACIP), the American Academy of Family Physicians (AAFP), the American College of Obstetricians and Gynecologists (ACOG), and the American College of Physicians (ACP).

Department of Health and Human Services Centers for Disease Control and Prevention

Footnotes

Recommended Adult Immunization Schedule—UNITED STATES - 2010

For complete statements by the Advisory Committee on Immunization Practices (ACIP), visit www.cdc.gov/vaccines/pubs/ACIP-list.html.

1. Tetanus, diphtheria, and acellular pertussis (Td/Tdap) vaccination

Tdap should replace a single dose of Td for adults aged 19 through 64 years who have not received a dose of Tdap previously.

Adults with uncertain or incomplete history of primary vaccination series with tetanus and diphtheria toxoid-containing vaccines should begin or complete a primary vaccination series. A primary series for adults is 3 doses of tetanus and diphtheria toxoid-containing vaccines; administer the first 2 doses at least 4 weeks apart and the third dose 6–12 months after the second; Tdap can substitute for any one of the doses of Td in the 3-dose primary series. The booster dose of tetanus and diphtheria toxoid-containing vaccine should be administered to adults who have completed a primary series and if the last vaccination was received ≥10 years previously. Tdap or Td vaccine may be used, as indicated.

If a woman is pregnant and received the last Td vaccination ≥10 years previously, administer Td during the second or third trimester. If the woman received the last Td vaccination < 10 years previously, administer Tdap during the immediate postpartum period. A dose of Tdap is recommended for postpartum women, close contacts of infants aged < 12 months, and all healthcare personnel with direct patient contact if they have not previously received Tdap. An interval as short as 2 years from the last Td is suggested; shorter intervals can be used. Td may be deferred during pregnancy and Tdap substituted in the immediate postpartum period, or Tdap can be administered instead of Td to a pregnant woman.

Consult the ACIP statement for recommendations for giving Td as prophylaxis in wound management.

2. Human papillomavirus (HPV) vaccination

HPV vaccination is recommended at age 11 or 12 years with catch-up vaccination at ages 13 through 26 years.

Ideally, vaccine should be administered before potential exposure to HPV through sexual activity; however, females who are sexually active should still be vaccinated consistent with age-based recommendations. Sexually active females who have not been infected with any of the four HPV vaccine types (types 6, 11, 16, 18 all of which HPV4 prevents) or any of the two HPV vaccine types (types 16 and 18 both of which HPV2 prevents) receive the full benefit of the vaccination. Vaccination is less beneficial for females who have already been infected with one or more of the HPV vaccine types. HPV4 or HPV2 can be administered to persons with a history of genital warts, abnormal Papanicolaou test, or positive HPV DNA test, because these conditions are not evidence of prior infection with all vaccine HPV types.

HPV4 may be administered to males aged 9 through 26 years to reduce their likelihood of acquiring genital warts. HPV4 would be most effective when administered before exposure to HPV through sexual contact.

A complete series for either HPV4 or HPV2 consists of 3 doses. The second dose should be administered 1–2 months after the first dose; the third dose should be administered 6 months after the first dose.

Although HPV vaccination is not specifically recommended for persons with the medical indications described in Figure 2, "Vaccines that might be indicated for adults based on medical and other indications," it may be administered to these persons because the HPV vaccine is not a live-virus vaccine. However, the immune response and vaccine efficacy might be less for persons with the medical indications described in Figure 2 than in persons who do not have the medical indications described or who are immunocompetent. Healthcare personnel are not at increased risk because of occupational exposure, and should be vaccinated consistent with age-based recommendations.

3. Varicella vaccination

All adults without evidence of immunity to varicella should receive 2 doses of single-antigen varicella vaccine if not previously vaccinated or the second dose if they have received only 1 dose, unless they have a medical contraindication.

Special consideration should be given to those who 1) have close contact with persons at high risk for severe disease (e.g., healthcare personnel and family contacts of persons with immunocompromising conditions) or 2) are at high risk for exposure or transmission (e.g., teachers; child-care employees; residents and staff members of institutional settings, including correctional institutions; college students; military personnel; adolescents and adults living in households with children; nonpregnant women of childbearing age; and international travelers).

Evidence of immunity to varicella in adults includes any of the following: 1) documentation of 2 doses of varicella vaccine at least 4 weeks apart; 2) U.S.-born before 1980 (although for healthcare personnel and pregnant women, birth before 1980 should not be considered evidence of immunity); 3) history of varicella based on diagnosis or verification of varicella by a healthcare provider (for a patient reporting a history of or presenting with an atypical case, a mild case, or both, healthcare providers should seek either an epidemiologic link with a typical varicella case or to a laboratory-confirmed case of evidence of laboratory confirmation, if it was performed at the time of acute disease); 4) history of herpes zoster based on diagnosis or verification of herpes zoster by a healthcare provider; or 5) laboratory evidence of immunity or laboratory confirmation of disease.

Pregnant women should be assessed for evidence of varicella immunity. Women who do not have evidence of immunity should receive the first dose of varicella vaccine upon completion or termination of pregnancy and before discharge from the healthcare facility. The second dose should be administered 4–8 weeks after the first dose.

4. Herpes zoster vaccination

A single dose of zoster vaccine is recommended for adults aged ≥ 60 years regardless of whether they report a prior episode of herpes zoster. Persons with chronic medical conditions may be vaccinated unless their condition constitutes a contraindication.

5. Measles, mumps, rubella (MMR) vaccination

Adults born before 1957 generally are considered immune to measles and mumps.

Measles component: Adults born during or after 1957 should receive 1 or more doses of MMR vaccine unless they have 1) a medical contraindication; 2) documentation of vaccination with 1 or more doses of MMR vaccine; 3) laboratory evidence of immunity; or 4) documentation of physician-diagnosed measles.

A second dose of MMR vaccine, administered 4 weeks after the first dose, is recommended for adults who 1) have been recently exposed to measles or are in an outbreak setting; 2) have been vaccinated previously with killed measles vaccine; 3) have been vaccinated with unknown type of measles vaccine during 1963–1967; 4) are students in postsecondary educational institutions; 5) work in a healthcare facility; or 6) plan to travel internationally.

Mumps component: Adults born during or after 1957 should receive 1 dose of MMR vaccine unless they have 1) a medical contraindication; 2) documentation of vaccination with 1 or more doses of MMR vaccine; 3) laboratory evidence of immunity; or 4) documentation of physician-diagnosed mumps.

A second dose of MMR vaccine, administered 4 weeks after the first dose, is recommended for adults who 1) live in a community experiencing a mumps outbreak and are in an affected age group; 2) are students in postsecondary educational institutions; 3) work in a healthcare facility; or 4) plan to travel internationally.

Rubella component: 1 dose of MMR vaccine is recommended for women who do not have documentation of rubella vaccination, or who lack laboratory evidence of immunity. For women of childbearing age, regardless of birth year, rubella immunity should be determined and women should be counseled regarding congenital rubella syndrome. Women who do not have evidence of immunity should receive MMR vaccine upon completion or termination of pregnancy and before discharge from the healthcare facility.

Healthcare personnel born before 1957: For unvaccinated healthcare personnel born before 1957 who lack laboratory evidence of measles, mumps, and/or rubella immunity or laboratory confirmation of disease, healthcare facilities should consider vaccinating personnel with 2 doses of MMR vaccine at the appropriate interval (for measles and mumps) and 1 dose of MMR vaccine (for rubella), respectively.

During outbreaks, healthcare facilities should recommend that unvaccinated healthcare personnel born before 1957, who lack laboratory evidence of measles, mumps, and/or rubella immunity or laboratory confirmation of disease, receive 2 doses of MMR vaccine during an outbreak of measles or mumps, and 1 dose during an outbreak of rubella.

Complete information about evidence of immunity is available at www.cdc.gov/vaccines/recs/provisional/default.htm.

6. Seasonal Influenza vaccination

Vaccinate all persons aged ≥ 50 years and any younger persons who would like to decrease their risk of getting influenza. Vaccinate persons aged 19 through 49 years with any of the following indications.

Medical: Chronic disorders of the cardiovascular or pulmonary systems, including asthma; chronic metabolic diseases, including diabetes mellitus; renal or hepatic dysfunction, hemoglobinopathies, or immunocompromising conditions (including immunocompromising conditions caused by medications or HIV); cognitive, neurologic or neuromuscular disorders; and pregnancy during the influenza season. No data exist on the risk for severe or complicated influenza disease among persons with asplenia; however, influenza is a risk factor for secondary bacterial infections that can cause severe disease among persons with asplenia.

Occupational: All healthcare personnel, including those employed by long-term care and assisted-living facilities, and caregivers of children age < 5 years.

Other: Residents of nursing homes and other long-term care and assisted-living facilities; persons likely to transmit influenza to persons at high risk (e.g., in-home household contacts and caregivers of children aged < 5 years, persons aged ≥ 50 years, and persons of all ages with high-risk conditions).

Healthy, nonpregnant adults aged < 50 years without high-risk medical conditions who are not contacts of severely immunocompromised persons in special-care units may receive either intranasally administered live, attenuated influenza vaccine (FluMist) or inactivated vaccine. Other persons should receive the inactivated vaccine.

7. Pneumococcal polysaccharide (PPSV) vaccination

Vaccinate all persons with the following indications.

Medical: Chronic lung disease (including asthma); chronic cardiovascular diseases; diabetes mellitus; chronic liver disease, cirrhosis; chronic alcoholism; functional or anatomic asplenia (e.g., sickle cell disease or splenectomy [if elective splenectomy is planned, vaccinate at least 2 weeks before surgery]); immunocompromising conditions including chronic renal failure or nephrotic syndrome; and cochlear implants and cerebrospinal fluid leaks. Vaccinate as close to HIV diagnosis as possible.

Other: Residents of nursing homes or long-term care facilities and persons who smoke cigarettes. Routine use of PPSV is not recommended for American Indians/Alaska Natives or persons aged < 65 years unless they have underlying medical conditions that are PPSV indications. However, public health authorities may consider recommending PPSV for American Indians/Alaska Natives and persons aged 50 through 64 years who are living in areas where the risk for invasive pneumococcal disease is increased.

8. Revaccination with PPSV

One-time revaccination after 5 years is recommended for persons with chronic renal failure or nephrotic syndrome; functional or anatomic asplenia (e.g., sickle cell disease or splenectomy); and for persons with immunocompromising conditions. For persons aged ≥ 65 years, one-time revaccination is recommended if they were vaccinated ≥ 5 years previously and were younger than aged < 65 years at the time of primary vaccination.

9. Hepatitis A vaccination

Vaccinate persons with any of the following indications and any person seeking protection from hepatitis A virus (HAV) infection.

Behavioral: Men who have sex with men and persons who use injection drugs.

Occupational: Persons working with HAV–infected primates or with HAV in a research laboratory setting.

Medical: Persons with chronic liver disease and persons who receive clotting factor concentrates.

Other: Persons traveling to or working in countries that have high or intermediate endemicity of hepatitis A (a list of countries is available at wwwn.cdc.gov/travel/contentdiseases.aspx).

Unvaccinated persons who anticipate close personal contact (e.g., household contact or regular babysitting) with an international adoptee from a country of high or intermediate endemicity during the first 60 days after arrival of the adoptee in the United States should consider vaccination. The first dose of the 2-dose hepatitis A vaccine series should be administered as soon as adoption is planned, ideally ≥ 2 weeks before the arrival of the adoptee.

Single-antigen vaccine formulations should be administered in a 2-dose schedule at either 0 and 6–12 months (Havrix), or 0 and 6–18 months (Vaqta). If the combined hepatitis A and hepatitis B vaccine (Twinrix) is used, administer 3 doses at 0, 1, and 6 months; alternatively, a 4-dose schedule, administered on days 0, 7, and 21–30 followed by a booster dose at month 12 may be used.

10. Hepatitis B vaccination

Vaccinate persons with any of the following indications and any persons seeking protection from hepatitis B virus (HBV) infection.

Behavioral: Sexually active persons who are not in a long-term, mutually monogamous relationship (e.g., persons with more than one sex partner during the previous 6 months); persons seeking evaluation or treatment for a sexually transmitted disease (STD); current or recent injection-drug users; and men who have sex with men.

Occupational: Healthcare personnel and public-safety workers who are exposed to blood or other potentially infectious body fluids.

Medical: Persons with end-stage renal disease, including patients receiving hemodialysis; persons with HIV infection; and persons with chronic liver disease.

Other: Household contacts and sex partners of persons with chronic HBV infection; clients and staff members of institutions for persons with developmental disabilities; and international travelers to countries with high or intermediate prevalence of chronic HBV infection (a list of countries is available at www.cdc.gov/travel/contentdiseases.aspx).

Hepatitis B vaccination is recommended for all adults in the following settings: STD treatment facilities; HIV testing and treatment facilities; facilities providing drug-abuse treatment and prevention services; healthcare settings targeting services to injection-drug users or men who have sex with men; correctional facilities; end-stage renal disease programs and facilities for chronic hemodialysis patients; and institutions and nonresidential daycare facilities for persons with developmental disabilities.

Administer or complete a 3-dose series of HepB to those persons not previously vaccinated. The second dose should be administered 1 month after the first dose; the third dose should be administered at least 2 months after the second dose (and at least 4 months after the first dose). If the combined hepatitis A and hepatitis B vaccine (Twinrix) is used, administer 3 doses at 0, 1, and 6 months; alternatively, a 4-dose schedule, administered on days 0, 7, and 21–30 followed by a booster dose at month 12 may be used.

Adult patients receiving hemodialysis or with other immuno-compromising conditions should receive 1 dose of 40 µg/mL (Recombivax HB) administered on a 3-dose schedule or 2 doses of 20 µg/mL (Engerix-B) administered simultaneously on a 4-dose schedule at 0, 1, 2 and 6 months.

11. Meningococcal vaccination

Meningococcal vaccine should be administered to persons with the following indications.

Medical: Adults with anatomic or functional asplenia, or persistent, or persistent complement component deficiencies.

Other: First-year college students living in dormitories; micro-biologists routinely exposed to isolates of *Neisseria meningitidis*; military recruits; and persons who travel to or live in countries in which meningococcal disease is hyperendemic or epidemic (e.g., the "meningitis belt" of sub-Saharan Africa during the dry season [December through June]), particularly if their contact with local populations will be prolonged. Vaccination is required by the government of Saudi Arabia for all travelers to Mecca during the annual Hajj.

Meningococcal conjugate vaccine (MCV4) is preferred for adults with any of the preceding indications who are aged ≤ 55 years; meningococcal polysaccharide vaccine (MPSV4) is preferred for adults aged ≥ 56 years. Revaccination with MCV4 after 5 years is recommended for adults previously vaccinated with MCV4 or MPSV4 who remain at increased risk for infection (e.g., adults with anatomic or functional asplenia). Persons whose only risk factor is living in on-campus housing are not recommended to receive an additional dose.

12. Selected conditions for which *Haemophilus influenzae* type b (Hib) vaccine may be used

Hib vaccine generally is not recommended for persons aged ≥ 5 years. No efficacy data are available on which to base a recommendation concerning use of Hib vaccine for older children and adults. However, studies suggest good immunogenicity in patients who have sickle cell disease, leukemia, or HIV infection or who have had a splenectomy. Administering 1 dose of Hib vaccine to these high-rick persons who have not previously received Hib vaccine is not contraindicated.

13. Immunocompromising conditions

Inactivated vaccines generally are acceptable (e.g., pneumococcal, meningococcal, influenza [inactivated influenza vaccine]) and live vaccines generally are avoided in persons with immune deficiencies or immunocompromising conditions. Information on specific conditions is available at www.cdc.gov/vaccines/pubs /acip-list.htm.

RECOMMENDED IMMUNIZATION SCHEDULE FOR PERSONS AGED 0 THROUGH 6 YEARS
UNITED STATES—2010

For those who fall behind or start late, see the catch-up schedule

FIGURE 3 Recommended Immunization Schedule for Persons Aged 0 Through 6 Years—United States, 2010

Vaccine	Birth	1 month	2 months	4 months	6 months	12 months	15 months	18 months	19–23 months	2–3 years	4–6 years
Hepatitis B[1]	Hep B	Hep B				Hep B					
Rotavirus[2]			RV	RV	RV[2]						
Diphtheria, Tetanus, Pertussis[3]			DTaP	DTaP	DTaP	*see footnote[3]*	DTaP				DTaP
Haemophilus influenzae type b[4]			Hib	Hib	Hib[4]	Hib					
Pneumococcal[5]			PCV	PCV	PCV	PCV					PPSV
Inactivated Poliovirus[6]			IPV	IPV		IPV					IPV
Influenza[7]						Influenza (Yearly)					
Measles, Mumps, Rubella[8]						MMR		*see footnote[8]*			MMR
Varicella[9]						Varicella		*see footnote[9]*			Varicella
Hepatitis A[10]						HepA (2 doses)					HepA Series
Meningococcal[11]											MCV

Range of recommended ages for all children except certain high-risk groups

Range of recommended ages for certain high-risk groups

This schedule includes recommendations in effect as of December 15, 2009. Any dose not administered at the recommended age should be administered at a subsequent visit, when indicated and feasible. The use of a combination vaccine generally is preferred over separate injections of its equivalent component vaccines. Considerations should include provider assessment, patient preference, and the potential for adverse events. Providers should consult the relevant Advisory Committee on Immunization Practices statement for detailed recommendations: **http://www/cdc.gov/vaccines/pubs/acip-list.htm**. Clinically significant adverse events that follow immunization should be reported to the Vaccine Adverse Event Reporting System (VAERS) at **http://vaers.hhs.gov** or by telephone, **800-822-7967.**

1. Hepatitis B vaccine (HepB). (Minimum age: birth) **At birth:**

- Administer monovalent HepB to all newborns before hospital discharge.

- If mother is hepatitis B surface antigen (HBsAg)-positive, administer HepB and 0.5 mL of hepatitis B immune globulin (HBIG) within 12 hours of birth.

- If mother's HBsAg status is unknown, administer HepB within 12 hours of birth. Determine mother's HBsAg status as soon as possible and, if HBsAg-positive, administer HBIG (no later than age 1 week).

After the birth dose:

- The HepB series should be completed with either monovalent HepB or a combination vaccine containing HepB. The second dose should be administered at age 1 or 2 months. Monovalent HepB vaccine should be used for doses administered before age 6 weeks. The final dose should be administered no earlier than age 24 weeks.

- Infants born to HBsAg-positive mothers should be tested for HBsAg and antibody to HBsAg 1 to 2 months after completion of at least 3 doses of the HepB series, at age 9 through 18 months (generally at the next well-child visit).

- Administration of 4 doses of HepB to infants is permissible when a combination vaccine containing HepB is administered after the birth dose. The fourth dose should be administered no earlier than age 24 weeks.

2. Rotavirus vaccine (RV). (Minimum age: 6 weeks)

- Administer the first dose at age 6 through 14 weeks (maximum age: 14 weeks 6 days). Vaccination should not be initiated for infants aged 15 weeks 0 days or older.

- The maximum age for the final dose in the series is 8 months 0 days

- If Rotarix is administered at ages 2 and 4 months, a dose at 6 months is not indicated.

3. Diphtheria and tetanus toxoids and acellular pertussis vaccine (DTaP). (Minimum) age: 6 weeks)

- The fourth dose may be administered as early as age 12 months, provided at least 6 months have elapsed since the third dose.

- Administer the final dose in the series at age 4 through 6 years.

4. *Haemophilus influenzae* type b conjugate vaccine (Hib). (Minimum age: 6 weeks)

- If PRP-OMP (PedvaxHIB or Comvax [HepB-Hib]) is administered at ages 2 and 4 months, a dose at age 6 months is not indicated.

- TriHiBit (DTap/Hib) and Hiberix (PRP-T) should not be used for doses at ages 2, 4, or 6 months for the primary series but can be used as the final dose in children aged 12 months through 4 years.

5. Pneumococcal vaccine. (Minimum age: 6 weeks for pneumococcal conjugate vaccine [PCV]; 2 years for pneumococcal polysaccharide vaccine [PPSV])

- PCV is recommended for all children aged younger than 5 years. Administer 1 dose of PCV to all healthy children aged 24 through 59 months who are not completely vaccinated for their age.

- Administer PPSV 2 or more months after last dose of PCV to children aged 2 years or older with certain underlying medical conditions, including a cochlear implant. See *MMWR* 1997;46(No. RR-8).

6. Inactivated poliovirus vaccine (IPV) (Minimum age: 6 weeks)

- The final dose in the series should be administered on or after the fourth birthday and at least 6 months following the previous dose.

- If 4 doses are administered prior to age 4 years a fifth dose should be administered at age 4 through 6 years. See *MMWR* 2009;58(30):829–830.

7. Influenza vaccine (seasonal). (Minimum age: 6 months for trivalent inactivated influenza vaccine [TIV]; 2 years for live, attenuated influenza vaccine [LAIV])

- Administer annually to children aged 6 months through 18 years.

- For healthy children aged 2 through 6 years (i.e., those who do not have underlying medical conditions that predispose them to influenza complications), either LAIV or TIV may be used, except LAIV should not be given to children aged 2 through 4 years who have had wheezing in the past 12 months.

- Children receiving TIV should receive 0.25 mL if aged 6 through 35 months or 0.5 mL if aged 3 years or older.

- Administer 2 doses (separated by at least 4 weeks) to children aged younger than 9 years who are receiving influenza vaccine for the first time or who were vaccinated for the first time during the previous influenza season but only received 1 dose.

- For recommendations for use of influenza A (H1N1) 2009 monovalent vaccine see *MMWR* 2009; 58(No. RR-10).

8. Measles, mumps, and rubella vaccine (MMR). (Minimum age: 12 months)

- Administer the second dose routinely at age 4 through 6 years. However, the second dose may be administered before age 4, provided at least 28 days have elapsed since the first dose.

9. Varicella vaccine. (Minimum age: 12 months)

- Administer the second dose routinely at age 4 through 6 years. However, the second dose may be administered before age 4, provided at least 3 months have elapsed since the first dose.

- For children aged 12 months through 12 years the minimum interval between doses is 3 months. However, if the second dose was administered at least 28 days after the first dose, it can be accepted as valid.

10. Hepatitis A vaccine (HepA). (Minimum age: 12 months)

- Administer to all children aged 1 year (i.e., aged 12 through 23 months). Administer 2 doses at least 6 months apart.

- Children not fully vaccinated by age 2 years can be vaccinated at subsequent visits.

- HepA also is recommended for older children who live in areas where vaccination programs target older children, who are at increased risk for infection, or for whom immunity against hepatitis A is desired.

11. Meningococcal vaccine. (Minimum age: 2 years for meningococcal conjugate vaccine [MCV4] and for meningococcal polysaccharide vaccine [MPSV4])

- Administer MCV4 to children aged 2 through 10 years with persistent complement component deficiency, anatomic or functional asplenia, and certain other conditions placing them at high risk.

- Administer MCV4 to children previously vaccinated with MCV4 or MPSV4 after 3 years if first dose administered at age 2 through 6 years. See *MMWR* 2009;58:1042–1043.

The Recommended Immunization Schedules for Persons Aged 0 through 18 years are approved by the Advisory Committee on Immunization Practices (**http://www.cdc.gov/vaccines/recs /acip**), the American Academy of Pediatrics (**http://www.aap .org**), and the American Academy of Family Physicians (**http ://www.aafp.org**).

Department of Health and Human Services • Centers for Disease Control and Prevention

RECOMMENDED IMMUNIZATION SCHEDULE FOR PERSONS AGED 7 THROUGH 18 YEARS
UNITED STATES—2010

For those who fall behind or start late, see schedule below and the catch-up schedule

FIGURE 4 Recommended Immunization Schedule for Persons Aged 7 Through 18 Years—United States, 2010

Vaccine	7–10 years	11–12 years	13–18 years
Tetanus, Diphtheria, Pertussis[1]		Tdap	Tdap
Human Papillomavirus[2]	*see footnote 2*	HPV (3 doses)	HPV series
Meningococcal[3]	MCV	MCV	MCV
Influenza[4]		Influenza (Yearly)	
Pneumococcal[5]		PPSV	
Hepatitis A[6]		HepA Series	
Hepatitis B[7]		Hep B Series	
Inactivated Poliovirus[8]		IPV Series	
Measles, Mumps, Rubella[9]		MMR Series	
Varicella[10]		Varicella Series	

Range of recommended ages for all children except certain high-risk groups

Range of recommended ages for catch-up immunization

Range of recommended ages for certain high-risk groups

This schedule includes recommendations in effect as of December 15, 2009. Any dose not administered at the recommended age should be administered at a subsequent visit, when indicated and feasible. The use of a combination vaccine generally is preferred over separate injections of its equivalent component vaccines. Considerations should include provider assessment, patient preference, and the potential for adverse events. Providers should consult the relevant Advisory Committee on Immunization Practices statement for detailed recommendations: **http://www.cdc.gov/vaccines/pubs/acip-list.htm**. Clinically significant adverse events that follow immunization should be reported to the Vaccine Adverse Event Reporting System (VAERS) at **http://www.vaers.hhs.gov** or by telephone, **800-822-7967.**

1. Tetanus and diphtheria toxoids and acellular pertussis vaccine (Tdap).

(Minimum age: 10 years for Boostrix and 11 years for Adacel)

- Administer at age 11 or 12 years for those who have completed the recommended childhood DTP/DTaP vaccination series and have not received a tetanus and diphtheria toxoid (Td) booster dose.
- Persons aged 13 through 18 years who have not received Tdap should receive a dose.
- A 5-year interval from the last Td dose is encouraged when Tdap is used as a booster dose; however, a shorter interval may be used if pertussis immunity is needed.

2. Human papillomavirus vaccine (HPV). (Minimum age: 9 years)

- Two HPV vaccines are licensed: a quadrivalent vaccine (HPV4) for the prevention of cervical, vaginal and vulvar cancers (in females) and genital warts (in females and males), and a bivalent vaccine (HPV2) for the prevention of cervical cancers in females.
- HPV vaccines are most effective for both males and females when given before exposure to HPV through sexual contact.
- HPV4 or HPV2 is recommended for the prevention of cervical precancers and cancers in females.
- HPV4 is recommended for the prevention of cervical, vaginal and vulvar precancers and cancers and genital warts in females.
- Administer the first dose to females at age 11 or 12 years.
- Administer the second dose 1 to 2 months after the first dose and the third dose 6 months after the first dose (at least 24 weeks after the first dose).
- Administer the series to females at age 13 through 18 years if not previously vaccinated.
- HPV4 may be administered in a 3-dose series to males aged 9 through 18 years to reduce their likelihood of acquiring genital warts.

3. Meningococcal conjugate vaccine (MCV4).

- Administer at age 11 or 12 years, or at age 13 through 18 years if not previously vaccinated.
- Administer to previously unvaccinated college freshmen living in a dormitory.
- Administer MCV4 to children aged 2 through 10 years with persistent complement component deficiency, anatomic or functional asplenia, or certain other conditions placing them at high risk.
- Administer to children previously vaccinated with MCV4 or MPSV4 who remain at increased risk after 3 years (if first dose administered at age 2 through 6 years) or after 5 years (if first dose administered at age 7 years or older). Persons whose only risk factor is living in on-campus housing are not recommended to receive an additional dose. See *MMWR* 2009;58:1042–1043.

4. Influenza vaccine (seasonal).

- Administer annually to children aged 6 months through 18 years.
- For healthy nonpregnant persons aged 7 through 18 years (i.e., those who do not have underlying medical conditions that predispose them to influenza complications), either LAIV or TIV may be used.
- Administer 2 doses (separated by at least 4 weeks) to children aged younger than 9 years who are receiving influenza vaccine for the first time or who were vaccinated for the first time during the previous influenza season but only received 1 dose.
- For recommendations for use of influenza A (H1N1) 2009 monovalent vaccine. See *MMWR* 2009;58(No. RR-10).

5. Pneumococcal polysaccharide vaccine (PPSV).

- Administer to children with certain underlying medical conditions, including a cochlear implant. A single revaccination should be administered after 5 years to children with functional or anatomic asplenia or an immunocompromising condition. See *MMWR* 1997; 46(No. RR-8).

6. Hepatitis A vaccine (HepA).

- Administer 2 doses at least 6 months apart.
- HepA is recommended for children aged older than 23 months who live in areas where vaccination programs target older children, who are at increased risk for infection, or for whom immunity against hepatitis A is desired.

7. Hepatitis B vaccine (HepB).

- Administer the 3-dose series to those not previously vaccinated.
- A 2-dose series (separated by at least 4 months) of adult formulation Recombivax HB is licensed for children aged 11 through 15 years.

8. Inactivated poliovirus vaccine (IPV).

- The final dose in the series should be administered on or after the fourth birthday and at least 6 months following the previous dose.
- If both OPV and IPV were administered as part of a series, a total of 4 doses should be administered, regardless of the child's current age.

9. Measles, mumps, and rubella vaccine (MMR).

- If not previously vaccinated, administer 2 doses or the second dose for those who have received only 1 dose, with at least 28 days between doses.

10. Varicella vaccine.

- For persons aged 7 through 18 years without evidence of immunity (See *MMWR* 2007;56[No. RR-4]), administer 2 doses if not previously vaccinated or the second dose if only 1 dose has been administered.

- For persons aged 7 through 12 years, the minimum interval between doses is 3 months. However, if the second dose was administered at least 28 days after the first dose, it can be accepted as valid.

- For persons aged 13 years and older, the minimum interval between doses is 28 days.

The Recommended Immunization Schedules for Persons Aged 0 through 18 Years are approved by the Advisory Committee on Immunization Practices.

http://www.cdc.gov/vaccines/recs/acip), the American Academy of Pediatrics (http://www.aap.org), and the American Academy of Family Physicians (http://www.aafp.org).

Department of Health and Human Service • Centers for Disease Control and Prevention

DEVELOPMENTAL ASSESSMENT: SCREENING FOR DEVELOPMENTAL DELAY AND AUTISM

Abbey Alkon

I. Introduction

A. General background

The prevalence of children with developmental and behavioral problems is estimated to be 12–16% in the United States (Hix-Small, Marks, Squires, & Nickel, 2007). In the 2007 National Survey of Children's Health, over 25% of children younger than 5 years of age were at risk for developmental and behavioral problems or social delays but fewer than one in five received the recommended screening (U.S. Department of Health and Human Resources, Health Resources and Services Administration, & Maternal and Child Health Bureau, 2009). Screening instruments help identify children with possible developmental delays or disorders who require follow-up or referrals to undergo a comprehensive assessment. Title V of the Social Security Act and the Individuals with Disabilities Education Improvement Act of 2004 reaffirm the mandate for child health professionals to provide early identification of, and intervention for, children with developmental disabilities through community-based collaborative systems. The Surgeon General in 2000 called for a healthcare system that responds to both the mental healthcare and physical healthcare needs of children. The Early and Periodic Screening, Diagnostic, and Treatment guidelines require that states provide regular health screenings and all medically necessary services to children and adolescents, including assessments of mental health development. The President's New Freedom Commission on Mental Health in 2003 included the goal for early mental health screening, assessment, and referral to services to be common practice and recommended that screening for mental disorders be included in primary health care and connect to treatment and support services. The American Academy of Pediatrics (AAP) provides guidelines for screening for developmental and behavioral problems as part of primary care (AAP Council on Children with Disabilities, AAP Section on Developmental Behavioral Pediatrics, Bright Futures Steering Committee, & AAP Medical Home Initiatives for Children with Special Needs Project Advisory Committee, 2006).

B. Primary care and screening

The AAP developed a policy statement "Identifying Infants and Young Children with Developmental Disorders: An Algorithm for Developmental Surveillance and Screening," which provides a strategy to incorporate into primary care ongoing developmental surveillance and screening of all children during preventive care visits (AAP Council on Children with Disabilities et al., 2006). The AAP recommends surveillance to be included in every visit and standardized screening to be included in well-child visits at 9, 18, 24, and 30 months of age. These recommendations are important because studies have shown that primary care practices fail to identify and refer 60–80% of children with developmental delays in a timely manner (Halfon et al., 2004). Although pediatric primary care practices are busy and primary care providers have a limited amount of time with children, children who are at risk for developing developmental and behavioral problems need to be identified early in life and referred for intervention services to prevent more serious problems later in life.

C. Why screen?

Administering standardized screening tests is more accurate than clinical impressions and thus is recommended at targeted ages to enhance the precision of developmental surveillance. Screening programs are provided to all children at risk for behavioral, developmental, and emotional problems. Children with positive screening tests may need to be referred for diagnostic testing because screening is not a diagnostic tool.

The goal of screening is to identify children who would benefit from early intervention services. Early intervention services for children with developmental problems have been shown to be extremely effective if children enter these programs at an early age (Glascoe,

2005a). Intervention programs can help identify children with behavior problems, autism, or developmental delays to help reduce the likelihood of future special education placement and increase the likelihood of future school success (Henderson & Strain, 2009; Johnson & Myers, 2007).

D. Where?

Screening is most effective when embedded in a preventive services system in primary care, where screening is part of a preventive services schedule coordinated with other guidance and screening activities, and where concerns and observations always lead to a within-office guidance process even if a referral to an outside agency or service is made.

The AAP recommends that all children have a "medical home," defined as care that is accessible, continuous, comprehensive, family-centered, coordinated, and compassionate (U.S. Department of Health and Human Services et al., 2009) but more than 4 out of 10 children do not have a medical home. Therefore, not all children are receiving the recommended screening in their primary care practices and new, innovative screening programs need to be developed through public health agencies.

E. Prevalence of disorders

At least one in every eight children has a developmental concern at some point during their childhood. Twelve to seventeen percent of all children have:

1. Speech or language delay

2. Mental retardation

3. Learning disability

4. Hearing loss

5. Emotional or behavioral concern

6. Delay in growth or development

The prevalence of autism spectrum disorders is estimated at about 1 in 110. The prevalence differs for boys (1 in 70) compared to girls (1 in 315) (CDC, 2009).

II. Developmental surveillance and screening algorithm

Figure 8-1 provides a flow chart algorithm with numbers and headings with associated explanations about providing surveillance and screening as part of preventive care visits (AAP Council on Children with Disabilities et al., 2006).

A. Pediatric patient at preventive care visit (#1)

The AAP recommends screening children at 9, 18, 24, and 30 months using a standardized screening tool.

B. Developmental surveillance (#2)

1. Definition

   a. Surveillance is the process of recognizing children who may be at risk of developmental delays. It is the process of gathering information about the family's well-being through report or observation, observing children's behavior, eliciting parents' concerns, and gathering data from medical history and current physical examination (Glascoe, 2005a).

   b. Surveillance is included in every well-child preventive care visit.

   c. Developmental surveillance alone, without screening, captures only 30% of children with delays and disabilities before the age of 5 years (www.first5ecmh.org).

   d. The components to surveillance are:

      i. Eliciting and attending to the parents' concerns about their child's development

      ii. Documenting and maintaining the child's developmental history

      iii. Making informed and accurate observations of the child's development

      iv. Identifying risk and protective factors for developmental delay

      v. Documenting the process and results of ongoing developmental surveillance and screening

C. Does surveillance demonstrate risk? (#3)

Any concerns raised by the parent or primary care provider during surveillance should be followed by the administration of a standardized screening tool. The screening should be done at a separate visit shortly after the surveillance initial visit.

D. Is this a 9-, 18-, or 30-month or prekindergarten visit? (#4)

A general developmental screen is recommended at the 9-, 18-, and 30-month and prekindergarten visits according to the current well-childcare guidelines Bright Futures: Guidelines for Health Supervision for Infants, Children and Adolescents (AAP, 2007). The AAP recommendations are based on recent research that credits standardized screening tools with capturing up to 80% of children with early developmental delays (http://www.first5ecmh.org). Autism screening is recommended for all children before they are 24 months of age (Johnson & Myers, 2007; Robins, 2008).

E. Administer screening tool (#5)

1. Definition

   a. Screening is the use of standardized tools to identify and refine that recognized risk (AAP Council on Children with Disabilities et al., 2006).

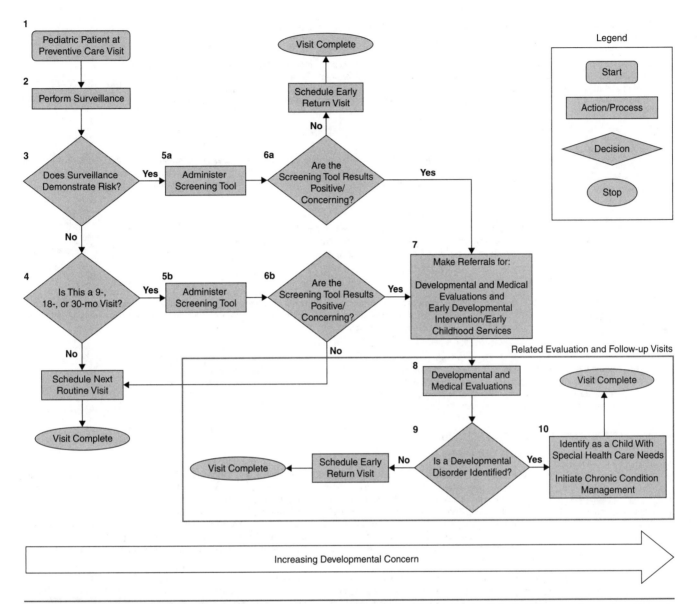

FIGURE 8-1a Developmental Surveillance and Screening Algorithm for Pediatric Primary Care. *(continues)*
Reproduced with permission from *Pediatrics*, Vol. 118, Pages 407–408, Copyright © 2006 by the AAP.

b. Assessments include gathering and synthesizing information across multiple domains, settings, and informants.

c. A list of selected screening tools is provided in Table 8-1.

F. Are the screening tool results positive? (#6)

Normal screening results provide an opportunity to focus on developmental promotion. If the results of the screening test are positive, explain the results to the parents and refer the child for further evaluation.

G. Referrals and evaluation (#7 and #8)

1. Initial referrals may be needed to rule out hearing and visual impairments, and then referrals for specific diagnostic tests are needed.

2. Evaluation is defined as a complex process aimed at identifying specific developmental disorders that are affecting a child.

3. Referrals for developmental and medical evaluations are needed and possibly referrals for early developmental intervention services.

H. Is a developmental disorder identified? (#9)

1. If a developmental disorder is not identified, then the child should be scheduled for frequent surveillance to follow areas of concern.

2. If a developmental disorder is identified, the child should be identified as a child with special healthcare needs, a diagnosis is made, and referrals for early intervention services are needed.

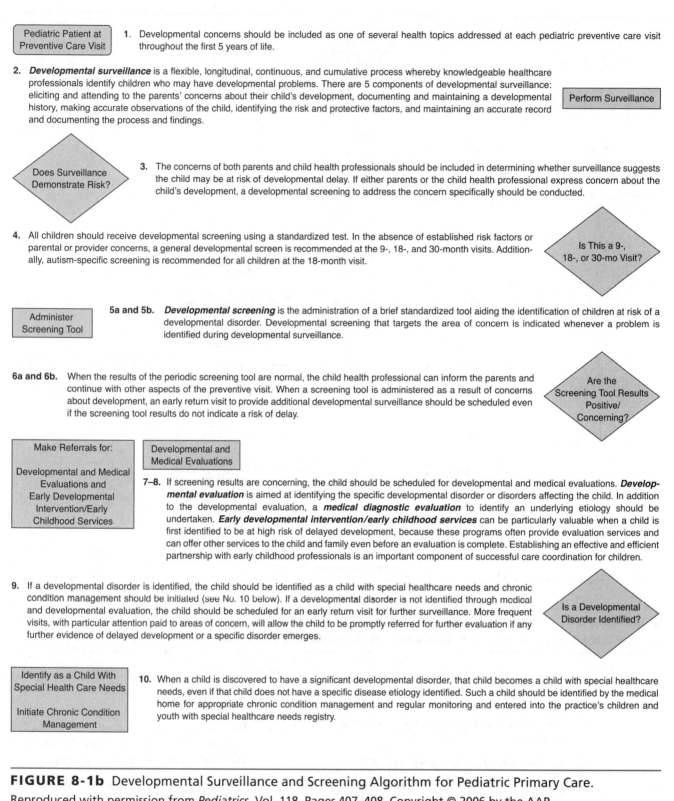

Pediatric Patient at Preventive Care Visit

1. Developmental concerns should be included as one of several health topics addressed at each pediatric preventive care visit throughout the first 5 years of life.

2. **Developmental surveillance** is a flexible, longitudinal, continuous, and cumulative process whereby knowledgeable healthcare professionals identify children who may have developmental problems. There are 5 components of developmental surveillance: eliciting and attending to the parents' concerns about their child's development, documenting and maintaining a developmental history, making accurate observations of the child, identifying the risk and protective factors, and maintaining an accurate record and documenting the process and findings.

Perform Surveillance

Does Surveillance Demonstrate Risk?

3. The concerns of both parents and child health professionals should be included in determining whether surveillance suggests the child may be at risk of developmental delay. If either parents or the child health professional express concern about the child's development, a developmental screening to address the concern specifically should be conducted.

4. All children should receive developmental screening using a standardized test. In the absence of established risk factors or parental or provider concerns, a general developmental screen is recommended at the 9-, 18-, and 30-month visits. Additionally, autism-specific screening is recommended for all children at the 18-month visit.

Is This a 9-, 18-, or 30-mo Visit?

Administer Screening Tool

5a and 5b. **Developmental screening** is the administration of a brief standardized tool aiding the identification of children at risk of a developmental disorder. Developmental screening that targets the area of concern is indicated whenever a problem is identified during developmental surveillance.

6a and 6b. When the results of the periodic screening tool are normal, the child health professional can inform the parents and continue with other aspects of the preventive visit. When a screening tool is administered as a result of concerns about development, an early return visit to provide additional developmental surveillance should be scheduled even if the screening tool results do not indicate a risk of delay.

Are the Screening Tool Results Positive/ Concerning?

Make Referrals for:

Developmental and Medical Evaluations and Early Developmental Intervention/Early Childhood Services

Developmental and Medical Evaluations

7–8. If screening results are concerning, the child should be scheduled for developmental and medical evaluations. **Developmental evaluation** is aimed at identifying the specific developmental disorder or disorders affecting the child. In addition to the developmental evaluation, a **medical diagnostic evaluation** to identify an underlying etiology should be undertaken. **Early developmental intervention/early childhood services** can be particularly valuable when a child is first identified to be at high risk of delayed development, because these programs often provide evaluation services and can offer other services to the child and family even before an evaluation is complete. Establishing an effective and efficient partnership with early childhood professionals is an important component of successful care coordination for children.

9. If a developmental disorder is identified, the child should be identified as a child with special healthcare needs and chronic condition management should be initiated (see No. 10 below). If a developmental disorder is not identified through medical and developmental evaluation, the child should be scheduled for an early return visit for further surveillance. More frequent visits, with particular attention paid to areas of concern, will allow the child to be promptly referred for further evaluation if any further evidence of delayed development or a specific disorder emerges.

Is a Developmental Disorder Identified?

Identify as a Child With Special Health Care Needs

Initiate Chronic Condition Management

10. When a child is discovered to have a significant developmental disorder, that child becomes a child with special healthcare needs, even if that child does not have a specific disease etiology identified. Such a child should be identified by the medical home for appropriate chronic condition management and regular monitoring and entered into the practice's children and youth with special healthcare needs registry.

FIGURE 8-1b Developmental Surveillance and Screening Algorithm for Pediatric Primary Care.
Reproduced with permission from *Pediatrics*, Vol. 118, Pages 407–408, Copyright © 2006 by the AAP.

I. Children with special healthcare needs: early intervention (#10)

1. Refer for early intervention services.

2. Coordination of services, monitoring progress and outcomes, and follow-up are needed.

III. Screening instruments

Table 8-1 lists a selected group of screening instruments that can be administered in a primary care office by the type of screening instrument, description of who completes the tool and why it is administered, age range, number of items, time for administration, psychometrics, languages available, how to purchase or obtain the tool, and primary references if available (AAP Council on Children with Disabilities et al., 2006; Glascoe, 2005a; Henderson & Strain, 2009; Ringwalt, 2008; Sosna & Mastergeorge, 2005). The tools were selected because they are designed to be administered to children less than 6 years of age, have a short administration time, have adequate reliability and validity, and are widely used in the field. The cultural relevance or ability to generalize the results of the instrument's psychometrics to other cultural groups is reported in the psychometrics column. The key references are included in the reference list in this chapter.

A. General development, including socioemotional tools

1. Ages and Stages Questionnaire, Third Edition (Squires & Bricker, 2009)

2. Behavior Assessment System for Children, Second Edition (Reynolds & Kamphaus, 2004)

3. Brigance Screens II (Glascoe, 2002 & 2005b)

4. Child Development Inventories (Doig, Macias, Saylor, Craver, & Ingram, 1999; Ireton, 1992)

5. Denver-II Developmental Screening Test* (Frankenburg, Camp, & Van Natta, 1971; Glascoe et al., 1992)

6. Devereux Early Childhood Assessment (LeBuffe & Naglieri, 2003)

7. Eyberg Child Behavior Inventory (Eyberg & Pincus, 1999)

8. Parents' Evaluation of Developmental Status (Glascoe, 2006)

* The Denver-II lacks adequate validation and overrefers or underdetects problems (Glascoe, 2005a).

B. Socioemotional screening tools

1. Ages and Stages Questionnaire: Social-Emotional (Squires, Bricker, & Twombly, 2002)

2. Brief Infant/Toddler Social Emotional Assessment (Briggs-Gowan, Carter, Irwin, Wachtel, & Cicchetti, 2004)

3. Pediatrics Symptom Checklist (Jellinek et al., 1999)

4. Preschool and Kindergarten Behavior Scales—Second Edition (Allin, 2004)

5. Vineland Social-Emotional Early Childhood Scales (Sparrow, Balla, & Cicchetti, 1998)

C. Autism screening tools

1. Modified Checklist for Autism in Toddlers (Robins & Dumont-Mathieu, 2006)

2. Pervasive Developmental Disorders Screening Test (Siegel, 2004)

3. In combination with a standardized screening tool, the following Diagnostic and Statistical Manual IV criteria for autism spectrum disorders can be applied for children younger than 3 years of age (Johnson, 2008; Johnson & Myers, 2007):

   a. Impairment in social interaction.
      i. Lack of spontaneous seeking to share enjoyment, interests, or achievements with other people (e.g., lack of pointing and showing)
      ii. Marked impairment in the use of multiple nonverbal behaviors, such as eye-to-eye gaze, facial expression, body postures, and gestures to regulate social interaction
      iii. Lack of social and emotional reciprocity

   b. Impairments in communication. Delay in or total lack of the development of spoken language (not accompanied by attempt to compensate using gestures or mime)

   c. Restricted repetitive and stereotyped patterns of behavior, interests, and activities

IV. Psychometrics (AAP Council on Children with Disabilities et al., 2006; Glascoe, 2005a; Henderson & Strain, 2009; Ringwalt, 2008; Sosna & Mastergeorge, 2005)

A. Characteristics of accurate screening tests

1. Sensitivity

   a. Definition: the accuracy of the test in identifying children suspected to be at risk for a developmental problem. Sensitivity is also seen as the percent of children with true problems correctly identified on a screening tool.

TABLE 8-1 Developmental Screening Tools

Screening Instrument	Description	Age Range	No. of Items	Time (administration; scoring)	Psychometric Properties	Language	Purchase/Obtainment Information	Key References
Multiple Developmental, Including Social-Emotional Screening Instruments								
Ages and Stages Questionnaire, Third Edition (ASQ-3)	Parent-completed questionnaire; series of 19 age-specific questionnaires screening communication, gross motor, fine motor, problem-solving, and personal adaptive skills; results in pass/fail score for domains	1–60 mo	30	10–15 adm, 2–3 score	Normed on 2008 children from diverse ethnic and socioeconomic backgrounds, including Spanish speaking; sensitivity: 0.70–0.90 (moderate to high); specificity: 0.76–0.91 (moderate to high)	English, Spanish, French, Korean	Brookes Publishing Co. http://www .brookespublishing.com/ Training at http://www.agesandstages .com/	Squires & Bricker (2009)
Behavior Assessment System for Children, Second Edition (BASC-2)	Parent or caregiver-completed questionnaire; Assesses behavioral and emotional functioning; measures adaptive and problem behaviors in school, home and community settings; Includes Teacher Rating Scale (TRS), Parent Rating Scale (PRS), self-report of personality, student observation, developmental history.	2–21 y	TRS: 100–139 PRS: 134–160	10–20 adm	Normed based on current US Census population characteristics. Internal consistency: acceptably high to strong results. Test-retest reliability, inter-rater reliability, and concurrent validity: moderate results.	English, Spanish	Pearson (PsychCorp) http://www .pearsonassessments.com/	Reynolds & Kamphaus (2004)

TABLE 8-1 Developmental Screening Tools *(continued)*

Screening Instrument	Description	Age Range	No. of Items	Time (administration) scoring)	Psychometric Properties	Language	Purchase/Obtainment Information	Key References
Brigance Screens II	Directly administered tool; series of 9 forms which screen articulation, expressive and receptive language, gross motor, fine motor, self-help, social-emotional, social skills and preacademic skills (when appropriate); for 0–23 mo, parent report	0–90 mo	8–10	10–15 adm	Normed on 1156 children from 29 clinical sites in 21 states; sensitivity: 0.70–0.80 (moderate); specificity: 0.70–0.80 (moderate)	English, Spanish	Curriculum Associates http://www.curriculumassociates.com/	Glascoe (2002), (2005)
Child Development Inventories (CDI) Infant Development Inventory (ID) Early Child Development Inventory (ECDI) Preschool Development Inventory (PDI)	Parent-completed questionnaire; measures social, self-help, motor, language, and general development skills; results in developmental quotients and age equivalents for different developmental domains; suitable for more in-depth evaluation	CDI: 15 mo–6 y ID: 0–18 mo ECDI: 18–36 mo PDI: 36–60 mo	300	30–50 adm	Normative sample included 568 children from south St Paul, MN, a primarily white, working class community; Doig et al included 43 children from a high-risk follow-up program, which included 69% with high school education or less and 81% Medicaid; sensitivity: 0.80–1.0. (moderate to high); specificity: 0.94–0.96 (high)	English	Pearson (PsychCorp) http://www.pearsonassessments.com/	Doig, Macias, Saylor, Craver, Ingram (1999); Ireton (1992)

(continues)

TABLE 8-1 Developmental Screening Tools (*continued*)

Screening Instrument	Description	Age Range	No. of Items	Time (administration scoring)	Psychometric Properties	Language	Purchase/Obtainment Information	Key References
Denver II Developmental Screening Test	Directly administered tool; designed to screen expressive and receptive language, gross motor, fine motor, and personal-social skills; results in risk category (normal, questionable, abnormal)	0–6 y	125	10–20 adm	Normed on 2096 term children in Colorado; not nationally representative; sensitivity: 0.56–0.83 (low to moderate); specificity: 0.43–0.80 (low to moderate)	English, Spanish	Denver Developmental Materials, Inc. http://www.denverii.com/	Glascoe, Byrne, Ashford, Johnson, Chang, Strickland (1992); Frankenburg, Camp, Van Natta (1971)
Devereux Early Childhood Assessment (DECA)	Parent/caregiver-completed questionnaire; screening initiative, self control, and attachment	2–5 y	53	10 adm	National normative sample of 2,000 children. Internal validity = 0.8 for parents, 0.88 for teachers. Test-retest reliability = 0.55 – 0.8 for parents, 0.68–0.91 for teachers. Inter-rater reliability = 0.59 – 0.77. Construct validity 0.65; Criterion validity 0.69.	English	Kaplan Early Learning Company http://www.kaplanco.com/	LeBuffe & Naglieri (1999)

TABLE 8-1 Developmental Screening Tools *(continued)*

Screening Instrument	Description	Age Range	No. of Items	Time (administration, scoring)	Psychometric Properties	Language	Purchase/Obtainment Information	Key References
Eyberg Child Behavior Inventory (ECBI)	Parent-completed. Assesses the current frequency and severity of disruptive behaviors in the home and school settings, as well as the extent to which parents and/or teachers find the behavior troublesome	2–16 y	36	5 adm, 5 score	Normative sample of 798 children (representative of 1992 census). Adequate validity and reliability studies. Test-retest reliability = 0.87 for intensity; 0.93 for problem. Inter-rater reliability: high to strong. Internal consistency = 0.98 for intensity; 0.96 for problem. Concurrent validity: Acceptably high to strong; Predictive validity is moderate; Discriminant validity = 0.8.	English	PAR, Inc. http://www.parinc.com/	Eyberg & Pincus (1999)
Parents' Evaluation of Developmental Status (PEDS)	Parent-interview form; designed to screen for developmental and behavioral problems needing further evaluation; single response form used for all ages; may be useful as a surveillance tool	0–8 y	10	2 to adm and score	Standardized with 771 children from diverse ethnic and socioeconomic backgrounds, including Spanish speaking; sensitivity: 0.74–0.79 (moderate); specificity: 0.70–0.80 (moderate)	English, Spanish, Vietnamese, Arabic, Swahili, Indonesian, Chinese, Taiwanese, French, Somali, Portuguese, Malaysian, Thai, Laotian	Ellsworth and Vandermeer Press, LLC http://pedstest.com/	Glascoe (2006)

(continues)

TABLE 8-1 Developmental Screening Tools (continued)

Screening Instrument	Description	Age Range	No. of Items	Time (administration, scoring)	Psychometric Properties	Language	Purchase/Obtainment Information	Key References
Socio-Emotional Screening Instruments								
Ages and Stages Questionnaire: Social-Emotional (ASQ-SE)	Parent/caregiver-completed questionnaire; screening self-regulation, compliance, communication, adaptive behaviors, autonomy, affect, and interaction with people	3–66 mo	30	10–15 adm, 1–3 score	Investigated with more than 3,000 questionnaires across the age intervals; reliability is 94%; validity is between 75% and 89%	English, Spanish	Brookes Publishing Co. http://www.brookes publishing.com/ Training at http://www .agesandstages.com/	Squires, Bricker, & Twombley (2002)
Brief Infant/Toddler Social Emotional Assessment (BITSEA)	Parent or caregiver forms; brief comprehensive screening instrument to evaluate social and emotional behavior	12–36 mo	42	5–7 adm	Clinical groups in the normative sample (n = 600) included young children who had delayed language, were premature, and those who had other diagnosed disorders. Not geographically representative. Internal consistency for Problem = 0.83 – 0.89; for Competence = 0.66 – 0.75. Test-retest reliability, inter-rater reliability, internal consistency: acceptably high to strong results. Concurrent validity: moderate results.	English, Spanish, French, Hebrew, Dutch	Pearson (PsychCorp) http://www .pearsonassessments. com/	Briggs-Gowan, Carter, Irwin, Wachtel & Cicchetti (2004)

TABLE 8-1 Developmental Screening Tools (continued)

Screening Instrument	Description	Age Range	No. of Items	Time (administration, scoring)	Psychometric Properties	Language	Purchase/Obtainment Information	Key References
Pediatric Symptom Checklist (PSC)	Parent or caregiver-completed questionnaire to identify emotional and behavioral problems. Identifies need for further evaluation.	4–16 years	35	10–15 minutes; Total score; clinical cut-off = 24 (4–5 year olds) and 28 (6–16 year olds)	Normative sample of middle and low SES. Test-retest reliability: high to strong; Internal consistency: high to strong; Predictive validity: moderate. Sensitivity: 80–95%; Specificity: 68–100%	English, Spanish, Japanese	www.dbpeds.org/pdf/psc.pdf	Jellinek, Murphy, Bishop, Pagano, Comer, & Kelleher (1999)
Preschool and Kindergarten Behavior Scales-Second Edition (PBKS-2)	Parent or caregiver-completed questionnaire; social skills scale includes social cooperation, social interaction, and social independence; problem behavior scale includes externalizing problems and internalizing problems	36–60 mo	76	12 adm	Normative sample of 3,317 children ages 3 through 6. Ethnicity, socioeconomic status, and special education classification of sample are similar to characteristics of U.S. population, based on 2000 census. Internal consistency is .96–.97. High concurrent validity. Inter-rater reliability: moderate results.	English, Spanish	Pro-Ed, Inc. http://www.proedinc.com/	Allin (2004)
Vineland Social-Emotional Early Childhood Scales (SEEC)	Parent or caregiver interview by licensed professional; assesses interpersonal relationships, play and leisure time, and coping skills; the social-emotional composite assess usual social-emotional functioning	0–71 mo	122	15–25 adm	Normative sample; nationally representative. Test-retest reliability and internal consistency; acceptably high to strong results; inter-rater reliability and concurrent validity: moderate results.	English	Pearson (PsychCorp) http://www.pearsonassessments.com/	Sparrow, Balla & Cicchetti (1998

(continues)

TABLE 8-1 Developmental Screening Tools (continued)

Screening Instrument	Description	Age Range	No. of Items	Time (administration, scoring)	Psychometric Properties	Language	Purchase/Obtainment Information	Key References
Autism Screening Instruments								
Modified Checklist for Autism in Toddlers —Revised (M-CHAT)-R	Parent-completed questionnaire designed to identify children at risk of autism from the general population	16–30 mo	23	5–10 adm	Standardization sample included 1293 children screened, 58 evaluated, and 39 diagnosed with an autistic spectrum disorder; validated using ADI-R, ADOS-G, CARS, DSM-IV; sensitivity: 0.85–0.87 (moderate); specificity: 0.93–0.99 (high)	English, Spanish, French, Chinese, Japanese, and other languages	First Signs, Inc. http://www.firstsigns.org/	Robins (2008); Robins & Dumont-Mathieu (2006)
Pervasive Developmental Disorders Screening Test (PDDST-II)	Parent-completed questionnaire designed to identify children at risk of autism from the general population	12–48 mo	22	10–20 adm	Validated using extensive multimethod diagnostic evaluations on 681 children at risk of autistic spectrum disorders and 256 children with mild-to-moderate other developmental disorders; no sensitivity/specificity data reported for screening of an unselected sample; sensitivity: 0.85–0.92 (moderate to high); specificity: 0.71–0.91 (moderate to high)	English, Spanish	Pearson (PsychCorp) http://www.pearsonassessments.com/	Siegel (2004)

b. Example: if the screening tool has 70% sensitivity, it means that 70% of the children who receive a positive screening result truly have a developmental problem.

c. Standards: 70–80% sensitivity is considered moderate and 90% or higher is strong.

2. Specificity

a. Definition: the accuracy of a test in identifying children who are not delayed. Specificity is also seen as the percent of children without true difficulties correctly identified by a negative result on a screening tool.

b. Example: if the test has 80% specificity, it means that 80% of the children screened who have a negative result have no developmental problem.

c. Standards: 80% or higher specificity is considered moderate to strong. This minimizes referrals for diagnostic tests for children with no developmental delays or problems.

3. Positive predictive value (PPV)

a. Definition: the percent of children who have a positive screening test result and actually have the diagnosis of a developmental problem. The PPV tells the clinician what a test result means for the individual child. PPV is frequently used by clinicians.

b. Example: if four out of five children have positive screening test results and are found to have a developmental problem, then the PPV is 80%. Therefore, for the screening test there is an 80% chance that the child actually has a developmental problem.

c. Standards: there is no agreed on standard for PPV. In reality, PPVs are rarely very high and can range between 30% and 50%.

4. Representative sample

Definition: the screening test should be standardized on a large nationally representative sample whose characteristics reflect those of the United States in terms of ethnicities and parents' level of education, income, and language spoken at home.

5. Reliability

The ability of a measure to produce consistent results. There are different types of reliability:

a. Test–retest reliability: the stability or consistency of results across different administrations.

b. Interrater reliability: the stability or consistency of results across different raters.

c. Internal consistency: the correlation across items on an instrument to show consistency or responses. Usually shown as the Cronbach's alpha coefficient.

6. Validity

The ability of a measure to discriminate between a child at a determined level of risk for delay and the rest of the population. There are many types of validity:

a. Concurrent validity: high correlation between the screening tool and a diagnostic measure with similar domains.

b. Discriminant validity: how well the screening tool distinguishes children with the problem or condition compared to those without the problem or condition.

c. Predictive validity: screening test results are compared to performance on diagnostic measures administered at a later time.

V. Conclusion

Routine screening at regular intervals helps identify children at risk for behavioral, developmental, and emotional problems and refer them for diagnostics tests and early intervention services. Children develop at different paces and surveillance and screening tests can help differentiate normal, intermittent changes in behavior from persistent challenging behaviors. In addition, screening tests can help identify children whose development has changed or whose developmental milestones have regressed (e.g., autism). Early identification of developmental, behavioral, and emotional problems during childhood may help children succeed in school, develop social relationships, and contribute to society.

VI. Clinician resources

1. AAP National Center of Medical Home Initiatives for Children with Special Needs (www.medicalhomeinfo.org). Resources developed by the AAP and pilot projects implementing the AAP algorithm for developmental screening, including policies and protocols, screening algorithms, and resources and tips on Medicaid billing. Includes parent resources.

2. *AAP policy statements on developmental screening* (http://aappolicy.aappublications.org).

3. AAP, Caring for Children with Autism Spectrum Disorders: A Resource Toolkit for Clinicians (http://www.aap.org/publiced/autismtoolkit.cfm). Includes identification, surveillance and screening tools, referrals, fact sheets, and family handouts.

4. AAP's Bright Futures (www.brightfutures.org/mental health). Provides health supervision guidelines and developmental, behavioral, and psychosocial screening and assessment tools used in the primary care. It includes questions to ask parents during the interview.

5. *Assuring Better Child Health and Development (ABCD Initiative)* (www.abcdresources.org). Research and resources promoting child health and development. Includes tools for clinicians and state resources.

6. *Centers for Disease Control and Prevention* (www.cdc.gov/ncbddd/child/devtool.htm). Overview of screening, including facts for medical providers with flow chart and diagram of staff responsibilities; child safety "developmental milestones" section (www.cdc.gov/ncbddd/chil); and autism and developmental screening section (www.cdc.gov/actearly)

7. Center on the Social and Emotional Foundations for Early Learning (http://www.vanderbilt.edu/scefel/index.html)

8. Developmental Screening Toolkit for Primary Care Providers (www.developmentalscreening.org). Resources developed by the Maternal and Child Health Bureau and Children's Hospital Boston for primary care providers implementing validated screening instruments into their practice. Includes information on screening tools, billing, and referrals. Includes billing issues and referral issues (www.developmentalscreening.org/billing_referring/billing_issues.htm).

9. *First Signs* (www.firstsigns.org/screening). Information for families on developmental screening and services.

10. *Ounce of Prevention Fund* (www.ounceofprevention.org). See *"Snapshots: Incorporating Comprehensive Developmental Screening into Programs and Services for Young Children."*

11. National Early Childhood Technical Assistance Center (www.nactac.org). See *"Developmental Screening and Assessment Documents."*

12. *The Commonwealth Fund* (www.commonwealthfund.org). Research on innovations on child health and development, including the work of the ABCD initiative and screening in primary care settings.

13. Technical Assistance Center of Social Emotional Intervention (http://www.challengingbehavior.org/)

REFERENCES

Allin, J. D. (2004). Book review: Preschool and kindergarten behavior scales-second edition. *Journal of Psychoeducational Assessment, 22*(1), 81–86.

American Academy of Pediatrics. (2007). *Bright futures: Guidelines for health supervision of infants, children, and adolescents* (3rd ed.). Elk Grove, IL: American Academy of Pediatrics.

American Academy of Pediatrics Council on Children with Disabilities, AAP Section on Developmental Behavioral Pediatrics, Bright Futures Steering Committee, & AAP Medical Home Initiatives for Children with Special Needs Project Advisory Committee. (2006). Identifying infants and young children with developmental disorders in the medical home: An algorithm for developmental surveillance and screening. *Pediatrics, 118*(1), 405–420.

Briggs-Gowan, M. J., Carter, A. S., Irwin, J. R., Wachtel, K., & Cicchetti, D. V. (2004). The brief infant-toddler social and emotional assessment: Screening for social-emotional problems and delays in competence. *Journal of Pediatric Psychology, 29*(2), 143–155.

Centers for Disease Control and Prevention. (2009). Prevalence of autism spectrum disorders: Autism and developmental disabilities monitoring network, United States, 2006. *Morbidity and Mortality Weekly Report, 58*(SS-10), 1–24.

Doig, K. B., Macias, M. M., Saylor, D. F., Craver, J. R., & Ingram, P. E. (1999). The child development inventory: A developmental outcome measure for the follow-up of the high risk infant. *Journal of Pediatrics, 135*, 358–362.

Eyberg, S., & Pincus, D. (1999). *Eyberg child behavior inventory (ECBI).* Odessa, FL: Psychological Assessment Resources.

Frankenburg, W. K., Camp, B. W., & Van Natta, P. A. (1971). Validity of the Denver developmental screening test. *Child Development, 42*, 475–485.

Glascoe, F. P. (2002). The Brigance Infant-Toddler Screen (BITS): Standardization and validation. *Journal of Developmental and Behavioral Pediatrics, 23*, 145–150.

Glascoe, F. P. (2005a). Screening for developmental and behavioral problems. *Mental Retardation and Developmental Disabilities Research Reviews, 11*, 173–179.

Glascoe, F. P. (2005b). *Technical report for the Brigance screens.* North Billerica, MA: Curriculum Associates.

Glascoe, F. P. (2006). *Parents' evaluation of developmental status (PEDS).* Nashville, TN: Ellsworth & Vandermeer Press.

Glascoe, F. P., Byrne, K. E., Ashford, L. G., Johnson, K. L., Chang, B., & Strickland, B. (1992). Accuracy of the Denver-II in developmental screening. *Pediatrics, 89*, 1221–1225.

Halfon, N., Regalado, M., Sareen, H., Inkelas, M., Reuland, C. P., Glascoe, F. P., & Olson, L. M. (2004). Assessing development in the pediatric office. *Pediatrics, 113*(6), 1926–1933.

Henderson, J., & Strain, P. (2009). *Screening for delays and problem behavior (roadmap to effective intervention practices).* Tampa, FL: University of Southern Florida.

Hix-Small, H., Marks, K., Squires, J., & Nickel, R. (2007). Impact of implementing developmental screening at 12 and 24 months in a pediatric practice. *Pediatrics, 120*(2), 381–389.

Ireton, H. (1992). *Child development inventory manual.* Minneapolis, MN: Behavior Science Systems.

Jellinek, M., Murphy, J., Little, M., Pagano, M., Comer, D., & Kelleher, K. (1999). Use of the Pediatric Symptom Checklist (PSC) to screen for psychosocial problems in pediatric primary care: A national feasibility study. *Archives of Pediatric and Adolescent Medicine, 153*(3), 254–260.

Johnson, C., & Myers, S. (2007). Identification and evaluation of children with autism spectrum disorders. *Pediatrics, 120*, 1183–1215.

Johnson, C. P. (2008). Recognition of autism before age 2 years. *Pediatrics in Review, 29*(3), 86–95.

LeBuffe, P., & Naglieri, J. (2003). *Devereux Early Childhood Assessment-Clinical Form* (DECA-C): Kaplan Early Learning Company, Lewisville, NC.

Reynolds, C., & Kamphaus, R. (2004). *Behavior Assessment System for Children* (BASC-II, Second Edition): Pearson (PsychCorp.), San Antonio, Texas.

Ringwalt, S. (2008). *Developmental screening and assessment instruments with an emphasis on social and emotional development for young children ages birth through five.* Chapel Hill, NC: The University of North Carolina, FPG Child Development Institute, National Early Childhood Technical Assistance Center.

Robins, D. (2008). Screening for autism spectrum disorders in primary care settings. *Autism, 12*(5), 537–556.

Robins, D., & Dumont-Mathieu, T. M. (2006). Early screening for autism spectrum disorders: Update on the Modified Checklist for Autism in Toddlers and other measures. *Journal of Developmental and Behavioral Pediatrics, 27*(Suppl. 2), S111–S119.

Siegel, B. (2004). *Pervasive Developmental Disorders Screening Test-II (PDDST-II): Early childhood screener for autistic spectrum disorders.* San Antonio, TX: Harcourt Assessment.

Sosna, T., & Mastergeorge, A. (2005). *The infant, preschool, family, mental health initiative: Compendium of screening tools for early childhood social-emotional development.* Sacramento, CA: California Institute for Mental Health.

Sparrow, S. S., Balla, D. A., & Cicchetti, D. V. (1998). *Vineland Social-Emotional Early Childhood Scales.* Circle Pines, MN: American Guidance Services, Inc.

Squires, J., & Bricker, D. (2009). *Ages and Stages Questionnaires, Third Edition (ASQ-3).* Baltimore, MD: Paul H. Brookes Publishing Co., Inc.

Squires, J., Bricker, D., & Twombly, E. (2002). *Ages and Stages Questionnaires: Social-Emotional.* Baltimore, MD: Paul H. Brookes Publishing Co., Inc.

U.S. Department of Health and Human Services, Health Resources and Services Administration, & Maternal and Child Health Bureau. (2009). *The National Survey of Children's Health 2007.* Rockville, MD: U.S. Department of Health and Human Services.

COMMON PEDIATRIC PRESENTATIONS

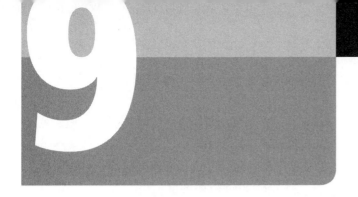

ATOPIC DERMATITIS IN CHILDREN

Karen G. Duderstadt and Nan Madden

I. Introduction and general background

A. Definition and overview

Atopic dermatitis (AD) is classified as an eczematous eruption of the skin in childhood. The term "eczema" is often used interchangeably with AD. Eczema means "flaring up," which describes the acute symptom complex of erythema, scaling, vesicles, inflamed papules, plaques, and crusts seen with AD (Goodhue & Brady, 2009). The protective barrier of the skin is impaired and undergoes stages of dryness; pruritus; inflammation; and increased susceptibility to bacterial, viral, and fungal infections. AD is often the initial manifestation of atopic disease in children. Children with severe AD have a higher risk of developing other atopic diseases.

B. Prevalence and incidence

AD, or atopic eczema, is the most common skin disorder in young children and affects approximately 10–20% of the pediatric population. It is increasing in prevalence in the United States and there has been a twofold to three-fold increase in the prevalence of AD in developing countries in the past 30 years (Leong, Boguniewicz, Howell, & Hamid, 2004). AD develops in 45% of affected children within the first 6 months of life, and in 60% of children by the first year of age. Allergic rhinitis develops in 50–80% of children with AD, and greater than 50% of children with AD develop asthma in adolescence or adulthood (Boguniewicz, 2005; Paller & Mancini, 2006).

AD occurs more commonly in urban populations, in smaller family units with higher socioeconomic status, and in families with less exposure to infectious agents and antigenic triggers than in families living in rural settings.

C. Etiology

The exact etiology or immune mechanism of AD is unknown. Children with AD have elevated serum IgE levels. Antigens activate T lymphocytes, which leads to an increase in interleukins and peripheral eosinophilia. The mechanism of scratching or rubbing the skin releases cytokines from the epidermal cells and perpetuates the inflammation (Paller & Mancini, 2006). About 75% of children with AD have a positive family history of the atopic disease indicating a genetic alteration as a causative factor.

II. Database (may include but is not limited to)

A. Subjective

1. History of the presenting illness and relevant past health history

    a. Feeding history: breast or formula fed
    b. When rash or lesions first appeared and on what areas of the body
    c. Has infant or child had periods without lesions or rash?
    d. Bathing routine? Soaps used?
    e. Sleep history? Quality of sleep and nighttime symptoms?
    f. Any known food or drug allergies?
    g. History of exposure to known allergens?
    h. What does the parent or child think about what makes the rash or lesions better or worse?
    i. Factors that lead to flares include (National Institute of Arthritis and Musculoskeletal and Skin Diseases, 2009):
        i.   Emotions: Especially anger, stress, and frustration.
        ii. Bacterial skin infections (exotoxins of *Staphylococcus aureus* may act as superantigens and stimulate activation of T cells and macrophages) (Fitzpatrick & Wolff, 2005).
        iii. Climate: Low humidity (but sometimes high humidity if it causes excessive perspiration) and a dry year-around climate. Ideal humidity for the home is 45–55%.

    iv.   Long or hot baths or showers.

    v.   Not using enough moisturizers after bath.

    vi.   Going from sweating to being chilled.

  j.   History of other atopic skin disease; hives or urticaria?

  k.   History of allergic rhinitis or asthma?

  l.   History of bacterial skin infections, herpes, fungal infections?

  m.   History of other chronic conditions or developmental delay?

2. Medication history

  a.   Over-the-counter medications used, topical and oral

  b.   Prescription medications used, topical and oral

  c.   Frequency of medication use, daily or with flares

  d.   In what areas are the medications applied?

  e.   Complementary or alternative medications or therapies?

  f.   Has child been on antibiotics in the past year?

3. Family history

  a.   Any family history of allergies, AD, eczema, allergic rhinitis, or asthma?

  b.   Siblings with atopic disease?

  c.   Known food allergies in parent or sibling?

4. Environmental history

  a.   Factors that trigger onset or exacerbation of AD are common but manifest differently in each individual (Figure 9-1).

5. Social history

  a.   Quality of life for children and families with AD. (Note: Quality of life is often diminished because of chronicity of condition, constant pruritus, and difficulty in identifying and avoiding triggers.)

6. Review of systems

  a.   Common constitutional signs and symptoms of AD include pruritus, age-specific patterns or distribution of skin involvement (Figure 9-2), sparing of diaper area in infants, and

---

FIGURE 9-1 Common Triggering Factors

TRIGGER	ASSOCIATED FINDINGS (may or may not include)
Food	Food items include eggs, peanuts, cow's milk, fish, shellfish, soy, and wheat.
	Food preservatives and food color may trigger allergies but no testing mechanism exists for these substances.
Decreased humidity	Cold seasons with reduced humidity often herald a flare for children with AD. Skin holds less moisture, dry skin becomes irritated, pruritus develops, and scratching begins.
Emotional stress	Physical and emotional stress can precipitate flares of AD. It is not causative but worsens the condition.
Aeroallergens	Most common trigger of aeroallergens: • Dust mites in household • Grass pollens • Animal dander • Molds
Temperature change and sweating	Increased scratching and rubbing caused by sudden change in temperature is common in infants and children with AD. Sweating particularly causes scratching and flares of AD.

Source: Habif, T. P. (2010). Atopic dermatitis. In T. P. Habif (Ed.), *Clinical dermatology: A color guide to diagnosis and therapy* (5th ed., pp. 154–180). Philadelphia, PA: Mosby/Elsevier.

sparing of groin and axillae in older children and adolescents; occasionally, irritability in infants with moderate-to-severe disease.

b. Skin, hair, and nails

   i. Dry skin (xerosis); erythema; occasional papules; vesicles; weeping lesions; and crusting

   ii. Chronic skin changes include hyperpigmentation on lighter skin; hypopigmentation on darker skin; lichenification or leathery, thickened skin; and scarring from scratching

c. Lymphadenopathy

   i. Enlarged lymph glands can be a common associated finding of children with AD, particularly in areas localized to exacerbations of AD or in children with associated bacterial, viral, or fungal infections.

d. Respiratory

   i. Pulmonary findings of wheezing are common in children with atopic disease and asthma is a common associated condition.

FIGURE 9-2   *Phases of Atopic Dermatitis in Children*

PHASES	CLINICAL FEATURES (may or may not include)
Infantile phase	Begins from birth to 6 months of age: • May begin on cheeks and progress to scalp, arms, trunk, and legs; generalized dry skin (xerosis) including scalp • Progresses to lateral extensor surfaces of arms and legs • Pruritus and itch-scratch-itch cycle develops • Acute phase with intense itching causing irritability in infant; vesicle formation, oozing, and crusting with excoriated areas on the skin • Hallmark sign is diaper area and groin are usually spared of lesions • May resolve by 2 years of age but can continue into childhood; symptoms may become milder as the child ages and disappear at adolescence or may continue throughout life
Childhood phase	Begins around 2 years of age: • Involves wrists, hands, neck, ankles, popliteal and antecubital spaces, commonly on flexural surfaces • Lesions tend to be dry, papular, circumscribed, scaly patches • Pruritus is often severe Chronic manifestations include: • Lichenification, thickening of skin causing leathery appearance • Hyperpigmentation • Scratch marks Often worse during winter dryness or summer heat.
Adult phase	Begins at puberty or ~12 years of age: • Most commonly involves flexural skin folds; bends of elbows and knees; face; neck; upper arms; back; and dorsa of the hands, feet, fingers, and toes • May be a new occurrence or reoccurrence of chronic condition Often postinflammatory hyperpigmentation and hypopigmentation disappear in adolescence or young adulthood.

Source: Paller A. S., & Mancini, A. J. (2006). Eczematous eruptions in childhood. In A. S. Paller & A. J. Mancini (Eds.), *Hurwitz clinical pediatric dermatology: A textbook of skin disorders of childhood and adolescence* (3rd ed., pp. 49–84). Philadelphia, PA: Saunders/ Elsevier.

B. Objective

7. Physical examination findings
    a. AD presents differently at different ages. There are three distinct phases of clinical features: (1) infantile phase, (2) childhood phase, and (3) adult phase (Figure 9-2).
    b. Associated features are often diagnostic in children and adolescents (Figure 9-3).
    c. Opportunistic infections are common in infants and children with AD (Figure 9-4).
    d. Additional physical examination findings of atopic disease:
        i. General appearance; pallor, allergic shiners, allergic salute, and xerosis
        ii. Head, eye, ear, nose, and throat: periorbital puffiness; tympanic membranes with effusion unilaterally or bilaterally; boggy nasal mucosa or erythematous turbinates with enlarged adenoids; and tonsilar hypertrophy, nonerythematous, nonexudative
        iii. Neck: enlarged lymph nodes (cervical, occipital, postauricular)
        iv. Chest: adventitious sounds such as wheezing

8. Supporting data from relevant diagnostic tests
    a. Diagnosis of AD is most often a clinical diagnosis and immunologic testing is reserved for moderate to severe disease (Table 9-1).
        i. A low accuracy of food allergy tests has been reported in children with AD
        ii. Diagnostic testing for skin allergies should be reserved for children who are

FIGURE 9-3 Conditions Associated with Atopic Dermatitis

ASSOCIATED CONDITIONS (may or may not include)	CLINICAL FEATURES
Dennie line or Dennie-Morgan fold	Extra grooves or accentuated lines seen below lower eyelids bilaterally; may result from chronic edema of the eyelids and skin thickening
Allergic shiners	Dark discoloration below lower eyelids in lighter skin; slate-gray discoloration in individuals with darker skin; a result of vascular stasis
Allergic salute	Crease over the nasal bridge or exaggerated linear nasal crease caused by frequent rubbing of nose or nasal tip; most often associated with allergic rhinitis but common in atopic children
Pityriasis alba	Hypopigmented, slightly elevated plaques; occasionally with fine scaling, irregular borders; nonpruritic; occurring most often on the face of young children; also may appear on the upper arms and thighs; ~2–4 cm in diameter round-to-oval, often occur in summer or fall
Keratosis pilaris	Most predominant on the lateral aspects of the upper arms, buttocks, and thighs; appears in early childhood and persists into adulthood; papular with plugged hair follicles and surrounding inflammation; characterized by redness on lighter skin
Nummular eczema	Coin-shaped lesions or plaques ~1 cm or greater in diameter; erythematous and formed by confluent papules or occasionally vesicles
Ichthyosis vulgaris	Transmitted as an autosomal-dominant trait; can be associated with AD but a separate disease; may occur as early as 3 months of age, but most common onset in later childhood; characterized by large scales on extensor surfaces of extremities, particularly on lateral aspect of the lower legs in plate-like scales; flexural surfaces are spared

Sources: Goodhue, J. G., & Brady, M. A. (2009). Atopic and rheumatic disorders. In C. E. Burns, et al., (Eds.), Pediatric primary care (4th ed., pp. 553–583). St. Louis, MO: Saunders/Elsevier; and Paller A. S., & Mancini, A. J. (2006). Eczematous eruptions in childhood. In A. S. Paller & A. J. Mancini (Eds.), Hurwitz clinical pediatric dermatology: A textbook of skin disorders of childhood and adolescence (3rd ed., pp. 49–84). Philadelphia, PA: Saunders/ Elsevier.

FIGURE 9-4   *Secondary Opportunistic Infection*

OPPORTUNISTIC INFECTIONS	ASSOCIATED FINDINGS (may or may not include)
Staphylococcus aureus	Erythematous with pustular, exudative lesions and crusting; the most common opportunistic infection in AD and recovered in 93% of patients with AD lesions, 79% from nares of atopic children
Streptococcus pyogenes	A less common opportunistic infection in children with AD than *S. aureus*; skin findings as above
Herpes simplex	Vesicles often become umbilicated; eczema herpeticum, rapid development of vesiculopustular lesions over the sites of dermatitis, can occur in individuals with AD
Viral molluscum contagiosum	Small, dome-shaped papules often with central umbilication; commonly affect trunk, axillae, and antecubital and popliteal fossae in 25% of children with AD

Source: Habif, T. P. (2010). Atopic dermatitis. In T. P. Habif (Ed.), *Clinical dermatology: A color guide to diagnosis and therapy* (5th ed., pp. 154–180). Philadelphia, PA: Mosby/Elsevier.

---

nonresponsive to traditional therapies or who may have gastrointestinal symptoms of AD

b.   At 6 months of age, 83% of children with severe AD show positive IgE sensitization to milk, eggs, and peanuts.

III. Assessment

A. *Determine the diagnosis*
   Differential diagnoses (Figure 9-5)

B. *Assess the severity of the disease*
   Scoring for Atopic Dermatitis is a clinical tool often used by dermatologists to assess the extent and the severity of AD in children, and to determine the effectiveness of the treatment regimen. The tool is available at http://dermnetnz.org/dermatitis/scorad.html

C. *Assess the significance of the problem to the child and family*

D. *Assess the family functioning and ability to follow the treatment regimen*

IV. Goals of clinical management

A. *Improve quality of life for children with AD and their families*

   1.   No nighttime awakening because of itching.

   2.   No daytime discomfort or itching.

TABLE 9-1 Common Laboratory Tests

Test	Definition	Clinical Implications	Comments
Skin prick test	Wheal response after skin prick with antigen	IgE-mediated food hypersensitivity	Often does not correlate with clinical manifestations in children with AD
Radioallergosorbent test	Circulating specific IgE	IgE-mediated food hypersensitivity	False-positive findings are common, particularly in older children

Source: Paller A. S., & Mancini, A. J. (2006). Eczematous eruptions in childhood. In A. S. Paller & A. J. Mancini (Eds.), *Hurwitz clinical pediatric dermatology: A textbook of skin disorders of childhood and adolescence* (3rd ed., pp. 49–84). Philadelphia, PA: Saunders/ Elsevier.

FIGURE 9-5   Common Differential Diagnosis of Atopic Dermatitis

CONDITION	ASSOCIATED FINDINGS (may or may not include)
Contact dermatitis	Irritant or allergic contact dermatitis is generally milder than AD; occurs on the cheeks and chin, extensor surfaces or diaper area of infants and young children; caused by harsh soaps, vigorous bathing, or saliva on cheek and chin area.
Seborrheic dermatitis	Greasy, yellow scales that involve the scalp, eyebrows, behind the ears, cheeks, and can spread to neck and chest area; generally nonpruritic. Often AD appears as seborrheic dermatitis subsides.
Psoriasis	Round, erythematous, well-marginated plaques; covered by grayish or silvery-white scales; ~1 cm or greater in diameter; commonly found on the scalp, elbows, knees, and lumbosacral area.
Scabies	Pruritic papules, nodules, vesiculopustules, and burrowing lesions; commonly occur on infants and young children; seen on trunk, between the fingers, wrists, ankles, axillae, waist, groin, palms of hands, and soles of feet; occasionally seen on the head of infants.

Source: Paller A. S., & Mancini, A. J. (2006). Eczematous eruptions in childhood. In A. S. Paller & A. J. Mancini (Eds.), *Hurwitz clinical pediatric dermatology: A textbook of skin disorders of childhood and adolescence* (3rd ed., pp. 49–84). Philadelphia, PA: Saunders/ Elsevier.

---

3. No missed school because of AD.

4. No missed workdays for the parents because of their child's symptoms.

B. *Prescribe medications that allow the minimum effective dose to prevent adverse reactions*

C. *Educate families so they understand and adhere to optimum skin care and medication regimens*

D. *Control environmental factors that may adversely affect the child's skin*
   (Note: Food avoidance is no longer first-line management or mainstay of treatment for AD.)

E. *Provide on-going emotional and medical support for children and their families*

V. Plan

A. *Develop an optimum skin care routine with the family. Instruct the family to use the following "soak and seal" technique:*
   1. Daily bath with warm water for about 10 minutes using a minimal amount of fragrance-free and dye-free gentle soap or cleanser that is formulated for sensitive skin. If the child is not too dirty, use soap only on hands, feet, armpits, and genital area, not all over the body.
      a. If the child complains of burning when sitting in a bathtub, the addition of one cup of table salt may make the bath more tolerable (Paller & Mancini, 2006).
   2. Gently pat away excess water, leaving skin slightly damp.
   3. If rash is present, apply skin medication to the rash on body and face with skin slightly damp and rub in well.
   4. After drying, apply a generous amount of moisturizing cream. This seals in the water from bathing and makes the skin less dry and itchy. Eucerin cream, Aquaphor™ ointment, and Cetaphil™ cream are effective products. Lotions are not recommended for adequate moisturizing in children with AD. Vegetable shortening can be used as an inexpensive moisturizer and sealer, and petroleum jelly is a good occlusive preparation, although not a moisturizer. This application should be done within 3 minutes of exiting the bath before water loss in the skin occurs from evaporation (Paller & Mancini, 2006).

5. When moisturizing products are not effective, some children may need a special preparation containing ammonium lactate or alpha-hydroxy acid lotion for maintenance care. These products have increased ability to hold water in the skin and the products may limit desquamation. However, they frequently cause burning of the affected skin and so should be used with caution with young children (Fitzpatrick & Wolff, 2005).

B. Avoid factors or allergic triggers that lead to flares

1. Irritants: things that may cause the skin to be red or itchy, or to burn

   a. Wash all new clothes before wearing to remove chemicals. Double rinse the child's laundry so that their skin is not in contact with residual detergent in clothing.

   b. Do not use fabric softeners.

   c. Avoid clothes made of wool and artificial fibers. Dress the child in loose fitting cotton clothes that allow air to pass freely to the skin.

   d. Avoid contact with harsh household cleaners. Use natural, environmentally safe products.

   e. Wear long pants and long sleeves when playing around irritating substances, such as sand, dirt, and plants.

   f. Eliminate the child's exposure to second-hand smoke because it can increase irritation and pruritus, and may also increase the tendency for the development of asthma (Paller & Mancini, 2006).

   g. Keep the child's fingernails short, smooth, and clean to help prevent skin irritation, infection, and damage caused by scratching. Explain to the family that when the child scratches the rash becomes worse and the skin becomes thicker.

2. Proved or suspected allergens

   a. Consider food allergy only in children who have reacted immediately to a certain food, and in infants and young children with moderate or severe uncontrolled AD, particularly with gastrointestinal symptoms or failure to thrive. (National Institute for Health and Clinical Excellence [NICE], 2007).

      i. Offer a 6- to 8-week trial of an extensively hydrolyzed protein formula as a substitute for cow's milk formula for bottle-fed infants younger than 6 months of age with moderate or severe AD. Refer to a dietary specialist if the baby needs to be on cow's milk–free diet for more than 8 weeks (Paller & Mancini, 2006).

      ii. Inform breastfeeding mothers that it is not known whether altering a mother's diet is effective in reducing symptoms. However, if a food allergy is strongly suspected consider a trial of elimination of the more allergenic foods, such as cow's milk, soy, wheat, tree nuts, peanuts, fish, and egg under dietary supervision.

   b. Consider inhalant allergy in children with seasonal flares, associated asthma, and allergic rhinitis, and in children older than 3 years of age with AD on the face. After 3 years of age, many children outgrow food allergies but become sensitive to airborne allergens, such as dust mites (Leong et al., 2004). Some children have shown improvement in symptoms when dust mites are controlled in their environment, especially in their bedroom:

      i. Eliminate floor coverings and curtains

      ii. Eliminate all upholstered furniture except the bed

      iii. Cover box springs, mattress, and pillows in plastic zippered covers or obtain allergy-proof covers

      iv. Eliminate clutter and limit the toys, especially stuffed animals

      v. Wash all bedcovers and stuffed animals at least once a week in hot water

      vi. Keep pets with fur or feathers out of the room because they attract dust

   c. Avoid only substances that are documented to cause an increase in symptoms. It is important not to deny children things unnecessarily, such as foods or outdoor activities.

   d. Most children with mild AD do not need diagnostic testing for skin allergies (NICE, 2007).

C. Treat symptoms when they occur

1. Topical corticosteroids are the therapeutic mainstay for AD. They not only suppress the inflammation and pruritus associated with AD, they may also have an effect on bacterial colonization (Boguniewicz & Nicol, 2002). Choosing which corticosteroid to prescribe depends on the severity and distribution of the lesions and the age of the child. Preparations are divided into seven groups based on relative potency, from very low preparations, such as hydrocortisone acetate, to very high preparations, such as clobetasol proprionate. Ointment-based preparations are more potent, more occlusive, and less drying than chemically equivalent cream-based agents. The most effective, but least potent, should be used

to prevent thinning of the skin. For children with mild-to-moderate disease, a group VII drug, such as hydrocortisone ointment 1% or 2.5%, is usually sufficient (Nicol, 2000). When corticosteroids are prescribed, consider the following:

a. Prescribe in adequate amounts to optimize control. Prescriptions that require frequent refills may lead to under-treatment or nonadherence.

b. Prescribe for application only once or twice a day.

c. Corticosteroids should be applied to areas of active lesions, not to clear skin for prophylaxis.

d. Consider the possibility of secondary bacterial or viral infection if the regular application of corticosteroids has not controlled the AD within 2 weeks.

e. Consider changing to a different topical corticosteroid of the same potency as an alternative to stepping up treatment if tachyphylaxis is suspected (NICE, 2007).

f. Do not use potent topical corticosteroids on the face or neck.

g. When inflammation is widespread avoid high-potency corticosteroids because of the risk of systemic adverse effects (Nicol, 2000).

h. Refer to a specialist if potent corticosteroids are needed for children younger than 12 months of age.

i. Explain to families that the benefits of topical corticosteroids outweigh the risks if applied correctly.

2. Topical calcineurin inhibitors are an option for treatment if the child's AD has not shown a satisfactory clinical response to adequate use of topical corticosteroids at the maximum strength and potency that is appropriate for the child's age and the area being treated (NICE, 2007). Both pimecrolimus cream 1% (Elidel) and tacrolimus ointment 0.03% and 0.1% (Protopic) are approved for treating AD in children 2 years of age and older.

a. Pimecrolimus is efficacious in children with mild-to-moderate AD.

b. Tacrolimus is appropriate for children with moderate-to-severe disease and its effectiveness has been compared to midpotency topical steroids.

c. Both medications are safe for use in the periorbital areas, and on the head, neck, and intertriginous area (Paller & Mancini, 2006).

d. A burning sensation may occur during the first few days of application in children with either medication, especially in children with more severe dermatitis.

e. Use sun protection when using either medication.

f. Because of the proved safety and effectiveness of calcineurin inhibitors, they are increasingly used as first-line therapy, with topical steroids used for flares (Boguniewicz, 2005).

3. Wet-wrap dressings reduce itching and inflammation by cooling the skin and improving penetration of topical corticosteroids for acute exacerbations. They also prevent excoriation from scratching. In the hospital, gauze is usually used for this procedure. At home, a method used for years at the National Jewish Medical and Research Center, Denver, Colorado, is a simpler approach. It uses wet clothing, such as long underwear and cotton socks, applied over an undiluted layer of topical corticosteroids with a dry layer of clothing on top (Boguniewitz & Nicol, 2002).

a. Use blankets to prevent chilling.

b. Should not be used for more than 7–14 consecutive nights (NICE, 2007).

4. Antihistamines are thought to have little direct effect on pruritus. However, the tranquilizing and sedating effects of sedating antihistamines, such as hydroxyzine, diphenhydramine, and doxepin, may provide symptomatic relief if given at bedtime. Ceterizine may have limited value, but it is also somewhat sedating. Nonsedating antihistamines are not effective in alleviating pruritus (Paller & Mancini, 2006).

a. Ensure that the medication does not interfere with the child's functioning during the daytime.

b. Topical antihistamines should be avoided because of possible local allergic reactions (Nicol, 2000).

5. Phototherapy could be considered for severe AD or when other management options have failed. Refer to a pediatric specialty clinic where staff is experienced in dealing with children.

6. Systemic corticosteroids should be avoided except in rare instances (Fitzpatrick & Wolff, 2005). Although effective for most patients with AD, the rapid rebound after discontinuation and high risk of potential side effects make their use impractical in children.

7. Treating flares of symptoms is an important area of patient education. Flares can occur at any time and the family should be prepared to step up treatment when needed.

a. Offer information on how to recognize flares.

b. Give written instructions, such as an Eczema Action Plan, on how to manage flares by stepping up treatment, and prescribe treatments accordingly.

   c. Treatment of flares should be started as soon as symptoms appear and should be continued for 48 hours after acute symptoms subside (NICE, 2007).

D. Treat complications

1. Bacterial superinfection with *S. aureus* is common in children with AD. First-generation cephalosporins, such as cephalexin, 25–50 mg/kg divided two or three times daily for 10 days, are commonly used, although in some communities it may be advisable to culture for methicillin-resistant *S. aureus* and then treat accordingly. The addition of one-quarter to one-eighth cup of chlorine bleach to a full tub of water, intermittent application of mupirocin ointment to the nares and hands of patients and caregivers daily for 3 weeks, and the use of a gentle antibacterial soap may decrease colonization (Paller & Mancini, 2006; Boguniewitz & Nicol, 2002). Control of pruritus and prevention of excoriation with proper skin care and medications also helps prevent cutaneous infections.

2. Herpes simplex virus infection (eczema herpeticum) is a potentially life-threatening complication.

   a. Considered if the following is observed:
     i. Areas of rapidly worsening and painful dermatitis
     ii. Systemic symptoms, such as fever, lethargy, or distress
     iii. Clustered blisters with the appearance of early stage cold sores
     iv. Punched-out erosions that are uniform in appearance and that may coalesce (NICE, 2007)
     v. Child's infected dermatitis fails to respond to antibiotic treatment and appropriate corticosteroids

   b. If suspected, treat immediately with systemic acyclovir and refer for same-day dermatologic advice.

   c. If there is involvement of the skin around the eyes refer for a same-day consultation with an ophthalmologist and dermatologist.

VI. Self-management

A. Patient and family education and home management of bathing and medication regimens are the key factor in determining

successful outcomes for children with AD. It is important to:

1. Involve the family in all treatment decisions. The family is likely to be more adherent with the treatment plans if they have been part of the decision-making process. Consider the family's cultural skin-care and bathing practices when discussing options.

2. Explain that AD often improves with time, but not all children grow out of the condition; at times it becomes worse as the child gets older.

3. Educate families regarding the avoidance of environmental, behavioral, or emotional factors that may trigger symptoms. Referral to a public health nurse or community health worker for an environmental assessment in the home may be helpful.

4. Clearly explain the quantity of moisturizer to use on the child's skin. Applying an insufficient amount of moisturizer is a common problem.

B. Families need comprehensive written and verbal information in their native language regarding maintenance therapy, when and how to step treatment up and down, how to treat flares, and how to recognize complications. All procedures, even the application of ointments, should be demonstrated.

C. Discuss complementary therapies with the family and explain that their effectiveness and safety for AD has not been adequately assessed (NICE, 2007).

VII. Psychosocial and emotional support

A. Considering the effect of AD on the quality of life of patients and their families, it is important to address possible psychosocial issues and to offer support:

1. Parents may feel guilty about the child's condition and they may be exhausted from sleep deprivation and from caring for the child's needs.

2. School-age children may be teased by their peers about the appearance of their skin and may also fall behind in their schoolwork because of absences.

3. Adolescents may be particularly self-conscious about their appearance and may be leading isolated lives.

B. *Refer the family and child to a local support group or for counseling if needed.*

C. *AD education resources:*

1. National Eczema Association Support Network: www.nationaleczema.org/support

2. National Jewish Medical and Research Center: www.nationaljewish.org

3. National Institute for Health and Clinical Excellence "Understanding NICE guidance— Information for patients and caregivers": www.nice.org.uk/CG57 (0870 1555 455)

4. National Eczema Society (UK): www.eczema.org (0870 241 3604)

5. Changing Faces: www.changingfaces.org.uk (0845 4500 275)

REFERENCES

Boguniewicz, M. (2005). Atopic dermatitis: Beyond the itch that rashes. *Immunology and Allergy Clinics of North America, 25,* 333–351.

Boguniewitz, M., & Nicol, N. (2002). Conventional therapies for atopic dermatitis. *Immunology and Allergy Clinics of North America, 22*(1), 107–121.

Fitzpatrick, T., & Wolff, K. (2005). *Fitzpatrick's color atlas and synopsis of clinical dermatology* (5th ed.). New York, NY: McGraw-Hill.

Goodhue, J. G., & Brady, M. A. (2009). Atopic and rheumatic disorders. In C. E. Burns et al., (Eds.), *Pediatric primary care* (4th ed., pp. 553– 583). St. Louis, MO: Saunders/Elsevier.

Habif, T. P. (2010). Atopic dermatitis. In T. P. Habif (Ed.), *Clinical dermatology: A color guide to diagnosis and therapy* (5th ed., pp. 154–180). Philadelphia, PA: Mosby/Elsevier.

Leong, D. Y. M., Boguniewicz, M., Howell, M. D., & Hamid, Q. A. (2004). New insight into atopic dermatitis. *Journal of Clinical Investigation, 113,* 651–657.

National Institute for Health and Clinical Excellence (NICE). (2007). *Atopic eczema in children (NICE clinical guideline 57).* London, UK: Author.

National Institute of Arthritis and Musculoskeletal and Skin Diseases Information Clearing House, National Institutes of Health. (2009). *Atopic dermatitis: Handout on health.* Bethesda, MD: Author. Full text available online: www.niams.nih.gov

Nicol, N. (2000). Managing atopic dermatitis in children and adults. *The Nurse Practitioner, 25* (4), 58–76.

Paller, A. S., & Mancini, A. J. (2006). Eczematous eruptions in childhood. In A. S. Paller & A. J. Mancini (Eds.), *Hurwitz clinical pediatric dermatology: A textbook of skin disorders of childhood and adolescence* (3rd ed., pp. 49–84). Philadelphia, PA: Saunders/ Elsevier.

Porth, C. M., & Matfin, G. (2009). *Pathophysiology: Concepts of altered health states* (8th ed.). Philadelphia, PA: Wolters Kluwer/Lippincott, Williams & Wilkins.

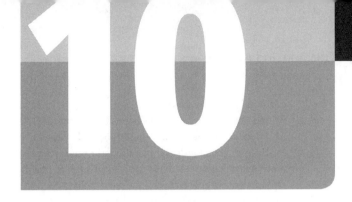

ATTENTION-DEFICIT/ HYPERACTIVITY DISORDER IN CHILDREN AND ADOLESCENTS

Naomi Schapiro

I. Introduction

Attention-deficit/hyperactivity disorder (ADHD) is one of the most common chronic conditions in childhood, and the most common of the chronic neuropsychiatric conditions (Merikangas et al., 2010). As a constellation of symptoms without distinctive physical or genetic markers (Steinhausen, 2009), there is some controversy as to whether or not ADHD is a distinctive disorder (Furman, 2008). Nevertheless, the major pediatric (American Academy of Pediatrics [AAP], 2000 & 2001) and child psychiatric (Pliszka & American Academy of Child and Adolescent Psychiatry [AACAP] Work Group on Quality Issues, 2007) organizations recognize both its existence and the benefits of diagnosing and treating this condition in childhood and adolescence. The advanced practice nurse (APN), working in either primary or specialty care, is well suited to detect, follow, refer, and manage children with ADHD (Vierhile, Robb, & Ryan-Krause, 2009).

II. Overview

A. Definitions

ADHD is defined by its features as a syndrome involving inattentiveness, hyperactivity, and impulsivity (Steinhausen, 2009). Diagnostic criteria for ADHD have been set historically by the Diagnostic and Statistical Manual for Mental Disorders (DSM). The current edition, DSM-IV-TR (American Psychiatric Association [APA], 2000) defines ADHD as "a persistent pattern of inattention and/or hyperactivity-impulsivity that is more frequently displayed and more severe than is typically observed in individuals of comparable development" (p. 85). The current diagnostic criteria also require that the individual has displayed some of these behaviors before age 7 years, and that they be present in at least two areas of the child's life, such as home and school. The DSM is currently under revision, with the DSM-V expected in 2013 (APA, n.d.). Proposed changes include age 12 as the upper limit for first appearance of symptoms, requiring only four symptoms for either inattention or hyperactivity for adolescents over 17 and adults, and an "inattentive restrictive" category for individuals who display no more than two characteristics of hyperactivity and impulsivity. Because current guidelines follow the DSM diagnostic criteria, it is important for the APN to become familiar with DSM-V criteria when they are published.

Current criteria require that the child display at least six inattentive behaviors or at least six impulsive or hyperactive behaviors, or six of a combination of inattentive and hyperactive–impulsive behaviors (APA, 2000). Examples of inattentive behaviors include difficulty in performing tasks that require sustained attention, distractibility, difficulty organizing tasks, forgetfulness, and appearing not to listen when spoken to directly. In adolescents and young adults, inattentive behaviors may involve procrastination, poor time management, and difficulty in multitasking (Katragadda & Schubiner, 2007). Examples of hyperactive or impulsive behaviors include fidgeting, leaving one's seat or running around in inappropriate settings, difficulty taking turns, blurting out answers, and acting as if "driven by a motor" (APA, p. 92). In adolescents and young adults, hyperactive behaviors may be more subtle, and impulsivity may manifest as impaired decision-making or impulsive driving errors (Katragadda & Schubiner). The presence of these behaviors must have a negative impact on the child's functioning in two areas (at home, at school, or with peers) to meet diagnostic criteria (Stein & Perrin, 2003). Although ADHD may manifest early in life, the behaviors previously mentioned are considered developmentally normal in preschool-age children, and the AAP guidelines for diagnosis and treatment of ADHD in primary care settings are for school-age children (AAP, 2000 & 2001). It may be prudent for the APN to refer younger children to behavioral or mental health specialists for diagnosis and initial treatment plans.

B. Incidence and prevalence

According to the 2006 National Health Interview Survey, 7% of United States children were reported by their parents to have been diagnosed with ADHD (Bloom, Cohen, & Freeman, 2007). Using part of the National Health and Nutrition Examination Survey sample, over 8% of children who were given a structured mental health diagnostic interview fit diagnostic criteria for ADHD (Merikangas et al., 2010). Only half of the children in this study with diagnosable mental health conditions had sought treatment with a mental health professional. Other studies indicate that prevalence is between 6 and 9% in children, and 3 and 5% in adults (Dopheide & Pliszka, 2009). The prevalence studies of coexisting conditions in children with ADHD come from samples of children referred to psychiatric care, and so should not be interpreted as being representative of all children: 35% of children with ADHD in referral samples have oppositional defiant disorder, 26% have conduct disorder, 26% have anxiety, and 18% have depressive disorders (Stein & Perrin, 2003). The APN should be aware of the need to be alert for coexisting conditions.

Some studies have shown that up to 60% of the behavioral problems of children with ADHD persist into adulthood (Schmidt & Petermann, 2009). In a 10-year longitudinal study of 110 boys with ADHD, Biederman, Petty, Evans, Small and Faraone (2010) found that 65% no longer met full diagnostic criteria for ADHD in adulthood, but 78% had higher rates of coexisting psychiatric conditions, family members with mood disorders, and educational or social impairments than the 105 controls without ADHD. In this same cohort, boys who were treated with stimulants had lower rates of psychiatric disorders and academic failure than boys with ADHD who were not treated (Biederman, Monuteaux, Spencer, Wilens, & Faraone, 2009). These findings reinforce the importance of early diagnosis and effective treatment for children and adolescents with ADHD.

C. Theories of pathophysiology

A recent review of etiology found that about 75% of the variance in ADHD could be explained by genetic factors (Steinhausen, 2009). However, this statement must be interpreted cautiously, because there were multiple potential genetic sites that might influence ADHD. In addition, most children with posited genetics factors did not have symptoms of ADHD, whereas many children with ADHD did not have any known genetic factors. The author of this review concluded that despite relatively simple diagnostic criteria, the label ADHD likely comprised "heterogeneous neurobiological disorders" (Steinhausen, p. 397). Theoretical descriptions of the specific core neurobiologic dysfunctions include (Dopheide & Pliszka, 2009; Tripp & Wickens, 2009): (1) deficits in behavioral inhibition, (2) executive function deficits, and (3) alterations in reinforcement mechanisms and sensitivity to delayed reinforcement. Dopamine, norepinephrine, and serotonin have been implicated in core symptoms, and stimulants may affect serotonin receptors and dopamine receptors (Tripp & Wickens).

III. Database: history

A. Chief complaint: referrals from parents, teachers, and family members

Parents may initiate care if they have noticed disruptive or attentional problems at home or at school, and are also frequently encouraged by school personnel to have their child evaluated for ADHD. The initiating symptoms, and motivation for seeking a diagnosis or treatment, are an important part of the history. Because specific behaviors are both part of the diagnostic criteria and help guide the treatment plan, it is important to have parents and children be as specific as possible about the core behavioral symptoms, and how they manifest in all the areas or domains of the child's life, particularly at home, at school, and with friends. Just as with a purely physical chief complaint, the APN can be guided in diagnosis by asking for the duration of the behaviors, specifically when they manifest (during which activities at home or which parts of the school day), any environmental characteristics or interventions that have made the behaviors better or worse, any associated problems, and any previous efforts by parents or teachers to manage the behaviors. For older adolescents and young adults, the functional impairment in school- and work-related settings may be the most salient part of the presenting complaint, and it may take skillful questioning to elicit the core behavioral symptoms that fit diagnostic criteria for ADHD, and the age at which they began to manifest (Katragadda & Schubiner, 2007).

Sleep problems, including sleep apnea, may result in daytime fatigue and inattention. Seizure disorders, especially absence seizures, may masquerade as inattention. Allergy symptoms, and the medications used to treat them, can also be related to inattention (Selekman, 2010). The APN's history should include questions about sleep, snoring, and nighttime awakening, and specific descriptions of inattentive behavior.

Children with hearing impairments or learning disabilities, such as reading disorders and receptive language delays, may also seem distractible and inattentive.

History should include questions about any unusual movements or habits, such as tics or obsessive–compulsive behaviors, which may coexist with ADHD.

B. Screening for ADHD

The AAP states that primary care clinicians may use ADHD-specific screening scales to aid in the diagnosis of ADHD (AAP, 2000; Stein & Perrin, 2003). The screening questionnaire in the AAP ADHD Toolkit, the Vanderbilt questionnaire (Wolraich et al., 2003), is available without cost on several websites in English and Spanish (Table 10-1). Broader questionnaires, such as the Achenbach Child Behavior Checklist, have not been found to be specific or sensitive enough for the diagnosis of ADHD in primary care settings (AAP, 2000), but may be used by psychiatric and mental health professionals as part of their assessment. Most clinical questionnaires for identifying ADHD include parent forms and teacher forms, and it is crucial to collect information directly from the child's teacher. Asking the parent to deliver and retrieve screening forms from the teacher saves the APN time and ensures that parents consent to the collection of this information.

C. Screening for coexisting psychiatric and behavioral issues

Screening questionnaires, such as the Vanderbilt or Conners forms, include questions whose positive answers raise the clinician's suspicion of coexisting oppositional, anxiety, or mood disorders. Unless the APN and collaborating clinicians within the practice are very experienced at diagnosing and managing mental health conditions in the primary care setting, children who may have coexisting conditions should be referred to mental health clinicians for diagnosis and comanagement. Children who are suffering the sequelae of family disruption, child abuse, or other traumas may exhibit distractibility, inattention, and fatigue from sleep problems related to anxiety or mood changes (Selekman, 2010).

TABLE 10-1 Screening Tools for ADHD

Name Contact	Cost	Individuals Screened	Languages	Additional Information
Vanderbilt Forms American Academy of Pediatrics http://www.aap.org/healthtopics/ADHD.cfm	$49.95	Parents Teachers	English Spanish	Screening forms Educational handouts Behavioral treatment guidelines
Vanderbilt Forms NICH-Q http://www.nichq.org/adhd_tools.html	No cost	Parents Teachers	English	Screening forms Educational handouts
Modified Vanderbilt Forms San Diego ADHD Project https://research.tufts-nemc.org/help4kids/forms.asp	No cost	Parents Teachers	English Spanish	Screening forms Educational handouts Links to behavioral treatment guidelines
Conners Forms http://downloads.mhs.com/mhs/ MHS_Catalogue_CA.pdf	$43/form up to $1,029 per software package	Parents Teachers Youth (8–18)	English Spanish	Screening—long and short forms
Barkley Forms and Questionnaires http://www.guilford.com/cgi-bin/cartscript.cgi ?page=pr/barkley3.htm&dir=pp/adhdr&cart_id=	$35	Parents Teachers Adults	English	Questionnaires School forms Interventions

Partial list of screening forms. Additional forms described in Pliszka, S., & AACAP Work Group on Quality Issues. (2007). Practice parameter for the assessment and treatment of children and adolescents with attention-deficit/hyperactivity disorder. *Journal of the American Academy of Child & Adolescent Psychiatry, 46,* 894–921.

D. Screening for learning disabilities

If the child's functioning at school indicates the possibility of both learning disabilities and ADHD, both evaluations should proceed. Most health insurance plans, private or public, do not cover learning evaluations, which must be requested by the parent from an overburdened public school system. Although these evaluations are legally required for children who may need special education services, parents may need assistance from the APN in advocating for them (Selekman & Vessey, 2010). For children who do not improve in academic performance within 1 or 2 months of ADHD diagnosis and treatment, the AACAP recommends an evaluation at that point for learning disorders (Pliszka & AACAP Work Group on Quality Issues, 2007).

IV. Database: physical examination

A. Overview

The physical examination in ADHD should help the APN eliminate potential physical causes of inattention, hyperactivity, and disruptive behavior, and any contraindications to medication that might be used to treat ADHD. There are no specific physical findings that confirm or rule out a diagnosis of ADHD.

B. Rule out potential physical causes of attentional issues and disruptive behavior

The physical examination should include a thorough head, eye, ear, nose, and throat examination; a cardiovascular evaluation; a thorough neurologic examination including documentation of any tics; and hearing and vision screening.

Many examiners look for signs of hyperthyroidism or hypothyroidism, anemia, or lead poisoning. However, these conditions typically present with more symptoms than just inattention or impulsivity (Pliszka & AACAP Work Group on Quality Issues, 2007). Most children with ADHD have a normal physical examination (Pliszka & AACAP Work Group on Quality Issues, 2007; Stein & Perrin, 2003), although some children may have "soft neurologic signs" (Gustafsson et al., 2009), demonstrating more clumsiness on tasks requiring cerebellar integration, such as rapid-finger or alternating hand tests, than most children of their age. A frankly abnormal neurologic examination should prompt a search for other diagnoses, additional testing, and referral.

Children with normal examinations do not need laboratory or other imaging tests (Pliszka & AACAP Work Group on Quality Issues, 2007; Stein & Perrin, 2003). In particular, hematocrit, blood lead levels, thyroid hormone tests, brain imaging studies, electroencephalograms, and continuous performance tests have not been found to be useful diagnostically (AAP, 2000).

However, some clinicians still ensure that the child has a normal hemoglobin and ferritin level, and may check both lead and thyroid hormone levels if there are concerns related to the history or examination. If the child also has symptoms of anxiety or mood disturbances, complete blood count, thyroid, lead, and metabolic panels may be indicated.

C. Monitor for possible cautions or contraindications to treatments

Recent concerns about possible cases of sudden death in children treated with stimulants for ADHD have prompted a call for screening all children with ADHD for cardiovascular disease before initiating treatment with medications (AAP & American Heart Association, 2008). This recommendation reinforces the need to take a history and perform a thorough physical examination to exclude cardiovascular disease. The joint statement recommends the clinician use judgment as to whether an electrocardiogram (ECG) should be done on any particular child before beginning medication to treat ADHD, but does not recommend universal use of premedication ECGs. In a clarification, Vetter and colleagues (2008) recommended that all children with a family history of such conditions as hypertrophic cardiomyopathy, prolonged QT interval, and Wolff-Parkinson-White syndrome, which carry an increased risk for sudden cardiac death, be evaluated by a cardiologist before beginning stimulant medication.

When a range of medications is being considered, consulting mental health professionals may ask for chemistry panels that could reassure prescribers about kidney function (creatinine and blood–urea–nitrogen) and a lack of liver inflammation (aspartate aminotransferase and alanine aminotransferase).

D. Neuropsychiatric conditions and ADHD: tic disorders

Between 3% and 6% of all school-age children exhibit chronic vocal or motor tics, lasting over 1 year, and fewer than 1% have Tourette syndrome. However, up to 55% of this group has ADHD as a coexisting condition, and the coexistence of tic disorders and ADHD may complicate treatment, as discussed later (Freeman, 2007; Schapiro, 2010). Although most children with tics can suppress them for a time in public settings, they may show up on examination.

V. Assessment

A. History and examination that support a diagnosis of ADHD

No coexisting mental or behavioral health conditions are present. The child may be treated in a primary care setting or comanaged with mental health and learning professionals.

B. History and examination that support a diagnosis of ADHD

Additional coexisting conditions exist, or the child is younger than 6. These children should be referred to mental health and learning professionals for more definitive diagnosis, and the APN may comanage. Coexistence of anxiety, mood disorders, or tic disorders may complicate treatment, and children with a family history of bipolar disorder may react poorly to stimulant medications, even if they themselves do not have coexisting conditions. Diagnosis of ADHD in children younger than school age may be beyond the scope of practice of primary care clinicians.

C. History and examination that do not support a diagnosis of ADHD

Refer to psychiatric or mental health professionals or neurology, as indicated by the findings

VI. Plan

Current practice guidelines recommend treating ADHD as a chronic condition, and recommend medication or psychosocial treatment, or both (AAP, 2001; Pliszka & AACAP Work Group on Quality Issues, 2007). The AAP (2001) in particular recommends the choosing of three to six target behaviors that the parent and child would specifically like to improve. The most recent review (Pliszka & AACAP Work Group on Quality Issues) found that behavioral interventions were generally less effective than medication, but could be used in addition or instead of medication depending on severity of ADHD and family preferences.

A. Behavioral approaches (American Academy of Pediatrics, 2001)

1. Psychoeducation
   a. Long-term developmental implications of ADHD
   b. Effects on self-esteem and strategies for positive parenting
   c. Goals of treatment
   d. Bringing in school personnel as part of the team
2. Parent behavioral training: 8–12 sessions to help parents work more effectively with their children, specifically using:
   a. Positive reinforcement (including point systems, token economy)
   b. Methods of negative reinforcement (e.g., cost response)
   c. Giving commands, shaping behavior effectively

B. Medication

1. Stimulant medications

   Although the exact mechanism of action is unclear, they affect core symptoms of ADHD in up to 75% of children if tried systematically (Pliszka & AACAP Work Group on Quality Issues, 2007) and are still considered first-line treatment by most clinicians (Table 10-2). All have potential side effects of appetite suppression; sleep disturbance (although this is also a core ADHD symptom); headaches; constipation; and irritability during the day as medication wears off. Stimulants can worsen anxiety or mania in children with anxiety or bipolar disorder, or in children with a family history of bipolar disorder. Although dextroamphetamine and mixed amphetamine salts are approved for children as young as 3, stimulants are not generally recommended in preschool age children, because they seem to have increased adverse effects, and may not be as effective as behavioral treatment in this age group. Extended-release medications can last anywhere from 6 to 12 hours, depending on the medication and absorption formulation. These medications obviate the need for mid-day dosing, may decrease irritability because the medication wears off more slowly, and may have less potential for abuse. They also offer coverage for after-school or after-work tasks, such as homework or driving (Dopheide & Pliszka, 2009; Pliszka & AACAP Work Group on Quality Issues; Taketomo, Hodding, & Kraus, 2009).

   a. Short-acting: rapid onset, duration of action 3–4 hours
      i. Advantages: dose clears system rapidly, effect rapid
      ii. Disadvantages: given two or three times a day, including mid-day; issues of convenience (parent, school personnel), training, safety, and child's embarrassment; and more reports of irritability as medication wears off
   b. Intermediate and long-acting medication
      i. Longer acting: 6–12 hours, no need for mid-day dose
      ii. May start long-acting directly, no need to start with short-acting first, except in very young children
      iii. May have slower onset, depending on formulation
      iv. May have decreased abuse potential relative to short-acting medication
      v. If slower, steady release, child may not "feel" that the medication is working as much as the short-acting or medication

TABLE 10-2 ADHD Medications: FDA Approved

Medication Class	Duration	Examples	Advantages	Disadvantages	Dosing
Stimulants	Short-acting (3–6 hr)	Methylphenidate Dextroamphetamine Dexmethylphenidate	Quick onset, ease of making dosage adjustments without changing prescription	Must be dosed mid-day to last through school or work day, higher abuse potential	Individualized, not mg/kg dosing, but starting dose adjusted to weight
	Medium-acting (4–8 hr)	Mixed amphetamine salts (sometimes listed as short-acting, however effects may last through school day)	May last during school day, lower abuse potential	Steady release of medications may be less effective than bursts of stimulants	Individualized, not mg/kg dosing, but starting dose adjusted to weight
	Long-acting, variable forms of absorption and release (8–12 hr)	Osmotic-controlled Release Oral delivery system (OROS) methylphenidate Methylphenidate –LA* Methylphenidate CD* Methylphenidate patch Dextroamphetamine XR Dexmethylphenidate XR* Mixed amphetamine salts XR* Lisdexamfetamine [†]	Lasts during entire school day, better coverage for driving, lower abuse potential	Cannot be crushed or altered, may affect sleep more	Dosing less flexible, conversion charts available from short-acting medications
Norepinephrine reuptake inhibitor	Long-acting, 24-hr effect, half-life 5–21 hr	Atomoxetine	24-hr coverage, low abuse potential, may be effective for depression	Extensive drug interactions, black box warnings regarding suicidality	Weight-based dosing for children < 70 kg
α_2-Agonist	Short- or long-acting (only extended-release FDA approved 2009), half-life 17 hr	Guanfacine Guanfacine ER	More effective for impulsivity and hyperactivity than for inattention	Rebound hypertension if withdrawn too quickly, some children complain of HA, somnolence, drug interactions	Start with 1 mg po daily, may increase in increments of 1 mg/wk, weight-based suggested upper limits

* Capsule may be opened and sprinkled on applesauce.

[†] Capsule may be opened and dissolved in water.

Sources: Dopheide, J. A., & Pliszka, S. R. (2009). Attention-deficit-hyperactivity disorder: An update. *Pharmacotherapy, 29*(6), 656–679; Pliszka, S., & AACAP Work Group on Quality Issues (2007). Practice parameter for the assessment and treatment of children and adolescents with attention-deficit/hyperactivity disorder. *J Am Acad Child Adolesc Psychiatry, 46*(7), 894–921; and Taketomo, C. K., Hodding, J. H., & Kraus, D. M. (2009). *Pediatric dosage handbook: 2009-2010* (16th ed.). Hudson, OH: Lexi-Comp. FDA prescribing information for guanfacine at http://www.accessdata.fda.gov/drugsatfda_docs/label/2009/022037lbl.pdf

released in several bursts, but literature shows equivalent effect

c. Absorption mechanisms available in long-acting medications (current available medications in parentheses accurate at time of publication)

    i. Osmotically released oral therapy: shorter release and nonabsorbable plastic shell contains some medication for later release; later onset; longer effect than spheroidal oral drug absorption system (methylphenidate)

    ii. Spheroidal oral drug absorption system: combination of immediate-release and longer-release beads; capsules may be opened up and sprinkled on food (methylphenidate, dexmethylphenidate)

    iii. Transdermal patch: releases medication over 9 hours; onset within 2 hours; duration 12 hours; applied on hip; site and patch changed daily (methylphenidate)

    iv. Prodrug, converted slowly to active drug, in intestines and liver; slower onset and 10 hours of active effect; lower abuse potential (lisdexamfetamine to dexamphetamine)

2. Nonstimulant medication

    a. Atomoxetine: affects norepinephrine receptors

        i. Slow onset, effects may not be felt for several weeks

        ii. 24-hour coverage, longest coverage

        iii. More acceptable to child and adolescent if first medication, rather than switching from stimulant (patient may not "feel" that medication is taking effect)

        iv. Some reports of liver toxicity, cleared through CYP2D6 pathway, half-life up to 21 hours in individuals with less active CYP2D6

        v. May increase effects of albuterol, sympathomimetic drugs in general

        vi. Black box warnings of suicidality

    b. α_2-Adrenergic agonists

        i. More effective for impulsivity than for inattention

        ii. Guanfacine approved for children 6 years and older in extended-release form only; clonidine used off-label

        iii. Clonidine patch available (off-label) when steady dose reached; medication must be tapered off slowly

        iv. Sometimes used for children with impulsive ADHD and tics (off-label for tics and aggression)

        v. Side effects: depression, headache, dizziness, fatigue, constipation, decreased appetite; rebound hypertension if discontinued suddenly; drug interactions

    c. Tricyclic antidepressants (off-label for ADHD): imipramine, nortriptyline, and desipramine

        i. Not considered first-line

        ii. May be effective for ADHD combined with other conditions, such as anxiety, tics, or enuresis

        iii. Many drug interactions (neuroleptics, selective serotonin reuptake inhibitors, H_2 blockers, combined hormonal contraceptives)

        iv. Rate of metabolism may decrease after puberty

        v. Side effects: anticholinergic; weight gain; cardiac arrhythmias (need premed ECG and repeat with increasing doses)

    d. Bupropion

        i. Off-label use for ADHD, Food and Drug Administration approved for depression, smoking cessation

        ii. Not approved for children younger than 18 years

        iii. Side effects: insomnia, fatigue, agitation, dry mouth, headaches, rash, and lower seizure threshold

        iv. Contraindicated if history of seizures, traumatic head injury, or eating disorders

C. General considerations about medication

1. Contraindications for stimulants

    a. Symptomatic cardiovascular disease (adults and children)

    b. Glaucoma

    c. Food and Drug Administration lists tics as a contraindication to stimulant medication; however, several studies of children with Tourette syndrome randomized to various treatment arms for ADHD showed no increase in tics with stimulant medicine

2. Tracking medication short-term effects

    a. Encourage systematic follow-up of ADHD core symptoms: designation of core symptoms and follow-up with parent, child, and school about effects of medication

b. Initial dose should be increased weekly until core symptoms show improvement or side effects increase

    i. Clinician and family should expect some loss of appetite during the dosing period for stimulants, with normal appetite before dose and after wearing off; lack of this effect may indicate subtherapeutic dose

    ii. Carefully monitor side effects if child is on nonstimulant medication or if taking additional medications

    iii. Check in weekly with parent and child by telephone or in office when starting medication and increasing dose. Stimulants are Schedule II medications: no refills by telephone and new prescriptions must be written and picked up when continuing these medications

    iv. Follow-up blood pressure, heart rate, and weight for stimulants; other medications as indicated (e.g., liver inflammation for atomoxetine)

c. Track adherence and diversion: especially an issue for adolescent and young adult patients, taking shorter-acting stimulant medication

d. Stimulant medication holidays

    i. Sometimes used or recommended on weekends and summer if core symptoms manageable outside of school; medication holidays are controversial

    ii. May increase side effects on restarting

    iii. May not be beneficial for adolescents, especially if they drive

3. Tracking medication long-term effects

a. Effects on academic and job performance and home and peer relationships

    i. Most documented benefits early in treatment (first 3 years) may be partly caused by more intensive management

    ii. May be more effective if started earlier in the course of ADHD

    iii. Interaction of ADHD and substance abuse is complex: in general, adolescents and adults with ADHD have higher rates of substance abuse compared to non-ADHD peers; effective treatment with stimulants seems to lower this risk while treatment is maintained

b. Emergence or persistence of any mood-related symptoms

c. Growth (height, weight) and blood pressure

d. Diversion or substance use issues: in-depth psychosocial screen for adolescents

D. Follow-up and indications for referral

1. Lack of expected improvement

    a. Most children respond to stimulants, but may require a switch in specific type or adjustments in dose

    b. Response to behavioral approaches

2. Coexisting learning, mood, or behavioral problems not improving or worsening

E. Parental/Patient Education

Encourage parental connection with other parents, peer support for children and youth, and community resources (Box 10-1)

BOX 10-1 Web Resources

National Institute of Child Health Quality
Caring for Children with ADHD: A Resource Toolkit for Clinicians
http://www.nichq.org/adhd_tools.html

American Academy of Pediatrics
Children's Health Topics—ADHD—with links to ADHD Toolkit
http://www.aap.org/healthtopics/ADHD.cfm

Developmental Behavioral Pediatrics Online
Materials related to screening and early identification of behavioral and mental health problems
http://www.dbpeds.org/

American Academy of Child and Adolescent Psychiatry
http://www.aacap.org/

Help4KidswithADHD
Tufts University site with resources in Spanish and English, including San Diego ADHD Project Screening Packets in Spanish and English, parent and teacher educational forms
https://research.tufts-nemc.org/help4kids/default.asp

Children and Adults with Attention Deficit Hyperactivity Disorder
http://www.chadd.org/

Adolescent Health Working Group
Behavioral Health Toolkit
Screening and treatment guidelines for providers, handouts for youth and parents, symptom and medication side effect tracking forms
http://www.ahwg.net/assets/library/98_behavioral-healthmodule.pdf

F. Long-term issues and transition to adulthood

1. Condition trajectory (Biederman et al., 2010; Katragadda & Schubiner, 2007)

    a. Initial presenting behavioral symptoms may diminish, functional impairments may improve or worsen

    b. Increasing appearance of coexisting conditions (anxiety, mood, conduct, substance abuse); may be mitigated by appropriate medication and behavioral treatment in childhood and adolescence

    c. Significantly increased risks of driving accidents, tickets, and impulsive errors, especially if not properly medicated

2. Long-term planning should begin with early adolescent and parent

    a. Skill building to increase confidence, offer alternatives to risky behavior, and aid in career planning (Jellinek, 2008)

        i. Reframing ADHD to highlight positive aspects of behavioral characteristics for appropriate careers

        ii. Jobs, chores to give youth a sense of accomplishment, instill work ethics

        iii. Focusing on strengths and interests

    b. Advocating for educational accommodations as needed, involving the adolescent as a self-advocate (Selekman, 2010)

    c. Shift to long-acting medication with decreased abuse potential and greater coverage for evening behaviors, especially driving

3. Transition to adult systems of care

    a. Adult providers are often unfamiliar with ADHD, relative to pediatric providers

    b. Loss of insurance coverage and difficulty continuing stimulant medications through publicly funded or indigent mental health care

        i. May be greatly mitigated through 2010 healthcare reforms

        ii. Decreased access to care affects educational and job trajectories

        iii. Severities of coexisting conditions may increase and risk of substance abuse increases without access to effective care

REFERENCES

American Academy of Pediatrics. (2000). Clinical practice guideline: Diagnosis and evaluation of the child with attention-deficit/hyperactivity disorder. *Pediatrics, 105,* 1158–1170.

American Academy of Pediatrics. (2001). Clinical practice guideline: Treatment of the school-aged child with attention-deficit/hyperactivity disorder. *Pediatrics, 108,* 1033–1044.

American Academy of Pediatrics, & American Heart Association. (2008). American Academy of Pediatrics/American Heart Association clarification of statement on cardiovascular evaluation and monitoring of children and adolescents with heart disease receiving medications for ADHD: May 16, 2008. *Journal of Developmental Behavioral Pediatrics, 29,* 335.

American Psychiatric Association. (n.d.). *DSM-5 development: Attention deficit/hyperactivity disorder.* Retrieved from http://www.dsm5.org/ProposedRevisions/Pages/proposedrevision.aspx?rid=383#

American Psychiatric Association. (2000). *Diagnostic and statistical manual of mental disorders* (Fourth, Text Revision Ed.). Washington, DC: Author.

Biederman, J., Monuteaux, M. C., Spencer, T., Wilens, T. E., & Faraone, S. V. (2009). Do stimulants protect against psychiatric disorders in youth with ADHD? A 10-year follow-up study. *Pediatrics, 124,* 71–78.

Biederman, J., Petty, C. R., Evans, M., Small, J., & Faraone, S. V. (2010). How persistent is ADHD? A controlled 10-year follow-up study of boys with ADHD. *Psychiatry Research, 177,* 299–304.

Bloom, B., Cohen, R. A., & Freeman, G. (2007). Summary health statistics for U.S. children: National health interview survey, 2006. *Vital Health Statistics 10*(234), 1–79.

Dopheide, J. A., & Pliszka, S. R. (2009). Attention-deficit-hyperactivity disorder: An update. *Pharmacotherapy, 29,* 656–679.

Freeman, R. D. (2007). Tic disorders and ADHD: Answers from a world-wide clinical dataset on Tourette syndrome. *European Child Adolescent Psychiatry, 16*(Suppl. 1), 15–23.

Furman, L. M. (2008). Attention-deficit hyperactivity disorder (ADHD): Does new research support old concepts? *Journal of Child Neurology, 23,* 775–784.

Gustafsson, P., Svedin, C. G., Ericsson, I., Linden, C., Karlsson, M. K., & Thernlund, G. (2009). Reliability and validity of the assessment of neurological soft-signs in children with and without attention-deficit-hyperactivity disorder. *Development Medicine and Child Neurology, 52,* 364–370.

Jellinek, M. (2008). ADHD treatments. Going beyond the meds. *Contemporary Pediatrics, 25*(5), 39–42, 44, 46.

Katragadda, S., & Schubiner, H. (2007). ADHD in children, adolescents, and adults. *Primary Care: Clinics in Office Practice, 34,* 317–341; abstract viii.

Merikangas, K. R., He, J. P., Brody, D., Fisher, P. W., Bourdon, K., & Koretz, D. S. (2010). Prevalence and treatment of mental disorders among US children in the 2001–2004 NHANES. *Pediatrics, 125,* 75–81.

Pliszka, S., & AACAP Work Group on Quality Issues. (2007). Practice parameter for the assessment and treatment of children and adolescents with attention-deficit/hyperactivity disorder. *J Am Acad Child Adolesc Psychiatry, 46,* 894–921.

Schapiro, N. A. (2010). Tourette syndrome and obsessive-compulsive disorder. In P. J. Allen, J. A. Vessey, & N. A. Schapiro (Eds.), *Primary care of the child with a chronic condition* (5th ed., pp. 795–814). St. Louis, MO: Mosby Elsevier.

Schapiro (Eds.), *Primary care of the child with a chronic condition* (5th ed., pp. 197–217). St. Louis, MO: Mosby Elsevier.

Schmidt, S., & Petermann, F. (2009). Developmental psychopathology: Attention deficit hyperactivity disorder (ADHD). *BMC Psychiatry, 9,* 58.

Selekman, J. (2010). Attention-deficit/hyperactivity disorder. In P. J. Allen, J. A. Vessey, & N. A.

Selekman, J., & Vessey, J. A. (2010). School and the child with a chronic condition. In P. J. Allen, J. A. Vessey, & N. A. Schapiro (Eds.), *Primary care of the child with a chronic condition* (5th ed., pp. 42–59). St. Louis, MO: Mosby Elsevier.

Stein, M. T., & Perrin, J. M. (2003). Diagnosis and treatment of ADHD in school-age children in primary care settings: A synopsis of the AAP practice guidelines. *Pediatrics in Review, 24,* 92–98.

Steinhausen, H. C. (2009). The heterogeneity of causes and courses of attention-deficit/hyperactivity disorder. *Acta Psychiatria Scandinavia, 120*(5), 392–399.

Taketomo, C. K., Hodding, J. H., & Kraus, D. M. (2009). *Pediatric dosage handbook: 2009–2010* (16th ed.). Hudson, OH: Lexi-Comp.

Tripp, G., & Wickens, J. R. (2009). Neurobiology of ADHD. *Neuropharmacology, 57,* 579–589.

Vetter, V. L., Elia, J., Erickson, C., Berger, S., Blum, N., Uzark, K., et. al. (2008). Cardiovascular monitoring of children and adolescents with heart disease receiving medications for attention deficit/hyperactivity disorder [corrected]: A scientific statement from the American Heart Association Council on Cardiovascular Disease in the Young Congenital Cardiac Defects Committee and the Council on Cardiovascular Nursing. *Circulation, 117,* 2407–2423.

Vierhile, A., Robb, A., & Ryan-Krause, P. (2009). Attention-deficit/hyperactivity disorder in children and adolescents: Closing diagnostic, communication, and treatment gaps. *J Pediatr Health Care, 23*(Suppl. 1), S5–S23.

Wolraich, M. L., Lambert, W., Doffing, M. A., Bickman, L., Simmons, T., & Worley, K. (2003). Psychometric properties of the Vanderbilt ADHD diagnostic parent rating scale in a referred population. *Journal of Pediatric Psychology, 28,* 559–567.

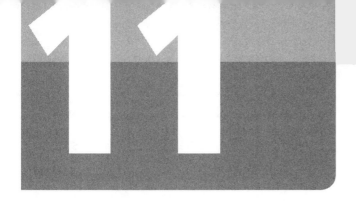

CHILDHOOD ASTHMA

Andrea Crosby, Nan Madden, and Shannon Thyne

I. Introduction and general background

A. Definition and overview

Asthma is a chronic lung disease causing narrowing of the airways. It is characterized by inflammation, bronchoconstriction, and mucus production, causing variable and recurring symptoms (National Heart, Lung, and Blood Institute, National Asthma Education and Prevention Program, & National Institutes of Health (NIH), 2007). Airway obstruction is generally partially or fully reversible (NIH).

B. Prevalence and incidence

Asthma onset often occurs during childhood (NIH, 2007). Over 10 million children (14%) younger than age 18 in the United States have ever been diagnosed with asthma (National Center for Health Statistics [NCHS], & Centers for Disease Control and Prevention [CDC], 2009). African American children and children from low-income families are more likely to have asthma (NCHS & CDC).

II. Database (may include but is not limited to)

A. Subjective

1. Past health history
   a. Prematurity (particularly with known lung disease).
   b. Hospitalization for respiratory syncytial virus infection.
   c. Wheezing in first years of life.
   d. Gastroesophageal reflux.
   e. Diagnoses from the "atopic triad": allergic rhinitis; asthma; and atopic dermatitis (eczema). The allergic component of asthma is much more prevalent and important in children.

2. Family history
   a. Asthma.
   b. Allergic rhinitis.
   c. Atopic dermatitis.

3. Occupational and environmental history
   a. Maternal smoking during pregnancy.
   b. Environmental exposure to tobacco smoke.
   c. Environmental exposure to toxin (through parental occupation, neighborhood of residence, and so forth).
   d. Home, school, or daycare exposure to environmental allergens (dust, animals, molds, and so forth).

4. Review of systems
   a. Constitutional signs and symptoms: nighttime awakening, poor sleep patterns, chronic cough, other problems related to poor sleep, sedentary lifestyle, and avoidance of physical activity.
   b. Pulmonary: wheezing, shortness of breath, nocturnal dry cough, exercise intolerance, and cough with exertion.
   c. Allergy symptoms: itchy eyes and nose, sneezing, and dry itchy skin.

B. Objective

1. Physical examination findings
   a. Increased respiratory rate.
   b. Skin: dry, erythematous patches and other symptoms of atopic dermatitis.
   c. Allergy-related findings: "allergic shiners" (dark circles under eyes) and "allergic salute" (crease across nose from chronic wiping).
   d. Ear, nose, and throat: boggy nasal turbinates, persistent ear effusions, and cobblestoning of posterior oropharynx from chronic postnasal drip.
   e. In acute flare, general state of alarm and anxiety because of "air hunger"; posturing (leaning forward to increase air entry); grunting; and inability to speak in full sentences.
   f. Pulmonary examination findings are most often normal when not in acute flare; however, many associated symptoms during flares.
      i. Prolonged expiratory phase
      ii. Wheezing (expiratory more common than inspiratory)

iii. Decreased air entry
iv. Use of accessory muscles
v. Cough (usually dry)

g. Abdomen: increased use of accessory muscles to improve air entry.

2. Supporting data from relevant diagnostic tests (further detailed under the Plan section)

a. Spirometry.
b. Allergy testing.
c. Radiology: chest radiograph.
d. Laboratory measures: complete blood count and arterial blood gas.

III. Assessment

A. *Differential diagnosis (NIH, 2007)*

1. Asthma

2. Allergic rhinitis

3. Sinusitis

4. Gastroesophageal reflux

5. Large airway obstruction

a. Foreign body in trachea or bronchus.
b. Vocal cord dysfunction.
c. Vascular rings or laryngeal webs.
d. Laryngotracheomalacia, tracheal stenosis, or bronchostenosis.
e. Enlarged lymph nodes or tumor.

6. Small airway obstruction

a. Bronchiolitis.
b. Cystic fibrosis.
c. Bronchopulmonary dysplasia.
d. Heart disease.

7. Habit cough

B. *Classify severity or control (Tables 11-1 and 11-2)*

1. Classify severity in a patient not currently on any controller medications, considering domains of both impairment and risk

a. Intermittent asthma.
b. Mild persistent asthma.
c. Moderate persistent asthma.
d. Severe persistent asthma.

2. Classify control in patients currently on a controller medication, considering domains of both impairment and risk

a. Well-controlled asthma.
b. Not well-controlled asthma.
c. Very poorly controlled asthma.

IV. Goals of clinical management

A. *Few or no daytime asthma symptoms*

B. *No nighttime awakenings caused by asthma symptoms*

C. *Normal spirometry*

D. *Ability to do normal physical activity and sports*

E. *Child should not miss school and care provider should not need to miss work*

V. Plan

A. *Diagnostic tests*

1. Spirometry

a. Obtain in children ages 5 years and older.
b. Forced expiratory volume in the first second of expiration, forced vital capacity, and forced expiratory flow, midexpiratory phase most useful in children.
c. Difficult to obtain accurate results in children, but trends over time can be helpful even if values remain in normal range.
d. Most often normal in children between asthma flares.
e. The comparison of the results of spirometry performed before and after the administration of a bronchodilator demonstrate obstruction and assess reversibility. An increase of greater than or equal to 12% in the forced expiratory volume in the first second of expiration shows significant reversibility and is diagnostic for asthma.

2. Chest radiograph

a. All children with asthma should have a baseline chest film to evaluate for structural abnormalities.
b. Can show hyperinflation, infiltrates, and bronchiolar cuffing.

3. Allergy skin testing

a. Allergy skin tests to detect specific IgE sensitization can be done on children of any age but it is more useful after the age of 2 years when positive reactions are more likely.
b. Test will not be accurate if antihistamine was taken recently.
c. Referral to a subspecialty clinic may be necessary for testing.

4. Specific IgE immunoassay (in vitro)

a. Tests for foods, airborne allergens, and known or possible triggers.

TABLE 11-1 Classifying Asthma Severity in Children 0–11 Years of Age

Components of Severity		Intermittent		Persistent Mild		Persistent Moderate		Persistent Severe	
		Ages 0–4	Ages 5–11	Ages 0–4	Ages 5–11	Ages 0–4	Ages 5–11	Ages 0–4	Ages 5–11
Impairment	Symptoms	≤ 2 d/wk		> 2 d/wk but not daily		Daily		Throughout the day	
	Nighttime awakenings	0	≤ 2×/mo	1–2×/mo	3–4×/mo	3–4×/mo	> 1×/wk but not nightly	> 1×/wk	Often 7×/wk
	Short-acting β₂-agonist use for symptom control (not prevention of EIB)	≤ 2 d/wk		> 2 d/wk but not daily		Daily		Several times per day	
	Inference with normal activity	None		Minor limitation		Some limitation		Extremely limited	
	Lung function (ages 5–11)	Normal FEV_1 between exacerbations FEV_1 > 80% predicted FEV_1/FVC > 85%		FEV_1 > 80% predicted FEV_1/FVC > 80%		FEV_1 = 60–80% predicted FEV_1/FVC = 75–80%		FEV_1 < 60% predicted FEV_1/FVC < 75%	
Risk	Exacerbations requiring oral systemic corticosteroids	0–1/year		**Children 0–4 years:** ≥ 2 exacerbations in 6 mo requiring oral systemic corticosteroids, or ≥ 4 wheezing episodes/1 year lasting > 1 d and risk factors for persistent asthma **Children 5–11 years:** ≥ 2/year					
		Consider severity and interval since last exacerbation. Frequency and severity may fluctuate over time. Relative annual risk may be related to FEV_1. Exacerbations of any severity may occur in patients in any severity category.							
Recommended Step for Initiating Therapy (see **Table 11-3** for recommended treatment steps)		Step 1		Step 2		Step 3 and consider short course of oral systemic corticosteroids			
		In 2–6 wk, depending on severity, evaluate level of asthma control that is achieved. If no clear benefit is observed in 4–6 wk, consider adjusting therapy or alternative diagnosis.							

Abbreviations: EIB = exercise-induced bronchospasm; FEV_1 = forced expiratory volume in the first second of expiration; FVC = forced vital capacity.

Source: U.S. Department of Health and Human Services, National Institutes of Health, National Heart, Lung, and Blood Institute. (2008). *National Asthma Education and Prevention Program Expert Panel Report 3: Guidelines for the diagnosis and management of asthma—Summary Report 2007* (pp. 40–42). NIH Publication Number 08-5846. Bethesda, MD: Author.

TABLE 11-2 Assessing Asthma Control and Adjusting Therapy in Children 0–11 Years of Age

Components of Control		Classification of Asthma Control					
		Well Controlled		Not Well Controlled		Very Poorly Controlled	
		Ages 0–4	Ages 5–11	Ages 0–4	Ages 5–11	Ages 0–4	Ages 5–11
Impairment	Symptoms	≤ 2 d/wk but not more than once on each day		>2 d/wk or multiple times on < 2 d/wk		Throughout the day	
	Nighttime awakenings	≤ 1×/mo		> 1×/mo	≥ 2×/mo	> 1×/wk	≥ 2×/wk
	Interference with normal activity	None		Some limitation		Extremely limited	
	Short-acting β_2-agonist use for symptom control (not prevention of EIB)	≤ 2 d/wk		> 2 d/wk		Several times per day	
	Lung function - FEV_1 (predicted) or peak flow personal best - FEV_1/FVC	N/A	> 80% / > 80%	N/A	60–80% / 75–80%	N/A	< 60% / < 75%
Risk	Exacerbations requiring oral systemic corticosteroids	0–1×/year		2–3×/year	≥ 2×/year	> 3×/year	≥ 2×/year
	Reduction in lung growth (ages 5–11)	Requires long-term follow-up					
	Treatment-related adverse effects	Medication side effects can vary in intensity from none to very troublesome and worrisome. The level of intensity does not correlate to specific levels of control but should be considered in the overall assessment of risk.					
Recommended Action for Treatment (see **Table 11-3** for treatment steps) The stepwise approach is meant to assist, not replace, clinical decision-making required to meet individual patient needs.		Maintain current step Regular follow-up every 1–6 mo Consider step-down if well controlled for at least 3 mo		Step-up 1 step	Step-up at least 1 step	Consider short course of oral systemic corticosteroids Step-up 1–2 steps	
				Before step-up: Review adherence to medication, inhaler technique, and environmental control. If alternative treatment was used, discontinue it and use preferred treatment for that step. Reevaluate the level of asthma control in 2–6 wk to achieve control, every 1–6 mo to maintain control. **Children 0–4 years old:** If no clear benefit is observed in 4–6 wk, consider alternative diagnosis or adjusting therapy. **Children 5–11 years old:** Adjust therapy accordingly. For side effects, consider alternative treatment options.			

Abbreviations: EIB = exercise-induced bronchospasm; FEV_1 = forced expiratory volume in the first second of expiration; FVC = forced vital capacity.

Source: U.S. Department of Health and Human Services, National Institutes of Health, National Heart, Lung, and Blood Institute. (2008). *National Asthma Education and Prevention Program Expert Panel Report 3: Guidelines for the diagnosis and management of asthma—Summary Report 2007* (pp. 40–42). NIH Publication Number 08-5846. Bethesda, MD: Author.

b. More expensive and less accurate than skin testing; however, not affected by recent doses of antihistamines.

c. Indicated if history of anaphylaxis to particular allergen.

d. Indicated if severe atopic dermatitis makes it difficult to find clear skin on which to perform the prick tests.

e. Requires blood draw.

5. Laboratory measures

a. Complete blood count: eosinophilia supportive of allergic component to child's asthma.

b. Arterial blood gas: in acute asthma flare, can show decreased oxygenation and retention of carbon dioxide, suggestive of impending respiratory failure.

B. Management

1. Environmental controls

a. Allergens: identify and minimize exposure to common allergens (dust mites, mold, animal dander, cockroaches, molds, and seasonal pollens).

i. Carpeting: harbors dust mites, and children like to play on the floor. Should be removed, or at least vacuumed frequently.

ii. Stuffed animals: try to limit to one or two stuffed toys, wash them in hot water every 2 weeks, or freeze and then place in the dryer.

iii. Allergen-proof mattress and pillow covers: for those with dust mite allergies.

iv. All bed linen should be washed in hot water and dried in a dryer every week.

b. Irritants (smoke, perfumes, or fumes from cleaning solutions).

i. Absolutely no one should smoke in the house or in a car with children, and those who choose to smoke outside should wear a smoking jacket that is never brought into the house.

ii. Use environmentally safe cleaning products and clean when the child is out of the home.

2. Medication (See Table 11-3)

a. Rescue medications are short-acting β-agonists (SABA) (albuterol HFA or levalbuterol HFA, also available in nebulized form). Give every 4 hours as needed for any signs of asthma, including coughing.

b. Controller medication.

i. Prescribe controller medications for any child with persistent asthma.

TABLE 11-3 Stepwise Approach for Managing Asthma Long Term in Children 0–11 Years of Age: Preferred Medications*

Intermittent Asthma	Persistent Asthma: Daily Medication				
Step 1	Step 2	Step 3	Step 4	Step 5	Step 6
	Ages 0–4				
SABA PRN	Low-dose ICS	Medium-dose ICS	Medium-dose ICS + LABA *or* montelukast	High-dose ICS + LABA *or* montelukast	High-dose ICS + LABA *or* montelukast + oral corticosteroids
	Ages 5–11				
	Low-dose ICS	Low-dose ICS + LABA, LTRA, or theophylline *or* medium-dose ICS	Medium-dose ICS + LABA	High-dose ICS + LABA	High-dose ICS + LABA + oral corticosteroids

Abbreviations: ICS = inhaled corticosteroids; LABA = long-acting β-agonists; LTRA = Leukotriene Receptor Antagonist.

* See NIH 2007 guideline for full details of stepwise treatment, including alternative therapies.

Source: U.S. Department of Health and Human Services, National Institutes of Health, National Heart, Lung, and Blood Institute. (2008). *National Asthma Education and Prevention Program Expert Panel Report 3: Guidelines for the diagnosis and management of asthma—Summary Report 2007* (pp. 40–42). NIH Publication Number 08-5846. Bethesda, MD: Author.

ii. Inhaled corticosteroids (ICS) are first-line treatment because they offer the best long-term control therapy (NIH, 2007).

iii. Start with a low-to-medium dose depending on the child's risk and severity of symptoms. If there is a response after 4–6 weeks, continue treatment for a total of 3 months. Then, step down to a lower dose if asthma is under control. Goal is to find minimal effective dose.

iv. Consider combining a long-acting β-agonist with the ICS for children who do not respond to the ICS alone. Also consider the addition of a leukotriene receptor antagonist if the child has symptoms of exercise-induced bronchospasm or a strong allergic component to their asthma.

v. If after 4–6 weeks there is no response to therapy, step up therapy or consider an alternative diagnosis.

c. Antihistamines.

i. Medication to decrease allergy symptoms, such as itchy eyes, frequent sneezing, or a scratchy throat or mouth, should also be considered. Besides interfering with a child's normal life and academic achievements, untreated allergies can make the asthma symptoms worse by causing bronchial smooth muscle contractions that quickly narrow the airways (Mahr & Sneth, 2005; NIH, 2007).

d. Omalizumab (Xolair).

i. Recommended for consideration for children older than 12 years of age who have severe allergic asthma (NIH, 2007).

ii. Omalizumab's major potential side effect is anaphylaxis, and is therefore administered in a specialist's office.

e. Oral systemic corticosteroids.

i. Short-course steroid "pulse" doses: used to decrease airway inflammation in moderate or severe exacerbations, or for patients who fail to respond promptly and completely to a SABA. Usually requires 3–10 days. No evidence that tapering "pulse" dose prevents relapse (NIH, 2007).

ii. Daily long-term use of oral steroids is a treatment of last resort, and is reserved for children with severe asthma who do not respond adequately to other controller medications.

3. Treat comorbid conditions

a. Treatment of the following conditions that are frequently seen with asthma may improve asthma control: rhinitis, sinusitis, gastroesophageal reflux, obesity, depression, and allergic bronchopulmonary aspergillosis.

b. Vaccinate all individuals with asthma for influenza. Refer patients with egg allergy to allergists for influenza vaccine skin testing.

c. When possible, young children should avoid contact with people who have viral respiratory infections, a common trigger and a major factor in the development, persistence, and possibly severity of asthma (NIH, 2007).

4. Encourage physical activity

If necessary, treat exercise-induced bronchospasm by use of a SABA before exercise. Increase or start a daily controller medication if exercise-induced symptoms persist, or if symptoms occur during daily activities.

5. Consider allergy immunotherapy

Referral may be appropriate if the child has mild-to-moderate asthma, and there is a correlation between their asthma symptoms and their exposure to allergens.

6. Involve the family and child (if old enough) in all treatment decision-making to encourage a partnership in the care and control of the child's asthma.

7. Follow-up

a. Patients with well-controlled asthma should be seen every 3–6 months, depending on the patient's past asthma history, the family's need for reinforcement and education, and social factors that might put the child at high risk.

b. At each follow-up visit reassess asthma control, adjust medications as needed, and review medication technique.

8. Referral to specialist

a. Child is a severe asthmatic.

b. Symptoms are not responding to appropriate treatment.

c. Child is candidate for immunotherapy or omalizumab therapy.

C. Patient and family education

1. Basic asthma education

a. Determine family's knowledge about asthma.

b. Show diagrams of the lungs and where they are located in the body to both the parent and child.

c. Explain that asthma is a chronic, inflammatory disease of the lungs. Although the child's asthma can be controlled and the child can lead a normal life, the asthma itself will not be cured. This is an important and difficult concept for some families and children to understand and accept.

2. Environmental controls

    Allergy and trigger reduction or avoidance (see the Management section)

3. Medications

    a. Explain the difference between rescue medication and controller medication. Lung diagrams showing normal lungs versus lungs affected by asthma, and then other diagrams showing the muscle-relaxing effect of bronchodilator versus the anti-inflammatory effects of controller medications can be very useful.

    b. Review the use of their asthma action plan and identification of symptoms (see the Self-Management Resources and Tools section).

    c. Demonstrate the proper use of spacer (with the appropriate-size mask for young children), inhalers, discus, and nebulizer.

    d. Address, if necessary, the family's concerns about their child's use of ICS. Long-term studies have shown that children reach predicted adult height despite ongoing use of inhaled steroids (Guill, 2004). If needed, point out that the risks of inadequately treated asthma include death.

    e. Teach methods of obtaining refills from a pharmacy.

4. Emergency care

    a. Use of medications for severe symptoms.
    b. When to call the medical provider.
    c. When to bring the child to the emergency room.

5. Follow-up telephone calls or emails

    a. Answer questions.
    b. Review the action plan.
    c. Review knowledge of emergency care of the child.
    d. Remind the family of follow-up appointments.

6. Educational tools

    a. Videos are another useful tool in patient education. Some people are more likely to watch a video in the clinic or office than to read educational materials at home.

    b. Written material should be available to those who are interested with consideration of the family's literacy level.

    c. Computer programs, peer education, and other school-based programs can be effective educational tools for school-aged children and adolescents.

7. Barriers to learning

    a. Family: No parent wants to think that their child may have a chronic disease so this can be very difficult emotionally for the parent to hear. Denial of the chronic nature of asthma is very common and frequently leads to nonadherence to medication routines and laxity in environmental controls.

    b. Patient: The child or teenager may also have difficulty accepting the diagnosis of asthma. After acknowledging this difficulty, naming famous athletes or celebrities who have controlled asthma might be reassuring.

8. Adherence

    a. Provide calendars with boxes for the parent or child to check when medicine has been given.

    b. Help the family or child coordinate the timing of taking their medication with another well-established habit, such as brushing their teeth.

    c. Remind the family and child that adherence helps them achieve their desired outcomes.

9. Goal setting: it might help for a child or teenager to set a goal for improvement. For example, they might set a very concrete goal, such as being able to blow out all the candles on their next pulmonary function test or being able to sleep all night without symptoms by the next office or clinic visit.

D. *Self-management resources and tools*

1. At home

    a. Asthma action plan.
        i. Complete a written asthma action plan, with a copy for any secondary home and for school or daycare.
        ii. To avoid confusion keep the medication regimen as uncomplicated as the child's condition allows.
        iii. Provide a new plan every time medication is changed

    b. Peak flow meter.
        i. Some motivated parents and patients find it helpful to monitor their child's asthma by using a peak flow meter twice a day. The purpose is to be able to detect or help recognize worsening symptoms by comparing the present reading with the child's best reading.
        ii. Observation of the child's symptoms is often more useful, because of inconsistent use of peak flow meters.

2. At child's school

    It is imperative that a school knows if a child has asthma, no matter how mild. Most schools require a written permission from the health provider and from the parent for the child to be able to use his or her rescue medication in school. Ensuring that the school has this permission should be part of the routine care of all children with asthma.

E. *Asthma education resources*

1. Allergy & Asthma Network Mothers of Asthmatics:
   www.breathville.org (1-800-878-4403)

2. American Academy of Allergy, Asthma and Immunology:
   www.aaai.org (1-414-272-6071)

3. American Lung Association:
   www.lungusa.org (1-800-586-4872)

4. Center for Disease Control and Prevention:
   www.cdc.gov/asthma (1-800-311-3435)

5. National Heart, Lung, and Blood Institute Information Center:
   www.nhlbi.nih.gov (1-301-592-8573)

6. National Jewish Medical and Research Center (Lung Line):
   www.nationaljewish.org (1-800-222-lung)

REFERENCES

Guill, M. F. (2004). Asthma update: Clinical aspects and management. *Pediatrics in Review, 25*(10), 338–342.

Mahr, T. A., & Sneth, K. (2005). Update on allergic rhinitis. *Pediatrics in Review, 25*(8), 284–289.

National Center for Health Statistics, & Centers for Disease Control and Prevention. (2009). *Summary health statistics for U.S. children: National health interview survey, 2008.* Retrieved from http://www.cdc.gov/nchs/data/series/sr_10/sr10_244.pdf

National Asthma Education and Prevention Program, & National Heart, Lung, and Blood Institute. (2009). *Expert panel report III: Guidelines for the diagnosis and management of asthma.* NIH publication no. 08-4051. Retrieved from www.nhlbi.nih.gov/guidelines/asthma/asthgdln.htm

National Heart, Lung, and Blood Institute, National Asthma Education and Prevention Program, & National Institutes of Health. (2007). *Expert panel report: Guidelines for the diagnosis and management of asthma.* Publication No. 97-4051. Bethesda, MD: Author.

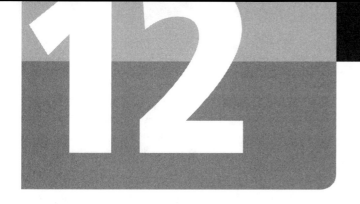

CHILDHOOD DEPRESSION

Damon Michael Williams

I. Introduction

A. General background

Clinical depression is a disease state with physical, emotional, and cognitive effects burdening children, adolescents, and adults. It is characterized by persistently low mood or loss of interest or pleasure such that the patient's subjective quality of life is lessened. Often, functional impairment in school, work, home, and relationships is also observed but is not a requisite for diagnosis. Subjective report of depressive symptoms by the patient as elicited by the clinician suffices; an important distinction in the evaluation of the adolescent or child whose parents may believe that the child "seems fine to me." Current research suggests genetic, biologic,[1] and environmental etiologic factors (Birmaher et al., 1996; Rao & Chen, 2009) in depression.

Despite clear evidence of familial transmission in the case of children and adolescents, it is unclear to what degree this is caused by genetic transmission, environmental influence, or some combination thereof (Rao & Chen, 2009). Regardless of causation, research suggests clinical depression is a relatively common occurrence in the pediatric population, with some estimates showing

adolescents mirroring adult lifetime prevalence rates of 15–25% (Birmaher et al., 1996; March et al., 2004; Rao & Chen). The single greatest risk factor for developing major depressive disorder (MDD) in childhood or adolescence is paternal or maternal loading for the disorder (Birmaher & Brent, 2007). Thus, subjective historical inquiry by the clinician should include any history of depression in the family, especially the child's parents.

Popular wisdom suggests that adolescents go through expectable "phases" of depression or irritability (Arnett, 1999). Although this may be true to a minor degree (Hines & Paulson, 2006), the typically developing child or adolescent should not go through an extended period of depression, irritability, or rebelliousness as a part of normative development. Therefore, any report by the parent, caretaker, or child of a prolonged period of irritability or oppositional behavior should trigger suspicion of depressive or other psychiatric illness and further inquiry by the provider.

B. Definition of clinical depression

In the clinical setting, diagnosis and assessment of the clinical syndromes defined by (or including) depressive features are guided by the 1994 text revision of the fourth edition of the *Diagnostic and Statistical Manual* published by the American Psychiatric Association (DSM-IV-TR). DSM-IV-TR includes the following syndromes, which have a depressive component:

1. MDD

2. Dysthymia

3. Depression, not otherwise specified

4. Bipolar affective disorder

5. Cyclothymia

Presentation of depressive illness in the pediatric population shows remarkable similarity to the adult population (Birmaher et al., 1996). These symptoms can include sad, low, or disinterested mood; loss of interest or pleasure in previously enjoyed activities and relationships (anhedonia); felt or observed decreased effectiveness at school; feelings of guilt; feelings of hopelessness; anorexia or hyperphagia; insomnia or hyperosomnia; or fatigue (American Psychiatric Association [APA], 1994). However, the primary care clinician evaluating the child or adolescent for depressive illness should keep in mind that mood may show more as "irritability" than sadness and the child may not report subjective change in appetite but instead show observable failure to make expected weight gains (APA, 1994).

MDD is the disease typically referred to when depression is spoken of generically. It is diagnosed based on the occurrence of one or more major depressive

---

[1] The neurobiology underlying depression is not well-understood, and continues to evolve. Current theories suggest more complicated and nuanced processes than the simplified vision of deficient serotonin or norepinephrine many were taught. These hypotheses are beyond the scope of this chapter. The reader is referred to an appropriate text, such as Stephen Stahl's "Essential Psychopharmacology: Neuroscientific Basis and Practical Applications, 2nd Edition" for a comprehensive overview of this area.

episodes (APA, 1994). A major depressive episode consists of 2 (or more) weeks of depressed mood or anhedonia and a minimum of four additional depressive symptoms (APA, 1994).

Dysthymia (also known as "minor depression") is similar in symptom profile to MDD but lacks its severity and demonstrates a course that is constant over a longer period of time without distinct episodes (APA, 1994). The presence of MDD and comorbid dysthymia identified in a single individual is commonly known as "double depression." The clinician should keep in mind that 5–10% of children and adolescents have depressive symptoms that are not severe enough to warrant diagnosis of a depressive syndrome, such as MDD or dysthymia, but that are debilitating to some degree nonetheless (Birmaher & Brent, 2007).[2] Additionally, of those children and adolescents with diagnosable depressive syndromes, 40–90% have other psychiatric disorders (Birmaher & Brent). Thus, the clinician should observe for any potential signs of other comorbid psychiatric illness, such as attention-deficit/hyperactivity disorder, anxiety disorders, and autism spectrum disorder.

Clinical depression is a major component of bipolar affective disorder, cyclothymia (a type of "minor" bipolar affective disorder as dysthymia is to MDD), and several other disease states and is the defining state of the unipolar depressive illnesses identified previously. Bipolar affective disorder and cyclothymia show periods of hypomanic or manic mood alternating with euthymic or depressed states. In the case of cyclothymia, symptoms occur over a period of at least 1 year. It is characterized by hypomanic symptoms that do not meet criteria for mania and depressive symptoms that do not meet criteria for major depressive episode (APA, 1994).

Children and adults with bipolar illness may present in a depressed, rather than elevated state. In these cases the clinician may diagnose unipolar depression rather than bipolar depression if inquiry is not made about mood and behavior over the lifetime of the patient rather than the limited course of the current episode alone. In cases of undiagnosed bipolar disorder, psychotropic medications (especially antidepressants) may precipitate hypomanic or manic mood or behavior when administered. Thus, the clinician evaluating clinical depression in the child, adolescent, or adult must always entertain the possibility of a bipolar illness presenting in its depressed phase, especially if antidepressant medication is being considered.

According to DSM-IV-TR, in diagnosing a depressive syndrome, symptoms caused by a general medical condition or substance must first be ruled out. Symptoms of MDD as described in DSM-IV-TR should be observed or elicited as appropriate and included in the database. In addition to depressed or irritable mood, these symptoms include anhedonia, fatigue, psychomotor agitation or slowing, feelings of worthlessness or guilt, decreased ability to think or concentrate, indecisiveness, unintentional weight changes, and suicidal ideation (APA, 1994). The reader is referred to DSM-IV-TR directly for complete diagnostic criteria. Note that DSM-IV-TR qualifies most of these symptom criteria as "most of the day, nearly every day" or "nearly every day" (APA).

II. Database guidelines (may include, but not limited to)

A. Subjective data

The primary care provider evaluating the child or adolescent is in an excellent position to evaluate for depression. The primary care provider usually has an established relationship with the child and family and some familiarity with the family dynamics and the child's developmental and other medical history, all essential components of a competent evaluation for pediatric depression. If this is not the case, the treating clinician should gather information from the child and parents about the family situation and the child's emotional, physical, and cognitive development and history since birth, including intrauterine conditions. Depending on age-appropriateness, pertinent negatives in the database may include history of the following elements.

1. Cardiovascular, seizure, endocrine, and metabolic problems, and chronic diseases, such as diabetes, physical impairments, or other relevant medical conditions

2. Medications, prescribed and over-the-counter

3. Developmental data
   a. Temperamental or developmental difficulties
   b. Behavioral problems

4. Education
   a. Academic difficulties ("How is school going for you?" "What kind of grades are you getting?")
   b. Learning disabilities

---

[2] In terms of the diagnostic nomenclature utilized by DSM-IV-TR, a patient with depressive symptoms that do not meet criteria for the MDD or dysthymia could be identified as having Depressive Disorder *Not Otherwise Specified (NOS)*.

5. Psychiatric history

   a. Self-injurious behavior, such as "cutting"

   b. Previous outpatient psychiatric treatment or inpatient psychiatric hospitalization

   c. Previous suicidal ideation (in the school-aged child this may be described as the desire to "disappear" or "not be here anymore")

   d. Previous suicide attempt (including type and lethality)

   e. Anxiety ("What worries you?" "Do you ever get so worried, you start to feel sweaty, like you can't breathe or are having an anxiety attack?")

   f. Hallucinations ("Besides my voice, do you hear anything or anyone else right now?" "Do you ever hear or see anything that other people cannot?")

   g. Do you ever have trouble paying attention or getting assignments completed?

   h. Do your parents or teachers complain about you being "fidgety"?

6. Substance use and abuse

   a. Cigarette, alcohol, marijuana, or other illicit or licit drug abuse

7. Social and family history

   a. Romantic relationships or break-ups ("Are you dating anybody?" rather than "Do you have a girlfriend/boyfriend?")

   b. Sexual debut

   c. Traumatic events ("Has anything happened recently that upset you and you think about a lot?")

   d. Sexual or physical abuse

   e. Family conflict (e.g., "How does your family get along?" "What's your relationship like with your parents?" "Is there any yelling or arguing in the household?")

   f. Peer relationships, including identifiable (namable) friends and peer support, and any peer bullying

B. Objective data

The mental status examination (MSE) is the psychiatric equivalent to the physical examination and it must be included in any evaluation of depressive illness or other psychiatric illness. However, the MSE does not substitute for the physical examination, if indicated to rule out organic factors in a depressive presentation or identify other comorbid medical illness.

Generally speaking, the MSE begins with gross physical observations and progresses to description of the internal cognitive and emotional processes as observed by the clinician in the course of the interview,

visit, or interaction, however brief. The MSE typically includes the following observations, adapted from Saddock and Saddock (2007):

1. General demeanor, response to clinician, and appearance (including remarkable identifiers) and grooming

2. Motor status: slowing, agitation, tremor, and hyperactivity

3. Speech: tone, volume, rate, rhythm, and production

4. Eye contact

5. Affect

6. Mood: the patient's direct report of how they feel in quotation marks (e.g., "sad," "tired," "bored," "none of your business," etc.)

7. Thought process

8. Thought content: includes suicidal and homicidal ideation, perceptual changes, or hallucinatory experience

9. Judgment

10. Insight

11. Some sources include impulsivity

III. Assessment

DSM-IV-TR provides clear diagnostic criteria for each syndrome involving depressed mood and guidance on differential diagnosis. The primary care clinician is encouraged to refer to DSM-IV-TR for complete diagnostic criteria and procedures.

No assessment of depressive illness in the child or adolescent is complete without assessment of suicide risk and any self-injurious behaviors. According to Gould, Greenberg, Velting, and Shaffer (2003), "Suicide was the third leading cause of death among 10- to 14-year-olds and 15- to 19-year-olds in the United States in 2000" (pp. 386–387). Risk of suicide and lethality must be assessed on an individual basis. Keeping this in mind, the clinician must be aware that the following factors (not listed in order of importance) confer higher risk for suicide attempt and completed suicide and may warrant emergent referral to a psychiatric provider or hospital emergency room (Gould et al.; Pelkonen & Marttunen, 2003):

1. Male gender

2. White race

3. Substance abuse or dependence

4. Posttraumatic stress disorder

5. Panic attacks

6. Prior suicide attempt or suicidal behavior

7. Poor interpersonal problem-solving ability

8. Aggressive–impulsive behavior

9. Same-sex sexual orientation

10. Family history of suicidal behavior

11. Parental psychopathology, particularly depression and substance abuse

12. Impaired parent–child relationship

13. Family violence and arguments

14. Precipitating incident or life stressors (e.g., interpersonal loss, legal problem, school change, being kicked out of school, disciplinary problems, physical changes, and so forth)

15. Physical abuse

16. Sexual abuse

17. Difficulties in school

18. Media coverage of suicide

19. Nonintact families of origin

20. Psychiatric disorder

21. Presence of plan

22. Intent to act on the plan

23. Access to means to execute the plan

A comprehensive review of assessment, evaluation, and treatment of suicidality in the child or adolescent is beyond the scope of this chapter. However, the reader is referred to the Academy of Child and Adolescent Psychiatry (ACAP)'s Practice Parameter on the topic. Included in this parameter is a more thorough treatment of risk factors, safety planning, national resources on suicide for the family and clinician, and a comparative review of suicide screening instruments for the child and adolescent, among other things. It is available for free from the ACAP website; a link is provided in the "Resources" section.

IV. Plan

A. Diagnostics

Diagnostic laboratory tests are not used to establish or rule out a diagnosis of depression. However, the following tests may be used to assess differentially an identifiable organic pathology (e.g., hypothyroidism or anemia) from a nonmedical depressive syndrome:

1. Thyroid-stimulating hormone

2. Complete blood count

3. Comprehensive metabolic panel

B. Treatment

1. Medications and the black box warning

   The Food and Drug Administration (FDA) issued a ruling in 2005 directing antidepressant manufacturers to include "black box" labeling identifying the possibility of increased suicidal ideation in children and adolescents up through age 24. The announcement of this black box warning was widely reported in the media. Since that time, there has been a marked drop in the prescription of first-line antidepressant treatment by primary care providers (Gibbons et al., 2007). The prudent clinician should continue circumspect prescribing and vigilant monitoring for increased suicidal ideation or behavior in the child or adolescent (through age 24) continuing on or initiated on antidepressant medication. However, considerable data continue to accumulate regarding the benefit of antidepressant treatment in children and adolescents, and the importance of early intervention and potential negative sequelae associated with failure to prescribe (Gibbons et al., 2007; Hammad, Laughren, & Racoosin, 2006; March et al., 2004). With this in mind, the primary care provider who has identified a child or adolescent with uncomplicated unipolar depression is encouraged to consider the benefits and risks with the family of cautiously initiating first-line antidepressant treatment.

   In addition to the potential risk of increased suicidal ideation and behavior, selective serotonin reuptake inhibitors (SSRIs), including escitalopram and fluoxetine, have significant gastrointestinal, nervous system, and sexual side effects, among others. Risk of various potential side effects (additional to suicidal ideation) must be reviewed with the child and their parents or guardians as part of the process for obtaining informed consent (Table 12-1). This medication guide may be helpful in assisting families through this process. Please see www.fda.gov for the most current version and other prescriber-directed medication advisories. The process of initiating first-line antidepressant treatment for the child or adolescent with uncomplicated unipolar depression may be done in tandem with referral to a pediatric psychiatric specialist.

TABLE 12-1 Revisions to Medication Guide

Medication Guide
Antidepressant Medicines, Depression and Other Serious Mental Illnesses, and Suicidal Thoughts or Actions

Read the Medication Guide that comes with your or your family member's antidepressant medicine. This Medication Guide is only about the risk of suicidal thoughts and actions with antidepressant medicines. **Talk to your, or your family member's, healthcare provider about:**
- all risks and benefits of treatment with antidepressant medicines
- all treatment choices for depression or other serious mental illness

What is the most important information I should know about antidepressant medicines, depression and other serious mental illness, and suicidal thoughts or actions?
1. **Antidepressant medicines may increase suicidal thoughts or actions in some children, teenagers, and young adults when the medicine is first started.**
2. **Depression and other serious mental illnesses are the most important causes of suicidal thoughts and actions. Some people may have a particularly high risk of having suicidal thoughts or actions.** These include people who have (or have a family history of) bipolar illness (also called manic-depressive illness) or suicidal thoughts or actions.
3. **How can I watch for and try to prevent suicidal thoughts and actions in myself or a family member?**
   - Pay close attention to any changes, especially sudden changes, in mood, behaviors, thoughts, or feelings. This is very important when an antidepressant medicine is first started or when the dose is changed.
   - Call the healthcare provider right away to report new or sudden changes in mood, behavior, thoughts, or feelings.
   - Keep all follow-up visits with the healthcare provider as scheduled. Call the healthcare provider between visits as needed, especially if you have concerns about symptoms.

Call a healthcare provider right away if you or your family member has any of the following symptoms, especially if they are new, worse, or worry you:
- thoughts about suicide or dying
- attempts to commit suicide
- new or worse depression
- new or worse anxiety
- feeling very agitated or restless
- Panic attacks
- trouble sleeping (insomnia)
- new or worse irritability
- acting aggressive, being angry, or violent
- acting on dangerous impulses
- an extreme increase in activity and talking (mania)
- other unusual changes in behavior or mood

What else do I need to know about antidepressant medicines?
- **Never stop an antidepressant medicine without first talking to a healthcare provider.** Stopping an antidepressant medicine suddenly can cause other symptoms.
- **Antidepressants are medicines used to treat depression and other illnesses.** It is important to discuss all the risks of treating depression and also the risks of not treating it. Patients and their families or other caregivers should discuss all treatment choices with the healthcare provider, not just the use of antidepressants.
- **Antidepressant medicines have other side effects.** Talk to the healthcare provider about the side effects of the medicine prescribed for you or your family member.
- **Antidepressant medicines can interact with other medicines.** Know all of the medicines that you or your family member takes. Keep a list of all medicine to show the healthcare provider. Do not start new medicines without first checking with your healthcare provider.
- **Not all antidepressant medicines prescribed for children are FDA approved for use in children.** Talk to your child's healthcare provider for more information.

This Medication Guide has been approved by the U.S. Food and Drug Administration for all antidepressants.

2. FDA-approved antidepressant agents

   Only two agents have FDA approval for use as antidepressants in children and adolescents: the SSRIs fluoxetine and escitalopram. Table 12-2 summarizes data on these agents. Note that sertraline, another SSRI, does not have FDA approval for use in the pediatric age group for depressive disorders. It does, however, have FDA approval for treatment of obsessive–compulsive disorder in children and adolescents age 6–17 years.

   After gaining appropriate consent, the clinician choosing to initiate antidepressant treatment in an uncomplicated case of unipolar depression should begin with the lowest dose possible and titrate in very slow intervals, generally not sooner than every 3–4 weeks. However, monitoring at more frequent intervals is recommended for children and adolescents receiving antidepressant medication. Increased vigilance is especially warranted when initiating, increasing, reducing, or otherwise changing dosage. The FDA recommends "at least weekly face-to-face contact with the prescriber during the first 4 weeks of treatment, then visits every other week for the next 4 weeks, then at 12 weeks, and as clinically indicated beyond 12 weeks" (Hughes et al., 2007, pp. 667–686).

   At a minimum, medication monitoring visits should include the following parameters:

   a. Patient's subjective response to the medication
   b. Objective evaluation of demeanor, energy, and affect
   c. Report of any adverse effects, including any changes in weight; sleep; behavior (activation); and sexual problems (adolescents). The clinician is referred to the manufacturer's literature for a comprehensive listing of drug side effects with frequency of occurrence.
   d. Dosing record and any difficulties with or obstacles to adherence, such as gastrointestinal complaints or sleep changes
   e. Suicidal ideation and self-harming behaviors
   f. Progress with psychiatric referral or response to psychotherapy or other nonpharmacologic treatments

3. Psychotherapy and combined treatment

   Psychotherapy either alone or combined with pharmacotherapy is effective in treating pediatric depression. Specifically, cognitive behavioral therapy (CBT) shows the strongest evidence for improved outcome (March et al., 2004; Weisz, McCarty, & Valeri, 2006). CBT, developed by Aaron Beck (and since elaborated by many other clinician-researchers), uses behavioral interventions, structured exercises, and talk therapy to change negative thinking. In the depressed child, CBT is thought to exert a therapeutic effect because it leads to restructuring of the negatively distorted cognitions that accompany and describe depressive illness.

   The best data concerning CBT and depression in the pediatric population come from the Treatment for Adolescents with Depression Study (TADS). The TADS is a highly powered 13-site, national study funded by the National Institute of Mental Health that tested three conditions in randomized-control trial design from spring through summer 2003 (March et al., 2004): fluoxetine alone, CBT alone, and fluoxetine plus CBT.

TABLE 12-2 Antidepressant Medications with FDA Approval for Use in the Pediatric Population

Proprietary Name	Generic Name	Generic Available	FDA Pediatric Indication	FDA Approval Granted	Dosage
Prozac	Fluoxetine hydrochloride	Yes	MDD, 8–18 years (also OCD, 7–17 years)	1/3/2003	Initial: 10–20 mg/day, depending on weight (initial dose in OCD is 10 mg)
Lexapro	Escitalopram	No	MDD, 12–17 years	3/19/2009	Initial: 10 mg once daily Recommended: 10 mg once daily Maximum: 20 mg once daily

Compiled by author from the U.S. Food and Drug Administration.

The study was conducted with the adolescent population, so conclusions should only be applied to that population. Among the conclusions reached by the TADS team:

a. "despite calls to restrict access to medications, medical management of MDD with fluoxetine, including careful monitoring for adverse events, should be made widely available, not discouraged" (March et al., 2004, p. 819).

b. "given incremental improvement in outcome when CBT is combined with medication and, as importantly, increased protection from suicidality, CBT also should be readily available as part of comprehensive treatment for depressed adolescents" (March et al., p. 819).

In addition to CBT, family therapy and interpersonal therapy are often used in the treatment of pediatric depression (Weisz et al., 2006). The clinician should keep in mind that all therapeutic interventions must be chosen on the basis of the child's particular context, family situation, and unique presentation.

C. Referral

Children and adolescents with depression and other psychiatric illness are optimally treated in the context of their families, school, and community within a developmental framework. Often the collateral contacts required for optimal assessment and treatment are not easily conducted within the confines of the 15-minute medical office visit. Thus, the primary care clinician should always feel free to consult with or refer to a pediatric psychiatric specialist. Referral or consultation should definitely be sought depending on severity, lethality, complexity, and comorbidity of the case. Cases in which emergent or urgent referral to a psychiatric colleague or hospital emergency room should be made include the following:

1. Suspected bipolar illness

2. Presence of suspected or identified suicidal ideation or behavior

3. Aggressive behavior

4. Comorbid or suspected psychiatric or medical illnesses

5. Comorbid or suspected substance abuse

6. Impaired parent–child functioning or other dysfunction in the family or support system

7. Significant pathology or history of suicide in the family

8. Comorbid or suspected learning disability

9. Any case in which the treating clinician desires consultation or believes that the presenting problem exceeds his or her scope or knowledge base to provide competent care

V. Self-management resources

A. For providers

1. Information on antidepressant use in children, adolescents, and adults with advisories from the FDA. http://www.fda.gov/Drugs/DrugSafety/InformationbyDrugClass/ucm096273.htm

2. A toolkit for child and adolescent depression treatment in primary care, developed from consensus guidelines. www.glad-pc.org

3. The general ACAP website also offers excellent educational material for families on a number of topics including medications and parameters for competent prescribing and evaluation in the child and adolescent population. http://www.aacap.org/cs/root/member_information/practice_information/practice_parameters/practice_parameters. Parameters are alphabetized.

B. For patients and families

1. http://wFacts for families: ww.aacap.org/cs/root/facts_for_families/facts_for_families

2. Depression resource center: http://www.aacap.org/cs/Depression.ResourceCenter

3. Children's health topics: Depression and suicide: http://www.aap.org/healthtopics/depression.cfm

4. Depression in children and adolescents: http://www.nami.org/Content/NavigationMenu/Mental_Illnesses/Depression/Depression_in_Children_and_Adolescents.htm

5. Child and adolescent mental health: http://www.nimh.nih.gov/health/topics/child-and-adolescent-mental-health/index.shtml

REFERENCES

American Psychiatric Association. (1994). *Diagnostic and statistical manual of mental disorders* (4th ed.). Washington, DC: Author.

Arnett, J. J. (1999). Adolescent storm and stress, reconsidered. *American Psychologist, 54*(5), 317–326.

Birmaher, B., & Brent, D. (2007). Practice parameter for the assessment and treatment of children and adolescents with depressive disorders. *Journal of the American Academy of Child & Adolescent Psychiatry, 46*(11), 1503–1526.

Birmaher, B., Ryan, N. D., Williamson, D. E., Brent, D. A., & Kaufman, J. (1996). Childhood and adolescent depression: A review of the past 10 years. Part II. *Journal of the American Academy of Child & Adolescent Psychiatry, 35*(12), 1575–1583.

Birmaher, B., Ryan, N. D., Williamson, D. E., Brent, D. A., Kaufman, J., Dahl, R. E., et al. (1996). Childhood and adolescent depression: A review of the past 10 years. Part I. *Journal of the American Academy of Child & Adolescent Psychiatry, 35*(11), 1427–1439.

Boylan, K., Romero, S., Birmaher, B. (2007). Psychopharmacologic treatment of pediatric major depressive disorder. *Psychopharmacology, 191*, 27–38.

Bridge, J. A., Iynegar, S., Slary, C. B., Barbe, R., Birmaher, B., Pincus, H., et al. (2007). Clinical response and risk for reported suicidal ideation and suicide attempts in pediatric antidepressant treatment: A meta-analysis of randomized controlled trials. *JAMA, 297*(15), 1683–1696.

Food and Drug Administration. (2007). FDA proposes new warnings about suicidal thinking, behavior in young adults who take antidepressant medications. Retrieved from http://test.fda.gov/NewsEvents/Newsroom/PressAnnouncements/2007/ucm1045580.htm

Gibbons, R. D., Brown, C. H., Hur, K., Marcus, S. M., Bhaumik, D. K., Erkens, J. A., et al. (2007). Early evidence on the effects of regulators' suicidality warnings on SSRI prescriptions and suicide in children and adolescents. *American Journal of Psychiatry, 164*, 1356–1363.

Gould, M. S., Greenberg, T., Velting, D. M., & Shaffer, D. (2003). Youth suicide risk and preventive interventions: A review of the past 10 years. *Journal of the American Academy of Child & Adolescent Psychiatry, 42*(4), 386–405.

Hammad, T. A., Laughren, T. P., & Racoosin, J. A. (2006). Suicidality in pediatric patients treated with antidepressant drugs. *Archives of General Psychiatry, 63*, 332–339.

Hammad, T. A., Laughren, T. P., & Racoosin, J. A. (2006). Suicide rates in short-term randomized controlled trials of newer antidepressants. *Journal of Clinical Psychopharmacology, 26*(2), 203–207.

Hines, A. R., & Paulson, S. E. (2006). Parents' and teachers' perceptions of adolescent storm and stress: Relations with parenting and teaching styles. *Adolescence, 41* (164), 597–614.

Hughes, C. W., Emslie, G. J., Crismon, M. L., Posner, K., Birhamer, B., Ryan, N., et al. (2007). Texas children's medication algorithm project: Update from the Texas consensus panel on medication treatment of childhood major depressive disorder. *Journal of the American Academy of Child & Adolescent Psychiatry, 46*(6), 667–686.

Jacobson, C. M., & Gould, M. (2007). The epidemiology and phenomenology of non-suicidal self-injurious behavior among adolescents: A critical review of the literature. *Archive of Suicide Research, 11*, 129–147.

Luby, J. L., Si, X., Belden, A. C., Tandon, M., Spitznagel, E. (2009). Preschool depression: Homotypic continuity and course over 24 months. *Archives of General Psychiatry, 66*(8), 897–905.

March, J., Silva, S., Petrycki, S., Curry, J., Wells, K., Fairbank, J., et al. (2004). Fluoxetine, cognitive-behavioral therapy, and their combination for adolescents with depression. *JAMA, 292*, 807–820.

March, J. S., Silva, S., Petrycki, S., Curry, J., Wells, K., Fairbank, J., et al. (2007). Treatment for Adolescents with Depression Study (TADS): Long-term effectiveness and safety outcomes. *Archives of General Psychiatry, 64*(10), 1132–1144.

March, J. S., & Vitiello, B. (2009). Clinical messages from the Treatment for Adolescents with Depression Study (TADS). *American Journal of Psychiatry, 166*, 1118–1123.

Pelkonen, M., & Marttunen, M. (2003). Child and adolescent suicide: Epidemiology, risk factors, and approaches to prevention. *Pediatric Drugs, 5*(4), 243–265.

Rao, U., & Chen, L. (2009). Characteristics, correlates, and outcomes of childhood and adolescent depressive disorders. *Dialogues in Clinical Neuroscience, 11*, 45–62.

Saddock, B. J., & Saddock, V. A. (2007). *Kaplan & Sadock's synopsis of psychiatry* (10th ed.). New York, NY: Lippincott, Williams & Wilkins.

Stahl, S. (2000). *Essential psychopharmacology: Neuroscientific basis and practical applications* (2nd ed.). New York, NY: Cambridge University Press.

Vitiello, B., & Swedo, S. (2004). Antidepressant medications in children. *New England Journal of Medicine, 350*, 1489–1491.

Weisz, J. R., McCarty, C. A., Valeri, S. M. (2006). Effects of psychotherapy for depression in children and adolescents: A meta-analysis. *Psychological Bulletin 132*(1), 132–149.

Whittington, C. J., Kendall, T., Fonagy, P., Cottrell, D., Cotgrove, A., Boddington, E. (2004). Selective serotonin reuptake inhibitors in childhood depression: Systematic review of the published versus unpublished data. *Lancet, 363*, 1341–1345.

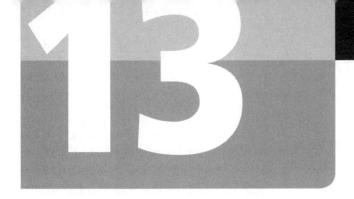

CHILD MALTREATMENT

Naomi Schapiro

I. Introduction

Child maltreatment encompasses physical, sexual, and emotional abuse and child neglect. Healthcare providers have legal, professional, and ethical responsibilities to assess children for maltreatment and to report suspected cases. Each of the 50 States, the District of Columbia, and territories, such as Puerto Rico, has its own definitions of child abuse and neglect, but all must conform to minimum Federal standards set in the Child Abuse Prevention and Treatment Act:

> Any recent act or failure to act on the part of a parent or caretaker, which results in death, serious physical or emotional harm, sexual abuse, or exploitation, or an act or failure to act which presents an imminent risk of serious harm (Child Abuse Prevention and Treatment Act; Child Welfare Information Gateway, 2007a).

Advanced practice nurses (APNs) can consult the website http://www.childwelfare.gov/systemwide/laws_policies /state/ for the specific definitions and reporting responsibilities in their own states.

The professional and ethical responsibilities to assess for, detect, and report child maltreatment are reinforced by a steadily accumulating body of literature on the myriad and long-lasting effects of these adverse events, including greater rates of depression and substance abuse, early onset of sexual activity, greater likelihood of becoming a teenage parent, and higher rates of type 2 diabetes mellitus and other adult chronic conditions (Dong et al., 2004; Flaherty et al., 2006; Stirling & Amaya-Jackson, 2008). In 2007, there were an estimated 3.2 million suspected cases of child abuse and neglect reported nationwide to child protective services (CPS). From these reports, an estimated 794,000 children were deemed to be victims of maltreatment, with a victimization rate of 10.6 per 1,000 children. An estimated 1,760 children died as a result of abuse or neglect, with

a rate of 2.34 deaths per 100,000 children. Death rates for infant boys were almost 19 per 100,000 and for infant girls 15 per 100,000 children (U.S. Department of Health and Human Services Administration on Children Youth and Families, 2009).

Assessing and responding to child maltreatment can be challenging for the APN, because the abuse or neglect may not be readily apparent and may not be the specific reason that the child is presenting for care. Epidemiologic risk factors for child maltreatment may be helpful in planning population-level interventions, but are not as helpful in the clinical setting, where the APN should always keep maltreatment in mind as part of the differential diagnosis (Schapiro, 2008). Child abuse and neglect involve injuries to children or failure to protect them from harm; maltreatment assessments and reports are made to protect children, not to punish "bad" parents (Dubowitz, 2009). Keeping the child in mind helps the APN to sort through what is often a confusing and emotion-laden picture.

Child maltreatment has been associated in the literature with a variety of risk factors including poverty; single parenthood; intimate partner violence; parental physical and mental illness; substance abuse; and child factors, such as disability, special healthcare needs, or temperamental mismatch with a parent (Dubowitz, 2002, 2009; Herrenkohl et al., 2008; Testa & Smith, 2009). Protective factors may include extended family cohesiveness; personal, financial, and community resources; religiosity; optimism on the part of the caregiver; and an engaging child (Dubowitz, 2002; Herrenkohl et al.). Although it is important for the APN to explore the resources and coping strategies of families who seem to have risk factors for maltreatment, it is also important to remember that child maltreatment can occur in families who do not have known risk factors. Research has shown that healthcare providers may underreport maltreatment in families they know well and assume to be stable (Jones et al., 2008).

A. Physical abuse

1. Definition and overview

    Broadly, physical abuse is an inflicted (nonaccidental) injury to a child that results in physical impairment. Mechanisms of injury may include biting, burning, kicking, striking, shaking, grabbing, stabbing, dragging, throwing, strangling, or poisoning. Legal definitions of reportable physical abuse vary widely from state to state (Child Welfare Information Gateway, 2007a).

2. Incidence and prevalence

    During 2007, 10.8% of victims of child maltreatment were physically abused. Physical abuse accounted for over 26% of child fatalities, and may have been a factor in an additional 35% of child deaths caused by maltreatment (U.S. Department of Health and Human Services Administration on Children Youth and Families, 2009). Lifetime prevalence estimates of severe physical abuse (not including hitting, slapping, or grabbing) from parental or self-reported surveys range from 5–35% (Gilbert, Widom et al., 2009). Widely differing definitions and overlap with nonabusive physical punishment make estimation of prevalence difficult.

B. Sexual abuse

1. Definition and overview

   Sexual abuse is defined under Federal law as the "the employment, use, persuasion, inducement, enticement, or coercion of any child to engage in, or assist any other person to engage in, any sexually explicit conduct or simulation of such conduct for the purpose of producing a visual depiction of such conduct; or the rape, and in cases of caretaker or inter-familial relationships, statutory rape, molestation, prostitution, or other form of sexual exploitation of children, or incest with children" (Child Welfare Information Gateway, 2008, p. 3). Sexual abuse may include fondling, deliberate exposure to sexual activity, and exposure to or involvement in pornography. In most states, consensual sexual activity of a minor with either an older minor or an adult may be reportable under sexual abuse laws (Sachs, Weinberg, & Wheeler, 2008).

2. Incidence and prevalence

   During 2007, 7.6% of child maltreatment victims were sexually abused (U.S. Department of Health and Human Services Administration on Children Youth and Families, 2009). Lifetime prevalence estimates range from 15–30% of girls and 5–15% of boys (Gilbert, Widom et al., 2009).

C. Psychologic or emotional abuse

1. Definition and overview

   Under Federal standards, psychologic abuse involves "a pattern of behavior that impairs a child's emotional development or sense of self-worth. This may include constant criticism, threats, or rejection, as well as withholding love, support, or guidance" (Child Welfare Information Gateway, 2008, p. 3). Emotional abuse is difficult to substantiate unless the child exhibits severe psychologic sequelae, and is also a component of other forms of child maltreatment, which impedes reporting and tracking of emotional abuse in itself. In some states, witnessing domestic violence may be considered a form of child abuse, whereas in others committing intimate partner violence in the presence of a child may result in an enhanced sentence or a requirement to pay for counseling for the child (Child Welfare Information Gateway, 2009).

2. Incidence and prevalence

   In 2007, 4.2% of child maltreatment victims were psychologically abused, and 13% were victims of multiple forms of maltreatment, which may have included psychologic abuse. Prevalence studies over childhood in developed countries range from 4–9% of children (Gilbert, Widom et al., 2009).

D. Neglect

1. Definition and overview

   As the most commonly reported form of child maltreatment, neglect has been understudied, yet its long-term consequences may be just as devastating as other forms of abuse (Gilbert, Kemp et al., 2009). Broadly, neglect involves the failure of a parent or caregiver to provide for a child's basic physical and emotional needs (Child Welfare Information Gateway, 2008), including food, clothing, shelter, educational needs, medical care, supervision, and emotional care. Although neglect may involve one instance of a dangerous failure to supervise or provide care, it also may result from the accumulation of smaller lapses over time, making assessment a challenge. The standard for reporting neglect involves the APN's suspicion of actual or imminent harm to a child (Schapiro, 2008). States vary widely in their specific definitions of neglect, with some including or excluding drug use, homelessness, or parental refusal of health care for their child for personal or religious reasons. In some states, failure to educate is covered under truancy rather than child abuse law (Child Welfare Information Gateway, 2007a). Poverty has been associated with child neglect, with increasing reports of neglect directly related to increasing unemployment, decreasing income, and stricter limits on welfare payments, independent of parenting characteristics (Slack, Holl, McDaniel, Yoo, & Bolger, 2004). There is a possibility that at least some of these increased reports reflect reporter perceptions (Jones et al., 2008).

2. Incidence and prevalence

   During 2007, 59% of child maltreatment victims in the United States were neglected, and less than 1% suffered from medical neglect (U.S. Department of Health and Human Services Administration on Children Youth and Families, 2009). Prevalence estimates range from 6–11.8% of children (Gilbert, Widom et al., 2009).

II. **Database** (may include but is not limited to)

A. *Subjective*

As with other sensitive subjects, history-taking about child maltreatment may be enhanced when written questionnaires are used in combination with direct questions by the practitioner (Gilbert, Kemp et al., 2009). Routinely asking questions about physical punishment or fighting, about forced or coerced sexual activity and inappropriate touching, and about general safety can send a message to the child and parent that these subjects are open topics of discussion during the visit, even if they do not answer them at first.

1. Chief complaint
   a. Injuries
      i. Detailed history of any new or old injuries: Is the injury consistent with the history?
      ii. History of similar injuries and general injury history.
      iii. Current or past history of delayed care for injuries.
      iv. History of seeking care for injuries at multiple facilities.
   b. Sudden changes in behavior
      Because children vary widely in temperament, and cultural influences may also affect their behavior in clinical settings, a sudden change in behavior is an important indicator of some kind of emotional trauma (including but not limited to child maltreatment): for example, the outgoing child who suddenly seems withdrawn, or the quiet child who suddenly seems driven by a motor.
   c. Sexual acting out
      Self-genital stimulation for pleasure, or masturbation, is a normal part of child development from toddlerhood through adolescence; children younger than school age may not have a well-developed sense of privacy and may masturbate in social settings considered inappropriate by adults. Sexual play between age mates, consisting of exploration of body parts and sexual jokes, is developmentally normal and not in itself a sign of sexual abuse (Fonseca & Greydanus, 2007). In a media-saturated society in which sexual images are widely available, discerning age-appropriate from inappropriate sexual knowledge may be difficult. However, some activities should raise a suspicion of sexual abuse:
      i. Sexual play involving penetration or use of objects.
      ii. Sexual play that closely mimics adult sexual activity.
      iii. Sexual play between children of different ages or across power gradients.
   d. Personal and social history and activities of daily living
      i. How does the parent describe the child? Red flags include obvious lack of enjoyment of the child, labeling the child as bad or inappropriate expectations for child's developmental stage.
      ii. Family routines and activities.
      iii. Methods of discipline used and their perceived effectiveness.
   e. Review of systems
      Recurrent headache, abdominal pain, or genitourinary discomfort may be related to somaticizing or actual recurrent injury. A thorough review of systems from both parent and child may be helpful in cases in which the history is confusing or inconsistent.

2. Situations that may heighten the risk of child maltreatment
   Children and families in these situations may need extra support, and should be asked how they are coping if they are experiencing any of the situations below (Dubowitz, 2009; Gilbert, Kemp et al., 2009; Kellogg, 2007):
   a. Sudden changes in family status
      Job loss, loss of health insurance, death, divorce, domestic violence, and parental illness, including mental health diagnoses, can all strain or overwhelm a parent's resources and ability to care for a child.
   b. Challenging stages in child development
      i. The inconsolable infant, the willful toddler, the school-age child with behavioral and learning difficulties, and normative developmental changes of adolescence can challenge all parents.
      ii. In some cases these typical challenges of parenting can exacerbate a stressed family system.
   c. Children who are difficult to care for
      This category encompasses a wide variety of conditions, from children with difficult temperaments to children with neuromuscular disabilities. Children who require a great deal of additional care or who are less able to give

the parent positive reinforcement for that care may be at greater risk for maltreatment.

3. Special considerations for taking histories from children about suspected maltreatment

   a. Toddlers and preschool-aged children

      i. Children under the age of 6 have limited vocabularies, a relatively undeveloped sense of time and sequence, and are best interviewed by a trained expert in child maltreatment.

      ii. Well-meaning parents and healthcare professionals can inadvertently feed the child information and unwittingly distort the story.

   b. School-age children

      i. School-age children have a developed sense of time and sequence. The challenge for the healthcare provider is to speak with the school-age child without the parent present.

      ii. If this is not possible, and the APN suspects maltreatment, a child abuse report may trigger a visit from a CPS worker to the child's school for a separate interview.

   c. Adolescents

      i. Adolescents may come in alone for care, and many clinics have established policies for taking written questionnaires and verbal histories from children over 12 without a parent in the room (see Chapter 7).

      ii. Each state has its own parameters for confidential services (Guttmacher Institute), and it is important to let the adolescent know which parts of the history are truly confidential and the APN's reporting responsibilities related to both sexual assault and consensual sexual activity between disparate-aged minors and between minors and adults (state statutory rape laws) (Sachs et al., 2008).

B. Objective

It is important to document any abnormal findings as thoroughly and accurately as possible, including measurement of injuries and drawings if appropriate. Photographic documentation may be useful if it conforms to local law enforcement standards for quality and chain of custody.

1. General overview of child's appearance and behavior

   The demeanor and behavior of the child or adolescent in the clinic can provide the APN with valuable information. However, it is important to

remember that the APN is just seeing a snapshot of the child in an artificial and sometimes stressful setting. Behavioral changes commonly seen in maltreated children may also occur after other adverse events of childhood, including death, incarceration or divorce of a parent, or sudden death of a close friend (Fairbank & Fairbank, 2009; Ford et al., 2000). Children may be overly compliant for their developmental age, may be withdrawn or attach readily to adults they do not know well, exhibit hypervigilance, or fail to seek comfort in the clinical setting from parents or caretakers (Child Welfare Information Gateway, 2007b).

2. Physical examination findings consistent with physical abuse (Table 13-1)

   a. Bruises are the most common injuries in physically abused children. Dating of bruises by appearance has been found to be unreliable (Bariciak, Plint, Gaboury, & Bennett, 2003). Bruising to the center of the face, ears, neck, back, buttocks, upper arms, and backs of the legs raise suspicions of inflicted injury, and any bruising in an infant, although bruising over bony prominences is more consistent with accidental injury (Kellogg, 2007).

   b. Burns may be inflicted or accidental. Accidental burns from hot objects, such as heaters or irons, may be difficult to distinguish from inflicted burns, because both have patterning. Splash burns, occurring for example when a toddler pulls a hot pot or cup off a surface, have typical and irregular formation, with the burn degree lessening as the liquid drips down the body. Immersion burns with a stocking or glove demarcation are more likely to be inflicted (Kellogg, 2007).

   c. Fractures are common in children, and distinguishing inflicted from accidental fractures can be difficult. Spiral fractures and metaphyseal fractures can be the result of inflicted or accidental trauma, and some pre-ambulatory infants in walkers have sustained accidental fractures (Kemp et al., 2008). The following findings on physical or radiologic examination should raise suspicions of physical abuse:

      i. Long bone fractures in a preambulatory infant.

      ii. Fractures in different stages of healing.

      iii. Rib fractures, especially posterior, in the absence of documented accidental trauma.

      iv. Bucket-handle or corner fractures (from shaking or squeezing).

d. Head trauma may be caused by shaking (coup–contra coup), striking, or throwing an infant, and are implicated in most cases of fatal physical abuse. Presentations may be acute or subtle, with children often misdiagnosed in emergency settings as suffering from a viral illness because of lethargy, vomiting, and poor feeding (Chiesa & Duhaime, 2009). The following findings can be associated with abusive head trauma:

i. Altered mental status.

ii. Retinal hemorrhages (requires dilated examination, pediatric ophthalmologist, and finding can be nonspecific).

TABLE 13-1 Physical Findings or Conditions that May Mimic Findings in Child Maltreatment

Findings	Etiology Related to Child Maltreatment	Possible Other Etiologies
Circular crusted plaques with red margins	Burns from cigarettes or other hot circular-tipped objects	Impetigo Iatrogenic: wart removal
Bullae	Inflicted burns	Accidental burns Bullous impetigo
Marked erythema with or without vesicles or bullae	Immersion burns	Staphylococcal scalded skin syndrome Toxic epidermal necrolysis
Red or hyperpigmented handprint	Slapping	In sun-exposed areas: phytophotodermatitis
Ecchymoses	Inflicted injury from punching or slapping	Accidental injury Clotting or bleeding disorders, chronic or acute (e.g., hemophilia vs. idiopathic thrombocytopenic purpura) Infants: birthmarks (Mongolian spots) Neonates: bruising from precipitous delivery
Black eye (eccorhymosis)	Inflicted injury from punching or slapping	Clotting disorders Accidental impact to forehead with movement of ecchymoses during healing Allergic "shiners"
Swollen red eyelid or orbital area	Fresh inflicted injury	Periorbital cellulitis
Scratches on wrists, popliteal spaces, back	Scratching, restraining child	Self-inflicted secondary to atopic dermatitis or neuropsychiatric conditions
Fractures inconsistent with history or child's developmental level; multiple fractures at different stages of healing	Grabbing, twisting, throwing	Pathologic fractures related to osteogenesis imperfecta or other bone abnormalities
Mucopurulent vaginal discharge in prepubertal girl	*Neisseria gonorrhea* or *Chlamydia trachomatis* infection	*Streptococcus pyogenes* or *Salmonella shigella* infection Intravaginal foreign body (e.g., toilet paper)
Clear, gray, or whitish vaginal discharge in early puberty	Nonspecific, or may indicate bacterial vaginosis, trichomoniasis	Physiologic leucorrhea common in Tanner stages 2 and 3
Anal fissure	Penetration (penis or foreign object)	Functional constipation
Weight loss or failure to thrive	Neglect	Metabolic, neuromuscular, or cardiac abnormalities, including malabsorption syndromes Depression Eating disorders

iii. Skull fractures and possibly additional long bone or rib fractures.

iv. Intracranial hemorrhages (also may be present in coagulopathies and other medical conditions).

e. Thoracoabdominal trauma: squeezing or punching may result in rib fractures, trauma to underlying structures, or abdominal trauma. Children may not have surface bruising, and the examination can be confounded by other injuries or concurrent head injury. Imaging studies, including computed tomography, may be indicated (Kellogg, 2007). Examination findings may include:

i. Decreased or absent bowel sounds.

ii. Guarding or abdominal muscle rigidity.

3. Physical examination findings consistent with sexual abuse

a. In examinations of sexually abused children, physical findings are rare (Heger, Ticson, Velasquez, & Bernier, 2002): over 90% of examinations of children who are evaluated for sexual abuse show no evidence of trauma or infection. Sexual abuse of prepubertal children most often consists of oral or digital contact. The elastic nature of genital and rectal tissues, added to delays in disclosure or examinations, contribute to the lack of findings (Adams et al., 2007). Some trauma to the genital area can occur accidentally, as with the asymmetric vulvar trauma consistent with straddle injuries. The APN who regularly examines the genital area of prepubertal girls during well-child examinations is more confident in distinguishing normal from abnormal findings (Schapiro, 2006). However, because apparently abnormal findings are often subtle, are difficult to determine without special magnification equipment (e.g., a colposcope), and can be caused by normal physiologic variations, they should be confirmed by an expert in sexual abuse examinations.

b. The following are findings that are consistent with sexual abuse:

i. Vaginal trauma: trauma may occur anywhere in the vulvar area, the periurethral or perihymenal tissue, or in the perineum, from either forceful digital penetration, use of objects, or penile penetration. The following are consistent with sexual abuse (Adams et al., 2007):

a. Acute trauma or notches or transactions of inferior hymenal tissue (caution: normally occurring redundant hymenal folds may appear to be notched).

b. Thin or absent hymenal tissue.

ii. Anorectal trauma: penetration may cause fissures, and repeated penetration may lead to laxity of the sphincter. The most common cause of anal fissures is large hard stools, so fissures in themselves are nonspecific. Laxity of the anal sphincter should raise suspicions of abuse, but may also be related to neurologic conditions.

iii. Penile trauma: penile trauma is an uncommon finding in sexual abuse, but may be associated with severe physical abuse.

iv. Sexually transmitted infections: most cases of vulvovaginitis in prepubertal children, including mucopurulent vaginal discharge, are caused by nonsexually transmitted infections, such as *Streptococcus pyogenes* and *Salmonella shigella*. Most cases of balanitis (inflammation of the foreskin) are also unrelated to sexual abuse. Gonorrhea and *Chlamydia* are rare in sexually abused prepubertal children (0.7–3.7%), and are more common in sexually abused teenagers whose rates of infection (14%) are higher than teenagers who report only consensual activity with peers (Bechtel, 2010). Vertical transmission of gonorrhea, *Chlamydia*, human papilloma virus, and herpes simplex virus are all possible (Adams et al., 2007). Ulcers or verrucous papules in the genital area should be cultured to test for herpes simplex virus and human papilloma virus typing.

4. Physical examination findings consistent with neglect

a. Physical signs of neglect may include evidence of generally poor hygiene, inadequate clothing, and failure to grow and gain weight as expected during childhood. These signs are nonspecific, because poor hygiene and inadequate clothing may also be caused by behaviors associated with pediatric neuropsychiatric conditions. Most cases of failure to thrive have a variety of causes, including congenital heart disease, malabsorption syndromes, neuromuscular disorders, and a variety of interactional failures between parent or caregiver and child (Black et al., 2006; Block & Krebs, 2005). These interactional failures may be related to neglect or to a parent's appropriate anxieties about a medically fragile child who does not respond easily to the parent's customary caretaking strategies.

b. A rare and puzzling form of maltreatment, pediatric condition falsification, also known as Munchausen syndrome by proxy (Pankratz,

2006; Stirling, 2007), involves elements of physical abuse, psychologic abuse, and child endangerment (often classified as neglect). In this form of maltreatment, parents induce symptoms of illness in their children, presenting them as victims of rare and serious medical conditions. The parent is typically a well-educated mother, often with training in a healthcare profession. Although uncommon, this form of maltreatment should be in the differential when children have repeated visits or hospitalizations for serious symptoms with negative diagnostic tests.

III. Assessment

Child maltreatment does not fit easily into a medical model or diagnostic algorithm in which one can "rule out" or "rule in" abuse or neglect. Many physical signs and behaviors associated with abuse are also associated with infections, serious chronic conditions, or variations of normal (Table 13-2). Children and their caretakers, for a variety of reasons, may withhold elements of the history that could, alone or considered together with physical findings, aid in the determination or elimination of child maltreatment as a likely explanation for a given clinical picture.

However, the APN's legal responsibility usually hinges on a reasonable suspicion or concern, rather than a firm or even likely diagnosis (Child Welfare Information Gateway, 2007a). The following elements should be carefully assessed when the APN suspects child maltreatment:

A. Safety

1. Is further testing or examination warranted by experts in child physical or sexual abuse?
   a. Fresh disclosure of sexual abuse or assault, especially involving penetration or exchange of body fluids (within 72 hours, or in some states up to 108 hours): the child or adolescent should be transported to a specialized center for forensic examination, usually an emergency room within the county where the abuse took place.
   b. Equivocal examination, for example an apparently abnormal genital examination, which warrants a specialized examination with magnification.
   c. Evaluation to determine if serious physical injuries are accidental or inflicted.

TABLE 13-2 Child Maltreatment: Associated Factors That May Trigger An Independent Report

Associated Factors	Specific Behaviors	Legal Implications
Domestic violence	Domestic violence committed in front of a child: injury to a child reportable under child abuse laws	Reportable in some states Adds to charges or sentencing of offender in some states Offender may have to pay for child's counseling
Substance abuse	Exposure of a child to substance abuse Manufacturing or using methamphetamine in front of a child Substance abuse affecting parenting ability Prenatal use of substances affecting a fetus Newborn testing positive for drugs of abuse	Specifically reportable in some states Providing substances to a child or failure to prevent access reportable in all states Some states have mandated follow-up for prenatally exposed newborns with evaluation by CPS before discharge
Poverty	Homelessness Failure to provide adequate food, clothing, shelter, health care	Homelessness reportable in some states, specifically excluded in others Inability to provide stable, adequate housing may be related to reporting in some states Some states have exemptions for personal or religious beliefs
Truancy	Failure to send child to school or provide home schooling, ensure child goes to school	Check individual state laws: in some states a violence of truancy; not under child protection laws

Source: Data from U.S. Department of Health and Human Services, Child Welfare Information Gateway, "State Statutes Search." Retrieved from http://www.childwelfare.gov/systemwide/laws_policies/state/

2. Is the child or adolescent safe to go home?

   a. Do the suspected injuries or overall physical condition warrant hospitalization?

   b. Is there a disclosure or suspicion of sexual abuse in the home or physical abuse with imminent danger to the child?

   c. Can the caretaker with the child keep or transport the child safely?

      i. Willingness or ability to protect the child.

      ii. Safe transport (e.g., intoxicated caregiver who drove to the clinic with the child).

   d. Will the disclosure or reporting of maltreatment put the child or caretaker at risk in the home?

      i. Family reactions to disclosure.

      ii. For adolescents, potential harsh punishment for disclosing behaviors associated with extrafamilial abuse (e.g., going to a forbidden party).

3. Are there potential safety issues for the APN in reporting?

   a. Suspected offending parent or caretaker in the clinic.

   b. Reactions of nonoffending parent or child or adolescent.

B. Need to report

1. Does the situation warrant mandatory reporting in the state in which the APN is practicing?

   a. Consultation with other clinic providers.

   b. Consultation with local child abuse reporting hotline.

2. How urgent is the report (related to safety issues above)?

   a. Immediate.

      i. Immediate safety issues.

      ii. Legal issues: evidence collection or documentation.

   b. End of the day (disclosures of past abuse, child and caretaker currently safe, sexual abuse outside of home beyond 72-hour period).

C. Are child's and family's immediate needs being met?

1. When suspected maltreatment is part of the family's chief complaint

   a. Determine their expectations for outcome regarding housing safety (e.g., shelter versus arrest of suspected offender, which is not always immediate).

   Further testing desired by child and family that may or may not be indicated.

2. If suspected maltreatment is not the chief complaint of the child or caregiver

   a. It is important for APN not to lose sight of child and family priorities, which may be equally or more urgent than the investigation of maltreatment.

   b. If a report is necessary, it may be easier to integrate into the child's and family's care if the family's priorities are respected.

IV. Plan

A. Diagnostic testing

1. Imaging: order in consultation with radiologist or child abuse specialist to determine occult, old, healing fractures.

2. Laboratory testing

   a. If there is fresh disclosure of sexual assault or abuse within time period for forensic evidence, examination and laboratory testing should be ordered by a specialized sexual abuse forensic testing center.

   b. Bacterial or viral cultures as indicated for skin lesions or discharge in anogenital area and the oropharynx.

   c. Serologic testing as indicated (HIV, RPR, hepatitis panels).

B. Management

1. Treat injuries or infections as indicated.

2. As indicated previously, refer any child or adolescent with sexual abuse or assault of less than 72 hours (or longer in some localities) to police and specialized child sexual abuse forensic team.

3. Make a child abuse report if maltreatment is suspected, following state and local procedures for verbal (telephone) and written reporting; usually both are required.

   a. Consider informing the parent about a report if it is safe for the provider to maintain trust in the therapeutic relationship.

   b. Involve the adolescent in making a report.

      i. In most states, reporting is required by law, regardless of the adolescent's wishes; in some states, the provider has discretion and the adolescent can decline to report sexual abuse or assault if the suspected offender is not a parent or caretaker (Sachs et al., 2008).

ii. Discuss APN legal responsibilities and the adolescent decision making about disclosing versus withholding information.

4. Arrange follow-up care

a. Counseling, if not arranged by law enforcement or CPS.

b. For suspected neglect, follow-up supports for family.

i. Practical and material (food banks, shelter assistance, transportation vouchers).

ii. Health supervision and support: public health nursing and health education.

c. Close clinic follow-up as indicated.

C. Patient education

Many states have excellent websites with parent and child educational material in multiple languages. The Child Welfare and Information Gateway http://www .childwelfare.gov/index.cfm is an excellent starting place for parent and provider education, with some materials available in Spanish.

REFERENCES

Adams, J. A., Kaplan, R. A., Starling, S. P., Mehta, N. H., Finkel, M. A., Botash, A. S., et al. (2007). Guidelines for medical care of children who may have been sexually abused. *J Pediatric and Adolescent Gynecology, 20,* 163–172.

Bariciak, E. D., Plint, A. C., Gaboury, I., & Bennett, S. (2003). Dating of bruises in children: An assessment of physician accuracy. *Pediatrics, 112,* 804–807.

Bechtel, K. (2010). Sexual abuse and sexually transmitted infections in children and adolescents. *Current Opinions in Pediatrics, 22,* 94–99.

Black, M. M., Dubowitz, H., Casey, P. H., Cutts, D., Drewett, R. F., Drotar, D., et al. (2006). Failure to thrive as distinct from child neglect. *Pediatrics, 117,* 1456–1458; author reply 1458–1459.

Block, R. W., & Krebs, N. F. (2005). Failure to thrive as a manifestation of child neglect. *Pediatrics, 116,* 1234–1237.

Chiesa, A., & Duhaime, A. C. (2009). Abusive head trauma. *Pediatric Clinics of North America, 56,* 317–331.

Child Abuse Prevention and Treatment Act (CAPTA). 42 U.S.C.A. § 5106g(2) (West Supp. 1998).

Child Welfare Information Gateway. (2007a). *Definitions of child abuse and neglect: State statutes series.* Retrieved from http://www.childwelfare .gov/systemwide/laws_policies/statutes/define.cfm.

Child Welfare Information Gateway. (2007b). *Recognizing child abuse and neglect: Signs and symptoms.* Retrieved from http://www.childwelfare .gov/pubs/factsheets/signs.cfm.

Child Welfare Information Gateway. (2008). *What is child abuse and neglect?* Retrieved from http://www.childwelfare.gov:80/pubs/factsheets /whatiscan.cfm

Child Welfare Information Gateway. (2009). *Child witness to domestic violence: Summary of state laws.* Retrieved from http://www.childwelfare .gov/systemwide/laws_policies/statutes/witnessdvall.pdf

Dong, M., Anda, R. F., Felitti, V. J., Dube, S. R., Williamson, D. F., Thompson, T. J., et al. (2004). The interrelatedness of multiple forms of childhood abuse, neglect, and household dysfunction. *Child Abuse and Neglect, 28,* 771–784.

Dubowitz, H. (2002). Preventing child neglect and physical abuse: A role for pediatricians. *Pediatrics in Review, 23,* 191–196.

Dubowitz, H. (2009). Tackling child neglect: A role for pediatricians. *Pediatric Clinics of North America, 56,* 363–378.

Fairbank, J. A., & Fairbank, D. W. (2009). Epidemiology of child traumatic stress. *Current Psychiatry Reports, 11,* 289–295.

Flaherty, E. G., Thompson, R., Litrownik, A. J., Theodore, A., English, D. J., Black, M. M., et al. (2006). Effect of early childhood adversity on child health. *Archives of Pediatrics and Adolescent Medicine, 160,* 1232–1238.

Fonseca, H., & Greydanus, D. E. (2007). Sexuality in the child, teen, and young adult: Concepts for the clinician. *Primary Care, 34,* 275–292; abstract vii.

Ford, J. D., Racusin, R., Ellis, C. G., Daviss, W. B., Reiser, J., Fleischer, A., & Thomas, J. (2000). Child maltreatment, other trauma exposure, and posttraumatic symptomatology among children with oppositional defiant and attention deficit hyperactivity disorders. *Child Maltreatment, 5,* 205–217.

Gilbert, R., Kemp, A., Thoburn, J., Sidebotham, P., Radford, L., Glaser, D., & MacMillan, H. L. (2009). Recognising and responding to child maltreatment. *Lancet, 373,* 167–180.

Gilbert, R., Widom, C. S., Browne, K., Fergusson, D., Webb, E., & Janson, S. (2009). Burden and consequences of child maltreatment in high-income countries. *Lancet, 373,* 68–81.

Guttmacher Institute. (n.d.). *Adolescents.* Retrieved from http://www .guttmacher.org/sections/adolescents.php

Heger, A., Ticson, L., Velasquez, O., & Bernier, R. (2002). Children referred for possible sexual abuse: Medical findings in 2384 children. *Child Abuse and Neglect, 26,* 645–659.

Herrenkohl, T. I., Sousa, C., Tajima, E. A., Herrenkohl, R. C., & Moylan, C. A. (2008). Intersection of child abuse and children's exposure to domestic violence. *Trauma Violence & Abuse, 9,* 84–99.

Jones, R., Flaherty, E. G., Binns, H. J., Price, L. L., Slora, E., Abney, D., Sege, R. D. (2008). Clinicians' description of factors influencing their reporting of suspected child abuse: Report of the child abuse reporting experience study research group. *Pediatrics, 122,* 259–266.

Kellogg, N. D. (2007). Evaluation of suspected child physical abuse. *Pediatrics, 119,* 1232–1241.

Kemp, A. M., Dunstan, F., Harrison, S., Morris, S., Mann, M., Rolfe, K., Maguire, S. (2008). Patterns of skeletal fractures in child abuse: Systematic review. *British Medical Journal, 337,* a1518.

Pankratz, L. (2006). Persistent problems with the munchausen syndrome by proxy label. *Journal of the American Academy of Psychiatry Law, 34,* 90–95.

Sachs, C. J., Weinberg, E., & Wheeler, M. W. (2008). Sexual assault nurse examiners' application of statutory rape reporting laws. *Journal of Emergency Nursing, 34,* 410–413.

Schapiro, N. A. (2006). Female genitalia. In K. Duderstadt (Ed.), *Pediatric Physical Assessment* (pp. 213–230). St. Louis, MO: Mosby.

Schapiro, N. A. (2008). Medical neglect of children: Reporting issues for nurse practitioners. *Journal for Nurse Practitioners, 4,* 531–534.

Slack, K. S., Holl, J. L., McDaniel, M., Yoo, J., & Bolger, K. (2004). Understanding the risks of child neglect: An exploration of poverty and parenting characteristics. *Child Maltreatment, 9,* 395–408.

Stirling, J., Jr. (2007). Beyond munchausen syndrome by proxy: Identification and treatment of child abuse in a medical setting. *Pediatrics, 119,* 1026–1030.

Stirling, J., Jr., & Amaya-Jackson, L. (2008). Understanding the behavioral and emotional consequences of child abuse. *Pediatrics, 122,* 667–673.

Testa, M. F., & Smith, B. (2009). Prevention and drug treatment. *Future of the Child, 19,* 147–168.

U.S. Department of Health and Human Services Administration on Children Youth and Families. (2009). *Child maltreatment 2007.* Retrieved from http://www.acf.hhs.gov/programs/cb/pubs/cm07/cm07.pdf

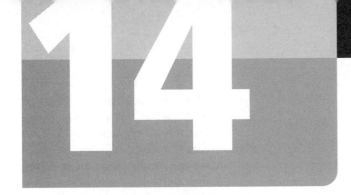

FAILURE TO THRIVE DURING INFANCY

Annette Carley

I. Introduction and general background

Failure to thrive (FTT) is a complex condition with multiple interacting causes manifesting as inadequate weight gain or consistent weight deceleration compared to age-appropriate norms. Weight is primarily affected when nutritional intake cannot support growth demands, although height and head circumference are affected by increasing malnutrition. Formerly labeled "organic" and "inorganic," FTT is now described in more useful terms based on its etiology: (1) inadequate caloric intake, (2) inadequate caloric absorption or use, or (3) excess caloric consumption. Regardless of the etiology, FTT may have long-term effects on cognitive and behavioral development, and create increased susceptibility to infection or long-term growth deficiency (Krugman & Dubowitz, 2003; Shah, 2002; Stephens, Gentry, Michener, & Kendall, 2008).

A. FTT from all causes

1. Overview

   The most common cause of FTT worldwide is poverty and poor access to adequate nutrition (Block, Krebs, Committee on Child Abuse and Neglect, & Committee on Nutrition, 2005). It occurs across all populations, although the risk is increased in impoverished urban and rural populations (Gahagan, 2006; Shah, 2002).

   a. In developed countries, it is also commonly associated with poor caretaking skills, reflecting a disparity between infant interactive and growth needs and caretaker attentiveness.

   b. FTT may be the sole clinical finding suggesting neglect or abuse.

   c. FTT accounts for up to 5% of pediatric hospitalizations (Stephens et al., 2008).

2. Prevalence and incidence

   a. FTT is usually identified during the first 2 years of life.

   b. It affects up to 10% of children in primary care settings, although only 1% of FTT in this group is caused by a recognized disorder, such as cardiac disease or inborn errors of metabolism (Block et al., 2005; Stephens et al., 2008).

   c. However, because there is a lack of consensus regarding criteria to establish the diagnosis (Olsen, 2006), this likely affects the reported incidence.

B. FTT caused by inadequate caloric intake

1. Overview

   FTT may be the result of poorly sustained nutrient availability, infant inability to consume adequate foods, or ineffective feeding interactions leading to decreased intake (the most common cause of FTT).

   a. Improper formula preparation, limited formula or food availability, insufficient breast milk production, or overuse of fruit juices at the expense of more nutrient-dense foods

   b. Motor feeding issues interfering with consuming adequate intake, such as inability to suck, chew, or swallow effectively

   c. Poor appetite

   d. Oral aversion

   e. Disturbed caregiver–infant interactions affecting feeding interest or success, including behavioral problems during the meal, caregiver inattention, or outright neglect (Corrales & Utter, 2005; Gahagan, 2006; Krugman & Dubowitz, 2003; Stephens et al., 2008). Some evidence supports an association with maternal depression (Stewart, 2007).

C. FTT caused by inadequate caloric absorption or use

1. Overview

   A number of genetic, structural, or functional conditions may create ineffective nutrient absorption or use, and must be recognized. Included among these conditions are:

   a. Celiac disease

   b. Cystic fibrosis

   c. Cow milk protein allergy

d. Vitamin or mineral deficiencies

e. Biliary atresia or hepatic dysfunction

f. Short gut syndrome

g. Genetic abnormalities, such as trisomy 13, 18, and 21

h. Short-stature syndromes including Russell-Silver syndrome, Turner syndrome, Down syndrome, hypothyroidism, hypophosphatemic rickets, growth hormone deficiency, and fetal alcohol syndrome

i. Metabolic disorders, such as glycogen storage disease and aminoacidopathies

j. Chronic vomiting

k. Gastroesophageal reflux

l. Chronic renal disease (Corrales & Utter, 2005; Gahagan, 2006; Krugman & Dubowitz, 2003; Stephens et al., 2008)

D. FTT caused by excess caloric consumption needs

1. Overview

Increased metabolic demands may interfere with growth, which may occur with such conditions as:

a. Chronic lung disease

b. Congenital heart disease

c. Chronic infection

d. Hyperthyroidism

e. Anemia

f. Diabetes

g. Renal tubular acidosis

h. Fever

i. Immunodeficiency

j. Malignancy

k. Intrauterine growth restriction (Corrales & Utter, 2005; Krugman & Dubowitz, 2003; Stephens et al., 2008)

II. Database (appropriate for the evaluation of FTT in developed countries; may include but is not limited to)

A. Subjective

1. History and review of systems

A thorough history is the most critical element in establishing the diagnosis, uncovering causes, and posing a therapeutic plan (Block et al., 2005; Corrales & Utter, 2005; Gahagan, 2006; Krugman & Dubowitz, 2003), and includes:

a. Past health history

   i. Prenatal history, including gravida and parity of mother, maternal weight gain during pregnancy, pregnancy complications, and prenatal care access

   ii. Birth history, including gestational age, weight, type of delivery, infant Apgar scores, and delivery complications

   iii. Neonatal history; including weight at discharge; complications; congenital disorders; and oral instrumentation, such as intubation

   iv. Early childhood history, including acute and chronic illness, hospitalizations, injuries, and developmental status

   v. Current history, including presenting complaint onset and duration and associated symptoms

   vi. Elimination history, including voiding and frequency and character of stools

b. Family history

   i. Age and health of parents, grandparents, and primary caretakers

   ii. Birth weight and height of parents and siblings

   iii. Congenital disorders; chronic illness; and mental health disorders, such as anxiety or depression

c. Social and environmental history

   i. Marital status and education of parents

   ii. Occupation and source of financial support and access to public assistance programs, such as WIC or food stamps

   iii. Type of housing and number of persons in household

   iv. Social or environmental concerns, such as unemployment, marital problems, abuse, and substance exposure

   v. Family and peer relationships, including physical and emotional closeness, communication, support, history of abuse or neglect, adaptive behaviors, positive social affect, and ability to ask for and receive support

   vi. Parenting skills, including previous experience caring for children, attendance at parenting classes, ability to interpret infant cues, daily routines, play activity with child, caretaking routines related to behavior, crying, and elimination

   vii. Disorganized or disruptive household environment, erratic family meals, and multiple caretakers

   viii. Caretaker concerns about growth and development

d. Nutrition history

   i. Maternal nutrition before, during, and after pregnancy, including number of meals per day, type, and amount of food and fluid intake

ii. Infant feeding history, including type of milk, volume and frequency of feedings, proper preparation of formula, strength of suck, burping, use of supplemental foods, and tolerance of food texture

iii. Obtain minimum 24-hour dietary recall

    a. For breastfed infants: frequency of feeding, duration of feeding, perceived satiety, strength of suck, single or two breasts at feeding, and maternal breast fullness before feeding and emptying after feeding

    b. For bottle-fed infants: frequency of feeding, duration of feeding, perceived satiety, strength of suck, and proper formula preparation

    c. For infant transitioning to solid foods: time of introduction of solids and foods self-fed by infant (Corrales & Utter, 2005; Gahagan, 2006; Locklin, 2005; O'Connor & Szekely, 2001).

e. Review of systems and clinical findings may reveal

    i. Dysmorphic features suggesting a syndrome, such as low-set ears, hypertelorism, or long philtrum

    ii. Pallor

    iii. Hair loss

    iv. Thin or wasted appearance, loose folds of skin

    v. Irritability

    vi. Sleepiness or easy fatigue

    vii. Poor eye contact or social smile

    viii. Delayed vocalization

    ix. Delayed motor development, including late rolling, sitting, crawling, or walking (Lucile Packard Children's Hospital, 2009; UPMC, 2009; Zamani, 2009).

B. Objective

1. Physical examination findings

    a. Establish a growth trend, including measuring and plotting head circumference, weight, and length (height) (Corrales & Utter, 2005; Gahagan, 2006).

        i. Most sources support weight less than fifth percentile or a downward growth trend crossing two percentile lines as meeting diagnostic criteria for FTT (Krugman & Dubowitz, 2003; Olsen, 2006).

        ii. Weight below third to fifth percentile on standardized curve or weight-to-height ratio, also known as Waterlow criteria, also used in determination of FTT

        iii. Using Waterlow criteria (Corrales & Utter, 2005)

            a. Mild FTT if 80–90% of expected weight-to-height

            b. Moderate FTT if 70–79% weight-to-height

            c. Severe FTT if less than 70% weight-to-height

        iv. Weight-to-age ratio is not recommended as the sole indicator because it does not accurately address those infants who are genetically or constitutionally small, or those born premature or small for gestational age; also known as Gomez criteria (Corrales & Utter, 2005; Krugman & Dubowitz, 2003; Olsen, 2006)

    b. Vital signs, including blood pressure

    c. Anthropometry studies, such as triceps skinfold or midarm muscle circumference, are not generally used, although they may aid in cases with associated edema (Corrales & Utter, 2005).

2. Observation and documentation of caregiver–child interactions

    a. Presence of eye contact, holding close to body, calling infant by name

    b. Observation during feeding

3. Supportive data from relevant diagnostic tests are rarely needed, although may be dictated by positive findings in the history (Stephens et al., 2008).

III. Assessment

A. Determine the diagnosis
Identify other causes of diminished growth, including those constitutionally small or genetically small.

B. Severity
Assess severity of the condition: severe malnutrition, dehydration, and suspected abuse are indications for hospitalization (Block et al., 2005; Gahagan, 2006; Stephens et al., 2008).

C. Significance
Assess significance of the problem to caregiver and family.

D. Motivation and ability
Determine caregiver and family willingness and ability to follow through with the treatment plan.

IV. Goals of clinical management

A. Screening or diagnosing FTT
Choose a practical, cost-effective approach to screening and diagnosis.

B. Treatment

Select a treatment plan that achieves appropriate growth and growth velocity, provides necessary micronutrients and macronutrients, and is individualized for the caregiver and child (Corrales & Utter, 2005).

C. Patient adherence

Select an approach that maximizes caretaker compliance.

V. Plan

A. Screening

Elicit a thorough history and perform a thorough physical examination; assess growth and development at all well-child visits

B. Diagnostic tests

Laboratory or radiographic tests are rarely necessary, because the diagnosis is generally apparent after review of history and physical examination findings. In addition to routine childhood screening at 6–18 months for iron deficiency and lead poisoning, supportive testing suggested by positive findings may include:

1. Urinalysis and urine culture, urine pH

2. Complete blood count with smear

3. Stool pH, reducing substances, and ova and parasites or occult blood

4. Sweat chloride

5. Tuberculosis testing: skin (Mantoux tuberculin skin test) or blood (interferon-gamma release assays)

6. Radiographic studies, including skeletal survey and bone age (CDC, 2010; Corrales & Utter, 2005; Gahagan, 2006; Stephens et al., 2008).

C. Management

1. FTT is a chronic process, and management continues long-term (Block et al., 2005).

2. Adequate growth is essential for survival, and interventions begin before completion of the diagnostic evaluation (Gahagan, 2006).

3. Most FTT cases can be managed on an outpatient basis, unless malnutrition is severe; hospitalization is indicated for evidence of severe dehydration, weight less than 70% of predicted weight-to-height, or suspected neglect or abuse (Block et al., 2005; Gahagan, 2006; Stephens et al., 2008).

4. A multidisciplinary approach is strongly encouraged, involving input from medicine, nursing, lactation specialists, pediatric nutritionist, physical therapy, behavioral psychology, and social services (Corrales & Utter, 2005; Locklin, 2005).

5. For breastfed infants efforts should support breastfeeding where possible, including:

   a. Breast pumping using dual-pump

   b. Considering galactalogues to increase milk production

   c. Encouraging maternal nutrition, fluids, and rest

   d. Developing strategies to modify maternal and environmental stress, and its negative impact on milk production

   e. Identifying sources of home and social support for breastfeeding

   f. If formula supplementation is deemed necessary to ensure sufficient nutrient intake, support the mother in efforts to resume or continue breastfeeding

6. For formula-fed infants efforts to optimize intake include:

   a. Increasing the number of feeds per day, with a goal of 100–120 kcal/kg/d

   b. Demonstrating techniques to awaken a sleepy feeder

   c. Reviewing formula preparation with the caretaker

7. For infants consuming solid foods, encourage self-feeding while ensuring adequate intake of nutritious foods and nutritionally competent choices of finger foods (Corrales & Utter, 2005; Gahagan, 2006).

8. Catch-up growth should be promoted until previous growth percentiles have been attained, which may necessitate increased protein intake and up to 20–30% increase in energy supply, in addition to provision of micronutrients. The refeeding plan is determined by the degree of malnutrition; however, caution must be exerted to avoid exceeding the child's absorptive capacity. Refeeding syndrome characterized by vomiting, diarrhea, metabolic disturbances, and circulatory collapse has been reported in cases of severe malnutrition treated overly aggressively. When encountered, caloric and protein provision may need to be reduced to normal levels for 1–2 weeks, and gradually increased to optimize catch-up growth (Corrales & Utter, 2005).

D. Client education

Offer ongoing caretaker support and education, and reinforce consistent effective nutritional practices at all office visits by:

1. Providing a supportive environment for parents to discuss concerns or conflicts related to the infant or home setting

2. Role modeling infant feeding, holding, and stimulation

3. Discussing normal development and infant behavior

4. Reinforcing proper nutritional practices, such as discussing caloric needs to optimize growth, demonstrating proper formula preparation, proposing a regular feeding schedule with written instructions, and directly assessing a feeding interaction

5. Maintaining ongoing contact with the caregiver and family, and modifying the nutritional plan accordingly

6. Referral to public health or home care nursing, as available in the community, for ongoing evaluation and support

E. Outcome

Most children with poor growth can demonstrate adequate improvement with intensive intervention. However, both cognitive and school outcomes of children with FTT are worse than their non-FTT counterparts, likely representing the cumulative effects of undernutrition and other environmental risks, such as inattention or lack of appropriate stimulation. These infants need ongoing developmental, behavioral, and growth monitoring to detect and manage long-term consequences of FTT (Gahagan, 2006).

VI. Resources

A. Patient–client education

The following resources provide online health library information for clients and professionals; see the reference list for appropriate links.

1. Children's National Medical Center, Washington, DC
   http://www.childrensnational.org/DepartmentsAnd Programs/default.aspx?Type=Dept&Id=376&Name =Failure to thrive (poor growth)

2. Lucile Packard Children's Hospital, Palo Alto, CA
   http://www.lpch.org/diseasehealthinfo/health library/growth/thrive.html

3. University of California, San Francisco Children's Hospital, San Francisco, CA
   http://www.ucsfchildcarehealth.org/pdfs/fact sheets/Failure to Thrive_en_0709.pdf

4. University of Pittsburgh Medical Center, Pittsburgh, PA
   http://www.upmc.com/HealthAtoZ/Pages/Health Library.aspx?chunkiid=11872

5. WebMD/eMedicine
   http://emedicine.medscape.com/article/985007 -overview

REFERENCES

Block, R. W., Krebs, N. F., Committee on Child Abuse and Neglect, & Committee on Nutrition. (2005). Failure to thrive as a manifestation of child neglect. *Pediatrics, 116*(5), 1234–1237.

Centers for Disease Control & Prevention (2010). Guidelines for screening for tuberculosis infection and disease during the domestic medical examination for newly arrived refugees. Retrieved from http://www .ced.gov/immigrantrefugeehealth/guidelines/domestic/tuberculosis -guidelines.html.

Corrales, K. M., & Utter, S. L. (2005). Growth failure. In P. Q. Samour & K. King, *Handbook of Pediatric Nutrition* (3rd ed., pp. 391–406). Sudbury, MA: Jones & Bartlett.

El-Baba, M. F., Bassali, R. W., Benjamin, J., & Mehta, R. (2009). *Failure to thrive.* Retrieved from http://emedicine.medscape.com/article /985007-overview

Gahagan, S. (2006). Failure to thrive: A consequence of undernutrition. *Pediatrics in Review, 27*(1), e1–11.

Krugman, S. D., & Dubowitz, H. (2003). Failure to thrive. *American Family Physician.* Retrieved from http://www.aafp.org/afp/20030901/879 .html

Locklin, M. (2005). The redefinition of failure to thrive from a case study perspective. *Pediatric Nursing, 31*(6), 474–479.

Lucile Packard Children's Hospital. (2009). *Failure to thrive.* Retrieved from http://www.lpch.org/diseasehealthinfo/healthlibrary/growth/thrive .html

O'Connor, M. E., & Szekely, L. J. (2001). Frequent breastfeeding and food refusal associated with failure to thrive. *Clinical Pediatrics, 40,* 27–33.

Olsen, E. M. (2006). Failure to thrive: Still a problem of definition. *Clinical Pediatrics, 45,* 1–6.

Shah, M. D. (2002). Failure to thrive in children. *Journal of Clinical Gastroenterology, 35,* 371–374.

Stephens, M. B., Gentry, B. C., Michener, M. D., & Kendall, S. K. (2008). What is the clinical workup for failure to thrive? *Journal of Family Practice, 57*(4), 264–266.

Stewart, R. C. (2007). Maternal depression and infant growth-a review of recent evidence. *Maternal & Child Nutrition, 3*(2), 94–107.

UPMC. (2009). *Failure to thrive.* Retrieved from http://www.upmc .com/HealthAtoZ/Pages/HealthLibrary.aspx?chunkiid=11872

Zamani, A. R. (2009). *Failure to thrive.* Retrieved from http://www.ucsf childcarehealth.org/pdfs/factsheets/Failure to Thrive_en_0709.pdf

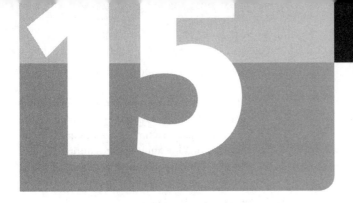

URINARY INCONTINENCE IN CHILDREN

Angel K. Chen

I. Introduction and general background

Urinary incontinence by definition is the involuntary loss of urine (Neveus et al., 2006). The bladder is responsible for the storage and emptying of urine. During infancy, this occurs as reflexive behavior by the complex pathway controlled by an "integration of sympathetic, parasympathetic, and somatic innervation that involves the lower urinary tract, the micturation center in the sacral spinal cord, the midbrain, and the higher cortical centers" (Hinds, 2005, p. 79). The infant also may not empty to completion (Feldman & Bauer, 2006). The cortical inhibitory pathway develops between 1 and 3 years of age, which inhibits bladder contraction and allows for voluntary control of the external sphincter (Feldman & Bauer, 2006). By age 4, a child has learned to control and coordinate the voiding process and can become dry between urination. The detrusor muscle (bladder wall muscle) is relaxed during the filling stage while the bladder neck remains closed to achieve continence. Once the bladder is full, the external sphincter relaxes while the detrusor muscle contracts during voiding to allow for complete emptying of the bladder. An estimated bladder capacity for a child over 2 years of age is approximately the child's age (in years) plus two (in ounces) up until puberty (Feldman & Bauer, 2006). However, a wide range of conditions or dysfunctions may cause either continuous or intermittent incontinence in children.

These same children may be at risk for a number of comorbidities including urinary tract infections (UTIs), stool retention, or encopresis because of behavioral patterns (Feldman & Bauer, 2006; Franco, 2007a). As one learns to contract the external sphincter muscle, it inhibits both detrusor contraction and stool motility, which can impact both systems. Chronic contraction of the sphincter muscle promotes further stool retention and distention, which may lead to decreased amplitude, reduced bladder contraction and activity (Franco, 2007a), and recurrent UTIs because of incomplete bladder emptying. In addition, a full rectum may exert pressure on the bladder, inducing bladder symptoms, such as sudden urgency or decreased bladder capacity, described as the "cross-talk" mechanism (Franco, 2007a).

Possible early childhood risk factors, such as developmental delays in motor, communication, and social skills, or even difficult temperament may contribute to a higher chance of daytime incontinence and soiling (Joinson, Heron, von Gontard, Butler, Golding, & Emond, 2008). Children with urinary incontinence have also been found to have social and psychologic distress that must be addressed at the same time (Butler & Heron, 2008; Feldman & Bauer, 2006). Although correction of incontinence may not alter internalizing problems, such as anxiety or obsessive–compulsive disorders, it does normalize the incidence of externalizing problems, such as conduct disorders (Glassberg & Combs, 2009). Our society has little tolerance for bladder and bowel incontinence; thus, children with such symptoms are at risk for further embarrassment and psychologic and emotional distress (Tobias, Mason, Lutkenhoff, Stoops, & Ferguson, 2008). Providers must handle both the initial work-up and routine follow-up with much sensitivity and respect for the child's self-esteem.

This chapter focuses on intermittent incontinence in children older than 5 years of age who are otherwise healthy and normal, both anatomically and neurologically. The assessment and management of both daytime and nighttime urinary incontinence (nocturnal enuresis) is discussed. There is also a brief review of the assessment and management of the common comorbid conditions of UTI, stool retention, and encopresis, and the psychologic, social, and cultural impact faced by children with these conditions. The chapter uses the standard terminology set forth by the International Children's Continence Society to standardize the language and avoid confusion among clinicians and researchers (Neveus et al., 2006).

A. Daytime incontinence

1. Definition and overview.

   Daytime urinary incontinence is the involuntary loss of urine while awake. It involves a wide array of clinical symptoms and causes, which differ by severity and reversibility. In addition, it may involve the maturation, functional, or behavioral process within the elimination cycle. Most commonly, children discover the power of controlling the external sphincter to postpone urination (by inhibiting the detrusor contraction), and thus eventually may reach a dyscoordination between the bladder and sphincter muscle control, or have a delay in maturation of the bladder sphincter coordination (Franco, 2007a), both of which lead to daytime urinary leakage. Furthermore, after repeated dyscoordination, the child may also have a difficult time relaxing the external sphincter muscle enough to void to completion, thus increasing the risk of UTI and causing even more uninhibited contractions of the bladder (Austin & Ritchey, 2000). Some of the major causes of daytime incontinence include:

a. Vaginal reflux and postvoid dribbling: involuntary leakage of urine immediately or within 10 minutes after voiding caused by urine trapped in the vagina during void; may cause skin irritation.

b. Overactive bladder and urge incontinence: increased detrusor contractions that lead to pelvic floor contraction; may or may not involve urinary frequency; high association with UTIs; associated with strong desire to void with tendency to perform classic postponing maneuvers ("potty dance," crossing legs fully, squatting with heel pressed into perineum, or penile grabbing) to externally contract the sphincter or compress urethra to temporarily relax the detrusor, postpone urination, or prevent urinary leakage.

c. Voiding postponement: typically with postponing maneuvers to postpone voiding, followed by a sudden urge to void.

d. Dysfunctional voiding: incomplete relaxation of external sphincter during voiding; verified by urodynamics or uroflow evaluation with staccato urinary flow pattern and prolonged voiding time with incomplete emptying of the bladder (elevated postvoid residual [PVR]); associated with increased risk for UTI.

e. Underactive bladder: low voiding frequency (three or less in 24-hour period) with need for intra-abdominal pressure (valsalva) to initiate, maintain, or complete voiding; caused by hypotonic detrusor muscle; large bladder volume with elevated PVR and increased risk for UTI.

f. Giggle incontinence (enuresis risoria): a rare condition with complete involuntary emptying of bladder that occurs during or after laughter; bladder normal while not laughing; seen in girls; methylphenidate has been shown to provide some improvement in symptoms (Berry, Zderic, & Carr, 2009).

g. Extraordinary daytime urinary frequency: frequent, small-volume voiding during the day only (> 1 time per hour with voided volume of < 50% estimated bladder capacity).

2. Prevalence and incidence.

Daytime urinary incontinence is generally considered a problem after 4 years of age (Feldman & Bauer, 2006). It may account for up to 40% of the visits in a pediatric urology clinic. In addition, dysfunctional voiding is associated with increased risk of UTIs, stool retention and encopresis, vesico-ureteral reflux, and psychologic distress (Feldman & Bauer, 2006; Hinds, 2005). Emotional stressors, such as sexual abuse, may sometimes trigger sudden dysfunctional voiding.

B. Nighttime incontinence (enuresis)

1. Definition and overview.

a. Nighttime incontinence, also known as enuresis, is the involuntary loss of urine in discrete episodes while asleep, occurring at least 2 nights per week (Butler, Heron, & The ALSPAC Study Team, 2006; Neveus et al., 2006). Enuresis is generally thought to be caused by nighttime polyuria, bladder overactivity, elevated arousal threshold, or reduced nighttime bladder capacity (Butler et al., 2006; Neveus et al., 2010; Robson, 2009). To better understand the type of nighttime incontinence, we further divide the children into subgroups based on symptoms or by onset of enuresis:

i. Monosymptomatic enuresis: enuresis as the sole symptom, without any bladder dysfunction or other lower urinary tract symptoms; the cause is thought to be immaturity of the brainstem, with fluctuation or decreased production of serum arginine vasopressin, which leads to increased nocturnal urine production (Glassberg & Combs, 2009).

ii. Nonmonosymptomatic enuresis: enuresis along with additional daytime lower urinary tract symptoms (e.g., daytime incontinence, frequency, and urgency); the cause is thought to be overactive bladder or even stool retention, or a combination of both (Franco, 2007a; Franco, 2007b).

iii. Primary enuresis: child has never been dry at night.

iv. Secondary enuresis: child has had dry nights for at least 6 consecutive months but now with reoccurrence of enuresis; may have similar presentation as primary enuresis with the difference in degree of constipation and age of toilet training

b. Additional causes of enuresis may include genetic factors; maturational delay; upper airway obstruction (rare); psychologic factors; UTI; or decreased nighttime bladder capacity. Severe stool retention may also lead to decreased bladder capacity. Secondary nonmonosymptomatic enuresis requires further work-up for neurologic involvement especially if unresponsive to traditional treatments for enuresis or stool retention (Bogan, 2005; Robson, 2009).

2. Prevalence and incidence.

Approximately 15–25% of 5 year olds have nocturnal enuresis despite cultural differences (Bogan, 2005; Feldman & Bauer, 2006). A small percentage of this age group still wet two or more times per week (Robson, 2009). Recent studies have found more children with nonmonosymptomatic enuresis than monosymptomatic enuresis (Neveus et al., 2010; Robson, 2009), although the literature is mixed on actual prevalence. Children with nonmonosymptomatic enuresis tend to have higher rates of comorbidity, including both bladder and bowel dysfunction (Butler et al., 2006). In addition, they tend to have more severe symptoms including more wet episodes per night, and more wet nights per week than those with monosymptomatic enuresis, because of persistent bladder overactivity throughout the night (Butler et al., 2006). The comorbid factors hinder the success of treatment for enuresis if left unresolved. The spontaneous cure rate in children is about 15% per year, depending on their culture. Approximately 2–3% of older adolescents and 1–2% of adults continue to experience nocturnal enuresis. This occurs more in boys than girls (Bogan, 2005; Robson, 2009). Although most children do outgrow enuresis, studies have shown reduced self-esteem in children with even just once per month enuresis. By providing treatment, self-esteem improves regardless of actual success of treatment (Robson, 2009). Another study by Butler and Heron (2006) reveals that 9-year-old children view enuresis as extremely stressful life events, even more stressful than physical illnesses. Insurance companies may pay for bed alarm treatment for children over 7 years of age with monosymptomatic enuresis (Aetna, 2009), but daytime symptoms must be ruled out initially. The decision about when to start treatment depends on how concerned and motivated is the child rather than on how concerned are the family or caregivers (Robson, 2009).

II. Database (may include but is not limited to)

A. Subjective

1. Detailed voiding and elimination history: most useful and most important (Table 15-1).

   a. History provides critical information.

   b. Direct questions at both child and parent because the child knows best what occurs during the day; parents have been found to be unreliable in stating the voiding and elimination history alone.

2. Past health history.

   a. Prenatal and birth history.

   b. Medical illnesses: significant congenital conditions especially of the genitourinary tract, heavy snoring.

   c. Surgical history: urologic or neurologic surgery.

   d. Obstetric and gynecological history: recent pregnancy.

   e. Growth and development: developmental milestones and any challenges or delays especially in neuromuscular area; attention-deficit/hyperactivity disorder; and school performance.

   f. Family history: renal or urologic diseases and history of enuresis.

   g. Diet: caffeine, soda, energy drinks, chocolate, or citrus intake (bladder irritants); fluid intake throughout the day and night; and fruit or fiber intake.

   h. Personal–social–psychologic history: traumatic events or history of abuse, family and social support, reaction to accidents, recent major changes in the family; temperament in general.

3. Review of systems (Table 15-1).

   a. General: self-esteem, mood, attitude, patterns of behavior, fatigue, weight loss.

   b. Musculoskeletal and neurologic: gait and changes in lower extremity sensation or control.

B. Objective

1. Physical examination findings (Table 15-2).

2. Supporting data from relevant diagnostic tests (Table 15-3); depends on work-up and management plan.

TABLE 15-1 Detailed Voiding and Elimination History Directed at Both Child and Parent

Category	Details
Voiding habits	Potty training process (age, approach, and length of time)
	Number of voids throughout the day or at school (0–3)
	Postponing behavior ("potty dance")
	Urgency or frequency (number of times per hour; can sit through a movie?)
	Intermittent versus smooth urine stream
	Use of abdominal pressure to void (Valsalva)
	Nocturnal polyuria
Daytime incontinence	Frequency: number of times wet per day or per week
	Amount and severity: dampness versus soaking accidents
	• number of pads or liners used per day
	Pattern: morning versus afternoon
	• weekday versus weekend
	Sudden wetting versus wet along the way to the bathroom
	Amount of time between voiding and wetting (immediately, 10 min, or 2 hr)
	Aware of wetting and change clothes independently?
	Previous treatment and results
Nighttime incontinence	Frequency: number of nights per week
	Amount and frequency: wet before or after midnight
	• number of times per night (1 or > 1)
	• soak through pull-ups or diapers
	Previous treatment and results; compliance or appropriate use?
	Age when initial nighttime wetting resolved (if applicable)
	Family history of delayed resolution of nighttime wetting
	Responsible for changing wet sheets or clothing
History of urinary tract infection	Bladder versus kidney infection
	Fever or other symptoms at presentation
	• symptoms after treatment
	Previous work-up
	Total number of infections, dates, and treatment
Elimination habits	Frequency of stooling in toilet
	Size, shape, and consistency of stool; clog the toilet?
	Staining on underwear versus complete soiling
	Postponing of stooling (withholding behavior)
	Chronic abdominal pain
	Water and fruit and fiber intake per day; evaluate timing of fluid intake
	Prior treatment and results
	Family history of constipation or infrequent stooling
Overall	Skin breakdown or rashes in perineum
	Awareness before or right after accident (urine or stool)?
	Which occurred first: urinary wetting or stool retention or soiling?
	Which is worse: daytime or nighttime wetting, or stool retention or soiling?
	Which is the child more motivated to correct?
	Which is the family more motivated to correct?
	Assess child's and family's readiness to address the issues

III. Assessment

A. Determine the diagnosis

1. Daytime urinary incontinence.

2. Nighttime urinary incontinence (enuresis).

3. Other conditions that may explain the patient's presentation.
   a. Rule out UTIs.
   b. Rule out constipation or stool retention.
   c. Rule out neurogenic bladder.
   d. Rule out diabetes insipidus or diabetes mellitus.
   e. Rule out ectopic ureter (typically continuous incontinence).

B. Severity

Assess the severity of the disease.

C. Significance

Assess the significance of the problem to the child and family.

D. Motivation and ability

1. Determine the child's motivation, willingness, and ability to follow the individualized treatment plan.

2. Provide individualized program and set realistic goals.

3. Provide frequent follow-up to monitor progress and sustain motivation.

TABLE 15-2 Physical Examination

System	Details
General	Assess self-esteem, attitude, and mood
Abdomen	Abdominal tenderness or distention Abdominal masses • kidneys and bladder • stool masses
Genitourinary	Overall hygiene Dampness or stool staining on underwear Tanner stage Anatomic abnormality Signs of skin breakdown or skin excoriation Signs of infection Male: urine pooled under foreskin; balanitis; or meatal stenosis Female: urine in introitus or perineum; discharge; or labial adhesion Active urine leakage at baseline versus with straining Rectum • stool staining around rectum • rectal fissures • sphincter tone and sensation; anal wink If positive stool symptoms then consider digital rectal examination for assessment of rectal tone, presence of fecal or solid mass, or hemoccult testing
Spine	Sacral dimple, pit, sinus tract Tuft of hair Hemangioma Subcutaneous lipoma Asymmetric gluteal crease
Neurologic	Gait Heel and toe walk Lower extremity muscle strength and tone Deep tendon reflexes Sensation in lower extremities

TABLE 15-3 Common Urologic Tests

Test	Definition	Clinical Implications	Comments
Urinalysis	Analysis of the urine by urine dipstick and when available, evaluation under the microscope with spun urine	Specific gravity • < 1.000 may reveal concentrating defect • > 1.020 may reveal dehydration and insufficient fluid intake Positive glucose on dipstick: rule out diabetes mellitus Positive protein on dipstick: repeat and rule out renal disease Positive leukocytes or nitrites on dipstick: proceed with microscopic evaluation and culture and sensitivity to rule out UTI	UTIs must be ruled out because they may be the cause of or the result of the incontinence Can exacerbate bladder symptoms
Urine culture and sensitivity	Cultured urine specimen to evaluate organism causing UTI and sensitivity to panel of antibiotics	Positive urine culture indicates UTI and requires treatment with antibiotics May follow with prophylactic antibiotics to prevent further infections until voiding dysfunction resolved	Method of obtaining specimen is important Use a catheterized specimen if not fully toilet trained to avoid contamination
Uroflowmetry	Noninvasive test measuring urinary flow rate, voiding pattern (degree of external sphincter relaxation), voiding volume, and time	Staccato flow (intermittent stream) indicates inability for sphincter to completely relax during voiding and may cause incomplete emptying in dysfunctional voiding Bell-shaped curve indicates proper sphincter relaxation during voiding Prolonged flow time with weak flow rate may indicated hypotonic bladder and detrusor contraction Best done with simultaneous pelvic floor electromyogram monitoring	Need to have at least half of estimated bladder capacity in the bladder to be effective Can be evaluated by listening and observing the urine flow if machine is not available
Bladder scan and PVR	Ultrasound of the bladder after voiding to determine residual urine within the bladder; noninvasive	Ideal goal of < 10% of expected bladder capacity Can detect bladder wall thickness (> 5 mm; caused by voiding dysfunction) and any masses within the bladder Useful as prognostic indicator Prevoid bladder volume is also helpful	

TABLE 15-3 Common Urologic Tests *(continued)*

Test	Definition	Clinical Implications	Comments
Renal bladder ultrasound	Ultrasound of the kidneys and bladder; noninvasive	Assess renal size and parenchyma, and any evidence of hydronephrosis Assess bladder volume, bladder wall thickness, and any masses within the bladder May see rectal distention (indicate stool retention)	Normal renal bladder ultrasound can also be reassuring to both families and provider
Kidneys, ureter, bladder radiograph	Plain film of kidneys, ureter, and bladder region	Assess degree of stool retention Assess for any spinal deformity	Complements clinical history and physical examination
Urodynamics	Invasive study involving urethral catheter and filling of bladder for evaluation of bladder pressure, compliance, detrusor and uninhibited contractions, and bladder capacity Also evaluates pelvic floor muscle coordination and condition of bladder at time of urinary leakage (if any) Fluoroscopic urodynamics also reveals VUR	Reserved for those without improvement or concern for neurogenic cause	Results may vary depending on how fast the bladder is filled and how cooperative is the patient
Spinal MRI	MRI of the spine to rule out tethered cord	Consider for those suspected of neurogenic bladder Should be MRI of entire spine	Children who require this work-up should also receive a full neurologic examination
Voiding cystourethrogram	Invasive fluoroscopic study with insertion of urinary catheter to fill the bladder and evaluate for signs of VUR; requires evaluation of voiding and PVR	Indicated if positive history of UTI to rule out VUR Also reveals bladder volume, bladder trabeculation, sphincter relaxation during voiding, urethra, and PVR Includes scout film (kidneys, ureter, bladder radiograph); reveals spinal deformity and degree of stool retention Incomplete relaxation of external sphincter during urination is seen as "spinning top urethra" in girls	Consider fluoroscopic urodynamics rather than voiding cystourethrogram only if the child has a history of incontinence and pyelonephritis

Abbreviations: UTI, urinary tract infection; PVR, postvoid residual; VUR, vesicourethral reflux; MRI, magnetic resonance imaging.

IV. Goals of clinical management

A. Screening or diagnosing

1. Choose a cost-effective approach for screening or diagnosing daytime and nighttime urinary incontinence in children.

2. Rule out other possible conditions causing urinary incontinence, which requires referral to a specialty service.

B. Treatment

1. Improve the patient's bladder and bowel health, including skin integrity.

2. Properly treat conditions with minimal use of medication (both in dose and length of treatment).

3. Decrease the prevalence of UTIs.

4. Improve the quality of life for both patient and family.

5. Prevent psychologic and emotional trauma caused by incontinence.

6. Foster a healthy and active lifestyle.

7. Empower the patient and family to manage bladder and bowel health.

C. Patient adherence

1. Select an approach that maximizes patient and family adherence, including positive reinforcement.

2. Provide close follow-up to maximize patient and family adherence.

V. Plan

A. Screening

Urinalysis or urine culture and sensitivities, if indicated, to rule out UTI and other abnormalities in the urine.

B. Diagnostic tests (Tables 15-3 and 15-4)

1. Voiding or elimination diary is both a diagnostic tool and treatment via the timed voiding and elimination process (Figure 15-1).

2. Uroflowmetry and bladder scan (if available) evaluate patient's voiding pattern and PVR; otherwise listen to urine flow for interruption or smooth flow.

3. Renal bladder ultrasound if positive for UTI or severe wetting.

4. Abdominal plain film if there is stool retention.

5. Voiding cystourethrogram if positive history of UTI; or may proceed with video urodynamics study, which includes fluoroscopic voiding cystourethrogram in addition to the urodynamics study of the bladder.

6. Urodynamics study and spinal magnetic resonance imaging if suspicion of neurogenic bladder for both day and nighttime incontinence or no improvement with initial treatment regimen of nonmonosymptomatic enuresis.

C. Management (includes treatment, consultation, referral, and follow-up care) (Tables 15-4, 15-5, and 15-6)

1. Daytime incontinence.

    a. Vaginal reflux and postvoid dribbling: sit on toilet with underwear all the way down by the ankles or sit backward on toilet to allow full abduction of legs during urination to avoid urine from back flowing into the vagina.

    b. Giggle incontinence and enuresis risoria: methylphenidate, 0.2–0.5 mg/kg orally daily for 2 months for trial:

        i. children less than 10 years of age: short-acting (4-hr) form used mid-morning

        ii. children more than 10 years of age: intermediate-acting (8-hr) form used before school (Berry, Zderic, & Carr, 2009)

    c. Valsalva voiding habits should be referred to pediatric urology for consultation and work-up.

2. Nighttime incontinence.

    a. Nonmonosymptomatic: start with treatment for daytime incontinence and address any other comorbid factors (e.g., stooling) before achieving nighttime continence.

    b. Monosymptomatic and primary nocturnal enuresis: choice of bed alarm or medication along with daytime treatment regimen if appropriate.

    c. Secondary nonmonosymptomatic nocturnal enuresis: if unresponsive to initial daytime treatment regimen, refer to pediatric urology for full work-up with renal bladder ultrasound, urodynamics, and spinal magnetic resonance imaging to rule out neurogenic bladder caused by possible tethered cord.

D. Client education

1. Information.

    Provide verbal and, preferably, written information regarding:

    a. Normal bladder and bowel functions, coordination of detrusor muscle with external sphincter muscle, and relationship between bladder and bowel functions.

TABLE 15-4 Urinary Incontinence Evaluation and Treatment Algorithm

		Presenting Symptoms				
		Daytime Wetting	Nighttime Wetting	Stool Retention or Encopresis	Hx of Urinary Tract Infection	Elevated Postvoid Residual on Bladder Scan
Step 1: Initial work-up or treatment	Antibiotic prophylaxis				X	X
	Timed voiding	X	X	X	X	X With double voiding
	Timed stooling	X	X	X	X	X
	Diary with rewards for attempts	X	X	X	X	X
	↑ Fluids, fruits, and fiber ⦸ Caffeine or sodas	X	X	X	X	X
	Polyethylene glycol (Miralax)			X Titrate accordingly		
	↓ Fluids after dinner		X			
	Renal bladder ultrasound	±			X ± further work-up	±
	Close follow-up	X	X	X	X	X
Step 2: Follow-up evaluation or treatment if still symptomatic (in addition to Step 1 intervention)	Review diary and modify regimen	X	X	X	X	X
	Uroflowmetry or postvoid residual (if available)	X	X	X	X	X
	Bed alarm		X			
	Desmopressin acetate DDAVP		X			
	Anticholinergic or antispasmotic Rx	X Only after strict time voiding and stooling regimen	±			Contraindicated
	Follow-up options	May consider other modalities	May consider other modalities		May come off Rx once symptom free	
Step 3: Without improvement despite treatment compliance	Referral for further work-up	Pediatric urology	Pediatric urology for urodynamics and spinal magnetic resonance imaging	Pediatric gastroenterology	Pediatric urology	Pediatric urology

FIGURE 15-1 Sample Voiding and Elimination Diary

Date _____

	Mon	Tues	Wed	Thurs	Fri	Sat	Sun
When you wake up							
Mid AM recess							
Lunch							
Mid PM (before leaving school)							
Dinner							
Bedtime							
Poop							
Dry Days							
Dry Nights							

Date _____

	Mon	Tues	Wed	Thurs	Fri	Sat	Sun
When you wake up							
Mid AM recess							
Lunch							
Mid PM (before leaving school)							
Dinner							
Bedtime							
Poop							
Dry Days							
Dry Nights							

Date _____

	Mon	Tues	Wed	Thurs	Fri	Sat	Sun
When you wake up							
Mid AM recess							
Lunch							
Mid PM (before leaving school)							
Dinner							
Bedtime							
Poop							
Dry Days							
Dry Nights							

TABLE 15-5 Management of Daytime and Nighttime Urinary Incontinence*

Step	Recommendation	Comments
Step 1: Initial work-up or treatment	Antibiotic prophylaxis if needed (see **Table 15-6**)	If positive for recurrent urinary tract infection or incomplete emptying, consider daily low-dose prophylactic antibiotics at the same time as timed voiding and stooling May consider • trimethoprim sulfamethoxazole • nitrofurantoin
	Timed voiding and double voiding	Initiated voiding every 1–2 hours during the day whether or not the child "feels the need"; approximately 6 times per day: first thing in the morning, mid-morning recess, lunch, mid-afternoon before coming home, dinner, and bedtime. If ↑ postvoid residual (> 10% estimated bladder capacity), perform double voiding by returning to void a few minutes after initial voiding; may consider antibiotic prophylaxis AVOID POSTPONING BEHAVIOR!
	Timed stooling	After a meal, typically dinner, sit on toilet for 10 minutes to attempt to have a bowel movement, and as needed (Walia, Mahajan, & Steffen, 2009) Avoid rushing through the attempt Use of stepstool to help with best posture in stooling
	Voiding and elimination diary (see **Figure 15-1**)	Document every voiding and elimination attempt each day, along with any dry days and nights May do a frequency–volume chart of shorter duration (i.e., 2-day) diary that includes fluid intake and volume voided Make note of size, shape, and consistency of stool
	Rewards system	Use the results on voiding–elimination diary to provide positive reinforcement Small treats, stickers, stamps, and privileges for voiding and elimination attempts rather than just for accident-free days and nights
	Dietary adjustments	Encourage fluids throughout the day (water best); avoid sodas and caffeinated beverages (Franco, 2007b) Increase fruit and fiber intake; natural best (Franco, 2007b) Age (in years) + 5 equal to number of grams of fiber per day (Walia, Mahajan, & Steffen, 2009)
	Stool retention and encopresis management (see **Table 15-6**)	If initial presentation with significant stool retention or encopresis, or on return with symptoms despite behavioral regimen, consider polyethylene glycol (Miralax 17 g/cap) for clean-out and maintenance regimen (Walia, Mahajan, & Steffen, 2009) May consider footstool to achieve best posture to relax external sphincter for stooling and voiding Refer to pediatric gastrointestinal service for further work-up if no improvement or gastrointestinal symptoms more severe than genitourinary symptoms Instruct families to expect 6–12 months of treatment, then wean therapy
	Fluid restriction (for nocturnal enuresis)	Avoid large amounts of fluids ingested at dinner and beyond Caution: children in afterschool sports activities require sufficient rehydration, thus significant fluid restriction may cause further dehydration Encourage fluid intake throughout the day
	Follow-up	Return to clinic in 1 month for close follow-up; best to maintain frequent contact especially if minor adjustments are necessary to behavior regimen

(continues)

TABLE 15-5 Management of Daytime and Nighttime Urinary Incontinence* *(continued)*

Step	Recommendation	Comments
Step 2: Follow-up evaluation or treatment	Reevaluate	On return, review voiding–elimination diary and symptoms since last visit Repeat uroflowmetry and postvoid residual; check if available If failed to comply with behavioral regimen, discuss barriers and possible ways to resolve barriers Continue with timed voiding, timed stooling, use of diary, and reward system
	Anticholinergic and antispasmodic medication (daytime incontinence or nonmonosymptomatic enuresis despite timed voiding) (see **Table 15-6**)	Use as adjunct to strict timed voiding for those with uninhibited bladder spasms and potentially increased functional bladder capacity May consider: • oxybutynin • tolteradine Second line of treatment for monosymptomatic enuresis or in conjunction with desmopressin acetate (DDAVP)
	Bed alarm system (monosymptomatic enuresis)	Consider for children greater than 6 years of age Choose loud sensor to wake child up at the beginning of accident at night; not the same as setting an alarm at a specific time of the night Sensor is attached to underwear and is activated by the wetting of the underwear Child needs to get up (or to be woken up) at the time of alarm activation to void, then reattach alarm Insurance may cover if other conditions are ruled out Should follow-up on results in 2–3 weeks; overall regimen for 2–3 months. If not effective, can consider pharmacologic regimen Pro: conditioning regimen; effective when used correctly in a motivated child and family (80%) Con: wakes up entire family with the loud sound; if soft then does not wake child up to void; relapse may occur after discontinuation
	Antidiuretic: desmopressin acetate (DDAVP) (monosymptomatic enuresis) (see **Table 15-6**)	First line of pharmacologic treatment for monosymptomatic enuresis
	Tricyclic antidepressant: imipramine (Tofranil) (see **Table 15-6**)	Third line of pharmacologic treatment for enuresis because of safety concerns
	Additional modalities: biofeedback	Consider biofeedback therapy to learn to relax sphincter and empty to completion; limited by child's ability to cooperate and follow directions (Franco, 2007b); "bladder stretching" exercises are not useful
	Other modalities (less evidence in the literature)	Alpha blocker therapy for overactive bladder Hypnosis Acupuncture Chiropractor Extracorporeal magnetic innervation therapy Botulinum A toxin for overactive bladder or sphincter dyssynergia (Franco, 2007b)
	Timed voiding and stooling regimen	Continue strict timed voiding and stooling along with medication trial
	Follow-up	Return in 1–2 months for follow-up and minor adjustments Continued support for patient and family Provide motivation in compliance with regimen Reminder regarding length of time required for full recovery
Step 3: Without improvement despite treatment compliance	Referral for further work-up	Pediatric gastroenterology if severe encopresis or stool retention Pediatric urology if recurrent urinary tract infection, persistent daytime or nighttime wetting, or suspicion of neurogenic bladder (require full work-up of renal bladder ultrasound, urodynamic study, spinal magnetic resonance imaging) Psychotherapy for emotional stressors to be assessed and treated

* Includes treatment, consultation, referral, and follow-up care.

TABLE 15-6 Common Urologic and Bowel Regimen Medication

Category	Indication and Mechanism of Action	Name	Dosage	Side Effects	Comments
Anticholinergic	1. Treat daytime incontinence caused by bladder overactivity (uninhibited contractions) 2. Second line of treatment for monosymptomatic enuresis or in conjunction with desmopressin acetate (DDAVP)	Oxybutynin	Daytime: 5 mg PO BID or TID dosing; or XL 10 mg PO daily Nighttime wetting: 5–10 mg PO QHS	Dry mouth, constipation, occasional initial drowsiness; do not use in hot weather because of reduced perspiration, which leads to facial flushing; possible mood changes	Contraindication: incomplete emptying
		Tolterodine	2 mg PO QHS		
Antidiuretic	Synthetic antidiuretic hormone to reduce urine output at night Consider for children > 6 years of age 30% respond fully; 40% partial response May use only for sleepovers or camp	Desmopressin acetate (DDAVP)	Dose: 0.2-mg tablet 1–3 tablet PO QHS (1 hour before bedtime); may use higher dose then taper down	Risk of hyponatremia (rare) with mostly nasal spray formulation (longer half-life); limit fluids after dinner	Contraindication: excessive fluid intake in evening, (+) headache, nausea, or vomiting
Antidepressant	Mechanism unknown; used rarely; 50% response rate	Imipramine	0.5–1.5 mg/kg/d given 1–2 hours before bedtime OR 25–50 mg PO QHS (50 mg for children > 9 years of age)	Daytime sedation, anxiety, insomnia, dry mouth, nausea, and personality changes	Overdose can cause fatal cardiac arrhythmias, hypotension, respiratory distress, and convulsions
Osmotic laxative	Induce catharsis by strong electrolyte and osmotic effect	Polyethylene glycol (Miralax)	Clean-out: 1.5 g/kg/d × 2 days (may split to BID dose) followed by daily maintenance dose and daily sit Maintenance: 2–11 years of age: 8.5 g (0.50 cap) in 4 oz of water per day > 12 years of age: 17 g (1 cap) in 8 oz of water per day; or 1 g/kg/d (titrate accordingly)	Nausea, vomiting, cramps	If no stooling, return to clean-out procedure and then maintenance Parents will titrate depending on stool output, consistency, and staining

(continues)

TABLE 15-6 Common Urologic and Bowel Regimen Medication *(continued)*

Category	Indication and Mechanism of Action	Name	Dosage	Side Effects	Comments
Antibiotic	Treatment of UTI; daily low dose prophylaxis for prevention of UTIs	Trimethoprim sulfamethoxazole	UTI Prophylaxis: 2 mg/kg/dose of TMP daily	Nausea, vomiting, Stevens-Johnson syndrome, rash	Contraindication: hypersensitivity to sulfa drug, trimethoprim, or components
		Nitrofurantoin	UTI Prophylaxis: 1–2 mg/kg/d as single daily dose; maximum 100 mg/d	Nausea, vomiting, anorexia, Stevens-Johnson syndrome, rash Avoid suspension; use capsule instead and sprinkle onto yogurt or ice cream Administer with food or milk	

Abbreviation: UTI, urinary Tract infection.

b. The disease process, including but not limited to signs and symptoms and underlying etiologies. Emphasize that this condition is neither the child's nor parent's fault and that the healthcare provider will work together to resolve issues. Provide encouragement and motivation throughout the recovery process (average 3–6 months or as long as the length of dysfunction).

c. Diagnostic tests that include a discussion about preparation, cost, the actual procedures, and after-care.

d. Management (rationale, action, use, side effects, associated risks, and cost of therapeutic interventions; and the need for adhering to long-term treatment plans).

2. Counseling.

a. Recommended if symptoms have contributed to emotional distress or social isolation.

b. If underlying issues contribute to the incontinence and encopresis, counseling or other psychotherapy may assist in addressing and correcting the issues.

VI. Self-management resources and tools

A. Patient and client education websites

1. www.Kidshealth.org.
   Part of Nemours Foundation's Center for Children's Health Media, Kidhealth.org is a website dedicated to providing health and safety information, and helpful tips, in both English and Spanish. Content is designed to specifically address parents, kids, and teenagers. Search "bedwetting" to retrieve helpful information.

2. www.Healthychildren.org.
   Sponsored by American Academy of Pediatrics. Contains health topics ranging from regular development to conditions, such as enuresis and constipation.

3. http://www.i-c-c-s.org.
   International Children's Continence Society official website. Includes resources for providers and patients on bladder and bowel dysfunction.

4. www.Bedwettingstore.com.
   Offers both resources and products to help manage daytime and nighttime urinary incontinence.

REFERENCES

Aetna, Inc. (2009). *Clinical policy bulletin: Nocturnal enuresis treatments.* Retrieved from http://www.aetna.com/cpb/medical/data/400_499/0431.html

Austin, P. F., & Ritchey, M. L. (2000). Dysfunctional voiding. *Pediatrics in Review, 21*(10), 336–341.

Berry, A. K., Zderic, S., & Carr, M. (2009). Methylphenidate for giggle incontinence. *The Journal of Urology, 182*(Suppl. 4), 2028–2032.

Bogan, P. A. (2005). Nocturnal enuresis. In L. Baskin & B. Kogan (Eds.), *Handbook of Pediatric Urology* (2nd ed., pp. 92–97). Philadelphia, PA: Lippincott Williams & Wilkins.

Butler, R., & Heron, J. (2008). An exploration of children's views of bedwetting at 9 years. *Child Care, Health and Development, 34*(1), 65–70.

Butler, R., Heron, J., & The ALSPAC Study Team. (2006). Exploring the differences between mono- and polysymptomatic nocturnal enuresis. *Scandinavian Journal of Urology and Nephrology, 40*(4), 313–319.

Feldman, A. S., & Bauer, S. B. (2006). Diagnosis and management of dysfunctional voiding. *Current Opinion in Pediatrics, 18*(2), 139–147.

Franco, I. (2007a). Overactive bladder in children. Part 1: Pathophysiology. *The Journal of Urology, 178*(3), 761–768.

Franco, I. (2007b). Overactive bladder in children. Part 2: Management. *The Journal of Urology, 178*(3), 769–774.

Glassberg, K. I., & Combs, A. J. (2009). Nonneurogenic voiding disorders: What's new? *Current Opinions in Urology, 19,* 412–418.

Hinds, A. (2005). Daytime urinary incontinence (in the otherwise healthy child). In L. Baskin & B. Kogan (Eds.), *Handbook of Pediatric Urology* (2nd ed., pp. 79–91). Philadelphia, PA: Lippincott Williams & Wilkins.

Joinson, C., Heron, J., von Gontard, A., Butler, U., Golding, J., & Emond, A. (2008). Early childhood risk factors associated with daytime wetting and soiling in school-age children. *Journal of Pediatric Psychology, 33*(7), 739–750.

Neveus, T., Eggert, P., Evans, J., Macedo, A., Rittig, S., Tekgül, S., . . . Robson, L. (2010). Evaluation of and treatment for monosymptomatic enuresis: A standardization document from the International Children's Continence Society. *The Journal of Urology, 183*(2), 441–447.

Neveus, T., von Gontard, A., Hoebeke, P., Hjälmås, K., Bauer, S., Bower, W., . . . Djurhuus, J. C. (2006). The standardization of terminology of lower urinary tract function in children and adolescents: Report from the Standardization Committee of the International Children's Continence Society. *The Journal of Urology, 176*(1), 314–324.

Robson, W. L. (2009). Clinical practice. Evaluation and management of enuresis. *The New England Journal of Medicine, 360*(14), 1429–1436.

Robson, W. L., Leung, A. K., & Van Howe, R. (2005). Primary and secondary nocturnal enuresis: Similarities in presentation. *Pediatrics, 115*(4), 956–959.

Tobias, N., Mason, D., Lutkenhoff, M., Stoops, M., & Ferguson, D. (2008). Management principles of organic causes of childhood constipation. *Journal of Pediatric Health Care, 22*(1), 12–23.

Walia, R., Mahajan, L., & Steffen, R. (2009). Recent advances in chronic constipation. *Current Opinion in Pediatrics, 21,* 661–666.

GYNECOLOGY

ABNORMAL UTERINE BLEEDING

Kim K. O'Hair, Geraldine Collins-Bride, and Fran Dreier

I. Introduction and general background

Abnormal uterine bleeding (AUB) is one of the most common presenting complaints in the health care of women. Changes in the menstrual cycle accounted for 19.1% of the 20.1 million visits to healthcare providers for gynecological conditions observed in a recent 2-year study (Nicholson, Ellison, Grason, & Powe, 2001). AUB is the indication for 25% of all gynecological surgical procedures in the United States (Jain & Santoro, 2005). Menorrhagia alone has been noted as the primary cause for 12% of referrals to gynecological specialty practices (Mohan, Page, & Higham, 2007).

AUB and dysfunctional uterine bleeding (DUB) are often regarded as synonymous; however, AUB refers to any bleeding pattern (frequency, duration, and amount of blood loss) that is different from the regular menstrual cycle and may be observed in both ovulatory and anovulatory women. DUB is a more limited term that characterizes AUB in anovulatory women. The potential differential diagnoses for AUB are numerous; may involve several systems; and can include pelvic infections, complications of pregnancy, benign pelvic abnormalities (e.g., polyps or leiomyomata) or genital pelvic malignancies, systemic diseases, coagulopathies, and iatrogenic causes (Table 16-1).

Menstruation, ovulation, and the coordinated sequence of endocrine signals that distinguish the menstrual cycle are the foundation for the regularity, predictability, and consistency of menses (Casablanca, 2008; Speroff & Fritz, 2005). Although an extensive explanation of the endocrinology of the menstrual cycle is beyond the scope of this discussion

and is available elsewhere (most notably in Speroff & Fritz [2005]), a summary of the basic events and organization of the normal menstrual cycle provides the background and the context for understanding AUB and DUB and the rationale supporting treatment options.

There are essentially three phases to a normal menstrual cycle: (1) the follicular phase, (2) ovulation, and (3) the luteal phase, all of which are managed by the hypothalamic-pituitary ovarian (HPO) axis, a complicated system of feedback between the hypothalamus, the pituitary, and the ovary (Speroff & Fritz, 2005; Star & Okasako, 2004). During the follicular phase, increasing levels of follicle-stimulating hormone cause the development and maturation of the dominant ovarian follicle, which in turn leads to increased production of estrogen and the proliferation of the endometrium. Increasing levels of estrogen also stimulate a surge of luteinizing hormone and ovulation occurs in response. After ovulation, the corpus luteum, which develops from the dominant ovarian follicle, continues to produce estrogen and also begins to produce progesterone. As this luteal phase progresses, the corpus luteum continues to enlarge, producing greater levels of progesterone and estrogen, and the endometrium becomes more organized in preparation for implantation. If conception does not occur, the corpus luteum regresses spontaneously on a predictable and stable timetable. With this regression, estrogen and progesterone levels drop rapidly and menstruation begins again (Albers, Hull, & Wesley, 2004; Casablanca, 2008; Speroff & Fritz, 2005). According to Speroff and Fritz (2005), "The sequence of events is so controlling that most ovulatory women have a pattern, volume, and duration of menstrual flow they recognize as their own and come to expect, very often accompanied by an equally consistent and predictable pattern of premenstrual molimina (bloating, breast tenderness, and mood swings)" (p. 548).

Alterations in menstrual patterns, especially those attributed to anovulation, are most common during adolescence and the perimenopause with the prevalence of anovulatory cycles greatest in women under the age of 20 and over the age of 40 (Jain & Santoro, 2005; Levine, 2006; Speroff & Fritz, 2005). However, AUB may occur at any time during the childbearing years and may involve any change in menstrual cycle frequency, duration, amount of flow, and bleeding between cycles. For postmenopausal women, AUB includes vaginal bleeding 12 months or more after the cessation of menses (the last menstrual period), or unpredictable bleeding in postmenopausal women who have been receiving hormone therapy for 12 months or more (Albers et al., 2004; Jain & Santoro, 2005). Most cases of DUB occur either at the end of the reproductive years (caused by waning ovarian activity), or during the early postmenarchal years, caused by immaturity of the HPO axis (Table 16-2).

TABLE 16-1 Etiologies of Abnormal Uterine Bleeding

Pregnancy and pregnancy-related conditions
- Abruptio placentae
- Ectopic pregnancy
- Miscarriage
- Placenta previa
- Trophoblastic disease
- Retained products of conception

Organic and pelvic tract pathology
- Endometriosis
- Neoplastic diseases: ovarian tumors
- Infections: salpingitis, cervicitis, endometritis, myometritis, pelvic inflammatory disease, tubo-ovarian abscess
- Benign anatomic abnormalities: adenomyosis, leiomyomata, polyps of the cervix or endometrium
- Premalignant lesions: cervical dysplasia, endometrial hyperplasia
- Malignant lesions: cervical squamous cell carcinoma, endometrial adenocarcinoma, estrogen- or testosterone-producing ovarian tumors, leiomyosarcoma
- Trauma: foreign body, abrasions, lacerations, sexual abuse or assault

Endocrine disorders
- Thyroid dysfunction
- Diabetes mellitus
- Hypothalamic dysfunction: habit changes, stress, anxiety, eating disorders, excessive weight loss, aggressive exercise, organic disease
- Polycystic ovary syndrome
- Pituitary diseases: hyperprolactinemia, acromegaly, pituitary adenoma
- Adrenal diseases: Cushing syndrome, Addison disease, tumors, congenital adrenal hyperplasia
- Obesity-related anovulatory abnormal uterine bleeding

Medications and iatrogenic causes
- Anabolic steroid use
- Aspirin and other prostaglandin synthetase inhibitors
- Anticoagulants
- Antipsychotics
- Corticosteroids
- Digitalis
- Phenytoin
- Propranolol
- Phenothiazines
- Butyrophenones
- Tranquilizers
- Tricyclic antidepressants
- Chemotherapeutic medications
- Herbal and other supplements: ginseng, ginko, soy
- Hormone replacement
- Intrauterine devices
- Oral contraceptives, subdermal or injectable hormones (estrogen and progesterone)
- Discontinuation of oral contraceptives
- Selective serotonin reuptake inhibitors
- Tamoxifen
- Thyroid replacement hormone

Systemic diseases and conditions
- Coagulation disorders: von Willebrand disease, idiopathic thrombocytopenia purpura, coagulation factor deficiencies and other thrombophilias, dysfibrogenemias
- Disorders that produce platelet deficiency: leukemia, severe sepsis, hypersplenism
- Increased endometrial fibrinolysins
- Hepatic disease
- HIV-related thrombocytopenia
- Systemic lupus erythematosus
- Aplastic anemia
- Renal disease

Sources: ACOG, 2001; Albers, Hull, & Wesley, 2004; Casablanca, 2008; Oriel & Schrager, 1999; Star & Okasako, 2004.

TABLE 16-2 Abnormal Uterine Bleeding Terminology

Term	Definition	ICD-9 Code
Amenorrhea	Absence of periods for a length of time equivalent to a total of at least three of the previous cycle intervals or 6 months	626.0
Primary amenorrhea	No menses ever in presence of normal growth and development in female > 16 years old	626.0
Secondary amenorrhea	Menses have ceased	626.0
Hypermenorrhea	Increased menstrual blood loss with normal cycle duration	626.2
Hypomenorrhea	Decreased blood flow during menses of normal length or shorter	626.1
Intermenstrual bleeding	Infrequent uterine bleeding of variable amounts occurring between normal periods	626.4
Menorrhagia	Unusually heavy bleeding; loss of > 80 ml of blood or > 7 days of flow at regular intervals	626.2
Metrorrhagia	Uterine bleeding of variable amounts at irregular but frequent intervals or between menses	626.6
Menometrorrhagia	Increased blood loss or duration of bleeding that occurs at irregular unpredictable intervals	626.2
Oliogomenorrhea	Menses length > 35 days	626.1
Polymenorrhea	Menses length < 21 days at regular interval	626.2
Postmenopausal bleeding	Bleeding that occurs > 1 year after menopause	627.1

Sources: Albers, Hull, & Wesley, 2004; Speroff & Fritz, 2005; Star & Okasako, 2004.

Other ICD-9 Codes That Can Be Used	Description
626.8	DUB, delayed, latent, protracted, retained and retrograde, suppression
626.4	Irregular menstrual cycle
626.9	Menstrual disorder/unspecified
626.5	Ovulation bleeding
626.7	Postcoital bleeding
627.2	Menopausal state
628.0	Anovulatory bleeding

A. Abnormal uterine bleeding

1. Definition and overview

   The characteristics of normal menstrual periods include duration of 4–6 days, an interval length of 24–35 days, and a volume of 20–80 mL of blood loss (Speroff & Fritz, 2005). Menstrual bleeding is considered abnormal if it persists for longer than 7 days (hypermenorrhea) or less than 2 days (hypomenorrhea); occurs more often than every 21 days (polymenorrhea); or exceeds a total blood loss of 80 mL (Table 16-2).

   In women of childbearing age, AUB includes any change in menstrual frequency, duration, or amount of flow, including bleeding between cycles (Albers et al., 2004; Star & Okasako, 2004). The most common causes of AUB in the United States are (Table 16-1)
   a. Pregnancy and pregnancy-related conditions
   b. Local pelvic conditions
   c. Endocrine disorders
   d. Systemic diseases
   e. Iatrogenic causes and medications
   f. Lifestyle factors

2. Prevalence and incidence

   AUB is a common reason that women seek care from their healthcare provider. Although there are many factors that cause AUB, the reason the patient enters the healthcare arena is her perception that her menstrual cycle has changed, that menstrual bleeding is either excessive or too little, or that some other characteristic of her pattern of bleeding has altered. The cause of AUB in premenopausal women can be ascertained in 50–60% of cases (Telner & Jakubovicz, 2007).

B. Dysfunctional uterine bleeding

1. Definition and overview

DUB is defined as excessive and prolonged uterine bleeding with no demonstrable organic origin, pelvic or extrapelvic. It is most often caused by abnormalities of endocrine origin, especially anovulation or oligo-ovulation (Casablanca, 2008). Often anovulation is caused by an immaturity of the feedback system of the HPO axis or as a result of the decrease in ovarian function at perimenopause, although it may occur at any time during the childbearing years (Albers et al., 2004). It is a diagnosis of exclusion, made after anatomic pathology, medical illnesses, and pharmaceutical causes have been excluded (Casablanca, 2008; Star & Okasako, 2004).

Women with anovulatory cycles undergo disrupted and unpredictable patterns of hormonal production that result in irregular and variable menstrual bleeding. These women are essentially in a continuous follicular phase because there is no stimulus for ovulation or subsequent luteal phase development. As a result, the endometrium is continually exposed to estrogen, with resulting proliferation. Ultimately, without the organizing support of the progesterone produced during the luteal phase, focal areas of the structurally fragile endometrium begin to break down, leading to an irregular pattern of menorrhagia and menometrorrhagia (Casablanca, 2008; Speroff & Fritz, 2005).

In some rare cases, DUB can be related to biochemical events affecting the endometrium. Excessive fibrinolytic activity and increased levels of plasminogen activator have each been identified in women with DUB and menorrhagia (Irvine & Cameron, 1999). DUB is often associated with the following conditions:

a. Perimenarchal or perimenopausal state
b. Hyperandrogenic: polycystic ovary syndrome, congenital adrenal hyperplasia, and androgen-producing tumor
c. Hypothydroidism
d. Hyperprolactinemia
e. Premature ovarian failure
f. Hypothalamic dysfunction: anorexia and bulimia
g. Persistent corpus luteum, luteal phase deficiency, decreased estrogen at ovulation, or increased endometrial fibrinolysins (Albers et al., 2004; Star & Okasako, 2004)

2. Prevalence and incidence

According to a recent Cochrane review, DUB is anovulatory in approximately 20% of cases and occurs most often at the extremes of reproductive life: soon after menarche (in early adolescence) and in the years before menopause (Hickey, Higham, & Fraser, 2009). Menarche is commonly followed by 5–7 years of relatively long cycles that gradually shorten over time to the common 28-day length. In the 8–10 years before menopause average cycle length and variability begin to increase as ovulation becomes more irregular and infrequent (Hickey et al., 2009; Jain & Santoro, 2005; Speroff & Fritz, 2005). Additionally, although approximately 10% of women with postmenopausal bleeding have endometrial cancer, approximately 12% of these cancers are diagnosed before menopause (Bignardi, Van den Bosch, & Condous, 2009).

DUB is the term applied to the abnormal bleeding patterns that occur in women secondary to anovulation or oligo-ovulation. All anatomic and medical diagnoses must be eliminated before the application of this term (Casablanca, 2008). Bleeding patterns are noncyclic and the flow may be heavy or light, with few if any moliminal symptoms (Albers et al., 2004; Casablanca, 2008; Star & Okasako, 2004). After all the underlying problems resulting in DUB are evaluated and addressed, medical treatment to reestablish cycle regularity and provide endometrial protection should be instituted (Albers et al., 2004).

II. Database (may include but is not limited to)

A. Subjective

1. Past medical history (Albers et al., 2004; Speroff & Fritz, 2005; Star & Okasako, 2004)

a. Obstetric history: gravidity and parity
   i. Dates and complications of previous pregnancies
   ii. Ectopic pregnancies and outcomes
   iii. Number of spontaneous and elective abortions and any adverse outcomes
   iv. Recent pregnancy, parturition, or fertility treatments
   v. Lactation status

b. Gynecological history
   i. Gynecological disorders and surgeries including evaluation, findings, and treatment

ii. Previous episodes of AUB including work-up and treatments

iii. Pap smear history including last Pap smear

iv. Sexually transmitted infections or upper reproductive tract infection (i.e., pelvic inflammatory disease, tubo-ovarian abscess, and so forth). Note dates and treatments.

v. Menstrual cycle history

    a. Age at menarche

    b. Last normal menstrual period

    c. Previous normal menstrual periods (preferably the previous three menses): usual cycle duration, flow, interval length, molinima symptoms (breast tenderness, bloating, mood changes, and dysmenorrhea)

    d. Date of onset of change in menses: rapid or gradual change

    e. Amount of flow: number of pads or tampons used and degree of saturation. Numerous studies to clarify amounts of blood lost have not been successful or practical and evaluation ultimately depends on the woman's perception of her blood loss (Irvine & Cameron, 1999; Jain & Santoro, 2005; Star & Okasako, 2004).

    f. Presence of intermenstrual bleeding, premenstrual or postmenstrual bleeding, and postcoital bleeding.

vi. Contraception history: methods, complications, and adverse outcomes

vii. Future fertility concerns

viii. Sexual history: sexual debut, sexual preference, number of lifetime sexual partners, and sexual practices

c. Medical history: medical illnesses (Table 16-1); general medical health; complete history of any and all medical problems including evaluation and treatments, ongoing and previous.

d. Surgical history: obstetric, gynecological, and endocrine surgical procedures particularly

e. Medication history: medications, vitamins, and supplements

f. Trauma: sexual assault or sexual abuse

g. Exposure history: radiation (i.e., breast cancer, thyroid cancer, pelvic malignancies, and so forth).

2. Family history

a. Gynecological problems: uterine, breast, ovarian malignancies, endometriosis, leiomyomata, and diethylstilbestrol exposure

b. Medical diseases: endocrine dysfunction, blood clotting disorders, and tuberculosis

3. Environmental and occupational hazards

4. Personal and social history

a. Education, occupation, social and family support systems, situational life stress, social and personal anxiety level, and cultural influences

b. Exercise: athletic training schedule

c. Habits: tobacco, alcohol, and recreational drugs

d. Nutrition: dietary status, food allergies and intolerances, and food preferences (i.e., vegan, lacto-ovo vegetarian)

e. Impact of AUB on lifestyle (sexual practices, deterrence of exercise, work time loss, and so forth)

5. Review of systems

a. Constitutional signs and symptoms: fatigue, weight gain or loss, weakness, malaise, hot or cold sensitivity, appetite change, headaches, obesity, and edema

b. Eyes: visual-field disturbances

c. Skin, hair, and nails: hair loss or unwanted hair growth, petechiae, bruising, jaundice, acne, acanthosis nigricans, and sweating

d. Cardiac: palpitations

e. Breast: galactorrhea and cyclical breast tenderness

f. Abdomen: nausea and bloating

g. Genitourinary: pelvic pain, dyspareunia, dysmenorrhea, hot flashes, night sweats, vaginal dryness, vaginal discharge, urinary frequency dysuria, and hematuria. Precipitating factors associated with AUB: (i.e., coitus, trauma, douching, exercise, diaphragm use, and the presence of a pessary)

h. Musculoskeletal: weakness

i. Neurologic: headaches, double vision (diploplia), and loss of vision

j. Hematologic: easy bruising and bleeding

B. Objective (physical examination)

A complete physical examination and assessment of the following systems is essential in the evaluation of a woman complaining of AUB. The following is appropriate for both AUB and DUB:

1. Vital signs: heart rate and blood pressure performed in standing, sitting, and lying positions; temperature; height; weight; and body mass index. A decrease in systolic blood pressure of at least 10 mm Hg or an increase of pulse by 20 beats per minute within 5 minutes of changing positions is considered ortho-static hypotension and if present may indicate hemodynamic instability. These patients should be evaluated in the emergency care setting (Levine, 2006).

2. General: body habitus, posture, stature, motor activity, gait, mood, affect, dress, grooming, and personal hygiene.

3. Hair: texture, hirsutism, pattern of loss if present (axillary, pubic, and scalp hair).

4. Eyes and ears: stare, lid lag, exophthalmos, and visual field abnormalities.

5. Neck: thyroid nodules or enlargement and lymph nodes.

6. Skin: pallor, jaundice, petechiae, ecchymoses, hematomas, palmar erythema, spider hemangiomata, dry or moist, warm or cold, rough or velvety, striae, acanthosis nigricans, acne, color of nail beds, and lesions.

7. Extremities: edema, perfusion, and wasting.

8. Cardiovascular: tachycardia and murmurs.

9. Lungs: hypoxia and accessory muscle use.

10. Breasts: development, galactorrhea, striae, masses, dimpling, retraction, and tenderness; concordance with developmental stage.

11. Abdomen: striae, ascites, hepatomegaly, splenomegaly, tenderness, male or female pattern escutcheon, inguinal nodes, uterine height if palpable.

12. Pelvis
    a. External genitalia: pubic hair distribution and developmental stage, clitoromegaly, lesions, edema, cysts, bruising, trauma, and atrophy
    b. Vagina: traumatic lesions, bruising, erythema, type of discharge, foreign bodies, and atrophy
    c. Cervix: polyps, eversion, ectopy, lesions, inflammation, erythema, mucopurulent discharge, cervical motion tenderness, atrophy, Chadwick's sign, and Hegar's sign
    d. Uterus: enlargement, contour, mobility, shape, consistency, tenderness, and masses
    e. Adnexae: masses and tenderness
    f. Rectum: masses and bleeding

13. Neurologic: Deep tendon reflexes, mental status exam (note mood, affect, and presence of anxiety or depression)

III. Assessment

A. Determine the appropriate diagnosis

1. Abnormal uterine bleeding.

2. Dysfunctional uterine bleeding.

3. Rule out complications of pregnancy in reproductive-age women.

4. Rule out malignancies in women in the postmenopause.

B. Assess for conditions that may underlie AUB (Table 16-1)

C. Assess severity of AUB and associated conditions

D. Assess significance of AUB to the patient and to family and significant others

E. Evaluate the ability of the patient to adhere to a treatment plan and follow-up

IV. Goals of clinical management

A. Choose a cost-effective approach for screening and evaluating AUB

B. Develop a treatment plan that addresses AUB and associated conditions, and returns the patient to stability and optimal health in a safe and effective manner

C. Determine, with the patient, a plan that enables adherence to treatment and follow-up and that is designed to reduce long-term complications of chronic anovulation

V. Plan

A. Diagnostic tests

As a general rule, the patient's age, reproductive status, and data from the history and physical examination guide decision-making regarding the appropriate diagnostic tests. Diagnostic testing is generally organized into three categories: (1) diagnostic tools, (2) initial testing, and (3) secondary or specialty-based testing.

1. Diagnostic tools.

    a. Menstrual calendars can be very helpful to establish bleeding patterns. Several on-line sites are available but usually include product advertisements and potentially biased information (e.g., *www.MyMonthlyCycles.com*). Counting pads or tampon number and degree of saturation is of limited use in evaluation of blood loss.

    b. Basal body temperature data and cervical mucus charting can be helpful to establish ovulation and mid-luteal phase serum progesterone assessment. An ovulation predictor kit data is simple to use and developed for patient ease, although this may be costly.

2. Initial testing (Table 16-3).

TABLE 16-3 Essential Initial Testing in the Investigation of Abnormal Uterine Bleeding

Test	Clinical Implications	Comments
Urine pregnancy test	A urine pregnancy test (qualitative β-human chorionic gonadotropin) should be performed on every woman of reproductive age. If positive, pelvic sonograms and serial quantitative α-human chorionic gonadotropin testing are appropriate to evaluate pregnancy-specific disorders and guide referral to an obstetrics specialty clinic if needed (Levine, 2006; Speroff & Fritz, 2005; Star & Okasako, 2004).	Pregnancy must first be considered in all premenopausal women
Complete blood count with differential	To assess the presence of significant anemia and thrombocytopenia.	Because the prevalence of blood dyscrasias (particularly von Willebrand diseases) in adolescents can be quite high (5–20%), and may present with heavy menstrual bleeding at menarche, routine screening for coagulation disorders is appropriate (ACOG, 2000; Levine, 2006).
Highly sensitive thyroid-stimulating hormone	An elevated thyroid-stimulating hormone is diagnostic of primary hypothyroidism	Thyroid disease is common in women. **See Chapter 66 for more information on diagnostic testing and treatment.**
Pap smear	For cervical cytology. Pap smears can also note estrogen deficiency states.	Endocervical and ectocervical sampling required for accuracy. **See Chapter 18 on cervical, vaginal, and vulvar cancer screening**
Endocervical cultures for *Neisseria gonorrhoeae (GC)* and *Chlamydia trachomatis*	As indicated for sexually active women	Urine testing for GC and *Chlamydia* is also acceptable.
Wet mount of vaginal secretions with normal saline and potassium hydroxide	Useful only if the woman is not bleeding heavily and vaginitis is suspected.	
Transvaginal ultrasonography of the pelvis	Indicated for: a. Determination of the presence of endometrial polyps or submucosal fibroids (Bignardi, Van den Bosch, & Condous, 2009). b. Measurement of the thickness of the endometrial lining. If the lining is 4 mm or less (and without pedicle artery sign), endometrial disease is very unlikely (Bignardi et al.). c. Evaluation for complications of pregnancy. d. Evaluation for adnexal masses and ovarian masses. e. Determination of adenomyosis and extent of tissue involvement. f. Evaluation for adnexal masses and ovarian masses. g. For evaluation of postmenopausal women on continuous hormone therapy, ultrasonography can be performed at any time.	Leiomyomas are very common, and abnormal uterine bleeding is the most common symptom if the leiomyoma is of submucosal origin, thus altering the endometrial lining. However, most leiomyomas are not the major cause of abnormal uterine bleeding and the evaluation of abnormal uterine bleeding should not necessarily cease with this finding. In the case of asymptomatic leiomyomas, treatment is not mandatory (Bignardi et al., 2009; Speroff & Fritz, 2005). Measurement of the thickness of the endometrial lining. If the lining is 4 mm or less (and without pedicle artery sign), endometrial disease is very unlikely (Bignardi et al., 2009). For women on cyclic hormone therapy, transvaginal ultrasound should occur after the progestin withdrawal bleed (Bignardi et al., 2009).

(continues)

TABLE 16-3 Essential Initial Testing in the Investigation of Abnormal Uterine Bleeding *(continued)*

Test	Clinical Implications	Comments
Hematologic Studies		
Coagulation panel: prothrombin time, partial thromboplastin time, bleeding time	Second-line testing when coagulation disorder is suspected	
Hormone assays: follicle-stimulating hormone, luteinizing hormone, estradiol, progesterone, prolactin	Indicated in perimenopausal women or those with suspected premature ovarian failure	**See Chapter 17 on amenorrhea** for a more in-depth discussion of all hormonal assay studies
Testosterone and DHEA-S	Indicated in the presence of hirsutism or virilization	
Ristocetin cofactor assay	For evaluation of suspected von Willebrand disease	Evaluation for von Willebrand disease is appropriate in adolescents, women with a worrisome family history, and in unexplained menorrhagia

Adapted from: ACOG, 2000; Albers, Hull, & Wesley, 2004; Bignardi, Van den Bosch, & Condous, 2009; Jain & Santoro, 2005; Speroff & Fritz, 2005; Star & Okasako, 2004.

3. Secondary and specialty-based testing: the following tests are often done by or in consultation with gynecology and women's health specialists:

   a. Biopsy of any suspicious vulvar, vaginal, or cervical lesion.

   b. Endometrial biopsy may be considered for women who are
      i. 40 years old or older
      ii. Obese
      iii. 30 years old or older with a significant history of anovulation or oligo-ovulation
      iv. Prolonged metrorrhagia
      v. Postmenopausal and not on hormone therapy
      vi. Postmenopausal and on hormone therapy for 12 months or more with unpredicted and unscheduled bleeding episodes (Albers et al., 2004; Jain & Santoro, 2005).

   c. Magnetic resonance imaging, sonohysterography, and computerized tomography may be used to evaluate adnexal, ovarian, and uterine masses, adenomyosis, and the presence of endometrial polyps.

   d. Hysteroscopy has long been the gold standard for evaluating the endometrium and is no longer exclusively performed in the operating room because newer technologies have expanded usage. Hysteroscopy allows for direct visualization of the endometrium:
      i. To assess for intrauterine adhesions
      ii. To assess and remove submucosal fibroids or endometrial polyps
      iii. To remove embedded intrauterine devices (IUDs)
      iv. To assess and biopsy any lesions for pathologic evaluation (Farquhar, Ekeroma, Furness, & Arroll, 2003; Bignardi et al., 2009).

   e. Hysterosalpingography is useful primarily in the setting of fertility evaluation where an assessment of tubal patency is required.

   f. Dilatation and curettage (D&C) is indicated for severe acute bleeding events where hypovolemia is present or where suspicion of malignancy is high. D&C is valuable for the removal of endometrial polyps and for histologic diagnosis when endometrial sampling has been unsuccessful or inadequate. D&C can also be a curative treatment for AUB.

B. **Treatment and management**

Treatment strategies directed toward specific bleeding patterns are for those women in which an organic, structural, or systemic illness has been ruled out. Most of the treatment strategies in this chapter address the management of DUB.

1. Acute hemorrhagic bleeding

   The patient with acute hemorrhagic bleeding, particularly in the presence of a positive pregnancy test or with orthostatic changes on physical examination, warrants urgent consultation or referral to gynecology or women's health service. Clinical management of such patients is beyond the scope of this discussion.

2. Acute heavy bleeding

    Medical management is usually sufficient. For women of reproductive age, once pregnancy status is confirmed as negative, the goal of therapy is to stabilize the endometrial lining; prevent recurrence; and establish regular, orderly, and synchronous bleeding patterns. Common drug therapies are discussed next.

    a. High-dose therapy: conjugated estrogens or ethinyl estradiol: 1.25 mg conjugated estrogen or 2 mg ethinyl estradiol by mouth every 4–6 hours for 24 hours, followed by 1.25 mg conjugated estrogen or 2 mg ethinyl estradiol daily for 7–10 days (American College of Obstetrics and Gynecology [ACOG], 2000; Hickey et al., 2009; Speroff & Fritz, 2005; Star & Okasako, 2004). Antiemetic therapy may be required to manage nausea from high-dose estrogen (Star & Okasako, 2004). High-dose estrogen therapy is recommended particularly when ultrasonography indicates a denuded and thin endometrium (Speroff & Fritz, 2005). A progestin withdrawal cycle must be planned after stabilization.

    b. Low-dose therapy: low-dose monophasic combination oral contraceptives (COC) taken by mouth daily two to three times a day for 5–7 days. The patient can continue on COC through the remainder of the cycle and will experience regular withdrawal bleeding after completing the pill pack. If desired, the patient may continue with COC to prevent anovulatory bleeding; otherwise she will experience regular COC withdrawal. High-dose estrogen therapy and COC are both contraindicated in any woman at risk of or with a personal or family history of thromboembolic events.

3. Chronic anovulatory bleeding

    Once pregnancy has been excluded, the goals for management of anovulatory bleeding are to eliminate acute bleeding, to prevent future episodes, and to reduce the patient's lifetime risk of complications arising from long-term anovulation by inducing or reestablishing regular patterns of menstrual bleeding (ACOG, 2000). Adherence issues may complicate treatment, because heavy bleeding may continue for several cycles after some treatment strategies have been initiated. Counseling the patient regarding treatment approaches and long-term goals improves adherence.

    For younger women, particularly adolescents and reproductive-age women to approximately 40 years of age, and for select perimenopausal women, treatment options include:

    a. Low-dose, monophasic COC: this treatment is contraindicated for women over 35 who smoke, women with evidence of vascular disease, or those with a personal or family history of thromboembolic events (ACOG, 2000; Star & Okasako, 2004).

    b. Medroxyprogesterone acetate (MPA), 10 mg by mouth daily for the first 10–14 days of each month for three to six cycles, with careful follow-up. Alternatively, continuing monthly cyclic MPA induces regular withdrawal and reduces the likelihood for long-term complications of anovulation (Speroff & Fritz, 2005; Star & Okasako, 2004). Other MPA regimens include:

        i. Norethindrone acetate, 5–10 mg orally once to three times a day for the first 10–14 days of each month (Star & Okasako, 2004).

        ii. Micronized progesterone, 200 mg orally twice a day for the first 10–14 days of each month (Hickey et al., 2009).

        iii. Depo-MPA (Depo-Provera®), 150 mg intramuscularly every 12 weeks (Hickey et al., 2009).

        iv. Levonorgestrel-releasing IUD (Mirena®) has been observed to reduce heavy menstrual bleeding by 75–95% and has been found to be more effective than norethindrone acetate (Lethaby, Irvine, & Cameron, 2003; Speroff & Fritz, 2005). This management option is also appropriate for patients with chronic illnesses that may cause anovulatory bleeding.

    c. For perimenopausal women the methods listed previously are all appropriate and should be carefully discussed with the patient to improve adherence. Additional contraceptive strategies for managing anovulatory bleeding include contraceptive vaginal ring releasing etonogestrel 120 µg/ethinyl estradiol 15 µg daily for 21 days each month; weekly transdermal contraceptive patch releasing norelgestromin 150 µg/ethinyl estradiol 20 µg daily; or subdermal implant releasing etonogestrel 68 µg over a 3-year period (Implanon®). For additional information on hormonal contraceptive management see Chapter 20 on Hormonal Contraception.

4. Metrorrhagia

    Hysteroscopy can provide both diagnosis and treatment (Farquhar et al., 2003). Observation and follow-up may be all that is needed. Ovulation predictor self-testing, basal body temperature charting, and cervical mucus sign charting can be used when needed for fertility awareness. Treatment is directed toward correction of underlying defect when organic pathology is discovered.

If pregnancy is not desired, premenstrual spotting can be addressed by cyclic monthly progestin during the luteal phase: MPA, 10 mg by mouth daily from Day 15 for 7–12 days (Star & Okasako, 2004). COC may be a more efficient means of management after any underlying pathology has been addressed.

Nonsteroidal anti-inflammatory drugs have been observed to reduce heavy menstrual flow in several studies, possibly by reducing prostaglandin levels in the endometrium by enzyme (cyclo-oxygenase) inhibition (Lethaby, Augood, Duckitt, & Farquhar, 2007; Speroff & Fritz, 2005). Counseling regarding the potential for gastrointestinal side effects should be provided:

a. Ibuprofen: 400 mg orally three times a day for the first 3 days of menses, or longer as needed.

b. Naproxen sodium: 275 mg by mouth four times a day for the first 3 days after a loading dose of 550 mg. May continue throughout the menstrual cycle.

c. Mefenamic acid: 500 mg by mouth three times day for the first 3 days of menses, or for the duration of the cycle, as needed.

5. Menorrhagia

a. COC may reduce heavy menstrual flow by promoting the development of an atrophic endometrium. Daily cyclic use (withdrawal every 28 days), sequential withdrawal (every 90 days), or continuous use may be considered as treatment strategies. The levonorgestrel-IUD is another viable option as are the other contraceptives discussed previously. Careful counseling improves adherence.

b. Gonadotropin-releasing hormone agonists, such as depot leuprolide (Lupron), 3.75 mg intramuscularly monthly or 11.25 mg every 90 days, or nafarelin, 0.2–0.4 mg intranasally twice a day, can be useful for short-term management of menorrhagia. These medications are most often used as a preoperative adjunctive therapy for women intending conservative (myomectomy or endometrial ablation) or definitive (hysterectomy) surgery for abnormal bleeding. The restoration of hemoglobin and iron stores by temporarily stopping heavy menstrual bleeding can reduce the need for intraoperative blood transfusion and attendant transfusion

risks (Speroff & Fritz, 2005). However, this therapy is limited to short-term use because of its expense and unpleasant side effects (menopausal vasomotor symptoms and bone loss).

c. Danazol: 200–400 mg by mouth daily for three cycles has been used in the past to inhibit ovulation, reduce serum estrogen levels, and promote endometrial atrophy. However, unpleasant side effects include acne; hirsutism; weight gain (2–4 kg); seborrhea; vasomotor symptoms (hot flashes and night sweats); mood changes (especially depression); and abnormal lipid profiles. Consultation with a specialist is warranted. For most women, long-term use is usually not acceptable (Speroff & Fritz, 2005; Star & Okasako, 2004).

d. Antifibrinolytic agents, in particular tranexamic acid, have been widely used elsewhere for management of menorrhagia. Doses of 1 gram every 6 hours for the first 4 days of the menstrual cycle are recommended, but gastrointestinal side effects and possible intermenstrual bleeding are common and may limit the usefulness of this therapy (Speroff & Fritz, 2005).

e. Surgical options:

i. D&C is most commonly considered in the acute care setting.

ii. Conservative management with endometrial ablation can be done with hysteroscopic guidance or with newer "blind" techniques. In all cases the goal is to prevent further menorrhagia by eliminating the endometrium. This is not indicated for women who desire further childbearing, who are menopausal, or who are at high risk of endometrial cancer. Because endometrial ablation can be done in the office or an out-patient surgical unit, it is less costly than hysterectomy, involves less risk of surgical complications, and requires less recovery time. It is appropriate for women with conditions that make them poor candidates for major surgery (Lethaby, Hickey, Garry, & Penninx, 2009; Speroff & Fritz, 2005).

iii. Hysterectomy remains the definitive treatment for menorrhagia and all abnormal bleeding patterns. It is appropriate for cases where treatment has failed or has been too noxious to tolerate, and where childbearing is no longer desired.

6. Postmenopausal bleeding

Both endometrial biopsy (EMB) and D&C provide information regarding the state of the endometrium, including evaluation for the presence of endometrial carcinoma. The pathologic examination of the sample identifies the presence of hyperplasia, atypia, polyps, and other endometrial lesions. The presence of atypia is of particular importance in determining an appropriate treatment plan (Speroff & Fritz, 2005). Endometrial sampling also provides information regarding the endometrium: the extent of disorganization, progestin or estrogen stimulation, atrophy, and phase determination (follicular versus luteal), each important in determining the treatment plan.

An initial transvaginal ultrasound (TVUS) finding of an endometrial lining less than or equal to 4 mm may reduce the need for endometrial sampling in some cases, but EMB together with TVUS establishes the most precise diagnosis (Farquhar et al., 2003). If atypia is not present, cyclic or daily progestin therapy with MPA or norethindrone acetate every month for 3 months may be considered. Close follow-up is strongly recommended and evaluation should be accelerated if abnormal bleeding patterns recur. The presence of atypia mandates specialty consultation for further evaluation. For postmenopausal women on hormone therapy, EMB findings can guide dose adjustments once endometrial pathology has been excluded.

C. Additional considerations and follow-up

1. All patients should be evaluated for anemia and treated as needed. Specialty referral should be instituted for
   a. Patients with suspected coagulation disorders
   b. When treatment fails or AUB is persistent or recurrent

2. Patients with acute bleeding require follow-up soon after initiation of therapy to evaluate for further bleeding or to evaluate for success of treatment.
   a. The schedule of follow-up care varies depending on the etiology and treatment of AUB and associated conditions.
   b. Assessment at regular intervals should be established as warranted (i.e., 3–6 months, or as needed).
   c. For leiomyomas, evaluation for symptoms and growth should be done every 6 months initially, although TVUS may not be required if symptoms remain unchanged.

D. Client education

1. Information: ACOG provides many educational pamphlets available on-line. Many websites providing support and information for specific disorders can be found on-line.

2. Counseling: detailed explanation of the etiologies of AUB, essential diagnostic tests, and treatment plans are imperative for patient understanding and adherence. Patient involvement in the decision-making process, inclusion of family members when desired, and consideration of cultural issues are essential for promoting adherence. The clinician should:
   a. Discuss all aspects of medications being considered as treatment options, including side effects, risks versus benefits, and expected outcomes (e.g., withdrawal bleeding after progestin therapy).
   b. Discuss all treatment options (medical versus surgical) and initiate referrals to specialists or surgeons.
   c. Consider associated issues, such as weight management, eating disorders, exercise issues, stress management, and management of chronic disorders. Referral for psychologic support may be necessary.

VI. Self-management resources and tools

The most important tool for the patient is the menstrual calendar (www.MyMonthlyCycles.com). Ovulation kits can also be helpful. Selected resources include

1. American Society for Reproductive Medicine (http://www.asrm.org/)

2. Harvard Women's Health Watch is a monthly publication providing information regarding issues in women's health written by the researchers and clinicians at Harvard Medical School (www.harvardwomenshealthwatch.org/)

REFERENCES

Albers, J. A., Hull, S. K., Wesley, R. M. (2004). Abnormal uterine bleeding. *American Family Physician, 69*(8), 1915–1926.

American College of Obstetrics and Gynecology (ACOG). (2000). Practice bulletin: Clinical management guidelines for obstetrician-gynecologists. Management of anovulatory bleeding. *International Journal of Gynaecology and Obstetrics, 72*(3), 263–271.

American College of Obstetrics and Gynecology (ACOG). (2001). Practice bulletin: Clinical management guidelines for obstetrician-gynecologists. Use of botanicals for management of menopausal symptoms. *Obstetrics and Gynecology, 96*(Suppl.), 1–11.

Bignardi, T., Van den Bosch, T., & Condous, G. (2009). Abnormal uterine bleeding and post-menopausal bleeding in the acute gynaecology unit. *Best Practice and Research Clinical Obstetrics and Gynaecology, 23*, 595–607.

Casablanca, Y. (2008). Management of dysfunctional uterine bleeding. *Obstetrics and Gynecology Clinics of North America, 35*, 219–234.

Farquhar, C., Ekeroma, A., Furness, S., & Arroll, B. (2003). A systematic review of transvaginal ultrasonography, sonohysterography and hysteroscopy for the investigation of abnormal uterine bleeding in premenopausal women. *Acta Obstetricia et Gynecologica Scandanivica, 82*, 493–504.

Hickey, M., Higham, J. M., & Fraser, I. (2009). Progestogens versus oestrogens and progestogens for irregular uterine bleeding associated with anovulation (Review). *Cochrane Database System Review, (4)*, CD001895.

Irvine, G. A., & Cameron, I. T. (1999). Medical management of dysfunctional uterine bleeding. *Ballière's Clinical Obstetrics and Gynaecology, 13*(2), 189–202.

Jain, A., & Santoro, N. (2005). Endocrine mechanisms and management of abnormal bleeding due to perimenopausal changes. *Clinical Obstetrics and Gynecology, 48*(2), 295–311.

Lethaby, A., Augood, C., Duckitt, K., & Farquhar, C. (2007). Nonsteroidal anti-inflammatory drugs for heavy menstrual bleeding (review). *Cochrane Database of Systematic Reviews* Issue (4), CD000400.

Lethaby, A., Hickey, M., Garry, R., & Penninx, J. (2009). Endometrial resection/ablation techniques for heavy menstrual bleeding. *Cochrane Database Systematic Reviews*, CD001501.

Lethaby, A., Irvine, G., & Cameron, I. (2003). Cyclical progestogens for heavy menstrual bleeding (review). *Cochrane Database of Systematic Reviews*, CD001016.

Levine, S. (2006). Dysfunctional uterine bleeding in adolescents. *Journal of Pediatric Adolescent Gynecology, 19*, 49–51.

Mohan, S., Page, L. M., & Higham, J. M. (2007). Diagnosis of abnormal uterine bleeding. *Best Practice & Research in Clinical Obstetrics and Gynaecology, 21*(6), 891–903.

Nicholson, W. K., Ellison, S. A., Grason, H., & Powe, N. R. (2001). Patterns of ambulatory care use for gynecologic conditions: A national study. *American Journal of Obstetrics and Gynecology, 184*(4), 523–530.

Speroff, L., & Fritz, M. A. (2005). Dysfunctional uterine bleeding. In L. Speroff and M. A. Fritz (Eds.), *Clinical gynecologic endocrinology and infertility* (7th ed., pp. 547–571). Philadelphia, PA: Wolters Kluwer/Lippincott Williams & Wilkins.

Star, W. L., & Okasako, J. Y. (2004). Abnormal uterine bleeding. In W. L. Star, L. L. Lommel, and M. T. Shannon (Eds.), *Women's primary health care: Protocols for practice* (2nd ed., pp. 12-3–12-12). San Francisco, CA: UCSF Nursing Press.

Telner, D. E., & Jakubovicz, D. (2007). Approach to diagnosis and management of abnormal uterine bleeding. *Canadian Family Physician, 53*, 58–64.

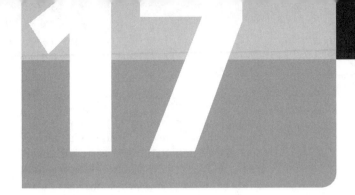

AMENORRHEA AND POLYCYSTIC OVARY SYNDROME

Pilar Bernal de Pheils

I. Introduction and general background

Amenorrhea is classified as primary or secondary. Primary amenorrhea is defined as the lack of initiation of menses by age 14 with concomitant lack of growth of secondary sexual characteristics, such as breast development. If growth of secondary sexual characteristics is present, this diagnosis may be delayed until age 16 (Speroff & Fritz, 2005). Some authorities advise initiating investigation for primary amenorrhea at age 15 as the upper limit and age 13 if there are no sexual characteristics (The Practice Committee of the American Society for Reproductive Medicine, 2006). Secondary amenorrhea is defined as a cessation of menses for more than 6 months, or a duration equivalent to three previous menstrual cycle intervals (Speroff & Fritz, 2005).

Distinguishing primary and secondary amenorrhea is important because the former encompasses a more extensive differential diagnosis that includes genetic or anatomic abnormalities. However, early categorization may lead to an unnecessary work-up (Speroff & Fritz, 2005).

Amenorrhea may result from disturbances at the level of the hypothalamus, pituitary, ovaries, uterus, or outflow tract. Polycystic ovarian syndrome (PCOS) is one of the most common causes of amenorrhea, with disturbances that involve the hypothalamic-pituitary-ovarian axis. Amenorrhea is physiologic during pregnancy, menopause, and in the postpartum period in lactating women.

A. Hypothalamic amenorrhea

1. Definition and overview

Hypothalamic amenorrhea is often used interchangeably with functional hypothalamic amenorrhea (FHA), the most common cause of amenorrhea in this category. In FHA, there is a decrease in gonadotropin-releasing hormone pulsatile secretion causing absent midcycle surges in luteinizing hormone secretion, failure to ovulate, and low serum estradiol concentrations. Low estrogen levels place the woman at risk for osteopenia and osteoporosis. Factors contributing to FHA include nutritional deficiencies, such as marked weight loss and crash dieting, malnutrition, or eating disorders (anorexia and bulimia); excessive exercise; and severe physical or emotional stress. However, in many women with FHA, no obvious precipitating factor is evident.

Untreated primary hypothyroidism can lead to hypothalamic amenorrhea (primary or secondary) by decreasing hypothalamic content of dopamine and increasing prolactin levels with or without resulting galactorrhea (Khawaja et al., 2006). Dopaminergic drugs (e.g., phenothiazines, antipsychotics, and antiemetic-gastrointestinal agents) may also be responsible for hypothalamic amenorrhea. Menses usually return to normal after discontinuation of medications.

2. Prevalence and incidence

Prevalence of adult-onset hypothalamic amenorrhea is 35.5% representing 20% of primary amenorrhea (Reindollar et al., 1986; Reindollar, Byrd, & McDonough, 1981). The "female athlete triad" is defined as amenorrhea, disordered eating, and osteoporosis or osteopenia. This syndrome is especially common in amenorrhea associated with ballet dancing. It is also prevalent in high school (Hoch et al., 2009) and college athletes (Beals & Hill, 2006).

B. Pituitary amenorrhea

1. Definition and overview

Prolactin-secreting tumors are responsible for most cases of amenorrhea attributed to the pituitary. Increased prolactin levels lead to anovulation and low ovarian estradiol levels, causing the same problems as seen in FHA. Hyperprolactinemia can cause galactorrhea. Most prolactinomas are small (< 10 mm in diameter), called microadenomas, and maintain normal pituitary function. Macroadenomas are

10 mm or larger and can exert mass effects causing headaches and vision changes. Prolactin-secreting tumors can be present in the premenarchal female and present as primary amenorrhea. Pituitary tumors should be suspected when patients have signs of acromegaly (excessive secretion of growth hormone). Cushing's disease, with excessive secretion of adenocorticotropic hormone and thyroid-stimulating hormone–secreting tumor, which causes secondary hyperthyroidism, are rare but potential causes of amenorrhea. Most of these tumors are associated with headaches and visual changes (Speroff & Fritz, 2005).

Hyperprolactinemia can also be caused by decreased clearance of dopamine in patients with chronic renal or liver impairment. Other causes of pituitary amenorrhea are Sheehan syndrome (severe postpartum hemorrhage causing acute infarction and necrosis of the pituitary gland) and empty sella syndrome. Lastly, hyperprolactinemia may be functional (idiopathic), found in about one-third of women (Speroff & Fritz, 2005).

2. Prevalence and incidence

Prolactin-secreting pituitary tumor (prolactinoma) is responsible for almost 20% of cases of secondary amenorrhea and is the most common pituitary etiology of amenorrhea (Reindollar et al., 1986). Pituitary disease is less common in primary amenorrhea, accounting for 5% of cases (Reindollar et al., 1981).

C. Amenorrhea originating from disorders of the ovaries

1. Definition and overview
   a. PCOS (discussed later as a separate category).
   b. Premature ovarian failure (POF) is defined as menopause before the age of 40. The average age of menopause is 51 with a range from 47–55. POF is best described as primary ovarian insufficiency because this condition may have periods of follicular development, ovulation, and menstrual bleeding followed by periods of hypoestrogenemia and anovulation. Causes of POF include autoimmune disorders, such as adrenal insufficiency and hypothyroidism; karyotypic abnormalities (Turner syndrome and mosaicism); and idiopathic causes. Radiotherapy and chemotherapy can also cause ovarian failure.
   c. Gonadal dysgenesis (karyotypic abnormalities as described previously) can present with primary or secondary amenorrhea.

2. Prevalence and incidence

Ovarian failure with normal chromosomes is more common than failure with abnormal karyotypes (Speroff & Fritz, 2005). Chromosomal abnormalities and gonadal dysgenesis are more common causes of primary amenorrhea than secondary amenorrhea (Reindollar et al., 1981).

D. Amenorrhea originating from disorders of the outflow tract or uterus

1. Definition and overview

End-organ abnormalities are rare in secondary amenorrhea. If present, the etiology is caused by Asherman syndrome, manifested clinically by very scant menstrual bleeding or amenorrhea. In almost all cases there is a history of uterine manipulation, such as a dilatation and curettage or other surgical procedures resulting in uterine scarring.

Congenital anomalies can lead to anatomic alterations in the genital tract, causing primary amenorrhea. These abnormalities include müllerian anomalies (vaginal septum or imperforate hymen) and müllerian agenesis (absence of the uterus and upper vagina). Ovaries are present as are secondary sex characteristics.

Androgen insensitivity is another etiology of primary amenorrhea. These patients are phenotypic females with some breast development, minimal axillary and pubic hair, external genitalia, blind vaginal canal, and absent uterus; however, they are genotypic males with testes, XY karyotype, and unresponsive androgen receptors but normal to high range of male testosterone levels.

2. Prevalence and incidence

Prevalence of Asherman syndrome is unknown (Berman, 2008). Müllerian abnormalities and complete androgen sensitivity are, with gonadal dysgenesis described previously, the most common causes of primary amenorrhea (Speroff & Fritz, 2005).

E. PCOS

1. Definition and overview

PCOS is one of the most common causes of anovulation. It is a syndrome, not a disease, reflecting multiple potential etiologies with variable clinical expression. Hallmarks of the syndrome are chronic anovulation, hyperandrogenism, and insulin resistance. Women with PCOS are frequently overweight (Vrbikova & Hainer, 2009). Regardless of obesity, insulin resistance is present, which poses risks for long-term metabolic sequelae and cardiovascular disease. Up to 30% of patients with PCOS also have metabolic syndrome (American College of Obstetrics and Gynecology [ACOG], 2009). Depression and anxiety in women with PCOS is increased independent of obesity (Jedel et al., 2010; Vrbikova & Hainer, 2009). Endometrial cancer may also be increased in women with PCOS because anovulation, central obesity, and diabetes are all risk factors for this cancer.

The 2003 Rotterdam PCOS Consensus Workshop Group (2004), redefined the diagnosis as the presentation of two of the following three criteria:

    a. Oligo-ovulation or anovulation (irregular cycles)

    b. Clinical or biochemical markers of hyperandrogenism

    c. Polycystic ovaries on ultrasonography and exclusion of other etiologies

The androgen society considers hyperandrogenism as essential to this diagnosis (ACOG, 2009).

PCOS remains a diagnosis of exclusion. Other conditions to be ruled out are hypothyroidism, hyperprolactinemia, ovarian or adrenal tumor, late-onset adrenal hyperplasia, and Cushing syndrome. Women with PCOS are at risk for infertility. If they become pregnant they are at an increased risk for gestational diabetes and hypertension (Altieri et al., 2010).

2. Prevalence and incidence

PCOS is frequently undiagnosed in the community. Its prevalence varies from a high of $17.8 \pm 2.8\%$ to a low of $10.2 \pm 2.2\%$ (March et al., 2010; Rotterdam PCOS Consensus Workshop Group, 2004).

II. **Database** (may include but is not limited to)

A. *Subjective*

1. Amenorrhea
   a. Past health history
      i. Medical illnesses (Table 17-1)
      ii. Surgical history: recent history of dilatation and curettage
      iii. Obstetric and gynecological: recent history of severe postpartum hemorrhage or oophorectomy
      iv. Exposure history: radiation or chemotherapy directed to the pelvic organs
      v. Medication history: dopamine adrenergic drugs or hormonal contraceptives (particularly oral contraceptives) (Table 17-1)

   b. Family history
      i. Delayed or absent puberty
      ii. POF
      iii. Fragile X syndrome, developmental or intellectual disabilities
      iv. Congenital abnormalities (e.g., Turner syndrome)
      v. Autoimmune disorders
   c. Occupational and environmental history
      i. Work-related exposures: radiation
   d. Personal and social history
      i. Severe stress, malnutrition, crash diet, excessive exercise
   e. Review of systems
      i. Constitutional symptoms: hot flushes or night sweats
      ii. Skin, hair, and nails: lanugo (anorexia)
      iii. Nose: anosmia (Kallmann syndrome)
      iv. Eyes: blurred vision if pituitary tumor (may be a late symptom in patients with macroadenomas)
      v. Breast: galactorrhea (hyperprolactinemia).
      vi. Genitourinary: oligomenorrhea (may precede amenorrhea), vaginal dryness if hypoestrogenic state, cyclical pelvic pain in primary amenorrhea
      vii. Endocrine: hot or cold sensitivity (suspect thyroid disease); fatigue polydypsia, polyphagia (pituitary disease)
      viii. Neurologic: headaches (may be a late symptom in patients with macroadenomas and other pituitary lesions) particularly associated with blurred vision; change in personality, report of marked mood changes (infiltrative pituitary lesions)

2. PCOS
   a. Ethnicity
      Consider congenital adrenal hyperplasia in women of Ashkenazi Jewish descent, Hispanics, Yugoslavs, Native American Inuits, Alaskans, or Italians (ACOG, 2009).
   b. Past health history
      i. Medical illnesses: metabolic syndrome may be present concomitantly or be the result of PCOS
      ii. Obstetric and gynecological history: menstrual irregularities and infertility or pregnancy complications (gestational diabetes and pregnancy-induced hypertension)
      iii. Mental illness: depression or anxiety
   c. Family history
      i. PCOS or other endocrinopathies

TABLE 17-1 Amenorrhea and PCOs Important Etiologies

Classification	Likely Etiology
Hypothalamic amenorrhea	Functional hypothalamic amenorrhea (common etiology for primary or secondary amenorrhea) <ul><li>Anorexia</li><li>Stress</li><li>Rapid weight loss</li><li>Excessive exercise</li><li>No precipitating event (idiopathic)</li></ul> Most likely presenting with primary amenorrhea <ul><li>Gonadotropin-releasing hormone deficiency, Kallmann syndrome if associated with anosmia</li></ul> Infiltrative lesions of the hypothalamus
Pituitary amenorrhea	Physiologic: breastfeeding Pathologic (pituitary): <ul><li>Prolactin-secreting hormone (most common)</li></ul> Other conditions <ul><li>Primary hypothyroidism</li><li>Cushing syndrome</li><li>Adrenocorticotropic hormone secreting hormone</li><li>Thyroid-stimulating hormone secreting tumor</li><li>Other tumors</li><li>Renal failure</li><li>Cirrhosis</li><li>Sheehan syndrome</li><li>Empty sella syndrome</li></ul>
Amenorrhea originating from disorders of the ovaries	Physiologic: menopause Pathologic: Local disturbance of ovarian conditions <ul><li>History of infection (tuberculosis, mumps)</li><li>History of radiation therapy or cytotoxic drugs</li><li>History of autoimmune disorders leading to premature ovarian failure</li></ul> Problems in gonadal development that can present either with primary or secondary amenorrhea <ul><li>Turner syndrome</li><li>Mosaicism</li></ul> Most likely explanation of secondary amenorrhea: Polycystic ovary syndrome–hyperandrogenism (caused by internal–external sources) Premature ovarian failure (common); supply of oocytes are depleted before age 40 <ul><li>Consider autoimmune disorders</li></ul>
Amenorrhea originating from disorders of the outflow tract	Abnormalities in the first compartment are rare in secondary amenorrhea If present, is caused by destruction of the endometrium, from dilatation and curettage resulting in uterine scarring (Asherman syndrome) Congenital anomalies can lead to anatomic alterations in the genital tract mostly causing primary amenorrhea <ul><li>Müllerian anomalies and agenesis (ovaries are present because they are not müllerian structures)</li><li>Complete androgen insensitivity (testicular feminization)</li></ul>

TABLE 17-1 Amenorrhea and PCOs Important Etiologies *(continued)*

Classification	Likely Etiology
Pharmacologic	Medications causing dopamine receptor blockade:
	Tranquilizers (phenothiazines derivates)
	Antipsychotics (risperidone)
	Antidepressants (desipramine, monoamine oxidase)
	Antihypertensive (methyldopa, reserpine, verapamil)
	Narcotics: opiates and heroin
	Gastrointestinal medications: metoclopramide (Reglan), cimetidine, domperidone
	Hormonal contraceptives (high-dose progestin)
	Danazol (androgen-like medication for endometriosis treatment)
Polycystic ovary syndrome	Unknown etiology. It is a syndrome, not a disease, reflecting multiple potential etiologies with variable clinical expression comprised of anovulation, hyperandrogenism, and insulin resistance

    d.   Personal and social history
        Waist and central obesity

    e.   Review of systems

        i.   Constitutional signs and symptoms: fatigue

        ii.   Skin and hair: acne, oily skin, acanthosis negricans (neck, axilla, under breast, or groins), hirsutism, and androgenic alopecia

        iii.   Genitourinary: irregular menses or amenorrhea

        iv.   Neurologic: depressive symptoms

B. Objective

    1.   Physical examination findings for both amenorrhea and PCOS (Table 17-2). Patient may also have a benign examination.

    2.   Supporting data from relevant diagnostic tests (Tables 17-3A–17-3C).

III. Assessment

A. Diagnosis

Diagnosis of amenorrhea is determined by its onset (primary or secondary); significant findings from the history physical examination; and the diagnostic tests discussed previously. Most prevalent etiologies encountered in primary care are as follows:

    1.   Primary or secondary amenorrhea caused by:

        a.   Hypothalamic etiology most likely functional hypothalamic

        b.   Pituitary etiology, most likely hyperprolactinemia or prolactinoma

        c.   Ovarian disorders, most likely POF in secondary amenorrhea or ovarian dysgenesis in primary amenorrhea (Turner syndrome and mosaicism)

        d.   Disorders of the outflow tract, most likely Asherman syndrome in secondary amenorrhea or müllerian agenesis or dysgenesis or complete androgen insensitivity in primary amenorrhea

        e.   PCOS

    2.   Other conditions that may explain the patient's presentation in PCOS are:

        a.   Thyroid disease (most likely primary hypothyroidism)

        b.   Late-onset adrenal hyperplasia

        c.   Androgen-producing tumor

        d.   Cushing disease

IV. Goals of clinical management

Select a treatment plan that helps the patient restore normalcy of her menstrual cycle and fertility, if she desires, and prevent long-term consequences of hypoestrogenic state or unopposed estrogen stimulation of the endometrium.

V. Plan

A. Diagnostic tests

Tables 17-3A–17-3C provide descriptions of relevant diagnostic studies.

    1.   All women late for their menses or with oligoamenorrhea should have a urine pregnancy test to rule out pregnancy.

    2.   Evaluation of the following diagnostic testing: prolactin, thyroid-stimulating hormone, and follicle-stimulating hormone (FSH) (Table 17-3A).

    3.   Some clinicians perform a progesterone withdrawal test in the initial evaluation of amenorrhea to determine endogenous estrogen status; others do not advocate for this test arguing poor sensitivity and specificity (ACOG, 2004; Speroff & Fritz, 2005).

TABLE 17-2 Physical Examination Findings and Likely Etiologies in Amenorrhea and PCOS*

Organ or System	Examination Findings	Likely Etiologies
Vitals	Increased blood pressure	High blood pressure may be present in pituitary diseases (e.g., Cushing disease); karyotype abnormalities (e.g., Turner syndrome); or associated with PCOS
Anthropometric measurements Body mass index	< 18.5 kg/m² – underweight or 25.0–29.9 kg/m² – overweight and > 30 kg/m² – obesity	Underweight may be present in functional hypothalamic amenorrhea (e.g., anorexia) Overweight or obesity may be present in PCOS or Cushing disease Waist circumference > 88 cm (35 in) is predictive of PCOS (Starr et al., 2004).
Height	Short stature	Consistent with Turner syndrome
General appearance	Mood affect, manner Change in personality, marked mood changes	Depression associated with PCOS Rare hypothalamic lesions
Hair	Excess terminal (thick pigmented) body hair in a male distribution, as seen in upper lip, sideburn area, chin, chest, inner thighs, lower back, lower abdomen, and buttocks Absent axillary and pubic hair Lanugo	PCOS Androgen-secreting tumor Thyroid disease Androgen insensitivity Anorexia
Skin	Acne, acanthosis negricans Dry, moist, warm, cold, rough Skin atrophy, easy bruisability, purple striae	Present in hypandrogenic, hyperinsulinemic states Thyroid disorders Cushing disease
Face	Moon face	Cushing disease
Eyes	Visual field defects Stare, lid lag, exophtamus	Pituitary tumor Hypothyroidism or Cushing disease
Neck	Thyroid enlargement Supraclavicular fat pads ("buffalo hump") Webbed neck	Thyroid disease Cushing disease Turner syndrome
Breast	Secretions and galactorrhea expressed from multiple ducts. Breast secretions under microscope reveal fat globules confirming galactorrhea. Undeveloped breast in primary amenorrhea	Occurs in 80% of patients with hyperprolactinemia Primary amenorrhea likely caused by karyotype abnormalities
Abdomen	Striae (purple) Inguinal nodes or masses Organomelia	Cushing disease Androgen insensitivity, where testes may be in a hernia (Speroff & Fritz, 2005) Growth hormone tumor (acromegaly)
Pelvic examination	Scant hair on mons pubis Vulvar or vaginal atrophy Clitoromegaly Imperforate hymen, vaginal pouch Enlarged ovaries	Androgen insensitivity Hypoestrogenic state as in premature ovarian failure Virilizing effect as in androgen tumor Müllerian abnormalities May be palpated if PCOS
Extremities	Wasting, edema Enlarged, swollen hands and feet increasing shoe and glove size	Cushing disease Acromegaly (rare)

Abbreviation: PCOS, polycystic ovary syndrome.

* Directed to organs and systems based on subjective information; examination may be benign.

TABLE 17-3A Essential Testing in the Investigation of Amenorrhea

Test	Definition	Clinical Implications	Comments
Urine pregnancy test	Measures the beta subunit of human chorionic gonadotropin hormone	Pregnancy is the most common cause of amenorrhea. This diagnosis must be ruled out in sexually active women before embarking on any additional work-up.	Pregnancy detection by urine human chorionic gonadotropin relative to the expected first day of menses (Wilcox et al., 2001) • Two days before (79%) • Seven days after (97%) • Eleven days after (100%)
Prolactin	Prolactin is produced by the lactotrophs of the anterior pituitary Serum prolactin elevation causes amenorrhea by inhibiting pulsatile gonadotropin-releasing hormone secretion. This inhibits follicle-stimulating hormone and luteinizing hormone secretion resulting in anovulation and low ovarian estrogen production Normal prolactin varies from 15 to 20 mcg	Prolactin levels measured > 50 mcg (or galactorrhea, or visual disturbances) deserves consultation to order a magnetic resonance image to rule out microadenoma or macroadenoma or other pituitary tumors or lesions (some practitioners would say 100 mcg) Prolactin < 100 mcg may be caused by dopamine agonist drugs, polycystic ovary syndrome, hypothyroidism, or functional (idiopathic); or may be caused by a microadenoma Prolactin > 150 mcg most likely indicates a prolactinoma (Casanueva et al. 2006)	Prolactin is best drawn fasting, early in the morning. Pregnancy, stress, intercourse, breast stimulation, and meals, can increase levels Prolactin may be mildly elevated in patients with polycystic ovary syndrome (Casanueva et al., 2006) or with long-standing hypothyroidism (Speroff & Fritz, 2005) If prolactin elevations are mild, repeat on a different day (Casanueva et al., 2006)
Highly sensitive thyroid-stimulating hormone	Measurement of thyroid-stimulating hormone: an anterior pituitary hormone that stimulates growth and function of thyroid cells	An elevated thyroid-stimulating hormone accompanying prolactin levels < 100 ng/ml is diagnostic of primary hypothyroidism (Speroff & Fritz, 2005)	Very few patients with amenorrhea or galactorrhea may have subclinical hypothyroidism that is not clinically apparent (Speroff & Fritz, 2005)
Follicle-stimulating hormone	Measures the amount of follicle-stimulating hormone produced by the anterior pituitary	Follicle-stimulating hormone ≥ 30 IU/L points to ovarian failure (premature ovarian failure) or insufficiency or gonadal dysgenesis in primary amenorrhea (with absent breast development in the latter case) a. Normal or low follicle-stimulating hormone concentrations indicate anovulation likely caused by hypothalamic or pituitary etiology in secondary amenorrhea, or polycystic ovary syndrome Müllerian dysgenesis in primary amenorrhea (anatomic defect)	Intermittent follicular development and normalization of follicle-stimulating hormone values may occur in premature ovarian failure
Progesterone challenge test	Useful in evaluating the status of estrogen production Administer progestins for 3–10 days. Bleeding is expected 2–7 days after discontinuation of the progestin (may bleed as late as 15 days later if ovulation triggered) Oral progestins available: Provera, 10 mg daily for 5–10 days, or micronized progesterone, 200 mcg at bedtime for 3–5 days	Progesterone challenge test is negative in patients who do not bleed after progestin withdrawal, which indicates lack of estrogen or end organ problems (Asherman syndrome) Progesterone challenge test is positive in patients who bleed 2–7 days after progestin withdrawal. This indicates that estrogen is being produced by the ovaries.	Some clinicians advocate the performance of progesterone challenge test to help in the interpretation of follicle-stimulating hormone values, and to assist in therapy decision making; need estrogen therapy for prevention of bone loss (Speroff & Fritz, 2005). Other clinicians do not advocate for the progesterone challenge test because of their stated false-positive and false-negative results (Fertility and Sterility, 2006)

TABLE 17-3B Second-Line Testing in the Investigation of Amenorrhea, including Tests Where Consultation or Referral is Suggested

Test	Definition	Clinical Implications	Comments
Abdominal–pelvic ultrasound	Ultrasound imaging to evaluate internal organs if unable to perform a pelvic examination, and particularly in the case of primary amenorrhea	Absent uterus, vaginal septum, or congenital absence of the vagina	Abdominal–pelvic sonogram may be useful to confirm the presence of a uterus and ovaries. Absent uterus and vagina is likely caused by müllerian dysgenesis or androgen insensitivity in primary amenorrhea.
MRI of the sella turcica to evaluate for prolactinomas (prolactin-secreting tumors) or other rare pituitary–hypothalamic tumors	The goal of imaging is to evaluate the possibility of a hypothalamic or pituitary lesion	In the case of a prolactinoma the image allows determination of a microadenoma or a macroadenoma (≤ 1 or > 1 cm, respectively) Abnormal imaging (or hyperprolactinemia) requires referral to a specialist	All women with high serum prolactin values (≥ 50 mcg/L; some practitioners would say > 100 mcg/L) should have imaging of the sella turcica (MRI) MRI is also indicated if galactorrhea, headaches, or visual field disturbances are present in the evaluation of amenorrhea MRI is indicated when delayed puberty and hypogonadism (Speroff & Fritz, 2005)
24-hour urine for free cortisol excretion if suspicion of Cushing disease	Tests to evaluate the possibility of Cushing disease	The urinary cortisol excretion should be unequivocally increased (threefold above the upper limit of normal for the assay) Mild elevations can be seeing in patients with polycystic ovary syndrome	Validity of the results depends on the collection of a complete 24-hour specimen and a reliable reference laboratory Other tests to rule out Cushing disease are indicated (e.g., rapid suppression test) under the care of a specialist
Karyotype evaluation	To evaluate for abnormal XY chromosomes in any woman diagnosed with premature ovarian failure, if younger than 30 years of age (Speroff & Fritz, 2005) To also evaluate fragile X syndrome permutations carriers	Mosaicism with a Y chromosome requires excision of gonadal areas Malignant tumor formation is highly possible with the presence of any testicular component within the gonad Permutation of fragile X syndrome can result in premature ovarian failure	Most gonadal tumors appear before 20 years of age. A significant number of cases appear between ages 20 and 30. None have been found above age 30 (Speroff & Fritz, 2005). The mechanism by which a permutation causes ovarian failure is not known
Saline-infusion hysterography or hysterosalpingogram	This imaging procedure allows for confirmation of Asherman syndrome	Presence of intrauterine synechiae	Hysteroscopy is used for the final diagnosis and treatment. Hysteroscopic lysis of adhesions is the main method of treatment

Abbreviations: MRI, magnetic resonance imaging; mcg., micrograms; ng, nano-grams; IU, international units

TABLE 17-3C Additional Tests in the Investigation of Polycystic Ovary Syndrome*

Test	Definition	Clinical Implications	Comments
Total and free testosterone	Serum testosterone provides the best estimate of androgen production. Total testosterone is more widely available and better standardized than free testosterone (free testosterone is the best estimate of bioavailable testosterone).	Testosterone values may be normal in women with PCOS Testosterone is in the male range in women with androgen insensitivity Total testosterone may be elevated (> 60 ng/dl), but is not required for the diagnosis of PCOS Values > 200 ng/dl are most likely caused by androgen-producing tumors	If free testosterone is performed, clinicians should be knowledgeable of local laboratory values because they vary greatly and the sensitivity and reliability are poor (ACOG, 2009). An elevation in free testosterone is the most sensitive test to establish the presence of hyperandrogenemia (Cho et al., 2008).
Dehydroepiandrosterone sulfate	A direct measurement of adrenal androgen activity. This test may be ordered to rule out androgen-secreting tumor.	Upper limit of normal is 350 ng/dl. It may vary by laboratory. It may also be mildly elevated in PCOS	It is most useful in the evaluation of rapid virilization, not as useful in common hirsutism (ACOG, 2009).
17-Hydroxy-progesterone	Serum blood test that evaluates adult-onset adrenal hyperplasia (caused by 21-hydroxylase deficiency).	Fasting, in the follicular phase: < 200 ng/dl excludes adult-onset adrenal hyperplasia	Limit test to high-risk women with hirsutism (Speroff & Fritz, 2005).
Pelvic ultrasound	To evaluate for presence of polycystic ovaries perform sonogram ideally days 3–5 of the menstrual cycle.	Polycystic ovaries are present when • 12 or more follicles are seen in one of the ovaries • Follicles measure 2–9 mm in diameter • Increase in ovarian volume > 10 ml	The appearance of polycystic ovaries is nonspecific. It can also be seen in women with normal hormonal function or with other androgen excess disorders. Hence it is not recommended solely for the evaluation of PCOS. If done, patients should not be on oral contraceptives because these medications can change the ovarian morphology.

Abbreviation: PCOS, polycystic ovary syndrome; ng, nano-grams

* PCOS is a diagnosis of exclusion. If initial testing for the investigation of amenorrhea and oligomenorrhea rules out other conditions the following tests are advised to rule out other hyperandrogenic conditions.

4. Diagnostic work-up in the adolescent with primary amenorrhea is based on the presence of breast development; secondary sexual characteristics; and the presence of the uterus and an intact outflow tract, likely determined with an ultrasound. If all are present and FSH is normal, the work-up should focus on the etiology of secondary amenorrhea. If there is no breast development and the FSH level is elevated, the probable diagnosis is gonadal dysgenesis. A karyotype should then be ordered. If the uterus or outflow tract is not present and the FSH

values are normal, then the diagnostic test should be directed to diagnose müllerian agenesis or androgen insensitivity syndrome. In the latter, circulating testosterone is in the male range and a karyotype confirms the presence of a Y chromosome.

5. Second-line diagnostic tests in the investigation of amenorrhea include tests where consultation and referral are suggested (Table 17-3B).

6. Magnetic resonance imaging (MRI) or computerized tomography scanning (not as sensitive but less

expensive) for the evaluation of a pituitary tumor in the setting of hyperprolactinemia, galactorrhea, or headaches and vision field changes.

7. Twenty-four–hour urine testing for free cortisol excretion if Cushing syndrome is suspected.

8. Serum insulinlike growth factor-1 if acromegaly is present.

9. Adrenal antibodies to 21-hydroxylase in the evaluation of autoimmune disorders leading to POF.

10. Karyotype, including fragile X testing, in any woman younger than 30 years of age diagnosed with POF (Speroff & Fritz, 2005), or for women presenting with primary amenorrhea.

11. Saline infusion hysterography or hysterosalpingogram, for the confirmation of intrauterine synechiae present in Asherman syndrome. Initial investigation of Asherman syndrome, in the setting of secondary amenorrhea and history of instrumentation, is performed by "priming" the uterus with 1 month of any low-dose combined oral contraceptive. Lack of withdrawal bleeding is highly suspicious of Asherman syndrome (Speroff & Fritz, 2005).

12. Abdominal and pelvic ultrasound to confirm the presence of the uterus.

13. There are no specific tests for the diagnosis of PCOS. Conditions that can mimic PCOS must first be excluded.

14. Women diagnosed with PCOS should have testing for the investigation of insulin resistance and metabolic abnormalities, including 2-hour oral glucose tolerance test and fasting lipids.

15. Additional testing to consider can be found in Table 17-3C.

B. Management

Therapeutic management of amenorrhea depends on its etiology, the goals of the woman including her desire for pregnancy, and the long-term consequences of her condition.

1. Hypothalamic amenorrhea

   a. Address the underlying condition and issues related to hypothalamic amenorrhea (e.g., eating disorders or excessive exercise) that may negatively impact ovulation and normal menstrual cycle. Cognitive behavioral therapy, designed to identify maladaptive attitudes toward eating and weight, and problem-solving strategies and coping skills to improve healthy eating behaviors have demonstrated

improvement of hypothalamic function (Berga et al., 2003).

   b. Begin oral replacement with estrogen to prevent osteoporosis. Any low-dose oral contraceptive method provides the necessary estrogen replacement in a woman during the reproductive years, in addition to providing contraception.

   c. Supplement with calcium and vitamin D to strengthen bone health.

   d. Refer to reproductive endocrinology if pregnancy is desired. Some women may respond to clomiphene citrate; most require gonadotropin-releasing hormone.

2. Pituitary amenorrhea

   a. In hyperprolactinemia and pituitary adenomas the treatment goal is to establish normal estrogen secretion, menstrual function, and tumor reduction if a macroadenoma. Therapy is indicated for all patients with macroadenoma and in most patients with microadenomas, particularly if there are bothersome symptoms and desired fertility, and for the prevention of osteoporosis (Casanueva et al., 2006). These patients may need trans-sphenoidal surgery or radiation therapy (Casanueva et al.). Women desiring fertility may need induction of ovulation, although in many cases pharmacologic management of hyperprolactenemia establishes ovulatory cycles.

   b. Dopamine agonists, such as bromocriptine and cabergoline, are the drug of choice for women with hyperprolactinemia and prolactinomas. These medications decrease the size of the prolactinomas, restore menstrual function and prolactin levels to normal, and ameliorate galactorrhea. Cabergoline is better tolerated, is more convenient, and has been demonstrated to be more effective in reduction of prolactin levels when used up to 2 years (Dekkers et al., 2010). Bromocriptine, however, has been used for many more years and is less expensive.

      i. If cost is an issue start with bromocriptine tablets, 2.5 mg at bedtime or half a pill twice a day, increasing levels weekly to the lowest possible that maintains normal prolactin levels, generally twice or occasionally three times a day dosing (Speroff & Fritz, 2005).

      ii. Side effects of bromocriptine are nausea, constipation, headache, faintness caused by orthostatic hypotension, headache, and nasal stuffiness. Side effects can be minimized by taking the pill at bedtime along with a snack, by increasing the dose slowly as described previously, or by administering the 2.5-mg tablet high into the vagina at bedtime avoiding the first pass through the liver and achieving therapeutic results at lower doses (Speroff & Fritz, 2005).

   iii. Cabergoline can be started at a dose of 0.5 mg, one-half to one tablet administered once or twice weekly. The dose is increased monthly until prolactin levels normalize. Doses over 3 mg per week are rarely necessary (Casanueva et al., 2006).

   iv. In a considerable proportion of patients, discontinuation of dopamine agonist medication results in resumption of symptoms, the tumor, and hyperprolactinemia.

c. Dopaminergic treatment may reestablish ovulation, even before the first normal menstruation. The woman needs contraception if she wants to prevent pregnancy (Casanueva et al., 2006).

d. Very few patients with microadenomas progress to larger tumors. Amenorrheic women with microadenomas do not need to be treated with dopamine agonist unless they want to become pregnant or they have bothersome galactorrhea. However, they need to be treated with estrogen and should have annual evaluations of serum prolactin. Request an MRI when prolactin rises significantly or symptoms of tumor expansion ensue (Casanueva et al., 2006). Estrogen should be provided with progestins. Any low-dose oral hormonal contraception can be recommended (Speroff & Fritz, 2005).

e. Calcium and vitamin D supplementation is advised in the amenorrheic patient for the prevention of osteoporosis.

f. Correct hypothyroidism.

g. Address hyperprolactinemia induced by medications. Review the patient medication profile for drugs that cause hyperprolactinemia and amenorrhea, such as dopamine agonist drugs and estrogen or danazol. Withdrawal of the drug for 72 hours, if able to do this safely, helps elucidate if the drug is responsible for hyperprolactinemia. MRI should be considered if this alternative is not feasible, particularly in patients with neurologic symptoms to rule out a pituitary lesion (Casanueva et al., 2006).

3. Ovarian disorders

a. Primary amenorrhea: refer patients diagnosed with Turner syndrome or mosaicism to a physician. Patients with Turner syndrome need a multidisciplinary approach for management including the approach for primary or secondary amenorrhea. It is critical to review with the woman in a sensitive manner the consequences of POF and the need for early estrogen to induce pubertal development in the case of primary amenorrhea and to protect bone health during the adult life (Bondy, 2007).

b. Secondary amenorrhea caused by POF

   i. Order a karyotype if woman is 30 years old or younger. Refer if the karyotype is abnormal. Malignant tumor formation within the gonad is associated in mosaicism with a Y chromosome. Removal of the gonadal areas is required (Speroff & Fritz, 2005).

   ii. In women younger than 35 consider an evaluation of autoimmune disorders.

   iii. Advise all women with POF to establish standard hormonal therapy with estrogen therapy. Therapy is advised at least until age 50 to prevent osteoporosis (Ostberg et al., 2007; Kalantaridou & Nelson, 2000). Progestin should be added to estrogen to protect the endometrium if there is an intact uterus. Hormonal treatment also reduces menopausal symptoms.

   iv. Women with POF commonly experience unpredictable and intermittent ovarian function (Rebar & Connolly, 1990). For women who wish to avoid pregnancy, offer any low-dose combined oral contraception instead of hormonal therapy because the estrogen doses in the hormonal therapy are not high enough to prevent pregnancy. The possibility of vasomotor symptoms during the cyclical hormone-free pill interval should be addressed.

   v. Refer women who desire pregnancy to an infertility specialist. Women with POF are candidates for ovum donation or adoption. Although rare, these women may become pregnant spontaneously (Check & Katsoff, 2006).

4. Disorders of the outflow tract

a. Primary amenorrhea

   i. Refer patients suspected of or diagnosed with androgen insensitivity to a specialist. Patients with this condition need removal of gonads to prevent the development of gonadal neoplasia. Gonadectomy is usually delayed until puberty in patients with complete androgen insensitivity syndrome.

These patients have a normal pubertal growth spurt and feminize at the time of expected puberty; tumors do not usually develop until after this time (Speroff & Fritz, 2005). These patients require psychologic counseling given that they have female phenotype and male karyotype (Speroff & Fritz, 2005).

ii. Refer patients diagnosed with müllerian abnormalities or agenesis to a specialist. Surgery is needed if there is vaginal outlet obstruction to allow passage of menstrual blood. Creation of a neovagina for patients with müllerian agenesis is usually delayed until the woman is emotionally mature and ready to participate in the postoperative care required to maintain vaginal patency (Speroff & Fritz, 2005).

b. Secondary amenorrhea: refer patients to a specialist if Asherman syndrome is suspected. Final diagnosis is made with hysteroscopy performed by lysis of adhesions during the diagnostic procedure (Speroff & Fritz, 2005).

5. PCOS

Treatment goals should be directed to control menstrual irregularities; management of hyperandrogenic manifestations (acne and hirsutism); infertility issues; and the long-term consequences of hyperinsulinemia.

a. Advise weight loss and regular exercise. Although the best treatment approach in obese PCOS patients remains to be defined, weight loss is the first-choice recommendation for the treatment of the clinical manifestations of PCOS, such as menstrual cycle irregularities, infertility, and hirsutism (Vrbikova & Hainer, 2009). A 5% weight loss has shown improvement in ovulatory cycles (ACOG, 2009).

b. Pharmacologic treatment for menstrual irregularities and hyperandrogenic manifestations include:

i. Any low-dose oral contraceptives, which may decrease bioavailable testosterone levels by 40–60% (ACOG, 2009; Sheehan, 2004).

ii. Metformin, although not approved by the Food and Drug Administration for PCOS management, is widely used for its anti-insulinic effects. The dose suggested to treat women with PCOS is 1,500–2,000 mg per day given in divided doses (De Leo et al., 2009). Metformin is preferred over other classes of anti-insulinic drugs because the medication tends to decrease weight (ACOG, 2009).

iii. Discuss contraception in women who do not desire pregnancy and are taking metformin because ovulation rates can improve with metformin.

c. Management of hirsutism can be additionally accomplished by:

i. Oral contraceptives: although the Food and Drug Administration has not approved them for the management of hirsutism, observational and nonrandomized studies have shown some benefit (ACOG, 2009).

ii. Antiandrogen medications: consult with a specialist for the prescription of these medications (ACOG, 2009). For spironolactone the usual dosage is 25–100 mg, twice a day. It may take up to 6 months to observe full clinical effect. A fifth of women on this medication may experience metrorrhagia if the dose is in the upper limit (Helfer, Miller, & Rose, 1988). Use cautiously in women with renal impairment because of hyperkalemia. Rarely, exposure has resulted in ambiguous genitalia in male infants. Offer mechanical hair removal (laser treatment).

d. Treatment to reduce risk of cardiovascular disease and diabetes.

e. Medical therapy for women with PCOS desiring pregnancy: the antiestrogen clomiphene citrate remains the drug of choice for ovulation induction. Discussion of ovulation induction is beyond the scope of this chapter.

C. Client education

1. Information: provide verbal and, preferably, written information regarding:

a. Risk-reduction strategies and screening for osteoporosis in women with hypothalamic and pituitary amenorrhea, and for metabolic syndrome and endometrial hyperplasia in women with PCOS.

b. The disease process: signs and symptoms and underlying etiologies.

c. Diagnostic tests: preparation, cost, the procedures, and after-care.

d. Medication management: rationale, action, use, side effects, associated risks, cost of therapeutic interventions, and the need for adhering to long-term treatment plans.

2. Counseling

Women interested in becoming pregnant should be counseled on possible therapeutic options and possible referral to reproductive and endocrinology specialists.

VI. Self-management resources and tools

A. Patient and client education

The Merck Source: Resource Library (2010) at http://www.mercksource.com includes education on amenorrhea under the title "Menstruation-absent," addressing definitions of primary and secondary amenorrhea, each with hyperlinks to the multiple etiologies. Additional education can be found at www.mayoclinic.com. The Mayo Clinic website includes definitions, symptoms, causes, preparing for appointments and tests, diagnosis, treatment, drugs, lifestyles issues, and home remedies.

B. Community support groups

Women with POF can consult the Premature Ovarian Failure Support group at www.posupport.org., created by the nonprofit organization The International Premature Ovarian Failure Support Group, Alexandria, VA (e-mail: info@pofsupport.org; tel. 703-913-4787).

REFERENCES

Altieri, P., Gambineri, A., Prontera, O., Cionci, G., Franchina, M., & Pasquali R. (2010). Maternal polycystic ovary syndrome may be associated with adverse pregnancy outcomes. *European Journal of Obstetrics, Gynecology and Reproductive Biology, 149*(1), 31–36.

American College of Obstetrics and Gynecology. (2004). Current evaluation of amenorrhea. *Fertility and Sterility, 82*(Suppl. 1), 266–272.

American College of Obstetrics and Gynecology. (2004). Revised 2003 consensus on diagnostic criteria and long-term health risks related to polycystic ovary syndrome. *Fertility and Sterility, 81*(1), 19–25.

American College of Obstetrics and Gynecology. (2009). ACOG Practice Bulletin No. 108: Polycystic ovary syndrome. *Obstetrics and Gynecology, 114*(4), 936–949.

Beals, K. A., & Hill, A. K. (2006). The prevalence of disordered eating, menstrual dysfunction, and low bone mineral density among US collegiate athletes. *International Journal of Sport Nutrition and Exercise Metabolism, 16*(1), 1–23.

Berga, S. L., Marcus, M. D., Loucks, T. L., Hlastala, S., Ringham, R., & Krohn, M. A. (2003). Recovery of ovarian activity in women with functional hypothalamic amenorrhea who were treated with cognitive behavior therapy. *Fertility and Sterility, 80*(4), 976–981.

Berman, J. M. (2008). Intrauterine adhesions. *Seminars in Reproductive Medicine, 26*(4), 349–355.

Bondy, C. A. (2007). Care of girls and women with Turner syndrome: A guideline of the Turner Syndrome Study Group. *The Journal of Clinical Endocrinology and Metabolism, 92*(1), 10–25.

Casanueva, F., Molitch, M. E., Schlechte, J. A., Abs, R., Bonert, V., Bronstein, M. D., et al. (2006). Guidelines of the Pituitary Society for the diagnosis and management of prolactinomas. *Clinical Endocrinology, 65*(2), 265–273.

Check, J. H., & Katsoff, B. (2006). Successful pregnancy with spontaneous ovulation in a woman with apparent premature ovarian failure who failed to conceive despite four transfers of embryos derived from donated oocytes. *Clinical and Experimental Obstetrics & Gynecology, 33*(1), 13–15.

De Leo, V., Musacchio, M. C., Palermo, V., Di Sabatino, A., Morgante, G., & Petraglia, F. (2009). Polycystic ovary syndrome and metabolic comorbidities: Therapeutic options. *Drugs Today, 45*(10), 763–775.

Dekkers, O. M., Lagro, J., Burman, P., Jørgensen, J. O., Romijn, J. A., & Pereira, A. M. (2010). Recurrence of hyperprolactinemia after withdrawal of dopamine agonists: Systematic review and meta-analysis. *The Journal of Clinical Endocrinology and Metabolism, 95*(1), 43–51.

Helfer, E. L., Miller, J. L., & Rose, L. I. (1988). Side-effects of spironolactone therapy in the hirsute woman. *The Journal of Clinical Endocrinology and Metabolism, 66*(1), 208–211.

Hoch, A. Z., Pajewski, N. M., Moraski, L., Carrera, G. F., Wilson, C. R., Hoffmann, R. G., . . . Gutterman, D. D. (2009). Prevalence of the female athlete triad in high school athletes and sedentary students. *Clinical Journal of Sport Medicine, 19*(5), 421–428.

Jedel, E., Waern, M., Gustafson, D., Landén, M., Eriksson, E., Holm, G., . . . Sterner-Victorin, E. (2010). Anxiety and depression symptoms in women with polycystic ovary syndrome compared with controls matched for body mass index. *Human Reproduction, 25*(2), 450–456.

Kalantaridou, S. N., & Nelson, L. M. (2000). Premature ovarian failure is not premature menopause. *Annals of the New York Academy of Sciences, 900*, 393–402.

Khawaja, N. M., Taher, B. M., Barham, M. E., Naser, A. A., Hadidy, A. M., Ahmad, A. T., . . . Ajlouni, K. M. (2006). Pituitary enlargement in patients with primary hypothyroidism. *Endocrine Practice, 12*(1), 29–34.

March, W. A., Moore, V. M., Willson, K. J., Phillips, D. I., Norman, R. J., & Davies, M. J. (2010). The prevalence of polycystic ovary syndrome in a community sample assessed under contrasting diagnostic criteria. *Human Reproduction, 25*(2), 544–551.

Ostberg, J. E., Storry, C., Donald, A. E., Attar, M. J., Halcox, J. P., & Conway, G. S. (2007). A dose-response study of hormone replacement in young hypogonadal women: Effects on intima media thickness and metabolism. *Clinical Endocrinology, 66*(4), 557–564.

Rebar, R. W., & Connolly, H. V. (1990). Clinical features of young women with hypergonadotropic amenorrhea. *Fertility and Sterility, 53*(5), 804–810.

Reindollar, R. H., Byrd, J. R., & McDonough, P. G. (1981). Delayed sexual development: A study of 252 patients. *American Journal of Obstetrics and Gynecology, 140*(4), 371–380.

Reindollar, R. H., Novak, M., Tho, S. P., & McDonough, P. G. (1986). Adult-onset amenorrhea: A study of 262 patients. *American Journal of Obstetrics and Gynecology, 155*(3), 531–543.

Rotterdam ESHRE/ASRM-Sponsored PCOS Consensus Workshop Group (2004). Revised 2003 consensus on diagnostic criteria and long-term health risks related to polycystic ovary syndrome. *Fertility and Sterility, 81*(1), 19–25.

Sheehan, M. T. (2004). Polycystic ovarian syndrome: diagnosis and management. *Clinical Medicine & Research, 2*(1), 13–27.

Speroff, L., & Fritz, M. C. (2005). *Clinical Gynecologic Endocrinology and Infertility* (7th ed.). Baltimore, MD: Lippincott Williams & Wilkins.

The Practice Committee of the American Society for Reproductive Medicine. (2004). Current evaluation of amenorrhea. *Fertility and Sterility, 82*(1), 266–72.

The Practice Committee of the American Society for Reproductive Medicine. (2006). Current evaluation of amenorrhea. *Fertility and Sterility, 86*(1), S148–S155.

Vrbikova, J., & Hainer, V. (2009). Obesity and polycystic ovary syndrome. *Obesity Facts, 2*(1), 26–35.

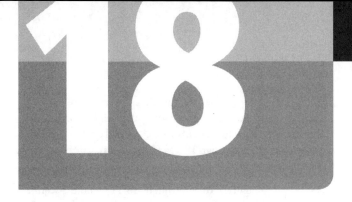

CERVICAL, VAGINAL, AND VULVAR CANCER SCREENING

Mary. M. Rubin and Lynn Hanson

I. Introduction and general background

A. Abnormal cytology

1. Intraepithelial neoplasia (IN), often referred to as dysplasia, is an abnormal precancerous change in cells as they mature. This abnormality can be found in multicentric areas of the lower genital tract, such as the cervix (CIN), vagina (VAIN), vulva (VIN), anus (AIN), and perianus. The natural history of the disease is unpredictable. Mediated by the immune system, the abnormality can regress, persist at the same level, or progress to malignancy.

2. The etiology of the condition is multifactorial, but the dominant agent is human papillomavirus (HPV) (Trottier & Franco, 2006). Over 100 different HPV types exist, but 14 types are considered oncogenic (Einstein, 2008). Worldwide, types 16 and 18 are responsible for 70% of cervical cancers (Parkin, 2006; World Health Organization, 2008). HPV is necessary for malignant cellular transformation, but other cofactors, such as age of first intercourse, number of sexual partners, other sexually transmitted infections (STIs), smoking, diet, stress, and host immunologic status all play a role (Winer et al., 2003). Persistence of high-risk HPV types is also required for progression to high-grade lesions (Kosiol et al., 2008; Trottier et al., 2009). The virus is for the most part sexually transmitted, and is responsible for other noncancerous conditions, such as genital warts (condyloma acuminata).

B. Screening guidelines

1. Screening guidelines for Pap smears have recently undergone major revision (American College of Obstetrics and Gynecology, 2009). The Pap test remains an important modality in determining the health of a woman's cervix, whether it is obtained by using the conventional Pap smear or the newer liquid-based test. It screens for both glandular and squamous cell abnormalities. The use of HPV testing in combination with cervical cytology is approved for screening women 30 years of age or older and as a reflex test in younger women who have atypical cells of undetermined significance reported on their results. Reflex testing involves submitting the cells determined to be atypical for a secondary analysis of the HPV DNA for the presence of high-risk HPV types. It is not necessary to test for low-risk types. HPV testing should not be used in women younger than 21 years, and if inadvertently done, positive results should not influence management.

2. According to the American College of Obstetricians and Gynecologists 2009 guidelines, the newest recommendations for initiation, frequency, and cessation of cervical screening are:

   a. Begin Pap test screening at age 21 and continue every 2 years through age 29.

   b. Women age 30 and older who have had three consecutive cervical cytology tests that are negative for intraepithelial lesions or malignancy may be screened every 3 years.

   c. Discontinuation of cervical cancer screening can be between the ages of 65 and 70 in women who have had three or more consecutive negative cytology test results and no abnormal results in the past 10 years.

   d. Women who have undergone a total hysterectomy for benign conditions and have not had prior CIN 2 (moderate dysplasia) or CIN 3 (severe dysplasia or carcinoma in situ) may discontinue Pap smear screening. The following conditions may increase a patient's risk for CIN and may necessitate more frequent Pap test screening:

      i. Women who have human immunodeficiency virus (HIV)

      ii. Women with other immunosuppressive conditions (e.g., organ transplantation)

      iii. Women who were exposed to diethylstilbestrol (DES) in utero

      iv. Women previously treated for CIN 2, CIN 3, or cancer.

3. With the introduction of the quadrivalent and bivalent HPV vaccines, screening guidelines for the vaccinated population will eventually be modified. At the present time the recommendation is to adhere to the current guidelines (Centers for Disease Control and Prevention, 2007).

C. Pap smear classifications

The Bethesda System Pap smear classification is currently the preferred method for reporting cytology results (Table 18-1). This system is used for cytologic evaluation for the cervix, vagina, and anus (Solomon & Nayar, 2004). Cytologic evaluation of the vulva is not very effective in securing cells that are able to be optimally evaluated because of the keratinized epithelium. The report encompasses the components of the specimen type, a statement of adequacy, a general categorization, the use of automated review or ancillary testing, and the interpretation of results. The following nomenclature is used for categorizing dysplasia or abnormality:

1. Atypical squamous cells of undetermined significance: refers to those samples where the cells are either equivocal or nondiagnostic for either benign conditions or squamous intraepithelial neoplasia.

2. Atypical squamous cells of undetermined significance cannot rule out high-grade: refers to the presence of cells that are not clearly high grade but it cannot be ruled out.

3. Low-grade squamous intraepithelial lesion: refers to any combination of HPV (cells characteristic of HPV); mild dysplasia; or CIN 1.

4. High-grade squamous intraepithelial lesion: refers to the presence of moderate to severe dysplasia; carcinoma in situ; or intraepithelial neoplasia grades 2 or 3 (CIN 2 or 3).

5. Squamous cell cancer or suspicious for squamous cell cancer

6. Atypical glandular cells of undetermined significance: refers to endocervical or endometrial cell abnormalities or glandular cells not otherwise specified for site. The range of abnormality can be reactivity (e.g., from an intrauterine device string); adenocarcinoma in situ; or adenocarcinoma.

D. Management of abnormal cytology

1. Triaging of each category of abnormal cytology is outlined in the algorithms developed at the 2006 consensus conference sponsored by the American Society for Colposcopy and Cervical Pathology (ASCCP) (Wright et al., 2007a). The evidence-based guidelines were developed by participants representing all disciplines involved in caring for patients with abnormal cytology (Figures 18-1 through 18-11) (Wright et al., 2007b).

2. Evaluation techniques: Throughout the algorithms (Figures 18-1 through 18-11) choices can be made as to repeating the Pap smear in a specified interval of time, performing HPV DNA testing, or proceeding to colposcopic evaluation. The high incidence of low-grade squamous intraepithelial lesion with a minor number of those cases progressing to high-grade squamous intraepithelial lesion has led to a conservative approach to managing adolescent and young women with abnormal cytology (Moscicki, 2008).

   a. Repeat Pap smear evaluation confirms the persistence or regression of abnormal cells over time.

   b. HPV DNA testing with hybridization techniques provides an opportunity to categorize the HPV virus into low-risk and high-risk types. Type-specific HPV testing is also available once the presence of high-risk HPV has been confirmed. Data show that the persistence of high-risk HPV is a risk factor for progression to high-grade intraepithelial neoplasia (Hager, 2009).

   c. Colposcopic evaluation with directed biopsy allows the clinician to visually assess the lower genital tract under high-power magnification and assess lesions according to color, borders, vessels, and surface. Colposcopically directed biopsies are obtained to determine the pathologic diagnosis of the lesions and guide the treatment and management strategies (Apgar, Brotzman, & Rubin, 2008).

   d. Endocervical sampling with a curette or a cytobrush is sometimes included in the colposcopic evaluation to further evaluate the endocervical canal. This occurs when glandular abnormality is present or the colposcopic evaluation was unsatisfactory and the squamocolumnar junction (the border where the squamous epithelium meets the columnar epithelium) was not completely visualized, thereby not establishing a normal endocervical canal.

   e. Endometrial sampling may also be included when abnormal glandular cells are present and the woman is older than 35 years or at risk for endometrial cancer. It may also be performed when atypical endometrial cells are found.

TABLE 18-1 2001 Terminology for the Bethesda System

Conventional versus liquid-based preparation
Specimen adequacy
Satisfactory for evaluation (describe presence or absence of endocervical transformation zone component and any other quality indicators)
Unsatisfactory for evaluation (specify reason)
Interpretation and results
Negative for intraepithelial lesion of malignancy
Organisms
• *Trichomonas vaginalis*
• Fungal organisms morphologically consistent with *Candida* sp.
• Shift in vaginal flora suggestive of bacterial vaginosis
• Bacteria morphology consistent with *Actinomyces* sp.
• Cellular changes consistent with herpes simplex virus
• Other nonneoplastic findings (optional to report)
• Reactive cellular changes associated with inflammation (includes typical repair), radiation, intrauterine contraception device
• Glandular cells status posthysterectomy
• Atrophy
Other
Endometrial cells (in a woman ≥ 40 years of age)
Epithelial cell abnormalities
Squamous cell
Atypical squamous cells
• Of undetermined significance
• Cannot exclude high-grade squamous intraepithelial lesion
Low-grade squamous intraepithelial lesion encompassing human papillomavirus/mild dysplasia/CIN 1
High-grade squamous intraepithelial lesion encompassing moderate and severe dysplasia, CIN 2, and CIN 3/CIS
With features suspicious for invasion (if invasion is suspected)
Squamous cell carcinoma
Glandular cell
Category reported as other
Atypical endocervical cells, endometrial cells, glandular cells
• Atypical glandular and endocervical cells, favor neoplastic
• Endocervical adenocarcinoma in situ
Adenocarcinoma
• Endocervical
• Endometrial
• Extrauterine
• Not otherwise specified
Other malignant neoplasms

Source: Solomon, D., & Nayar, R. (Eds.). (2004). *The Bethesda System for reporting cervical cytology: Definitions, criteria and explanatory notes* (2nd ed.). New York, NY: Springer-Verlag.

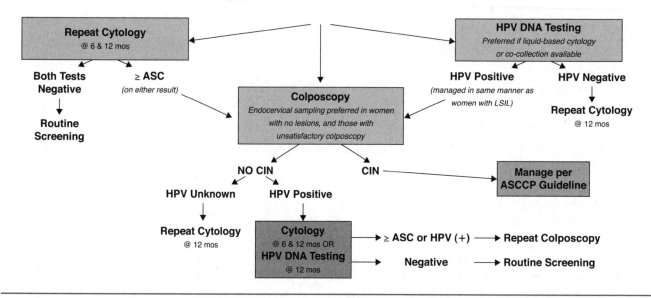

FIGURE 18-1 Management of Women with Atypical Squamous Cells of Undetermined Significance (ASC-US)

Source: Reprinted from *The Journal of Lower Genital Tract Disease,* Vol. 11, Issue 4, with the permission of ASCCP American Society for Colposcopy and Cervical Pathology 2007. No copies of the algorithms may be made without the prior permission of ASCCP.

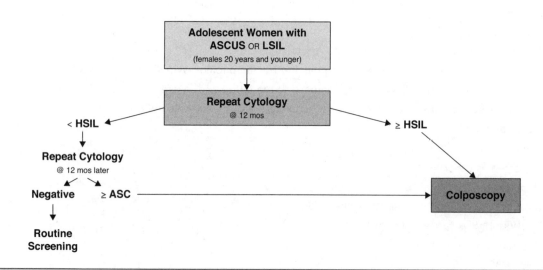

FIGURE 18-2 Management of Adolescent Women with Either Atypical Squamous Cells of Undetermined Significance (ASCUS) or Low-Grade Squamous Intraepithelial Lesion (LSIL)

Source: Reprinted from *The Journal of Lower Genital Tract Disease,* Vol. 11, Issue 4, with the permission of ASCCP American Society for Colposcopy and Cervical Pathology 2007. No copies of the algorithms may be made without the prior permission of ASCCP.

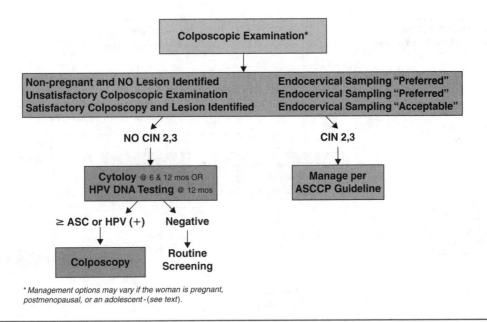

FIGURE 18-3 Management of Women with Low-Grade Squamous Intraepithelial Lesion (LSIL)

Source: Reprinted from *The Journal of Lower Genital Tract Disease,* Vol. 11, Issue 4, with the permission of ASCCP American Society for Colposcopy and Cervical Pathology 2007. No copies of the algorithms may be made without the prior permission of ASCCP.

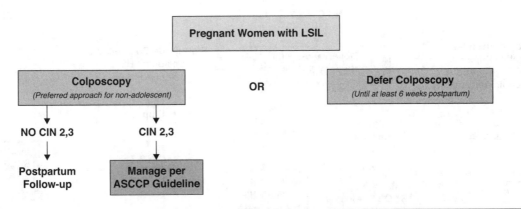

FIGURE 18-4 Management of Pregnant Women with Low-Grade Squamous Intraepithelial Lesion

Source: Reprinted from *The Journal of Lower Genital Tract Disease,* Vol. 11, Issue 4, with the permission of ASCCP American Society for Colposcopy and Cervical Pathology 2007. No copies of the algorithms may be made without the prior permission of ASCCP.

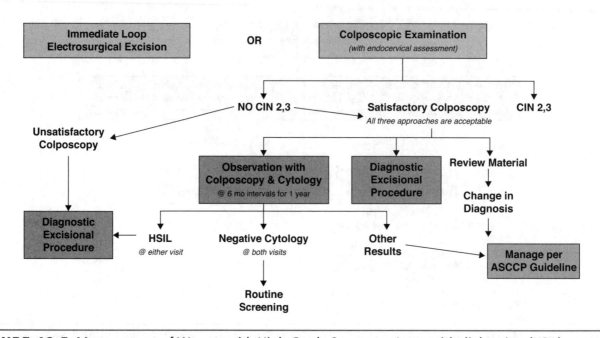

FIGURE 18-5 Management of Women with High-Grade Squamous Intraepithelial Lesion (HSIL)

Source: Reprinted from *The Journal of Lower Genital Tract Disease,* Vol. 11, Issue 4, with the permission of ASCCP American Society for Colposcopy and Cervical Pathology 2007. No copies of the algorithms may be made without the prior permission of ASCCP.

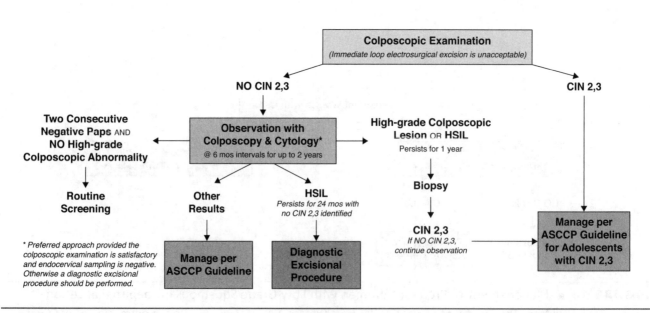

FIGURE 18-6 Management of Adolescent Women (20 Years and Younger) with High-Grade Squamous Intraepithelial Lesion (HSIL)

Source: Reprinted from *The Journal of Lower Genital Tract Disease,* Vol. 11, Issue 4, with the permission of ASCCP American Society for Colposcopy and Cervical Pathology 2007. No copies of the algorithms may be made without the prior permission of ASCCP.

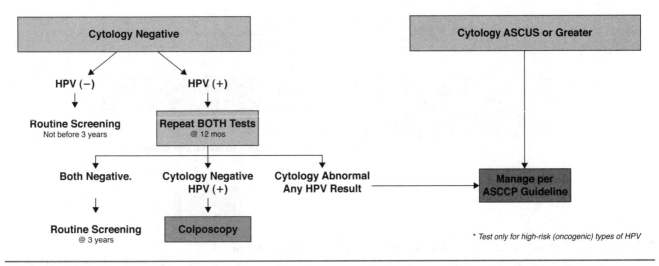

FIGURE 18-7 Cytology

Source: Reprinted from *The Journal of Lower Genital Tract Disease,* Vol. 11, Issue 4, with the permission of ASCCP American Society for Colposcopy and Cervical Pathology 2007. No copies of the algorithms may be made without the prior permission of ASCCP.

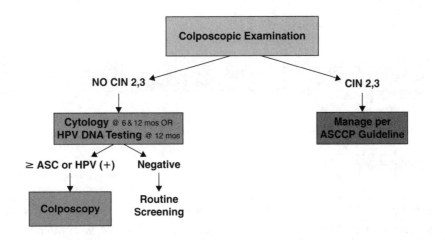

FIGURE 18-8 Management of Women with Atypical Squamous Cells: Cannot Exclude High-Grade SIL (ASC-H)

Source: Reprinted from *The Journal of Lower Genital Tract Disease,* Vol. 11, Issue 4, with the permission of ASCCP American Society for Colposcopy and Cervical Pathology 2007. No copies of the algorithms may be made without the prior permission of ASCCP.

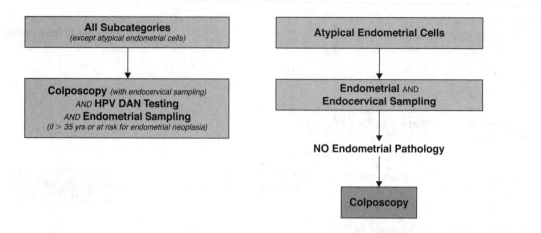

FIGURE 18-9 Initial Workup of Women with Atypical Glandular Cells (AGC)

Source: Reprinted from *The Journal of Lower Genital Tract Disease,* Vol. 11, Issue 4, with the permission of ASCCP American Society for Colposcopy and Cervical Pathology 2007. No copies of the algorithms may be made without the prior permission of ASCCP.

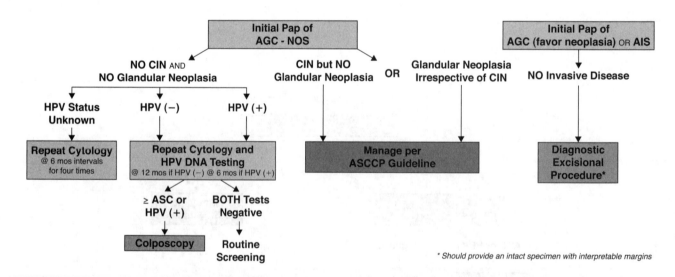

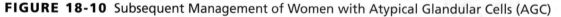

FIGURE 18-10 Subsequent Management of Women with Atypical Glandular Cells (AGC)

Source: Reprinted from *The Journal of Lower Genital Tract Disease,* Vol. 11, Issue 4, with the permission of ASCCP American Society for Colposcopy and Cervical Pathology 2007. No copies of the algorithms may be made without the prior permission of ASCCP.

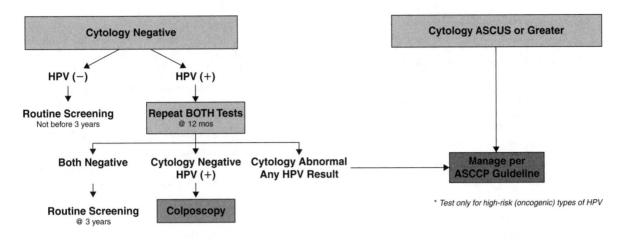

FIGURE 18-11 Use of HPV DNA as an Adjunct to Cytology for Cervical Cancer Screening in Women 30 Years and Older

Source: Reprinted from *The Journal of Lower Genital Tract Disease,* Vol. 11, Issue 4, with the permission of ASCCP American Society for Colposcopy and Cervical Pathology 2007. No copies of the algorithms may be made without the prior permission of ASCCP.

II. Database (may include but is not limited to)

A. Subjective

1. Past health history

    a. Medical illnesses: immune disorders including HIV, systemic lupus erythematosus, organ transplant, or blood dyscrasias.

    b. Medication history: medications that affect immune response (e.g., prednisone), hormone therapy, or anticoagulant or aspirin therapy.

    c. Allergy history: iodine or shellfish.

    d. Surgical history: hysterectomy and excisional or ablative treatment.

    e. Obstetric and gynecological history: parity, current or recent pregnancy, desire for future pregnancy, history of intraepithelial neoplasia, condylomata, abnormal cytology or positive HPV testing, menstrual history, history of STIs, history of DES exposure, HPV vaccination.

2. Family history: gynecological cancers

3. Personal and social history: age at onset of sexual activity; number of sexual partners; birth control method and condom use; sexual preference; and tobacco, alcohol, and drug use.

4. Review of systems

    a. General health.

    b. Psychosocial: ability to understand disease and relation to sexual activity, depression, anxiety, and guilt or shame.

    c. Reproductive: presence of pruritis; vulvar, vaginal, or anal pain; dyspareunia; abnormal bleeding; abnormal anogenital growths; and vaginal discharge or odor.

B. Objective

1. External: gross inspection of vulvar and perianal skin, noting presence of condylomata, ulcers, pigmented lesions, leukoplakia, microtears, inflammation, atrophy, raised lesions; colposcopic inspection noting acetowhite epithelium with or without vessel patterns, such as punctation, mosaic, or atypical vessels; and Lugol's nonstaining lesions (avoid if allergic to iodine).

2. Speculum examination: gross inspection of cervix and vagina noting discharge, inflammation, atrophy, leukoplakia, ulcers, and raised lesions; colposcopic examination noting location of squamocolumnar junction, acetowhite epithelium with or without vessel patterns, and Lugol's nonstaining lesions (Ferris, Cox, O'Connor, Wright, & Forester, 2004).

3. Supporting data from relevant diagnostic tests, including wet smear and KOH, cytology and histology, and HPV test.

III. Assessment

A. Determine the diagnosis
Genital warts, AIN, VIN, VAIN, CIN, AIS, or invasive cancer

B. Determine the severity and location

1. Low-grade: mild dysplasia (intraepithelial neoplasia Grade I)

2. High-grade: moderate (intraepithelial neoplasia Grade 2)

3. Severe or carcinoma in situ (intraepithelial neoplasia Grade 3)

4. Unifocal versus multifocal, exocervical, endocervical, vaginal, or vulvar.

C. Significance

Assess the significance of the diagnosis to the patient and significant others.

D. Motivation and ability

Determine the patient's willingness and ability to follow the treatment plan.

IV. Goals of clinical management

The choice of treatment is influenced by a number of factors, including the patient's preference; age; parity; the location, extent, degree of abnormality; cost of treatment; the limitations of the healthcare facility to provide certain treatments; the patient's desire for future fertility; the patient's ability to understand and follow the treatment protocol; and probability of patient follow-up. The dose and duration of treatment should be determined by referring to product guidelines.

A. Screening for the purpose of diagnosing or preventing cervical, vaginal, and vulvar cancer.

Anal and perianal intraepithelial neoplasia are also a growing concern but are not covered in this chapter. Choose a cost-effective approach for screening or diagnosing HPV, precancerous, and cancerous lesions.

B. Treatment

Select a treatment plan that reduces symptoms and prevents progression.

C. Patient adherence

Select an approach that maximizes patient adherence.

V. Plan

A. Screening

Screening for cervical, vaginal, and vulvar cancer is influenced by the age of the patient, the onset of sexual activity, the presence of immunosuppressive diseases or medications, history of DES exposure (Rubin, 2007), history of abnormal cytology or positive HPV tests, and the presence of risk factors for acquiring STIs.

B. Diagnostic tests

May include cervical cytology, HPV DNA testing, anal cytology, biopsy, endocervical curettage, cervical cultures for gonorrhea and *Chlamydia*, wet smear and KOH, and urine human chorionic gonadotropin.

C. Management

1. Treat vaginitis, STIs, vaginal atrophy, and dermatosis.

2. Treat genital warts: trichloroacetic acid 0.5%, imiquimod (Aldara) 5% cream, 5-fluorouracil (Efudex) 3–5%, and sinecalechin (Veregen); cryotherapy with liquid nitrogen or cryoprobe; surgical excision; laser therapy; or interferon alfa-2b (Intron).

3. Treat VIN: wide local excision, laser therapy, skinning vulvectomy, imiquimod (Aldara) 5%, 5-fluorouracil 2–5%, cryotherapy, or observation.

4. Treat VAIN: 5-fluorouracil 2–5%, laser therapy, surgical or electrosurgical excision, or observation.

5. Treat CIN: follow ASCCP Guidelines for HPV, premalignant and malignant lesions (Figures 18-1 through 18-11). HPV vaccination as indicated.

D. Client education

1. Concerns and feelings
   a. Discuss the emotional impact of HPV-associated disease on the patient's self esteem, body image, and feelings of trust and safety with her sexual partner.
   b. Discuss concerns about cancer and fertility (Ferris et al., 2003; Rubin & Tripsas, 2010).

2. Information
   a. Discuss smoking cessation, healthy diet and lifestyle, safer sex, partner transmission, and HPV in pregnancy.
   b. Discuss the relationship between HPV and cancer, and the need for ongoing follow-up (refer to ASCCP guidelines).
   c. Discuss diagnostic tests including colposcopy, biopsy, and endocervical curettage.
   d. Discuss treatments and side effects.
   e. Discuss HPV vaccination benefits and limitations.

3. Resources and tools
   a. http://www.asccp.org
   b. http://www.cdc.org./std/hpv
   c. http://www.asha.org/hpv/publications.cfm
   d. http://www.cancer.org
   e. http://www.analcancerinfo.ucsf.edu

REFERENCES

American College of Obstetricians and Gynecologists. (ACOG). (2009). ACOG practice bulletin No 109: Cervical cytology screening. *Obstetrics and Gynecology, 114*(6), 1409–1420.

Apgar, B., Brotzman, G., & Rubin, M. (2008). Principles and technique of the colposcopic exam. In B. Apgar, G. Brotzman, & M. Spitzer (Eds.). *Colposcopy Principles and Practice: An Integrated Textbook and Atlas* (2nd ed., pp. 101–125). Philadelphia, PA: W.B. Saunders.

Centers for Disease Control and Prevention. (2007). Quadrivalent human papilloma vaccine. *Morbidity and Mortality Weekly Reports, 56*, 1–24.

Einstein, M. (2008). Acquired immune response to oncogenic human papillomavirus associated with prophylactic cervical cancer vaccine. *Cancer Immunology and Immunotherapy, 157*(4), 443–451.

Ferris, D., Cox, J., O'Connor, D., Wright, C., & Forester, J. (2004). *Modern Colposcopy Textbook and Atlas* (2nd ed.). Dubuque, IA: Kendall/ Hunt Publishing.

Ferris, D., Gilman, P., Lopez, A., Litaker, M., Miller, J., & Macfee, S. (2003). Psychological effects of women experience before and after a colposcopic examination and primary care appointment. *Journal of Lower Genital Tract Disease, 7*(2), 89–94.

Hager, W. D. (2009). Human papillomavirus infection & prevention in the adolescent population. *Journal of Pediatric & Adolescent Gynecology, 22*(4), 197–204.

Kosiol, J., Lindsay, L., Pimenta, J., Poole, C., Jenkins, D., & Smith, J. (2008). Persistence of human papillomavirus infection and cervical neoplasia: A systematic review and meta analysis. *American Journal of Epidemiology, 168*(2), 123–137.

Moscicki, A. B. (2008). Conservative management of adolescents with abnormal cytology and histology. *Journal of National Comprehensive Cancer, 6*(1), 101–106.

Parkin, D. M. (2006). The global health burden of infection-associated cancers in the year 2002. *International Journal of Cancer, 118*(12), 3030–3044.

Rubin, M. (2007). Antenatal exposure to DES: Lessons learned . . . concerns for the future. *Obstetrical and Gynecological Survey, 62*(8), 1–7.

Rubin, M., & Tripsas, C. (2010). Uncertainty, coping strategies and adaptation in women with human papillomavirus (HPV) on Papanicolaou smears. *Journal of Lower Genital Tract Disease, 14*(3), 81–89.

Soloman, D., & Nayar, R. (2004.) *The Bethesda system for reporting cervical cytology: Definitions, criteria, and explanatory notes.* New York: Springer.

Trottier, H., & Franco, E. L. (2006). The epidemiology of genital human papillomavirus infection. *Vaccine, 24*(Suppl. 1), S1–S15.

Trottier, H., Mahmud, S., Lindsay, L., Quint, W., Weiting, S., Schuind, A., & Franco, E. (2009). Persistence of an incident human papillomavirus infection and timing of cervical lesions in previously unexposed young women. *Cancer Epidemiologic Biomarkers Prevention, 8*, 854–862.

Winer, R. L., Lee, S. K., Hughes, J. P., Adam, D. E., Kiviat, N. B., & Koutsky, L. A. (2003). Genital human papillomavirus infection: Incidence and risk factors in a cohort of female university students. *American Journal of Epidemiology, 157*(3), 218–226.

World Health Organization. (2008). *Human papillomavirus and cervical cancer.* Retrieved from http://www.who.int/immunization/topics /hpv/en/

Wright, T. C., Massad, S., Dunton, C., Spitzer, M., Wilkinson, E., & Solomon, D. (2007a). 2006 American Society for Colposcopy and Cervical Pathology–sponsored Consensus Conference. *American Journal of Obstetrics & Gynecology, 97*(4), 346–355.

Wright, T. C., Massad, L. S., Dunton, C. J., Spitzer, M., Wilkinson, E. J., & Solomon, D. (2007b). 2006 American Society for Colposcopy and Cervical Pathology-sponsored Consensus Conference. 2006 consensus guidelines for the management of women with cervical intraepithelial neoplasia or adenocarcinoma in situ. *Journal of Lower Genital Tract Disease, 11*(4), 102–222.

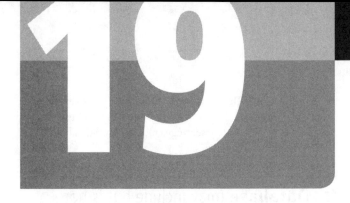

FEMALE AND MALE STERILIZATION

Janis Luft

I. Introduction and general background

Thirty-nine percent of reproductive age couples desiring contraception use sterilization, making this the most commonly used form of contraception in the United States (Pollack, Carignan, & Jacobstein, 2004).

Female sterilization describes a number of surgical procedures intended to physically prevent sperm from uniting with and fertilizing an egg. Sterilization surgeries can include the removal of the uterus (hysterectomy). However, the more typically performed, less invasive procedures involve disrupting fallopian tubal patency. Tubal ligation, either by excision of a portion of the tube or by electrocautery, or tubal occlusion through the use of surgical clips or rings are generally performed via laparoscopy. Tubal occlusion using fallopian inserts (Essure®, Adiana®) can be done hysteroscopically through the cervix, thus avoiding surgical incision. All of these procedures effectively end a woman's fertility. More than three quarter of a million women use these methods annually. Vasectomy is the male form of sterilization. About a half a million men a year choose this permanent form of contraception. A vasectomy is a minor surgical procedure that is performed under local anesthesia. One or two small incisions are made in the scrotum and the vas deferens is ligated, cauterized, or occluded, thus preventing sperm from admixing with semen.

A. Tubal ligation

1. Definition and overview

   a. Sterilization is a permanent form of contraception that is 99.96% effective.

   b. Laparoscopy can be performed under general, regional, or local anesthesia with sedation. Fallopian tubes can be ligated, cauterized, or clamped.

   c. Mini-laparotomy involves a small abdominal incision and requires general anesthesia. Salpingectomy (removal of the fallopian tubes) or any of the previously mentioned procedures can be performed using mini-laparotomy.

2. Benefits

   a. Both surgeries provide immediate and permanent contraception.

   b. Highly effective with an overall 10-year failure rate of 1.85% in the United States.

   c. Extremely safe with rare operative complications.

   d. Covered benefit of Medi-Cal and Medicaid programs

3. Risks and disadvantages

   a. There are no absolute contraindications to these procedures, but people with certain health conditions, such as obesity, pelvic adhesions, diabetes, or severe cardiac or lung disease, may not be ideal surgical candidates.

   b. General anesthesia may be required.

   c. A 30-day waiting period postcounseling and postconsenting is required by federal Medicaid guidelines.

B. Transcervical tubal occlusion

1. Definition and overview

   These procedures are done via hysteroscopy and involve placing foreign objects into the horns of the uterus, causing scarring and occlusion of the fallopian tubes. These are done using local anesthesia only, require no incision, and thus can be done in an outpatient setting. Both Food and Drug Administration approved methods require an appropriately trained clinician. Accurate insertion of the devices can fail in as many as one in seven placements. Verification of tubal occlusion requires hysterosalpingogram 3 months after placement of the occluding devices.

   a. Essure®: this device resembles a tiny coil spring. After placement, there is a delay in efficacy until tubal fibrosis occurs (typically 3 months) during which alternate contraception must be used.

   b. Adiana®: this system uses radio signals that are directed at the fallopian tubes to create a lesion in each tube. A tiny piece of soft silicone is then inserted into each fallopian tube. Twelve weeks is typically required before tissue growth is sufficient to provide tubal occlusion.

2. Benefits

a. Hysteroscopy precludes the need for a surgical incision. There is less risk of infection and faster recovery time. It may be a better choice for women who are not ideal candidates for even minimally invasive pelvic surgery.

b. There is no need for general or regional anesthesia. Generally only paracervical block or mild oral or intravenous sedation is used, and thus it can be done in an outpatient setting.

c. It is highly effective; 5-year efficacy is 99.74% (Hastings-Tolsma, Nodine, & Teal, 2006).

d. It is covered by Medi-Cal and most Medicaid programs.

3. Risks and disadvantages

a. There is a delay in the efficacy of these methods of 3 months or more to allow for sufficient tubal fibrosis to take place. A hysterosalpingo-gram is required to ensure that the tubes are occluded. Other methods of contraception (but not an intrauterine device) must be used in the 3-month interim between the procedure and ensurance of tubal fibrosis.

b. The provider must be trained in the use and placement of these devices.

c. Certain uterine malformations (e.g., bicornuate uterus) may preclude proper placement of the devices.

d. Women must be at least 6 weeks postpartum.

e. A 30-day waiting period postcounseling and postconsenting is required by federal Medicaid guidelines.

C. Vasectomy

1. Definition and overview

Vasectomy is male sterilization accomplished by severing the vas deferens, thus preventing sperm from entering the ejaculate.

2. Benefits

a. Provides permanent contraception with low failure rates.

b. Requires local anesthesia and can be done in the outpatient setting.

c. Covered by Medi-Cal and most Medicaid programs.

3. Risks and disadvantages

a. It can take up to 3–6 months to achieve complete aspermia. Effective contraception must be used until ejaculate tests negative for the presence of sperm. Most vasectomy "failures" occur within the first 3 months after the procedure.

b. There is postprocedure pain and swelling.

c. A 30-day waiting period postcounseling and postconsenting is required by federal Medicaid guidelines.

II. Database (may include but is not limited to)

A. Subjective

1. Gynecological, urologic, medical, and psychosocial history

a. Patient desires permanent sterilization.

b. They have considered and declined other contraceptive options.

c. There are no medical contraindications to the procedure that would incur high surgical risk.

B. Objective

1. Complete gynecological and urologic examination; negative pregnancy test for women.

2. Absence of psychiatric or mental disability.

III. Assessment

A. Patient is a candidate for sterilization

1. According to federal guidelines, candidate must be at least 21 years of age.

2. Mentally competent.

3. Women not currently pregnant.

4. No medical contraindications to procedure.

B. Understands and accepts the permanent nature of the procedure and is prepared to end childbearing.

IV. Plan

A. Client education

1. Information and counseling

a. Before undergoing sterilization, patients must be sure that they no longer want to bear children and will not want to bear children in the future, even if life circumstances change. Information must also be provided about the many effective contraceptive choices available.

b. Discuss risks, benefits, discomforts, and recovery times associated with various procedures.

c. Review follow-up testing as appropriate. Discuss plan for and provide interim contraception as needed.

2. Consenting
   a. In California, clinicians are required to provide a copy of the sterilization booklet published by the Department of Health Services. In other states, check the state Department of Health for similar requirements.
   b. Obtain informed consent. Federal Medicaid guidelines require written consent signed at least 30 days and no more than 180 days before the planned procedure for patients receiving public funding. A copy must be placed in the medical record and a copy provided to the patient.
   c. Assure the patient of his or her right to revoke consent at any time.

V. Self-management resources

1. *The American Congress of Obstetricians and Gynecologists, Sterilization for men and women:*
   http://www.acog.org/publications/patient_education/bp011.cfm

2. *Planned Parenthood, Sterilization for women (tubal ligation)*
   http://www.plannedparenthood.org/health-topics/birth-control/sterilization-women-4248.htm

3. *Planned Parenthood, Vasectomy:*
   http://www.plannedparenthood.org/health-topics/birth-control/vasectomy-4249.htm

REFERENCES

Hastings-Tolsma, M., Nodine, P., & Teal, S. B. (2006). Essure: hysteroscopic sterilization. *Journal of Midwifery & Womens Health, 51*(6), 510–513.

Palmer, S. N., & Greenberg, J. A. (2009). Transcervical sterilization: A comparison of essure permanent birth control system and adiana permanent contraception system. *Reviews in Obstetrics & Gynecology, 2*(2), 84–92.

Pollack, A. E., Carignan, C. S., & Jacobstein, R. (2004). Female and male sterilization. In R. A. Hatcher, J. Trussell, F. Stewart, A. E. Nelson, W. Cates, F. Guest, & D. Kowal (Eds.), *Contraceptive Technology* (18th rev. ed., pp. 531–573). New York, NY: Ardent Media.

Sokal, D. C., & Labrecque, M. (2009). Effectiveness of vasectomy techniques. *Urologic Clinic of North America 36*, 317–329.

The ESHRE Capri Workshop Group. (2009). Female contraception over 40. *Human Reproduction Update, 15*(6), 599–612.

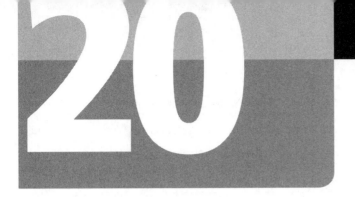

HORMONAL CONTRACEPTION

Lynn Hanson

I. Introduction and general background

Hormonal contraception is used extensively and successfully throughout the world for family planning. When used properly, it is highly effective and safe. The most common form of hormonal contraception is the combined oral contraceptive (COC) pill. Other forms include the progestin-only pill (POP; Minipill), transdermal contraceptive patch, vaginal contraceptive ring, medroxyprogesterone acetate (Depo-Provera®) injection, progesterone implant (Implanon®), and levonorgestrel intrauterine system (LNG-IUS; Mirena®). Levonorgestrel alone or in a COC pill is used as the emergency contraception pill (ECP) (this should not be used as a regular method of contraception). All of these methods contain a form of progestin alone or in combination with an estrogen. The mechanism of contraception is primarily supplied by the progestin, through thickening of the cervical mucus, change in fallopian tube motility, inhibition of ovulation, and sperm capacitation, and in some cases endometrial atrophy. The addition of estrogen can further inhibit ovulation, and may alter the endometrial lining to prevent implantation. Estrogen helps to prevent breakthrough bleeding and maintain normal cycle patterns (Nelson, 2007).

Many factors must be weighed in determining if hormonal contraception is appropriate for a patient. Certain medical conditions present contraindications or relative contraindications to hormone use (Tables 20-1, 20-2, 20-4, and 20-5). Patient compliance and tolerance of side effects may be required. Efficacy may be of primary importance to a woman where pregnancy is contraindicated for medical or personal reasons. Time to return of fertility may be

important. Cost may be prohibitive for some patients. High-risk sexual behavior should also be considered, because many patients are less likely to use condoms when using hormonal contraception, placing them at higher risk for sexually transmitted diseases. Comfort with and ease of use of the method must also be considered. See Appendix 20-1 for a comparison of oral contraceptives.

A. Combined hormonal contraception

Combined hormonal contraception (CHC) includes methods that contain both estrogen and a progestin. These include the COC pill, transdermal patch, and vaginal ring. Combined injectable contraceptives are not currently available in the United States. CHC has many advantages beyond prevention of pregnancy. Dysmenorrhea and menorrhagia are often significantly reduced, and menstrual cycle regularity is improved. Symptoms and severity of endometriosis may be reduced, and fertility preserved. Premenstrual syndrome and migraine headaches are often improved but may also be increased. Many women benefit from a reduction in incidence of ovarian cyst problems when using estrogen-containing methods. Symptoms related to polycystic ovary syndrome, such as acne and hirsutism, often improve. Lighter menstrual cycles contribute to lower incidence of iron deficiency anemia. CHC is associated with a decrease in ectopic pregnancy, pelvic inflammatory disease (PID), and benign breast disease. In perimenopausal women, use of estrogen-containing methods may reduce hot flashes, vaginal dryness, and bone loss. Finally, ovarian, endometrial, and colorectal cancer risk is reduced in users of CHC.

Much data has been collected about the safety of the COC pill, and although less is available about the safety of the patch and ring, they seem to have a similar profile. The World Health Organization (WHO) 2009 Medical Eligibility Criteria provides detailed information on hormonal contraceptive safety, and is available on the WHO website (www.who.int/reproductive health). Tables 20-1 and 20-2 list contraindications and relative contraindications to initiating CHC adapted from the WHO guidelines, and Table 20-3 lists conditions where CHC may be used with possible need for additional monitoring. Items with asterisks may fall into one or another category; the reader is directed to the full text of the WHO publication for detail.

1. COC pill

   COC pills have been in use for almost 50 years. When used correctly, the failure rate is 0.3% in perfect use, and 8% in typical use (Trussell, 2007). There are many different combinations of estrogen- and progestin-containing pills marketed today. Most contain ethinyl

TABLE 20-1 Absolute Contraindications to Starting Combined Hormonal Contraceptives

Breastfeeding, < 6 weeks postpartum

Smoking in woman 35 years or older, and 15 or more cigarettes per day

Multiple risks factors for arterial cardiovascular disease*

Hypertension if vascular disease is present, or systolic 160 or more and diastolic 100 or more

History of DVT/PE, acute DVT/PE, or on anticoagulant therapy for DVT/PE

Major surgery with prolonged immobilization

Known thrombogenic mutations (factor V Leiden, prothrombin mutation, protein S, protein C, and antithrombin deficiencies)

Current and history of ischemic heart disease

Cerebrovascular accident

Complicated valvular heart disease (pulmonary hypertension, risk of atrial fibrillation, or history of subacute bacterial endocarditis)

Systemic lupus erythematosus with positive or unknown antiphospholipid antibodies

Migraine with aura at any age

Breast cancer currently or in past 5 years

Diabetes with nephropathy, neuropathy, retinopathy, or other vascular disease, or diabetes of > 20 years' duration*

Cirrhosis (severe, decompensated)

Viral hepatitis, acute or flare*

Liver tumor (malignant or hepatocellular adenoma)

*Indicates overlap with Category III list, see WHO text for discussion.
Source: Adapted from 2009 WHO Guidelines, Category IV.

TABLE 20-2 Relative Contraindications to Starting Combined Hormonal Contraceptives

Breastfeeding, ≥ 6 weeks or < 6 months postpartum (primarily breastfeeding)

Postpartum ≤ 21 days

Smoking in woman 35 years or older, and < 15 cigarettes per day

Multiple risk factors for cardiovascular disease*

Hypertension with systolic 140–159 or diastolic 90–99, or history of hypertension where blood pressure cannot be evaluated, or adequately controlled blood pressure where blood pressure can be evaluated

Hyperlipidemia (according to type, severity, and other cardiovascular risk factors)*

Migraine without aura and 35 years or older

Breast cancer in past and no evidence of current disease for 5 years

Diabetes with nephropathy, neuropathy, retinopathy, or other vascular disease, or diabetes of > 20 years' duration*

Gallbladder disease if current or symptomatic and medically treated

Cholestasis related to use of combined hormonal contraceptives in past

Viral hepatitis, acute or flare*

Antiretroviral therapy with retonavir-boosted protease inhibitors

Anticonvulsant therapy with phenytoin, carbamazepine, barbiturates, primodone, topiramate, oxcarbazepine, and lamotrigine

Antimicrobial therapy with rifampicin or rifambutin therapy

*Indicates overlap with Category IV or II list, see WHO text for discussion.
Source: Adapted from 2009 WHO Guidelines, Category III.

TABLE 20-3 Initiate Combined Hormonal Contraceptives, May Need to Monitor

Age 40 years or older

Breastfeeding and ≥ 6 months postpartum

Smoking and < 35 years old

Obesity (≥ 30 kg/m² body mass index)

Hypertension during pregnancy

Family history of DVT/PE

Major surgery without prolonged immobilization

Superficial thrombophlebitis

Hyperlipidemia*

Valvular heart disease if uncomplicated

Systemic lupus erythematosus without severe thrombocytopenia or immunosuppressive treatment

Migraine headache without aura and < 35 years old

Vaginal bleeding without explanation before evaluation

Cervical intraepithelial neoplasia or cervical cancer awaiting treatment

Breast mass, awaiting diagnosis

Diabetes, nonvascular (insulin or noninsulin dependent)

Gallbladder disease, asymptomatic or treated by cholecystectomy

Cholestasis, related to pregnancy

Benign liver tumor, focal nodular hyperplasia

Sickle cell disease

Antiretroviral therapy with nonnucleoside reverse transcriptase inhibitors

*Indicates overlap with Category III list, see WHO text for discussion.

Source: Adapted from 2009 WHO Guidelines, Category II.

TABLE 20-4 Absolute Contraindications to Progestogen-Only Contraceptives

Breast cancer currently or in past 5 years

Puerperal sepsis (LNG-IUS)

Immediate postseptic abortion (LNG-IUS)

Unexplained vaginal bleeding before evaluation (LNG-IUS)

Gestational trophoblastic disease (LNG-IUS*)

Cervical cancer, awaiting treatment (LNG-IUS)

Endometrial cancer (LNG-IUS)

Uterine fibroids or other anatomic abnormalities that distort the uterine cavity (LNG-IUS)

Current pelvic inflammatory disease (LNG-IUS)

Current purulent cervicitis or chlamydia or gonorrhea infection (LNG-IUS)

Pelvic tuberculosis (LNG-IUS)

Where individual methods in parentheses, contraindication exists only for these methods. Where no parentheses, contraindication exists for all methods.

*Indicates overlap with Category III list, see WHO text for discussion.

Source: Adapted from 2009 WHO Guidelines, Category IV.

TABLE 20-5 Relative Contraindications to Progestogen-Only Contraceptives

Breastfeeding and < 6 weeks postpartum (POP, Depo-provera®, Implanon®)

Breastfeeding and < 4 weeks postpartum (LNG-IUS)

Multiple risks factors for atrial cardiovascular disease (Depo-provera®)

Hypertension with vascular disease or systolic ≥ 160, diastolic ≥ 100 (Depo-provera®)

Acute DVT/PE

Ischemic heart disease, current or history of (Depo-provera®)

Stroke (Depo-provera®)

Systemic lupus erythematosus with positive antiphospholipid antibodies (all) or severe thrombocytopenia (Depo-provera®)

Vaginal bleeding without explanation (Depo-provera®, Implanon®)

Gestational trophoblastic disease (LNG-IUS*)

Breast cancer in past, and no evidence of current disease for 5 years

Ovarian cancer (LNG-IUS)

Increase risk of STIs (LNG-IUS*)

AIDS (LNG-IUS*)

Diabetes with nephropathy, neuropathy, or retinopathy (Depo-provera®)

Cirrhosis (severe, decompensated)

Liver tumor (malignant or hepatocellular adenoma)

Antiretroviral therapy with nucleoside reverse transcriptase inhibitors (LNG-IUS*)

Antiretroviral therapy with nonnucleoside reverse transcriptase inhibitors (LNG-IUS*)

Antiretroviral therapy with retonavir-boosted protease inhibitors (POP, LNG-IUS*)

Anticonvulsant therapy with phenytoin, carbamazepine, barbiturates, primidone, topiramate, or oxcarbazepine (POP)

Antimicrobial therapy with rifampicin or rifabutin therapy (POP)

Where individual methods in parentheses, contraindication exists only for these methods. Where no parentheses, contraindication exists for all methods.
*Indicates overlap with Category IV or II list, see WHO text for discussion.
Source: Adapted from 2009 WHO guidelines, Category III.

estradiol, whereas a few of the higher estrogen pills contain mestranol. A new COC pill containing the natural estrogen estradiol is on the horizon (Nelson, 2010). The dosage of ethinyl estradiol ranges from 20 to 50 mcg, although doses above 35 mcg are rarely used. Eight synthetic progestins are in use in the United States ranging in dosage from 0.1 to 1 mg. The combination of estrogen and progestin define the efficacy and characteristics of the COC pill.

All COC pills have four biologic activities: (1) endometrial activity (defined as the percentage of breakthrough bleeding in the third cycle of use); (2) estrogenic activity; (3) progestational activity; and (4) androgenic activity (Dickey, 2007). The side effects experienced by many pill users relate to these activities, and may be reduced by switching to COC pills with different biologic profiles (Pharmacist's Letter/Prescriber's Letter, 2007). For instance, breast swelling and tenderness, nausea, mood changes, and fluid retention resulting in weight gain or headaches are related to the estrogen effect, and may

be relieved by switching to a pill with greater progestational activity. COC pills with greater progestational activity may cause weight gain from appetite stimulation, increased varicosities, increased vaginal discharge including moniliasis, and mood changes. Pills with high androgenic activity can cause acne, hirsutism, and increased libido. Two excellent pocket guides for quick reference for COC pill selection are *Managing Contraceptive Pill Patients* (Dickey) and *A Pocket Guide to Managing Contraception* (Zieman et al., 2007–2009).

Additionally, different COC pill combinations have varying effects on high-density lipoprotein and low-density lipoprotein cholesterol, thus affecting the potential for serious complications, such as venous thrombosis (VTE) and cardiovascular disease (CVD). This effect is mainly related to the dose of estrogen, and only slightly to the type of progestin (Nelson, 2007). This should be considered when choosing COCs for users with other risk factors for VTE and CVD (e.g., older age, smoking, diabetes, hypertension, obesity, and family history of VTE or CVD).

After COC pills are initiated, patients must be counseled about the symptoms of serious or potentially serious side effects, and the possible need for immediate discontinuation. These include:

a. Loss or distortion of vision (retinal artery thrombosis).
b. Severe chest pain (myocardial infarction).
c. Hemoptysis (pulmonary embolism).
d. Severe unilateral leg pain, swelling, and redness (VTE, thrombosis).
e. Severe persistent headaches, unilateral numbness, weakness or tingling, and slurring of speech (stroke).
f. Abdominal pain (thrombosis, myocardial infarction, pulmonary embolism, and gall bladder or liver disease). Patients who develop migraine headaches with aura after starting COC pills should be switched to a progestin-only method.

COC pills may be monophasic, with each pill containing the same dose, or multiphasic, with pill weeks containing varying doses of estrogen and progestin. Most COC pills have 21 active pills, and seven inactive or "placebo" pills, allowing for regular menstrual cycling. Several newer formulations extend the active pill days to reduce menstrual flow and related problems. Some have 24 days of active pills, and 3 days of placebos. The shortened pill-free interval improves pill efficacy and lessens withdrawal bleeding (Endrikat et al., 2001; Spona et al., 1996). Others have 84 days of active pills, followed by 7 days of placebos. One COC pill formulation is continuous with no placebo days. Extended COC pill use is ideal for women who suffer from menstrual-related problems, or who have conditions, such as endometriosis, that are suppressed by COC pill use.

There is no medical necessity for withdrawal bleeding (Miller & Notter, 2001). Women may experience breakthrough bleeding with extended COC pill use and should be counseled that this is not harmful. COC pills offer advantages and disadvantages. COC pills are often preferred by women who feel most comfortable with an oral as opposed to transdermal or vaginal delivery system. However, failure rates are often higher, because timely and consistent dosing requires discipline and motivation. Because of the variety of pill types, more options are available for managing side effects. Many COC pills are now sold generically, thus reducing the cost. A woman may choose to start COC pills in one of three ways:

a. Quick start allows her to take her first pill on the day she receives the prescription, increasing compliance and reducing the risk of subsequent pregnancy. A pregnancy test should be performed at the time of her visit, and if indicated, emergency contraception should be given, followed by initiation of the first COC pill no later than the next day. She should use a back-up method for the first 7 days, and return for a urine pregnancy test in 2–3 weeks if pregnancy before starting the COC pill is a possibility.
b. First day start is another option. The user begins her COC pill on the first day of her menses. This approach reduces the risk of ovarian follicle development in the first cycle, thus reducing the risk of pregnancy.
c. Sunday start requires the user to start her first pill on the Sunday after her menstrual cycle begins. Many women find it is easier to remember to start a new pill cycle on a Sunday, and enjoy the lower likelihood of bleeding on the weekend. However, this approach has the disadvantage of possible ovarian follicle formation, so a back-up method should be used for the first 7 days.

2. Transdermal patch

There is one transdermal patch currently marketed under the name Ortho-Evra®. It contains norelgestromin and ethinyl estradiol in a three-layered adhesive polyester patch. The hormonal dose is absorbed through the skin, thus bypassing the liver and gastrointestinal system. A new patch is applied once a week for 3 weeks, followed by a patch free-week, during which withdrawal bleeding will likely occur. The transdermal patch is equivalent to COC pills in efficacy in women who weigh less than 198 pounds (Zieman et al., 2002). Additionally, ease of use improves compliance, although pregnancy rates for women over 198 pounds are slightly higher. Care must be taken to ensure that the patch is completely adhered, because partial or complete separation from the skin has occurred. Although fewer long-term data are available for the patch, it seems to provide similar advantages, risks, and side effects as the COC pill. Serum levels of ethinyl estradiol are higher in patch users by 60% compared to users of a 35-mcg pill, but it is unclear whether this increases the risk of VTE (Nanda, 2007). Some users of the patch have experienced localized reactions, including rash and skin irritation at the site of application. Women with dermatologic conditions may not be candidates for patch use. The same options for starting COC pills are available for patch users; backup methods should be used for Quick start and Sunday start options. Management of missed or late patches depends on the week of use; manufacturer instructions should be given to the user.

3. Vaginal contraceptive ring

The vaginal contraceptive ring (Nuvaring®) is a soft, flexible ring made of ethylene vinyl acetate that releases ethinyl estradiol and etonogestrel (a metabolite of desogestrel) in a low and steady dose. It is worn in the vagina for 3 weeks, and removed for 1 week to allow for withdrawal bleeding. The hormones are absorbed transvaginally, and like the patch, bypass the liver and gastrointestinal system. Circulating levels of hormone are lower than in the transdermal patch or COC pill, and do not fluctuate throughout the day. Cycle control is often better than with the COC pill, and there are relatively few side effects (Bjarnadottir, Tuppurainen, & Killick, 2002).

Efficacy is comparable to the transdermal patch and COC pill, but similar to patch use, compliance is improved. Users are subject to the same advantages, risks, and side effects as with the other combined hormonal methods, but additionally some users experience vaginal discomfort and discharge. The ring may inadvertently be removed with intercourse, so care should be taken to check for its presence post-coitus. When initiating ring use, it is recommended that the first ring be inserted any time within the first 5 days of onset of menses, with back-up contraception for the first 7 days.

B. Progestin-only contraception

Progestin-only contraception is an option for women who cannot take estrogen because of medical contra-indications or estrogen-related side effects. Progestin can be taken orally (POP); by injection (medroxy-progesterone acetate); by implant (Implanon®); or through an intrauterine system (LNG-IUS). Each has its advantages, risks, and potential side effects. The only absolute contraindication to progestin use is current or recent breast cancer, although additional absolute contraindications exist for the LNG-IUS (Table 20-4). Relative contraindications to progestin and its delivery systems are listed in Table 20-5. Table 20-6 lists conditions where progestin and its delivery systems may be used but may require monitoring. As with Tables 20-1, 20-2, and 20-3, these tables are adapted from the WHO Medical Eligibility Criteria guidelines. When individual methods, noted in parentheses, are not specified, contra-indications and cautions apply to all progestin methods.

1. POP

The POP contains either norgestrel or norethin-drone, and no estrogen. The POP has a perfect use failure rate of 0.3%, and a typical use failure rate of 8%, and requires diligent pill-taking (pill must be taken within 3 hours of same time every day). It is often prescribed during lactation, ideally beginning 6 weeks postpartum. The main action of the POP is to thicken the cervical mucus; ovulation may or may not be inhibited. Therefore, ovarian cysts are more likely to occur with the POP than with the COC pill (Tayob, Adams, Jacobs, & Guillebaud, 1985). Without the cycle-regulating effect of estrogen, irregular bleeding (breakthrough bleeding, amenorrhea, or shortened cycles) can occur. There are no placebo pills; active pills are taken every day. If POPs are started within 5 days of the first day of menses, backup contraception is not necessary. If started at other times in the cycle, a pregnancy test should be done, and a backup method used for 2 days. POPs are in general more expensive than COC pills, and less effective in controlling medical conditions, such as dysmenorrhea, acne, and hir-sutism. POPs protect against uterine and ovarian cancer, PID, and benign breast disease.

2. Injectable progestin (Depo-provera®)

Depo-provera® (depo Medroxyprogesterone ace-tate), 150 mg, is given by intramuscular injec-tion every 11–13 weeks. A subcutaneous dose of 104 mg is also available for self administration. Medroxyprogesterone acetate is highly efficacious, with a failure rate of 0.3–3%. It is discreet and convenient, and can be used by women with con-traindications to estrogen. Medroxyprogesterone acetate suppresses the follicle-stimulating hormone and luteinizing hormone surge, resulting in ovula-tion suppression. Additionally, it thickens the cervi-cal mucus, thins the endometrium, and slows tubal motility. Disadvantages include irregular or heavy bleeding; amenorrhea; weight gain; depression; unfavorable lipid changes in some women; and decrease in bone density, which is largely revers-ible (Kaunitz, Arias, & McClung, 2008). Users should be encouraged to take calcium supplements and exercise regularly. Additionally, there can be a delay in return of fertility averaging 10 months from last injection. Medroxyprogesterone acetate is contraindicated in women with breast cancer, and should be used with caution in women with CVD and risk factors for CVD, liver disease, and vaginal bleeding without explanation. Advantages include convenience; high efficacy; possible decreased menorrhagia and dysmenorrhea; and a reduction in PID, endometrial cancer, fibroids, sickle cell anemia crises, and seizures. Medroxyprogesterone acetate should be initiated any time during the first 7 days of onset of menstruation, or at any time if the candidate is not pregnant. A backup method should be used for 7 days if injection occurs outside of the first 7 days of the cycle.

TABLE 20-6 Initiate Progestogen-Only Contraceptives, May Need to Monitor

Menarche to < 18 years, or > 45 years old (Depo-provera®)

Menarche to < 20 years or nulliparous (LNG-IUS)

Following second-trimester abortion (LNG-IUS)

Past ectopic pregnancy (POP)

Obesity and menarche to < 18 years old (Depo-provera®)

Multiple risk factors for arterial cardiovascular disease (POP, LNG-IUS, Implanon®)

History of hypertension where blood pressure cannot be measured

Adequately controlled hypertension where blood pressure can be evaluated (Depo-provera®)

Hypertension with systolic 140–159 or diastolic 90–99 (Depo-provera®)

Hypertension with systolic ≥ 160 or diastolic ≥ 100, or vascular disease present (POP, LNG-IUS, Implanon®)

History of DVT/PE, or DVT/PE on anticoagulant therapy, or major surgery with prolonged immobilization

Known thrombogenic mutations (factor V Leiden, prothrombin mutation, protein S, protein C, and antithrombin deficiencies)

Current and history of ischemic heart disease (POP, LNG-IUS, Implanon®)

Stroke (POP, LNG-IUS, Implanon®)

Known hyperlipidemias

Complicated valvular heart disease (LNG-IUS)

Systemic lupus erythematosus with severe thrombocytopenia (POP, LNG-IUS, Implanon®)

Systemic lupus erythematosus and on immunosuppressive treatment, or without other conditions

Migraine headache without aura and any age (Depo-provera®, LNG-IUS, Implanon®)

Migraine headache with aura and any age

Irregular vaginal bleeding and heavy or prolonged vaginal bleeding (POP, Depo-provera®, Implanon®)

Unexplained vaginal bleeding (POP)

Cervical intraepithelial neoplasia (Depo-provera®, Implanon®, LNG-IUS)

Cervical cancer awaiting treatment (Depo-provera®, Implanon®)

Breast mass, awaiting diagnosis

Cervical stenosis or laceration (LNG-IUS)

Past pelvic inflammatory disease and no subsequent pregnancy (LNG-IUS)

Increased risk of STIs, or current STI infection (excluding gonorrhea or *Chlamydia*) (LNG-IUS*)

Vaginitis, including trichomonas and bacterial vaginosis (LNG-IUS)

HIV infection (LNG-IUS)

AIDS (LNG-IUS*)

Diabetes, nonvascular, noninsulin or insulin-dependent

Diabetes with nephropathy, retinopathy, or neuropathy (POP, LNG-IUS, Implanon®)

Diabetes with other vascular disease or > 20 years' duration (POP, Implanon®, LNG-IUS)

Gallbladder disease, current or treated, symptomatic or asymptomatic

History of cholestasis related to COC use

Benign liver tumors, focal nodular hyperplasia

Antiretroviral therapy with nucleoside reverse transcriptase inhibitors (LNG-IUS*)

Antiretroviral therapy with nonnucleoside reverse transcriptase inhibitors (POP, Implanon®, LNG-IUS*)

Antiretroviral therapy with retinovir-boosted protease inhibitors (Implanon®, LNG-IUS*)

Anticonvulsant therapy with phenytoin, carbamazepine, barbiturates, primidone, topiramate, or oxycarbazepine (Implanon®)

Antimicrobial therapy with rifampicin or rifabutin therapy (Implanon®)

Where individual methods in parentheses, relative risk exists only for these methods. Where no parentheses, relative risk exists for all methods.
*Indicates overlap with Category III list, see WHO text for discussion.
Source: Adapted from 2009 WHO guidelines, Category II.

3. Implants (Implanon®)

Implanon® is a single implant containing etonogestrel in an ethylene vinyl acetate capsule. It is inserted under the skin of the nondominant upper arm by a trained clinician (training can be obtained through a company-sponsored training session). Implanon® is a highly effective form of birth control, with a 0.05% failure rate. It is effective for at least 3 years; efficacy is not dependent on user compliance. Its mechanism of action is to thicken the cervical mucus, suppress ovulation, and cause atrophy of the endometrium. It is discrete, and can be easily removed at any time with a single incision. Among the advantages of Implanon® is reduction in menstrual flow and cramping, rapid reversibility of fertility, and high acceptability and continuation. Disadvantages include irregular bleeding, amenorrhea, and pain or infection at implant site postinsertion. Implanon ® can be inserted at any time in the cycle, if pregnancy has been ruled out. If inserted within the first 7 days of onset of menses, no additional contraception is needed; otherwise, backup should be used for 7 days. Fertility is restored within 3–6 weeks of removal in 94% of women. Initially cost is high, but if spread out over 3 years of use, it can be less expensive than many other hormonal options.

4. Levonorgestrel intrauterine system (LNG-IUS)

LNG-IUS (Mirena®) is an intrauterine system containing levonorgestrel in a capsule molded to a polyethylene T-shaped device. The progestin is released directly into the uterine cavity, with only a small amount of systemic absorption. The amount of plasma concentration is lower than for implants and POPs, but the contraceptive effect remains high. Two strings are attached to the base, and extend through the cervix into the vagina. The strings allow users to check for the presence of the device and facilitate removal. LNG-IUS is effective for at least 5 years, with failure rates at 0.14% in the first year, and 0.71% by the fifth year. A total of 2–10% are expelled in the first year of use, often without the awareness of the user (it is important to teach the patient to check for her strings regularly). Mechanism of action is through thickening of the cervical mucus, inhibition of sperm capacitation, suppression of the endometrium, and in some cases suppression of ovulation. It is discrete and well tolerated.

Noncontraceptive benefits include decrease in menstrual flow and pain, and in risk of endometrial cancer. LNG-US has been used in the treatment of women with menorrhagia, endometriosis, adenomyosis, and fibroids. Disadvantages include pain with and after insertion, especially in nulliparous women; infection postinsertion (0.1%); perforation of uterus at the time of insertion (less than 0.1%); spontaneous expulsion; irregular spotting and bleeding (usually limited to first 6 months); amenorrhea; ovarian cyst problems; and rare side effects, such as headaches, acne, mood changes, and back and abdominal cramping. The cumulative risk for PID for users of LNG-US is 0.8% over a 5-year period, and is higher in women younger than age 25 (Anderson, Odlind, & Rybo, 1994).

Cervical cultures for *Chlamydia* and gonorrhea should be performed before insertion, and women should be counseled to use condoms with new or high-risk partners. The insertion process requires clinician training. It can be inserted immediately after abortion or delivery, and if inserted within the first 7 days of menstrual onset, no backup method is needed. It can be inserted at other times in the menstrual cycle if pregnancy is ruled out. Backup contraception should be used for 7 days. Cost of the LNG-IUS is high, but if used for 5 years the overall cost is lower than other hormonal methods.

C. ECP

ECP provides the only postcoital method of contraception; thus, it is an excellent option after unplanned intercourse, after rape, or after contraceptive failure (condom breakage, missed COC pills or POPs, delay of more than 14 days in getting medroxyprogesterone acetate injection, delay of 2 or more days in starting a new ring or patch cycle). Prepackaged ECP contains progestin only; they are Plan B One-Step, which contains 1.5 mg of levonorgestrel taken once, and Next Choice®, which contains two pills of 0.75 mg of levonorgestrel taken 12 hours apart (these can also both be taken at once). CHC pills containing at least 100 mcg of ethinyl estradiol and 100 mcg of norgestrel or 0.5 mg levonorgestrel can also be used in two doses taken 12 hours apart (Yuzpe method). This approach may cause nausea and vomiting; antinausea medication may be prescribed. Although no absolute contraindications exist for ECPs, those containing only progestin are safer, more effective, and have fewer side effects, and should be used when possible.

ECPs have varying actions depending on the phase of the cycle in which they are taken. They may disrupt normal follicular maturation; interfere with corpus luteum function; or alter the endometrium, cervical mucus, and tubal transport. The first dose should be taken immediately, or within 120 hours of unprotected intercourse (72 hours is mandated by package insert, although it has been shown to be effective at the longer interval). Plan B and Next Choice® reduce the risk of pregnancy by 89%; combined estrogen and progesterone pills reduce the risk by 75%. Efficacy is dependent on what phase in the woman's cycle she takes the ECP, and how many hours have elapsed since intercourse. ECP may cause early or later menstrual flow. If no bleeding occurs within 3 weeks of taking the dose, a pregnancy test should be performed. ECP should not be used as a primary birth control method, because it is less effective than other methods. However, all patients using CHC methods, POP, medroxyprogesterone acetate, and nonhormonal contraceptives should be advised to obtain ECP as a backup method ahead of need. Pharmacies provide ECP to patients 18 and older without a prescription. Patients under the age of 18 should be given a prescription.

II. **Database** (may include but is not limited to)

A. *Subjective*

1. Combined Hormonal Contraceptive (CHC)
   a. Medical illnesses
   b. Family history (especially deep VTE and pulmonary embolism)
   c. Personal and social history
   d. Age
   e. Parity and desire for future fertility
   f. Breastfeeding, postpartum (in nonbreastfeeding women)
   g. Postabortion
   h. Smoking
   i. Sexual history: recent history of unprotected intercourse, current risk for sexually transmitted disease
   j. Previous contraceptive use: satisfaction, compliance, problems
   k. Preference for and comfort with different hormone delivery systems
   l. Tolerance of side effects: weight change, breast tenderness, bleeding irregularities, melasma and chloasma, nausea, headaches, libido changes, mood swings, vaginal discharge (vaginal contraceptive ring)
   m. Financial constraints
   n. Current medication use
   o. Menstrual history: age of menarche, character of menses, date of last menstrual period

2. Progestin-only contraception
   a. Medical illness
   b. Family illness
   c. Personal and social history
   d. Age
   e. Parity and desire for future fertility
   f. Breastfeeding, postpartum
   g. Postabortion
   h. Smoking
   i. Sexual history: recent history of unprotected intercourse, current risk for sexually transmitted disease
   j. Previous contraceptive use and satisfaction, compliance, problems
   k. Preference for and comfort with different hormonal delivery systems (e.g., not fearful of needles and willing to return for repeat)
   l. Injections (medroxyprogesterone acetate), willing to undergo a minor procedure (LNG-IUS, Implanon®)
   m. Tolerance of side effects: menstrual cycle disturbances; weight gain (medroxyprogesterone acetate); breast tenderness; mood changes; and possible local inflammation and infection (Implanon)®
   n. Financial constraints
   o. Current medications
   p. Menstrual history: age of menarche, character of menses, and date of last menstrual period
   q. Noncontraceptive benefits: scant or no menses (less anemia); decreased menstrual problems; decreased risk of endometrial and ovarian cancer; decreased risk of PID and fibroids; decreased pain from endometriosis; and fewer seizures and sickle cell crises (medroxyprogesterone acetate)

3. ECP
   a. Age
   b. Date of last menstrual period
   c. Time of unprotected intercourse
   d. Medical conditions
   e. Contraceptive methods used and nature of failure or misuse
   f. Occurrence of rape

B. *Objective*

1. CHC
   a. Blood pressure and weight
   b. Breast examination
   c. Speculum and pelvic examination (not required unless symptomatic)
   d. Pap smear and testing for sexually transmitted diseases as indicated
   e. Assessment for skin conditions (patch use)
   f. Pregnancy test

2. Progestin-only contraception
   a. Blood pressure and weight
   b. Breast examination
   c. Speculum examination with Pap smear and cultures for gonorrhea and *Chlamydia* (LNG-IUS), assess for cervical stenosis (LNG-IUS)

d. Pelvic examination (required for LNG-IUS and if symptomatic)

e. Pregnancy test

3. ECP

Pregnancy test

III. Assessment

A. CHC

1. No medical contraindications to estrogen or progestin

2. Nonsmoker (if older than age 35)

3. Not breastfeeding

4. Noncontraceptive benefits: decreased acne and hirsutism; less endometrial and ovarian cancer; decreased benign breast disease; improved cycle control; suppression of endometriosis; less gonorrheal PID; improvement in premenstrual syndrome and perimenopausal symptoms; decreased anemia; fewer ovarian cyst problems; possible reduction in such diseases as polycystic ovary syndrome, rheumatoid arthritis, uterine fibroids, seizure and asthma episodes, colorectal cancer, and osteoporosis; possible improvement of lipid profile.

5. Normotensive

6. No breast masses

7. No lifestyle barriers: need for discretion; difficulty remembering to use method; difficulty with storage or access; need for protection against sexually transmitted infections; financial constraints; desire for rapid return to fertility (delayed in some COC users)

8. No skin rashes (patch)

9. No physical or psychologic limitations with vaginal insertion or removal (ring)

10. Willing to tolerate side effects

B. Progestin-only contraception

1. No medical contraindications to progestin or vehicle for progestin

2. Noncontraceptive benefits: reduction in menstrual flow and pain, migraine headaches and ovarian cyst formation (Implanon®)

3. Appropriate when estrogen contraindicated (smoker, hypertension, lactation, or migraine headache)

4. No breast masses

5. No lifestyle barriers: need for discretion (POP); difficulty remembering to use method (POP);

difficulty with storage or access; need for protection against sexually transmitted infections; financial constraints; desire for rapid return to fertility (medroxyprogesterone acetate); and intolerance of irregular bleeding

6. Obesity (medroxyprogesterone acetate, and transdermal patch)

7. High efficacy desired (medroxyprogesterone acetate, Implanon®, and LNG-IUS)

8. No PID, *Chlamydia*, gonorrhea, or cervical or uterine anomalies (LNG-IUS)

9. Willing to tolerate discomfort of delivery (Implanon®, and medroxyprogesterone acetate)

10. Willing to tolerate side effects

C. ECP

1. Within window of effective use (120 hours from unprotected intercourse versus 72 hours mandated in package insert)

2. Willing to tolerate side effects (Yuzpe method)

IV. Goals of clinical management

A. Screen for contraindications to contraceptive method

B. Management and patient adherence

1. Select appropriate contraceptive method; discuss risks, benefits, and costs.

2. Provide counseling and tools to increase compliance. Discuss smoking cessation and prevention of sexually transmitted infections with all methods of contraception.

V. Plan

A. Screening and diagnostic tests

In addition to Pap smear and sexually transmitted infection testing, may include mammogram, pelvic ultrasound (rule out fibroids or other anomalies), lipid testing (if family history of premature CVD), fasting blood sugar (if family history of diabetes), Leiden factor V.

B. Management and patient adherence

1. COC pills

a. Choose any low-dose (≤ 35 mcg) pill. If patient has polycystic ovary syndrome, hirsutism, or acne, choose pill with low androgenic activity. Choose monophasic pill if cycle suppression planned.

b. Select starting option (first day, quick start, Sunday start) based on patient desire, compliance, and willingness to use backup.

c. Select cycling pattern based on patient desire and medical indications (endometriosis, dysmenorrhea, and menstrual migraines).

d. May cycle every 6–9 weeks, or may use continuously (no cycling).

e. May choose prepackaged extended cycle pills or skip placebo pills.

f. Discuss possible side effects and option for changing pill type, breakthrough bleeding, and lack of withdrawal bleeding.

g. **Review warning signs (ACHES):**
   i. Abdominal pain
   ii. Chest pain
   iii. Headaches
   iv. Eye problems
   v. Severe leg pain

h. Discuss compliance (take at same time every day); tips for remembering pills (e.g., set alarm, put near toothbrush); what to do if pill missed; when to use backup.

i. Provide prescription for ECP if patient younger than 18 and suggest older patients obtain ECP ahead of time.

j. Discuss interactions with medications (certain antiretroviral therapy, certain anticonvulsant therapy, rifampicin, St. John's wort may interfere with efficacy; most antibiotics do not lower effectiveness).

2. Transdermal patch

a. Select starting option (same as for COC pills)

b. Discuss patch placement
   i. Place on clean, dry, skin of lower abdomen, buttock, upper arm, or upper back without rash or abrasion; rotate sites
   ii. Avoid use of body lotions and oils; can be worn in shower and bath, during exercise and swimming

c. Discuss compliance including daily patch inspection; tips for remembering patch removal and replacement dates; what to do if dates missed (patch effective for 2 extra days); when to use backup.

d. Discuss side effects, warning signs (ACHES).

e. Provide prescription for replacement patch if patch dislodged.

f. Provide prescription for ECP if patient younger than 18; suggest older patients obtain ECP ahead of time.

g. Dispose of used patch in product package to avoid environmental contamination.

3. Vaginal contraceptive ring

a. Instruct to insert first ring within first 5 days of onset of menses, or at anytime if not pregnant (use backup for 7 days).

b. When possible, have patient insert and remove ring at time of examination to demonstrate comfort and ease of insertion.

c. Ring is usually worn during intercourse, but can be removed before intercourse if replaced within 3 hours. If worn with intercourse, check for presence in vagina postcoitus.

d. Dispose of used ring in product package.

e. Discuss side effects and warning signs (ACHES).

f. Discuss compliance; tips for remembering insertion and removal dates; what to do if dates missed (ring offers 1 extra week of efficacy); and backup.

g. Provide prescription for ECP if patient younger than 18; suggest older patients obtain ECP ahead of time.

4. POP

a. Begin first pill at any time during the first 5 days of menses, or begin at any time if not pregnant (use backup for 2 days). May begin immediately if postpartum (6 weeks if breastfeeding) or postabortion.

b. Discuss compliance; tips for remembering to take pills; what to do if pill missed or late by 3 or more hours (use backup for at least 48 hours).

c. Manage side effects: for amenorrhea, rule out pregnancy, then reassure. For irregular bleeding, rule out underlying pathology, then reassure. Explain that bleeding is likely to improve within 3 months. For heavy bleeding, nonsteroidal anti-inflammatory medications (NSAID) for 3-day course may be beneficial.

d. Discuss interactions with medications (see COC pills).

e. Provide prescription for ECP if patient younger than 18.

5. Injectable progestin

a. Provide first injection within 7 days of onset of menses (no backup method needed) or at any time if not pregnant (use backup for 7 days). Medroxyprogesterone acetate may be given within 7 days postpartum and immediately postabortion.

b. Inject 150 mg intramuscularly deeply into deltoid or gluteus maximus.

c. Schedule subsequent injections every 11–12 weeks. If more than 13 weeks from previous injection, test for pregnancy. Assess for weight gain and depression.

d. Review potential side effects: weight gain, depression, severe headaches, heavy bleeding, and amenorrhea.

e. Manage bleeding problems. For heavy bleeding, rule out underlying pathology, then may provide NSAIDs (800 mg ibuprofen every 8 hours for 3 days) or conjugated estrogen (2.5, 1.25, or 0.625 mg one to four times a day for 4–6 days), or COC pills for 1–2 months. For spotting or breakthrough bleeding, rule out underlying pathology, reassure, or treat as for heavy bleeding. For amenorrhea, test for pregnancy if indicated and reassure.

f. Discuss delayed return to fertility of up to 1.5 years.

g. Discuss bone health; recommend 1,000–1,200 mg of calcium daily and 1,000 iu of vitamin D_3 daily, discuss weight-bearing exercise.

h. Provide prescription for ECP if patient younger than 18; suggest older patients obtain ECP in advance.

6. Implants

a. Implanon® should be inserted by a trained practitioner according to manufacturer guidelines. It may be inserted within 7 days of onset of menses (no backup method needed) or at any time in the cycle if not pregnant (backup should be used for 7 days).

b. Discuss possible side effects: irregular bleeding and infection or abscess at insertion site.

c. Manage side effects: for amenorrhea, perform pregnancy test, then reassure. For spotting or breakthrough bleeding, rule out underlying pathology, then treat as for medroxyprogesterone acetate. For arm pain and swelling, rule out infection, then treat with icepacks and NSAIDs. For infection without abscess, treat with oral antibiotics, and recheck in 24–48 hours. For abscess, treat with antibiotics, drain pus, and remove implant.

d. Remove implant according to manufacturer guidelines after 3 years, or as desired by patient. Discuss rapid return to fertility with patient.

7. LNG-IUS

a. Insertion of LNG-IUS should be performed by a trained clinician, according to manufacturer guidelines. The system can be inserted within the first 7 days of onset of menses; no backup method is needed. It may be inserted at other times if pregnancy is excluded; use backup for 7 days.

b. Cervical dilation may be necessary, either with graduated dilators, or misoprostol, 200-µg tablet placed in the vagina or buccal cavity 1–2 hours before insertion. Patients can be premedicated with ibuprofen or with a paracervical block.

c. Patients should be observed postinsertion for adverse events, including signs of perforation and vasovagal reaction.

d. Advise NSAIDs for postinsertion pain.

e. Patients may be scheduled for a follow-up visit in 2 months to assess for presence of strings and for side effects; return sooner if problems.

f. Discuss side effects, including menstrual changes, and warning signs of expulsion and infection. Teach patient how to check for strings.

g. Discuss signs of PID, including prolonged heavy bleeding, unusual discharge, pelvic pain, fever and chills, and dysparunia. If PID is diagnosed, treat with antibiotics.

8. ECP

a. All women who are using COC pills and POPs, rings, patch, and nonhormonal contraception should be advised to have ECP available.

b. Advise patients to purchase ECP in advance. Plan B One-Step and Next Choice® are more effective than COC pills.

c. Write prescription for patients younger than 18.

d. Provide ECP to all patients if unprotected intercourse has occurred within 120 hours; review directions for taking ECP.

e. Discuss possible side effects (nausea and vomiting with COC pills; may prescribe antiemetic to take 1 hour before first dose; not needed with Plan B).

f. Discuss possible changes in menstrual cycle post-ECP (early or delayed menses). Recommend pregnancy test if no menses in 3 weeks.

g. Report rape; provide or refer for trauma services.

h. Discuss prevention of sexually transmitted disease, offer testing.

i. Advise no teratogenic effect if pregnancy occurs.

j. Advise no prolonged contraceptive effect after ECP dose, may begin new cycle of CHC or POC immediately.

k. Discuss contraceptive compliance, reason for contraceptive failure if indicated.

REFERENCES

Anderson, K., Odlind, V., & Rybo, G. (1994). Levonorgestrel-releasing and copper releasing (Nova-T) intrauterine devices during five years of use: A randomized comparative trial. *Contraception, 49,* 56–72.

Bjarnadottir, R. I., Tuppurainen, M., & Killick, S. R. (2002). Comparison of cycle control with a combined contraceptive vaginal ring and oral levonorgestrel/ethinyl estradiol. *American Journal of Obstetrics and Gynecology, 186,* 389–395.

Dickey, R. P. (2007). *Managing Contraceptive Pill Patients* (13th ed.). New Orleans, LA: EMIS Medical Publishers.

Endrikat, J., Cronin, M., Gerlinger, C., Ruebig, A., Schmidt, W., & Düsterberg, B. (2001). Open, multicenter comparison of efficacy, cycle control, and tolerability of a 23-day oral contraceptive regimen with 20 microg ethinyl estradiol and 150 microg desogestrel. *Contraception, 64*(3), 201–207.

Kaunitz, A. M., Arias, R., & McClung, M. (2008). Bone density recovery after depot medroxyprogesterone acetate injectable contraception use. *Contraception, 77,* 67–76.

Miller, L., & Notter, K. M. (2001). Menstrual reduction with extended use of combination oral contraceptive pills: Randomized controlled trial. *Obstetrics and Gynecology, 98*(5 Pt 1), 771–778.

Nanda, K. (2007). Contraceptive patch and vaginal contraception. In R. A. Hatcher, J. Trussell, A. L. Nelson, W. Cates, F. H. Stewart, & D. Kowal (Eds.), *Contraceptive Technology* (19th rev. ed., pp. 271–295). New York, NY: Ardent Media.

Nelson, A. L. (2007). Combined oral contraceptives. In R. A. Hatcher, J. Trussell, A. L. Nelson, W. Cates, F. H. Stewart, & D. Kowal (Eds.), *Contraceptive Technology* (19th rev. ed., pp. 193–270). New York, NY: Ardent Media.

Nelson, A. L. (2010). A new OC with a new estrogen, a new progestin, and a new indication. *The Female Patient, 35*(1), 36–38.

Pharmacist's Letter/Prescriber's Letter. (2007) *Comparison of Oral Contraceptives.* Stockton: Therapeutic Research Center, CA..

Spona, J., Elstein, M., Feichtinger, W., Sullivan, H., Lüdicke, F., Müller, U., . . . Dusterberg, B. (1996). Shorterpill-free interval in combined oral contraceptives decreases follicular development. *Contraception, 54*(2), 71–77.

Tayob, Y., Adams, J., Jacobs, H. S., & Guillebaud, J. (1985). Ultrasound demonstration of increased frequency of functional cysts in women using progestogen-only oral contraception. *British Journal of Obstetrics and Gynaecology, 92,* 1003–1009.

Trussell, J. (2007). Contraceptive efficacy. In R. A. Hatcher, J. Trussell, A. L. Nelson, W. Cates, F. H. Stewart, & D. Kowal (Eds.), *Contraceptive Technology* (19th rev. ed., pp. 747–826). New York, NY: Ardent Media.

World Health Organization, Department of Reproductive Health and Research. (2009). *Medical Eligibility Criteria for Contraceptive Use* (4th ed.). Geneva: Author.

Zieman, M., Guillebaud, J., Weisberg, E., Shangold, G. A., Fisher, A. C., & Creasy, G. W. (2002). Contraceptive efficacy and cycle control with the Ortho Evra/Evra transdermal system: The analysis of pooled data. *Fertility and Sterility, 77*(Suppl. 2), S13–S18.

Zieman, M., Hatcher, R. A., Cwiak, C., Darney, P. D., Creinin, M. D., & Stosur, H. R. (2007–2009). *A Pocket Guide to Managing Contraception.* Tiger, GA: Bridging the Gap Foundation.

APPENDIX 20–1: COMPARISON OF ORAL CONTRACEPTIVES

TABLE 1 Comparison of Oral Contraceptives (Updated September 2009)

Products[a]	Manufacturer	Estrogen	Progestin	Comments
LOW-DOSE MONOPHASIC PILLS				
Aviane-28 Lessina Levlite Lutera Sronyx	Teva Teva Bayer Watson Watson	EE 20 mcg	Levonorgestrel 0.1 mg	Low estrogen; low progestin; low androgen.[14] Low estrogen dose may cause more spotting and less margin of error for missed pills. Good choice to minimize risk of estrogen side effects like nausea, breast tenderness, etc.[6]
Junel 1/20 Junel Fe 1/20 Loestrin-21 1/20 Loestrin Fe 1/20 Microgestin 1/20 Microgestin Fe 1/20	Teva Teva Warner Chilcott Warner Chilcott Watson Watson	EE 20 mcg	Norethindrone 1 mg	Low estrogen; high progestin; medium androgen.[13, 14] Low estrogen dose may cause more spotting and less margin of error for missed pills. Good choice to minimize risk of estrogen side effects like nausea, breast tenderness, etc.[6]
Levora Nordette-28 Portia-28	Watson Teva Watson	EE 30 mcg	Levonorgestrel 0.15 mg	Low estrogen; medium progestin; medium/high androgen.[13, 14] Good choice to minimize estrogen side effects like nausea, breast tenderness, etc. Good choice to minimize spotting and/or breakthrough bleeding.[6]
Cryselle-21 Cryselle-28 Low-Ogestrel-21 Low-Ogestrel-28 Lo/ Ovral-28	Teva Teva Watson Watson Wyeth	EE 30 mcg	Norgestrel 0.3 mg	Low estrogen; medium progestin; medium/high androgen.[13, 14] Good choice to minimize estrogen side effects like nausea, breast tenderness, etc; and to minimize spotting and/or breakthrough bleeding.[6]
Junel 1.5/30 Junel Fe 1.5/30 Loestrin 1.5/30-21 Loestrin Fe 1.5/30 Microgestin 1.5/30 Microgestin Fe 1.5/30	Teva Teva Warner Chilcott Warner Chilcott Watson Watson	EE 30 mcg	Norethindrone acetate 1.5 mg	Low estrogen; high progestin; high androgen.[13,14] Good choice to minimize estrogen side effects like nausea, breast tenderness, etc. [6]
Apri Desogen Ortho-Cept Reclipsen	Teva Organon Ortho Watson	EE 30 mcg	Desogestrel 0.15 mg	Low estrogen; high progestin; low androgen.[13,14] Increased risk of DVT with desogestrel over other progestins (controversial data).[1] Good choice to minimize spotting and/or breakthrough bleeding; and to minimize androgenic effects. Has favorable lipid profile. [6]

TABLE 1 Comparison of Oral Contraceptives (Updated September 2009) *(continued)*

Products[a]	Manufacturer	Estrogen	Progestin	Comments
LOW-DOSE MONOPHASIC PILLS *(continued)*				
Yasmin Ocella	Bayer Teva	EE 30 mcg	Drospirenone 3 mg	Low estrogen; progestin potency unclear; anti-androgenic and antimineralocorticoid activity.[6,23] Does not appear to cause cyclic fluid retention. May be good choice for women with PMS, premenstrual dysphoric disorder, acne, hirsutism, or PCOS.[6] Can increase potassium: avoid in renal/hepatic dysfunction or renal insufficiency. Check potassium during first cycle if another potassium-sparing drug (NSAID, ACE inhibitor, angiotensin receptor blocker, potassium-sparing diuretic, aldosterone antagonist) is given.[3]
Kelnor 1/35 *Zovia 1/35*	Teva Watson	EE 35 mcg	Ethynodiol diacetate 1 mg	Medium estrogen; high progestin; low androgen.[13,14] Good choice to minimize androgenic effects.[6]
Ortho-Cyclen-28 *MonoNessa* *Sprintec*	Ortho Watson Teva	EE 35 mcg	Norgestimate 0.25 mg	Medium estrogen; low progestin; low androgen.[13,14] Good choice to minimize spotting and/or breakthrough bleeding and to minimize androgenic effects. Has favorable lipid profile.[6]
Necon 1/50	Watson	Mestranol 50 mcg	Norethindrone 1 mg	Medium estrogen; medium progestin; medium androgen.[13,14]
Ovcon-35 *Balziva* *Femcon Fe* chewable *Zenchent*	Warner Chilcott Teva Warner Chilcott Watson	EE 35 mcg	Norethindrone 0.4 mg; total of 8.4 mg/cycle.[6]	Medium estrogen; low progestin; low androgen.[13,14] Good choice to minimize androgenic effects. Has favorable lipid profile.[6]
Brevicon-28 *Modicon-28* *Necon 0.5/35* *Nortrel 0.5/35*	Watson Ortho Watson Teva	EE 35 mcg	Norethindrone 0.5 mg; total of 10.5 mg/cycle.	Medium estrogen; low progestin; low androgen.[13,14] Good choice to minimize androgenic effects. Has favorable lipid profile.[6]
Necon 1/35-28 *Norinyl 1+35-28* *Nortrel 1/35-28* *Ortho-Novum 1/35-28*	Watson Watson Teva Ortho	EE 35 mcg	Norethindrone 1 mg; total of 21 mg/cycle.[6]	Medium estrogen; medium/high progestin; medium androgen.[6,13]
HIGH-DOSE MONOPHASIC PILLS [b]				
Ovcon-50	Warner Chilcott	EE 50 mcg	Norethindrone 1 mg	High estrogen; medium progestin; medium androgen.[13,14]
Ogestrel 0.5/50-28	Watson	EE 50 mcg	Norgestrel 0.5 mg	High estrogen; high progestin; high androgen.[13,14]
Zovia 1/50-28	Watson	EE 50 mcg	Ethynodiol diacetate 1 mg	High estrogen; high progestin; medium/high androgen.[13,14]

(continues)

TABLE 1 Comparison of Oral Contraceptives (Updated September 2009) *(continued)*

Products[a]	Manufacturer	Estrogen	Progestin	Comments
BIPHASIC PILLS				
Mircette *Kariva* Desogestrel/ethinyl estradiol	Duramed Teva Watson	EE 20 mcg × 21 days, placebo × 2 days, 10 mcg × 5 days	Desogestrel 0.15 mg × 21 days	Low estrogen; high progestin; low androgen.[13,14] Shorter hormone-free interval may help menstrual migraine, dysmenorrhea, PMS. Increased risk of DVT with desogestrel over other progestins.[1]
Necon 10/11	Watson	EE 35 mcg	Norethindrone 0.5 mg × 10 days, 1 mg × 11 days.	High estrogen; medium progestin; low/medium androgen.[13,14] Poor cycle control compared with levonorgestrel triphasic pill.[5]
TRIPHASIC PILLS				
Estrostep Fe *Tilia Fe*[f] *Tri-Legest Fe*	Warner Chilcott Watson Teva	EE 20 mcg × 5 days, 30 mcg × 7 days, 35 mcg × 9 days	Norethindrone 1 mg × 21 days	Low estrogen; high progestin; medium androgen.[13,14] FDA-labeled for acne. Good choice to minimize estrogen side effects like nausea, breast tenderness, etc; and to minimize spotting and/or breakthrough bleeding. [6]
Ortho Tri-Cyclen Lo *Tri Lo Sprintec*	Ortho Watson	EE 25 mcg × 21 days	Norgestimate 0.18 mg × 7 days, 0.215 mg × 7 days, 0.25 mg × 7 days.	Low estrogen; low progestin; low androgen.[13,14] Good choice to minimize spotting, breakthrough bleeding, and androgenic effects. Has favorable lipid profile.[6]
Cyclessa *Velivet* Desogestrel/ethinyl estradiol	Schering-Plough Teva Watson	EE 25 mcg × 21 days	Desogestrel 0.1 mg × 7 days, 0.125 mg × 7 days, 0.15 mg × 7 days.	Low estrogen; high progestin; low androgen.[23] First triphasic pill with desogestrel. Increased risk of DVT with desogestrel over other progestins. Better cycle control and less weight gain than *Ortho-Novum 7/7/7*. [15]
Enpresse *Trivora*	Teva Watson	EE 30 mcg × 6 days, 40 mcg × 5 days, 30 mcg × 10 days	Levonorgestrel 0.05 mg × 6 days, 0.075 mg × 5 days, 0.125 mg × 10 days. Total of 1.925 mg/cycle.[6]	Medium estrogen; low progestin; low/medium androgen.[13,14] Better cycle control than with norethindrone biphasic pill (*Ortho-Novum 10/11*).[5]
Ortho Tri-Cyclen *TriNessa* *Tri-Sprintec*	Ortho Watson Teva	EE 35 mcg × 21 days	Norgestimate 0.18 mg × 7 days, 0.215 mg × 7 days, 0.25 mg × 7 days.	Medium estrogen; low progestin; low androgen.[13,14] FDA-labeled for treatment of acne.
Aranelle *Leena* *Tri-Norinyl*	Teva Watson Watson	EE 35 mcg × 21 days	Norethindrone 0.5 mg × 7 days, 1 mg × 9 days, 0.5 mg × 5 days. Total of 15 mg/cycle.[6]	Medium estrogen; medium progestin; low/medium androgen.[6,13,14]
Ortho-Novum 7/7/7 *Nortrel 7/7/7* *Necon 7/7/7*	Ortho Teva Watson	EE 35 mcg × 21 days	Norethindrone 0.5 mg × 7 days, 0.75 mg × 7 days, 1 mg × 7 days. Total of 15.75 mg/cycle.[6]	Medium estrogen; medium progestin; low/medium androgen.[6,13,14]

TABLE 1 Comparison of Oral Contraceptives (Updated September 2009) *(continued)*

Products[a]	Manufacturer	Estrogen	Progestin	Comments
EXTENDED-CYCLE PILLS				
Loestrin-24 Fe	Warner Chilcott	EE 20 mcg × 24 days	Norethindrone 1 mg × 24 days	Low estrogen; high progestin; medium androgen.[13, 14] Low estrogen dose may cause more spotting and less margin of error for missed pills. Good choice to minimize risk of estrogen side effects like nausea, breast tenderness, etc.[6] 24/4-day cycle combination may be helpful for women wanting to stay on a 28-day cycle, but minimize duration of withdrawal bleeding and menstrual-related symptoms.
LoSeasonique	Duramed	EE 20 mcg × 84 days, 10 mcg × 7 days	Levonorgestrel 0.1 mg × 84 days	A low dose version of *Seasonique*. [25]
Seasonale *Jolessa* *Quasense*	Duramed Teva Watson	EE 30 mcg × 84 days	Levonorgestrel 0.15 mg × 84 days	84-day active pills then 7-day pill-free interval. More intermenstrual bleeding and/or spotting than with 28-day cycle; total days of bleeding and/or spotting similar.[9] May allow women to experience menstruation-related symptoms less frequently.[1,6]
Seasonique	Duramed	EE 30 mcg × 84 days, 10 mcg × 7 days	Levonorgestrel 0.15 mg × 84 days	84-day active pills then 7-day low-dose estrogen instead of placebo pills. Extended cycle and lack of hormone-free interval may help menorrhagia, dysmenorrhea, menstrual migraine, and PMS.[1,19]
Yaz	Bayer	EE 20 mcg × 24 days	Drospirenone 3 mg × 24 days	FDA-approved for premenstrual dysphoric disorder and moderate acne. Follows 24/4-day cycle and contains ingredients of *Yasmin*, but with lower estrogen dose (20 mcg EE compared to 30 mcg EE in *Yasmin*). Also see *Yasmin* comments.
CONTINUOUS-CYCLE PILLS				
Lybrel	Wyeth	EE 20 mcg	Levonorgestrel 90 mcg	Active pill taken every day (NO pill-free interval).[22] Breakthrough bleeding/spotting common initially and decreases with continued use. May allow women to experience menstruation-related symptoms less frequently.[1,6]

(continues)

TABLE 1 Comparison of Oral Contraceptives (Updated September 2009) *(continued)*

Products[a]	Manufacturer	Estrogen	Progestin	Comments
PROGESTIN-ONLY PILLS[c]—"Mini-pill"				
Camila *Errin* *Jolivette* *Micronor* *Nor-QD* *Nora-BE*	Teva Teva Watson Ortho Watson Watson	Not applicable	Norethindrone 0.35 mg	Irregular menses, but overall blood loss reduced. Preferred over COCs in women who are breastfeeding.[1]
EMERGENCY CONTRACEPTION				
Plan B *Next Choice*	Duramed Watson	Not applicable	Levonorgestrel 0.75 mg tablets × 2	For prevention of pregnancy for women who present within 72 hours of unprotected intercourse or contraceptive failure. Traditional FDA-approved regimen consists of 2 tablets with the first tablet taken as soon as possible within 72 hours and the second tablet taken 12 hours later.[20,26] Alternatively taking both tablets at once is equally effective and is recommended by some experts.[1] *Plan B* can be considered for a woman who presents within 5 days of unprotected or inadequately protected sexual intercourse; however, it's more effective the earlier it is taken.[1] *Plan B* is about 89% effective if used within 3 days after sex.[20]
Plan B One-Step	Duramed	Not applicable	Levonorgestrel 1.5 mg tablet	One tablet for prevention of pregnancy for women who present within 72 hours of unprotected intercourse or contraceptive failure. Similar efficacy and adverse effects as *Plan B*.[10]

[a]These products are grouped together by hormone content for the purpose of clinical equivalence. This grouping is not an indication of therapeutic equivalence for purposes of substitution as defined by the FDA's Orange Book. For therapeutic equivalence, consult the Orange Book.[17]

[b] Avoid pills with more than 35 mcg of ethinyl estradiol in hypertensive women; lower doses of estrogen can be used in non-smoking women age 35 years or younger who have well–controlled hypertension, and no evidence of end-organ vascular disease [Level B]. Also avoid pills with more than 35 mcg of ethinyl estradiol in women with controlled hyperlipidemia; use alternative contraceptive if LDL cholesterol >160 mg/dL or multiple additional risk factors for coronary heart disease [Level C].[7]

[c]The American College of Obstetrics and Gynecology considers progestin-only contraceptives to be safer than combined oral contraceptives for women with: migraine headache [Level B]; smoker over 35 years old [Level A]; history of thromboembolic disease [Level A]; less than two weeks postpartum; hypertension with vascular disease or over 35 years of age; diabetes with vascular disease or over 35 years of age; systemic lupus erythematosus with vascular disease, nephritis, or antiphospholipid antibodies [Level B]; hypertriglyceridemia.[7] Combined oral contraceptives are contraindicated in coronary artery disease, congestive heart failure, and cerebrovascular disease; a progestin-only contraceptive may be an appropriate alternative for women with these conditions [Level C]. Combined oral contraceptives may be considered for women with migraine who do not have focal neurologic signs, do not smoke, are otherwise healthy, and are younger than 35 years old [Level B]. Progestin-only contraceptives can be started immediately postpartum. They are the preferred form of hormonal contraception in women who are breastfeeding; combined oral contraceptives can be considered when milk flow is well-established [Level A].[7]

[f] *Tilia Fe* has same NDA as *Estrostep Fe*.

Abbreviations: COC = combined oral contraceptives; DVT = deep vein thrombosis; EE = ethinyl estradiol; PCOS = polycystic ovary syndrome.

Pharmacist's Letter / Prescriber's Letter ~ P.O. Box 8190, Stockton, CA 95208 ~ Phone: 209-472-2240 ~ Fax: 209-472-2249

www.pharmacistsletter.com ~ www.prescribersletter.com

TABLE 2 Hormonal Alternatives to Oral Contraception

Brand Name	Manufacturer	Estrogen	Progestin	Failure Rate[d]	Comments
Depo-Provera CI Medroxyprogesterone Acetate Injection	Pfizer Sicor	None	Medroxyprogesterone acetate 150 mg	0.3%	IM injection once every 3 months. Long duration of action may be inappropriate for some women. Noncontraceptive benefits in women with sickle cell disease. May decrease risk of seizures in women with epilepsy. May decrease bone mineral density.[6,7]
Depo-SubQ Provera 104	Pfizer	None	Medroxyprogesterone acetate 104 mg	N/A	SC injection once every 3 months. FDA approved for use as a contraceptive in December 2004 and for management of pain associated with endometriosis in March 2005. Efficacy similar to *Depo-Provera* and medroxyprogesterone injections, but at lower doses. Long-term adverse effects similar to *Depo-Provera*.
Implanon	Schering-Plough	None	Etonogestrel (release rate varies over time)	N/A	Implantable (subdermal) rod. Provides contraception for up to 3 years. Failure rate = < 1 pregnancy per 100 women using *Implanon* for 1 year. Effectiveness rate in very overweight women unknown.[21]
Mirena	Bayer	None	Levonorgestrel 20 mcg/day for 5 years	0.1%	Intrauterine device (IUD). In October 2009, approved to treat heavy menstrual bleeding in women who use IUDs for contraception.[24]
NuvaRing	Schering-Plough	Ethinyl estradiol 15 mcg/day	Etonogestrel (active form of desogestrel) 0.12 mg/day	0.3%	Vaginal ring that is left in for 3 weeks and removed for 1 week. May have higher incidence of vaginal discharge than pills.
Ortho Evra	Ortho	Ethinyl estradiol 35 mcg/day (Release rate extrapolated from Canadian product monograph which shows identical pharmacokinetic data for *Evra* [Canada] and *Ortho Evra* [U.S.])	Norelgestromin (active form of norgestimate) 200 mcg/day (Release rate extrapolated from Canadian product monograph which shows identical pharmacokinetic data for *Evra* [Canada] and *Ortho Evra* [U.S.])	0.3%	Transdermal patch applied weekly (for 3 weeks, then week 4 is patch-free).[9] Application site reactions. Cycle control poor in 20% of women in first cycle. More breast discomfort in first 2 cycles than with combined oral contraceptive. Body weight > 90 kg may increase risk of unintended pregnancy. Has been used continuously with 9 active patches in a row followed by 7-day patch-free interval.[1] Compliance may improve compared with combined oral contraceptive.[16]

Users of this document are cautioned to use their own professional judgment and consult any other necessary or appropriate sources prior to making clinical judgments based on the content of this document. Our editors have researched the information with input from experts, government agencies, and national organizations. Information and Internet links in this article were current as of the date of publication.

[d]Unintended pregnancy in first year of perfect use.[1]

Levels of Evidence

In accordance with the trend towards Evidence-Based Medicine, we are citing the **LEVEL OF EVIDENCE** for the statements we publish.

Level	Definition
A	High-quality randomized controlled trial (RCT)
	High-quality meta-analysis (quantitative systematic review)
B	Nonrandomized clinical trial
	Nonquantitative systematic review
	Lower quality RCT
	Clinical cohort study
	Case-control study
	Historical control
	Epidemiologic study
C	Consensus
	Expert opinion
D	Anecdotal evidence
	In vitro or animal study

Adapted from Siweck J, et al. How to write an evidence-based clinical review article. *Am Fam Physician* 2002;65:251–258.

Project Leaders in preparation of this Detail-Document: *Jill Allen, Pharm.D., BCPS (original document), Melanie Cupp, Pharm.D., BCPS (November 2007 update), Neeta Bahal O'Mara, Pharm.D., BCPS (September 2009 update).*

REFERENCES

1. Zieman M, Hatcher RA, Cwiak C, et al. Managing Contraception for Your Pocket 2007–2009 edition. http://www.managingcontraception.com/shopping/mcpocket.pdf. (Accessed September 16, 2009).
2. Seibert C, Barbouche E, Fagan J, et al. Prescribing oral contraceptives for women older than 35 years of age. *Ann Intern Med* 2003;138:54–64.
3. Product information for *Yasmin*. Bayer Healthcare Pharmaceuticals, Inc. Wayne, NJ 07470. May 2003.
4. Van Vliet HA, Grimes DA, Helmerhorst FM, Schulz KF. Biphasic versus monophasic oral contraceptives for contraception (Cochrane Review). In: The Cochrane Library, Issue 3, 2003. Oxford: Update Software.
5. Van Vliet HA, Grimes DA, Helmerhorst FM, Schulz KF. Biphasic versus triphasic oral contraceptives for contraception (Cochrane Review). In: The Cochrane Library, Issue 3, 2003. Oxford: Update Software.
6. Hatcher RA, Trussell J, Stewart F, et al. Contraceptive Technology: 18th Revised Edition. New York, NY: Ardent Media, Inc, 2004.
7. American College of Obstetrics and Gynecology Committee on Practice Bulletins-Gynecology. ACOG Practice Bulletin. The use of hormonal contraception in women with coexisting medical conditions. Number 18, July 2000. *Int J Gynaecol Obstet* 2001;75:93–106.
8. FDA. Birth control guide (2009). http://www.fda.gov/downloads/ForConsumers/ByAudience/ForWomen/FreePublications/UCM164655.pdf. (Accessed October 9, 2009).
9. Product information for *Ortho Evra*. Ortho-McNeil. Raritan, NJ 08869. July 2009.
10. Product information for *Plan B One-Step*. Duramed Pharmaceuticals, Inc. Pomona, NY 10970. July 2009.
11. Cachrimanidou AC, Hellberg D, Nilsson S, et al. Long-interval treatment regimen with a desogestrel-containing oral contraceptive. *Contraception* 1993;48:205–216.
12. Vercellini P, Frontino G, De Giorgi O et al, Continuous use of an oral contraceptive for endometriosis-associated recurrent dysmenorrhea that does not respond to a cyclic pill regimen. *Fertil Steril* 2003;80:560–563.
13. Darney PD. OC Practice guidelines: Minimizing side effects. *Int J Fertil* 1997;42 (suppl 1):158–169.
14. Facts and Comparisons, Inc. eFacts monograph on oral contraceptives. Available online at: http://www.efactsweb.com. (Accessed September 15, 2009).
15. Kaunitz AM. Efficacy, cycle control, and safety of two triphasic oral contraceptives: *Cyclessa* (desogestrel/ethinyl estradiol) and *Ortho-Novum 7/7/7* (Norethindrone/ethinyl estradiol). *Contraception* 2000;61:295–302.
16. Audet MC, Moreau M, Koltun WD, et al. Evaluation of contraceptive efficacy and cycle control of a transdermal contraceptive patch vs an oral contraceptive. *JAMA* 2001;18:2347–2354.
17. United States Food and Drug Administration. Approved Drug Products with Therapeutic Equivalence Evaluations (Orange Book Query). http://www.fda.gov/cder/orange/default.htm. (Accessed September 16, 2009).
18. American Society of Health-system Pharmacists. AHFS Drug Information 2009. Bethesda, MD.
19. Product information for *Seasonique*. Duramed Pharmaceuticals. Pomona, NY 10970. May 2006.

20. Product information for *Plan B*. Duramed Pharmaceuticals. Pomona, NY 10970. July 2009.
21. Product information for *Implanon*. Organon. Roseland, NJ 07068. February 2009.
22. Product information for *Lybrel*. Wyeth. Philadelphia, PA 19101. September 2008.
23. Hardman JL. Contraception. In: Koda-Kimble MA, Young LY, Kradjan WA, Guglielmo BJ, eds. Applied Therapeutics: the clinical use of drugs. 8th ed. Philadelphia: Lippincott Willliams & Wilkins. 2005.
24. Product information for *Mirena*. Bayer HealthCare. Wayne, NJ 07470. October 2009.
25. Product information for *LoSeasonique*. Duramed. Pomona, NY 10970. October 2008.
26. Product information for *Next Choice*. Watson Labs. Corona, CA 92880. November 2009.

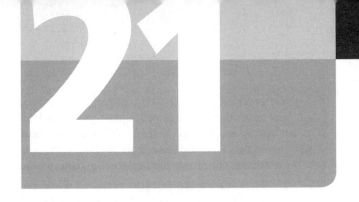

MENOPAUSE TRANSITION

Priscilla Abercrombie

I. Introduction and general background

Menopause is the result of the natural decline in the hormones produced in the ovaries. As hormone levels decrease, a number of symptoms may emerge, although their presentation and severity varies greatly from woman to woman. Menopause is a retrospective diagnosis made after complete cessation of the menstrual period for 12 consecutive months (Speroff & Fritz, 2005). The average age of menopause is 51.4 years old. Women who smoke reach menopause 1.74 years earlier than nonsmokers (McKinlay, Bifano, & McKinlay, 1985). Menopause usually occurs between the mid-40's and the mid-50's. The menopause transition is not only a time marked by physiologic changes; there are also important developmental changes that occur at this time of life. During this transition, women face such issues as the meaning of midlife and aging; role and purpose in life; and changes in interpersonal relationships (children, spouse, and parents) (Deeks, 2002). The experience of the menopause transition is thought to be influenced by sociocultural background. Women with a negative attitude toward the menopause seem to report more symptoms (Forshaw & Hunter, 2010). This chapter addresses the management of the major symptoms experienced by women during the menopause transition.

A. Other definitions

1. Surgical menopause occurs when both ovaries are surgically removed (bilateral oophorectomy).

2. Medical menopause can be induced by the use of certain drugs, such as gonadotropin-releasing hormone antagonists, or treatments, such as chemotherapy or radiation therapy.

3. Premature ovarian failure is the loss of ovarian function before the age of 40 years.

B. Vasomotor changes

1. Definition and overview: Symptoms range from flushing or warmth in the face and upper body to sweating and chills. Hot flashes can lead to severe sleep disturbances in some women. Hot flashes typically begin when cycles become irregular.

2. Etiology: Hot flashes stem from declining levels of estradiol affecting the hypothalamic temperature regulating center. This results in altered thermoregulation, although the exact mechanism is unknown.

3. Prevalence and incidence: The prevalence of vasomotor symptoms varies from 35–50% in peri-menopause to 30–80% in postmenopause (National Institutes of Health [NIH] Consensus Statement, 2005). High body mass index and early age of menopause are risk factors for vasomotor symptoms. They usually end 1–2 years after menstruation has ceased but can continue for 5 years or more.

C. Urogenital atrophy

1. Etiology and definition: Decreasing estrogen levels lead to a decrease in the production of vaginal lubrication and loss of vaginal elasticity and thickness of the epithelium (Speroff & Fritz, 2005). As a result, women experience symptoms of vaginal dryness that can lead to painful sexual intercourse (dyspareunia).

2. Prevalence and incidence: In a cohort study involving over 1,000 women, 50% experienced problematic vaginal dryness and 40% of the sexually active women had dyspareunia (Huang et al., 2010).

D. Menstrual cycle disturbances

Disturbances in the menstrual cycle are a hallmark sign of the menopausal transition. Fluctuations in hormone levels lead to variations in cycle length and menstrual flow. Periods of amenorrhea caused by anovulatory cycles can be followed by heavy and prolonged menstrual bleeding. Menstrual cycle length eventually increases especially in the year preceding cessation of menses. During the perimenopause transition follicle-stimulating hormone (FSH) and estradiol levels rise (Speroff & Fritz, 2005), whereas luteinizing hormone (LH) levels remain normal. Although FSH levels can be high, ovarian follicular development is unpredictable, thus the use of contraceptive methods is encouraged to prevent unwanted pregnancy. In the postmenopause, FSH and LH levels remain high and estrogen is low. Dysfunctional uterine bleeding may occur because of the hormonal fluctuations. Abnormal menstrual bleeding may be a symptom of endometrial hyperplasia or cancer. Further evaluation with endometrial biopsy may be warranted.

    a. Menorrhagia is excessive or prolonged bleeding. Gynecological conditions, such as fibroids, endometrial polyps, adenomyosis, and anovulation, contribute to menorrhagia.

    b. Menometrorrhagia is irregular excessive bleeding.

    c. Intermenstrual bleeding is bleeding that occurs between menstrual periods. It may be a symptom of endometrial hyperplasia or cancer.

    d. Persistent abnormal vaginal bleeding, suspected unopposed estrogen, and postmenopausal bleeding should be investigated further.

E. Mood and cognition

There is limited evidence that changes in ovarian function are the cause of depression, anxiety, or irritability during the menopause transition (NIH Consensus Statement, 2005). Women who experience vasomotor symptoms and insomnia are more at risk for depression (Gyllstrom, Schreiner, & Harlow, 2007). Women with a history of depression especially during reproductive events may be more vulnerable to relapse during perimenopause. Mood symptoms are experienced by approximately 11–21% of perimenopausal women and 8–38% of postmenopausal women.

Difficulty thinking, forgetfulness, and other cognitive disturbances are frequently reported during the menopause transition. Existing studies have not been able to separate the effects of aging from the effects of menopause (NIH Consensus Statement, 2005). Episodic memory performance declines with age, although the natural menopause transition is not associated with changes in episodic memory (Henderson, 2009). More research is needed to understand whether estrogen may be beneficial when initiated after surgical menopause or earlier in midlife. In a large longitudinal study, hormone therapy (HT) with conjugated equine estrogen did not prevent dementia or cognitive decline in women older than age 65 years (Coker et al., 2009). HT was associated with adverse effects on cognition persisting years after therapy in this group of women.

F. Sexual functioning

Population-based studies show a decline in many aspects of sexual functioning in conjunction with a decline in estradiol levels, not androgen levels (Dinnerstein, 2003). In one Australian study, during perimenopause scores indicating sexual dysfunction rose from 42% to 88%. Sexual function in midlife women is a complex issue that is not only affected by hormonal changes but by many other factors, such as premorbid sexual functioning, personality, educational level, stress, physical and psychologic health status, partner health status, and the woman's feelings toward her partner. The level of distress experienced as a result of the sexual problems should also be assessed. Sexual dysfunction can be categorized into disorders of desire, arousal, orgasm, or pain.

1. Hypoactive sexual desire disorder is a lack of desire for sexual activity and lack of responsiveness to sexual stimulation. Decreased sexual desire is a relatively common problem for women. About 24–43% of women complain of low sexual desire. It can become particularly problematic for women during life transitions, such as pregnancy, postpartum, and menopause.

2. Sexual aversion disorder: intermittent or persistent avoidance of sexual contact with a partner because of fear or loathing of such an experience.

3. Sexual arousal disorder: intermittent or persistent inability to attain or maintain adequate sexual excitement. Sexual thoughts that typically produce somatic changes, such as vaginal lubrication or swelling, are absent.

4. Orgasmic disorder: intermittent or persistent difficult or inability to attain orgasm after sufficient stimulation and arousal.

5. Sexual pain disorder: dyspareunia, vaginismus, non-coital sexual pain.

II. Database (may include but is not limited to)

A. Subjective: menopause transition

1. Past medical history: cardiovascular disease, stroke, venous thromboembolism (VTE), hypertension, hyperlipidemia, thyroid disease, depression or anxiety, liver disease, obesity, prolactinoma, and anorexia.

2. Surgical history: hysterectomy with bilateral oophorectomy.

3. Obstetric and gynecological history

    a. Obstetric: pregnancies, deliveries, abortions, and postpartum issues

    b. Contraception and family planning: current and past use, experience with hormonal contraception

    c. Urinary: recurrent cystitis, interstitial cystitis, overactive bladder, and urinary incontinence

    d. Gynecological: vulvar disease, vulvar pain disorders, abnormal uterine or vaginal bleeding, cervical cancer screening, uterine fibroids, endometriosis, dysfunctional uterine bleeding, and ovarian cysts

e. Sexually transmitted infections
f. Anatomic issues: organ prolapse, stenosis, scarring, cervical mass, pain, and Asherman syndrome
g. Cancer: gynecological and breast malignancies; history of treatment with surgery, radiation, chemotherapy and/or drugs

4. Sexual history
   a. Sexual experience or inexperience
      i. Sexual orientation and gender identity
      ii. Baseline and current receptivity to sex play
      iii. Assess current pattern and explore why pattern has changed
      iv. Discuss disparity between patient and partner's desire
      v. Assess nonpartner-initiated sexual expression (masturbation, erotic dreams, and sexual thoughts) and trauma history (history of sexual abuse or assault)

5. Exposure history: environmental exposures that affect hormone production.

6. Medication history: medications that affect hormone production (antipsychotics, contraceptives, gonadotropin-releasing hormone antagonists, and so forth).

7. Family history: age of menopause, breast and ovarian cancer, and osteoporosis.

8. Occupational and environmental history.

9. Personal social history: religious or cultural considerations, current or past relationship issues, and perception of menopause.

10. Review of systems
    a. Constitutional signs and symptoms: fatigue and hot flashes
    b. Genitourinary: heavy menses or amenorrhea, intermenstrual spotting, dysuria, urinary incontinence, dyspareunia, vaginal dryness, decreased sexual arousal or orgasm, and postcoital bleeding
    c. Musculoskeletal: joint stiffness or pain, myalgias
    d. Neurologic: lethargy, depressed mood, moodiness, decreased libido, and poor short-term memory

B. Objective
1. Physical examination findings
   a. Vasomotor changes: may witness flushing, normal thyroid
   b. Urogenital atrophy (Castelo-Branco, Cancelo, Villero, Nohales, & Julia, 2005).
   c. Visual inspection changes seen in vaginal epithelium is the most common diagnostic indicator:
      i. Vaginal pH greater than 4.5
      ii. Pale dry vaginal tissues with decreased rugae
      iii. Shrinkage of labia minora, check for lesions, inflammation, and friability
   d. Inspect for urethral caruncle, prolapse or polyps, and atrophy
   e. Thinning of pubic hair
   f. Cystocele or rectocele
   g. Menstrual cycle disturbances: menstrual flooding at time of examination, intermenstrual spotting on examination, cervical mass or stenosis, uterine fibroids, and ovarian cysts and adnexal mass
   h. Mood and cognition: inappropriate affect, depressed or anxious affect, crying, and poor cognition during interview
   i. Sexual functioning:
      i. Cotton swab Q-tip test to rule out vulvodynia
      ii. Assess pelvic floor muscles to rule out pelvic floor muscle dysfunction
      iii. Vulvar lesions
      iv. Tightening of introitus secondary to atrophic changes or other vulvar conditions

III. Assessment

A. *Determine the diagnosis; menopause transition is diagnosed based on chronologic age, menstrual cycle history, and menopausal symptoms*

B. *Other conditions to consider based on symptoms and examination findings*

1. Vasomotor symptoms
   a. Cardiovascular disease
   b. Hyperthyroidism
   c. Pheochromocytoma
   d. Cancer
   e. Effect of medications

2. Urogenital atrophy
   a. Urinary incontinence
   b. Urinary tract infection
   c. Vulvar disease

3. Menstrual cycle disturbances
   a. Causes of secondary amenorrhea: hyperprolactinemia or prolactinoma, pregnancy, hypothalamic dysfunction, thyroid disease, prolapsed fibroid, cervical mass or stenosis,

and Asherman syndrome (see Chapter 17 on amenorrhea).

   b. Abnormal vaginal bleeding: endometrial hyperplasia and unopposed estrogen, endometrial or cervical cancer, endometrial polyps, adenomyosis, pregnancy, and Spontaneous abortion (SAB) (see Chapter 16 on abnormal uterine bleeding).

4. Mood and cognition

   a. Depression and anxiety disorders

   b. Dementia and Alzheimer disease

   c. Hyperthyroidism

5. Sexual dysfunction

   a. Anxiety and depression disorders

   b. Vulvar disease, vulvar pain disorder, and pelvic floor muscle dysfunction

   c. Sexual abuse history

C. *Severity: assess the severity of the symptoms and transition*

1. The menopausal rating scale can be found at http://www.menopause-rating-scale.info/.

2. See the review of instruments to measure quality of life during the menopause transition (Zollner, Acquadro, & Schaefer, 2005).

D. *Significance: assess the significance of the transition to the patient and significant others*

IV. Goals of clinical management

A. *Alleviate symptoms of the menopause transition that impact quality of life*

B. *Rule out abnormalities*

C. *Prevent major causes of morbidity and mortality*

1. Osteoporosis

2. Cardiovascular disease and stroke

3. Cancer: lung, breast, and colorectal

V. Plan

A. *Screening*

1. See Chapter 37 on healthcare maintenance of the adult for age-appropriate physical examination and screening test recommendations.

B. *Diagnostic testing based on symptoms*

1. For abnormal bleeding: endometrial biopsy, pelvic ultrasound, complete blood count, and thyroid-stimulating hormone (see Chapter 16 on abnormal uterine bleeding for a more in-depth discussion).

2. For amenorrhea: pregnancy test, prolactin, thyroid-stimulating hormone, and FSH (see Chapter 17 on amenorrhea for more in-depth discussion).

3. For mood and cognition symptoms: screen for depression and dementia.

4. For sexual dysfunction symptoms: consider baseline free testosterone levels, lipid profile, and liver enzyme levels. Especially important before initiating testosterone therapy.

C. *Management*

The results of multiple clinical trials including the Women's Health Initiative and the Heart and Estrogen/progestin Replacement Study have influenced HT prescribing practices. Guidelines developed by the North American Menopause Society (NAMS) and the American Congress of Obstetricians and Gynecologists (ACOG) recommend HT for perimenopausal or postmenopausal women with moderate to severe symptoms (ACOG, 2008; NAMS, 2010). The lowest effective dose should be given over the shortest duration as possible (< 5 years) close to the time of menopause. HT should not be used for the prevention of cardiovascular disease. HT has been shown to reduce postmenopausal bone fractures but should not be used for this purpose alone unless alternative therapies have failed. Suggestions for management of the following symptoms include:

1. Vasomotor changes: HT is the most effective treatment for vasomotor symptoms and is recommended for women who are experiencing moderate to severe hot flashes.

   a. Contraindications: history of breast cancer, heart disease, VTE, hypertension or stroke, and undiagnosed vaginal bleeding

   b. Risks: there is an increased risk of ischemic stroke, VTE, and breast cancer with HT.

2. Estrogen therapy: there are multiple types of estrogen available in many doses and formulations including pills, creams, lotions, and patches. Observational data suggest transdermal administration of estrogen may decrease the risk of VTE (Canonico et al., 2007). It may also be more advantageous in the setting of hypertension, gallbladder disease, and diabetes but more research is needed. Low-dose regimens include 0.3-mg conjugated estrogens or 0.5-mg oral micronized estradiol, and 0.014- to 0.0025-mg oral or transdermal 17β-estradiol patch (NAMS, 2010). An alternative is to prescribe 20 mcg of ethinyl estradiol.

3. Progestogen therapy: women with an intact uterus should receive progestogen in addition to estrogen to prevent endometrial hyperplasia. Progestins

seem to attenuate the beneficial effects of estrogen on lipids. Oral micronized progesterone may be more advantageous because it seems to have little or no effect on lipids (Writing Group for the PEPI Trial, 1995). Progestogens may worsen depression.

a. Low-dose progestogens: 1.5-mg oral medroxy-progesterone acetate, 0.1-mg oral norethindrone acetate, 0.5-mg oral drospirenone, and 50- to 100-mg oral micronized progesterone

b. Dosing regimens: the advantages, disadvantages, and the patient's preferences should be taken into account when prescribing HT.
   i. Daily administration of both estrogen and progestogen.
   ii. Intermittent progestogen with daily estrogen. The progestogen could be given on days 1–14 each month. At this time there are inadequate data to support the use of long-cycle regimens, such as progestogen, every 3 months, vaginal administration of progesterone, levonorgestrel-releasing intrauterine system, or low-dose estrogen without progestogen (NAMS, 2010).

c. Discontinuing therapy: There is a 50% risk of symptoms recurring after HT is discontinued (NAMS, 2008). Recurrence of vasomotor symptoms is similar whether tapered or if cessation is abrupt.

4. Bioidentical HT: bioidentical hormones are thought to more closely mimic the hormones normally found in the female body. There are three different types of estrogen produced in the body: (1) E_2 or estradiol is produced primarily during the reproductive years, (2) E_1 or estrone is produced primarily after menopause, and (3) E_3 or estriol is produced primarily during pregnancy. Each form of estrogen works differently throughout the body. It is thought that estriol may be protective against breast cancer but it has not been well studied. Progesterone is also naturally found in the body.

a. There is insufficient evidence at this time that bioidentical estrogens are safer or more beneficial than other synthetic hormones (Boothby & Doering, 2008). That being said, there is mounting evidence that estradiol and micronized progesterone may have some beneficial effects over other synthetic hormones (Holtorf, 2009; Moskowitz, 2006).

b. There are Food and Drug Administration (FDA)–approved bioidentical hormones available by prescription. Estradiol comes in many different forms including pills, patches, creams, lotions, and vaginal products. Oral progesterone is also available.

c. Compounded hormones are non-FDA approved prescription hormones that are prepared by a compounding pharmacist. By compounding the hormones, pharmacists are able to provide a wide range of dosages and formulations that are not available from pharmaceutical companies. In 2008, the FDA sent warning letters to seven compounding pharmacies for making false claims about the safety and effectiveness of bioidentical hormonal replacement therapy.

d. There is no evidence that salivary or blood hormone testing should be used to adjust hormone levels (Boothby & Doering, 2008). NAMS has made a statement against the use of compounded hormones and salivary testing. More information is available on their website: http://www.menopause.org/bioidentical.aspx

5. Nonhormonal drugs: reviews of randomized controlled trials show evidence for the efficacy of many nonhormonal therapies for the treatment of vasomotor symptoms (Cheema, Coomarasamy, & El-Toukhy, 2007; Nelson et al., 2006). The drugs include selective serotonin reuptake inhibitors, serotonin-norepinephrine reuptake inhibitors, clonidine, and gabapentin. These drugs are less effective than HT but are a good alternative for women who are not candidates for HT. Most of these drugs have been studied in women with breast cancer, not women experiencing naturally occurring menopause, and were found to be safe for use.

a. Paroxetine: 10–25 mg daily. Side effects of selective serotonin reuptake inhibitors include dry mouth, insomnia, sedation, decreased appetite, constipation, and decreased libido. Severe withdrawal syndrome if discontinued abruptly.

b. Venlafaxine: 37.5 or 75 mg daily. May cause heavy uterine bleeding, galactorrhea, or mastodynia. The evidence for the effectiveness of fluoxitine is mixed.

c. Gabapentin: 900 mg daily. Side effects include somnolence, fatigue, dizziness, and palpitations.

d. Clonidine: 0.1–0.4 mg daily. Side effects include drowsiness, dry mouth, constipation, hypertension, insomnia, postural hypotension, and reaction to skin patch. Discontinue slowly to reduce dose to avoid rebound hypertension, headaches, and agitation.

e. None of these drugs are FDA approved for the treatment of hot flashes.

f. As with prescribing any drug be aware of drug interactions, contraindications for use, and side effects.

6. Alternative treatments

 a. A review of double-blind randomized clinical trials using black cohosh (*Cimicifuga racemosa*) for the treatment of menopausal symptoms did not show that it was consistently effective, although a benefit could not be excluded (Borrelli & Ernst, 2008).

   i. Study doses ranged from 20 to 80 mg twice daily

   ii. Mechanism of action is unknown but unlikely hormonal. A systematic review of the clinical evidence for the safety of black cohosh found that clinical studies suggest that it is safe, although case reports including liver toxicity have been reported (Borrelli & Ernst, 2008). The U.S. Pharmacopeia also reviewed the case reports and concluded that dietary supplements containing black cohosh should have a cautionary statement on the label: One should discontinue use and consult a healthcare practitioner if there is a liver disorder or if symptoms of liver trouble develop, such as abdominal pain, dark urine, or jaundice (Mahady et al., 2008). Baseline and periodic evaluation of liver enzymes when prescribing black cohosh may be prudent.

 b. Soy isoflavones: a review of studies found mixed results in the efficacy of soy isoflavones in reducing vasomotor symptoms (Jacobs, Wegewitz, Sommerfeld, Grossklaus, & Lampen, 2009).

 c. Herbs and supplements thought to be ineffective for the treatment of hot flashes include red clover (*Trifolium pratenese*), ginseng (*Panax ginseng*), vitamin E, evening primrose oil, and dong quai (*Angelica sinensis*).

 d. A review of acupuncture for the treatment of menopausal symptoms found it to be associated with a reduction in the number of hot flashes (Borud & White, 2010). Further research is needed to confirm these findings.

7. Multiple lifestyle strategies are suggested but there has been little research done to support their efficacy.

 a. Regulation of core body temperature
 b. Regular exercise
 c. Relaxation techniques
 d. Paced breathing
 e. Weight loss
 f. Smoking cessation

8. Urogenital atrophy

 a. Vaginal dryness or dyspareunia related to atrophy (See Sturdee & Panay, 2010).

   i. Vaginal estrogen (Archer, 2010)

     a. Low-dose vaginal tablets, rings, and creams are equally effective.

     b. Less systemic and endometrial effects with low-dose vaginal estradiol tablets and estriol-containing formulations. Low-dose vaginal estrogen therapy does not generally require a progestogen (NAMS, 2010).

     c. Doses of greater than 1-mg conjugated ethinyl estradiol are more likely to cause systemic side effects and endometrial hyperplasia.

     d. Safe for most women because of little systemic effect but has not been adequately studied in women with breast cancer (Al-Baghdadi & Ewies, 2009).

     e. May be of some benefit for women with urge incontinence (NAMS, 2010)

     f. May reduce the risk of recurrent urinary tract infection (Perrotta, Aznar, Mejia, Albert, & Ng, 2008)

     g. Estriol is a weaker estrogen and is well absorbed from vaginal mucosa but must be ordered from a compounding pharmacist. Usually given as 1 mg/g nightly for 2 weeks then twice weekly.

 b. Vaginal moisturizers
 c. Lubricants for sexual intercourse
 d. Maintain sexual activity: women who are sexually active have less vaginal atrophy
 e. There is mounting evidence that DHEA suppositories improve vaginal atrophy, sexual pain and sexual desire. Usually given as 12.5 mg ovule.

9. Urinary frequency, urgency, or incontinence (see Chapter 23 on urinary incontinence in women).

 a. These symptoms may not be related to estrogen deficiency and often are not relieved with the administration of estrogen alone
 b. Refer for urogynecology assessment

10. Mood and cognition

 a. Depression

   i. If accompanied by other menopausal symptoms consider HT

   ii. Psychotherapy referral

   iii. Antidepressants

 b. Cognition: consider referral for neuropsychiatric assessment

11. Sexual dysfunction: See Al-Azzawi et al. (2010) for a review of therapeutic options for postmenopausal women with sexual dysfunction. Consider a referral to a sex therapist or sexologist. For decreased desire

    a. Treat contributing psychologic (e.g., depression) or underlying medical conditions
    b. Change or discontinue medication contributing to decreased desire
        i. The use of testosterone in women with disorders of sexual desire is controversial.
        ii. The role of testosterone therapy in postmenopausal women: position statement of The North American Menopause Society (2005) states that postmenopausal women who are distressed by decreased sexual desire and have no other known cause (physical or psychological) are candidates for testosterone therapy.
        iii. Point by point rebuttal to NAMS guidelines is available (Traish, Guay, & Spark, 2007)
        iv. Research has shown that the addition of an androgen to estrogen therapy demonstrated a significant positive incremental effect on sexual functioning in women (Cochrane Review, 2005)
        v. Side effects: decreased high-density lipoprotein, acne, hirsutism, clitoral enlargement, voice deepening, weight gain, menstrual irregularities, and probable increased breast cancer risk
        vi. Benefits: increased clitoral sensitivity, vaginal lubrication, and libido
        vii. Contraindications: history of breast or uterine cancer, liver disease, and cardiovascular disease
        viii. Consider initiating therapy if below normal or low normal free testosterone. Transdermal formulations preferred. Counsel regarding risks and benefits of therapy.
            a. Combination product (Estratest) (less lipid changes)
            b. Methyltestosterone, 0.25–1.25 mg daily: can compound in 1-ml syringe; apply to genitals 0.25 mg/d, then switch to oral if effective
            c. Natural testosterone, 5 mg/g cream: apply 1 g three times per week to lower abdomen, mons pubis, inner thigh, or buttocks
                i. Micronized oral testosterone, 5 mg twice a day
                ii. Testosterone is not FDA approved for sexual dysfunction in women
            d. Results seen in 6–12 weeks, may first experience erotic dreams.
            e. Reevaluation at 3 months: monitor testosterone levels before and after therapy for supraphysiologic levels, lipid profile, and liver enzymes; monitor symptoms and side effects
                i. Goal: free testosterone levels in upper normal range
                ii. Continued therapy: taper to lowest effective dose, monitor lipids and liver enzymes at 3 months then one to two times per year
            f. Discuss sexual issues when a new medication is prescribed, presurgery and postsurgery for bilateral oophorectomy
            g. Consider lifestyle issues: boredom with sexual routine (give permission for experimentation); stress (importance of relaxation); and children (privacy and relationship time)
            h. Directed resexualization: take 20 minutes three times a week for erotic literature; exercises that increase blood flow to genitals, such as biking; masturbation; and be aware of sexual cues

12. Herbal alternatives include: American ginseng (*Panax quinquefolius*), damiana (*Turnera aphrodisiaca*), and wild oats milky seed (*Avena sativa*). Although there is a long history of traditional use of herbs for decreased sexual desire, there is little research evidence to support their use.

13. Disorders of arousal
    a. Over-the-counter products include L-arginine (oral), Zestra
    b. Enhance stimulation and eliminate routine: use erotic materials, masturbation, encourage communication during sex; use vibrators, varying positions, times of day or places, and make a date for sex

14. Sexual pain disorder
    a. Provide distraction techniques (helps with anxiety, increasing relaxation): erotic or nonerotic fantasy, Kegel exercises with sex, background music, or videos or television
    b. Encourage noncoital behaviors: sensual massage, sensate-focus exercises, oral or noncoital stimulation with or without orgasm

15. Client education

    a. Concerns and feelings: discuss menopause transition as a normal physiologic and developmental process that affects each woman uniquely

    b. Information: provide verbal and preferably written information regarding the menopause transition, diagnostic tests, and management strategies

16. Nutrition

    a. Seven to nine servings of fresh fruits and vegetables

    b. Plentiful use of grains and beans for 25–30 g of fiber daily

    c. Healthy fats: monounsaturated (olive oil, canola oil, avocados, and so forth) and polyunsaturated fats and omega 3 fatty acids (flaxseed, fish, walnuts, and so forth)

    d. Protein primarily from fish, poultry, and beans

    e. Calcium from dark green vegetables and nonfat dairy to meet the need of 1,200 mg/day

17. Physical activity

    a. Weight-bearing exercise for bone strength: walking, dancing, and jump rope

    b. 30 minutes of aerobic exercise at least 5 days per week

    c. Flexibility training, such as yoga, to decrease falls two to three times per week

    d. Strength training to improve muscle mass two to three times per week

18. Spiritual life

    a. Participate in activities that bring purpose and meaning to life

    b. Take time for reflection

      i. Journaling

      ii. Women's group

      iii. Walks in nature

      iv. Religious activities: prayer, meditation, and ritual

      v. Reflective questions:

        a. What keeps you going? What sustains you?

        b. Where do you find meaning and purpose in life?

        c. Where do you find joy?

        d. What or whom do you turn to when you get down?

VI. Self-management resources and tools

A. Patient education

1. NAMS: http://www.menopause.org/Consumers.aspx

2. ACOG: http://www.acog.org/publications/patient_education/bp047.cfm

3. Association of Reproductive Health Professionals: http://www.arhp.org/topics/menopause

VII. Clinical practice guidelines

A. American Association of Clinical Endocrinologists:
http://www.aace.com/pub/guidelines/

B. NAMS:
http://www.menopause.org/

C. NIH state-of-the-science conference statement on the management of menopause-related symptoms.

REFERENCES

Al-Azzawi, F., Bitzer, J., Brandenburg, U., Castelo-Branco, C., Graziottin, A., Kenemans, P., . . . Zahradrnik, W. (2010). Therapeutic options for postmenopausal female sexual dysfunction. *Climacteric, 13*(2), 103–120.

Al-Baghdadi, O., & Ewies, A. (2009). Topical estrogen therapy in the management of postmenopausal vaginal atrophy: An up-to-date overview. *Climacteric, 12,* 91–105.

American College of Obstetrics and Gynecology. (2008). ACOG committee opinion no. 420, November 2008: Hormone therapy and heart disease. *Obstetrics and Gynecology, 112*(5), 1189–1192.

Archer, D. (2010). Efficacy and tolerability of local estrogen therapy for urogenital atrophy. *Menopause, 17*(1), 194–203.

Boothby, L. A., & Doering, P. L. (2008). Bioidentical hormone therapy: A panacea that lacks supportive evidence. *Current Opinion in Obstetrics and Gynecology, 20*(4), 400–407.

Borrelli, F., & Ernst, E. (2008). Black cohosh (Cimicifuga racemosa): A systematic review of adverse events. *American Journal of Obstetrics and Gynecology, 199*(5), 455–466.

Borrelli, F., & Ernst, E. (2008). Black cohosh (Cimicifuga racemosa) for menopausal symptoms: A systematic review of its efficacy. *Pharmacological Research, 58*(1), 8–14.

Borud, E., & White, A. (2010). A review of acupuncture for menopausal problems. *Maturitas, 66*(2), 131–134.

Canonico, M., Oger, E., Plu-Bureau, G., Conard, J., Meyer, G., Lévesque, H., . . . ESTHER Study Group. (2007). Hormone therapy and venous thromboembolism among postmenopausal women: Impact of the route of estrogen administration and progestogens: The ESTHER study. *Circulation, 115*(7), 840–845.

Castelo-Branco, C., Cancelo, M., Villero, J., Nohales, F., & Julia, M. (2005). Management of post-menopausal vaginal atrophy and atrophic vaginitis. *Maturitas, 525,* 546–552.

Cheema, D., Coomarasamy, A., & El-Toukhy, T. (2007). Non-hormonal therapy of post-menopausal vasomotor symptoms: A structured evidence-based review. *Archives in Gynecology and Obstetrics, 276*(5), 463–469.

Coker, L. H., Espeland, M. A., Rapp, S. R., Legault, C., Resnick, S. M., Hogan, P., . . . Shumaker, S. A. (2009). Postmenopausal hormone therapy and cognitive outcomes: The Women's Health Initiative Memory Study (WHIMS). *The Journal of Steroid Biochemistry and Molecular Biology, 118*(4-5), 304–310.

Deeks, A. (2002). Is this menopause? Women in midlife-psychosocial issues. *Australian Family Physician, 33*(11), 889–893.

Dinnerstein, L., Alexander, J. & Kotz, K. (2003). The menopause and sexual functioning: A review of population-based studies. *Annual Review of Sex Research, 14*, 64–82.

Forshaw, M., & Hunter, M. (2010). The impact of attitudes towards the menopause on women's symptom experience: A systematic review. *Maturitas, 65*, 28–36.

Gyllstrom, M. E., Schreiner, P. J., & Harlow, B. L. (2007). Perimenopause and depression: Strength of association, causal mechanisms and treatment recommendations. *Best Practice & Research Clinical Obstetrics & Gynaecology, 21*(2), 275–292.

Henderson, V. W. (2009). Aging, estrogens, and episodic memory in women. *Cognitive and Behavioral Neurology, 22*(4), 205–214.

Holtorf, K. (2009). The bioidentical hormone debate: Are bioidentical hormones (estradiol, estriol, and progesterone) safer or more efficacious than commonly used synthetic versions in hormone replacement therapy? *Postgraduate Medicine, 121*(1), 73–85.

Huang, A., Moore, E. E., Boyko, E. J., Scholes, D., Lin, F., Vittinghoff, E., . . . Fihn, S. D. (2010). Vaginal symptoms in postmenopausal women: Self reported severity, natural history, and risk factors. *Menopause, 17*(1), 121–126.

Jacobs, A., Wegewitz, U., Sommerfeld, C., Grossklaus, R., & Lampen, A. (2009). Efficacy of isoflavones in relieving vasomotor menopausal symptoms: A systematic review. *Molecular Nutrition & Food Research, 53*(9), 1084–1097.

Mahady, G. B., Dog, T. L., Barrett, M. L., Chavez, M. L., Gardiner, P., Ko, R., . . . Sarma, D. N. (2008). United States pharmacopeia review of the black cohosh case reports of hepatotoxicity. *Menopause, 15*(4), 628–638.

McKinlay, S. M., Bifano, N. L., & McKinlay, J. B. (1985). Smoking and age at menopause in women. *Annals of Internal Medicine, 103*(3), 350–356.

Moskowitz, D. (2006). A comprehensive review of the safety and efficacy of bioidentical hormones for the management of menopause and related health risks. *Alternative Medicine Review, 11*(3), 208–223.

National Institutes of Health state-of-the-science conference statement on management of menopause-related symptoms. (2005). *NIH consensus and state-of-the-science statements, 22*(1), 1–38.

Nelson, H. D., Vesco, K., Haney, E., Fu, R., Nedrow, A., Miller, J., . . . Humphrey, L. (2006). Nonhormonal therapies for menopausal hot flashes: Systematic review and meta- analysis. *Journal of the American Medical Association, 295*(17), 2057–2071.

North American Menopause Society. (2005). The role of testosterone therapy in postmenopausal women: Position statement of the North American Menopause Society. *Menopause, 12*(5), 496–511; quiz 649.

North American Menopause Society. (2010). Estrogen and progestogen use in postmenopausal women: 2010 position statement of the North American Menopause Society. *Menopause, 17*(2) 242–255.

Perrotta, C., Aznar, M., Mejia, R., Albert, X., & Ng, C. W. (2008). Oestrogens for preventing recurrent urinary tract infection in postmenopausal women. *The Cochrane Database of Systematic Reviews, 2*, CD005131.

Somboonporn, W., Davis, S., Seif, M. W., & Bell, R. (2005). Testosterone for peri- and postmenopausal women. *Cochrane Database of Systematic Reviews.* 2005 Oct 19;(4):CD004509

Speroff, L., & Fritz, M. (2005). Menopause and perimenopause transition. In L. Speroff & M. Fritz, *Clinical Gynecologic Endocrinology and Infertility* (7th ed., pp. 621–688). Philadelphia, PA: Lippincott Williams & Wilkins.

Sturdee, D. & Panay, N. (2010). Recommendations for the management of postmenopausal vaginal atrophy. *Climacteric, 13*, 509–522.

Traish, A., Guay, A. T., & Spark, R. F. (2007). Are the endocrine society's clinical practice guidelines on androgen therapy in women misguided? A commentary. *The Journal of Sexual Medicine, 4*(5), 1223–1234; discussion 1234.

The Writing Group for the PEPI Trial. (1995). Effects of estrogen or estrogen/progestin regimens on heart disease risk factors in postmenopausal women. The Postmenopausal Estrogen/Progestin Interventions (PEPI) Trial. *Journal of the American Medical Association, 273*(3), 199–208.

Zollner, Y. F., Acquadro, C., & Schaefer, M. (2005). Literature review of instruments to assess health-related quality of life during and after menopause. *Quality of Life Research, 14*(2), 309–327.

NONHORMONAL CONTRACEPTION

Kimberley Chastain

I. Introduction and general background

Nonhormonal contraception is a form of family planning used by couples during coitus or postcoitally to prevent pregnancy without the use of exogenous hormones. It includes barrier methods that can be used by either the male or female partner placed before genital contact; spermicides, placed inside the vagina moments or minutes before genital contact; the ParaGard® intrauterine contraceptive (IUC), placed inside a woman's uterus by her provider in advance or in some cases up to 5 days after unprotected intercourse as emergency contraception (EC); and natural family planning (NFP), which are learned behaviors and include fertility awareness methods (FAM), and the lactational amenorrhea method (LAM).

Nonhormonal contraception can be an appropriate option for most women, although most of the methods, excluding the IUC and strict NFP, have effectiveness rates that are lower than those containing hormones. Still, many women or couples prefer to use nonhormonal methods for a variety of reasons including but not limited to contraindication to hormones, reduced side effect profile, past experience, religious beliefs, and personal values. Advantages of nonhormonal contraception include little or no side effects for most methods, low long-term cost, no clinic visit required for several of the methods, and in all cases near immediate effectiveness and an immediate return to fertility once the method is stopped. With all of the methods discussed in this chapter, a patient should also be offered the EC pill or a prescription as a back-up in case of user or method failure. The EC pill is discussed in a separate chapter.

Choosing a method of family planning is a multifaceted process. Patients need current, factual information about all methods of contraception and must be allowed to participate fully in the decision-making process. Efficacy rate is an important component in choosing a contraceptive method. In this chapter, efficacy rates are reported rather than failure rates. Terms used to identify these rates are "perfect use" and "typical use." Perfect use refers to the number of women out of 100 who prevent pregnancy in 1 year's time with correct and consistent use of the method, reported as a percentage rate. Typical use refers to the percentage of women out of 100 who do not use the method consistently or correctly each time and over 1 year still avoid pregnancy (Trussell, 2008).

A. Barrier methods

A barrier method of contraception is one that is designed to physically prohibit sperm from entering the vagina or the uterus during intercourse. The current barrier methods available in the United States include the male condom, the female condom, the diaphragm, the FemCap, and the sponge. Effectiveness rates increase when combined with a spermicidal agent, such as nonoxynol-9, discussed in a later section.

1. Male condom

The condom is a barrier method of contraception designed to prevent sperm from entering the vagina. Made of latex, polyurethane, or lambskin, male condoms come in a variety of textures, colors, and sizes, and with or without spermicide and with or without lubrication, each intended to improve user acceptance of the method. Additionally, they are available with or without reservoir tips, designed to help prevent spillage of the ejaculate and are therefore usually recommended. Male condoms are placed on a man's erect penis before genital contact with a partner. Condom use instructions should be carefully followed because correct placement and removal are essential to avoid pregnancy. Perfect use efficacy rate for the male condom is 98%, whereas typical use rate is 85% (Trussell, 2008).

One of the major advantages of using either latex or polyurethane male condoms for contraception is that they also help prevent sexually transmitted infections (STIs) including HIV (World Health Organization [WHO], 2000). However, although lambskin condoms protect equally as well against pregnancy as other condoms, they do not protect against most STIs or HIV. Other advantages to condoms include cost (male condoms are relatively inexpensive compared with other methods); the ability to offer men a role in contraception; the lack of physical examination or prescription requirement; ready availability over the counter; and a low side effect profile. Additionally, they can be used simultaneously with every other available birth control method except the female condom. Disadvantages include possible allergies or sensitivities to latex; reduction in sexual spontaneity; need for cooperation by the partner; and the possibility for breakage or slipping off, resulting in method failure.

2. Female condom

Currently, there is only one female condom approved by the Food and Drug Administration (FDA) for use in the United States. Formerly known as the "Reality," the second-generation female condom is called the FC2®, and is produced by the Female Health Company. Made of synthetic nitrile, the FC2® has a flexible inner ring that facilitates insertion into the vagina, with a second outer ring designed to hold it in place and cover part of the vulva. Perfect use of the female condom confers a 95% efficacy rate, compared with 79% with typical use in the first year (Trussell, 2008).

Advantages to using the female condom include the fact that it is relatively inexpensive (although more expensive than the male condom), and is available over the counter without an examination or prescription. Additionally, it reduces the risk of STIs including HIV in laboratory testing (French et al., 2003), giving women an opportunity to actively play a role in preventing HIV and STI transmission during intercourse. Disadvantages are that it can be somewhat awkward to place correctly and can become dislodged easily. Of note is that the female condom should not be used simultaneously with a male condom, because they can stick to one another, causing one or both to slip off or tear.

3. Contraceptive sponge

The contraceptive sponge was first introduced to the US market as the Today® Sponge in 1983. However, after multiple production stops and starts, it was reintroduced most recently in May of 2009 by Mayer Laboratories. The polyurethane sponge acts as a physical barrier to sperm by trapping them within the sponge before they can enter the cervix. Additionally, the sponge contains the spermicide nonoxynol-9 for added protection. Before insertion, the sponge must be moistened with water to activate the spermicide. It is then placed deep inside the vagina, with the concave side toward the cervix up to 24 hours before intercourse. The sponge must be left in place a minimum of 6 hours after intercourse to ensure that all sperm

are immobilized. The sponge should not be left in the vagina longer than 30 hours because of the risk of toxic shock syndrome. Perfect use efficacy rates for the contraceptive sponge are 91% for nulliparous women and 80% for parous women, whereas typical use yields efficacy of 84% for nulliparous and 68% for parous women (Trussell, 2008).

Advantages to using the sponge are that it is readily available over the counter and does not require a prescription or examination. Disadvantages include risk of sensitivity or allergy to nonoxynol-9 and the fact that it must be moistened with water before insertion, requiring advance preparation. The only absolute contraindications to use are current cervical cancer or women at high risk for HIV (WHO, 2009) because of the nonoxynol-9 component (see the section on spermicides).

4. Diaphragm

The diaphragm is one of the first female-worn barrier methods to be used in the United States. The diaphragm is a physical barrier made of either latex or silicone in the shape of a dome surrounded by a flexible "spring" rim, designed to be placed deep inside the vagina blocking the cervix entirely. Diaphragms are available in several different rim styles and diameters ranging from 55 to 95 mm. Because of the wide range of female anatomic differences, the diaphragm style and size must be fit for the patient during a pelvic examination by a trained provider. To use the diaphragm, a woman should check for integrity before insertion. A dime-sized amount of spermicidal jelly or cream is placed in the cup side of the dome and extra spermicide is placed around the rim. Pinching the diaphragm in half, the user places it deep inside her vagina making sure to completely cover the entire cervix, requiring both education and practice. The diaphragm must be kept in the vagina for at least 6 but no more than 24 hours after intercourse. Spermicide must be reinserted vaginally with every new act of intercourse while the diaphragm is in place. Perfect use effectiveness rate for the diaphragm is 94%, whereas typical use is 84% (Trussell, 2008).

Advantages to the diaphragm are that it can be placed well in advance of sexual intercourse (≤ 24 hours); it is discrete; and it is relatively inexpensive considering that each one lasts up to 2 years, with the only additional cost being extra spermicide. Additionally, it has been observed that the diaphragm may reduce the risk of human papillomavirus transmission (by blocking the cervix) and therefore lower the risk of cervical dysplasia (Cates & Raymond, 2007). Disadvantages are that it is available by prescription only, and must be fit in the clinic by a provider. It should normally be replaced every 2 years, but refitting is required after any full-term pregnancy, second-trimester abortion, or a weight gain or loss of 20% or more. Although not contraindicated, diaphragms should be used with caution in women with a history of repeated urinary tract infections. Absolute contraindications include women with current cervical cancer and those women at high risk for HIV (WHO, 2009) because of the necessary spermicide use.

5. FemCap

Because former contraceptive cervical caps, such as the Prentif and Lea's Shield®, have gone by the wayside, the FemCap is currently the only cap available on the US market. Approved by the FDA in March of 2003, the current version is a small silicone device shaped similarly to a sailor's cap, designed to cover the cervix and be held in place by the muscular walls of the vagina. The major difference between the current and original FemCap device introduced in 1999 is that it now includes a strap for easier removal. The FemCap comes in three diameter sizes; small (22 mm) for nulligravida women; medium (26 mm) for women with prior pregnancies that resulted in only abortion or cesarean delivery; and large (30 mm) for parous women with a history of vaginal delivery. Although not required, fit is best determined by a provider to check sizing in the clinic because of differences in female anatomy regardless of parity.

FemCap must be used along with a spermicidal jelly, placed both in the "bowl" of the cap and around its "brim." It is then placed by the user with its concave side directly over her cervix up to 42 hours before intercourse, and ideally at least 15 minutes before full female sexual arousal. Very few studies on effectiveness rates are available, but estimates are 92% with typical use (FemCap, 2010). Like the diaphragm and sponge, the FemCap must be left in place at least 6 hours after intercourse; however, it can be left in place for a full 48 hours if necessary.

Advantages of the FemCap are that it is non-latex, is discrete, and can be placed well ahead of sexual intercourse. Disadvantages are that it requires a prescription, sizing and fit are best done by an experienced provider, and it must be replaced every year or after any new pregnancy. The only absolute contraindications to use of the FemCap are current cervical cancer or women at high risk for HIV (WHO, 2009) because of the use of a spermicide.

B. Spermicides

Contraceptive spermicides are formulations of either a gel, foam, cream, suppository, or film base that have an added surface-active chemical to kill sperm. The only currently approved spermicidal chemical in the United States is nonoxynol-9. If a spermicidal formulation is correctly inserted into the vagina before intercourse, the efficacy rate for perfect use is 85%, whereas typical use is 71% (Trussell, 2008). Following package instructions is essential because of the fact that each formulation may require different amounts of time to dissolve or disperse to be effective. Spermicidal formulations require reinsertion after 1 hour and after each act of intercourse. They are commonly used with barrier methods, such as male and female condoms; come already imbedded in the sponge; and are recommended as standard practice with diaphragms and the FemCap to achieve full efficacy rates.

Advantages of spermicides are that no examination or prescription is required, they are readily available over the counter, they are relatively inexpensive, they provide lubrication during sex, and they increase efficacy of other methods. Disadvantages are that they can be somewhat messy, suppositories or film may require up to 15 minutes to dissolve, and some people experience allergies or irritation with use.

Additionally, studies have shown that there is a possible increased risk of genital ulceration or epithelial disruption from the use of nonoxynol-9, which could actually facilitate STI transmission including HIV, especially in frequent users (considered more than two times per day) (WHO, 2002). For women who are at low risk for STIs, spermicides remain a good contraception option.

C. Copper T 380-A intrauterine contraceptive (ParaGard®)

1. IUC as long-acting reversible contraceptive

Approved by the FDA in 1984, the Copper T 380-A, also known as the ParaGard®, is an IUC made of polyethylene shaped like a "T," wrapped in fine copper wire. Placed inside a woman's uterine cavity through the cervix by a trained provider, the IUC is considered a long-acting reversible contraceptive (LARC), and is highly effective at preventing pregnancy. Two monofilament threads (strings) are attached to the base of the device, and extend through the cervix into the vaginal cavity. The strings are provided to facilitate removal, but are also a convenient way for the patient to check for the presence of her IUC monthly by feeling for them with her finger. Because there is nothing for the patient to do after receiving the IUC to activate it, perfect use and typical use efficacy rates are similar at 99.4% and 99.2%, respectively (Trussell, 2008). This difference results from a perfect user checking her "strings" regularly at home and being more aware of spontaneous expulsion than a typical user. The ParaGard® works primarily by preventing sperm from fertilizing an egg by increasing copper ions, enzymes, prosta-glandins, and macrophages in uterine fluid, both altering transport and affecting the sperm and egg, ultimately preventing fertilization (Grimes, 2007).

Despite the high effectiveness and reversibility, the United States has some of the lowest IUC user prevalence rates of any country (Population Reference Bureau, 2008). This may be caused by several common misconceptions. Although IUCs that were on the market before the 1980s had a design flaw that caused an increased prevalence of pelvic infection, current studies of today's IUCs show no increased incidence or only a slight increased incidence of infection in the first 30 days after insertion. Additionally, IUCs decrease the risk of ectopic pregnancy and are safe in nulliparous women (Grimes, 2007).

An ideal candidate for the IUC is any woman looking for a highly effective, long-term, reversible method and who is able to tolerate minor discomfort with insertion. Absolute contraindications to the use of the ParaGard® according to the WHO (category 4) include current untreated chlamydia or gonorrhea; current pelvic inflammatory disease (or infection within the last 3 months); known cervical cancer that has yet to be treated; known endometrial cancer; known pelvic tuberculosis; persistent gestational trophoblastic disease; endometritis or septic abortion in the past 3 months; physical distortion of the uterine cavity, such as fibroids that would prevent proper placement; and undiagnosed suspicious, abnormal vaginal bleeding (WHO, 2009). Allergy to copper or history of Wilson disease are also contraindications.

Advantages of the IUC include high effectiveness, reversibility, and relatively low cost. Although initial cost may seem high, if used for at least 2 years, the ParaGard® is the most cost-effective contraceptive on the US market (Trussell et al., 1995). Currently, the ParaGard® IUC is approved for use up to 12 years, at which time it can be removed and replaced immediately by another, if desired. Insertion can be done at any time during a woman's menstrual cycle (including the postpartum period) as long as pregnancy is reliably excluded. It has been shown to be highly safe and effective when inserted immediately postaspiration abortion (Goodman et al., 2008). Another advantage of the IUC is that there is nothing for the patient to remember at home other than checking her strings. Disadvantages include an increase in menstrual bleeding and cramping in the first several cycles, possible spontaneous expulsion (rate is less than 1 per 1,000), and rare insertion risks including perforation and infection.

2. IUC as EC

    First reported in 1976, the ParaGard® IUC is the most highly effective method of postcoital EC available today. When placed within 5 days of unprotected intercourse, the ParaGard® has an efficacy rate of over 99% compared with only 75–89% for the EC pills (Trussell et al., 1995). It is recommended as an appropriate method of EC for all women who meet the standard criteria for ParaGard® IUC insertion and have none of the contraindications as listed in the previous section (American College of Obstetricians and Gynecologists, 2005).

    Once an existing pregnancy has been ruled out by a good history and a high-sensitivity urine pregnancy test, the patient may have the ParaGard® IUC placed immediately by a trained provider in the same normal manner. Aside from the fact that it is highly effective as an EC, a great advantage to this method is that it is excellent for women who also desire long-term contraception, because it can confer up to another 12 years of protection. Disadvantages are the same as listed for ParaGard® as a LARC method.

D. Natural family planning (NFP)

NFP methods are for the most part behavioral methods of contraception requiring body awareness, self-control, education, and commitment. Methods include FAM and the LAM. Coitus interruptus (or withdrawal) and abstinence can also be considered methods of NFP and both can be incorporated into the other methods, although neither is discussed in this chapter.

1. Fertility awareness (FAM)

    FAM is the practice of detecting and interpreting a woman's fertile ovulation period and avoiding all intercourse during that time. Two ways of identifying this fertile window are through either calendar-based or symptom-based methods. Simple periodic abstinence based on misinformation or guesswork without formal instruction regarding "safe" times yields an overall typical use rate of only about 75% (Trussell, 2008). However, actual FAMs depend on careful instruction, understanding, and strict adherence. If a specific method is adhered to correctly, perfect use rates have been shown to be very successful.

    Calendar methods involve keeping track of the menstrual cycle and include the calendar rhythm method, with a 91% perfect use rate, and the standard days method, with a 95% perfect use rate. The calendar rhythm method involves tracking menstrual cycles for 6–12 months and using a simple mathematical formula to calculate fertile days, whereas the standard days method uses a tool called CycleBeads® for keeping track of fertile days, and is ideal for low-literacy patients (Trussell, 2008). These methods along with the basal body temperature method, of which there are no reliable data for effectiveness rate, have been largely replaced in favor of newer methods that use other physical signs of fertility, such as cervical secretions (Pallone & Bergus, 2009). The "two-day method" and the "ovulation method" confer a 96% and 97% effectiveness, respectively (Trussell, 2008), whereas the "symptothermal method," using a combination of basal body temperature and cervical mucus, has a perfect use rate of 98% (Trussell, 2008).

Teaching these methods can take considerably more time than teaching other methods of contraception, with an estimated 4–6 hours for a woman to learn the necessary skills (Jennings, Arevalo, & Kowal, 2007). Therefore, it is important that referrals to specialized instructors be provided if none are available in the clinical setting, or to encourage literate couples to read at least one or two books on the method of choice before beginning.

Advantages of FAMs are that there are no health risks or side effects, they can be acceptable for couples with religious concerns about other contraceptive methods, they can increase body awareness, and they are either free or very low cost. Additionally, some of the methods can be used in reverse for couples wanting to plan a pregnancy. Disadvantages are primarily that learning a method takes time and effort, and using it requires considerable commitment and self-control. Additionally, many of the methods cannot be reliably used by women with irregular cycles or a vaginal infection, those who have recently reached menarche, those approaching menopause, those in the immediate postpartum period or while breastfeeding, or if they have recently discontinued hormonal contraceptive. Finally, there is no protection against STIs with FAM.

2. Lactational Amenorrhea Method (LAM)

LAM is a very effective method of NFP but is limited to the 6 months postpartum period for women meeting specific criteria. A woman must have had no return to menses since giving birth; be breastfeeding almost exclusively, with less than 10% of infant calories from supplements; feed at least every 4 hours during the day, and at least every 6 hours at night; and be "pumping" for an effectiveness rate of 98% to be achieved. However, if she pumps even part of her milk, the rate is reduced to 95% (Pallone & Bergus, 2009).

II. Database (may include but is not limited to)

A. Subjective

1. Barrier methods

   a. Medical illnesses: current cervical cancer (FemCap) and history of urinary tract infections (diaphragm)

   b. Personal and social history
      i. Gravida and para (FemCap and sponge)
      ii. Allergies: (male and female) latex, nonoxynol-9 (condoms, FemCap, diaphragm, sponge, and spermicide)
      iii. Sexual history: recent history of unprotected intercourse and current risk of STI
      iv. Previous contraceptive use and satisfaction, compliance, or problems
      v. Preference for and comfort with method
      vi. Tolerance of side effects: potential allergy or sensitivity to latex or nonoxynol-9
      vii. Financial constraints

2. Spermicides

   a. Personal and social history
      i. Allergies: (male and female) nonoxynol-9
      ii. Sexual history: current risk of STI
      iii. Previous contraceptive use and satisfaction, compliance, or problems
      iv. Preference for and comfort with method
      v. Tolerance of side effects: potential skin irritation or ulceration

3. Cu T380-A IUC

   a. Medical illnesses (cervical or endometrial cancer, history of Wilson disease, pelvic tuberculosis, pelvic inflammatory disease, endometritis or septic abortion in past 3 months, or persistent gestational trophoblastic disease)

   b. Personal and social history
      i. Allergies (to copper)
      ii. Postpartum (first 48 hours best, or wait 4 weeks after delivery for insertion)
      iii. Postabortion (immediate insertion appropriate)
      iv. Sexual history: recent history of unprotected intercourse (last 5 days for EC) and current risk for STI
      v. Previous contraceptive use and satisfaction, compliance, or problems
      vi. Preference for and comfort with method (i.e., can tolerate insertion process including minor pain or discomfort)

vii. Tolerance of side effects: possible increased bleeding or menstrual cramping in first several cycles

viii. Financial constraints

4. NFP

   a. Medical illnesses

   b. Personal and social history

      i. Postpartum

      ii. Breastfeeding

      iii. Sexual history: current risk for STI

      iv. Previous contraceptive use and satisfaction and compliance problems

      v. Preference for, comfort with, and expressed ability to learn and strictly adhere to chosen FAM or LAM

   c. Menstrual history and problems: length and regularity of cycles, recent menarche, or approaching menopause

   d. Current and recent medications (i.e., hormonal contraceptives)

B. **Objective**

1. Barrier methods

   a. Screening or testing for STIs as indicated

   b. Speculum examination with screening Pap if not up to date to rule out cervical cancer

   c. Pelvic examination and sizing for diaphragm; fitting for FemCap

2. Spermicides
   Screening and testing for STIs as indicated

3. Cu T 380-A IUC as LARC or EC

   a. Pregnancy test

   b. Screening for STIs

   c. Speculum examination with Pap if not up to date to rule out cervical cancer

   d. Pelvic examination to determine size, shape of uterus, and position of fundus; "sounding" to measure length of uterine cavity (minimum 6 cm required)

4. NFP
   Screening and testing for STIs as indicated

III. Assessment

A. **Needs**
Determine the current and future childbearing plans of the patient.

B. **Significance**
Determine the significance of an unplanned pregnancy to the patient.

C. **Motivation and ability**
Determine the patient's willingness and ability to correctly and consistently use the method of choice.

D. **Meets criteria**
No contraindications to the method of choice.

IV. Goals of clinical management

A. **Desired outcomes met**

1. Patient provided with methods that support his or her family planning needs; pregnancy prevention, planning, and spacing as desired

2. Screening, diagnosis, and treatment of any STIs or other infections

B. **Patient adherence**
Select an approach that maximizes patient adherence and satisfaction

V. Plan

A. **Screening for all methods**

1. STI, human papilloma virus, and Pap screening as indicated. Major authorities including the United States Preventative Services Task Force recommend *Chlamydia* and gonorrhea screening for all sexually active women 25 years of age and younger, and men and women in geographically high-risk areas. Additionally, screening for HIV and syphilis is recommended for all men and women engaging in high-risk sexual behavior (United States Preventative Services Task Force, 2004).

B. **Management (includes treatment, consultation, referral, and follow-up care)**

1. Barrier methods

   a. Provide method of choice in office or by prescription

   b. Follow-up for resizing of diaphragm after weight gain or loss of 20 pounds or more, or after vaginal childbirth

   c. Follow-up for refitting of new FemCap after any pregnancy beyond first trimester

2. Spermicides

   a. Provide in office or direct patient to convenient locations for purchase

   b. Have patient return to clinic for evaluation if vaginal or penile ulceration noted to rule out pathology

   c. Provide EC pills or a prescription

3. Cu T 380-A IUC

    a. Insert IUC at office visit per protocols

    b. Follow-up with clinic visit in 2 to 3 months for postinsertion to check for expulsion and trim strings if desired by patient

    c. Return to clinic for evaluation if extended, heavy menses or amenorrhea

4. NFP

    a. Refer to well-trained individuals for instruction if not experienced or comfortable with teaching methods

    b. Encourage follow-up to reinforce learning

    c. Support and encourage breastfeeding moms who choose LAM and refer to lactation specialist if necessary

    d. Provide EC pills or prescription

C. Client education

1. Information: provide verbal and written information regarding

    a. Risk reduction and screening

    b. Action, use, side effects, associated risks, and importance of adherence

2. Counseling

    a. Encourage full client participation in the contraceptive selection process; ideally meet with both patient and partner

    b. Discuss benefits and risks of all available methods

    c. Discuss possible outcomes and choices if user or method failure occurs

    d. Discuss risk factors for STIs

    e. Document discussion on patient records

VI. Self-management resources and tools

A. Patient and client education

Both of these sites have excellent patient information and interactive tools that allow the user to filter and search through different options to find the right method for them.

    a. Planned Parenthood Federation of America website at www.plannedparenthood.org has full color pictures and detailed information about all available contraception. They also have an interactive tool called "My Method" that can be reached directly by going to: https://www.plannedparenthood.org/all-access/my-method.

    b. The Association of Reproductive Health Professionals site at www.arhp.org has patient information and an interactive tool that can be reached directly at: http://www.arhp.org/methodmatch.

REFERENCES

American College of Obstetricians and Gynecologists. (ACOG). (2005). ACOG Practice Bulletin No. 59. *Obstetrics & Gynecology, 105*, 223–232.

Cates, W., & Raymond, E. (2007). Vaginal barriers and spermicides. In R. A. Hatcher, J. Trussell, A. L. Nelson, W. Cates, F. H. Stewart, & D. Kowal (Eds.), *Contraceptive Technology* (19th ed., pp. 317–335). New York, NY: PDR Network, LLC.

FemCap. (2010). *Natural birth control for health-conscious women.* Retrieved from http://www.femcap.com/

French, P. P., Latka, M., Gollub, E. L., Rogers, C., Hoover, D. R., & Stein, Z. A. (2003). Use-effectiveness of the female versus male condom in preventing sexually transmitted disease in women. *Sexually Transmitted Disease, 30*, 433–439. Retrieved from http://www.cdc.gov/mmwr/

Goodman, S., Hendlish, C., Benedict, M., Reeves, M., Pera-Floyd, A., & Foster-Rosales, S. (2008). Increasing intrauterine contraception use by reducing barriers to post-abortal and interval insertion. *Contraception, 78*(2), 136–142.

Grimes, D. (2007). Intrauterine devices (IUDs). In R. A. Hatcher, J. Trussell, A. L. Nelson, W. Cates, F. H. Stewart, & D. Kowal (Eds.), *Contraceptive Technology* (19th ed., pp. 117–143). New York, NY: PDR Network, LLC.

Jennings, V., Arevalo, M., & Kowal, D. (2007). Vaginal barriers and spermicides. In R. A. Hatcher, J. Trussell, A. L. Nelson, W. Cates, F. H. Stewart, & D. Kowal (Eds.), *Contraceptive technology* (19th ed., pp. 317–335). New York, NY: PDR Network, LLC.

Meyers, D., Wolff, T., Gregory, K. Marion, L., Moyer, V., Nelson, H., & USPSTF. (2008). *USPSTF Recommendations for STI Screening.* Originally published in *American Family Physician, 77*, 819–824. Rockville, MD: Agency for Healthcare Research and Quality.

Pallone, S., & Bergus, G. (2009). Natural family planning. *Journal of the American Board of Family Medicine, 22*, 147–157.

Population Reference Bureau. (2008). *Statistics on IUC (lowest preference).* Retrieved from http://www.prb.org/Datafinder/Topic/Bar.aspx?sort=v&order=d&variable=49

Trussell, J. (2008). Contraceptive efficacy. In R. A. Hatcher, J. Trussell, A. L. Nelson, W. Cates, F. H. Stewart, & D. Kowal (Eds.), *Contraceptive Technology* (19th ed., pp. 747–826). New York, NY: PDR Network, LLC.

Trussell, J., & Ellerston, C. (1995). Efficacy of emergency contraception. *Fertility Control Review, 4*, 8–11.

Trussell, J., Leveque, J. A., Koenig, J. D., London, R., Borden, S., Henneberry, J., & Wysocki, S. (1995). The economic value of contraception: A comparison of 15 methods. *American Journal of Public Health, 85*, 494–503.

United States Preventative Services Task Force. (2004). *USPSTF Recommendations for STI Screening.* AHRQ. Retrieved from http://www.ahrq.gov/clinic/uspstf08/methods/stinfections.htm

World Health Organization. (2000). *Effectiveness of Male Latex Condoms in Preventing Sexually Transmitted Infections Including HIV.* Retrieved from http://www.who.int/reproductivehealth/topics/rtis/male_condom/en/index.html

World Health Organization. (2002). *Nonoxynol-9 Ineffective in Preventing HIV Infection.* Retrieved from http://www.who.int/mediacentre/news/releases/who55/en/index.html

World Health Organization. (2009). *Medical Eligibility Criteria for Contraceptive Use* (4th ed.). Geneva, Switzerland: Department of Reproductive Health and Research. Retrieved from www.who.int/reproductivehealth

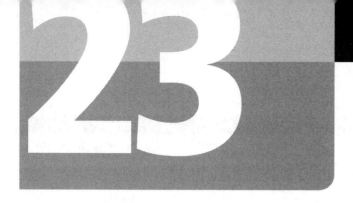

URINARY INCONTINENCE IN WOMEN

Janis Luft

I. Introduction and general background

Involuntary loss of urine, or urinary incontinence (UI), affects more than 13 million American women, 25% of whom are of reproductive age and up to 50% of whom are postmenopausal (Anger, Saigal, Litwin, & Urologic Diseases of America Project, 2006; Hannestad, Rortveit, Sandvik, & Hunskaar, 2000; Melville, Katon, Delaney, & Newton, 2005). The condition is associated with a profound adverse impact on quality of life and a higher risk of falls, fractures, nursing home admissions, and social isolation. Each year, consumers spend more than $30 billion on incontinence, including $20 billion in out-of-pocket costs for incontinence management. Yet, UI among adult women is a frequently unrecognized and undertreated problem.

A. Types of UI

UI classification is based on clinical presentation and severity. The primary circumstances leading to leakage of urine determine the type of incontinence. Most patients seen in the ambulatory care setting with UI present with stress, urge, or mixed UI (Table 23-1).

1. Stress UI

   The involuntary loss of urine as a result of physical stress or increased abdominal pressure from coughing, sneezing, straining, or exercise.

2. Urge incontinence and overactive bladder

   a. Urge incontinence (UUI) describes the loss of urine associated with a strong urge or need to void. Urinary frequency and nocturia are a frequent part of the clinical presentation of

this condition. Some patients report nocturnal enuresis.

   b. Women with overactive bladder (OAB) can be characterized as having wet or dry OAB. Wet OAB includes episodes of UUI. Women with dry OAB experience frequency, urgency, or nocturia but manage to avoid accidents with various behavioral strategies (e.g., limiting fluids, voiding often, and avoiding dietary bladder irritants).

3. Mixed incontinence

   Women with mixed incontinence have symptoms of both stress and urge incontinence, although one or the other condition may predominate.

4. Overflow incontinence

   Bladder outlet obstruction or hypocontractility of the detrussor muscle can cause incomplete bladder emptying. An abnormally full bladder can overspill resulting in overflow incontinence. This is a less common bladder dysfunction in women.

5. Functional incontinence

   This is urine loss that occurs because of factors exogenous to the lower urinary tract, such as diminished cognition or limited ambulation.

6. Reflex incontinence or neurogenic bladder

   Incontinence associated with neurologic dysfunction (e.g., multiple sclerosis or spinal cord injury). This can occur without warning or sensory awareness.

B. Prevalence

The prevalence of UI types varies according to age and underlying health status. Stress incontinence is more common in younger, ambulatory women, whereas urge and mixed incontinence increase with age and other health conditions. The proportion of women with UI varies widely (from 2% to 55%) depending on the definitions researchers used and the populations they surveyed. Researchers in the United States followed 64,000 women for at least 2 years in the Nurses' Health Study. The 2-year incidence of UI was 13.7%, but the 2-year remission rate (i.e., the percentage of women who reported leaking at least once a month at baseline and no leaking on follow-up) was 13.9% (Townsend et al., 2007). This surprising result underscores the dynamic nature of UI as a clinical condition.

C. Risk factors

1. Nonmodifiable: age, race or ethnicity, and possibly genetics.

2. Potentially modifiable: pregnancy, vaginal delivery, other obstetric events, and hysterectomy.

3. Modifiable or preventable: obesity, diabetes, smoking, chronic cough, and constipation.

TABLE 23-1 Differential Diagnosis of Urinary Incontinence in Women

Type	Presentation	Timing	Volume
Stress	Leakage associated with greater abdominal pressure from coughing, sneezing, straining, or exercise	Immediate	Small to moderate
Urge	Leakage occurs with a strong urge or need to void	Delayed	Drops to large
Mixed	Combination of stress and urge incontinence; one or the other may predominate	Varies	Varies

II. Initial evaluation

Initial evaluation of UI begins with a thorough medical, surgical, obstetric, and gynecological history and a complete list of the patient's medications. Clinicians can use a three-part screening tool to determine the type of incontinence (Table 23-2). These questions reliably correlate with clinical findings.

A. Subjective

1. Urinary symptoms
   a. Timing, frequency, severity, and precipitants of incontinence episodes
   b. Number of daytime and nighttime urinations
   c. Urinary diary (Table 23-3)
2. Amount and nature of fluid intake
3. Bowel habits (e.g., constipation, diarrhea, or straining)

B. Objective

1. Although not a prerequisite to diagnosis and the initiation of nonsurgical treatment for UI, the following may provide data that aid in individualization of treatment or assist in the management of UI refractory to treatment
   a. Assess for genital atrophy
   b. Directed pelvic examination to assess for prolapse or other pathology, such as a pelvic mass
2. Simple neurologic examination: mental status and sensory and motor function of the perineum and lower extremities

TABLE 23-2 Initial Screening for Urinary Incontinence

1. **During the last 3 months, have you leaked urine (even a small amount)?**
   ❏ Yes ❏ No

2. **During the last 3 months, did you leak urine (*check all that apply*):**
   ❏ a. When you were performing some physical activity, such as coughing, sneezing, lifting, or exercise?
   ❏ b. When you had the urge or the feeling that you needed to empty your bladder, but you could not get to the toilet fast enough?
   ❏ c. Without physical activity and without a sense of urgency?

3. **During the last 3 months, did you leak urine most often (*check only one*):**
   ❏ a. When you were performing some physical activity, such as coughing, sneezing, lifting, or exercise?
   ❏ b. When you had the urge or the feeling that you needed to empty your bladder, but you could not get to the toilet fast enough?
   ❏ c. Without physical activity and without a sense of urgency?
   ❏ d. About equally as often with physical activity as with a sense of urgency?

Type of Urinary Incontinence Is Based on Responses to Question 3	
Responses to Question 3	**Type of Incontinence**
a. Most often with physical activity	Stress only or stress predominant
b. Most often with the urge to empty the bladder	Urge only or urge predominant
c. Without physical activity or a sense of urgency	Other cause only or other cause predominant
d. About equally with physical activity and a sense of urgency	Mixed

Source: Brown, J. S., Bradley, C. S., Subak, L. L., Richter, H. E., Kraus, S. R., Brubaker, L., et al. (2006). The sensitivity and specificity of a simple test to distinguish between urge and stress urinary incontinence. *Annals of Internal Medicine, 144,* 715–723. Reprinted with permission.

TABLE 23-3 Urinary Diary*

Time	Urinate in Toilet	Leaking Accident	Reason for Accident	Fluid Intake	
				Type	Amount
6 A.M.					
7 A.M.					
8 A.M.					
9 A.M.					
10 A.M.					
11 A.M.					
12 NOON					
1 P.M.					
2 P.M.					
3 P.M.					
4 P.M.					
5 P.M.					

INSTRUCTIONS

1. In the 1st column mark an (x) every time you urinate into the toilet.
2. In the 2nd column, mark an (x) every time you accidentally leaked urine.
3. If an accident occurred, indicate the reason or circumstances surrounding the accident, for example, "coughed, bent over, sudden urge."
4. Under "Fluid Intake" describe the type (coffee, tea, juice, etc.) and amount (a cup, 1 quart, etc).
5. Circle the time when you went to bed and when you got up in the morning.
6. Record number and type of pads used.
7. Under Notes write any additional information you would like to include. For example, type and dose of medication you may be on for your urinary incontinence.

*Actual diary contains 24 rows labeled for each hour.

III. Assessment

A. Determine the diagnosis
The screening tool found in Table 23-2 can be used to determine the initial diagnosis of UI type (Table 23-1).

B. Severity
Assess the severity of the condition.
1. Number and types of pads or hygienic products used
2. Psychologic distress and depression associated with the condition (e.g., limitation to travel, time with family, social isolation, fear of odor or accidents, restriction of exercise)
3. Disruption of sleep

C. Significance
Assess the significance of the problem to the patient and significant others.

D. Motivation and ability
1. Determine the patient's goals for treatment (e.g., reduction in incontinent episodes vs. complete dryness, fewer daytime urinations, or less nocturia).
2. Determine the patient's preferences for treatment (e.g., behavioral modification, medication, combination of these, or other treatment options).
3. Determine the patient's willingness and ability to follow the treatment plan.

IV. Goals of clinical management

A. Screening or diagnosing UI
Choose a cost-effective approach for screening or diagnosing UI that is compatible with the patient's goals and preferences.

B. Treatment

Select a treatment plan that achieves the patient's objectives for bladder control in a safe and effective manner.

C. Patient adherence

Select an approach that maximizes patient adherence.

V. Plan

A. Screening

Although an extremely common chronic condition in women, UI is underreported by patients and unaddressed by many clinicians (Brown et al., 1999). Primary or women's healthcare providers can effectively screen patients by simply asking about issues of bladder control or using the simple questionnaire provided in Table 23-2.

B. Diagnostic tests (Table 23-2)

1. Incontinence Questionnaire
2. A urinary diary that the patient keeps for 1–3 days (Table 23-3)
3. A dipstick urinalysis to rule out underlying infection
4. Postvoid residual urine to rule out overflow incontinence
5. Urodynamic testing measures detrusor function, bladder capacity and compliance, and sensation to void. Although such testing may be useful in evaluating patients with complex symptoms or voiding dysfunction, it is unnecessary in all patients with incontinence before proceeding to treatment based on clinical presentation.

C. Management (includes treatment, consultation, referral, and follow-up care)

1. Nonpharmacologic management
   a. Bladder training helps patients reestablish voluntary bladder control. Patients learn how to void on a set schedule, beginning with about 30–60 minutes between voids and then slowly increasing the interval to 3 or 4 hours (Table 23-5)
   b. Relaxation and urge suppression techniques effectively suppress the strong urge to void that is associated with urge UI (Table 23-6).
   c. Pelvic floor muscle exercises or Kegel exercises strengthen the muscles of the pelvic floor and improve urethral pressure and inhibit involuntary detrusor contractions (Table 23-6).
   d. Biofeedback uses electromyography or manometry to help patients learn pelvic floor muscle exercises through directed instructions as they receive feedback in the form of dynamic graphs or tones that reinforces their actions. This modality can help women isolate pelvic muscles and improve the efficacy of pelvic floor muscle exercises.
   e. Weight loss has been shown to improve continence symptoms (Subak et al., 2005; Subak et al., 2009). As little as 3–5% weight loss has been shown to reduce weekly incontinence episodes by 50–60%.
   f. Diet modification can be helpful. Some patients find that elimination of "bladder triggers," such

TABLE 23-4 Medications for Overactive Bladder

Short-acting oral agents	Oxybutynin (Ditropan®), 5 mg	0.50–1 tablet two to four times a day
	Tolterodine (Detrol®), 1 and 2 mg	1 tablet twice daily (start with 2 mg and decrease to 1 mg if severe side effects)
	Trospium chloride (Sanctura®), 20 mg	1 tablet twice daily on an empty stomach
Extended-release oral agents	Oxybutynin ER (Ditropan XL®), 5–15 mg	1 tablet daily
	Tolterodine ER (Detrol LA®), 2 and 4 mg	1 capsule daily (start with 4 mg and decrease to 2 mg if severe side effects)
	Darifenacin (Enablex®), 7.5 and 15 mg	1 tablet daily
	Solifenacin (VesiCare®), 5 and 10 mg	1 tablet daily
	Fesoterodine (Toviaz®), 4 and 8 mg	1 tablet daily
Transdermal agents	Oxybutynin transdermal patch (Oxytrol)®, 3.9 mg/day	1 patch on dry skin (hip, abdomen, or buttocks) every 3–4 days
	Oxybutynin transdermal gel 10% (Gelnique®), 100 mg/g	1 sachet daily to dry, intact skin on the abdomen, upper arms or shoulders, or thighs

NOTES

Contraindications: Narrow-angle glaucoma or severe liver or kidney disease.

Side effects: Dry mouth and constipation are the most common. Adjust dose to balance drug effectiveness versus side effects.

Alternative: Imipramine, 10 mg, at bedtime and adjust as often as weekly. Adjust per the patient's urinary diary and symptoms to a maximum of 100 mg at bedtime. Use with caution in the elderly because of hypotension or cognitive impairment.

as caffeine, alcohol, spicy foods, and concentrated citrus, can reduce urinary urgency and frequency. Overhydration and underhydration should be discouraged. Fluid intake sufficient to maintain "lemon juice" colored urine is ideal.

2. Pharmacologic treatment options

A growing number of medications are available to treat UUI, urgency, and frequency, and nocturia (Table 23-4). Generally, these agents, which inhibit the bladder's contractile activity, have an anticholinergic or antimuscarinic effect. Although they provide excellent symptom relief and reduce weekly incontinent episodes by 15–60%, they may also cause bothersome side effects, such as dry mouth, constipation, drowsiness, and blurred vision (Nygaard & Heit, 2009). Sustained-release medications may cause fewer side effects.

Medical treatment of stress UI has been largely unsuccessful. There are no pharmaceutical agents for the treatment of SUI on the US market.

Treatment of incontinence with estrogen is not recommended. Two large randomized, controlled trials (the Women's Health Initiative and the Heart and Estrogen Replacement Study) demonstrated an increase in the prevalence of UI with the use of both estrogen-only and combined hormone-replacement therapy on stress, urge, and mixed UI (40–50% over a 4-year period and 20–60% at 12 months) (Hendrix et al., 2005; Grady et al., 2001).

3. Treatment requiring referral to a continence specialty practice

a. Pessaries: well-fit incontinence ring or incontinence dish pessaries can relieve the symptoms of stress UI. The pessary compresses the urethra against the upper posterior portion of the symphysis pubis and elevates the bladder neck. This causes an increase in outflow resistance and corrects the angle between the bladder and the urethra.

TABLE 23-5 Bladder Retraining

Bladder retraining is a behavioral treatment for urinary incontinence that uses scheduled toileting to help you relearn normal bladder function. The purpose of bladder retraining is to

(a) increase the amount of time between emptying your bladder.

(b) increase the amount of fluids your bladder can hold.

(c) diminish the sense of urgency and/or leakage associated with your problem.

Keeping the diary of your bladder activity is very important. This helps us to determine the correct starting interval for you and to monitor your progress throughout your program.

INSTRUCTIONS

1. Empty your bladder as soon as you get up in the morning. This begins your retraining schedule.

2. Go to the bathroom every _____.

   Wait the full amount of time before you urinate again *AND* when it is your scheduled time, be sure to empty your bladder even if you feel no urge to urinate. Follow the schedule during waking hours ONLY. During the night time go to the bathroom only if you awaken and find it necessary.

3. A helpful hint: When the urge to urinate is felt before the next designated time, use the "urge suppression" technique described on the pink handout, or try relaxation techniques like deep breathing. Focus on relaxing all other muscles. If possible, sit down until the sensation passes. If the urge is suppressed, adhere to the schedule. If you cannot suppress the urge, wait 5 minutes then slowly make your way to the bathroom; then re-establish the schedule. Repeat this process each time an urge is felt.

4. When you have accomplished this goal, gradually increase the time between emptying your bladder by 15 minute intervals. Try to increase your interval each week, but you will be the best judge of how quickly you can advance to the next step. The time between each urination is increased until you reach a 3- to 4-hour voiding interval.

5. It should take between 6 and 12 weeks to accomplish your goal. Don't be discouraged by set-backs. You may find you have good days and bad days. As you continue bladder retraining you will start to notice more and more good days, so keep practicing.

6. You will hasten your success by doing your pelvic muscle exercises faithfully every day. Your diaries will help you see your progress and identify your problem times.

7. If you need more help, medication or other treatments are available and may be useful.

TABLE 23-6 Urge Suppression

Urge incontinence is the loss of urine when you have a strong desire to urinate and are unable to reach a bathroom in time. The urge is a signal that it is time to urinate. Your goal is to maintain bladder control until you reach a toilet. A normally functioning bladder can wait until the appropriate opportunity to empty, an unstable bladder cannot.

For a person with urge incontinence, *rushing* to the bathroom when you have a strong urge to urinate is the worst thing you can do. Rushing actually causes bladder irritability to increase and interferes with your ability to concentrate on controlling your bladder. When urgency strikes, you should use the "urge suppression" technique to maintain control.

1. Stop all movement immediately and stand still. Sit down if possible. Remaining still increases your ability to stay in control.

2. Squeeze your pelvic floor muscles quickly and tightly several times. Do not relax the muscles fully between these very quick squeezes. Squeezing your pelvic floor muscles this way signals the bladder to relax and increases your feeling of being in control.

3. Take a deep breath and relax. Shrug your shoulders and let them go limp. Release the tension in the rest of your body.

4. Concentrate on suppressing the urge feeling. Some women find distraction an effective technique.

5. When the strong urgency subsides, walk *slowly and calmly* to the bathroom. If the urge begins to build again, repeat the above steps. You can also try contracting your muscles as you walk to the bathroom.

Remember: going to the bathroom is not an emergency!!

b. Electrical stimulation
   i. Vaginal or rectal electrical stimulation uses an internal sensor to deliver electrical currents at preset frequencies. Higher frequency causes involuntary levator ani contractions that improve pelvic floor tone and assist in learning to contract these muscles at will. Lower frequencies are used to blockade the sacral nerve plexus, reducing detrusor irritability.
   ii. Percutaneous tibial nerve stimulation is used to treat OAB. A fine-needle electrode is inserted into the lower, inner aspect of the leg, slightly cephalad to the medial malleolus. The goal is to send stimulation through the tibial nerve. The needle electrode is connected to an external pulse generator that delivers an adjustable electrical pulse that travels to the sacral plexus via the tibial nerve. The treatment protocol requires once-a-week treatments for 12 weeks, roughly 30 minutes per session.

c. Surgical treatments
   i. Multiple surgical options are available to treat stress incontinence. The most common sling procedure is the tension-free vaginal tape, in which the surgeon places a narrow piece of polypropylene mesh under the mid-urethra and passes it through the anterior abdominal wall behind the pubic bone. A more recent variation on tension-free vaginal tape is the transobturator tape.
   ii. Patients whose stress incontinence results from intrinsic sphincter deficiency may benefit from urethral bulking agents, such as collagen (Contigen®) and carbon-coated beads (Durasphere®), which are injected transurethrally as an outpatient surgery.
   iii. Sacral nerve stimulation, also called sacral nerve neuromodulation (InterStim®) therapy is a reversible treatment for people with UUI caused by OAB who do not respond to behavioral treatments or medication. InterStim® is a surgically implanted neurostimulation system that sends mild electrical pulses to the S3 sacral nerve root, a nerve that influences bladder control.
   iv. Botox® (botulinum toxin A) injection into the detrusor muscle is an option for neurogenic or idiopathic UUI unresponsive to conservative measures. Botox® is injected into numerous sites in the bladder wall using a cystoscope. The toxin works by inactivating proteins involved in neurotransmitter release from nerve terminals. As neurotransmitter levels decrease, underlying muscle spasm may be diminished or ablated. The Food and Drug Administration has not yet approved Botox® for this use, but studies have been encouraging and approval is expected in the near future.

v. Bladder augmentation is infrequently used and reserved for people with UUI who do not benefit from bladder retraining or medication. This procedure increases the capacity of a small, hyperactive, or nonresilient bladder by adding bowel segments or by reducing the muscle-squeezing ability of the bladder.

D. Client education

1. Information
   Provide verbal and, preferably, written information regarding
   a. Prevalence, morbidity, cost, and available treatments for UI.
   b. Modifiable risk factors for UI, such as obesity, diabetes, and smoking.
   c. Management rationale, action, use, side effects, associated risks, and cost of therapeutic interventions; and the need for adhering to long-term treatment plans.

2. Counseling
   a. Weight loss counseling and advice as needed.
   b. Management of diabetic glucose levels.
   c. Avoidance of constipation.
   d. Decision making regarding elective pelvic surgery.

VI. Self-management resources and tools

A. Patient and client education

1. National Institute for Diabetes, Digestive and Kidney Diseases (NIDDK)

   The NIDDK is a division of the National Institutes of Health. According to their website, "the NIDDK conducts and supports research on many chronic and costly diseases affecting the public health. Several diseases studied by the NIDDK are among the leading causes of disability and death in the Nation; all affect seriously the quality of life of those suffering from them." Both patient and provider literature is available on their website (www2.niddk.nih.gov)

2. UCSF Women's Continence Center website (www.ucsf.edu/wcc)

   The UCSF Women's Continence Center website provides information about women's UI, pelvic floor prolapse, and treatment options. Downloadable diaries and handouts are available for public use.

B. Community support groups

1. National Association for Continence (NAFC)

   Founded in 1982, the NAFC was originally known as Help for Incontinent People. Today, the renamed National Association for Continence is the largest private consumer organization dedicated to educating and advocating for people with bladder and pelvic floor dysfunction. The NAFC provides educational resources, healthcare referrals, public education, and personal support for those with incontinence (www.nafc.org or 1-800-BLADDER).

2. The Simon Foundation

   The mission statement of the Simon Foundation is that of "bringing the topic of incontinence out into the open, removing the stigma surrounding incontinence, and providing help and hope for people with incontinence, their families, and the health professionals who provide their care." The organization provides public education materials (www.simonfoundation.org).

REFERENCES

Anger, J. T., Saigal, C. S., Litwin, M. S., & Urologic Diseases of America Project. (2006). The prevalence of urinary incontinence among community dwelling adult women: Results from the National Health and Nutrition Examination Survey. *Journal of Urology, 175,* 601–604.

Brown, J., Grady, D., Ouslander, J. G., Herzog, A. R., Varner, R. E., & Posner, S. F. (1999). Prevalence of urinary incontinence and associated risk factors in postmenopausal women. Heart & Estrogen/Progestin Replacement Study (HERS) Research Group. *Obstetrics & Gynecology, 94,* 66–70.

Grady, D., Brown, J. S., Vittinghoff, E., Applegate, W., Varner, E., Snyder, T., & HERS Research Group. (2001). Postmenopausal hormones and incontinence: The Heart and Estrogen/Progestin Replacement Study. *Obstetrics & Gynecology, 97,* 116–120.

Hannestad, Y. S., Rortveit, G., Sandvik, H., & Hunskaar, S. (2000). A community-based epidemiological survey of female urinary incontinence: The Norwegian EPINCONT study. Epidemiology of Incontinence in the County of Nord-Trøndelag. *Journal of Clinical Epidemiology, 53,* 1150–1157.

Hendrix, S. L., Cochrane, B. B., Nygaard, I. E., Handa, V. L., Barnabei, V. M., Iglesia, C., et al. (2005). Effect of estrogen with and without progestin on urinary incontinence. *Journal of the American Medical Association, 293,* 935–948.

Melville, J. L., Katon, W., Delaney, K., & Newton, K. (2005). Urinary incontinence in U.S. women: A population-based study. *Archives of Internal Medicine, 165,* 537–542.

Nygaard, I. E., & Heit, M. (2009). Stress urinary incontinence. *Obstetrics & Gynecology, 104,* 607–620.

Subak. L. L., Whitcomb, E., Shen, H., Saxton, J., Vittinghoff, E., & Brown, J. S. (2005). Weight loss: A novel and effective treatment for urinary incontinence. *Journal of Urology, 174,* 190– 195.

Subak, L. L., Wing, R., West, D. S., Franklin, F., Vittinghoff, E., Creasman, J. . . . PRIDE Investigators. (2009). Weight loss to treat urinary incontinence in overweight and obese women. *New England Journal of Medicine, 360,* 481–490.

Townsend, M. K., Danforth, K. N., Lifford, K. L., Rosner, B., Curhan, G. C., Resnick, N. M., . . . Grodstein, F. (2007). Incidence and remission of urinary incontinence in middle-aged women. *American Journal of Obstetrics & Gynecology, 197(2),* 167.e1-5.

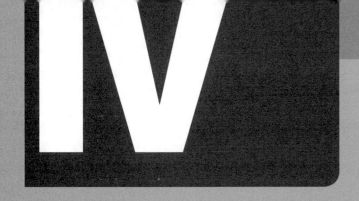

IV

OBSTETRIC HEALTH MAINTENANCE
AND PROMOTION

THE INITIAL PRENATAL VISIT

Rebekah Kaplan

I. Definition and background

Pregnancy is a time of great physical and emotional changes in a woman's life. Careful, regular monitoring during pregnancy can reassure the mother-to-be and detect variations from a normal pregnancy.

The basic components of prenatal care include early and continuing risk assessment, health promotion and education, and medical and psychosocial interventions and follow-up. Not only is a pregnancy a time when most women are unusually open to making positive lifestyle changes, but prenatal care offers the clinician an opportunity to develop a relationship with women over the duration of the pregnancy (Enkin, 2001).

Although current evidence shows that the standard model of individual prenatal care visits does not show positive effects on decreasing the rates of low-birth-weight infants or preterm delivery, the variety of components of care helps practitioners to identify risks for a woman and family in many aspects of her life and initiate appropriate interventions (Fiscella, 1995; Vintzileos, Ananth, Smulian, Scorza, & Knuppel, 2002). The objectives for guiding prenatal care are focused on

- Nonintervention: the reproductive cycle is a normal and essentially healthy process.
- Consideration of the patient as a member of the healthcare team.
- Patient education appropriate to age, culture, and needs including anticipatory guidance and nutrition.
- Promotion of self-esteem and empowerment.
- Individualization of care: respecting cultural background, sexual orientation, and patient priorities (Walker, McCully, & Vest, 2001).

The initial prenatal visit includes a health history, with a special focus on prior pregnancies and pertinent details of relevant medical, surgical, and psychosocial history, followed by a complete physical examination. Additional baseline data are gathered through routine laboratory work (Walker, McCully, & Vest, 2001).

II. Database (may include, but is not limited to)

A. Subjective

1. History of the current pregnancy
   a. Pregnancy symptoms: nausea, vomiting, fatigue, sore breasts, headache, and fetal movement
   b. Problems: vaginal bleeding and excessive vomiting
   c. Feelings about pregnancy: planned or wanted

2. Information for dating of pregnancy
   a. Past menstrual history: menarche, cycle interval, length of flow, and amount of flow
   b. Last normal menstrual period: sureness of date; length of flow; previous menstrual period if last period not normal; and any factors that potentially interfere with duration of cycle or ovulation (e.g., hormonal contraceptives, other medications).
   c. Dates and results of home pregnancy testing
   d. Symptoms of pregnancy including onset and evolution, and fetal movement
   e. Previous ultrasound (Hunter, 2009). (Box 24-1)

3. Obstetric history
   a. Total number of pregnancies: abortions (spontaneous and therapeutic) and number of living children
   b. Deliveries: date; mode of delivery (vaginal birth, cesarean, or vacuum or forceps assisted); gestational age; gender; birth weight; length of labor; anesthesia; pregnancy weight gain; spontaneous or induced labor
   c. Pregnancy complications: preterm labor, gestational diabetes, preeclampsia, pregnancy-induced hypertension, small for gestational age, large for gestational age, and cholestasis of pregnancy
   d. Delivery complications: previous cesarean section and indication, shoulder dystocia, postpartum hemorrhage, third- or fourth-degree laceration

BOX 24-1 Establishing a Due Date

Dating the pregnancy is an essential part of the first prenatal visit. The practitioner must take into consideration all the information for dating the pregnancy and establish a best estimate of the delivery date (EDD). For most women a sure and "normal" last menstrual period (LMP) is the most useful method. Calculate the EDD based on LMP by using a gestational wheel or Naegle's rule (LMP + 7 days − 3 months, based on 28-day cycle). Use an ultrasound EDD if first-trimester ultrasound dates differ by more than 5–7 days or second-trimester dates differ by more than 10 days.

Accuracy of Dating

- In vitro fertilization ± 1 day
- Ovulation indication ± 3 days
- Single intercourse record/insemination ± 3 days
- Basal body temperature record ± 4 days
- Ultrasound 7–10 weeks (crown-rump length) ± 5 days
- "Regular" and certain LMP with 28-day cycle ± 10–14 days
- Second-trimester ultrasound (1 ± 7–14 days
- Third-trimester ultrasound 14–28 days
- First-trimester physical examination ± 2 weeks
- Second-trimester physical examination ± 4 weeks
- Third-trimester physical examination ± 6 weeks

Source: Adapted from Hunter, L. A. (2009). Issues in pregnancy dating: Revisiting the evidence. *Journal of Midwifery & Women's Health, 54*(3), 184–190.

---

      cardiovascular, thyroid, hepatitis, anemia, tuberculosis, seizures, and psychiatric illnesses
    c. Allergies: medications, other
    d. Surgeries or hospitalizations

6. Family history: significant illnesses with genetic risk, such as diabetes, hypertension, renal disease, cancer, cardiovascular disease, blood disorders, multiple gestation, congenital or chromosomal abnormalities, and substance abuse

7. Social history
    a. Country of origin (immigration worries)
    b. Current living situation
    c. Support
    d. Financial stability
    e. Insurance/Women, Infants and Children (WIC) program
    f. Food access
    g. Occupation and work safety (exposure to hazards: chemical, biologic, or physical)
    h. Intimate partner violence
    i. History of violence or sexual abuse
    j. Toxic habits (cigarettes, alcohol, drugs, current and past use)
    k. HIV risk factors
    l. Educational level (reading level, years of schooling, how they learn best)

8. Nutritional history
    a. Prepregnancy weight and basal metabolic index
    b. Weight gain or loss
    c. Current diet: restrictions (vegetarian or lactose intolerant); adequate protein; calcium; grains; fruits and vegetables

B. Objective

1. Baseline data: height, weight, blood pressure, and urinalysis

2. Complete physical examination
    a. Head, ears, eyes, nose, and throat
    b. Teeth
    c. Skin
    d. Neck and thyroid
    e. Breasts
    f. Heart
    g. Chest and lungs
    h. Abdomen: including uterine size or fundal height and fetal heart tones (after 10 weeks)
    i. Neurologic: deep tendon reflexes
    j. Extremities
    k. Pelvic examination
        i. External genitalia
        ii. Vagina: discharge

---

    e. Postpartum complications: infection, wound issues, depression, or mastitis
    f. Neonatal or newborn complications

4. Gynecological history
    a. Sexually transmitted infections including herpes simplex virus of patient or partner
    b. Fibroids
    c. Gynecological surgery
    d. Abnormal Pap smears and related loop electrosurgical excision procedure or cone procedures

5. Medical history
    a. Present medications: prescriptions, over the counter, or supplements
    b. Significant illnesses: asthma, diabetes, hypertension, frequent urinary tract infections,

   iii. Cervix: polyps, dilation of os, length, consistency, and position

   iv. Uterus: size, position, and symmetry

   v. Adnexa: difficult to palpate after 12 weeks

   vi. Rectum: note hemorrhoids

   vii. Pelvimetry if indicated

      a. Assessment: subpubic arch, bispinous diameter, diagonal conjugate, inclination of sidewalls, bituberous diameter, anteroposterior diameters of the midpelvis.

      b. Classification: gynecoid, android, anthropoid, platypoid, and mixed pelvic type.

III. Assessment

A. Estimated gestational age and date of delivery: size (S)/dates (D) relationship (S = D, S < D, or S > D)

B. Problems identified from history, physical examination, or existing laboratory data

C. Role assessment: are problems appropriate for consultation or advanced practice clinician management

IV. Plan

A. Diagnostic and laboratory screening (Boxes 24-2 and 24-3)

B. Therapeutic interventions and medications

1. Prenatal vitamins

2. Other vitamins or supplementation as indicated by history or nutritional assessment

   a. Iron, 325 mg daily if anemic (hemoglobin < 10, hematocrit < 32) (Graves & Barger, 2001).

   b. Vitamin D$_3$ (Cannell & Hollis, 2008)

   c. Fish oil: omega 3 fatty acids (Holland, Smith, Saarem, Saugstad, & Drevon, 2003)

   d. Calcium if dietary intake less than 1,200 mg daily (including prenatal vitamin)

3. Prescriptions (assess safety in pregnancy): clinicians need to be mindful of the US Food and Drug Administration risk category for drugs during pregnancy when prescribing medications for the pregnant woman. Categories include

   a. No risk of harm to the fetus (A)

   b. No risk seen in animals, but no controlled studies in women; probably little risk (B)

BOX 24-2 Laboratory Data

Initial screening "routine"

- Complete blood count with platelets and mean corpuscular volume
- Maternal blood type with antibody screen
- Hepatitis B surface antigen
- Rubella immunity
- Syphilis serology (RPR or VDRL)
- HIV antibody offer
- Urine culture and sensitivity
- Pap smear if due

Initial screening "risk based" based on population served or individual risk

- Hepatitis C antibody
- Varicella immunity if antibody unknown
- Purified protein derivative (tuberculosis skin test)
- Toxoplasmosis
- Early glucose load test
- Tay-Sachs disease
- Cystic fibrosis
- Hemoglobin electrophoresis
- Wet mount
- Gonorrhea and chlamydia if indicated

BOX 24-3 Timing of Diagnostic and Screening Tests Offered Women Before 20 Weeks

This may vary by location and what is available

- First-trimester blood screen (10–13 weeks)
- Nuchal translucency screening ultrasound (11–14 weeks)
- Second-trimester or quadruple marker blood screen (15–20 weeks)
- If indicated: ultrasound (first trimester) and chorionic villus sampling (10–13 weeks)
- Amniocentesis (15–20 weeks)
- Fetal survey/screening ultrasound (18–20 weeks, routine in many practices)

c.   Animal studies may show some risk to fetus; studies in women unavailable. Give only if benefit outweighs risk (C)

d.   Positive evidence of human fetal risk, but benefits may be acceptable in life-threatening situation (D)

e.   Known fetal abnormalities (X)

C. *Patient education (Figure 24-1)*

1.   Options for prenatal screening and diagnosis offered, reviewed, and discussed

2.   Nutrition and exercise

3.   Substance use and abuse

4.   Over-the-counter medications

5.   Food safety (e.g., listeria, mercury, and pasteurization)

6.   Teratogens

7.   Workplace safety and exposure

8.   Safer sex

9.   Prenatal care and compliance

10.   Women, Infant and Children Program (WIC): federally funded special supplemental food assistance program for low income women, infants, and children

11.   Danger signs

12.   Community resources

13.   Physiologic and emotional changes

14.   Sexuality during pregnancy

15.   Fetal growth and development

16.   Common discomforts of pregnancy

D. *Consultation and referrals (could include)*

1.   Genetic counseling for advanced maternal age; family history of genetic disorder, developmental delays and cardiovascular defects; as indicated by ethnic background, multiple miscarriages, consanguinity and exposure to potential teratogens.

2.   Ancillary services: social worker, nutritionist, health educator, prenatal classes, psychiatry as needed or desired

3.   Community resources (e.g., WIC feeding program, public health nurse, smoking cessation, community-based organizations)

4.   Medical consultation and referral (obstetric) (Box 24-4)

E. *Follow-up*

1.   Patient should return per the return visit schedule guideline. This should be flexible, individualized, and depend on parity and risk (Box 24-5).

2.   Patient should return to a physician if she is assessed to be high risk per guidelines or for consultation around a specific problem (see Chapter 28 on guidelines for medical consultation during pregnancy).

V. Internet resources

A. *American College of Nurse Midwives Consumer Education website:*
There is information regarding pregnancy advice, parenting, and women's health including easy to use patient education handouts from the "Share with Women Series" (http://www.mymidwife.org/).

B. *March of Dimes:*
Information is available for providers and patients in both written and audio–video formats in English and Spanish on pregnancy, birth, and newborn development and care (http://www.marchofdimes.com/).

C. *National Women's Health Information Center:*
This is a US Department of Health and Human Services women's health information website. There are numerous fact sheets on all aspects of women's health including pregnancy in both Spanish and English (http://www.womenshealth.gov).

D. *Childbirth Connection:*
This organization promotes evidenced-based maternity care and helps women and providers to make informed decisions. There are numerous patient education, pregnancy, and childbirth resources (http://www.childbirthconnection.org/).

E. *American College of Obstetrics and Gynecology:*
There are limited numbers of patient education handouts available by provider request (http://www.acog.org/).

FIGURE 24-1 OB Provider Education Flow Sheet

First and Second Trimester

❑ Received First-Trimester Packet

❑ Received Second-Trimester Packet

❑ Centering offered   ❑ Accepted   ❑ Declined   Why? _____

_____

❑ Orientation to clinic, CNM service, clinic _____

❑ Dental referral _____

Common discomforts:

Back pain _____   N/V _____

Constipation _____   Dizziness _____

HA _____   Round ligament pain _____

SOB _____   Urinary frequency _____

Other: _____

Food and drug safety _____

Dating/sonogram _____

Fetal growth and dev _____

Exercises in preg (back care, stretching, yoga, keeping fit) _____

Fetal movement _____

Additional education:

_____

_____

Method of infant feeding _____

Breastfeeding:

❑ Received breastfeeding class info

Breastfeeding experience _____

Benefits of breastfeeding _____

Exclusive breastfeeding 6 mo _____

Method of contraception _____

❑ Consent signed   ❑ Attended TL class

S/sx preterm labor (UCs, VB, LOF or ROM, pelvic pressure) _____

Danger signs (fever, VB, severe abd pain, dysuria) _____

(continues)

FIGURE 24-1 OB Provider Education Flow Sheet (continued)

Third Trimester
❏ Received Third-Trimester Packet
❏ Gave CB class info
❏ Attended CB class

Labor and delivery:

Birth plan _____

Relaxation techniques _____

Pain control options _____

Fetal monitoring methods _____

Early labor comfort measures _____

Support people in labor _____

S/Sx labor (UCs, bloody show, ROM) _____

PPD & Tdap vaccination _____

Breastfeeding:

❏ Attended breastfeeding class

Early initiation of breastfeeding _____

Skin to skin/rooming in _____

Infant feeding cues _____

Latch _____

Colostrum/milk production _____

Breastfeeding and returning to work _____

Breastfeeding resources _____

Baby care:

Experience with baby care _____

Help with baby at home _____

Sibling rivalry _____

Preparing for baby at home _____

Calming your baby _____

Car seat _____

Additional education: _____

_____

_____

Fetal movement _____

Kick counts _____

_____

Danger signs: general (VB, ROM, sev abd pain, decr FM, fever) _____

Danger signs: preeclampsia (HA, scotoma, RUQ or epig pain) _____

BOX 24-4 *Medical Conditions Requiring Transfer of Care to High-Risk Obstetric Clinic*
(These may differ in different settings)

Maternal conditions

- Chronic hypertension diagnosed before pregnancy
- Active or uncontrolled seizure disorder
- Severe asthma (hospitalization or requiring systemic steroids during pregnancy)
- Cardiac disease (except asymptomatic mitral valve prolapse)
- Pulmonary hypertension
- Platelet count less than 100,000
- Deep vein thrombosis
- Sickle cell disease
- Lupus, scleroderma, or any connective tissue disease
- Cancer
- Active tuberculosis
- Active viral hepatitis
- HIV positive
- Hyperthyroidism
- Diabetes: Type I and Type II
- Multiple gestation

BOX 24-5 *Visit Schedule Guidelines*

Frequency of prenatal visits

- 1–28 weeks – every 4 weeks
- 28–36 weeks – every 2–3 weeks
- 36+ weeks – every week

Reduced visit schedule

One visit during each gestational age or age range (approximately eight visits)

- 6–8 weeks
- 14–16 weeks
- 24–28 weeks
- 32 weeks
- 36 weeks
- Weekly from 38 weeks

REFERENCES

Cannell, J., & Hollis, B. (2008). Use of vitamin D in clinical practice. *Alternative Medicine Review 13*(1), 6–20.

Fiscella, K. (1995). Does prenatal care improve birth outcomes? A critical review. *Obstetrics & Gynecology, 85*(3), 468–479.

Graves, B. W., & Barger, M. K. (2001). A conservative approach to iron supplementation during pregnancy. *Journal of Midwifery and Women's Health, 45*(3), 163–166; 159–163 (for N282A).

Helland, I. B., Smith, L., Saarem, K., Saugstad, O. D. & Drevon, C. A. (2003). Maternal supplementation with very-long-chain n-3 fatty acids during pregnancy and lactation augments children's IQ at 4 years of age. *Pediatrics, 111*(1), 39–44.

Hunter, L. A. (2009). Issues in pregnancy dating: revisiting the evidence. *Journal of Midwifery & Women's Health, 54*(3), 184–190.

Vintzileos, A., Ananth, C. V., Smulian, J. C., Scorza, W. E., & Knuppel, R. A. (2002). The impact of prenatal care on neonatal deaths in the presence and absence of antenatal high-risk conditions. *American Journal of Obstetrics and Gynecology, 186*(5), 1011–1016.

Walker, D. S., McCully, L., & Vest, V. (2001). Evidence-based prenatal care visits: When less is more. *Journal of Midwifery and Women's Health, 46*(3), 146–151.

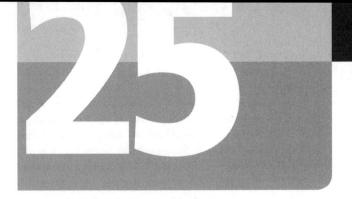

PRENATAL GENETIC SCREENING

Deborah Anderson and Amy J. Levi

I. Introduction and general background

Genetic screening tests for chromosomal abnormalities, single gene defects, and structural birth defects are now available to all pregnant women.

A. Prenatal screening for trisomies 21 and 18 and open neural tube defects

Second-trimester maternal serum screening for fetal aneuploidy and fetal open neural tube defects has been available for over two decades. More recently, advances in genetic screening tools have made it possible for all women to have noninvasive genetic screening during the first trimester of pregnancy. Combining first- and second-trimester screening strategies rather than using single-method testing yields higher-risk detection rates.

Several optional first- and second-trimester screening strategies are available to assess risk for trisomy 21 (Down syndrome) and trisomy 18, and open neural tube defects. The tests use serum biochemical markers and fetal ultrasound to refine and improve risk assessment beyond standard population-based risk assessments. Timing of screening and interpretation of results may vary slightly according to differing laboratory and practice guidelines.

1. First-trimester screening

First-trimester screening begins with maternal serum testing between 10 and 13 weeks 6 days gestational age (California Prenatal Screening Program, 2009). The biochemical markers assessed are pregnancy-associated plasma protein A and human chorionic gonadotropin. First-trimester serum testing is followed with an ultrasound measurement of fetal nuchal translucency (NT) between 11 weeks 2 days and 14 weeks 2 days gestation (California prenatal screening program). The combination of the first-trimester serum test and NT measurement can further refine a woman's risk for trisomies 21 and 18.

NT refers to measurement of a clearly demarcated fluid-filled space behind the fetal neck that is present in all fetuses. A normal measurement is less than or equal to 3 mm. Skill at obtaining NT measurement requires training for a standardized method of measurement; therefore, this screening tool may not be available in all communities. NT measurement alone has a detection rate for trisomy 21 of 64–70% with a 5% false-positive rate. Detection rates improve and can further revise risk assessment when combined with first-trimester serum testing. NT measurement may be useful with multiple pregnancies because serum screening is not as sensitive in twin or triplet gestations. Women with NT measurements 3 mm or greater should be offered diagnostic testing, additional genetic testing, targeted ultrasound, or echocardiogram, because increased results are associated with other fetal structural anomalies, such as congenital heart defects, diaphragmatic hernias, skeletal dysplasias, and other genetic syndromes (Driscoll & Gross, 2009).

2. Second-trimester screening

The most widely used test for second-trimester screening is the quad marker serum examination that screens for trisomies 21 and 18, and determines risk for open neural tube defects. A maternal blood specimen is obtained between 15 and 20 weeks (16–18 weeks optimum). The "quad screen" tests for four biochemical markers: alpha fetoprotein, human chorionic gonadotropin, unconjugated estriol, and dimeric inhibin-A. The quad marker screen can be interpreted alone or combined with first-trimester serum testing or NT measurement for improved risk detection rates.

3. Serum integrated screening

Serum integrated screening combines first-trimester blood test results with second-trimester (quad marker) blood test results. This may be useful when NT measurements cannot be obtained because of timing, patient wishes, or where NT programs are not available. Serum integrated screening provides a higher sensitivity and lower false-positive rate compared to the single first- or second-trimester serum screen.

4. Full integrated screening

The greatest sensitivity for risk detection for trisomies 21 and 18 is determined when combining NT results with first- and second-trimester blood test results. Open neural tube defect risk rates remain the same as with serum integrated screening.

B. Carrier screening for recessive conditions

Prenatal genetic screening includes serum testing for a variety of genetic diseases. Carrier screening identifies carriers of targeted genetic diseases that are found to have increased prevalence in certain ethnic groups. Table 25-1 lists genetic diseases for which screening is recommended and the patient populations that carry an increased risk for these disorders.

Genetic screening may also be performed for parents with family histories of these disorders. Inherited disorders for which carrier screening is currently recommended are cystic fibrosis, Tay-Sachs disease, Canavan disease, familial dysautonomia, α-thalassemia, β-thalassemia, and sickle cell anemia (Norton, 2008). When both partners are genetic carriers of these or other inherited disorders, genetic counseling is recommended to review options for possible confirmatory diagnostic testing and education.

The American College of Obstetricians and Gynecologists (ACOG, 2005) recommends that cystic fibrosis carrier screening also be offered to all women planning a pregnancy or seeking prenatal care regardless of ethnicity or family history. Test sensitivity and carrier risk vary among different ethnic groups. Negative test results may reduce but do not eliminate the risk of being a cystic fibrosis carrier.

II. Database

A. Subjective

1. Age. According to ACOG guidelines (ACOG, 2007), all women regardless of age should have the option for genetic screening or diagnostic testing. Advanced maternal age (35 years old) alone is no longer used as a determining factor for who is offered prenatal diagnostic testing. Prenatal screening tests do not detect other forms of aneuploidy that occur with advancing maternal age, such as trisomy 13 and Klinefelter syndrome; these may be detected with diagnostic testing, such as chorionic villus sampling or amniocentesis.

2. Last menstrual period. If unsure, order an ultrasound to determine gestational age. All screening tests are sensitive to gestational age.

3. Genetic and obstetric history. Identify any genetic risk factors. If positive for chromosome abnormalities, genetic disorders, or congenital malformation, offer referral to genetic counselor or a perinatal specialist. Further counseling may alter a woman's choices for prenatal screening and testing.

4. Determine whether the woman desires prenatal testing. Factors to be considered if women choose to have or decline testing include
   a. Gestational age at first visit
   b. Genetic history and family history
   c. Obstetric history
   d. Number of fetuses
   e. NT availability
   f. Test sensitivity and limitations
   g. Desire for testing
   h. Risks of diagnostic procedures
   i. Options for early termination

B. Objective

1. Confirm gestational age

2. If ultrasound dating is available, include crown-rump length on laboratory form for dating in first trimester and biparietal diameter in second trimester. Including ultrasound dating reduces the false-positive rate and increases the detection rate of open neural tube defects.

3. If after the test the expected date of delivery is changed based on a discrepancy of more than 10 days by ultrasound, the laboratory must be informed of the date change for reinterpretation of test results.

TABLE 25-1 Ethnicity-Based Recommendation for Carrier Screening

Patient Population	Inherited Genetic Disorder
All	Cystic fibrosis
Cajun, French-Canadian	Tay-Sachs disease
Ashkenazi Jewish	Tay-Sachs, Canavan disease, familial dysautonomia
African, African-American	Sickle cell anemia
Southeast Asian	α-Thalassemia, β-thalassemia
Mediterranean	β-Thalassemia

III. Assessment

A. *Patient chooses prenatal genetic screening (note specific type of screening that is desired).*

B. *Patient declines prenatal genetic screening.*

IV. Plan

A. *Screening or diagnostic testing*

1. Offer prenatal screening to all women.

2. Timing of the first-trimester serum screen, NT, and quad marker testing are limited by gestational age.

   a. First-trimester serum screen: 10 to 13 weeks 6 days intrauterine pregnancy (may vary with practice site)

   b. NT ultrasound: 11 weeks 2 days to 14 weeks 2 days (may vary with practice site)

   c. Quad marker: 15–20 weeks

   d. Fill out the appropriate laboratory forms including the best dating parameters, gestational age at time of test, and current weight

3. Document woman's acceptance or refusal of genetic screening tests. Some states require a standardized signed accept/decline form for first-trimester serum screen, NT, or quad marker.

B. *Counseling regarding tests and results*

1. Inform the woman that these tests provide individual risk assessment and are not diagnostic tests. These screening tests do not detect all fetal chromosomal anomalies and neural tube defects.

2. Review risk detection rates and false-positive rates of screening strategies.

3. Women may opt to have diagnostic testing without prenatal screening, or screening without further diagnostic testing.

4. When reviewing serum integrated or full integrated screening results with women, it is preferred to communicate the numerical risk assessment of the final analysis rather than a positive or negative result. It may be useful to compare their screening risk to their age-related risk.

C. *Consultation and referral*

If results indicate a risk greater than that of the age-related risk, refer to a genetic counselor for further counseling regarding interpretation of results, recommendations for follow-up examinations, possible diagnostic testing, and follow-up and supportive counseling.

REFERENCES

American College of Obstetricians and Gynecologists. (2005, December). Committee Opinion Number 325. Update on carrier screening for cystic fibrosis. *Obstetrics & Gynecology, 106*(6), 1465–1458.

American College of Obstetricians and Gynecologists. (2007). Practice Bulletin Number 77. Screening for fetal chromosomal abnormalities. *Obstetrics & Gynecology, 109*(1), 217–227.

California Prenatal Screening Program. (2009). Genetic Disease Screening Program. Richmond, CA: California Department of Public Health. http://www.cdph.ca.gov/programs/pns/pages/default.aspx

Driscoll, D. A., & Gross, S. J. (2009). Screening for fetal aneuploidy and neural tube defects. *Genetics in Medicine, 11*(11), 818–821.

Norton, M. E. (2008). Genetic screening and counseling. *Current Opinion in Obstetrics and Gynecology, 20*(2), 157–163.

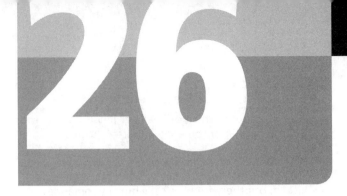

THE RETURN PRENATAL VISIT

Rebekah Kaplan and Margaret Hutchison

I. Definition and background

The purpose of return prenatal visits is to evaluate the progress of the pregnancy through ongoing health, nutritional, and psychosocial assessments. Referrals within the healthcare system and assistance with movement toward positive health behavior changes are also integral parts of the prenatal care process. The frequency and content of prenatal visits can be tailored to the specific needs of each client (medical risk factors, psychosocial needs, and parity).

The format of care delivery may also vary depending on the site. Although most prenatal care in the United States is still structured around one-on-one visits with a medical care provider, there is increasing use of group-based prenatal care models, most notably CenteringPregnancy. For sites using CenteringPregnancy, care is moved out of the examination room and into a group space, and cohorts of 8–12 women go through pregnancy together. Women receive medical assessment, health education, and social support within the group space during each of 10 sessions. Table 26-1 provides a summary of CenteringPregnancy session content (Baldwin, 2006).

II. Database

A. Subjective

1. Gestational age
2. Estimated delivery date: review dating
3. Problems or concerns since her last visit (e.g., uterine activity, change in vaginal discharge, or psychosocial issues)

4. Follow-up on problems from previous visit (e.g., nausea, back pain, and fetal position)
5. Follow-up on problems from "problem list" (e.g., Was medication taken for urinary tract infection? Was *Monilia* resolved?)
6. Danger signs (e.g., bleeding, pain, fetal movement, leaking of fluid, or intimate partner violence): The Family Violence Prevention Fund recommends screening for intimate partner violence and abuse at each prenatal visit (Table 26-2).
7. History review (age, current pregnancy, obstetric, medical, family, psychosocial, and nutrition)
8. Consults: Results and management plans (physician, social worker, public health nurse, and so forth)

B. Objective

1. Vital signs and urine
   a. Weight
   b. Blood pressure
   c. Urinalysis: if indicated to screen for preeclampsia or urinary tract infection (evidence does not support routine urine screening in low-risk women [Alto, 2005])
2. Laboratory data
   a. Results for current problems (e.g., urine dip or wet mount)
   b. Are laboratory values up-to-date? (e.g., chest radiograph after a positive purified protein derivative, third-trimester testing for group B streptococcus) (Table 26-3)
3. Physical examination
   a. General appearance (e.g., new striae or signs of depression)
   b. Abdominal examination
      i. Fundal height: measure by landmarks before 22–24 weeks, then with measuring tape (from the superior border of the symphysis pubis to the fundus)
      ii. Leopold's maneuvers (position and presentation) after 32–36 weeks
      iii. Estimated fetal weight after 36 weeks
   c. Fetal heart rate
      i. Doppler 9–12 weeks
      ii. Fetoscope 18–20 weeks
      iii. Ultrasound after 6–7 weeks (if indicated)
   d. Other physical examination as indicated by patient problems or concerns (e.g., costovertebral angle tenderness or vaginal discharge)

TABLE 26-1 CenteringPregnancy®: Overview of Session Content*

Session 1: 14–18 weeks gestational age (GA)
- Self-care skills (blood pressure [BP], weight, charting)
- Learning about Centering
- Nutrition
- Personal goals

Session 2: 18–22 weeks GA
- Nutrition follow-up
- Common discomforts of pregnancy

Session 3: 22–26 weeks GA
- Stress reduction
- Beginning to think about infant feeding

Session 4: 26–28 weeks GA
- Contraception
- Sexuality
- Personal safety
- Preterm labor

Session 5: 28–30 weeks GA
- Overview of childbirth

Session 6: 30–32 weeks GA
- More about the birth process and options

Session 7: 32–34 weeks GA
- Caring for the newborn
- Siblings
- More about the birth process

Session 8: 34–36 weeks GA
- Relaxation measures
- Support systems
- Postpartum period

Session 9: 36–38 weeks GA
- Thoughts and concerns about birth process, postpartum, parenting
- Sharing birth stories (return of women who have delivered)

Session 10: 38–40 weeks GA
- More birth stories
- Reviewing plans for taking care of self and family

* This list is considered the "core content" of CenteringPregnancy®, and includes health education, nutrition, and psychosocial topics. Exact content and session flow may vary based on population and group needs.

TABLE 26-2 Abuse Assessment Screen

1. Have you ever been emotionally or physically abused by your partner or someone important to you?

   ❏ YES ❏ NO

2. Within the last year, have you been hit, slapped, kicked, or otherwise physically hurt by someone?

   ❏ YES ❏ NO

   If YES, by whom? _____

   Total number of times: _____

3. Since you've been pregnant, were you hit, slapped, kicked, or otherwise physically hurt by someone?

   ❏ YES ❏ NO

   If YES, by whom? _____

   Total number of times: _____

Source: Family Violence Prevention Fund: http://endabuse.org

TABLE 26-3 Timing of Testing for Women Without Significant Medical Risk Factors

Initial visit (see Chapter 24, Initial Prenatal Visit)
8–20 weeks

- 10–13 weeks: offer first-trimester blood screening test
- 11^2–14^2 weeks: offer ultrasound for nuchal translucency
- 15–20 weeks: offer second-trimester blood screening test

Diagnostic testing if indicated

- 10–13 weeks: chorionic villae sampling
- 15–20 weeks: amniocentesis
- 18–20 weeks: fetal survey screening ultrasound as needed
- 26–28 weeks: complete blood count, 1-hour glucose load test, antibody screen if rhesus factor negative; if indicated, venereal disease reference laboratory, HIV
- 32–36 weeks: if indicated, repeat sexually transmitted infection testing
- 35–37 weeks: group beta streptococcus (GBS) culture

III. Assessment

A. *Gestational age: identify any size and dates discrepancy*

B. *Differential diagnosis for any identified abnormal physical examination or laboratory findings (e.g., anemia, preterm labor, or urinary tract infection)*

C. *Determine appropriateness of weight gain and nutritional status (Tables 26-4 and 26-5)*

D. *Determine prenatal educational needs*

E. *Identify psychosocial issues (e.g., food insecurity, immigration problems, housing, or social isolation)*

IV. Plan

A. *Laboratory*

1. Laboratory or diagnostic testing (Table 26-3)

2. Other laboratory tests needed related to physical examination findings (e.g., urine culture, chlamydia test, or anemia work-up)

3. Follow-up on any previous abnormal laboratory studies

B. *Medication*

1. Refill prenatal vitamins as necessary

2. Supplementation: calcium, fish oil, vitamin D_3, and iron if deficient; treatment of specific problems (e.g., urinary tract infection or vaginitis)

C. *Education and counseling*

1. Patient concerns

2. Current laboratory data

3. Weight gain and diet

4. Teaching appropriate to gestational age and patient needs (Figure 26-1)

5. Danger signs of pregnancy (e.g., spontaneous abortion, preterm labor, and preeclampsia)

6. Emotional preparation for motherhood

7. Exercise, stress management, and behavior modification

D. *Refer for consultation or antepartum fetal evaluation*

1. Refer any patients as indicated for physician consultation or transfer of care (see Chapter 28 on Guidelines for Medical Consultation and Referral During Pregnancy)

2. Initiate and refer for fetal evaluation and antenatal testing if indicated (Table 26-6)

E. *Update problem list*

1. Add or resolve any outstanding problems or concerns

F. *Follow-up visit*

1. This should be flexible and individualized based on patient needs, parity, and risk following a standard or reduced visit schedule reviewed in Chapter 24, the Initial Prenatal Visit.

2. Post dates (Table 26-7)

TABLE 26-4 Recommended Pattern of Weight Gain for Pregnancy

First trimester 1.1–4.4 lb

Rates for second and third trimester
- Underweight: 1 lb/wk (1–1.3)
- Normal weight: 1 lb/wk (0.8–1)
- Overweight: 0.6 lb/wk (0.5–0.7)
- Obese (all classes): 0.5 lb/wk (0.4–0.6)

2–4 lb a month

Source: Institute of Medicine. (2009). *Report brief. Weight gain during pregnancy: Reexamining the guidelines*

TABLE 26-5 Daily Dietary Needs for Normal-Weight Women

Second and third trimester: 300 additional calories a day (e.g., 8 oz 1% milk, one hardboiled egg, and one apple)
- Protein: 60 g (teenagers, 75–80 g)
- Grains: 6 oz
- Vegetables: 2.5 cups
- Fruit: 2 cups
- Calcium: 1,000 mg

FIGURE 26-1 *Prenatal Care Flow Sheet*

8–14 Weeks	15–20 Weeks	20–28 Weeks
LABS/TESTS	**LABS/TESTS**	**LABS/TESTS**
Sono/dating	Expanded MSAFP (Quad marker)	CBC, glucose load test (26–28 weeks)
Blood type, Rh, antibody screen CBC, Hgb elec	Sono fetal survey (19–20 weeks)	HIV, RPR (if indicated)
RPR, rubella, varicella (by hx or titers), HIV, PPD, HBsAg	Flu vaccine (Oct–May)	
Urine C+S, urine dip screening		
Pap (if due), GC/*Chlamydia*		
First-trimester diagnostic screen		
Nuchal translucency		
SELECTIVE TESTING	**SELECTIVE TESTING**	**SELECTIVE TESTING**
Early glucose load test	Amniocentesis	3–hour glucose tolerance test
Hepatitis C	Early glucose load test	Antibody screen
Urine toxicology screen	Urine toxicology screen	Rhogam at 28 weeks
BV screening	CXR (if +PPD)	
CF, Ashkenazi screening	Urine C+S	
Genetic screening based on FHx	HBV vaccine (high-risk behaviors)	
Refusal of blood products consent	Level 2 ultrasound, fetal echo	
EDUCATION	**EDUCATION**	**EDUCATION**
Orientation to clinic/service	Breastfeeding benefits	Signs/symptoms PTL
Expect Parents Club referral	Exclusive breast milk 6 months	Contraception
Danger signs	BF class referral	Danger signs
Common discomforts	Fetal movement and quickening	Fetal movement
Nutrition, weight gain and exercise	Exercise in pregnancy	VBAC/TOL discussion
Genetic testing options	Common discomforts	PPTL class referral (PPTL papers can be signed after 17 weeks)
OTC/Rx med use	Danger signs	Breastfeeding benefits
Toxic habits counseling		Exercise in pregnancy
Dental services information		Attended breastfeeding class ❏
		Attended Expectant Parents Club ❏

FIGURE 26-1 *Prenatal Care Flow Sheet* (continued)

28–32 Weeks	32–37 Weeks	37–41 Weeks
LABS/TESTS	**LABS/TESTS**	**LABS/TESTS**
Optional/Indicated	GBS (35–37 weeks)	**Optional/Indicated**
Antenatal testing		Antenatal testing: NST/AFI (after 41 weeks)
Kick counts	**Optional/Indicated**	
	Antenatal testing	
	Disability	
EDUCATION	**EDUCATION**	**EDUCATION**
Contraception	Early initiation of breastfeeding	Pain control options
BCM _____	Skin to skin and rooming in	Signs and symptoms labor
Consent signed ❏	Latch	Managing early labor at home
Attended PPTL class ❏	Infant feeding cues	Danger signs
VBAC/TOL consent ❏	BF and returning to work	Going past due date (induction 41–42 weeks)
Signs and symptoms of PTL	Colostrum and milk production	Attended Labor Prep Class ❏
Other danger signs	BF resources	Pain control preference
Newborn procedures	Circumcision	
Referral to birth prep class ❏	Danger signs	
	Signs and symptoms labor	Support system
	Infant car seat and baby supplies	
	Last chance for PPTL papers	
	Reinsert the box after PPTL	

Source: Community Health Network of San Francisco, Department of Public Health.

TABLE 26-6 Antepartum Fetal Evaluation

Conditions posing risk for fetal compromise include, but are not limited to:

- Postterm pregnancy; hypertensive disease; fetal growth restriction; diabetes; previous unexplained stillbirth; decreased fetal movement; increased unexplained maternal serum alpha fetoprotein; increased serum human chorionic gonadotropin; cholestasis of pregnancy; twins with discordant growth; preterm premature rupture of membranes; oligohydramnios; unexplained severe polyhydramnios; rhesus factor isoimmunization; active substance abuse; lupus; gastroschisis; and medical problems (e.g., cardiac disease, hyperthyroidism)

Initiation of testing

- Begin testing at the gestational age at which the provider is willing to intervene to save the life of the fetus balanced with the age at which one would expect to detect abnormal testing (generally 34–36 weeks)

Methods of testing

- Fetal movement assessments (kick counts)
- Nonstress test
- Amniotic fluid index
- Vibroacoustic stimulation
- Biophysical profile
- Contraction stress test

First line:

No consistent evidence suggests that formal kick counts decrease incidence of intrauterine fetal demise, although the method is widely used in practice for higher-risk pregnancies (Darby-Stewart, Strickland, & Jamieson, 2009).

Second line:

Modified biophysical profile: nonstress test plus amniotic fluid index.

If modified biophysical profile is not reassuring consult for biophysical profile, Doppler flow studies, and induction of labor after a contraction stress test

TABLE 26-7 Postdates Pregnancy*

Management

- Review of dating criteria
- Leopold's for good estimation of fetal weight
- Examine cervix; Bishops score greater than 5 is favorable
- Consider sweeping membranes at 38–41 weeks
- Consider alternative methods of induction

Education

- Counsel risks and benefits of induction versus expectant management

Follow-up

- Biweekly antenatal testing (NST, AFI) by 41 weeks gestation
- Kick counts should be initiated at 40–41 weeks

* Gestation of 42 weeks or more (although 41 weeks may be considered postterm in some settings).

REFERENCES

Alto, W. A. (2005). No need for glycosuria/proteinuria screen in pregnant women. *The Journal of Family Practice, 54*(11), 978–983.

Baldwin, K. A. (2006). Comparison of selected outcomes of centering pregnancy versus traditional prenatal care. *Journal of Midwifery & Women's Health, 51*(4), 266–272.

Darby-Stewart, A. L., Strickland, C. & Jamieson, B. (2009). Do abnormal fetal kick counts predict intrauterine death in average-risk pregnancies? *The Journal of Family Practice, 58*(4), 220a–220c.

Institute of Medicine. (2009). *Report brief. Weight gain during pregnancy: Reexamining the guidelines.* Washington DC: National Academies Press.

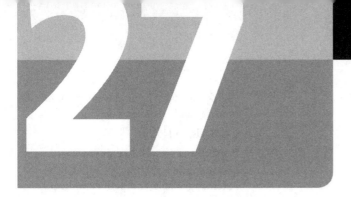

THE POSTPARTUM VISIT

Jenna Shaw-Battista

I. Introduction and general background

The postpartum period is a time of tremendous physical and emotional change for new mothers. Although women experience the most profound adaptations during this 6–8 week period, their partners, older children, and extended family also experience significant transitions. The goals of family-centered postpartum care include the identification, management, and resolution of abnormal physical, psychologic, and psychosocial adaptations. Additionally, postpartum care involves lactation supervision and contraceptive counseling, if appropriate, for individual women. Furthermore, new mothers appreciate opportunities to discuss their experience of childbirth, although there are few data to guide the format or content of these conversations (Rowan, Bick, & Bastos, 2007). Postpartum visits also serve as a transition from obstetric to primary health care, and provide opportunities to initiate or resume routine health screening and maintenance activities.

This chapter uses the subjective, objective, assessment, and plan note format to outline essential elements of postpartum care, which should be customized for individual women. The timing, number, and content of postpartum visits necessarily vary. Women are typically examined daily during their inpatient postpartum stay, and scheduled for outpatient follow-up 4–6 weeks later as recommended by the American Academy of Pediatrics and the American College of Obstetricians and Gynecologists (2007). Women may be examined more frequently if they experienced complications of parturition; possess significant risk factors for adverse postpartum conditions; or require atypical follow-up for other reasons, such as breastfeeding difficulties, management of

chronic health conditions, or timing of birth control initiation. Appointment reminders or incentives may increase postpartum visit attendance, and prove particularly useful in the care of high-risk populations (e.g., adolescents or women with mood disorders) (MacArthur et al., 2003; Stevens-Simon, O'Connor, & Bassford, 1994). In high-risk populations, perinatal outcomes may also be improved with home visits or referrals to postpartum educational programs or peer support groups among other interventions (Shaw, Levitt, Wong, & Kaczorowski, 2006). In addition to considerations of women's health status and risk factors, the time elapsed since childbirth should inform the type of screening, intervention, education, and referrals to be provided.

II. Database (may include but is not limited to)

A. Subjective data

These data may be gleaned from postpartum patient interviews or review of medical records if available

1. History of medical conditions or antenatal complications requiring follow-up (e.g., thyroid disorder, hypertension, preexisting or gestational diabetes mellitus)

2. Description of the woman's intrapartum experience, including date and method of delivery, complications, and her understanding and feelings about events

3. General well-being and psychologic status should be assessed by screening for

   a. Excessive fatigue, which interferes with self and infant care

   b. Depression or mania, anhedonia, excessive crying, insomnia, anxiety, hypervigilance, or thoughts of harming self or infant

   c. Report of feeling generally unwell (e.g., fever, chills, or malaise)

   d. Inability to cope with demands of new role

4. Sexuality, including satisfaction, libido, resumption of sexual activity, need for contraception, and altered self-perception

5. Family and social integration

   a. Relationship with partner

   b. Sibling and grandparent adjustment

   c. Bonding with infant

   d. Plans to start or return to work outside the home

6. Review of systems (screen for)
   a. Breasts
      i. Breast or nipple pain
      ii. Masses noted
      iii. Concerns about insufficient breast milk or infant feeding
   b. Abdomen
      i. Abdominal or uterine pain or cramping that has increased since delivery or is unrelieved with pain medication
      ii. Report of pain, redness, odor, or discharge at the site of a cesarean incision
   c. Pelvis, genitals, and lochia
      i. Pelvic pain, particularly over the symphysis pubis or coccyx
      ii. Vaginal, vulvar, or perineal pain that has increased since delivery or is unrelieved by pain medication, with or without edema
      iii. Excessive or prolonged bleeding (e.g., fills pad in < 1–2 hours, large recurrent clots, or lochia beyond 6 weeks postpartum)
      iv. Foul-smelling lochia
      v. Resumption of menses
   d. Elimination
      i. Urinary or fecal incontinence
      ii. Urinary retention
      iii. Constipation
      iv. Dysuria
      v. History of intrapartum or postpartum bladder catheterization, or other risk factors for urinary tract infection
   e. Extremities
      i. Calf pain, heat, or redness
      ii. Edema that increases or persists beyond 7 days postpartum, particularly if unilateral

B. *Objective data*
   1. General well-being and psychologic status: observe affect, eye contact, and general appearance
   2. Family integration: observe interactions between mother, child, and family members present
   3. Weight and vital signs
   4. Head and neck
      a. Thyroid gland: palpate for size and nodularity
      b. Lymph nodes: palpate for size and tenderness
   5. Breasts
      a. Observe size, color, and symmetry
      b. Palpate for tenderness, masses, and warmth
      c. Observe infant position and latch during breastfeeding if appropriate
   6. Abdomen
      a. Inspect and palpate for masses, tenderness, uterine involution, and diastasis recti

b. Check surgical site for closure, pain, masses, exudates, and erythema if applicable

7. Pelvis, genitals, and lochia
   a. Palpate over symphysis pubis or coccyx if report of pain
   b. External genitalia and perineum: inspect for symmetry, excoriation, and varicosities; assess laceration for approximation and healing; visualize the amount and appearance of lochia
   c. Pelvic and rectal examination as indicated
      i. Vagina: assess for uterine prolapse, cystocele, or rectocele; assess for leakage of urine; check the strength of pelvic musculature during a Kegel exercise
      ii. Uterus: assess position, size, and tenderness
      iii. Cervix: assess os appearance and closure
   d. Rectum: assess for hemorrhoids, fissures, fistulas, masses, and stool

8. Elimination
   a. Palpation of stool during pelvic and rectal examinations if performed
   b. Evidence of urinary or fecal incontinence (e.g., visualization of urine or stool, or excoriation of periurethral or perianal tissue)
   c. Suprapubic pain on palpation

9. Extremities
   a. Assess for calf pain, heat, or redness on inspection and palpation
   b. Homan's sign
   c. Assess for hyperreflexia, with or without clonus, in women with a history of hypertensive disorder in pregnancy, particularly in the first 3–7 days when risk of eclamptic seizure is elevated
   d. Assess for edema that increases or persists beyond 7 days postpartum, particularly if unilateral

III. Assessment

Assessment should incorporate subjective and objective data, and address the woman's physical, emotional, and social postpartum adaptation.

IV. Plan

A. *Diagnostics*
   1. Laboratory testing as indicated by history, subjective data, or examination, for example
      a. Urine dipstick to assess for protein or nitrites
      b. Urine culture and sensitivity to rule out urinary tract infection
      c. Complete blood count to assess for infectious processes or anemia

d. Wet mount

e. Testing for *Chlamydia*, gonorrhea, and other sexually transmitted infections

f. 2-hour, 75-g oral glucose tolerance test performed 6–12 weeks after delivery for women with diagnosis of gestational diabetes

2. Health screening as indicated

a. Pap smear

b. Occult fecal blood

c. Mammography

B. Treatment and follow-up

1. Visits: daily inpatient postpartum visits are standard, with outpatient follow-up 4–6 weeks later. Early or frequent outpatient visits or telephone consultations may be indicated among women with adverse health conditions or risk factors for postpartum complications.

2. Medications and therapeutics

a. Continue daily prenatal vitamins or multivitamin during lactation

b. Other medications as warranted by subjective and objective data (e.g., stool softener, analgesics and antibiotics)

c. Anti-D immune globulin within 72 hours of birth for rhesus factor negative women with infants who are rhesus factor positive

d. Vaccinations (e.g., rubella or varicella for women without immunity)

e. Contraception

C. Patient education

1. Address questions and concerns of the woman and her family, which often include

a. Return to normal daily activities, exercise, and work

b. Infant care (e.g., feeding; pediatric visits; and safety measures, such as sleeping arrangements and car seats)

c. Sexual health and dysfunction

i. Sexual practices, libido, arousal, and orgasm

ii. Changes in psychologic aspects of sexuality (e.g., differences related to parenting a newborn or breastfeeding)

iii. Dyspareunia, frequently related to genital laceration or inadequate lubrication

a. Return of fertility and menses

b. Contraception

c. Optimal pregnancy interval: although conclusive data are lacking, women should be advised that maternal and neonatal outcomes are improved when pregnancies are 18–60 months apart (Conde-Agudelo, Rosas-Bermúdez, & Kafury-Goeta, 2007)

d. Counseling about nutrition and exercise is essential in the postpartum period and should include

i. Encouragement to achieve and maintain a normal body mass index to reduce immediate and long-term health risks

ii. Advice that regular exercise may prevent or reduce depressive symptomatology (Daley, Macarthur, & Winter, 2007)

iii. Nutritional supplementation specific to the postpartum period, such as iron supplementation following postpartum hemorrhage and anemia.

iv. Essential fatty acids intake, which may minimize incidence and severity of postpartum depression in women or optimize brain development in infants (Freeman, 2009; Genuis & Schwalfenberg, 2006; Sontrop & Campbell, 2006)

2. Additional health maintenance counseling should include

a. Resumption of routine gynecological and primary care

b. Breast self-examination

c. If urinary or fecal incontinence is present, women should be advised they occur in 30% and 10% of postpartum women, respectively. Pelvic floor muscle training, pessary fitting, and surgical intervention may be discussed if tincture of time and simple Kegel exercises do not result in improved symptoms within 1–2 months postpartum (Dumoulin & Hay-Smith, 2010)

D. Consultation and referral

1. Local public health programs, visiting nurses associations, lactation consultants, and postpartum doulas may have services for the evaluation, monitoring, and treatment of select maternal physical and psychosocial problems, and infant concerns.

2. Conditions that warrant medical consultation or referral include, but are not limited to

a. Endometritis

b. Infection or dehiscence of surgical site

c. Infection or wound dehiscence at site of perineal laceration

d. Excessive or prolonged vaginal bleeding

e. Breast abscess

f. Postpartum depression, mania, or psychosis

g. Postpartum thyroiditis

h. Suspected child abuse or neglect (notify pediatrician and child protective services)

i. Chronic medical conditions requiring follow-up, if outside of the nurse-practitioner or nurse-midwife scope of practice

REFERENCES

American Academy of Pediatrics, American College of Obstetricians and Gynecologists. (2007). *Guidelines for Perinatal Care* (6th ed.). Washington, DC: American College of Obstetricians and Gynecologists.

Conde-Agudelo, A., Rosas-Bermúdez, A., Kafury-Goeta, A. C. (2007). Effects of birth spacing on maternal health: A systematic review. *American Journal of Obstetrics and Gynecology, 96*(4), 297–308.

Daley, A. J., Macarthur, C., & Winter, H. (2007). The role of exercise in treating postpartum depression: A review of the literature. *Journal of Midwifery & Women's Health, 52*(1), 56–62.

Dumoulin, C., & Hay-Smith, J. (2010). Pelvic floor muscle training versus no treatment, or inactive control treatments, for urinary incontinence in women. *The Cochrane Database of Systematic Reviews,* (1), CD005654.

Freeman, M. P. (2009). Omega-3 fatty acids in major depressive disorder. *The Journal of Clinical Psychiatry, 70*(Suppl. 5), 7–11.

Genuis, S. J., & Schwalfenberg, G. K. (2006). Time for an oil check: The role of essential omega-3 fatty acids and maternal and pediatric health. *Journal of Perinatology, 26,* 59–65.

MacArthur, C., Winter, H. R., Bick, D. E., Lilford, R. J., Lancashire, R. J., Knowles, H., . . . Gee, H. (2003). Redesigning postnatal care: A randomised controlled trial of protocol-based midwifery-led care focused on individual women's physical and psychological health needs. *Health Technology Assessment, 7*(37), 1–98.

Rowan, C., Bick, D., & Bastos, M. H. (2007). Postnatal debriefing interventions to prevent maternal mental health problems after birth: Exploring the gap between the evidence and UK policy and practice. *Worldviews on Evidence-based Nursing, 4*(2), 97–105.

Shaw, E., Levitt, C., Wong, S., & Kaczorowski, J. (2006). Systematic review of the literature on postpartum care: Effectiveness of postpartum support to improve maternal parenting, mental health, quality of life, and physical health. *Birth, 33*(3), 210–220.

Sontrop, J., & Campbell, M. K. (2006). Omega-3 polyunsaturated fatty acids and depression: A review of the evidence and a methodological critique. *Preventative Medicine, 42*(1), 4–13.

Stevens-Simon, C., O'Connor, P., & Bassford, K. (1994). Incentives enhance postpartum compliance among adolescent prenatal patients. *Journal of Adolescent Health, 15*(5), 396–399.

GUIDELINES FOR MEDICAL CONSULTATION AND REFERRAL DURING PREGNANCY

Jenna Shaw-Battista

Despite a continuum of medical and obstetric risk, pregnant women are frequently dichotomized as being at "low" or "high" risk for suboptimal perinatal outcomes. There is little disagreement as to what constitutes a normal pregnancy in a healthy parturient, and nurse practitioners and nurse midwives routinely provide independent care for these low-risk women. At the other end of the spectrum are women for whom exclusive physician care and referral to perinatology or neonatology are immediately indicated.

For women with one or more moderate risk factors, decisions about consultation and referral to medical providers are influenced by many factors including the clinical experience, skill set, and scope of practice of the clinicians involved. These gray areas in clinical decision-making necessarily involve consideration of state and federal regulatory language, institutional policy, collaborative practice protocols, research findings, and community standards, in addition to a childbearing family's preferences for care (Avery, 2000; Bailey, Jones, & Way, 2006). In some circumstances, nurse practitioners and nurse midwives collaborate with physician colleagues to care for pregnant women with moderate- or high-risk conditions, including selected disorders of the endocrine, cardiovascular, hematologic, neurologic, musculoskeletal, pulmonary, gastrointestinal, and renal systems; and specific psychiatric diagnoses; infectious diseases; malignancies; and abnormal diagnostic testing (Office of Technology Assessment, 1986).

Perinatal risk factors and antepartum complications include, but are not limited to

    a. Habitual abortions: three or more consecutive miscarriages less than 12 weeks gestation

    b. Previous classical cesarean section or other uterine surgery

    c. Prenatal diagnosis of minor or major fetal anomalies

    d. Multiple gestation

    e. Fetal malpresentation

    f. Postdates pregnancy ($\geq$ 41–42 weeks gestation)

    g. Preterm labor or ruptured membranes before term (12–36 weeks gestation)

    h. Premature rupture of membranes at term

    i. Polyhydramnios or oligohydramnios

    j. Abnormal placentation (e.g., previa or accreta)

    k. Unexplained second- and third-trimester bleeding

    l. Rhesus factor sensitization or other IgG antibody sensitization

    m. Hypertensive disorders in pregnancy (essential or gestational hypertension, preeclampsia, or eclampsia)

    n. Hemolysis, elevated liver enzymes, and low platelets syndrome

    o. Idiopathic thrombocytopenic purpura

    p. Cholestasis of pregnancy

    q. Preexisting or gestational diabetes mellitus

    r. Selected anemias or hemoglobinopathies

        i. Hemoglobin less than 10 g/dl, not responsive to iron therapy

        ii. Sickle cell crisis

        iii. Thalassemias

    s. Selected maternal infections with potential fetal sequelae (e.g., human immunodeficiency virus, cytomegalovirus, parvovirus, rubella, syphilis, toxoplasmosis, primary herpes infection, or presence of genital lesions at term)

    t. Additional maternal illnesses (e.g., severe asthma requiring hospitalization during pregnancy, autoimmune disorders, cardiac disease other than asymptomatic mitral valve prolapse, renal disease or recurrent urinary tract infections, or thyroid disorders)

Interprofessional practices benefit from written policies regarding methods and types of consultation and referral. These and other strategies to encourage communication and collaboration may facilitate a common understanding of clinicians' scopes of practice and improve patient outcomes (Bailey et al., 2006; Brooten et al., 2005; Zwarenstein, Goldman, & Reeves, 2009). Interprofessional guidelines for obstetric care frequently describe comanagement of pregnant patients with specific moderate-risk factors. Varied levels of consultation may be delineated, with or without direct physical assessment and documentation of collaborative management plans by the medical consultant. When pregnant women experience complications that require ongoing medical or obstetric management, referral rather than consultation is indicated. These high-risk patients may return to the nurse practitioner or nurse midwife caseload for pregnancy care if their condition stabilizes and collaborative care is mutually agreeable.

For many women, risk status and provider type are determined by the severity rather than presence of a specific condition. For example, nurse practitioners and nurse midwives may collaboratively care for women with gestational diabetes who can maintain euglycemia with diet and exercise or oral hypoglycemic agents, but refer to physician care if insulin becomes necessary (Avery, 2000; Jacobson et al., 2005; Nicholson et al., 2009). Similarly, collaborative practice guidelines may suggest transfer of care when women require antihypertensive medications, but endorse comanagement of women with mild gestational hypertension or preeclampsia (Chummun, 2009). These details, and other specifics of clinical protocols and collaborative practice agreements, necessarily differ among practice sites. Variation also occurs over time as interprofessional practices evolve in response to changes in clinician members, patient populations, and supportive data (Bailey et al., 2006; Zwarenstein et al., 2009).

Regardless of the indication for collaborative care, comanagement must include ongoing communication among providers to ensure patient safety (Bailey et al., 2006; Brooten et al., 2005; Zwarenstein et al., 2009). The structure of interprofessional communication varies among sites but typically includes periodic clinical conversations about specific patients and management plans via telephone or in person. Similarly, interprofessional practices may use regularly scheduled meetings to discuss their high-risk patient caseload. This formalizes the comanagement process and ensures timely review of patients' evolving health status. These communications should be documented in the medical record in addition to standard written consultant reports and routine charting following clinical encounters. See Figure 28-1 for an algorithm for medical consultation and referral during pregnancy.

REFERENCES

Avery, M. D. (2000). Diabetes in pregnancy: The midwifery role in management. *Journal of Midwifery & Women's Health, 45*(6), 472–480.

Bailey, P., Jones, L., & Way, D. (2006). Family physician/nurse practitioner: Stories of collaboration. *Journal of Advanced Nursing, 53*(4), 381–391.

Brooten, D., Youngblut, J., Blais, K., Donahue, D., Cruz, I., & Lightbourne, M. (2005). APN-physician collaboration in caring for women with high-risk pregnancies. *Journal of Nursing Scholarship, 37*(2), 178–184.

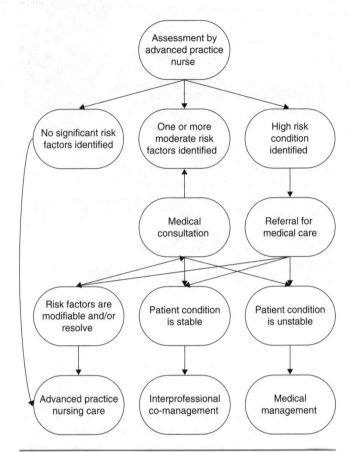

FIGURE 28-1 Algorithm for Medical Consultation and Referral During Pregnancy

Chummun, H. (2009). Hypertension: A contemporary approach to nursing care. *British Journal of Nursing, 18*(13), 784–789.

Jacobson, G. F., Ramos, G. A., Ching, J. Y., Kirby R. S., Ferrara, A., & Field, D. R. (2005). Comparison of glyburide and insulin for the management of gestational diabetes in a large managed care organization. *American Journal of Obstetrics and Gynecology, 193*(1), 118–124.

Nicholson, W., Bolen, S., Witkop, C. T., Neale, D., Wilson, L., & Bass, E. (2009). Benefits and risks of oral diabetes agents compared with insulin in women with gestational diabetes: A systematic review. *Obstetrics and Gynecology, 113*(1), 193–205.

Office of Technology Assessment. (1986). *Health Technology Case Study 37. Nurse Practitioners, Physician Assistants, and Certified Nurse-Midwives: A Policy Analysis.* Washington, DC: Congress of the United States.

Zwarenstein, M., Goldman, J., & Reeves, S. (2009). Interprofessional collaboration: Effects of practice-based interventions on professional practice and healthcare outcomes. *The Cochrane Database of Systematic Reviews, 3,* CD000072.

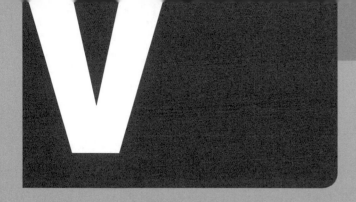

V

COMMON OBSTETRIC PRESENTATIONS

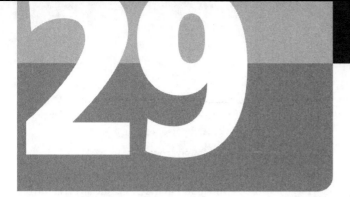

ANEMIA IN PREGNANCY

Laurie Jurkiewicz

I. Introduction and general background

Anemia refers to an insufficient red blood cell supply and is characterized by a significant reduction in hemoglobin (Hgb) and red blood cells as measured by laboratory indices. Hgb combines with oxygen to form oxyhemoglobin. This binding of Hgb and oxygen occurs in the lungs and separates in the tissue capillaries to supply the surrounding cells with oxygen. Iron, proteins, B vitamins, and folic acid are essential nutrients in Hgb synthesis. Severe anemia in pregnancy is associated with an increased risk of spontaneous abortion, low birth weight, preterm birth, and fetal death (Brabin, Hakimi, & Pelletier, 2001). Persistent severe anemia increases the risk of maternal mortality (Sifakis & Pharmakides, 2000).

During pregnancy, the blood volume increases by about 50% to meet the demands of increased circulation of the placenta and maternal fetal tissue. This increase in intravascular volume starts at 6 weeks, peaks at about 28–34 weeks, and levels off during the last 6 weeks of pregnancy. Because plasma volume expansion is faster and greater than red blood cell production, there is a lowering of the Hgb and hematocrit referred to as "physiologic anemia." If there is no significant blood loss during the intrapartal period, the Hgb and hematocrit typically return to normal at about 6 weeks postpartum.

The most common causes of anemia in pregnancy are iron deficiency, hemoglobinopathies, and folic acid deficiency. Determining the proper diagnosis is dependent on the laboratory evaluation of Hgb (Hgb electrophoresis) and the mean corpuscular volume (MCV). It is common to have a combination of different anemias, confusing the clinical picture. Therefore, it may be necessary to test the father of the baby

(FOB) for potential anemia and Hgb variation and conduct iron studies to determine the exact etiology of the anemia.

A. Iron deficiency anemia

Iron deficiency anemia is common in pregnancy, accounting for about 75% of nonphysiologic anemia. The physiology is described by an increased demand on iron stores during pregnancy not only for Hgb synthesis but also for fetal liver storage to meet the needs of the infant in the first 6 months of life. The demand for iron increases in the second half of the pregnancy because of the increased red cell mass and the demands of the growing fetus. It is more prevalent in African American, low-income, and adolescent pregnant women (Graves & Barger, 2001; Laubach & Bendell, 2008).

Classically, there is a low Hgb and hematocrit, normal Hgb electrophoresis, and decreased MCV. Although it is common practice to recommend iron supplement of 30 mg daily to all pregnant women for the prevention of iron deficiency anemia, the United States Preventive Services Task Force (2006) found poor evidence for or against the use of daily iron supplementation for the nonanemic pregnant woman. However, treatment of a diagnosed iron deficiency anemia is indicated.

B. Hemoglobinopathies

Anemia in pregnancy is less commonly caused by hemoglobinopathies, genetic variations to the Hgb itself. The most prevalent among them include α-thalassemia, β-thalassemia, and sickle cell anemia. Women who are carriers for either a thalassemia or sickle cell trait often have a mild anemia, microcytosis, and an abnormal Hgb profile. Women who are found to be carriers and whose partner is also a carrier of either a thalassemia or sickle cell trait should have genetic counseling because of the risk of fetal hemoglobinopathy. Women who either have a thalassemia or sickle cell disease may have profound anemia with considerable neonatal morbidity and therefore should be cared for by a specialist in obstetrics and hematology.

C. Folic acid deficiency

Folic acid deficiency causes a megaloblastic anemia, which is most commonly seen in association with iron deficiency. It is more prevalent in women with low income, closely spaced pregnancies, and in adolescent pregnant women (Laubach & Bendell, 2008). Folic acid deficiency increases a woman's risk of neural tube defects in the fetus. Therefore, the Centers for Disease Control and Prevention (1998) and the United States Preventative Task Force (May 2006) recommend folic acid, 400 mcg of supplementation, before, during, and after pregnancy.

II. **Database** (may include, but is not limited to)

A. Subjective

1. Risk factors

    a. Demographic history: although sickle cell disease primarily affects those of African descent, it is also found in women of Saudi Arabian, Mediterranean, and Caribbean ancestry (Modell & Darlison, 2008). Women from the Mediterranean, Africa, Southeast Asia, Middle East, and the Indian Subcontinent and American-born blacks are at higher risk for thalassemias. Given the increased number of multiethnic couples, ethnicity is not always a good predictor of hemoglobinopathy risk (ACOG, 2008). African Americans, adolescents, and women of low socioeconomic status are at increased risk of iron and folic acid deficiencies (Graves & Barger, 2001; Laubach & Bendell, 2008).

    b. Medical history: history of recent surgery, chronic infection or disease, chronic anemia, frequent blood donation, known hemoglobinopathies, parasitic infection, and anticonvulsant therapy.

    c. Obstetric history: closely spaced pregnancies, multiple gestation, and poor weight gain.

2. Review of symptoms: weakness, fatigue, syncope, vertigo, dizziness, shortness of breath, chest pain, irritability, brittle nails, food cravings, cold intolerance, pallor, irregular heartbeat, and headaches are often asymptomatic.

B. Objective

1. Physical examination: lymphadenopathy; hepatosplenomegaly (indicate hemolysis); and bone tenderness (could indicate anemia caused by metastatic cancer).

2. Abnormal indices for Hgb and hematocrit:

	(g/dl)/(%)
First trimester	< 11/33
Second trimester	< 10.5/32
Third trimester	< 11/33
Postpartum	< 12/37.7

    African American women have lower Hgb values normally. Therefore, it is recommended to lower the Hgb cutoff by 0.8 g/dl (Institute of Medicine, 1993).

3. Serum ferritin: ≤ 10 mcg/L suggests an iron deficiency anemia (Ravel, 1995).

4. Transferrin saturation: < 15% suggests an iron deficiency anemia (Ravel, 1995).

5. Zinc protoporphyrin or free erythrocyte protoporphyrin: > 40 mcg/ml suggests iron deficiency anemia or lead poisoning.

6. MCV: normal 80–100 fL

    a. < 80 indicates thalassemia or iron deficiency.

    b. > 100 indicates megaloblastic anemia; further studies need to be done to confirm a folic acid deficiency (Ravel, 1995).

7. Hgb electrophoresis

    a. Normal adult values are HgbA > 95%, HgbA$_2$ ≤ 3.5%, Hgb F < 2% (Ravel, 1995).

    b. HgbA$_2$ ≤ 3.5% and MCV < 80 fL suggest α-thalassemia or iron deficiency.

    c. HbgA$_2$ > 3.5%, Hgb F > 2%, and MCV 80 fL suggest β-thalassemia, unless coexisting iron deficiency.

    d. Abnormal Hgb type (e.g., Hbg S, C, D, or E): presence indicates trait carrier or disease.

8. Serum folate: in general, may not be very useful for diagnosis of anemia caused by folic acid deficiency; normal range, 3–15 ng/ml (Ravel, 1995).

9. Red blood cell folate: < 149 ng/ml suggests folic acid deficiency. Red blood cell folate is a more reliable test than serum folate for diagnosing folic acid deficiency (Ravel, 1995).

10. See Chapter 42 for a discussion on additional laboratory studies (Figure 29-1).

III. Assessment

1. Rule out iron deficiency anemia

2. Rule out α-thalassemia

3. Rule out β-thalassemia

4. Rule out sickle cell trait

5. Rule out folic acid deficiency

6. Rule out anemia of chronic disease

7. Rule out lead poisoning

IV. Plan

1. Iron deficiency anemia

    a. Encourage intake of iron-rich foods: lean red meat, poultry, egg yolks, beans, dried fruit, dark leafy greens, broccoli, asparagus, or infusion of dried nettle.

    b. Review foods that interfere with iron absorption: coffee, tea, soda, dairy, and antacids.

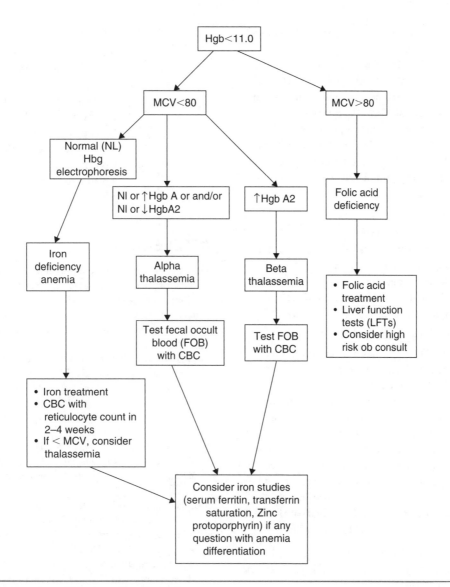

FIGURE 29-1 Laboratory Workup for Anemia

c. Ferrous sulfate therapy, 325 mg (65 mg elemental iron) daily to twice daily, depending on severity of anemia treatment, in addition to prenatal vitamins. A 4-week trial of iron supplementation for mild anemia before a definitive diagnosis of iron deficiency anemia with iron studies is an acceptable initial intervention. If the follow-up complete blood count (CBC) is normal, it is reasonable to assume the anemia was caused by a deficiency in iron.

d. Discuss ways to increase iron intake and absorption: take with juice with vitamin C and in-between meals.

e. Review side effects of supplementation: constipation, nausea, bloating, black tarry stool, and abdominal cramps.

f. If iron is poorly tolerated because of side effects, consider switching to ferrous fumarate, 325 mg, or ferrous gluconate, 325 mg.

g. Keep iron tablets out of reach of children, because they can be fatal if ingested in quantities of only 10–20 pills.

h. If the patient has mild anemia, consider intermittent dosing (120 mg elemental iron one to two times weekly).

i. Consider informing the patient of the availability in health food stores of Floridex Liquid Iron Supplement. Floridex has very little elemental iron, and thus is better tolerated. However, it may not be as effective in treating anemia.

j. Elemental iron interferes with zinc absorption, so zinc supplementation (25 mg, which is the amount found in prenatal vitamins) is recommended.

k. Repeat CBC and reticulocyte count in 2–4 weeks after initiation of treatment. An increased reticulocyte count confirms that the patient is taking iron supplementation.

l. If no improvement despite iron supplementation, get lead level to rule out lead poisoning.

m. Obtain medical consultation if Hgb is less than 9 g/dl despite initiation of therapy or if anemia is chronic.

2. Thalassemia

a. If laboratory values suggest a thalassemia, the father (FOB) should be tested: CBC and Hgb electrophoresis.

b. Genetic counseling and prenatal diagnosis referral if the FOB has an abnormal CBC and Hgb evaluation.

3. Sickle cell trait

a. Test FOB if he has not yet been tested: CBC and Hgb electrophoresis.

b. If FOB is found to be a sickle cell trait carrier, refer to genetics for counseling regarding the risk of sickle cell disease in the neonate.

c. Urine culture and sensitivity screening every trimester should be done, because pregnant women who are a carrier for sickle cell trait have an increased risk of urinary tract infection (Pastore, Savitz, & Thorp, Jr., 1999).

d. If the couple already has a child with sickle disease, refer to genetics for counseling.

4. Folic acid deficiency

a. Start high-dose folic acid supplementation (4 mg daily).

b. Discuss a diet rich in folic acid.

c. Conduct iron studies to rule out coexisting iron deficiency anemia.

d. Offer genetic counseling and referral to prenatal diagnosis for amniocentesis to rule out neural tube defects.

5. Anemia of chronic disease

If all other causes of anemia are ruled out and anemia of chronic disease is suspected, a consult with the obstetrician is indicated for further work-up and plan of treatment.

6. Lead poisoning

a. Investigate the patient's possible lead exposures (exposure to lead-based paint, lead-contaminated dust, and lead-contaminated residential soil) (US Environmental Protection Agency, 2010).

b. Refer patient to the public health department to help with investigation of lead exposure.

c. Consult with the obstetrician to evaluate for a plan of treatment (e.g., need for therapeutic administration of a chelating agent).

REFERENCES

American College of Obstetricians and Gynecologists. (ACOG, 2008). ACOG Practice Bulletin No. 95: Anemia in pregnancy. *Obstetrics & Gynecology, 112*(1), 201–207.

Brabin, B. J., Hakimi, M., & Pelletier, D. (2001). An analysis of anemia and pregnancy-related maternal mortality. *The Journal of Nutrition, 131,* 604S.

Centers for Disease Control and Prevention. (1998). Recommendations to prevent and control iron deficiency in the United States. *Morbidity and Mortality Weekly Report, 47,* 1–29.

Graves, B. W., & Barger, M. K. (2001). A "conservative" approach to iron supplementation during pregnancy. *Journal of Midwifery & Women's Health, 46*(3), 159–160.

Institute of Medicine. (1993). *Iron Deficiency Anemia: Recommended Guidelines for the Prevention, Detection, and Management Among U.S. Children and Women of Childbearing Age.* Washington, DC: Institute of Medicine.

Laubach, J., & Bendell, J. (2008). Hematologic changes of pregnancy. In R. Hoffman, H. Heslop, B. Furie, E. Benz, Jr., P. McGlave, L. Silberstein & S. Shattil. *Hematology: Basic Principles and Practice* (5th ed., pp. 2385–2396). Philadelphia, PA: Churchill Livingstone.

Modell, B., & Darlison, M. (2008). Global epidemiology of haemoglobin disorders and derived service indicators. *Bulletin of the World Health Organization, 86,* 480.

Pastore, L. M., Savitz, D. A., & Thorp, Jr., J. M. (1999). Predictors of urinary tract infection at the first prenatal visit. *Epidemiology, 10,* 282.

Ravel, R. (1995). *Clinical laboratory medicine: Clinical application of laboratory data.* St. Louis, MO: Mosby.

Sifakis, S., & Pharmakides, G. (2000). Anemia in pregnancy. *Annals of the New York Academy of Sciences, 900,* 125.

United States Environmental Protection Agency. (2010, May 19). *Lead in paint, dust and soil.* Retrieved from http://www.epa.gov/lead/.

United States Preventative Task Force. (2006, May). *Screening for iron deficiency anemia—including iron supplementation for children and pregnant women.* Retrieved from http://www.ahrq.gov/clinic/uspstf/uspsiron.htm.

BIRTH CHOICES FOR WOMEN WITH A PREVIOUS CESAREAN DELIVERY

Rebekah Kaplan

I. Introduction and general background

With the rate of cesarean delivery in the United States rapidly rising, increasing numbers of women are faced with the choice of whether to have a repeat cesarean or a trial of labor (TOL) and attempt a vaginal birth after a cesarean (VBAC). Cesarean delivery rates in the United States have risen by 53% from 1996 to 2007, reaching 32.8%, the highest rate ever reported in the United States (Hamilton et al., 2010).

For most of the 20th century, women who had a primary cesarean were advised to have subsequent cesarean deliveries. In 1980, the National Institute of Child and Human Development and the National Center for Health Care Technology examined the evidence for this practice and outlined recommendations for offering women a TOL. From 1980 to 1996 VBAC rates increased, but from 1996 to 2006 rates steadily declined from 28.3% to 8%. Interestingly, for those women who choose to have a TOL the rates of successful VBAC have remained steady at about 74%.

In 2010 the National Institutes of Health (NIH) addressed the issue of declining availability and low VBAC rates at the Consensus Development Conference on Vaginal Birth After Cesarean. Their recommendation was that institutions offer TOL as an option to women with previous low transverse cesarean sections (LTCS) (NIH, 2010). The American Academy of Family Physicians (Wall et al., 2005),

American College of Nurse Midwives (2010) and American College of Obstetricians and Gynecologists (AGOG Bulletin 115, 2010) have made the same recommendation.

When helping women and families make the decision about their preferred mode of delivery, the practitioner must assess the woman's desires, her candidacy for TOL and review the risks and benefits, and complete a consent form. Choices may be institution-specific and a provider should know who in the obstetric community offers VBAC as an option.

II. Data collection

First visit

1. Document the reason for previous cesarean and events surrounding the birth. These include

    a. Reason for prior cesarean (e.g., emergency cesarean birth for nonreassuring fetal heart tracing, placenta previa, arrest of descent, or breech presentation)

    b. Emergent versus nonemergent surgery

    c. Gestational age and fetal weight

    d. Stage of labor (cervical dilation and station) and length of labor

    e. Fetal position, if possible (e.g., posterior)

    f. Where surgery was performed: a small clinic or major hospital

    g. Type of physician performing surgery (obstetrician, gynecologist, or general practitioner)

    h. Future TOL: Did the physician advise the patient whether or not she could attempt a TOL in the future? (Table 30-1)

2. Note desired family size

3. Assess type of scar: on physical abdominal examination, assess transverse or vertical skin scar

4. Attempt to obtain an operative report (Table 30-2)

III. Risks and benefits of TOL versus repeat cesarean delivery

A. Uterine rupture

Evidence shows that the risk of uterine rupture for all women with a previous LTCS is 0.3%. The risk of a uterine rupture for a woman choosing a TOL is 0.47% (0.28–0.77%) (Guise et al., 2010). If a woman has had a previous vaginal birth either before or after her cesarean birth this rate drops. If the prior cesarean was done

TABLE 30-1 VBAC Success Rates

Indication for Cesarean	% Success
Failure to progress	60–65%
Nonrecurring conditions (placenta previa, breech)	74–89%
Fetal intolerance of labor	69–73%
Body mass index > 40	52–70%
(see Internet VBAC success calculator for individual risk)	

TABLE 30-2 Relative Contraindications for Trial of Labor

- Previous cesarean birth with a uterine incision in the upper part of the uterus ("classical" incision), or low transverse uterine incision with an extension into the upper part of the uterus (active segment)
- Uterine surgery other than a low transverse cesarean delivery
- Previous uterine rupture
- More than two previous uterine scars (many institutions state one)
- Medical or obstetric complication that precludes vaginal birth
- Inability to perform emergency cesarean birth

within 24 months of the birth, the risk of rupture is slightly higher. Women with a history of two prior LTCS have about a 2% risk of uterine rupture. If labor is being induced the rate of rupture increases to 1.5% and if labor is being induced at more than 40 weeks, the risk of rupture increases to 3.2%. Labor augmentation does not seem to increase risk of uterine rupture. There have been no reported maternal deaths caused by uterine rupture. Approximately 6% of uterine ruptures result in neonatal death (NIH, 2010).

Although the literature on uterine rupture is imprecise and inconsistent, existing studies indicate that 370 (study numbers range from 213–1,370) elective caesarean deliveries need to be performed to prevent one symptomatic uterine rupture (Guise et al., 2004).

B. Risk for future pregnancies

1. Placenta accreta

   Women with multiple cesareans have an increased rate of placenta accreta and hysterectomy with each subsequent cesarean birth (incidence of placenta accreta from one previous cesarean to five: 3%, 11%, 40%, 61%, and 67%) (Silver et al., 2006).

2. Placenta previa

   The incidence of placenta previa significantly increases in women with each additional cesarean delivery occurring in 9% who have one prior cesarean delivery, 17% who have two prior cesarean deliveries, and 30% in women who have three or more cesarean deliveries (NIH, 2010).

C. Maternal mortality

Overall estimates of maternal death number are 4 per 100,000 for women who undergo a TOL versus 13 per 100,000 for a repeat elective cesarean birth (Guise et al., 2010).

D. Maternal morbidity

Cesarean deliveries are associated with a 10% risk of morbidity including increased risk of infection (endometritis, urinary tract, or wound); thromboembolism; hysterectomy (2%); larger blood loss and severe postpartum hemorrhage (7.3%); blood transfusion; and surgical injury (e.g., injury to the bladder, ureter, or bowel). Women who have a repeat cesarean are more at risk for deep vein thrombosis than in the TOL group, although the risk of hysterectomy, blood transfusion, and infection are similar in both groups (Guise et al., 2010). There is no difference in long-term effects of urinary incontinence in women who have a VBAC versus cesarean birth, although mild incontinence may be higher in the short-term for women who have a VBAC (Press, Klein, & von Dadelszen, 2006). Evidence shows lower rates of maternal morbidity in TOL patients with higher predicted VBAC success rates (> 70%) (Grobman et al., 2009).

E. Neonatal mortality

Studies show that the neonatal mortality rate is higher for TOL at 1.3 per 1,000 compared to elective repeat cesarean at 0.5 per 1,000. The neonatal mortality rate for all first time mothers is 1 per 1,000 (Smith, Pell, Cameron, & Dobbie, 2002; Guise et al., 2010). For women with term pregnancies who have no reported medical risks or complications evidence shows that there is equal or greater risk of neonatal mortality for women undergoing repeat cesarean births compared to VBAC (Menacker, MacDorman, & Declercq, 2010). Neonatal death rates are higher in settings where emergent cesarean sections cannot be performed.

F. Neonatal morbidity

Evidence indicates that infants born by cesarean have higher rates of respiratory distress syndrome, persistent pulmonary hypertension, transient tachypnea of the newborn, and need for oxygen and ventilator support than do infants born vaginally (NIH, 2010). Rates of hypoxic–ischemic encephalopathy in one study were 8 per 10,000 in the TOL group and none in the repeat cesarean group (Landon et al., 2004).

G. *Postpartum period*

Women recover more quickly, have less postpartum pain, and have shorter hospital stays after a vaginal birth versus an operative birth. Women who have cesareans not only have a longer recovery but also delayed mother–infant interaction, lower rates of breastfeeding, and more difficulty establishing breastfeeding. The maternal rehospitalization rate within 30 days is 2.3 times higher in women with a cesarean birth (Declercq et al., 2007) (Table 30-3).

IV. Assessment

Establish if the patient is a candidate for TOL

TABLE 30-3 Factors for VBAC Success

Positive factors

- Maternal age < 40
- Prior vaginal delivery (especially VBAC)
- Favorable cervical factors
- Presence of spontaneous labor
- Nonrecurring indication for previous cesarean (e.g., breech, previa)
- Greater maternal height

Negative factors

- Increased number of prior cesarean deliveries
- Gestational age > 40 weeks
- Birth weight > 4,000 g
- Induction or augmentation of labor (63% success)
- Maternal obesity (body mass index > 30)
- Increased interpregnancy weight gain
- Gestational diabetes
- Maternal disease (e.g., hypertension)

V. Plan

A. *Attempt to obtain an operative report.*

B. *Educate on risks and benefits of repeat cesarean versus TOL: consider patient desires, factors for success, and previous experience.*

C. *Establish the patient's choice.*

D. *Have the patient sign consent for her birth choice (Figure 30-1).*

E. *If the patient has an unknown scar, consult with a physician.*

F. *For those choosing TOL: discuss with the client the care during her birth (continuous fetal monitoring, intravenous or saline lock). Consult per site guidelines. With induction of labor, the risk of uterine rupture increases and VBAC success decreases. If induction is indicated the patient needs to be recounseled.*

G. *For patients choosing a cesarean delivery: Consult with the physician obstetric team to schedule a cesarean at 39 weeks except for those with prior classical scars.*

1. Good dating: 39 weeks

2. Two prior cesareans: 39 weeks

3. Known classical scar consider delivery at 36 weeks

VI. Internet resources for providers, patients, and families

A. *VBAC Success Calculator* (http://www.bsc.gwu.edu/mfmu/vagbirth.html): Enter data, such as maternal age, height, weight, ethnicity, and historical factors, to calculate the predicted chance of VBAC (based on Grobman et al., 2007).

B. *Childbirth Connection* (http://www.childbirthconnection.org/): Organization promoting evidenced-based maternity care and helping women and providers make informed decisions. Several sections regarding VBAC decision-making.

C. *NIH Consensus Development Conference on Vaginal Birth After Cesarean: New insights* (http://consensus.nih.gov/2010/vbac.htm).

FIGURE 30-1 Sample Birth Choices after Cesarean Birth—Patient Information and Choice Form

COMMUNITY HEALTH NETWORK
OF SAN FRANCISCO
Birth Choices After Cesarean Birth—Patient Information and Choice Form
Page 1 of 2

NAME _____

DOB _____

MRN _____

PCP _____

Patient ID / Addressograph _____

Even though you had a cesarean birth before, you may choose to try a vaginal birth or choose another cesarean birth for this pregnancy. There are both risks and benefits to trying a vaginal birth or choosing another cesarean. We want you to have the information that you need to make your choice. We want you and your baby to be healthy and we want you to feel good about your choice.

Please read the information below and talk about it with your provider.

1. VAGINAL BIRTH ADVANTAGES
Mothers who have vaginal births usually have less pain after the baby is born. Most recover faster and are able to go home sooner. There is less chance of getting an infection or needing a blood transfusion. Also, babies who go through labor have less breathing problems at birth. Finally, having a vaginal birth avoids the risks of having another cesarean (see number 4).

Many women who had a cesarean can try a vaginal birth. Your chances of being able to have a vaginal birth depend on why you needed a cesarean before. Reasons that had to do with the baby, like breech position (bottom first) or having twins, might not happen again. Reasons that have to do with your body, like a small pelvis, could make a vaginal birth less likely. About 75% of women who had a cesarean before are able to have a vaginal birth with their next pregnancy.

When you are in labor, your family or close friends can be with you. We will give you pain medicine if you want. We will watch you and your baby closely during labor. Sometimes the baby cannot be born through the vagina. If this happens, we will recommend another cesarean. Many women, however, try for a vaginal birth and are successful.

2. CESAREAN BIRTH ADVANTAGES
The main advantage of choosing another cesarean is that you have less risk of having the scar on your uterus open during labor (see number 3). If you decide to have a cesarean, you avoid the chance of having labor and then still needing a cesarean. This could happen if your labor does not progress or if the baby shows signs of stress during labor. Women who try to have a vaginal birth but then need a cesarean during labor may have more surgical problems than women who choose a cesarean before labor begins. Also, if you choose to have another cesarean, you probably will not have labor pains.

3. VAGINAL BIRTH RISKS
There is a small chance that the scar on your uterus from your cesarean could open up during labor. The risk of this happening depends on where your uterus was cut during your cesarean. If the scar from your cesarean is in the lower part of your uterus, the risk of it opening during labor is less than 1% (1 in 200). If you have had more than one cesarean or if your cesarean was recent (less than 2 years ago), the risk will be slightly increased that the scar could open during labor. If the scar is in the upper part of your uterus, there is much more risk that it could open in labor (as high as 10%). If you have a scar in the upper part of the uterus, we don't think you should try a vaginal birth.

Continue on page 2 of 2.

COMMUNITY HEALTH NETWORK
OF SAN FRANCISCO
Birth Choices After Cesarean Birth - Patient Information and Choice Form
Page 2 of 2

NAME _____

DOB _____

MRN _____

PCP _____

Patient ID / Addressograph _____

Continued from page 1 of 2

3. (Continued from previous page.)
If your provider does not know where your uterus was cut, your risk of the scar opening during labor appears to be the same as those with a scar in the lower part of your uterus (<1%) as most women have cesareans with lower uterine scars. However, it could be as high as 10% if the scar is in the upper part of your uterus.

If the scar on your uterus does open, you might need an emergency cesarean. You could bleed a lot and need a blood transfusion (blood from another person). You also could need a hysterectomy (removal of your uterus). There is a small chance that your baby or you could be injured or die.

4. CESAREAN BIRTH RISKS
If you are able to have a vaginal birth you can avoid some of the risks of a cesarean. For every 100 women who choose a cesarean, about 10 will have a problem. Two women get a wound infection, 6 get a fever, 1 needs a blood transfusion, and less than 1 will have an injury to her intestines, bladder or blood vessels. For every 1,000 women who have a cesarean, about 2 will need a hysterectomy (removal of uterus), usually because of bleeding. The more times you have a cesarean, the more likely you are to have one of these problems.

A cesarean can also cause scarring around the uterus. This scarring can make your next surgery more difficult. In another pregnancy, it can cause problems with the placenta and serious bleeding in a future pregnancy. Rarely, cesareans can weaken the uterus and the scar can open during another pregnancy.

5. I know I can change my choice at any time.

> **Put your initials next to your choice.**

> _____ I choose to try a vaginal birth.

> _____ I choose another cesarean.

I understand the information on this paper. I talked to my pregnancy care provider about this information. I had all of my questions answered.

Patient signature: _____   _____   Date: _____
                          Print name   Signature

Counseling Provider: _____   _____   Date: _____
                           Print name   Signature

Translator (if applicable): _____   _____   Date: _____
                                 Print name   Signature

REFERENCES

ACOG Practice bulletin no. 115, (2010). Vaginal birth after previous cesarean delivery. *Obstetrics & Gynecology, 116*(2 Pt 1), 450–463.

American College of Nurse Midwives (2010). American College of Nurse-Midwives Responds to ACOG's 2010 VBAC recommendations. News Release. http://www.midwife.org/acnm/files/ccLibraryFiles/Filename/000000000075/ACNMResponsetoVBACBulletin_082610FINAL.pdf

Declercq, E., Barger, M., Cabral, H. J., Evans, S. R., Kotelchuck, M., Simon, C. . . . Heffner, L. J. (2007). Maternal outcomes associated with planned primary cesarean births compared with planned vaginal births. *Obstetrics & Gynecology, 109*(3), 669–677.

Grobman, W. A., Lai, Y., Landon, M. B., Spong, C. Y., Leveno, K. J., Rouse, D. J. . . . Mercer, B. M. (2007). Development of a nomogram for prediction of vaginal birth after cesarean delivery. *Obstetrics & Gynecology, 109*(4), 806–812.

Grobman, W. A., Lai, Y., Landon, M. B., Spong, C. Y., Leveno, K. J. . . . Rouse, D. J. (2009). Can a prediction model for vaginal birth after cesarean also predict the probability of morbidity related to a trial of labor? *American Journal of Obstetrics and Gynecology, 200*(1), 56e1-56e6.

Guise, J., Denman, M. A., Emeis, C., Marshall, N., Walker, M., Fu, R. . . . McDonagh, M. (2010). Vaginal birth after cesarean: New insights on maternal and neonatal outcomes. *Obstetrics & Gynecology, 115*(6), 1267–1278.

Guise, J. M., McDonagh, M. S., Osterweil, P., Nygren, P., Chan, B. K., & Helfand, M. (2004). Systematic review of the incidence and consequences of uterine rupture in women with previous caesarean section. *British Medical Journal, 329*(7456), 19–25.

Hamilton, B. E., Martin, J. A., Ventura, S. J. CDC Division of Vital Statistics (2010). Births: preliminary data for 2008. *National Vital Statistics Report, 58*(16) 1–18. http://www.cdc.gov/nchs/data/nvsr/nvsr58/nvsr58_16.pdf

Landon, M. B., Hauth, J. C., Leveno, K. J., Spong, C. Y., Leindecker, S. . . . Moawad, A. H. (2004). Maternal and perinatal outcomes associated with a trial of labor after prior cesarean delivery. *The New England Journal of Medicine, 351*(25), 2581–2589.

Menacker, F., MacDorman, M. F., & Declercq, E. (2010). Neonatal mortality risk for repeat cesarean compared to vaginal birth after cesarean (VBAC) deliveries in the United States, 1998–2002 birth cohorts. *Maternal and Child Health Journal, 14*(2), 147–154.

National Institutes of Health Consensus Development Conference statement: vaginal birth after cesarean: new insights. March 8–10, 2010. (2010). *Obstetrics & Gynecology, 115*(6), 1279–1295.

Press, J., Klein, M. C., & von Dadelszen, P. (2006). *Mode of delivery and pelvic floor dysfunction: A systematic review of the literature on urinary and fecal incontinence and sexual dysfunction by mode of delivery.* Retrieved from http://www.medscape.com/viewprogram/4989.

Silver, R. M., Landon, M. B., Rouse, D. J., Leveno, K. J., Spong, C. Y. . . . Thom, E. A. (2006). Maternal morbidity associated with multiple repeat cesarean deliveries. *Obstetrics & Gynecology, 107*(6), 1226–1232.

Smith, G. C., Pell, J. P., Cameron, A. D., & Dobbie, R. (2002). Risk of perinatal death associated with labor after previous cesarean delivery in uncomplicated term pregnancies. *Journal of the American Medical Association, 287*(20), 2684–2690.

Wall, E., Roberts, R., Deutchman, M., Hueston, W., Ireland, B., & Atwood, L. (2005). Practice Guidelines: Trial of Labor after Cesarean Delivery. *American Family Physician, 72*(10), 2126–2134.

COMMON DISCOMFORTS OF PREGNANCY

Cynthia Belew and Jamie Meyerhoff

I. Introduction to common discomforts of pregnancy

The normal physiologic changes of pregnancy affect all major body systems and can cause a number of uncomfortable symptoms. The degree of discomfort experienced by the individual woman is impacted by many factors, including diet; exercise; genetics; personal self-care habits (e.g., obtaining adequate sleep); mood; body image; level of stress; and social support. The pregnant client likely experiences less stress if she understands the physiologic basis of the symptoms and has knowledge regarding which symptoms are normal and which require an evaluation by a healthcare provider. In addition, knowledge regarding self-care measures to prevent or relieve discomforts may increase her sense of autonomy and control. It is, therefore, a primary responsibility of the healthcare provider to provide anticipatory guidance and education about the physiologic basis and treatment of common discomforts of pregnancy.

Women with multiple or severe symptoms should be screened for depression, because depression can increase symptoms and, conversely, multiple symptoms may increase the risk of developing depression (Kamysheva, Wertheim, Skouteris, Paxton, & Milgrom, 2009). Poor quality of sleep also may contribute to the development of physical complaints and depressive symptoms, and may be correlated with preterm birth (Strange, Parker, Moore, Strickland, & Bliwise, 2009). Pregnant women ought to be encouraged to prioritize adequate sleep and be provided education regarding sleep hygiene practices.

II. Musculoskeletal

Hormonal changes of pregnancy cause relaxation of ligaments throughout the body. The resulting increased mobility of pelvic joints and widening of the sacroiliac and symphyseal joints facilitate childbirth, but may lead to pelvic instability and pain. Biomechanical factors also contribute to pregnancy discomforts. The growing uterus moves the center of gravity forward, pulls the spine into lordosis, and strains the lower back. In most cases pain resolves within 4 weeks after delivery.

Two types of lumbopelvic pain are common during pregnancy. Low back pain (LBP) is musculoskeletal pain experienced in the area of the lumbar spine. Pelvic girdle pain (PGP) is musculoskeletal pain experienced in the sacroiliac area, the symphysis pubis, or gluteal area, possibly with radiation to the posterior thigh. LBP and PGP may occur concurrently (Vermani, Mittal, & Weeks, 2009). Both LBP and PGP may be provoked by any sustained posture or activity, including prolonged sitting, standing, or walking. PGP generally is more debilitating than LBP (Gutke, Oberg, & Ostgaard, 2006). Women with PGP may report a "catching" sensation in the leg while walking and may report that pain is aggravated by twisting, standing on one leg, climbing stairs, and turning in bed.

Many treatments target both LBP and PGP; differences in approach are specified next and in Table 31-1.

A. Prevention

The woman with strong abdominal, back, gluteal, and pelvic muscles may be less likely to develop lumbopelvic pain of pregnancy (Bewyer, Bewyer, & Messenger, 2009). Several studies show that physical fitness exercises before pregnancy may reduce a woman's risk of developing back pain in pregnancy (Vermani et al., 2009). A tailored exercise program during pregnancy was shown to be effective in preventing LBP (Mørkved, Salvesen, Schei, Lydersen, & Bø, 2007). Individualized exercise programs are generally more effective than group training or no treatment.

Workplace restrictions may significantly impact a woman's risk. Because sustained sitting, standing, or walking may provoke pain, a pregnant woman benefits from the freedom to change activities and positions frequently. Research shows that pregnant women who have job autonomy and the ability to take breaks at work experience less back pain, whereas those working in jobs that necessitate staying in a confined area experience more back pain (Cheng, 2009).

B. Database (may include but is not limited to)

The distribution of pain is the most useful history item for diagnosis. The presence of "red flag" signs and symptoms indicates the possibility of disk herniation and

273

TABLE 31-1 Differential Diagnosis and Management of Pelvic Pain and Low Back Pain in Pregnancy

	Subjective	Physical Examination	Imaging	Treatment
Low back pain	Lumbar pain, worse with forward flexion	Negative PPPPT	Not indicated	Water aerobics
				Group exercise for abdominal, back, and pelvic strength
				Acupuncture
				Osteopathic manipulation
				Exercise: pelvic tilt
				Abdominal support garments
Pelvic girdle pain	Sacroiliac pain May radiate to posterior thigh May involve symphysis pubis or gluteal area	Positive PPPPT	Not indicated	Nonelastic pelvic belt to increase stability of sacroiliac joint Individualized pelvic stabilizing and core strengthening exercises
Cauda equina syndrome (severe nerve compression)	Rapid onset of bilateral radiating pain Lower extremity numbness and weakness Numbness of perineum, inner thigh, back of legs Bladder or bowel dysfunction	Supine straight leg raise elicits radiating pain to ipsilateral foot on flexion of hip	Immediate MRI	Orthopedic consultation If stable: bedrest and muscle relaxants If deteriorating: surgery

Source: Adapted from Smith, M. W., Marcus, P. S., & Wurtz, L. D. (2008). Orthopedic issues in pregnancy. *Obstetrical & Gynecological Survey, 63*(2), 103–111; Vermani, E., Mittal, R., & Weeks, A. (2009). Pelvic girdle pain and low back pain in pregnancy: A review. *Pain Practice, 10*(1): 60–71.

requires immediate consultation and possibly magnetic resonance imaging of the spine (Table 31-2).

1. Subjective
   a. Signs or symptoms of preterm labor
   b. Signs or symptoms of pyelonephritis
   c. Events preceding onset
      i. Recent or past history of physical trauma
      ii. History of similar pain
      iii. Anxiety or depression
      iv. Patterns of activity throughout the day
   d. Location and characteristics of pain
      i. Radiation: bilateral or unilateral to thigh or foot
      ii. Pattern of pain: intermittent or constant
      iii. Postures or movements that provoke or alleviate pain
      iv. Quality: sharp, aching, dull; intensity
      v. Level of impact on function and patterns of pacing activity during the day
      vi. Self-treatment, coping strategies, pain beliefs, remedies, and over-the-counter medications

2. Objective
   a. Digital cervical examination to rule out pre-term labor if indicated (see Chapter 35 on prenatal care and preterm labor)
   b. Test for costovertebral angle tenderness to rule out pyelonephritis
   c. Observe gait and ability to change positions; observe distress level
   d. Palpate over the sacroiliac, lumbar, symphysis, and gluteal regions (may help to identify pain distribution to differentiate between LBP and PGP; may also rule out structural abnormalities)
   e. Do a posterior pelvic pain provocation test to differentiate PGP from LBP
      i. The patient lies supine with hips flexed to 90 degrees.
      ii. The examiner applies pressure on the flexed knee in the longitudinal axis of the femur while stabilizing the pelvis with the other hand resting on the opposite anterior superior iliac spine.

TABLE 31-2 Musculoskeletal Red Flag
Symptoms Requiring Consultation or Referral

- Sudden onset of incapacitating back or leg pain, especially pain radiating from the spine along a dermatone bilaterally
- Numbness of perineum, inner thighs, or backs of legs
- Bladder or bowel dysfunction, decreased rectal sphincter tone
- Localized neurologic symptoms (symptoms limited to one nerve root dermatome)
- Decreased muscle strength and sensitivity
- Structural deformity
- Altered DTRs
- Localized neurology (symptoms limited to one nerve root dermatome)

   iii. If this maneuver produces deep pain in the gluteal region, the test is positive and supports a diagnosis of PGP.

  f. Perform the supine active straight leg raise (SLR) test to identify the possibility of disk herniation with nerve compression. If the SLR elicits pain radiating in a dermatomal pattern or if there is numbness or leg weakness, carry out the following tests: reflexes (Achilles or knee), sensation of lateral and medial sides of feet and toes, and strength testing of the big toe during extension.

  g. Imaging studies, such as magnetic resonance imaging, are recommended only when there are multiple red flags (Albert, Ostgaard, Sturesson, Stuge, & Vleeming, 2008).

3. Differential diagnosis
   a. Pregnancy-related LBP or PGP
   b. Preterm labor
   c. Pyelonephritis
   d. Muscle strain caused by trauma
   e. Sciatica
4. Management
   a. Maternity support garments
     i. For PGP, a nonelastic pelvic belt stabilizes the sacroiliac joints and may provide pain relief (Damen, Mens, Snijders, & Stam, 2006). It is most effective when at the level of the greater trocanters.
     ii. Physiotherapists recommend that it be worn for short periods of time rather than continuously (Albert et al., 2008; Chow et al., 2009).

   iii. PGP is less likely than LBP to respond to exercise classes. The abdominal lift garment may be the most beneficial type of maternity support garment for LBP (Albert et al., 2008).

  b. Exercise
     i. Group exercise focused on increasing strength and flexibility and water exercise have been shown to decrease LBP in the second part of pregnancy (Garshasbi & Zadeh, 2005).
     ii. Gentle exercise at home may be helpful, including the pelvic tilt, knee pull, curl-up, lateral SLR, and pelvic floor exercises.
     iii. For PGP, pelvic stabilizing exercises given by a physical therapist are effective (Vleeming, Albert, Ostgaard, Sturesson, & Stuge, 2008).

  c. Workplace modification: a provider's letter to the employer recommending regular rest breaks and movement outside of confined working areas may be beneficial for some women.

  d. Medication for pregnancy-related LBP and PGP
     i. Acetaminophen may not be more effective than placebo for LBP and PGP of pregnancy (Vermani et al., 2009).
     ii. Nonsteroidal anti-inflammatory drugs are not recommended in the last trimester of pregnancy because of risk of premature closure of the ductus arteriosos and risk of oligohydramnios.
     iii. Opioids: Occasional use of small doses of opioids (e.g., codeine) is sometimes indicated in severe cases of pain. Opioid use in late pregnancy can cause respiratory depression in the newborn and, with long-term use, withdrawal effects in the newborn (Vermani et al., 2009).

5. Referrals and self-management resources
   a. European guidelines consider evidence sufficient to recommend the following for PGP: exercise, individualized physical therapy, massage, acupuncture, osteopathic manipulation, and chiropractic care (Albert et al., 2009).
   b. Useful on-line resources include the Association of Chartered Physiotherapists in Women's Health (www.acpwh.org) and the Pelvic Instability Network Support (http://pelvicgirdle pain.com).

6. Patient education (adapted from acpwh.org)
   a. Teach pertinent anatomy and physiology and reassure that pelvic and back pain are a normal

part of pregnancy for many women, likely to resolve in the weeks after birth.

    b. Provide guidance regarding appropriate pacing of activity and rest.

        i. Be as active as possible within the limits of pain. Staying active can reduce pain and improve function (Krismer & van Tulder, 2007).

        ii. Avoid fatigue by taking frequent rest breaks.

        iii. Avoid being in one posture for a prolonged time.

        iv. Avoid activities that worsen pain. Encourage sitting down to put on pants and shoes.

    c. Advise supportive shoes and avoidance of heels.

    d. Recommend placement of one pillow between the knees and one under the abdomen when sleeping side-lying (Faulkner, Thomas, Nicklin, & Pollock, 1989).

III. Gastrointestinal tract

Elevated levels of progesterone during pregnancy facilitate maintenance of the pregnancy by relaxing the uterine muscle. However, smooth muscle relaxation decreases gastric and intestinal motility, leading to nausea, dyspepsia, and constipation. Mechanical pressure from the enlarging uterus contributes to heartburn. Management of common gastrointestinal tract discomforts of pregnancy, such as nausea, heartburn, and constipation, proceeds in a step-wise algorithm that begins with lifestyle and dietary modifications, and gentle natural remedies. Pharmaceutical treatment is reserved for persistent or severe symptoms. This conservative approach is recommended because of the benign nature of common gastrointestinal tract discomforts of pregnancy and the fact that safety data for most pharmaceuticals in pregnancy is not of high quality. Limited evidence shows that pharmaceutical antiemetic drugs are not associated with fetal anomalies.

The Canadian organization Motherisk, a clinical research and teaching program at The Hospital for Sick Children, has an excellent on-line resource (www.motherisk.org). They provide information both to pregnant and lactating women and to healthcare professionals regarding risks to the fetus from maternal exposure to drugs, chemicals, diseases, radiation, and environmental agents. They maintain several helplines, including one dedicated to questions regarding nausea and vomiting of pregnancy (NVP).

A. Nausea and vomiting of pregnancy

    1. Definition and clinical implications

    NVP is considered to be a result of hormonal changes. Fifty to eighty percent of all pregnant women experience NVP. Typically, symptom onset is around 5 weeks from the last menstrual period, with resolution at 11–14 weeks gestation. In a subset of women, symptoms may persist until 18 weeks, and 5% of pregnant women have nausea throughout pregnancy. If onset of symptoms occurs at a gestational age of 10 weeks or greater, the etiology is not likely to be pregnancy.

NVP is a normal part of most pregnancies. Although NVP may significantly impact a woman's daily life, it is benign. The presence of NVP is associated with favorable pregnancy outcomes, including a lower risk of miscarriage, perinatal death, low birthweight, and preterm birth. The reduced maternal nutrient intake that commonly occurs during the first trimester in women with NVP seems to cause complex hormonal and metabolic changes that actually enhance placental growth (Huxley, 2000). It is also proposed that NVP serves a protective evolutionary function, causing women to avoid foods that may cause harm to the embryo (Sherman & Flaxman, 2002). Most women make up for first trimester weight loss by gaining more weight later in pregnancy.

In contrast, hyperemesis gravidarum (HG) can pose serious risks, and is a more debilitating condition. On the continuum from severe NVP to HG, HG is defined as symptoms that lead to weight loss of more than 5% of prepregnancy body weight, hypokalemia, and dehydration or ketonuria. HG may require hospitalization. Holmgrem and colleagues review the management of HG (Holmgrem, Aagaard-Tillery, Silver, Porter, & Varner, 2008). HG requires medical management because it can be associated with serious sequelae, such as micronutrient deficiency or Wernicke's encephalopathy, if not properly managed (Dodds, Fell, Joseph, Allen, & Butler, 2006).

If heartburn exists concurrent with NVP, pharmacologic treatment of the heartburn is shown to decrease symptoms of NVP (Gill, Maltepe, Mastali, & Koren, 2009).

B. Database (may include but is not limited to)

    1. Subjective data

        a. Timing of onset, pattern, and frequency of nausea and vomiting

        b. Triggers and coexisting gastric reflux

        c. Eating habits and self-treatment

        d. Red flags for gallbladder disease and HELLP syndrome (hemolysis, elevated liver enzymes, and low platelets)

            i. Epigastric pain, right upper quadrant pain, or coffee grounds emesis

            ii. Upper abdominal pain in a pattern of biliary colic (episodes of sharp, intense pain after meals or at night lasting 30 minutes to 3 hours, or radiation to back or right shoulder) may indicate gallbladder disease.

iii. The "PUQE" (pregnancy-unique quantification of emesis/nausea) index may be used to evaluate severity. The woman's subjective experience of the impact of symptoms on her life is an important consideration and may override the PUQE score (King & Murphy, 2009) (Table 31-3).

2. Objective data

   a. Weight loss
   b. Urinalysis: ketones and specific gravity
   c. Signs of dehydration: tachycardia, dry mucosa, and sunken eyes
   d. If severe symptoms are present: order an electrolyte panel and an obstetric ultrasound to rule out twin gestation or trophoblastic disease (molar pregnancy)
   e. If onset of symptoms occurs in third trimester: rule out HELLP syndrome with complete blood count (CBC) and platelets even if symptoms are not severe
   f. If symptoms suggest gallbladder disease: CBC, lipase, liver enzymes, and abdominal ultrasound

3. Differential diagnosis

   a. Dehydration
   b. Ketonuria
   c. Electrolyte imbalance
   d. HG
   e. HELLP syndrome (third trimester)
   f. Gallbladder, liver, or pancreatic disease
   g. Fatty liver of pregnancy (rare)

4. Management

   Women commonly find that one therapeutic measure works well for a few days but then becomes less effective. Knowledge about multiple treatments is beneficial to switch tactics as needed.

5. Education

   Reassure that mild to moderate symptoms do not have a negative effect on fetal growth and development. Discuss dietary and lifestyle changes.

6. Hydration and nutrition

   a. Avoid dehydration by sipping small amounts of water frequently (as little as an ounce every 15 minutes). Large volumes of fluid may provoke nausea.
   b. Drink fluids between meals instead of with meals.
   c. Eat small amounts of food every 1–3 hours. Low blood sugar provokes nausea. Eat a high-protein snack at bedtime.
   d. Keep dry crackers at the bedside and eat a few before rising in the morning.
   e. Avoid spicy or fatty foods.

7. Trigger avoidance: triggers are highly individual but may include

   a. Strong odors, stuffy rooms, or bus travel.
   b. The sight or smell of certain foods.
   c. Brushing teeth (avoid within 1–2 hours after eating and use small amounts of a low-foaming toothpaste or brush without toothpaste).
   d. Multivitamins: continue to take multivitamin if possible, because it may decrease symptoms, but if taking multivitamin aggravates nausea, discontinue and replace with 600 mcg of folic acid. Resume multivitamin at a later gestational age when NVP resolves. A multivitamin without iron may be more easily tolerated.

TABLE 31-3 Pregnancy-Unique Quantification of Emesis and Nausea Index

1. On the average day, for how long do you feel nauseated or sick to your stomach?				
> 6 hr	4–6 hr	2–3 hr	≤ 1 hr	Not at all
(5 points)	(4 points)	(3 points)	(2 points)	(1 point)
2. On an average day, how many times do you vomit or throw up?				
≥ 7 hr	5–6	3–4	1–2	None
(5 points)	(4 points)	(3 points)	(2 points)	(1 point)
3. On an average day, how many times do you have retching or dry heaves without bringing anything up?				
≥ 7 hr	5–6	3–4	1–2	None
(5 points)	(4 points)	(3 points)	(2 points)	(1 point)
Total score (sum of replies to 1, 2, and 3): mild NVP, ≤ 6; moderate NVP, 7–12; severe NVP, ≥ 13.				

Source: Reprinted from Lacasse, A., Rey, E., Ferreira, E., et al., (2008). Validity of a modified Pregnancy-Unique Quantification of Emesis and Nausea (PUQE) scoring index to assess severity of nausea and vomiting of pregnancy. *American Journal of Obstetrics and Gynecology, 198*(1), 71.e3; with permission from Elsevier.

8. Therapeutic
   a. Alternative and complementary
      i. The Canadian Motherisk reports that 61% of women with NVP report use of complementary and alternative remedies but only 8% of women had discussed these remedies with their healthcare provider (Hollyer, Boon, Georgousis, Smith, & Einarson, 2002).
      ii. Ginger, chamomile, fennel seed, raspberry leaf, and mint are all used traditionally in a tea or tincture for gastric upset. These herbs are regarded as safe by the Canadian Motherisk group (Mills, Duguoa, Perri, & Koren, 2006) and the German Commission E (Blumenthal, Goldberg, & Brinckmann, 2000). Both are authoritative expert panels dealing with the topic of herb safety.
   b. Evidence exists supporting the effectiveness and safety of the following therapies:
      i. Acupressure wrist bands (Seabands, Travel-eze) worn continuously over the P6 acupuncture point (Can Gürkan & Arslan, 2008).
      ii. Ginger capsules, 250 mg orally four times a day (Bryer, 2005)
      iii. Vitamin B$_6$, 25 mg orally three times a day. Avoid excessive doses, which may cause peripheral neuropathy (Keller, Frederking, & Layer, 2008).
   c. Intravenous fluid therapy: Intravenous fluid therapy with normal saline, alone or in combination with pharmaceuticals, typically causes an improvement of symptoms for several days. Some women choose it as a primary management strategy, receiving hydration every few days as needed (King & Murphy, 2009). Avoid dextrose-containing fluids, because they may precipitate Wernicke encephalopathy, a rare but serious complication, in a woman with thiamine deficiency. The addition of thiamine is recommended for the prevention of Wernicke encephalopathy. Potassium chloride may be added as needed.
9. Pharmacotherapy (Table 31-4.)
   a. Dopamine antagonists
      i. Metoclopramide is the drug of choice for many providers. Recent research examining more than 3,400 first-trimester exposures found no association with any of several adverse outcomes (Matok et al., 2009). In a comparison of promethazine and metoclopramide, Tan and colleagues found similar effectiveness but metoclopramide had fewer side effects (Tan, Khine, Vallikkannu, & Omar, 2010).
      ii. Metoclopramide and other dopamine antagonists may cause extrapyramidal symptoms or dystonic reactions. Promethazine and prochlorpemazine cause sedation, which may be difficult for women to tolerate.
      iii. Evidence supports both the safety and effectiveness of Bendectin (doxylamine, 10 mg, and pyridoxine, 10 mg, three to four times a day) despite its removal from the market after lawsuits and alleged teratogenic effects (McKeigue, Lamm, Linn, & Kutcher, 1994).
      iv. Ondansetron (Zofran) is expensive. Anecdotal reports support its effectiveness. A randomized control trial reported it was not more effective than low-dose promethazine (6.25 or 12.5 mg) for women with HG (Moser, Caldwell, & Rhule, 2006).
      v. See the management algorithm in Figure 31-1.
10. Follow-up
    a. Send to labor and delivery for rehydration and medication as needed.
    b. Increase the frequency of prenatal visits to once or twice weekly until symptoms diminish.

IV. Heartburn

A. Definition

Heartburn, also known as gastroesophageal reflux disease, is a normal part of most pregnancies. Symptoms are usually mild to moderate. Lifestyle and dietary modifications accompanied by safe home remedies and simple antacids are effective in providing relief. Pregnancy seems to be protective against esophagitis and gastric ulcer disease, and these conditions are uncommon during pregnancy (Cappell, 2003). Even severe symptoms of gastroesophageal reflux disease usually resolve soon after birth.

B. Database *(may include but is not limited to)*

Red flag symptoms and signs help in the differentiation of benign heartburn from more serious medical conditions. Gallbladder disease and, in the third trimester, HELLP syndrome must be ruled out. HELLP syndrome may or may not present with hypertension (Sibai & Stella, 2009). Red flag symptoms and signs require immediate consultation.

TABLE 31-4 Pharmacotherapy for NVP

Generic Name (Trade Name)	Dosage	Major Side Effects
Antihistamines		
Diphenhydramine (Benadryl®)	50–100 mg q 4–6 hr PO/IM/IV For treatment of dystonic reaction: 50 mg IV	Drowsiness
Doxylamine (Unisom®)*	12.5 mg BID PO or 125 mg in morning and 25 mg at night	
Trimethobenzamide (Tigan®)	200 mg IM/PR q 6–8 hr	Drowsiness
Dopamine antagonists		
Metoclopramide (Reglan)	1–2 mg/kg IV (dilute in 50 ml IVF) or 5–10 mg Q 8 hours PR/IM	Agitation, anxiety, acute dystonic reactions*
Prochlorperazine (Compazine®)	5–10 mg PO/IV/IM q 6–8 hr or 25 mg rectal suppository BID/prn for breakthrough vomiting with other medications)	Sedation, anticholinergic effects, EPS
Promethazine (Phenergan®)	12.5–25 mg PO/IV/IM/PR q 4–6 hr	Sedation, anticholinergic effects, dystonic reactions*
Serotonin (5-HT3) antagonists		
Ondansetron (Zofran®)*	4–8 mg PO q 6–8h 4–8 mg IV q 12 hr, given over 15 min	Headache
Other		
Inapsine (Droperidol®)	0.625–2.5 mg IV over 15 min then 1.25 mg or 2.5 mg IM as needed, can be given IV continuously at 1–1.25 mg/h	Dystonic reactions,* prolonged QT syndrome
Pyridoxine (vitamin B$_6$)	25 mg TID. Consider combining with doxylamine	
Zingiber officinale (ginger)	Capsules: 250–500 mg TID-QID Not to exceed 1.5 g in 24 hr	

* Give 50 mg diphenhydramine before dose to prevent extrapyramidal reactions

Source: Reprinted from King, T. L., & Murphy, P. A. (2009). Evidence-based approaches to managing nausea and vomiting in early pregnancy. *Journal of Midwifery & Women's Health, 54*(6), 435; with permission from Elsevier.

1. Subjective
   a. Typical symptoms of gastric acid reflux during pregnancy include
      i. Burning in the upper abdomen or mid-chest.
      ii. Discomfort associated with eating or with a recumbent position.
      iii. Typically worsens as the pregnancy progresses.
      iv. Relieved by antacids.
   b. Red flag symptoms of gallbladder disease
      i. Episodes of sharp, intense right upper quadrant pain similar to heartburn; occurs after meals or at night, lasting 30 minutes to 2 hours.
      ii. Belching or indigestion commonly co-occur
   c. Red flag symptoms of HELLP include
      i. Right upper quadrant, mid-epigastrium, or retrosternal pain
      ii. Nausea, vomiting, and malaise

2. Objective
   a. Physical examination
      i. Assess for red flag signs of HELLP
      ii. Right upper quadrant or mid-epigastrium tenderness
      iii. May or may not present with hypertension
3. Assessment
   a. Normal gastric reflux of pregnancy. This diagnosis is based on symptoms alone.
   b. Rule out liver, gallbladder, and pancreatic disease.
   c. Rule out HELLP if in third trimester
   d. Diagnostic laboratory tests
      i. CBC with platelets if symptoms include red flags for HELLP
      ii. Liver function tests, lipase, and bilirubin, if clinically suspicious for gallbladder disease, HELLP, or other liver disease.
4. Management
   Lifestyle modifications and antacids are the first-line therapy for gastric reflux in pregnancy. If these

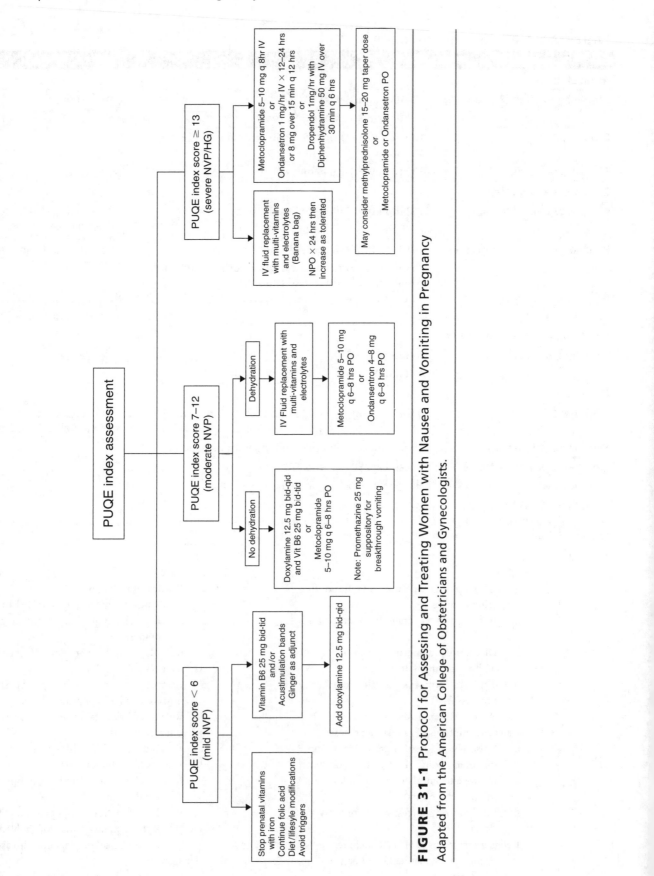

FIGURE 31-1 Protocol for Assessing and Treating Women with Nausea and Vomiting in Pregnancy

Adapted from the American College of Obstetricians and Gynecologists.

are not effective, histamine 2 (H_2) receptor antagonists can be used. Proton pump inhibitors are usually reserved for women with severe symptoms. The promotility agent, metoclopramide, may also be used.

a. Lifestyle modification
  i. Avoid aggravating foods, which may include fatty or spicy foods, caffeinated or carbonated beverages, chocolate, alcohol, citrus, tomato products, peppermint, or ginger.
  ii. Do not drink more than one cup of fluid with meals.
  iii. Eat small frequent meals; avoid eating for 2–3 hours before lying down
  iv. When lying down, lie on the left side. Reflex is less frequent compared with right-side recumbent or supine position (Ali, Roberts, & Tierney, 2009).
  v. Elevating the head of bed 4–6 inches with bricks or blocks is shown to decrease esophageal acid exposure.
  vi. Smoking cessation.
b. Remedies
  i. Almonds: many women report that chewing 8–10 raw almonds thoroughly, repeated several times daily as needed, effectively reduces heartburn.
  ii. Herbs for heartburn and gastritis
  iii. Expert opinion and traditional use supports the benefit and safety of marshmallow root (Althea) and the inner bark of slippery elm (Ulmas rubra) for heartburn and gastritis (Romm, 2010). They contain mucilage (insoluble polysaccharides), which absorbs acid and sooths irritated or inflamed mucosa (Deters et al., 2010).
    a. Slippery elm
      i. Commercially prepared lozenges (sold for use for sore throat) two to three at a time, up to 12 per day.
      ii. One teaspoon of powdered herb stirred into oatmeal, applesauce, juice, or hot water.
    b. Marshmallow root
      i. One ounce of dried herb steeped for at least 30 minutes in one quart of hot water, strain, sip throughout the day as needed, up to three cups daily.
    c. Chamomile
      i. Chamomile (Matricaria recutita) has gastric protective, anti-inflammatory and antispasmodic effects (McKay & Blumberg, 2006) and is shown in randomized controlled trials to have effectiveness for anxiety (Amsterdam et al., 2009) and infant colic (Savino, Cresi, Castagno, Silvestro, & Oggero, 2005).
      ii. Tea of ginger, chamomile, linden (lime flower), mint, fennel seed, individually or in combination, are used for gastric upset (Romm, 2010).
    d. Dandelion root tea (one to three cups sipped throughout the day) or tincture (20–40 drops diluted in a small amount of water three times daily).
      i. Dandelion root is contraindicated if there are painful gallstones (acute biliary colic) or cholecystitis.
c. Pharmaceuticals
  i. Calcium or magnesium-containing antacids are effective in most cases and recommended as the first-line treatment (Tytgat et al., 2003).
    a. Excessive use of calcium carbonate (> 2 g/day) can result in milk alkali syndrome (hypercalcemia and alkalosis, which can cause renal damage).
    b. Although some advocate the benefits of calcium carbonate as an antacid because it also provides supplemental calcium, in reality calcium carbonate contains only 40% elemental calcium and has poor bioavailability (Sipponen & Harknen, 2010).
  ii. Medications to avoid (Mahadevan & Kane, 2006)
    a. Sodium bicarbonate (large amounts can cause metabolic acidosis and fluid overload)
    b. Magnesium trisilicates (Gaviscon®)
    c. Bismuth (Pepto-Bismol®, Kaopectate)
    d. Aluminum-containing antacids
    e. Alka Seltzer® (contains aspirin, sodium bicarbonate)
      i. Antacids should be taken at a different time than iron.
      ii. For moderate–severe gastroesophageal reflux with a lack of relief from the previously mentioned treatments, consider:
        a. Sucralfate, 1 g orally before meals and at bedtime

b. Metoclopramide (Reglan®), 10–15 mg orally before meals and at bedtime, four times a day

c. H_2 receptor antagonists.

   i. Cimetidine or ranitidine are the preferred H_2 receptor antagonists (Mahadevan & Kane, 2006).

   ii. Theoretical concerns exist regarding H_2 receptor antagonists in pregnancy. Histamine is involved in the relaxation and contraction of placental vessels. H_2 receptor blockage with famotidine is shown to significantly inhibit the relaxation phase. This could have implications for the development of preeclampsia. Uterine contractility is also impacted by H_2. Although researchers have not specifically explored the impact of H_2 antagonists on preeclampsia or preterm labor, it may be wise to minimize the use of these drugs during pregnancy (Mills, Taggart, Greenwood, Baker, & Wareing, 2007).

d. For moderate to severe gastric reflux that does not respond to the previously mentioned treatments

   i. Proton pump inhibitors (PPIs) (Gill, O'Brien, Einarson, & Koren, 2009).

   ii. Omeprazole (Prilosec®) is recommended as the PPI of choice (Mahadevan & Kane, 2006).

   iii. A recent meta-analysis reported that the use of PPIs during pregnancy was not associated with an increased risk of birth defects, spontaneous abortions, or preterm delivery (Gill et al., 2009). However, other significant adverse effects are associated with acid inhibitor use, especially PPIs.

e. Adverse effects of acid-inhibitors.

   i. Gastric acid is necessary for the destruction of pathogenic organisms and for absorption of minerals and vitamin B_{12}. PPIs are associated with an increased risk of gastroenteritis, *Clostridium difficile* disease, and pneumonia (Ali et al., 2009). Long-term use of PPIs is associated with hypomagnesemia (Kuipers), impaired calcium homeostasis, and increased risk of hip fracture (Corley, Kubo, Zhao, & Quesenberry, 2010). The detrimental effects of PPIs may not be seen with antacids because antacids only impact gastric acidity for approximately 1 hour.

   ii. Acid-suppressant medications may also contribute to food allergy and asthma (Untersmayr & Jensen-Jarolim, 2008). Maternal use of gastric acid inhibitors is associated with a 50% increased risk in asthma in the offspring (Dehlink, Yen, Leichtner, Hait, & Fiebiger, 2009).

   iii. Rebound acid hypersecretion occurs after use of PPIs (Waldum, Qvigstad, Fossmark, Kleveland, & Sandvik, 2010).

5. Follow-up
   a. Increase frequency of visits based on response to treatment
   b. Nutritionist referral
   c. Physician consultation for persistent severe symptoms unresponsive to treatment

REFERENCES

Albert, H. B., Ostgaard, H. C., Sturesson, B., Stuge, B., & Vleeming, A. (2008). European guidelines for the diagnosis and treatment of pelvic girdle pain. *European Spine Journal, 17*(6), 794–819.

Ali, T., Roberts, D. N., & Tierney, W. M. (2009). Long-term safety concerns with proton pump inhibitors. *The American Journal of Medicine, 122*(10), 896–903.

Amsterdam, J. D., Li, Y., Soeller, I., Rockwell, K., Mao, J. J., & Shults, J. (2009). A randomized, double-blind, placebo-controlled trial of oral Matricaria recutita (chamomile) extract therapy for generalized anxiety disorder. *Journal of Clinical Psychopharmacology, 29*(4), 378–382.

Bewyer, K. J., Bewyer, D. C., & Messenger, D. (2009). Pilot data: Association between gluteus medius weakness and low back pain during pregnancy. *The Iowa Orthopaedic Journal, 29*, 97–99.

Blumenthal, M., Goldberg, A., & Brinckmann, J. (2000). *Herbal Medicine: Expanded Commission E Monographs.* Newton, MA: Integrative Medicine Communications.

Bryer, E. (2005). A literature review of the effectiveness of ginger in alleviating mild-to-moderate nausea and vomiting of pregnancy. *Journal of Midwifery & Women's Health, 50*(1), e1–e3.

Can Gürkan O., & Arslan, H. (2008). Effect of acupressure on nausea and vomiting during pregnancy. *Complementary Therapy Clinical Practice, 14*(1), 46–52.

Cappell, M. S. (2003). Gastric and duodenal ulcers during pregnancy. *Gastroenterology Clinics of North America, 32*(1), 263–308.

Cheng, P. L., Pantel, M., Smith, J. T., Dumas, G. A., Leger, A. B., Plamondon, A. . . . McGrath, M. J. (2009). Back pain of working pregnant women: identification of associated occupational factors. *Applied Ergonomics, 40*(3), 419–423.

Chow, D. H., Chung, J. W., Ho, S., Lao, T., Li, Y., & Yu, W. (2009). Effectiveness of maternity support belts in reducing low back pain during pregnancy: A review. *Journal of Clinical Nursing, 18*(11), 1523–1532.

Corley, D. A., Kubo, A., Zhao, W., & Quesenberry, C. (2010). Proton pump inhibitors and histamine-2 receptor antagonists are associated with hip fractures among at-risk patients. *Gastroenterology, 139*(1), 93–101.

Damen, L., Mens, J. M., Snijders, C. J., & Stam, H. J. (2006). The mechanical effect of a pelvic belt in patients with pregnancy-related pelvic pain. *Clinical Biomechanics, 21*(2), 122–127.

Dehlink, E., Yen, E., Leichtner, A. M., Hait, E. J., & Fiebiger, E. (2009). First evidence of a possible association between gastric acid suppression during pregnancy and childhood asthma: A population-based register study. *Clinical and Experimental Allergy, 39*(2), 246–253.

Deters, A., Zippel, J., Hellenbrand, N., Pappai, D., Possemeyer, C., & Hensel, A. (2010). Aqueous extracts and polysaccharides from marshmallow roots (Althea officinalis L.): Cellular internalisation and stimulation of cell physiology of human epithelial cells in vitro. *Journal of Ethnopharmacology, 127*(1), 62–69.

Dodds, L., Fell, D. B., Joseph, K. S., Allen, V. M., & Butler, B. (2006). Outcomes of pregnancies complicated by hyperemesis gravidarum. *Obstetrics & Gynecology, 107*(2), 285–292.

Faulkner, K., Thomas, I. L., Nicklin, J., & Pollock, H. (1989). Evaluation of a maternity cushion (Ozzlo pillow) for backache and insomnia in late pregnancy. *The Australian & New Zealand Journal of Obstetrics & Gynaecology, 29*(2), 133–138.

Garshasbi, A., & Zadeh, S. F. (2005). The effect of exercise on the intensity of low back pain in pregnant women. *International Journal of Gynecology and Obstetrics, 88*(3), 271–275.

Gill, S. K., Maltepe, C., Mastali, K., & Koren, G. (2009). The effect of acid-reducing pharmacotherapy on the severity of nausea and vomiting of pregnancy. *Obstetrics and Gynecology International*, Epub July 1, 2009, 585269, 1–4.

Gill, S. K., O'Brien, L., Einarson, T. R., & Koren, G. (2009). The safety of proton pump inhibitors (PPIs) in pregnancy: A meta-analysis. *The American Journal of Gastroenterology, 104*(6), 1541–1545.

Gutke, A., Oberg, B., & Ostgaard, H. C. (2006). Pelvic girdle pain and lumbar pain in pregnancy: A cohort study of the consequences in terms of health and functioning. *Spine, 31*(5), e149–e155.

Holmgren, C., Aagaard-Tillery, K. M., Silver, R. M., Porter, T. F., & Varner, M. (2008). Hyperemesis in pregnancy: an evaluation of treatment strategies with maternal and neonatal outcomes. *The American Journal of Obstetrics and Gynecology,198*(1):56.e1–e4.

Hollyer, T., Boon, H., Georgousis, A., Smith, M., & Einarson, A. (2002). The use of CAM by women suffering from nausea and vomiting during pregnancy. *BMC Complementary and Alternative Medicine, 2*, 5.

Huxley, R. (2000). Nausea and vomiting in early pregnancy—it's role in placental development. *Obstetrics & Gynecology, 95*(5), 779–782.

Kamysheva, E., Wertheim, E. H., Skouteris, H., Paxton, S. J., & Milgrom, J. (2009). Frequency, severity, and effect on life of physical symptoms experienced during pregnancy. *Journal of Midwifery & Women's Health, 54*(1), 43–49.

Keller, J., Frederking, D., & Layer, P. (2008). The spectrum and treatment of gastrointestinal disorders during pregnancy. *Nature Clinical Practice Gastroenterology & Hepatology, 5*(8), 430–443.

King, T. L., & Murphy, P. A. (2009). Evidence-based approaches to managing nausea and vomiting in early pregnancy. *Journal of Midwifery & Women's Health, 54*(6), 430–444.

Krismer, M., & van Tulder, M. (2007). Strategies for prevention and management of musculoskeletal conditions: Low back pain (nonspecific). *Best Practice & Research Clinical Rheumatology, 21*(1), 77–91.

Lacasse, A., Rey, E., Ferreira, E., et al., (2008). Validity of a modified Pregnancy-Unique Quantification of Emesis and Nausea (PUQE) scoring index to assess severity of nausea and vomiting of pregnancy. *American Journal of Obstetrics and Gynecology, 198*(1), 71.e3.

Mahadevan, U., & Kane, S. (2006). American Gastroenterological Association institute technical review on the use of gastrointestinal medications in pregnancy. *Gastroenterology, 131*(1), 283–311.

Matok, I., Gorodischer, R., Koren, G., Sheiner, E., Wiznitzer, A., & Levy, A. (2009). The safety of metoclopramide use in the first trimester of pregnancy. *New England Journal of Medicine, 360*(24), 2528–2535.

McKay, D. L., & Blumberg, J. B. (2006). A review of the bioactivity and potential health benefits of chamomile tea (Matricaria recutita L.). *Phytotherapy Research, 20*(7), 519–530.

McKeigue, P. M., Lamm, S. H., Linn, S., & Kutcher, J. S. (1994). Bendectin and birth defects: I. A meta-analysis of the epidemiologic studies. *Teratology, 50*(1), 27–37.

Mills, E., Duguoa, J., Perri, D., & Koren, G. (2006). *Herbal medicines in pregnancy and lactation: An evidence-based approach.* New York, NY: Taylor & Francis.

Mills, T. A., Taggart, M. J., Greenwood, S. L., Baker, P. N., & Wareing, M. (2007). Histamine-induced contraction and relaxation of placental chorionic plate arteries. *Placenta, 28*(11-12), 1158–1164.

Mørkved, S., Salvesen, K. A., Schei, B., Lydersen, S., & Bø, K. (2007). Does group training during pregnancy prevent lumbopelvic pain? A randomized clinical trial. *Acta Obstetricia et Gynecologica Scandinavica, 86*(3), 276–282.

Moser, J. D., Caldwell, J. B., & Rhule, F. J. (2006). No more than necessary: Safety and efficacy of low-dose promethazine. *The Annals of Pharmacotherapy, 40*(1), 45–48.

Romm, A. (2010). *Botanical Medicine for Women's Health.* St. Louis, MO: Churchill Livingstone Elsevier.

Savino, F., Cresi, F., Castagno, E., Silvestro, L., & Oggero, R. (2005). A randomized double-blind placebo-controlled trial of a standardized extract of Matricariae recutita, Foeniculum vulgare and Melissa officinalis (ColiMil) in the treatment of breastfed colicky infants. *Phytotherapy Research, 19*(4), 335–340.

Sherman, P. W., & Flaxman, S. M. (2002). Nausea and vomiting of pregnancy in an evolutionary perspective. *American Journal of Obstetrics and Gynecology, 186*(Suppl. 5), S190–S197.

Sibai, B. M., & Stella, C. L. (2009). Diagnosis and management of atypical preeclampsia-eclampsia. *American Journal of Obstetrics and Gynecology, 200*(5), 481–487.

Sipponen, P., & Harkonen, M. (2010). Hypochlorhydric stomach: A risk condition for calcium malabsorption and osteoporosis. *Scandinavian Journal of Gastroenterology, 45*(2), 133–138.

Smith, M. W., Marcus, P. S., & Wurtz, L. D. (2008). Orthopedic issues in pregnancy. *Obstetrical & Gynecological Survey, 63*(2), 103–111.

Strange, L. B., Parker, K. P., Moore, M. L., Strickland, O. L., & Bliwise, D. L. (2009). Disturbed sleep and preterm birth: A potential relationship? *Clinical and Experimental Obstetrics & Gynecology, 36*(3), 166–168.

Tan, P. C., Khine, P. P., Vallikkannu, N., & Omar, S. Z. (2010). Promethazine compared with metoclopramide for hyperemesis gravidarum: A randomized controlled trial. *Obstetrics and Gynecology, 115*(5), 975–981.

Tytgat, G. N., Heading, R. C., Müller-Lissner, S., Kamm, M. A., Schölmerich, J., Berstad, A., Fried, M., . . . Briggs A. (2003). Contemporary understanding and management of reflux and constipation in the general population and pregnancy: A consensus meeting. *Alimentary Pharmacology & Therapeutics, 18*(3), 291–301.

Untersmayr, E., & Jensen-Jarolim, E. (2008). The role of protein digestibility and antacids on food allergy outcomes. *The Journal of Allergy and Clinical Immunology, 121*(6), 1301–1308; quiz 1309.

Vermani, E., Mittal, R., & Weeks, A. (2009). Pelvic girdle pain and low back pain in pregnancy: A review. *Pain Practice, 10*(1), 60–71.

Vleeming, A., Albert, H. B., Ostgaard, H. C., Sturesson, B., & Stuge, B. (2008). European guidelines for the diagnosis and treatment of pelvic girdle pain. *European Spine Journal, 17*(6), 794–819.

Waldum, H. L., Qvigstad, G., Fossmark, R., Kleveland, P. M., & Sandvik, A. K. (2010). Rebound acid hypersecretion from a physiological, pathophysiological and clinical viewpoint. *Scandinavian Journal of Gastroenterology, 45*(4), 389–394.

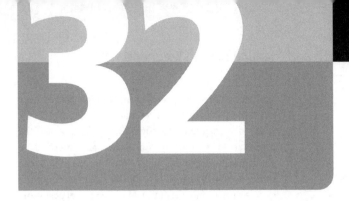

GESTATIONAL DIABETES MELLITUS: EARLY DETECTION AND MANAGEMENT IN PREGNANCY

**Maribeth Inturrisi,
Julio Diaz-Abarca,
and JoAnne M. Saxe**

I. Introduction and general background

Normal pregnancy can be viewed as a progressive condition of insulin resistance, hyperinsulinemia, and mild postprandial hyperglycemia. The mild postprandial hyperglycemia serves to increase the amount of time that maternal glucose levels are elevated above the basal glucose levels after a meal, thereby increasing the flux of ingested nutrients from mother to the fetus and enhancing fetal growth.

During the fasting state (5 hours after food intake), the metabolic processes are relatively the same as the nonpregnant state except that they proceed at an accelerated rate. Because of the hormones of pregnancy, by 10 weeks the fasting blood sugar in the pregnant woman is lower than in a nonpregnant woman. However, in the fed state these same hormones cause a resistance to the cellular uptake of glucose by insulin-sensitive tissue–muscle and fat. This pattern of insulin resistance tends to parallel the growth of the fetal–placental unit and levels of hormones secreted by the placenta. In normal individuals, pancreatic β cells respond to insulin resistance by increasing their insulin output resulting in normal circulating glucose levels.

The fetus does most of its growing during the latter two-thirds of pregnancy. During this time, the fetus is constantly feeding but the mother is alternately fasting and feeding. Glucose is transported across the placenta from the mother by facilitated diffusion. The concentration of glucose within the fetus is lower than maternal glucose.

Insulin does not cross the placenta. The fetus synthesizes its own insulin starting at about 9 weeks of gestation. The fetal β cells, which synthesize insulin for the fetus, respond to both an increase in glucose and amino acids. Spikes in maternal glucose cause spikes in fetal insulin production.

A. Gestational diabetes mellitus: definition and overview

Gestational diabetes mellitus (GDM) has been defined as any degree of glucose intolerance with onset or first recognition during pregnancy with most cases resolving after delivery. Women with GDM cannot overcome the insulin resistance created by these changes in carbohydrate metabolism mediated by placental hormones. These women may increase their insulin production but cannot do so enough to maintain normoglycemia. They may begin to exhaust already impaired β cells, thus accelerating the impairment. It is estimated that women with an abnormal oral glucose tolerance test (OGTT) in pregnancy have at baseline (nonpregnant) impaired function in at least 30–50% of their β cells.

Their fetuses produce insulin in response to the circulating glucose levels. Fetal β cells, in turn, hypertrophy in utero initiating a cascade of abnormal metabolic processes resulting in fetal overgrowth and fetal hyperinsulinemia in the short term and in the long term insulin resistance and early β cell failure (Hillier et al., 2007).

The International Association of Diabetes and Pregnancy Study Groups Consensus Panel (IADPSGCP), including the American Diabetes Association (ADA), recommend that high-risk women (women who are overweight or African-American, Asian/Pacific Islander, East Indian, Hispanic, or Native American) who are found to have diabetes at their initial prenatal visit with the use of standard diagnostic criteria receive a diagnosis of overt, not gestational diabetes (ADA, 2010). In addition, in March 2010, the IADPSGCP set forth global recommendations to change the way GDM is diagnosed. These recommendations are based on data from the randomized prospective double-blinded Hyperglycemia and Adverse Pregnancy Outcomes study (HAPO). The research subjects were 25,000 women from around the globe (The HAPO Study Cooperative Research Group, 2008).

Treatment of gestational diabetes has been shown to reduce serious perinatal morbidity, such as fetal death, macrosomia, birth injury, preeclampsia, and neonatal complications (Crowther et al., 2005; Landon et al., 2009). GDM is optimally managed by referral to a multidisciplinary health education team trained and skilled in the management of diabetes during pregnancy.

B. Prevalence and incidence

Approximately 7% of all pregnancies in the United States (ranging from 1 to 14%) are complicated by diabetes. Although 90% of these pregnant women have GDM, a growing number of women (over 8%) have preexisting type 2 diabetes mellitus (Baptiste-Roberts et al., 2009). As the ongoing epidemic of obesity and the increased ethnic diversity in the United States (African-American, Asian/Pacific Islander, East Indian, Hispanic, and Native American populations) has led to more type 2 diabetes in women of childbearing age, the number of pregnant women with undiagnosed type 2 diabetes has increased.

II. Database (may include but is not limited to)

A global method of diagnosing diabetes has been developed from the results of the HAPO Study (The HAPO Study Cooperative Research Group, 2008). A writing committee from the IADPSGCP (2010) translated the results into a clinical practice guideline for diagnosing diabetes during pregnancy. Both the new method and the current method of diagnosing diabetes are presented.

A. Subjective

1. Screen all women for risk factors for undiagnosed type 2 diabetes and prediabetes at the first prenatal visit

   a. Past health history
      i. Medical illnesses: prediabetes; gestational diabetes; obesity (body mass index > 30); and polycystic ovary syndrome
      ii. Obstetric and gynecological history: macrosomia, unexplained stillbirth, and malformed infant
      iii. Medications: any medications that adversely affect glucose levels (e.g., corticosteroids and progesterone)
   b. Family history of overt diabetes among first-degree relatives
   c. Personal and social history: high-risk ethnic group (African American, American Indian, Hispanic/Latina, Asian/Pacific Islander, South-East Asian, and East Indian, Native American)

2. In the presence of the high-risk factors noted previously, IADPSGCP suggest that women be screened at first booking (preferably with the prenatal panel) to identify undiagnosed prediabetes or diabetes. They also suggest that it may be cost effective in some populations to universally screen women at the first prenatal visit (Figure 32-1). A glycosylated hemoglobin (HbA_{1C}) is the preferred screen by some but any method to diagnose diabetes supported by the ADA can be used (Figure 32-1). If the early screening is negative, obtain OGTT at 24–28 weeks of gestation. IADPSGCP also suggests that it may be beneficial to simply screen all women at first booking.

3. If any risk factors are present, screen using 1-hour 50-g glucose challenge test (GCT) (current protocol) or HbA_{1C} (IADPSGCP Protocol) as soon as possible (this is an early screen).

III. Assessment

A. If the early screening is negative, test at 24–28 weeks, then complete the following protocol

1. Step one
   a. Administer 50 g nonfasting GCT
   b. Any level greater than or equal to 140 mg/dl requires additional follow-up

2. Step two
   a. If the result of the 1-hour screening test is 140–179 mg/dl, order a 3-hour 100-g OGTT
   b. If the glucose loading test is equal to or greater than 180 mg/dl, order a stat fasting blood

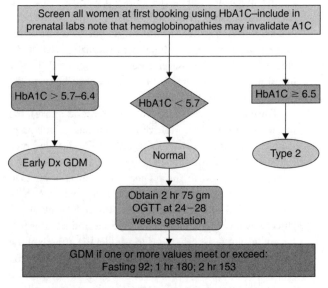

Diagnosing GDM and type 2 during pregnancy algorithm (adapted from IADPSGCP, 2010)

Screen all women at first booking using HbA1C–include in prenatal labs note that hemoglobinopathies may invalidate A1C

HbA1C > 5.7–6.4 → Early Dx GDM

HbA1C < 5.7 → Normal

HbA1C ≥ 6.5 → Type 2

Normal → Obtain 2 hr 75 gm OGTT at 24–28 weeks gestation

GDM if one or more values meet or exceed: Fasting 92; 1 hr 180; 2 hr 153

FIGURE 32-1 Algorithm for Diagnosing Diabetes in Pregnancy
Adapted from IADPSGCP, 2010.

glucose (FBG); if the value is less than 95 mg/dl, perform an OGTT.

i. If FBG value is equal to or greater than 95 mg/dl, do not perform the OGTT; treat as GDM. No OGTT is needed.

ii. Elevated FBG of equal to or greater than 95 mg/dl is diagnostic of GDM. No OGTT is needed.

iii. Any value 200 or above after an OGTT is diagnostic of GDM.

iv. Two values equal to or above cut points = GDM (cut points: FBG, 95 mg/dl; 1-h, 180 mg/dl; 2-h, 155 mg/dl; 3-h, 140 mg/dl) (IADPSGCP Protocol, 2010) (see Figure 32-2).

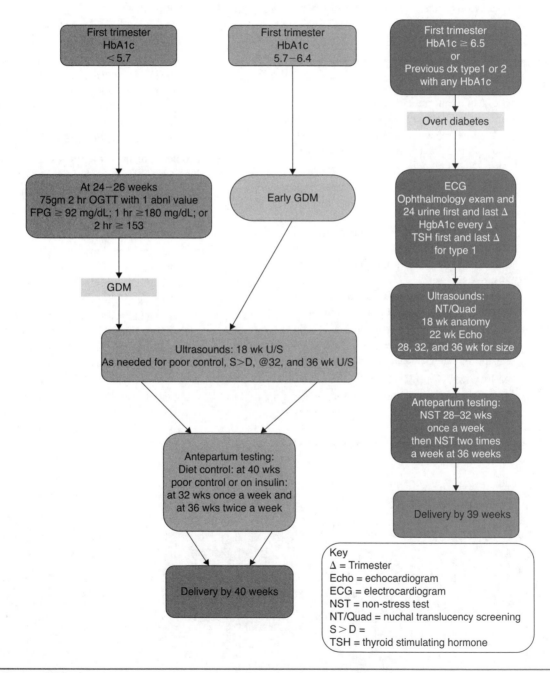

FIGURE 32-2 Hyperglycemia in Pregnancy Management Algorithm

Source: California Diabetes and Pregnancy Program, Sweet Success Region 1 & 3, 2010.

B. *One step process: administer 75-g 2-hour glucose tolerance test (OGTT) to all pregnant women not already diagnosed with diabetes (no GCT)*

1. If one value is equal to or greater than the cut points, the GCM diagnosis is confirmed.

2. Cut points: fasting, 92 mg/dl; 1-h, 180 mg/dl; 2-h, 153 mg/dl

3. Note that this test can be stopped as soon as an abnormal value occurs. It can be scheduled with the third trimester laboratory tests at 26–27 weeks.

IV. Plan

For women who achieve normoglycemia with diet and exercise (also known as GDMA1), educate patients concerning healthy lifestyle behaviors that result in successful self-management of GDM (American Association of Diabetes Educators, 2010).

A. *Successful behaviors*

1. Healthy eating

   a. Refer for education to a registered dietitian concerning healthy eating during pregnancy complicated by diabetes and follow-up every 1–3 weeks.

   b. Prepregnant body mass index should be determined at first visit. Weight gain recommendation is accordingly determined. Weight gain should be followed closely and plotted on the appropriate California Pregnancy Weight Graph (Figure 32-3) (ACOG, 2005).

2. Staying active: recommend and monitor regular exercise of at least 30 minutes per day, such as brisk walking 10 minutes after each meal (ACOG, 2002; California Diabetes and Pregnancy Program, 2008)

3. Monitoring

   a. Review the target blood sugar range (fasting < 90 mg/dl; 1-h post start of meal < 130 mg/dl).

   b. Instruct patient on self-monitoring of blood glucose using home glucometer, test strips, and finger-sticking device.

   c. Teach how to record blood glucose results (Hawkins et al., 2009; California Diabetes and Pregnancy Program, 2008).

4. Healthy coping

   a. Have woman rate her level of stress, discuss coping strategies, refer as needed.

   b. Use a standardized depression screening tool for pregnant women (e.g., Edinburgh Pregnancy Depression Scale [American Academy of Pediatrics, 2010]) in the early third trimester. Note that women with diabetes are at greater risk for depression (ACOG, 2006).

5. Problem solving: teach signs and symptoms of hyperglycemia and hypoglycemia, prevention, and treatment (California Diabetes and Pregnancy Program, 2008).

6. Reducing risks

   a. Review habits, such as smoking, alcohol, and drugs.

   b. Educate concerning tests of fetal well-being. Although kick counts at 28 weeks may be reassuring to the pregnant woman, this assessment has not been shown to predict fetal distress or deaths in average-risk pregnancies (Darby-Stewart, Strickland, & Jamieson, 2009).

   c. If clinically indicated (size greater than dates, poor blood glucose control, refusal of medication) obtain ultrasound at 32–35 weeks. A woman can be allowed a trial of labor for fetus weighing less than 4,500 g (ACOG, 2001).

FIGURE 32-3 *Resources for Professionals*

The prenatal weight gain charts have been updated. The recommended weight at the 13 weeks gestation line is modified because of new guidance from the Institute of Medicine.

- The forms are located at http://www.cdph.ca.gov/pubsforms/forms/Pages/MaternalandChildHealth.aspx .
- CDPH 4472 B1 Prenatal Weight Gain Grid: Pre-pregnancy Underweight Range
- CDPH 4472 B2 Prenatal Weight Gain Grid: Pre-pregnancy Normal Weight Range
- CDPH 4472 B3 Prenatal Weight Gain Grid: Pre-pregnancy Overweight Range
- CDPH 4472 B4 Prenatal Weight Gain Grid: Pre-pregnancy Obese Weight Range

For proper viewing please print CDPH 4472 B1, CDPH 4472 B2 , CDPH 4472 B3 , and CDPH 4472 B4

d. Nonstress tests are not done unless there is the presence of increased blood pressure, macrosomia, history of intrauterine fetal demise, decreased fetal movement, intrauterine growth restriction, poor blood glucose control, taking glucose-lowering medications, or other indications until patient reaches 40 weeks. To continue pregnancy beyond 40 weeks, obtain nonstress test and amniotic fluid index test biweekly (California Diabetes and Pregnancy Program, 2008).

7. Taking medications: if blood glucose values exceed targets (fasting three times in a week, post meal six times in a week consider insulin or oral agent once diet and exercise have been optimized). May require referral to a high-risk program (California Diabetes and Pregnancy Program, 2008). When medication is added to treatment the type of GDM is GDMA2.

B. Postpartum management of GDMA1

1. Test with the 75-g OGTT (fasting plus 2 h postprandial) at 4–6 weeks (ACOG, 2009; The HAPO Study Cooperative Research Group, 2007).

2. Educate patients to get checked for diabetes every year (baby's birthday as a reminder) (The HAPO Study Cooperative Research Group, 2007 & 2008).

3. Preconception and contraception planning. Avoid progesterone-only birth control methods, such as medroxyprogesterone (Depoprovera), etonogestrel (Implanon), and progesterone-only pills because these have been found to increase the conversion rate of GDM to type 2 diabetes in Hispanic women who were breastfeeding (The HAPO Study Cooperative Research Group, 2007; California Diabetes and Pregnancy Program, 2008).

4. Strongly encourage breastfeeding (The HAPO Study Cooperative Research Group, 2007).

C. Resources for patients

1. American Diabetes Association:
   (800) 342-2383,
   www.diabetes.org

2. American Association of Diabetes Educators:
   (800) 338-DMED,
   www.aadenet.org

3. Centers for Disease Control and Prevention. Division of Diabetes Translation:
   (877) 232-3422,
   www.cdc.gov/diabetes

4. Sweet Success: California's Diabetes and Pregnancy Program:
   www.cdph.ca.gov/programs/cdapp

REFERENCES

American Academy of Pediatrics. (2010). Edinburgh postnatal depression scale. *Developmental Pediatrics Online.* Retrieved from http://www.dbpeds.org/articles/detail.cfm?TextID=485

American Association of Diabetes Educators. (2010). *AADE 7 self-care behaviors.* Retrieved from http://www.diabeteseducator.org/ProfessionalResources/AADE7/

American College of Obstetricians and Gynecologists. (2001). ACOG Practice Bulletin. Clinical management guidelines for obstetrician-gynecologists. Number 30, September 2001 (replaces Technical Bulletin Number 200, December 1994). Gestational diabetes. *Obstetrics & Gynecology, 98*(3), 525–538.

American College of Obstetricians and Gynecologists. (2002). ACOG Committee opinion. Number 267, January 2002: Exercise during pregnancy and the postpartum period. *Obstetrics & Gynecology, 99*(1), 171–173.

American College of Obstetricians and Gynecologists. (2005). ACOG Committee Opinion Number 315, September 2005. Obesity in pregnancy. *Obstetrics & Gynecology, 106*(3), 671–675.

American College of Obstetricians and Gynecologists. (2006). ACOG Committee Opinion No. 343: Psychosocial risk factors: Perinatal screening and intervention. *Obstetrics & Gynecology, 108*(2), 469–477.

American College of Obstetricians and Gynecologists. (2009). ACOG Committee Opinion No. 435: Postpartum screening for abnormal glucose tolerance in women who had gestational diabetes mellitus. *Obstetrics & Gynecology, 113*(6), 1419–1421.

American Diabetes Association. (2010). Position Statement: Diagnosis and classification of diabetes mellitus. *Diabetes Care, 32*(Suppl.), S63–S69.

Baptiste-Roberts, K., Barone, B. B., Gary, T. L., Golden, S. H., Wilson, L. M., Bass, E. B., & Nicholson, W. K. (2009). Risk factors for type 2 diabetes among women with gestational diabetes: A systematic review. *American Journal of Medicine, 122*(3), 207–214, e4.

California Diabetes and Pregnancy Program. (2008). *Sweet success diabetes and pregnancy pocket guide for providers.* San Diego, CA: State of California: Department of Public Health, Maternal and Child Health Division.

California Diabetes and Pregnancy Program. (2010). *Sweet success hyperglycemia in pregnancy management algorithm.* State of California: Department of Public Health, Maternal and Child Health Division, Region 1 & 3.

Crowther, C., Hiller, J., Moss, J., McPhee, A., Jeffries, W., & Robinson, J. (2005). Effect of treatment of gestational diabetes mellitus on pregnancy outcomes from the Australian carbohydrate intolerance study in pregnant women (ACHOIS) trial. *New England Journal of Medicine, 352*(24), 2477–2486.

Darby-Stewart, A. L., Strickland, C., & Jamieson, B. (2009). Do abnormal fetal kick counts predict intrauterine death in average-risk pregnancies? *The Journal of Family Practice, 58*(4), 220a–220c.

Hawkins, J. S., Casey, B. M., Lo, J. Y., Moss, K., McIntire, D. D., & Leveno, K. J. (2009). Weekly compared with daily blood glucose monitoring in women with diet-treated gestational diabetes. *Obstetrics & Gynecology, 113*(6), 1307–1312.

Hillier, T. A., Pedula, K. L., Schmidt, M. M., Mullen, J. A., Charles, M. A., & Pettitt, D. J. (2007). Childhood obesity and metabolic imprinting: The ongoing effects of maternal hyperglycemia. *Diabetes Care, 30*(9), 2287–2292.

International Association of Diabetes and Pregnancy Study Groups Consensus Panel (IADPSGCP), The HAPO Study Cooperative

Research Group, Metzger, B. E., Gabbe, S. G., Persson, B., Buchanan, T. A., Catalano, P. A. . . . Damm, P. (2010). International Association of Diabetes and Pregnancy Study Groups recommendations on the diagnosis and classification of hyperglycemia in pregnancy. *Diabetes Care, 33*(3), 676–682.

Landon, M. B., Spong, C. Y., Thom, E., Carpenter, M. W., Ramin, S. M. . . . Casey, B. (2009). A multicenter, randomized trial of treatment for mild gestational diabetes. *New England Journal of Medicine, 361*(14), 1339–1348.

The HAPO Study Cooperative Research Group, Metzger, B. E., Buchanan, T. A., Coustan, D. R., de Leiva, A., Dunger, D. B. . . . Hadden, D. R. (2007). Summary and recommendations of the fifth international workshop-conference on gestational diabetes mellitus. *Diabetes Care, 30*(Suppl. 2), S251–S260.

The HAPO Study Cooperative Research Group, Metzger, B. E., Lowe, L. P., Dyer, A. R., Trimble, E. R., Chaovarinder, U. . . . Coustan, D. R. (2008). Hyperglycemia and adverse pregnancy outcomes. *New England Journal of Medicine, 358*(19):1991–2002.

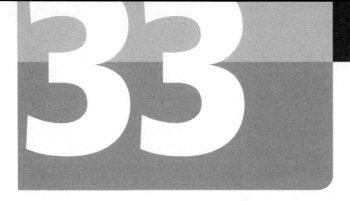

PREECLAMPSIA

Jenna Shaw-Battista

I. Introduction and general background

Preeclampsia occurs in 2–8% of pregnancies and is diagnosed in the presence of proteinuria and gestational hypertension (American College of Obstetricians and Gynecologists, 2002; National High Blood Pressure Education Program, 2000). Proteinuria is typically defined as greater than or equal to 300 mg of protein in a 24-hour urine specimen. Gestational hypertension occurs after 20 weeks and is defined as a systolic blood pressure reading of greater than or equal to 140 mm Hg or diastolic blood pressure of greater than or equal to 90 mm Hg, observed on at least two occasions greater than 6 hours apart. Preeclampsia and gestational hypertension may be superimposed on chronic hypertension. About 25% of women with gestational hypertension later develop proteinuria (i.e., preeclampsia).

When mild gestational hypertension or preeclampsia is diagnosed at or near term, significant perinatal complications are unlikely. Mild preeclampsia is not associated with increased perinatal death, preterm birth, small for gestational age infants, or placental abruption (Sibai, 2003). However, maternal and neonatal morbidities are likely to result from severe gestational hypertension or preeclampsia, particularly before 32–35 weeks of gestation.

A combination of hypertension and proteinuria indicates progression of the disease process, as does end-organ involvement evidenced by abnormal laboratory values, physical examination findings, and patient symptomatology. Preeclampsia is progressive and may induce eclamptic seizures, which are strongly associated with poor perinatal outcomes including maternal and fetal death (Sibai, 2005).

The etiology of preeclampsia–eclampsia is largely unknown, although abnormal placentation is implicated as are immunologic factors and inflammatory vascular processes. There are no preventative measures with demonstrable efficacy in both low- and high-risk women. However, some study findings suggest that oral calcium supplementation may reduce incidence among women with poor dietary intake and risk factors for the disease (Rath & Fischer, 2009; Sibai, 1998 & 2003). Similarly, low-dose aspirin therapy during the first 16–24 weeks of gestation may be marginally efficacious at preventing recurrence among women with a history of the disorder (Rath & Fischer, 2009; Sibai, 1998 & 2003). Although these measures do not seem to exert a significant protective effect, particularly in mixed-risk populations, in select individuals they may reduce disease morbidity if not incidence.

Similarly, early detection and management can reduce adverse perinatal outcomes and may improve long-term cardiovascular health (Sibai, 2003). Preeclampsia–eclampsia is associated with increased relative risks for chronic hypertension, ischemic heart disease, venous thromboembolism, stroke, and mortality 5–15 years after the affected pregnancy (Bellamy, Casas, Hingorami, & Williams, 2007).

II. Database (may include but is not limited to)

A. Subjective

Assess for the presence of risk factors.

1. Past health history
   a. Medical illnesses: obesity and chronic renal, vascular, or autoimmune disease, such as essential (chronic) hypertension, diabetes, systemic lupus erythematosus, and antiphospholipid syndrome
   b. Obstetric and gynecological history: first pregnancy, extremes of childbearing age, and multiple gestation

2. Family history: hypertensive disorder in pregnancy

3. Personal and social history: African American descent

4. Review of systems
   a. Constitutional signs and symptoms: complaint of feeling unwell (e.g., fatigued, malaise, dizzy, light-headed, anxious, or confused)
   b. Skin: unexplained ecchymosis
   c. Eyes: visual disturbances including blurred vision, "spots," "stars," "flashing lights," or blindness (indicative of retinal detachment)
   d. Respiratory and cardiovascular: shortness of breath or dyspnea (may indicate concomitant pulmonary edema); increased swelling, particularly facial or periorbital

e. Gastrointestinal: pain in the right upper quadrant of the abdomen, heartburn, nausea or vomiting

f. Genitourinary: decreased urinary output, decreased fetal movement, vaginal bleeding (may indicate abruption placentae resulting from severe hypertension)

g. Neurologic: headaches, particularly new onset; increased severity or frequency. Headaches associated with preeclampsia are often frontal or occipital. Paresthesia of hands, feet, or extremities (may accompany significant edema); report of seizure; or loss of consciousness

B. Objective

1. Vital signs

    a. Blood pressure greater than or equal to 140/90 mm Hg on at least two occasions more than 4–6 hours apart. Blood pressure should be measured with the woman in an upright or sitting position using an appropriately sized sphygmomanometer cuff. The cuff length should be at least 1.5 times the circumference of the woman's upper arm and the cuff bladder should cover at least 80% of the arm circumference (American College of Obstetricians and Gynecologists, 2002).

    b. Rapid and excessive weight gain (> 2 pounds per week)

2. Skin examination: petechiae, ecchymosis, or jaundice (may be present with hemolysis or thrombocytopenia)

3. Cardiovascular examination: generalized edema, particularly facial or periorbital, with or without pitting

4. Abdominal examination

    a. Liver may be enlarged

    b. Right upper quadrant abdominal pain

5. Genitourinary and pelvic examination

    a. Proteinuria: more than 1+ protein on macrourinalysis with a clean, midstream sample

    b. Fundal height less than expected for gestational age

6. Neurologic examination: hyperreflexia, with or without clonus

III. Assessment

A. Determine the diagnosis

The diagnosis of preeclampsia requires gestational hypertension and proteinuria. If criteria are not met, the differential diagnosis should include but is not limited to impending or atypical preeclampsia, chronic or gestational hypertension, liver or renal disease, and substance use (Stella & Sibai, 2009). Similarly, HELLP syndrome should be considered, especially when hemolysis (H), elevated liver enzyme levels (EL), or low platelet counts (LP) are observed.

B. Severity

The American College of Obstetricians and Gynecologists (2002, p. 68) describes preeclampsia as severe if one or more of the following criteria are met

1. Blood pressure of greater than or equal to 160 mm Hg systolic or greater than or equal to 110 mm Hg diastolic on two occasions at least 6 hours apart while the patient is on bed rest.

2. Proteinuria of greater than or equal to 5 g in a 24-hour urine specimen, or greater than or equal to 3+ on macro-urine analysis of two random urine samples collected via clean catch or catheter at least 4 hours apart.

3. Oliguria of less than 500 ml in 24 hours.

4. Cerebral or visual disturbances

5. Pulmonary edema or cyanosis

6. Epigastric or right upper quadrant abdominal pain

7. Impaired liver function

8. Thrombocytopenia

9. Fetal growth restriction

IV. Plan

A. Diagnostic tests

1. Repeat blood pressure assessment

    After a 10–30 minute rest period with the patient in an upright or sitting position, use an appropriately sized sphygmomanometer cuff to repeat the blood pressure assessment. Two or more elevated readings, greater than 6 hours apart, are diagnostic of gestational hypertension.

2. Obtain clean midstream urine sample.

    Assess for more than 1+ protein on macro-urinalysis if not previously done. Consider culture and sensitivity to rule out urinary tract infection if proteinuria is present.

3. Initiate 24-hour urine collection to assess for proteinuria if the urine dipstick is greater than 1+ protein and patient is hypertensive.

    Twenty-four hour urine samples with greater than or equal to 300–499 mg of protein are indicative of mild preeclampsia, whereas greater than or equal to

500 mg is suggestive of severe disease (American College of Obstetricians and Gynecologists, 2002).

Serum protein/creatinine ratio is currently being investigated as a proxy for proteinuria assessment via burdensome 24-hour urine collection. A protein/creatinine ratio greater than or equal to 600 mg/g is highly predictive of proteinuria but any level greater than or equal to 150 mg/g should be evaluated further using 24-hour urine specimens (Papanna, Mann, Kouids & Glantz, 2008).

4. Order serum complete blood count with platelets, and liver function panel including aspartate aminotransferase, alanine aminotransferase, serum protein, and creatinine. Although commonly ordered, uric acid has a 33% positive predictive value and is not a useful diagnostic tool (American College of Obstetricians and Gynecologists, 2002). With abnormal liver function and significant proteinuria (particularly ≥ 500 mg on 24-hour specimen) severe preeclampsia is present and women should be evaluated for elevated transaminase and oliguria (< 500 ml urine output in 24 h).

B. Treatment and follow-up

1. Fetal surveillance and management (American College of Obstetricians and Gynecologists, 2002; National High Blood Pressure Education Program, 2000)

   a. In cases of mild preeclampsia, weekly nonstress tests or biophysical profiles are recommended. Biweekly testing should be ordered for severe preeclampsia, oligohydramnios, and suspected fetal growth restriction before formal diagnosis. In these circumstances, immediate consultation and referral are indicated and delivery may be expedited.

   b. Ultrasound assessments of fetal growth and amniotic fluid indices are recommended at less than or equal to 3-week intervals.

2. Maternal surveillance and management (American College of Obstetricians and Gynecologists, 2002; National High Blood Pressure Education Program, 2000)

   a. There is no consensus about appropriate blood pressure surveillance, although evaluation every 1–7 days is commonly performed.

   b. In cases of mild preeclampsia without worsening symptomatology, laboratory testing may be repeated weekly. If disease stage and progression are questionable, diagnostics may be repeated at shorter intervals.

   c. If liver function studies worsen and/or platelet counts decrease over time, diagnose severe preeclampsia and order coagulation studies.

   d. In cases of severe preeclampsia, medical consultation and referral are immediately indicated. Inpatient maternal surveillance may be initiated, and the delivery may be expedited.

   e. Antihypertensive agents are commonly prescribed although supportive data are few, particularly for mild preeclampsia (Sibai, 2003). Antihypertensive agents may reduce disease progression but there is little evidence that perinatal outcomes are improved (Magee et al., 2009; Sibai, 2003). Severe hypertension (blood pressure ≥ 160/110) should be treated, particularly in women who are remote from term (Magee et al., 2009; Sibai, 2003).

   f. There is no compelling evidence that bed rest effectively reduces disease progression or improves perinatal outcomes. However, the left lateral recumbent position may optimize uterine, placental, and fetal circulation and should be encouraged, particularly if significant edema is present.

   g. Consider home blood pressure monitoring and recording if women with mild preeclampsia are being managed on an outpatient basis.

   h. During return visits

      i. Review and record home blood pressure readings if previously ordered

      ii. Assess current blood pressure

      iii. Perform macro-urinalysis to detect the presence of proteinuria; consider using a urine sample obtained via bladder catheter

      iv. Repeat laboratory diagnostics as previously described

      v. Evaluate fundal height and fetal heart tones

      vi. Assess for edema, liver enlargement, and hyperreflexia

      vii. Review fetal movement, danger signs and symptoms, and parameters for acute reevaluation

      viii. Ongoing medical consultation about evolving patient condition and collaborative management plan

      ix. Ensure patient has appointments for subsequent fetal and maternal surveillance as previously described

C. Patient education

1. Teach the woman how to perform kick counts twice daily after 28 weeks gestation. Instruct her to notify providers if fewer than 10 fetal movements are felt in a 2-hour period, preferably when she is at rest following a meal.

2. If home blood pressure monitoring is initiated, teach the woman how to use the machine and

record values. Instruct her to immediately report critical values ($\geq 160/110$ mm Hg).

3. Discuss self-care including nutrition, hydration, stress management, and relaxation.

4. Provide anticipatory guidance about disease progression and both immediate and long-term sequelae.

5. Review research that supports vaginal delivery at term for women with mild preeclampsia and provide anticipatory guidance regarding induction of labor. For women with severe preeclampsia, discuss data favorably comparing induction of labor to scheduled cesarean section and encourage individualized care-planning with medical providers (American College of Obstetricians and Gynecologists, 2002).

D. Consultation and referral

Refer to Chapter 28, Guidelines for Medical Consultation and Referral During Pregnancy. Physician consultation is indicated for suspected or documented preeclampsia of any severity. In some interprofessional practices, mild gestational hypertension and preeclampsia are independently managed by nurse-practitioners or nurse-midwives with physician consultation, or collaboratively managed on either an inpatient or outpatient basis. Severe preeclampsia generally warrants immediate referral to physician care within a maternal–fetal medicine specialty service.

REFERENCES

American College of Obstetricians and Gynecologists. (2002). ACOG practice bulletin. Diagnosis and management of preeclampsia and eclampsia, Number 33. *International Journal of Gynecology and Obstetrics, 77*(1), 67–75.

Bellamy, L., Casas, J. P., Hingorami, A. D., & Williams, D. (2007). Preeclampsia and risk of cardiovascular disease and cancer in later life: Systematic review and meta-analysis. *British Medical Journal (Clinical Research Edition), 335*(7627), 974–982.

Magee, L. A., Abalos, E., von Dadelszen, P., Sibai, B., Walkinshaw, S. A., & CHIPS Study Group (2009). Control of hypertension in pregnancy. *Current Hypertension Reports, 11*(6), 429–436.

National High Blood Pressure Education Program. (2000). Report of the National High Blood Pressure Education Program working group on high blood pressure in pregnancy. *American Journal of Obstetrics and Gynecology, 183*(1), S1–S22.

Papanna, R., Mann, L. K., Kouids, R. W., & Glantz, J. C. (2008). Protein/creatinine ratio in preeclampsia. *Obstetrics & Gynecology, 112*(1), 135–144.

Rath, W., & Fischer, T. (2009). The diagnosis and treatment of hypertensive disorders of pregnancy: New findings for antenatal and inpatient care. *Deutsches Ärzteblatt International, 106*(45), 733–738.

Sibai, B. M. (1998). Prevention of preeclampsia: A big disappointment. *American Journal of Obstetrics & Gynecology, 179*, 1275–1278.

Sibai, B. M. (2003). Diagnosis and management of gestational hypertension and preeclampsia. *Obstetrics & Gynecology, 102*(1), 181–192.

Sibai, B. M. (2005). Diagnosis, prevention, and management of eclampsia. *Obstetrics & Gynecology, 105*(2), 402–410.

Stella, C. L., & Sibai, B. M. (2009). Diagnosis and management of atypical preeclampsia-eclampsia. *American Journal of Obstetrics and Gynecology, 200*(5), 481–487.

PRENATAL GENETIC DIAGNOSIS

Deborah Anderson and Amy J. Levi

I. Introduction and general background

Invasive prenatal diagnosis allows for the identification of fetal chromosomal abnormalities. It is available to all pregnant women regardless of age. A woman's decision to have prenatal diagnosis is a very personal decision and is based on many factors. Considerations may include the anticipated risk that the fetus will have an abnormality, gestational age of the fetus, previous obstetric history, risk of pregnancy loss from an invasive procedure, feelings about having a child with a chromosomal abnormality, and beliefs about termination. Chorionic villus sampling (CVS) and amniocentesis are the most common methods of invasive prenatal diagnosis.

A. Chorionic villus sampling

Under ultrasound guidance, a small sample of the placenta is obtained through a transcervical or transabdominal route.

1. Timing of test: 9 completed weeks of gestation to 14 weeks of gestation

2. Risks

    a. Risk rates approach or may be the same as amniocentesis (see amniocentesis).

    b. Amniotic fluid leak or infection, vaginal bleeding, or cell culture failure.

3. Benefits

    a. Because CVS is generally performed in the first trimester it allows for earlier diagnosis compared to amniocentesis.

    b. Results are usually available 1–2 weeks after the procedure.

B. Amniocentesis

Under ultrasound guidance a small amount of amniotic fluid is aspirated via a transabdominal puncture of the uterus and amnion.

1. Timing of test: 15–20 weeks gestation

2. Risks

    a. Procedure-related loss is 1 in 300–500, depending on provider.

    b. Amniotic fluid leakage or rupture, transient vaginal spotting, chorioamnionitis, rare needle injury to fetus, and failure of amniotic fluid cell culture.

3. Benefits

    a. Results are usually available 1–2 weeks after the procedure.

    b. Cytogenetic diagnostic accuracy is greater than 99%.

C. Cordocentesis (also known as percutaneous umbilical blood sampling)

With cordocentesis fetal blood sampling is obtained with puncture of the umbilical vein under ultrasound guidance. It is used to further evaluate abnormal chromosomal findings and is rarely needed.

1. Risks: procedure-related pregnancy loss rate is less than 2%

2. Benefits: karyotype analysis of fetal blood is available in 7–10 days

II. Database

A. Subjective

1. Identify genetic indications for prenatal diagnosis

    a. Chromosomal abnormality in previous offspring, parent, or close relative

    b. Structural anomalies identified by ultrasound examination

    c. History of previous fetus or child with any chromosome abnormality

    d. Parental carrier of chromosome translocation or chromosome inversion

    e. Parental aneuploidy or mosaicism for aneuploidy

    f. Abnormal prenatal screening test results

    g. Both parents are carriers of mendelian conditions, such as cystic fibrosis, hemophilia, muscular dystrophy, or hemoglobinopathies

    h. Both parents are carriers of inborn errors of metabolism, such as Tay-Sachs disease, mucopolysaccharidoses, or peroxisomal diseases

i. Age: according to American College of Obstetricians and Gynecologists guidelines (2007), all women regardless of age should have the option for genetic screening or diagnostic testing. Advanced maternal age (35 years old) alone is no longer used as a determining factor for who is offered invasive prenatal diagnostic testing. Prenatal screening tests do not detect other forms of aneuploidy that occur with advancing maternal age, such as trisomy 13 and Klinefelter syndrome; these may be detected with invasive testing, CVS, or amniocentesis.

B. Objective
1. Dating by ultrasound confirms estimated date of delivery.

III. Assessment

A. Patient desires CVS or amniocentesis

B. Patient declines CVS or amniocentesis

IV. Plan

A. Diagnosis
1. Refer women who choose CVS or amniocentesis for procedure during appropriate time periods.

B. Education
1. Review the risks and benefits of procedures and compare to screening tests.
2. For women with positive results, refer for further genetic counseling.
3. Consider referral to social workers, parent support networks, clergy, and therapeutic counselors for further support and information.

C. Medication
1. Rh-negative nonsensitized women need $Rh_o(D)$ immune globulin (RhoGam) administration after CVS or amniocentesis.

REFERENCE

American College of Obstetricians and Gynecologists. (2007, December). ACOG Practice Bulletin Number 88. Invasive prenatal testing for aneuploidy. *Obstetrics & Gynecology, 110*(6), 1459–1467.

PRETERM LABOR MANAGEMENT

Mary Barger

I. Introduction and general background

Prematurity, which occurs in one out of eight births in the United States, is the leading cause of infant and neonatal mortality. The birth of a premature infant can lead to long-term health consequences, such as cerebral palsy and lung, hearing, and vision problems, and new evidence shows an increase in adult diseases, such as cardiovascular disease and diabetes. Unfortunately, there are large differences in the burden of prematurity by race and ethnicity with African Americans having the highest rate. Premature births (PTB) have a large economic impact of healthcare costs averaging more than $50,000 in medical costs per premature infant and 10 times the medical expenses in the first year of life compared to term infants (Behrman & Butler, 2007).

A. Definition

A PTB is any birth that occurs after 20 weeks gestation and before 37 completed weeks of gestation. PTB are further classified into "very PTB," which are those that occur before 32 completed weeks of gestation, and "late PTB," between 34 and 36 weeks gestation.

B. Prevalence and incidence

Over the last 25 years in the United States the PTB rate has increased nearly 40% to its present rate of 12.7%, 5% points higher than the Healthy People 2010 goal of 7.6% (Hamilton, Martin, & Ventura, 2009). Some of this increase is caused by the increasing number of multiple births (2.4% in 1992 to 3.3% in 2005), because 50% of twins and more than 90% of higher-order multiple pregnancies result in a preterm birth (Hamilton et al., 2009). Another source of the increase is a larger number of late

PTB, which have accounted for the shifting of the distribution of gestational ages at birth by a full week less (Martin, Kirmeyer, Osterman, & Shepherd, 2009). There are significant race and ethnicity differences for PTB, with African Americans having a 70% higher rate than Asians, who have the lowest rate (18.3% and 10.7%, respectively).

Two-thirds of PTB are spontaneous and the other one-third is for indicated reasons. It has been noted that as the rate of indicated late PTB increased, the rate in stillbirths has decreased.

II. Database (may include but is not limited to)

A. Subjective

1. Reproductive history

   a. Previous PTB: risk of PTB in a subsequent pregnancy after one previous PTB in a singleton pregnancy is 15%, which increases to 33% with two previous PTBs and is 24% if a woman had a term pregnancy followed by a PTB (Adams, Elam-Evans, Wilson, & Gilbertz, 2000). This is the most important risk factor for PTB.

   b. One or more second-trimester abortions

2. Gynecological history

   a. Presence of a uterine malformation

   b. Previous cervical cone biopsy or excision with loop electrosurgical excision procedure

   c. In utero exposure to diethylstilbestrol

3. Medical history which puts a woman more at risk for indicated preterm birth

   a. Diabetes, not well controlled especially pre-conception

   b. Hypertension

   c. Asthma, if chronic

   d. Seizure disorder

4. Pregnancy history and personal habits for the respective pregnancy

   a. Multiple gestation

   b. Polyhydramnios or oliogohydramnios

   c. Abdominal surgery after 18 weeks gestation or cervical surgery

   d. Vaginal bleeding in more than one trimester

   e. Pregnancy as a result of assisted reproductive technology

   f. Presence of a fetus with a congenital anomaly

   g. Interpregnancy interval of less than 6 months

   h. Body mass index less than 19

i. Smoking more than 10 cigarettes a day
j. Cocaine use
k. Febrile illness
l. High social stress
m. Cervical length on mid-trimester ultrasound less than 15–25 mm

5. Presence of signs or symptoms of preterm labor

a. Uterine contractions that are frequently painless
b. Back pain, constant or intermittent
c. Menstrual-type cramping
d. Pelvic pressure
e. Change in vaginal discharge
f. Vaginal spotting or bleeding (bloody show)

B. Objective

1. Note if febrile

2. Palpate abdomen and uterus for tenderness and presence of contractions

3. Perform gentle speculum examination to obtain fetal fibronectin (fFN) specimen (this must be done before any examination of the cervix and other vaginal or cervical cultures)

4. Check cervix for position; consistency; dilation; effacement (length); and station of presenting part

5. Assess urine for nitrites and leukocytes; and culture and sensitivity if with signs and symptoms of preterm labor.

III. Assessment

A. At risk for preterm labor

B. Threatened preterm labor

IV. Plan

A. Women at risk for preterm labor

1. Screen all pregnant women for asymptomatic bacteriuria at initial presentation and treat if positive urine culture to prevent pyelonephritis

2. If body mass index is less than 19, ensure the woman knows the recommended weight gain in pregnancy and refer to a nutritionist if needed

3. Ensure women eat a Mediterranean-type diet low in fat and processed food, rich in fruits and vegetables, and two servings of fatty fish a week or take omega-3 supplements of 1–1.5 g/d. Women eating this way decreased their risk of PTB at 90% (Khoury, Henriksen, Christophersen, & Tonstad, 2005).

4. Ensure women have adequate levels of vitamin D either through sun exposure or supplementation. Prevalence of inadequate vitamin D (< 20 ng/mL) in pregnant women in the United States ranges between 13% for whites and 80% for non-Hispanic blacks (Ginde, Sullivan, Mansbach, & Camargo Jr., 2010). A recent randomized clinical trial showed a 50% reduction in PTB in pregnant women supplemented with 4,000 IU of vitamin D_3 compared to those taking the current recommended amount of 400 IU per day (Hollis & Wagner, 2009).

5. Offer screening to women with a prior PTB at initial visit for bacterial vaginosis and treat as indicated. Note that the US Preventive Services Task Force recommends against screening asymptomatic low-risk women but states the evidence is conflicting for high-risk women, although it will probably cause no harm (US Preventive Services Task Force, 2008).

6. Refer women who smoke to a smoking cessation program.

7. Refer women using cocaine for drug treatment.

8. Consult after the first prenatal visit regarding prophylactic progesterone therapy on women with a history of a previous PTB in a singleton pregnancy (ACOG Committee Opinion, 2008).

9. Obtain a second-trimester ultrasound for cervical length. Consult with a physician if the cervix is less than 25 mm (Crane & Hutchens, 2008).

10. Perform cervical examinations at visits starting at 28 weeks or at the time preterm labor started in a previous pregnancy or with symptoms.

B. Women with signs and symptoms of preterm labor

1. Obtain a clean catch urine and complete a macro-urinalysis and micro-urinalysis with culture and sensitivity, if indicated, to rule out a urinary tract infection.

2. Perform an abdominal examination for contractions and tenderness; use a toco monitor to detect the presence of contractions, if available in the setting.

3. Depending on setting

a. Refer to a birthing unit for further evaluation

b. If the woman will be observed in the ambulatory setting

    i. First, obtain a posterior fornix sample for fFN

    ii. Obtain a sample for group B streptococcus, if not previously obtained, and other samples as indicated for vaginal infections

    iii. Then, perform a digital cervical examination

    iv. Observe the woman and after 2 hours recheck her cervix

        a. If she meets the criteria for preterm labor, refer her to a birthing unit for further evaluation with fFN swab that was obtained.

        b. Diagnostic criteria for preterm labor

            i. Gestational age 20–36 weeks, and

            ii. Documented regular contractions, and

            iii. One of the following: rupture of membranes, documented cervical change, cervical dilation greater than or equal to 2 cm or cervical effacement greater than or equal to 80%.

c. If no cervical change and no uterine contractions after a 2-hour observation, then educate regarding the signs and symptoms of preterm labor and criteria for calling the healthcare provider.

REFERENCES

ACOG Committee Opinion. (2008). Use of progesterone to reduce preterm birth. *Obstetrics & Gynecology, 112,* 963–965.

Adams, M. M., Elam-Evans, L. D., Wilson, H. G., & Gilbertz, D. A. (2000). Rates of and factors associated with recurrence of preterm delivery. *Journal of the American Medical Association, 283,* 1591–1596.

Behrman, R., & Butler, A. S. (Eds.). (2007). *Preterm birth: Causes, consequences, and prevention.* Institute of Medicine committee on Understanding Premature Birth and Assuring Healthy Outcomes. Washington, DC: National Academies Press.

Crane, J. M., & Hutchens, D. (2008). Transvaginal sonographic measurement of cervical length to predict preterm birth in asymptomatic women at increased risk: A systematic review. *Ultrasound Obstetrics and Gynecology, 31,* 579–587.

Ginde, A. A., Sullivan, A. F., Mansbach, J. M., & Camargo Jr., C. A. (2010). Vitamin D insufficiency in pregnant and non-pregnant women of childbearing age in the U.S. *American Journal of Obstetrics and Gynecology, 202,* e1–e8.

Hamilton, B. E., Martin, J. A., & Ventura, S. A. (2009). Births: Preliminary data from 2007. *National Vital Statistics Report, 57,* 1–23.

Hollis, B. W., & Wagner, C. L. (2009). Randomized trial of vitamin D and perinatal outcomes. In the *14th Workshop on Vitamin D.* October 4-8, 2009. Brugge, Belgium.

Khoury, J., Henriksen, T., Christophersen, B., & Tonstad, S. (2005). Effect of a cholesterol-lowering diet on maternal, cord, and neonatal lipids, and pregnancy outcome: A randomized clinical trial. *American Journal of Obstetrics and Gynecology, 193,* 1292–1301.

Martin, J. A., Kirmeyer, S., Osterman, M., & Shepherd, R. A. (2009). Born a bit too early: Recent trends in late preterm births. *NCHS Data Brief, 24,* 1–8.

US Preventive Services Task Force. (2008). Screening for bacterial vaginosis in pregnancy to prevent preterm delivery: US Preventive Services Task Force recommendation statement. *Annals Internal Medicine, 148,* 214–219.

URINARY TRACT INFECTION: PREVENTION AND MANAGEMENT IN PREGNANCY

Mary Barger

I. Introduction and general background

Both the physiologic and anatomic pregnancy changes in the urinary tract make it easier for bacteria from the bladder to ascend into the kidneys. Clinically, this means that pregnant women with bacteria in their bladders, whether symptomatic (cystitis) or asymptomatic (asymptomatic bacteriuria [ASB]), are more prone to pyelonephritis. This may pose a problem in pregnancy because pyelonephritis may be a risk factor for preterm labor. Bacteria in urine of pregnant women were found to be a risk factor for both preterm birth and increased perinatal mortality in the Comprehensive Perinatal Study (Zinner & Kass, 1971; Naeye, 1979) and more recently in a population-based study of nearly 200,000 births (Mazor-Dray, Levy, Schlaeffer, & Sheiner, 2009). However, a Cochrane review of 14 randomized trials comparing antibiotic treatment to placebo for ASB in pregnancy, of which the overall quality of the studies was rated as poor, showed antibiotic therapy to be effective in prevention of pyelonephritis (odds ratio, 0.23; 95% confidence interval, 0.13–0.41) and reduced the low birthweight rate (odds ratio, 0.66; 95% confidence interval, 0.49–0.89) but did not show a difference in preterm births (Smaill & Vasquez, 2007).

A. Asymptomatic bacteriuria

ASB is defined by a mid-stream urine culture with 100,000 colonies/mL of a single organism or 100 or more colonies from urine obtained from a catheter specimen without any accompanying cystitis symptoms. It occurs in 4–6% of childbearing women (Hooton et al., 2000). Women with a history of recurrent or persistent urinary tract infections (UTIs), diabetes, low socioeconomic status, and who are multiparous are at increased risk for ASB. In pregnancy, 25–40% of women with untreated ASB develop pyelonephritis.

B. Urinary tract infection

The presence of a UTI in pregnancy meets the definition of a "complicated UTI" because of the increased risk for it to develop into pyelonephritis. Therefore, a pregnant woman presenting with cystitis symptoms, pyuria, and who has 100 or more colonies/mL of a single organism on a mid-stream urine culture should be treated using the management strategies for a complicated UTI (e.g., using longer doses of antibiotics and following-up with a urine culture for a test of cure).

II. Database (may include but is not limited to)

A. Subjective

1. Medical history
   a. UTI: number and precipitating factors (e.g., associated with coitus)
   b. Pyelonephritis
   c. Urinary tract abnormality (e.g., single kidney or displaced kidneys)
   d. Diabetes
   e. Immunosuppression
   f. Sickle cell hemoglobinopathy, especially with other risk factors. Note that although women with sickle cell are at increased risk for pyelonephritis, newer data show that they are not at increased risk for ASB (Thurman, Steed, Hulsey, & Soper, 2006).

2. Reproductive history
   a. Parity
   b. Pyelonephritis in a previous pregnancy
   c. UTI in a previous pregnancy

3. Presence of signs or symptoms of cystitis
   a. Abrupt onset of urinary frequency and dysuria
   b. Suprapubic or low back pain

c. Flank pain (unusual)

d. Presence of vaginal discharge or irritation (decreases the likelihood of cystitis)

4. Presence of signs of pyelonephritis: signs of cystitis plus at least one of the following

a. Fever and chills

b. Nausea and vomiting

c. Flank pain

B. Objective

1. For diagnosis of ASB: culture urine on all pregnant women at 12–16 weeks or with initial prenatal visit if later (Lin & Fajardo, 2008).

2. Women presenting with UTI symptoms

a. Assess temperature and maternal pulse

b. Palpate abdomen and uterus for tenderness and presence of contractions

c. Check for costovertebral angle tenderness

d. Complete a macro-urinalysis for nitrites, leukocytes, and blood

e. Send urine for culture and sensitivity (C&S)

f. Depending on history, perform speculum examination to rule out urethritis from a vaginal infection

III. Assessment

A. Rule out ASB

B. Rule out cystitis

C. Rule out possible pyelonephritis

D. Rule out vaginal infection

IV. Plan

A. Women without ASB on initial culture do not need a rescreening later in pregnancy unless they have a urinary tract anomaly or history of pyelonephritis.

B. Women with ASB (≥ 100,000 colonies/mL and no cystitis symptoms)

1. Treat with appropriate antibiotic for 3–7 days after initial culture

2. Repeat urine C&S 1–2 weeks after treatment.

3. If culture is positive, then retreat for 7–10 days.

4. Rescreen at a minimum of each trimester.

5. Women with group B streptococcus on an ASB urine culture should be considered group B streptococcus positive and do not need a vaginal or rectal screen in the third trimester.

C. Women with UTI (≥ 100 colonies/mL of a single organism per milliliter, cystitis symptoms, and pyuria)

1. Treat with the appropriate antibiotic for at least 3–7 days.

2. Repeat urine C&S 1–2 weeks after treatment.

3. Initiate suppressive therapy for women with two or more treatments in pregnancy; typically nitrofurantoin, 50–100 mg at bedtime, or cephalexin, 250–500 mg at bedtime.

D. Women with suspected pyelonephritis

1. Consult with a physician

2. Refer to a birthing unit for assessment and parenteral antibiotic treatment

3. Ensure the woman receives UTI suppressive therapy for remainder of the pregnancy

E. Women with a history of recurrent UTIs temporally related to coitus

These women should be offered postcoital prophylaxis because it has been shown to decrease the rate of UTIs (Hooton, Besser, Foxman, Fritsche, & Nicolle, 2004). Typically, prophylaxis is a single dose of cephalexin, 250 mg, or nitrofurantoin, 50 mg, taken postcoitally.

F. Patient education for prevention of UTIs

1. Encourage adequate fluid intake

2. Educate on the importance of voiding frequently and voiding after coitus

3. Especially for women with a history of UTIs or ASB, encourage drinking 8 oz of cranberry juice daily (Wing, Rumney, Preslicka, & Chung, 2008).

REFERENCES

Hooton, T. M., Besser, R., Foxman, B., Fritsche, T. R., & Nicolle, L. E. (2004). Acute uncomplicated cystitis in an era of increasing antibiotic resistance: A proposed approach to empirical therapy. *Clinical Infectious Diseases, 39,* 75–80.

Hooton, T. M., Scholes, D., Stapleton, A. E., Roberts, P. L., Winter, C., Gupta, K. . . . Stamm, W. E. (2000). A prospective study of asymptomatic bacteriuria in sexually active young women. *New England Journal of Medicine, 343,* 992–997.

Lin, K., & Fajardo, K. (2008). Screening for asymptomatic bacteriuria in adults: Evidence for the U.S. preventive services task force reaffirmation recommendation statement. *Annals of Internal Medicine, 149,* W20–W24.

Mazor-Dray, E., Levy, A., Schlaeffer, F., & Sheiner, E. (2009). Maternal urinary tract infection: Is it independently associated with adverse pregnancy outcome? *Journal of Maternal, Fetal, and Neonatal Medicine, 22*(2), 124–128.

Naeye, R. L. (1979). Causes of the excessive rates of perinatal mortality and prematurity in pregnancies complicated by maternal urinary tract infection. *New England Journal of Medicine, 300,* 819–823.

Smaill, F., & Vasquez, J. C. (2007). Antibiotics for asymptomatic bacteriuria in pregnancy. *Cochrane Database of Systematic Reviews,* CD000490.

Thurman, A. R., Steed, L. L., Hulsey, T., & Soper, D. E. (2006). Bacteriuria in pregnant women with sickle cell trait. *American Journal of Obstetrics and Gynecology, 194*(5), 1366–1370.

Wing, D. A., Rumney, P. J., Preslicka, C. W., & Chung, J. H. (2008). Daily cranberry juice for the prevention of asymptomatic bacteriuria in pregnancy: A randomized, controlled pilot study. *Journal of Urology, 180*(4), 1367–1372.

Zinner, S. H., & Kass, E. H. (1971). Long-term (10 to 14 years) follow-up of bacteriuria of pregnancy. *New England Journal of Medicine, 285,* 820–824.

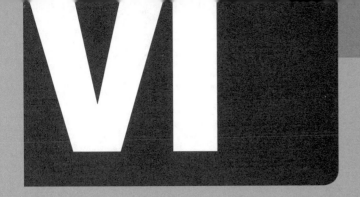

VI

ADULT HEALTH MAINTENANCE
AND PROMOTION

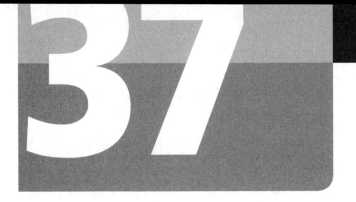

HEALTHCARE MAINTENANCE OF THE ADULT

Hattie C. Grundland and JoAnne M. Saxe

I. Introduction and general background

The goals of healthcare maintenance (HCM) are to promote health and prevent disease. Health counseling topics, screening tests, immunizations, and prophylactic medications are types of preventative services with the potential to improve a patient's health and well-being.

Recommendations for preventative services must be made selectively based on the unique qualities of the individual and the effectiveness of the therapy. Tailoring services to the individual is a complex process that involves (1) an assessment of the patient's general and specific risks, (2) an assessment of the willingness and ability of the patient to adopt a lifestyle or behavior change, and (3) delivering evidence-based counseling about the benefits and limitations of the recommended preventative service (Rodnick & Shore, 2007). Although there are many professional societies and voluntary agencies that make preventative service recommendations, the US Preventive Service Task Force offers a comprehensive resource that evaluates the quality of evidence supporting specific preventative services (U.S. Department of Health and Human Services, 2010).

The increase in number of recommended services in recent years and the complex decision making around who is an appropriate candidate for these services contribute to the challenge of preventative care delivery. Additionally, the needs of prevention care often compete with the needs of a patient's active health problems. System-based approaches to providing preventative care services have proved to be an effective tool in improving the delivery of preventative care services. A number of studies have shown improved rates of immunization and screening services with clinic implementation of systematic patient reminders. A 2009 randomized controlled trial evaluating interventions to promote screening for colon cancer found mailed patient reminders were an effective tool to increase colorectal cancer screening rates among adults in a primary care setting (Sequist, Zaslavsky, Marshall, Fletcher, & Ayanian, 2009).

This chapter is devoted to the HCM of adult populations. It should be noted that older adolescent populations often receive care in adult clinic settings. For these patients, preventative service recommendations specific to adolescent populations may be more appropriate, and these recommendations are defined in Chapter 7, entitled the 12 to 21 Years of Age Interval Visit.

II. Database

A. Subjective

1. Pertinent past health history
   a. Past medical illnesses and injuries
   b. Surgeries and hospitalizations
   c. Psychiatric conditions
   d. Obstetric and gynecological history
   e. Medications
   f. Allergies
   g. Environmental exposure and travel history
   h. Immunization history
   i. Transfusion and parenteral exposures

2. Family history

3. Occupational history: past and current employment (titles and duration of each position; hours, tasks, and responsibilities; exposures; protective equipment; relationships with coworkers and superiors; and job satisfaction)

4. Personal and social history
   a. Health-related behaviors (tobacco use, alcohol and drug use, physical activity, nutrition, sleep, dental care, safety belt use, and sexual activity and behavior)
   b. Major life events
   c. Stress and emotional well-being and coping strategies
   d. Relationships
   e. Education
   f. Future goals

g. Personal safety and home hazards (violence, fire alarms, or guns in the home)

h. Perception of health and illness as indicators for behavior change (Figure 37-1)

5. Review of systems

B. Objective

1. The extent of the physical examination should be determined by the patient's

a. General risk factors (age, biological sex, gender identity, and ethnicity)

b. Specific risk factors (as determined by past medical history, family history, occupational history, and personal and social history)

III. Assessment

A. *Identify the patient's general and specific health risks.*

B. *Determine the patient's current health status.*

C. *Determine the patient's motivation to change health-damaging behaviors or promote and maintain health-promoting behavior (see Figure 37-1).*

D. *Delineate the patient's ability to accomplish and master adult developmental milestones.*

FIGURE 37-1 Assessing a Patient's Readiness for Behavior Change

Counseling interventions regarding patient lifestyle and healthy behaviors begin with an assessment of the patient's recognition of unhealthy behavior and an assessment of the patient's readiness to make health-directed changes. Readiness to change is one of many frameworks designed to help the primary care provider choose an interviewing approach that will be most meaningful to the patient. The Transtheoretical Model defines behavior change as a process that occurs in stages (Huddleston, 2009). These stages, often referred to as "stages of change," help the clinician understand why certain patients are more or less successful at changing behavior and which motivational interviewing strategies may help the patient move closer to changing unhealthy behaviors (Walley & Roll, 2007).

Stage of Change	Definition	Patient Approach
Precontemplation	The patient has not recognized the behavior as unhealthy or they are not ready to change the behavior even though they know they should	• Inform and educate the patient about the unhealthy behavior and health consequences • Advise the patient to change the behavior
Contemplation	The patient understands their behavior is unhealthy but is ambivalent about making a change	• Elicit reasons for ambivalence • Weigh the pros and cons and address the patient's concerns • Individualized feedback on negative effects of the unhealthy behavior
Preparation	The patient makes a decision to change the behavior	• Commend the decision to change • Assist in choice of treatment or referral
Action	The patient is active in some change of the behavior	• Support the changes made and provide encouragement to sustain the changes
Maintenance	The patient has made behavior change and is stable	• Recognize the patient's commitment and continued struggle to maintain the healthy behavior • Anticipate difficulties that may challenge maintenance • Address relapse

Sources: Prochaska, J. O., Norcross, J. C., & Diclemente, C. C. (1994). *Changing for good.* New York, NY: Avon Books; and Walley, A. Y., & Roll, F. J. (2007). Principles of caring for alcohol and drug users. In T. E. King & M. B. Wheeler (Eds.). *Medical management of vulnerable and underserved patients: Principles, practice and populations* (1st ed., pp. 341–350). New York, NY: McGraw-Hill.

IV. Plan

A. Screening and secondary prevention tests

1. Screen for diseases and conditions based on the patient's risk profile.

2. Follow Table 37-1 for general screening test recommendations.

B. Management

1. Refer to Figure 37-2 for the recommended adult immunization schedule from the Centers for Disease Control and Prevention or see http://www.cdc.gov/vaccines/

2. Follow the institution's prescribing/furnishing/drug ordering guidelines if prescribing or furnishing chemoprophylaxis.

TABLE 37-1 Screening Test Recommendations

Screening Recommendation	Who to Screen	Screening Test and Frequency	Additional Considerations
Abdominal aortic aneurysm	Males aged 65–75 who have ever smoked	Ultrasonography, one-time screening	Smoking history of at least 100 cigarettes; lifetime
Alcohol misuse	Adult males and females	Many screening tools available (i.e., AUDIT, CAGE). Alcohol abuse and alcoholism website has tools available: http://www.niaa.niaaa.nih.gov// The best interval for screening is unknown.	Risky; hazardous drinking defined as > 7 drinks/wk or > 3 drinks per occasion for females and > 14 drinks/wk or > 4 drinks per occasion for males
Breast cancer	Females between the ages of 50 and 74 years of age	Mammography every 2 years	There is insufficient evidence to recommend for or against yearly clinical breast examination or teaching self breast examination
Cervical cancer	Females age 21 or 3 years after beginning sexual activity, whichever comes first	Cytologic screening with conventional cytology (Pap smear) or liquid-based cytology methods, every 1–3 years	May discuss discontinuing screening in females older than 65 if adequate recent screening was normal
Chlamydial infection	Females ≤ 24 years of age who are sexually active and older women at increased risk	Nucleic acid amplification test; annual screening for women at increased risk should be considered	There is insufficient evidence to recommend routine screening for men
Colorectal cancer	Males and females 50–75 years of age	Annual high-sensitivity fecal occult blood testing or sigmoidoscopy every 5 years combined with high-sensitivity fecal occult blood testing every 3 years or colonoscopy every 10 years	Routine screening in adults 76–85 should be made on an individual basis
Depression	All adults given appropriate diagnosis, treatment, and follow-up can be offered	Many screening tools available (e.g., Patient Health Questionnaire); the best interval for screening is unknown	Screening by asking two questions may be as effective as formal screening tools: "Over the past 2 weeks, have you felt down, depressed or hopeless?" "Over the past 2 weeks, have you felt little interest or pleasure in doing things?"
Diabetes, type 2	All adults with sustained blood pressure > 135/80	Fasting plasma glucose, hemoglobin A_{1c}, or 2-hour postload plasma glucose; the best interval for screening is unknown	Fasting plasma glucose has more reproducible results and is easier and faster to perform Diabetes defined as fasting plasma glucose level ≥ 126 mg/dl on separate visit screening (ADA, 2009)

(continues)

TABLE 37-1 Screening Test Recommendations *(continued)*

Screening Recommendation	Who to Screen	Screening Test and Frequency	Additional Considerations
Gonorrhea infection	All sexually active females at increased risk	Nucleic acid amplification test; the best interval for screening is unknown	Risk factors include females and males and ≤ 25 with history of prior sexually transmitted infection, new or multiple sex partners, inconsistent use of barrier methods, sex workers, drug use, and increased community prevalence of gonorrhea infections
High blood pressure	All adults 18 years and older	Sphygmomanometer every 2 years if blood pressure ≤ 120/80 mm Hg and yearly if systolic 120–139 mm Hg or diastolic 80–90 mm Hg	Hypertension defined as blood pressure ≥ 140/90 mm Hg found on ≥ 2 or more visits over a period of 1 to several weeks
High cholesterol	Males ≥ 35 and 20–35 years of age at increased risk for coronary heart disease Females ≥ 20 years of age if at increased risk for heart disease	Total cholesterol and high-density lipoprotein on fasting or nonfasting visits; screen every 5 years or with increased frequency if lipid levels close to levels requiring treatment; may decrease frequency of screening if repeated screening levels are normal	Increased risk for coronary heart disease: diabetes, prior history of coronary heart disease or noncoronary atherosclerosis, family history of coronary heart disease in males ≤ 50 and females ≤ 60 years of age, tobacco use, hypertension, and body mass index ≥ 30
HIV infection	All adults at risk for HIV	Enzyme immune assay followed by confirmatory Western blot or immunofluorescent assay or rapid HIV antibody; the best interval for screening is unknown	Increased risk includes men who have sex with men, multiple sex partners with inconsistent use of barrier methods, sex workers, those with past or present sex partners who are HIV$^+$, blood transfusion between 1978 and 1985, and those who request an HIV test
Obesity	All adults	Body mass index; the best interval for screening is unknown	Obesity defined as body mass index ≥ 30
Osteoporosis	Females ≥ 65 and ≥ 60 and older at increased risk	Dual-energy x-ray absorptiometry measured at femoral neck; the best interval for screening is unknown	Consider screening every 2 years in females of average risk
Prostate cancer	The current evidence is insufficient to assess the benefit of screening males < 75 Not recommended for men 75 years and older	Prostate-specific antigen and digital rectal examination	Males < 75 may desire screening after a discussion of the potential but uncertain benefits and risks of prostate cancer screening with prostate-specific antigen
Syphilis	Adults at increased risk	Venereal Disease Research Laboratory or Rapid Plasma Reagin; the best interval for screening is unknown	Increased risks include men who have sex with men, engaging in high-risk sex behavior, sex workers including exchanging sex for drugs, and adults in correctional facilities
Tobacco use	All adults	Ask about tobacco use; regular, systematized screening systems increase clinician intervention rates	Many approaches for behavioral counseling (Figure 37-1)

Source: U.S. Department of Health and Human Services. (2010). Guide to clinical preventive services. Retrieved from http://www.ahrq.gov/clinic/pocketgd1011/gcp10s1.htm; and USPSTF, (2009).

RECOMMENDED ADULT IMMUNIZATION SCHEDULE
UNITED STATES—2011

Note: These recommendations *must* be read with the footnotes (on pages 312–314) that follow containing number of doses, intervals between doses, and other important information.

VACCINE ▼	AGE GROUP ▶	19–26 years	27–49 years	50–59 years	60–64 years	¥65 years
Influenza[1,*]		1 dose annually				
Tetanus, diphtheria, pertussis (Td/Tdap)[2,*]		Substitute 1-time dose of Tdap for Td booster; then boost with Td every 10 years				Td booster every 10 years
Varicella[3,*]		2 doses				
Human papillomavirus (HPV)[4,*]		3 doses (females)				
Zoster[5]					1 dose	
Measles, mumps, rubella (MMR)[6,*]		1 or 2 doses		1 dose		
Pneumococcal (polysaccharide)[7,8]		1 or 2 doses				1 dose
Meningococcal[9,*]		1 or more doses				
Hepatitis A[10,*]		2 doses				
Hepatitis B[11,*]		3 doses				

*Covered by the Vaccine Injury Compensation Program

For all persons in this category who meet the age requirements and who lack evidence of immunity (e.g., lack documentation of vaccination or have no evidence of previous infection)

Recommended if some other risk factor is present (e.g., based on medical, occupational, lifestyle, or other indications)

No recommendation

FIGURE 37-2a Recommended Adult Immunization Schedule, by Vaccine and Age Group

VACCINE ▼	INDICATION ▶ Pregnancy	Immunocompromising conditions (excluding human immunodeficiency virus [HIV])[3,5,6,13]	HIV infection[3,6,12,13] CD4 T lymphocyte count <200 cells/μL	¥200 cells/μL	Diabetes, heart disease, choronic lung disease, chronic alcoholism	Asplenia[12] (including elective splenectomy) and persistent complement component deficiencies	Chronic liver disease	kidney failure, end-stage renal disease, receipt of hemodialysis	Health-care personnel
Influenza[1,*]		1 dose inactivated (TIV) annually							1 dose TIV or LAIV• annually
Tetanus, diphtheria, pertussis (Td/Tdap)[2,*]	Td	Substitute 1-time dose of Tdap for Td booster; then boost with Td every 10 years							
Varicella[3,*]	Contraindicated			2 doses					
Human papillomavirus (HPV)[4,*]		3 doses through age 26 years							
Zoster[5]	Contraindicated			1 dose					
Measles, mumps, rubella[6,*]	Contraindicated			1 or 2 doses					
Pneumococcal (polysaccharide)[7,8]		1 or 2 doses							
Meningococcal[9,*]		1 or more doses							
Hepatitis A[10,*]		2 doses							
Hepatitis B[11,*]		3 doses							

*Covered by the Vaccine Injury Compensation Program

For all persons in this category who meet the age requirements and who lack evidence of immunity (e.g., lack documentation of vaccination or have no evidence of previous infection)

Recommended if some other risk factor is present (e.g., on the basis of medical, occupational, lifestyle, or other indications)

No recommendation

• live attenuated influenza vaccine (LAIV)

FIGURE 37-2b Vaccines That Might Be Indicated for Adults Based on Medical and Other Indications

Department of Health and Human Services Centers for Disease Control and Prevention

Footnotes

Recommended Adult Immunization Schedule—UNITED STATES - 2011

For complete statements by the Advisory Committee on Immunization Practices (ACIP), visit www.cdc.gov/vaccines/pubs/ACIP-list.html.

1. Influenza vaccination

Annual vaccination against influenza is recommended for all persons aged 6 months and older, including all adults. Healthy, nonpregnant adults aged less than 50 years without high-risk medical conditions can receive either intranasally administered live, attenuated influenza vaccine (FluMist), or inactivated vaccine. Other persons should receive the inactivated vaccine. Adults aged 65 years and older can receive the standard influenza vaccine or the high-dose (Fluzone) influenza vaccine. Additional information about influenza vaccination is available at http ://www.cdc.gov/vaccines/vpd-vac/flu/default.htm.

2. Tetanus, diphtheria, and acellular pertussis (Td/Tdap) vaccination

Administer a one-time dose of Tdap to adults aged less than 65 years who have not received Tdap previously or for whom vaccine status is unknown to replace one of the 10-year Td boosters, and as soon as feasible to all 1) postpartum women, 2) close contacts of infants younger than age 12 months (e.g., grandparents and child-care providers), and 3) health-care personnel with direct patient contact. Adults aged 65 years and older who have not previously received Tdap and who have close contact with an infant aged less than 12 months also should be vaccinated. Other adults aged 65 years and older may receive Tdap. Tdap can be administered regardless of interval since the most recent tetanus or diphtheria-containing vaccine.

Adults with uncertain or incomplete history of completing a 3-dose primary vaccination series with Td-containing vaccines should begin or complete a primary vaccination series. For unvaccinated adults, administer the first 2 doses at least 4 weeks apart and the third dose 6–12 months after the second. If incompletely vaccinated (i.e., less than 3 doses), administer remaining doses. Substitute a one-time dose of Tdap for one of the doses of Td, either in the primary series or for the routine booster, whichever comes first.

If a woman is pregnant and received the most recent Td vaccination 10 or more years previously, administer Td during the second or third trimester. If the woman received the most recent Td vaccination less than 10 years previously, administer Tdap during the immediate postpartum period. At the clinician's discretion, Td may be deferred during pregnancy and Tdap substituted in the immediate postpartum period, or Tdap may be administered instead of Td to a pregnant woman after an informed discussion with the woman.

The ACIP statement for recommendations for administering Td as prophylaxis in wound management is available at http://www.cdc.gov /vaccines/pubs/acip-list.htm.

3. Varicella vaccination

All adults without evidence of immunity to varicella should receive 2 doses of single-antigen varicella vaccine if not previously vaccinated or a second dose if they have received only 1 dose, unless they have a medical contraindication. Special consideration should be given to those who 1) have close contact with persons at high risk for severe disease (e.g., health-care personnel and family contacts of persons with immunocompromising conditions) or 2) are at high risk for exposure or transmission (e.g., teachers; child-care employees; residents and staff members of institutional settings, including correctional institutions; college students; military personnel; adolescents and adults living in households with children; nonpregnant women of childbearing age; and international travelers).

Evidence of immunity to varicella in adults includes any of the following: 1) documentation of 2 doses of varicella vaccine at least 4 weeks apart; 2) U.S.-born before 1980 (although for health-care personnel and pregnant women, birth before 1980 should not be considered evidence of immunity); 3) history of varicella based on diagnosis or verification of varicella by a health-care provider (for a patient reporting a history of or having an atypical case, a mild case, or both, health-care providers should seek either an epidemiologic link with a typical varicella case or to a laboratory-confirmed case or evidence of laboratory confirmation, if it was performed at the time of acute disease); 4) history of herpes zoster based on diagnosis or verification of herpes zoster by a health-care provider; or 5) laboratory evidence of immunity or laboratory confirmation of disease.

Pregnant women should be assessed for evidence of varicella immunity. Women who do not have evidence of immunity should receive the first dose of varicella vaccine upon completion or termination of pregnancy and before discharge from the health-care facility. The second dose should be administered 4–8 weeks after the first dose.

4. Human papillomavirus (HPV) vaccination

HPV vaccination with either quadrivalent (HPV4) vaccine or bivalent vaccine (HPV2) is recommended for females at age 11 or 12 years and catch-up vaccination for females aged 13 through 26 years.

Ideally, vaccine should be administered before potential exposure to HPV through sexual activity; however, females who are sexually active should still be vaccinated consistent with age-based recommendations. Sexually active females who have not been infected with any of the four HPV vaccine types (types 6, 11, 16, and 18, all of which HPV4 prevents) or any of the two HPV vaccine types (types 16 and 18, both of which HPV2 prevents) receive the full benefit of the vaccination. Vaccination is less beneficial for females who have already been infected with one or more of the HPV vaccine types. HPV4 or HPV2 can be administered to persons with a history of genital warts, abnormal Papanicolaou test, or positive HPV DNA test, because these conditions are not evidence of previous infection with all vaccine HPV types.

HPV4 may be administered to males aged 9 through 26 years to reduce their likelihood of genital warts. HPV4 would be most effective when administered before exposure to HPV through sexual contact.

A complete series for either HPV4 or HPV2 consists of 3 doses. The second dose should be administered 1–2 months after the first dose; the third dose should be administered 6 months after the first dose.

Although HPV vaccination is not specifically recommended for persons with the medical indications described in Figure 2, "Vaccines that might be indicated for adults based on medical and other indications," it may be administered to these persons because the HPV vaccine is not a live-virus vaccine. However, the immune response and vaccine efficacy might be less for persons with the medical indications described in Figure 2 than in persons who do not have the medical indications described or who are immunocompetent.

5. Herpes zoster vaccination

A single dose of zoster vaccine is recommended for adults aged 60 years and older regardless of whether they report a previous episode of herpes zoster. Persons with chronic medical conditions may be vaccinated unless their condition constitutes a contraindication.

6. Measles, mumps, rubella (MMR) vaccination

Adults born before 1957 generally are considered immune to measles and mumps. All adults born in 1957 or later should have documentation of 1 or more doses of MMR vaccine unless they have a medical contraindication to the vaccine, laboratory evidence of immunity to each of the three diseases, or documentation of provider-diagnosed measles or mumps disease. For rubella, documentation of provider-diagnosed disease is not considered acceptable evidence of immunity.

Measles component: A second dose of MMR vaccine, administered a minimum of 28 days after the first dose, is recommended for adults who 1) have been recently exposed to measles or are in an outbreak setting; 2) are students in postsecondary educational institutions; 3) work in a health-care facility; or 4) plan to travel internationally. Persons who received inactivated (killed) measles vaccine or measles vaccine of unknown type during 1963–1967 should be revaccinated with 2 doses of MMR vaccine.

Mumps component: A second dose of MMR vaccine, administered a minimum of 28 days after the first dose, is recommended for adults who 1) live in a community experiencing a mumps outbreak and are in an affected age group; 2) are students in postsecondary educational institutions; 3) work in a health-care facility; or 4) plan to travel internationally. Persons vaccinated before 1979 with either killed mumps vaccine or mumps vaccine of unknown type who are at high risk for mumps infection (e.g. persons who are working in a health-care facility) should be revaccinated with 2 doses of MMR vaccine.

Rubella component: For women of childbearing age, regardless of birth year, rubella immunity should be determined. If there is no evidence of immunity, women who are not pregnant should be vaccinated. Pregnant women who do not have evidence of immunity should receive MMR vaccine upon completion or termination of pregnancy and before discharge from the health-care facility.

Health-care personnel born before 1957: For unvaccinated health-care personnel born before 1957 who lack laboratory evidence of measles, mumps, and/or rubella immunity or laboratory confirmation of disease, health-care facilities should 1) consider routinely vaccinating personnel with 2 doses of MMR vaccine at the appropriate interval (for measles and mumps) and 1 dose of MMR vaccine (for rubella), and 2) recommend 2 doses of MMR vaccine at the appropriate interval during an outbreak of measles or mumps, and 1 dose during an outbreak of rubella. Complete information about evidence of immunity is available at http://www.cdc .gov/vaccines/recs/provisional/default.htm.

7. Pneumococcal polysaccharide (PPSV) vaccination

Vaccinate all persons with the following indications:

Medical: Chronic lung disease (including asthma); chronic cardiovascular diseases; diabetes mellitus; chronic liver diseases; cirrhosis; chronic alcoholism; functional or anatomic asplenia (e.g., sickle cell disease or splenectomy [if elective splenectomy is planned, vaccinate at least 2 weeks before surgery]); immunocompromising conditions (including chronic renal failure or nephrotic syndrome); and cochlear implants and cerebrospinal fluid leaks. Vaccinate as close to HIV diagnosis as possible.

Other: Residents of nursing homes or long-term care facilities and persons who smoke cigarettes. Routine use of PPSV is not recommended for American Indians/Alaska Natives or persons aged less than 65 years unless they have underlying medical conditions that are PPSV indications. However, public health authorities may consider recommending PPSV for American Indians/Alaska Natives and persons aged 50 through 64 years who are living in areas where the risk for invasive pneumococcal disease is increased.

8. Revaccination with PPSV

One-time revaccination after 5 years is recommended for persons aged 19 through 64 years with chronic renal failure or nephrotic syndrome; functional or anatomic asplenia (e.g., sickle cell disease or splenectomy); and for persons with immunocompromising conditions. For persons aged 65 years and older, one-time revaccination is recommended if they were vaccinated 5 or more years previously and were aged less than 65 years at the time of primary vaccination.

9. Meningococcal vaccination

Meningococcal vaccine should be administered to persons with the following indications:

Medical: A 2-dose series of meningococcal conjugate vaccine is recommended for adults with anatomic or functional asplenia, or persistent complement component deficiencies. Adults with HIV infection who are vaccinated should also receive a routine 2-dose series. The 2 doses should be administered at 0 and 2 months.

Other: A single dose of meningococcal vaccine is recommended for unvaccinated first-year college students living in dormitories; microbiologists routinely exposed to isolates of *Neisseria meningitidis*; military recruits; and persons who travel to or live in countries in which meningococcal disease is hyperendemic or epidemic (e.g., the "meningitis belt" of sub-Saharan Africa during the dry season [December through June]), particularly if their contact with local populations will be prolonged. Vaccination is required by the government of Saudi Arabia for all travelers to Mecca during the annual Hajj.

Meningococcal conjugate vaccine, quadrivalent (MCV4) is preferred for adults with any of the preceding indications who are aged 55 years and younger; meningococcal polysaccharide vaccine (MPSV4) is preferred for adults aged 56 years and older. Revaccination with MCV4 every 5 years is recommended for adults previously vaccinated with MCV4 or MPSV4 who remain at increased risk for infection (e.g., adults with anatomic or functional asplenia, or persistent complement component deficiencies).

10. Hepatitis A vaccination

Vaccinate persons with any of the following indications and any person seeking protection from hepatitis A virus (HAV) infection:

Behavioral: Men who have sex with men and persons who use injection drugs.

Occupational: Persons working with HAV-infected primates or with HAV in a research laboratory setting.

Medical: Persons with chronic liver disease and persons who receive clotting factor concentrates.

Other: Persons traveling to or working in countries that have high or intermediate endemicity of hepatitis A (a list of countries is available at http://www.cdc.gov/travel/contentdiseases.aspx).

Unvaccinated persons who anticipate close personal contact (e.g., household or regular babysitting) with an international adoptee during the first 60 days after arrival in the United States from a country with high or intermediate endemicity should be vaccinated. The first dose of the 2-dose hepatitis A vaccine series should be administered as soon as adoption is planned, ideally 2 or more weeks before the arrival of the adoptee.

Single-antigen vaccine formulations should be administered in a 2-dose schedule at either 0 and 6–12 months (Havrix), or 0 and 6–18 months (Vaqta). If the combined hepatitis A and hepatitis B vaccine (Twinrix) is used, administer 3 doses at 0, 1, and 6 months; alternatively, a 4-dose schedule may be used, administered on days 0, 7, and 21–30, followed by a booster dose at month 12.

11. Hepatitis B vaccination

Vaccinate persons with any of the following indications and any person seeking protection from hepatitis B virus (HBV) infection:

Behavioral: Sexually active persons who are not in a long-term, mutually monogamous relationship (e.g., persons with more than one sex partner during the previous 6 months); persons seeking evaluation or treatment for a sexually transmitted disease (STD); current or recent injection-drug users; and men who have sex with men.

Occupational: Health-care personnel and public-safety workers who are exposed to blood or other potentially infectious body fluids.

Medical: Persons with end-stage renal disease, including patients receiving hemodialysis; persons with HIV infection; and persons with chronic liver disease.

Other: Household contacts and sex partners of persons with chronic HBV infection; clients and staff members of institutions for persons with developmental disabilities; and international travelers to countries with high or intermediate prevalence of chronic HBV infection (a list of countries is available at http://wwwn.cdc.gov/travel/contentdiseases .aspx).

Hepatitis B vaccination is recommended for all adults in the following settings: STD treatment facilities; HIV testing and treatment facilities; facilities providing drug-abuse treatment and prevention services; health-care settings targeting services to injection-drug users or men who have sex with men; correctional facilities; end-stage renal disease programs and facilities for chronic hemodialysis patients; and institutions and nonresidential day-care facilities for persons with developmental disabilities.

Administer missing doses to complete a 3-dose series of hepatitis B vaccine to those persons not vaccinated or not completely vaccinated. The second dose should be administered 1 month after the first dose; the third dose should be given at least 2 months after the second dose (and at least 4 months after the first dose). If the combined hepatitis A and hepatitis B vaccine (Twinrix) is used, administer 3 doses at 0, 1, and 6 months; alternatively, a 4-dose Twinrix schedule, administered on days 0, 7, and 21 to 30, followed by a booster dose at month 12 may be used.

Adult patients receiving hemodialysis or with other immunocompromising conditions should receive 1 dose of 40 µg/mL (Recombivax HB) administered on a 3-dose schedule or 2 doses of 20 µg/mL (Engerix-B) administered simultaneously on a 4-dose schedule at 0, 1, 2, and 6 months.

12. Selected conditions for which *Haemophilus influenzae* type b (Hib) vaccine may be used

1 dose of Hib vaccine should be considered for persons who have sickle cell disease, leukemia, or HIV infection, or who have had a splenectomy, if they have not previously received Hib vaccine.

13. Immunocompromising conditions

Inactivated vaccines generally are acceptable (e.g., pneumococcal, meningococcal, influenza [inactivated influenza vaccine]) and live vaccines generally are avoided in persons with immune deficiencies or immunocompromising conditions. Information on specific conditions is available at http://www.cdc.gov/vaccines/pubs/acip-list.htm.

These schedules indicate the recommended age groups and medical indications for which administration of currently licensed vaccines is commonly indicated for adults ages 19 years and older, as of January 1, 2011. For all vaccines being recommended on the adult immunization schedule: a vaccine series does not need to be restarted, regardless of the time that has elapsed between doses. Licensed combination vaccines may be used whenever any components of the combination are indicated and when the vaccine's other components are not contraindicated. For detailed recommendations on all vaccines, including those used primarily for travelers or that are issued during the year, consult the manufacturers' package inserts and the complete statements from the Advisory Committee on Immunization Practices (http:// www.cdc.gov /vaccines/pubs/acip-list.htm).

---

3. Diet and exercise prescriptions as indicated by the patient's age, risk profile, health status, and patient readiness.

C. *Patient and family education*

1. Provide health counseling information in verbal or written format as needed based on the needs identified in the HCM assessment. For patients with cognitive impairment always involve the family or caregivers in this process.

2. See Table 37-2 for general health counseling and education topics.

D. *Self-management resources*

1. Offer, if appropriate, self-management resources noted in Table 37-2 to assist the patient and family with making lifestyle changes. The noted resources have a Flesch-Kincaid reading score of grade 8 or less.

TABLE 37-2 Health Counseling and Health Education Recommendations

Periodic Health Counseling	Self-Management Resources
Tobacco prevention and cessation	*You can quit smoking: support and advice from your prenatal care provider (English version)* (U.S. Department of Health and Human Services, 2008a) http://www.ahrq.gov/clinic/tobacco/prenatal.pdf
	You can quit smoking: support and advice from your prenatal care provider (Spanish version) (U.S. Department of Health and Human Services, 2008b). http://www.ahrq.gov/clinic/tobacco/prenatalsp.pdf
Alcohol and illicit drug use, abuse, and avoidance	*National Institute of Drug Abuse Infofacts: Science based facts on drug abuse and addiction (English version)* (National Institute on Alcohol Abuse and Alcoholism, 2010a) http://www.drugabuse.gov/infofacts/Infofaxindex.html
	National Institute of Drug Abuse Infofacts: Science based facts on drug abuse and addiction (Spanish version) (National Institute on Alcohol Abuse and Alcoholism, 2010b) http://www.drugabuse.gov/nidaespanol.html
	U.S. adult drinking patterns (National Institute on Alcohol Abuse and Alcoholism, 2004) http://pubs.niaaa.nih.gov/publications/Practitioner/CliniciansGuide2005/clinicians_guide17.htm
Sexual behavior and sexually transmitted disease prevention	*Sexually transmitted diseases: Fact sheets (English version)* (Centers for Disease Control and Prevention, 2010a). http://www.cdc.gov/std/healthcomm/fact_sheets.htm
	Sexually transmitted diseases: Fact sheets (Spanish version) (Centers for Disease Control and Prevention, 2010b) http://www.cdc.gov/std/Spanish/default.htm
Nutrition	*The practical guide: Identification, evaluation, and treatment of overweight and obesity in adults* http://www.nhlbi.nih.gov/guidelines/obesity/prctgd_c.pdf
Physical activity*	*Physical activity: An introduction (videostream)* (Centers for Disease Control and Prevention, 2008). http://www.cdc.gov/physicalactivity/everyone/guidelines/adults.html
	The practical guide: Identification, evaluation, and treatment of overweight and obesity in adults http://www.nhlbi.nih.gov/guidelines/obesity/prctgd_c.pdf
Violence prevention	*Understanding elder maltreatment* (Centers for Disease Control and Prevention, 2009e) http://www.cdc.gov/violenceprevention/pdf/EM-FactSheet-a.pdf
	Understanding intimate partner violence (Centers for Disease Control and Prevention, 2009f) http://www.cdc.gov/violenceprevention/pdf/IPV_factsheet-a.pdf
	Understanding sexual violence (Centers for Disease Control and Prevention, 2009g) http://www.cdc.gov/violenceprevention/pdf/SV_factsheet-a.pdf
	Understanding suicide (Centers for Disease Control and Prevention, 2009h) http://www.cdc.gov/violenceprevention/pdf/Suicide-FactSheet-a.pdf

(continues)

TABLE 37-2 Health Counseling and Health Education Recommendations *(continued)*

Periodic Health Counseling	Self-Management Resources
Injury prevention (motor vehicle occupant restraints and alcohol avoidance while driving)	*Home and recreational injuries* (Centers for Disease Control and Prevention, 2009c) http://www.cdc.gov/HomeandRecreationalSafety/index.html *Motor vehicle safety* (Centers for Disease Control and Prevention, 2009d) http://www.cdc.gov/Motorvehiclesafety/index.html
Occupational health	*Stress at work* (Centers for Disease Control and Prevention, 1999) http://www.cdc.gov/niosh/docs/99-101/pdfs/99-101.pdf *Violence on the job (videostreams)* (Centers for Disease Control and Prevention, 2004) http://www.cdc.gov/niosh/docs/video/violence.html
Aspirin chemoprophylaxis (myocardial infarction reduction assessment in men age 45–79 and ischemic stroke reduction in women age 55–79)	Heart disease: educational materials for patients (Centers for Disease Control and Prevention, 2009b) http://www.cdc.gov/heartdisease/materials_for_patients.htm Stroke: educational materials for patients (Centers for Disease Control and Prevention, 2010c) http://www.cdc.gov/stroke/materials_for_patients.htm
Breast cancer chemoprophylaxis (discuss with women at high risk for breast cancer)	*Breast cancer* (Centers for Disease Control and Prevention, 2009a) http://www.cdc.gov/cancer/breast/basic_info/treatment.htm

Source: USPSTF, 2009.

*The USPSTF concludes that the evidence is insufficient to recommend for or against counseling in this area in primary care settings.

REFERENCES

American Diabetes Association. (2009). *Executive summary: Standards of medical care in diabetes.* Retrieved from http://care.diabetesjournals.org/content/33/Supplement_1

Centers for Disease Control and Prevention. (1999). *Stress at work.* Retrieved from http://www.cdc.gov/niosh/docs/99-101/pdfs/99-101.pdf

Centers for Disease Control and Prevention. (2004). *Violence on the job (videostreams).* Retrieved from http://www.cdc.gov/niosh/docs/video/violence.html

Centers for Disease Control and Prevention. (2008). *Physical activity: An introduction (videostream).* Retrieved from http://www.cdc.gov/physicalactivity/everyone/guidelines/adults.html

Centers for Disease Control and Prevention. (2009a). *Breast cancer.* Retrieved from http://www.cdc.gov/cancer/breast/basic_info/treatment.htm

Centers for Disease Control and Prevention. (2009b). *Home and recreational injuries.* Retrieved from http://www.cdc.gov/HomeandRecreationalSafety/index.html

Centers for Disease Control and Prevention. (2009c). *Heart disease: Educational materials for patients.* Retrieved from http://www.cdc.gov/heartdisease/materials_for_patients.htm

Centers for Disease Control and Prevention. (2009d). *Motor vehicle safety.* Retrieved from http://www.cdc.gov/Motorvehiclesafety/index.html.

Centers for Disease Control and Prevention. (2009e). *Understanding elder maltreatment.* Retrieved from http://www.cdc.gov/violenceprevention/pdf/EM-FactSheet-a.pdf

Centers for Disease Control and Prevention. (2009f). *Understanding intimate partner violence.* Retrieved from http://www.cdc.gov/violenceprevention/pdf/IPV_factsheet-a.pdf

Centers for Disease Control and Prevention. (2009g). *Understanding sexual violence.* Retrieved from http://www.cdc.gov/violenceprevention/pdf/SV_factsheet-a.pdf

Centers for Disease Control and Prevention. (2009h). *Understanding suicide.* Retrieved from http://www.cdc.gov/violenceprevention/pdf/Suicide-FactSheet-a.pdf

Centers for Disease Control and Prevention. (2011). *Adult immunization schedule.* Retrieved from http://www.cdc.gov/vaccines/recs/schedules/adult-schedule.htm

Centers for Disease Control and Prevention. (2010a). *Sexually transmitted diseases: Fact sheets (English version).* Retrieved from http://www.cdc.gov/std/healthcomm/fact_sheets.htm

Centers for Disease Control and Prevention. (2010b). *Sexually transmitted diseases: Fact sheets (Spanish version).* Retrieved from http://www.cdc.gov/std/Spanish/default.htm

Centers for Disease Control and Prevention. (2010c). *Stroke: Educational materials for patients.* Retrieved from http://www.cdc.gov/stroke/materials_for_patients.htm

Gorin, S. S., & Arnold, J. (Eds.) (2006). *Health promotion in practice.* San Francisco, CA: Jossey-Bass.

Huddleston, J. S. (2009). Health promotion and behavior change. In A. J. Lowenstein, L. Foord-May, & J. C. Romano (Eds.), *Teaching strategies for health education and health promotion. Working with patients, families and communities* (1st ed., pp. 299–328). Sudbury, MA: Jones and Bartlett.

National Institute on Alcohol Abuse and Alcoholism. (2004). *Patient education materials: U.S. adult drinking patterns.* Retrieved from http://pubs.niaaa.nih.gov/publications/Practitioner/CliniciansGuide2005/clinicians_guide17.htm

National Institute on Alcohol Abuse and Alcoholism. (2009). *A pocket guide for alcohol screening and brief intervention (2005)*. Retrieved from http://pubs.niaaa.nih.gov/publications/Practitioner/pocketguide/pocket_guide.htm

National Institute on Alcohol Abuse and Alcoholism. (2010a). *National Institute of Drug Abuse Infofacts: Science based facts on drug abuse and addiction (English version)*. Retrieved from http://www.drugabuse.gov/infofacts/Infofaxindex.html

National Institute on Alcohol Abuse and Alcoholism. (2010b). *National Institute of Drug Abuse Infofacts: Science based facts on drug abuse and addiction (Spanish version)*. Retrieved from http://www.drugabuse.gov/nidaespanol.html

National Institutes of Health. (2000). *The practical guide: Identification, evaluation, and treatment of overweight and obesity in adults*. Retrieved from http://www.nhlbi.nih.gov/guidelines/obesity/prctgd_c.pdf

Prochaska, J. O., Norcross, J. C., & Diclemente, C. C. (1994). *Changing for good*. New York, NY: Avon Books.

Rodnick, J., & Shore, W. B. (2007). *The database*. San Francisco, CA: University of California, San Francisco Press.

Sequist, T. D., Zaslavsky, A. M., Marshall, R., Fletcher, R. H., Ayanian, J. Z. (2009). Patient and physician reminders to promote colorectal cancer screening: A randomized controlled trial. *Archives of Internal Medicine, 169*(4), 364–371.

U.S. Department of Health and Human Services. (2008a). *You can quit smoking: Support and advice from your clinician (English version)*. Retrieved from http://www.ahrq.gov/clinic/tobacco/tearsheet.pdf

U.S. Department of Health and Human Services. (2008b). *You can quit smoking: Support and advice from your clinician (Spanish version)*. Retrieved from http://www.ahrq.gov/clinic/tobacco/tearsheetsp.pdf

U.S. Department of Health and Human Services. (2010). Guide to clinical preventive services. Retrieved from http://www.ahrq.gov/clinic/pocketgd1011/gcp10s1.htm

Walley, A. Y., & Roll, F. J. (2007). Principles of caring for alcohol and drug users. In T. E. King & M. B. Wheeler (Eds.). *Medical management of vulnerable and underserved patients: Principles, practice and populations* (1st ed., pp. 341–350). New York, NY: McGraw-Hill.

HEALTHCARE MAINTENANCE FOR ADULTS WITH DEVELOPMENTAL DISABILITIES

Geraldine Collins-Bride and Clarissa Kripke

I. Introduction and general background

People with developmental disabilities (DDs) often have complex health issues that may be compounded by challenges with communication, mobility, sensory processing, and behavioral disorders. They experience higher rates of adverse health conditions, such as epilepsy and neurologic disorders, dermatologic problems, fractures and orthopedic problems, gastrointestinal disorders, cardiovascular disorders, behavioral and psychiatric disorders, and sensory disorders (Krahn, Hammond, & Turner, 2006). Individuals with DDs experience health disparities across a number of domains. In the context of disability, a healthcare disparity is a population with a difference in health status not directly attributable to the condition leading to or associated with the disability. Disparities are caused by differences in access to medical care. The current healthcare system presents an array of structural deficits that severely limit its ability to provide appropriate care for this vulnerable population. These deficits include:

- Lack of clinicians who are knowledgeable and skilled in the treatment of adults with DDs.
- Lack of regular health assessment and care.
- Lack of coordination among provider teams.

- Limited availability of services in places where patients with DDs live and reside.
- Lack of clear policies regarding consent, medical stabilization, and sedation. Lack of research and proven care guidelines (Harder and Company Community Research, 2008).

Disparities in preventive health care for individuals with DDs have gained attention in the literature. Numerous publications note the gap in preventive health screening for people with DDs compared to the general population (US Public Health Service [USPHS], 2001; Havercamp, Scandlin, & Roth, 2004; Krahn, Hammond, & Turner, 2006). In the 2001 Surgeon General's report, *Closing the Gap: A National Blueprint to Improve the Health of Persons with Mental Retardation*, it was noted that "individuals with mental retardation are more likely to receive inappropriate and inadequate treatment, or be denied health care altogether." Six goals and action steps were set forth in this document. Two of those goals are targeted in this chapter: to increase knowledge and understanding about DDs and to train healthcare providers to provide appropriate care (USPHS, 2001).

Life expectancy for individuals with DDs has increased significantly over the past several decades as people with DDs have moved from institutional settings to community-based care. Currently, most adults with DDs live in the community in their own homes, with their families, or in group homes. Some lead very independent lives and others are supported by a variety of service providers (healthcare advocates, independent living coaches, or case managers) and caregivers including family members, home health workers, and board and care home staff. The current life expectancy for older adults with intellectual disability (ID) is 66.1 years. The life expectancy of younger adults with DDs approaches that of the general population (Horwitz, Kerker, Owens, & Zigler, 2000). With the rise in life expectancy comes the increased risk for chronic diseases. Many of the chronic illnesses acquired by elders with DDs are similar to those seen in the general population, such as cardiovascular disease, cancers, pulmonary disease, diabetes, and renal diseases. Although individuals with DDs do have an increased incidence of respiratory, gastrointestinal, and musculoskeletal problems, it is imperative that the healthcare practitioner not focus solely on these conditions and perform routine screening for other chronic diseases.

Transition of care from the child-oriented to the adult healthcare system is a particularly challenging and vulnerable time for patients, families, and clinicians. Clinicians who serve children have accumulated a wealth of information about the individual and often have a well-established, trusting relationship with the patient and the family or caregivers. Clinicians who serve adults are rarely trained in this field and often do not have the resources to provide the range of services required to provide comprehensive care. It is not uncommon for pediatric healthcare providers to continue to provide care for individuals with DDs well beyond the age of 21 (American Academy of Pediatrics, American Academy of Family Physicians, & American College of Physicians, 2011).

A. Definition of DD

DD as defined by the Developmental Disabilities Assistance and Civil Rights Act of 2000 is a severe, chronic disability caused by physical or mental impairments manifesting before the age of 22 and is likely to continue indefinitely. These impairments cause limitations in three or more of the following categories: self-care, learning, receptive and expressive language, mobility, self-direction, capacity for independent living, and economic self-sufficiency (Developmental Disabilities Assistance and Bill of Rights, 2000). Many states define DD according to specific diagnoses and have different age cut-offs. All states must have a mechanism of delivering support and services to individuals meeting the state requirements for DD, although the structure of each system is left to the individual state. Both Federal and State statutes have been established to determine when a developmental problem is severe enough to constitute a disability. Clinicians can refer individuals to the local or regional developmental resource center for an eligibility consultation or determination if the situation arises or if the individual is not currently enrolled in services.

There is a strong self-advocacy movement in the disability rights community that has fought hard to dispel the old notion that individuals with disabilities are limited in their capacity to contribute meaningfully and be fully included in society. People with disabilities have the same rights to lead productive, independent lives. This inclusion includes the right to access appropriate and high-quality healthcare services.

B. Overview of common syndromes seen in primary care

1. Intellectual Disability (ID) (formerly mental retardation)

   ID is a "disability characterized by significant limitations both in intellectual functioning (reasoning, learning, problem solving) and in adaptive behavior, which covers a range of everyday social and practical skills. This disability originates before the age of 18" (American Association on Intellectual and Developmental Disabilities, 2010). Etiologies of ID include genetic abnormalities; intrauterine factors (asphyxia, maternal infections, and substance use); perinatal factors (hypoxic ischemic encephalopathy, sepsis, and prematurity); and

postnatal causes, such as childhood infections, environmental toxins, trauma, and severe malnutrition. Alcohol exposure during pregnancy is the toxin most clearly linked to ID. The common thread in the etiology of ID is brain dysfunction, caused by varying degrees of abnormal brain development or damage to the developing brain. The prevalence of ID is approximately 3%, with most (80%) in the mild range. With increased severity of ID, there is a higher incidence of nonverbal communication, resistive behavior, and significant health problems. Given these factors, individuals with severe ID are at particular risk for not receiving regular preventive health screening and lifestyle counseling.

2. Cerebral palsy

   Cerebral palsy (CP) is a term used to describe a

   > group of chronic conditions affecting body movement and muscle coordination. It is caused by damage to one or more specific areas of the brain, usually occurring during fetal development; before, during, or shortly after birth; or during infancy. Thus, these disorders are not caused by problems in the muscles or nerves. Instead, faulty development or damage to motor areas in the brain disrupts the brain's ability to adequately control movement and posture.

   'Cerebral' refers to the brain and 'palsy' to muscle weakness/poor control. Cerebral palsy itself is not progressive (i.e., brain damage does not get worse); however, secondary conditions, such as muscle spasticity, can develop which may get better over time, get worse, or remain the same. Cerebral palsy is not communicable. It is not a disease and should not be referred to as such. Although cerebral palsy is not 'curable' in the accepted sense, training and therapy can help improve function" (United Cerebral Palsy, 2011).

   The prevalence of CP is 2.1–3.3 per 1,000 live births with higher rates seen in males and African Americans (Yeargin-Allsopp, 2010). The greatest risk factor for CP is prematurity with an estimated one in three very low birth weight children (< 1,500 g) eventually diagnosed with CP. CP occurs as a consequence of the perinatal course because of poorly regulated cerebral blood flow. Spastic diplegia (greater involvement in the legs than the arms) is the type of CP most commonly associated with prematurity with hallmark findings of periventricular leukomalacia commonly seen on CT. Hemiplegic (one side of the body) CP is almost always caused by an in-utero or perinatal stroke, which should raise concerns about possible familial hypercoagulable disorders. Other etiologies for CP include chromosomal and brain abnormalities, genetic and metabolic disturbances, infection, and trauma.

Individuals with CP frequently have problems with spasticity, mobility, dystonia, dysarthria, swallowing, and gastroesophageal reflux. Individuals with hemiplegic CP most commonly have normal intelligence and do not have problems with speech and are not at increased risk for aspiration, gastroesophageal reflux disease, and other problems common to individuals with more widespread involvement. The impairments that result from CP may "become more disabling as the person ages or they may accelerate the aging process" (Svien, Berg, & Stephenson, 2008). Symptoms of fatigue, depression, impaired mobility, and musculoskeletal problems frequently worsen with aging. Mortality studies suggest that individuals with CP have high rates of cardiovascular and respiratory disease with aspiration pneumonia as the leading cause of death across all age groups of individuals with CP (Svien et al., 2008).

3. Autism spectrum disorders

Autism spectrum disorders (ASD) are neurodevelopmental conditions of unclear etiology that are classified according to the *Diagnostic and Statistical Manual IV* criteria to include atypical development in three major areas: (1) communication, (2) social interaction, and (3) behavior. The hallmark of all of the ASDs (autism, pervasive developmental disorders not otherwise specified, and Asperger syndrome) is atypical social interaction and differences in learning and sensory integration. People on the autism spectrum have a wide range of function and many have special interests or skills. While some people on the autism spectrum are highly verbal or skilled in writing and mechanical skills, challenges with communication can include atypical development such as speech delays, difficulty with articulation and noncommunicative speech. Social interaction can include differences in social or emotional reciprocity, difficulty developing friendships and peer relationships or unusual use of multiple nonverbal communication behaviors. Behaviors seen in ASD often include repetitive movements (or "stims", narrow focus on specific interests or activities, and difficulties with change or transitions (Johnson & Myers, 2007).

The prevalence of ASD continues to rise throughout the world with recent estimates of 1 in 110 children (Centers for Disease Control and Prevention, 2009). ASD is four times more common in boys. The incidence of intellectual impairment is much lower than previously estimated with less than 50% of individuals with ASDs showing ID once appropriate testing is done. Many individuals with ASD experience sensory integration problems and may be extremely hypersensitive to sounds or stimuli in the environment. Sensory processing differences should be explored to learn how to increase the comfort of people with autism in medical environments and during the physical examination. Many people with autism also have seizure disorders and associated mental health conditions, such as anxiety and depression. Although individuals with ASD may experience the same range of health problems as the general population, the communication and behavioral features of this condition often require accommodations to deliver quality care in primary care settings. These accommodations might include preparation about the visit or examination ahead of time and the use of a timer to indicate the start and stop of the examination.

4. Genetic disorders

A comprehensive genetics work-up can reveal the cause of DD in 40–60% of individuals. One of the most common and well characterized of these genetic disorders is Down syndrome, a chromosomal disorder with an estimated incidence of 1 in 750. The risk for Down syndrome rises with increasing maternal age with women over 40 years having an incidence of 1 in 105 live births (Kozma, 2008). The distinguishing characteristics of Down syndrome include facial dysmorphology (dysmorphic indicates an abnormal appearance), muscle hypotonia, and ID of varying degrees. Numerous medical problems are seen with Down syndrome including visual and hearing impairments, obesity, sleep apnea, hypothyroidism, cardiac and respiratory diseases, and early onset Alzheimer disease. There are well-established healthcare guidelines for following individuals with Down syndrome (Cohen, 1999; Sullivan et al., 2011).

A relatively new technology, microarray comparative genomic hybridization (CGH), has added greatly to the ability to find the underlying genetic defect in various DDs. This technology can show small duplications and deletions in the chromosomes that were previously undetectable. It is estimated that approximately 20% of individuals with ID with previously unidentified causes have these small deletions and duplications. Given the advances in today's genetic testing, it may be helpful to refer adults with unidentified ID for a genetics evaluation for further diagnostic testing. References for learning about other common (Fragile X and Klinefelter syndromes) and less common genetic syndromes can be found at the end of this chapter.

5. Epilepsy

Epilepsy refers to a group of conditions that are characterized by the recurrent disturbance of cerebral function (seizures) caused by excessive neuronal discharges in the brain occurring in a paroxysmal manner. An epileptic seizure occurs when the cerebral cortex is rendered hyperexcitable (because of an increase in excitatory neurotransmission, a decrease in inhibitory neurotransmission, or a disturbance in brain circuitry) by any of a number of causes including metabolic disturbances, injuries, strokes, tumors, and developmental abnormalities. For further discussion of epilepsy, see Chapter 54.

II. Database (may include but is not limited to)

A. Subjective

It can be challenging to obtain an accurate and comprehensive history on individuals with DDs, especially when the individual has communication or cognitive impairments. To gather a comprehensive and accurate view of the patient, historical data must be obtained from a variety of sources including caregivers, case managers, ID and DD nurses, and medical record review.

In some systems, a structured health interview and examination tool is being used to collect and document important past and current health issues. An example of such a tool can be found at http://www.cddh.monash.org/disability-health-assessment.html. This yearly health assessment form is a component of many healthcare delivery models for adults with DDs throughout the world, although not consistently in use in the United States. These health assessment forms have been well studied and capture key information on functional, behavioral, developmental, and psychosocial issues pertinent to adults with DDs (Lennox et al., 2007). Regardless of the type of data collection tool used for the history and physical examination, when possible, the healthcare provider should allow extra time for appointments when seeing individuals with DDs. It can also be helpful to schedule visits at regular or more frequent intervals to address the complexities of the patient's healthcare issues. Flexibility and creativity are often required to ensure a successful office visit. Home visits or visits in community settings can be very effective ways to provide care. Such strategies as desensitization, telephone conferences with caregivers, and obtaining assistance from health advocates or case

managers can allow the visit to proceed more smoothly. Always attempt to prepare the individual for the appointment and enlist support from a trusted caregiver. For severely agitated patients, presedation with a low dose of benzodiazepines, such as lorazepam, 0.5–1 mg, may be indicated. Caregivers should always be advised to give a test dose of the medication at home first to determine the timing of peak effect and dose, and because some patients have been known to experience a paradoxical reaction where agitation actually increases rather than decreases.

1. Pertinent past medical history, as outlined in Chapter 37, with a focus on the following additional data

    a. Etiology of DD with review of pediatric records and medical summary when possible. Note previous developmental and genetic evaluations (Sullivan et al., 2011). Note any history of institutionalizations.

    b. Previous medical illnesses, noting history of
        i. Epilepsy: frequency of seizures, medications, use of seizure tracking logs, and emergency management plan.
        ii. Gastroesophageal reflux disease: previous work-up, treatment, and *Helicobacter pylori* testing.
        iii. Constipation: unrecognized or untreated constipation can be a significant cause of morbidity and mortality. Note previous work-up and treatment.
        iv. Visual impairment: use of eyeglasses or contact lenses and date of last ophthalmology examination.
        v. Hearing impairment: use of hearing devices and date of last audiology examination.
        vi. Sensory integration problems: note problems with sounds, touch, taste, and sensation, which may impact the ability to perform a physical examination. Document recommendations from caregivers, family, and others about the best methods of approaching individuals with sensory integration problems.

    c. Communication: document the patient's usual method of communication (verbal, written, sign language, or gestures) and use of augmentative devices.

    d. Mobility and neuromotor function: note if the patient is ambulatory or nonambulatory, use of adaptive equipment, and how much time per day is spent using the equipment. Note how the person transfers if non–weight bearing and what assistance is needed for transfers (equipment, such as a Hoyer lift; staff or family and how many are needed). Note fine and gross motor skills, spasticity, and changes in motor tone, either increased or decreased.

e. Swallowing and feeding: episodes of choking or coughing with eating, history of aspiration, pneumonia, last swallowing study, and speech therapy treatments.

f. Bowel and bladder function: constipation, urinary incontinence or retention, and use of diapers or other incontinence supplies.

g. Dental health issues: caries, periodontal disease, and gingival hyperplasia. Inquire about ongoing dental care, cleanings and need for presedation before dental visits.

h. Mental health issues: depression, posttraumatic stress disorder, and anxiety are the most common disorders with rates similar to the general population. There is a much lower incidence of psychotic disorders, although antipsychotic medication is often overprescribed to control behavior. Ask specifically how symptoms manifest themselves. Some patients may be capable of verbally expressing mood symptoms and others may express symptoms as a change in behavior. Behavior needs to be interpreted developmentally. For example, a person with an intellect similar to a 3 year old may have imaginary friends and tantrum when frustrated. This behavior is appropriate to the person's intellectual development and is not an indication of a mental illness.

i. Medications: polypharmacy is a significant issue, with multiple medications often used to treat the same health problem. This is an especially common and ineffective practice used in the treatment of aggressive or difficult behaviors. It is important to note the indications and duration of use for all medications with attention to any side effects, drug interactions, and medication efficacy.

j. Immunization status: in addition to the primary vaccination series and scheduled boosters, note if the patient has received vaccines for hepatitis A and B, pneumococcal, and seasonal flu.

k. History of injuries or falls

l. History of abuse or victimization. This is especially prevalent in those individuals with IDs but it is also seen with high frequency in all individuals with disabilities (Sobsey & Doe, 1991).

m. History of resistive or challenging behavior. *Behavior is always a form of communication.* Difficult behaviors are not part of the disability but rather a means of communication for a patient with neurocognitive disorders. Difficult behaviors that are new or a change from the individual's usual level of functioning may signify an undiagnosed medical or psychiatric problem or may be a sign of a mismatch between a person's needs and the services and supports they are receiving or the environments in which they live and work. New behaviors always warrant a medical evaluation. Note previous medical and psychiatric evaluation of behavior change. Document behavioral, environmental, and pharmacologic therapies used for treatment.

2. Family history, with emphasis on developmental and genetic disorders

3. Occupational history: people with DDs work in a variety of settings from traditional companies to sheltered workshops and "day programs" run by community organizations serving people with DDs. Inquire about a job coach or other personnel support present at work. Obtain specific details about job tasks to screen for repetitive motion injuries. Ask about job satisfaction and relationships with coworkers.

4. Personal and social history

a. Housing status and level of independence: note if the patient lives independently and what support is required for independent living, such as in home support services, independent living coaches, or case management support. Include type of housing (apartment, family, or residential care home), noting how many individuals live in the home and ratio of staff/caregivers needed to provide a safe environment.

b. Relationships and social support network: note significant relationships with family, friends, and life partners. Inquire about the quantity and quality of social contact and relationships.

c. Future goals: note desired future personal, educational, and occupational goals.

5. Habits

a. Nutrition

b. Exercise and activity

c. Tobacco, alcohol, and substance use

d. Sleep

e. Sexual activity

6. Interdisciplinary healthcare team members: note each team member's name and contact information, which may include a case manager, nurse, dentist, pharmacist, physical therapist, occupational therapist, speech and language therapist, psychotherapist, and medical specialists (Figure 38-1).

❖ Interdisciplinary health care team chart

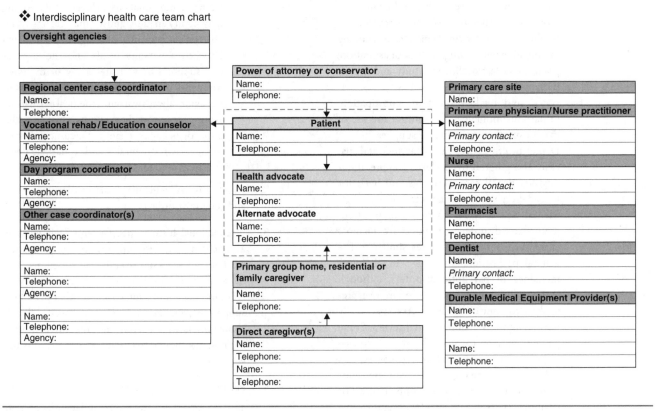

FIGURE 38-1 Interdisciplinary Health Care Team Chart
Source: Office of Developmental Primary Care (UCSF).

B. *Objective*

1. Perform an annual physical examination with blood pressure, height, weight, and Body Mass Index (New York State Office of Mental Retardation and Developmental Disabilities, 2009). The physical examination is particularly important for patients with cognitive and communication impairments, where subjective symptoms may be difficult to elicit (Figure 38-2).

2. Pay particular attention to a careful oral examination given the frequency of dental disease (Glassman et al., 2003).

3. Perform annual office-based vision and hearing screening examinations (New York State Office of Mental Retardation and Developmental Disabilities, 2009; Sullivan et al., 2011).

4. Document the patient's baseline, typical behavior, and method of communication.

5. Schedule a separate appointment dedicated solely to the gynecologic examination. Extra time is needed for the pelvic examination because these examinations can be challenging for providers and

for women with disabilities (Figure 38-3). Another excellent resource for healthcare providers is "Table Manners and Beyond: The Gynecologic Exam for Women with Developmental Disabilities and Other Functional Limitations" from Breast Health Access for Women with Disabilities (www.bhawd.org/sirefiles/tblMrs/cover.html).

III. Assessment

A. *Identify the patient's general and specific health risk profile. If the cause of the DD is unknown or unclear, consider a referral to genetics for an evaluation (Sullivan et al., 2011).*

B. *Recognize health habits that benefit from lifestyle modification*

C. *Ascertain additional members of the interdisciplinary health team that would be beneficial to improve the healthcare plan (Figure 38-1).*

FIGURE 38-2 Exam Room Etiquette

You may need to provide support to communicate with a patient with a developmental disability. Communication may take more thought and planning. Assess whether your patient uses spoken language, if not, they may use other forms of language, such as sign language, written language, or augmentative and alternative communication. Even people who do not use language can communicate through behavior, facial expressions, and sounds. Listening to your patient may require using more of your senses. Below are some ideas, but ask your patient and their caregivers what works best for them.

- Order an interpreter if spoken English is not the patient's primary language.
- Use person-first language (unless your patient prefers something else).
- Talk directly to your patient in an adult voice and listen attentively for your patient to respond and to finish. If your patient appears to be thinking, wait quietly.
- A patient may have better receptive than expressive language. Match the complexity of language to the person's ability.
- If your patient is not using words to communicate, then use non-verbal communication strategies, such as demonstrations, pictures, touch, gestures, and facial expressions.
- People with social communication challenges, such as autism, may not be able to interpret facial expressions and gestures and therefore may benefit from concrete, literal explanations.
- Get your patient's attention before speaking to them.
- Check for understanding by repeating and asking your patient to repeat.
- If necessary, use short, concrete questions that require yes or no answers.
- If necessary, ask questions that can be answered non-verbally. For example, "Show me how you say yes."
- Sit at eye level and treat wheelchairs as personal space. Don't touch a wheelchair without permission.
- Before helping, offer assistance and wait for a response and instructions.
- Offer to shake hands even if your patient has limited use of hands or an artificial limb.
- Identify yourself and others to people with visual disabilities and indicate to whom you are speaking.
- It is okay to use common idioms that refer to vision or hearing such as, "Have you heard about . . ." or "See the light . . .".

Used with permission from the Office of Developmental Primary Care, Department of Family & Community Medicine, University of California, San Francisco.

D. Determine the support needed for medical decision making and informed consent for diagnostic testing and procedures. Document whether the individual has a power of attorney or a legal decision maker for healthcare decisions. Although many individuals with IDs and DDs require the support of families and caregivers for decision making, it is important to remember that people with IDs and DDs have the right to make decisions about their lives and their health care. For individuals who lack capacity for decision making and have no identified decision-making support, the state Developmental Disability Service can be contacted for procedures to support medical decision making for diagnostic, treatment, or emergency decisions.

E. Assess the patient and caregiver's assets, barriers, and resources needed for implementing recommendations.

IV. Plan

A. Diagnostics (screening and secondary prevention tests)

1. Screen for diseases and conditions based on the patient's risk profile.

2. Screen for diseases and conditions specific to the patient's underlying DD or known specific

FIGURE 38-3 Tips for a Successful Pelvic Exam

For many women with intellectual disabilities, pelvic exams can be frightening and potentially uncomfortable. If the situation permits, focus the first visit on history and relationship building alone. The following may be helpful to reduce both the patient's and the provider's anxiety about the pelvic examination:

- Get to know your patient before attempting a pelvic exam.
- Educate the patient and caregivers about the exam.
- Don't assume that a pelvic exam will be any more difficult or uncomfortable for a person with a disability than for anyone else. You don't know until you try.
- Women with disabilities, including those with intellectual disabilities, can and do have sex.
- Use anatomy models with visual demonstration before the visit.
- Allow extra time (this is a must!).
- Encourage your patient to bring a supportive person to the appointment.
- If needed, locate the cervix manually.
- The anatomy of women with disabilities is often normal. However, it may be helpful to have several different pediatric and adult sized speculums available.
- Pelvic exams can be done in a variety of positions. You may need assistants to hold a flashlight or help the patient maintain a comfortable position.
- Use a soothing voice, deep breathing, visualization and praise.
- Consider pelvic ultrasound if bimanual exam is not possible.
- Consider using a short acting benzodiazepine for pre-sedation before a pelvic exam for women who have anxiety, spasticity or agitation. Consider a test dose at home prior to the visit. Ask the caregiver to carefully document the patient's reaction, as well as the peak action of the medication.
- Consider doing the exam under conscious sedation or general anesthesia especially if the patient has a scheduled surgical or dental procedure under anesthesia. Other exams, such as echocardiograms, labs, EKG, hearing tests, etc., can be coordinated at the same time.

Used with permission from the Office of Developmental Primary Care, Department of Family & Community Medicine, University of California, San Francisco.

developmental syndrome. For specific screening and diagnostic test recommendations see Table 38-1.

B. Treatment

1. For general health, see Chapter 37.

2. For recommendations targeted towards individuals with DDs, see Table 38-1.

3. For immunizations: see the Centers for Disease Control Recommended Adult Immunization Schedule, Figure 2. Vaccines that might be indicated for adults based on medical and other indications are available at http://www.cdc.gov/mmwr/PDF /wk/mm5901-Immunization.pdf.

4. For bone health: advise adequate calcium and vitamin D supplementation (1,500 mg/d) for those patients with a high-risk profile for osteoporosis (mobility impairments, long-term use of antiepileptic or antipsychotic medications, Down syndrome, CP, Prader-Willi syndrome, history of fractures, history of amenorrhea, and cigarette smoking) (New York State Office of Mental Retardation and Developmental Disabilities, 2009).

5. For mental health: review common stress management strategies with patients and caregivers. Prompt referral for psychologic counseling or psychiatry for signs and symptoms of mental illness.

6. For oral health: to reduce dental caries and gingival disease an expert dental panel recommends

   a. Brushing teeth twice daily for 2 minutes with a fluoridated toothpaste containing triclosan.

   b. Using xylitol for 5 minutes, three times per day. If the patient tolerates chewing, use chewing gum. If chewing is not possible, use a dissolved lozenge, spray, mint, or lollipop.

   c. Consulting with a dentist regarding fluoride varnishes, rinses, and chlorhexidine rinses (Glassman et al., 2003).

TABLE 38-1 Healthcare Maintenance Guidelines for Adults with Developmental Disabilities

NOTE: Health problems that are seen more frequently in this population and require additional attention by healthcare providers are highlighted in the shaded area.

Health Problem	19 – 40 Years	40 – 65 Years	65 Years and Older
Abuse & Neglect	Identify and evaluate unexplained physical and/or behavioral signs and symptoms at each visit. These signs might include some of the following: unexplained bruising, falls, injuries, weight loss, depression and behavior changes.		
Alcohol & Substance Abuse	Screen yearly.		
Breast Cancer (Women)			
Clinical Breast Exam	Perform yearly breast exam every two to three years.[4] Routine screening with clinical breast exam not recommended.[22]	For ages 40–65 screen with clinical breast exam yearly.[4] Start screening at age 50 with yearly clinical breast exam.[22]	Perform clinical breast exam every one to two years if life expectancy is greater than or equal to five years[21]
Mammography	Routine screening with mammography not recommended.[22]	Order screening mammography yearly.[4] Women ages 40–49 routine mammogram not recommended.[22]	Order screening mammography every two years until age 74. At age 75, consider stopping routine screening if patient has significant medical problems that threaten life expectancy.[22] Order screening mammography every one to two years if life expectancy is greater than or equal to five years.[21]
BRCA	For women with a family history associated with increased risk for BRCA1 or BRCA2 gene mutations, consider referral for genetic counseling and evaluation.[20] **Comments** *Family history is often difficult to obtain in this population. Individual decision-making is critical. Inform women and caregivers of potential benefits and consequences of breast cancer screening.* *Consider clinical breast exam as women with intellectual disabilities may not understand the significance of changes or have the skills to communicate changes they notice. Also, women with sensory or neuromuscular problems may have difficulty performing an accurate self-exam.* *Consider genetic testing for the BRCA-A gene for women who have a strong family history and are unable to do a mammogram.[20]*		
Cervical Spine Atlanto-Axial Instability	Perform an annual neurologic examination for signs and symptoms of spinal cord injury for patients with Down syndrome.[1] Order Cspine x-ray with lateral flexion and extension if symptoms develop, such as: changes in behavior or activity, changes in hand preference or urinary incontinence. If this is the first Cspine, also order an anteroposterior view. **Comments** *Consider screening cervical spine films prior to participation in athletics.*		

(continues)

TABLE 38-1 Healthcare Maintenance Guidelines for Adults with Developmental Disabilities *(continued)*

NOTE: Health problems that are seen more frequently in this population and require additional attention by healthcare providers are highlighted in the shaded area.

Health Problem	19 – 40 Years	40 – 65 Years	65 Years and Older
Cervical Cancer (Women)	Individualized decision-making depending on patient risk and sexual history. No consensus, but major groups recommend the following:		
	Before age 21, avoid pap smear screening regardless of sexual activity. At age 21, begin pap smear screening. Ages 21–29 screen every two years, then every three years for women with three consecutive normal paps.[3] Perform pap smear within three years after first sexual intercourse or by age 21, whichever comes first. Pap every one to three years.[22, 19]	Perform pap smear screening every three years for women with three consecutive normal paps.[3] Perform pap smear screening every one to three years.[22, 19]	At age 65[22], or age 70[4], consider discontinuing pap smear screening if the patient has had three or more documented, consecutive normal tests.
	Comments *See Breast Health Access for Women with Disabilities (BHAWD): "Table Manners and Beyond: The Gynecological Exam for Women with Developmental Disabilities and Other Functional Limitations": www.bhawd.org/sitefiles/TblMrs/cover.html* *See "Tips for a Successful Pelvic Exam": http://lfamilymedicine.medschool.ucsf.edulodpcldocs/pdf/practice_pearlsltips_for_a_successful_pelvic_exam.pdf*		
Chlamydia	Screen annually for sexually active women through age 26.[6]	For patients age 40 and older, since there is no data, individualized decision-making is appropriate.	
	Comments *Patients may not reliably report sexual activity or symptoms.*		
Cholesterol & Lipid Disorders	Order a fasting lipid panel every five years. More frequently if patient is taking atypical antipsychotic medications or has diabetes.[22]		
Colorectal Cancer	—	At age 50, screen with one of the following strategies: 1. Colonoscopy every ten years. 2. Flexible sigmoidoscopy every five years. 3. Fecal Occult Blood Test (FOBT) annually plus flexible sigmoidoscopy every three years. 4. FOBT annually. (UPSTF 2002, ASGE 2006, AAFP 2008).[10]	
	Comments *Depending on the patient's co-morbidities, anesthesia risk may outweigh the benefits of colonoscopy.* *Patients with mobility disorders, spasticity, and/or cognitive impairment may require hospital admission the day prior to testing with colonoscopy and sigmoidoscopy for professional assistance with the bowel preparation.*		

TABLE 38-1 Healthcare Maintenance Guidelines for Adults with Developmental Disabilities *(continued)*

NOTE: Health problems that are seen more frequently in this population and require additional attention by healthcare providers are highlighted in the shaded area.

Health Problem	19 – 40 Years	40 – 65 Years	65 Years and Older
Dental Disease	Perform an annual oral exam.		
	Refer to dentist for regular dental care including cleaning every six months or as recommended by the dentist.		
	Pay special attention to dental and gum health in persons with certain syndromes, such as Cornelia de Lange, Cerebral Palsy, Down, Prader-Willi, Turner, Rett, Williams and Tuberous Sclerosis.[16]		
Comments	*Patients with developmental disabilities are at high risk for periodontal disease for numerous reasons, including: difficulty maintaining hygiene, lack of access to regular dental care, syndrome-specific susceptibilities and medications.*		
	In some patients unable to tolerate office exams and treatment, hospital dentistry under anesthesia may be indicated. Other necessary diagnostic testing should be considered while patient is sedated.		
Depression	Screen annually or sooner for behaviors or emotions that may indicate depression.[16]		
Comments			
	Patients with developmental disabilities may have difficulty recognizing and communicating symptoms such as depressed mood, anxiety, and sadness. Mental health symptoms are often expressed in physical or behavioral changes. It is critical that healthcare providers obtain information about the patient's usual level of functioning, skills and behavior in order to assess the potential for mental health disorders.		
	See Diagnostic Manual-Intellectual Disabilities for more in-depth discussion on assessment.[11]		
Diabetes	Screen at least every three years until age 45. Screen annually after age 45 and annually for patients on antipsychotic medication and those with syndromes associated with diabetes, such as Prader-Willi, Klinefelter, Turner and Down.[16]		
Comments			
	Individualized decision-making about screening is appropriate for other individuals with developmental disabilities.		
	See American Diabetes Association. Consensus Statement on Antipsychotic Drugs and Obesity and Diabetes: http://care .diabetesjournals.org/content/27/2/596.full?ijkey=8499e4a1017d5491d7d7bb66d30b77013a2397c8&keytype2=tf_ipsecsha		
Fall Risk	For all ages: evaluate as part of the annual physical examination including an evaluation of the medication profile for drugs that may impact balance and/or gait. Screen more frequently if there is a change in gait/balance or for individuals at high risk, such as those who have a history of two or more falls in the previous year.[16]		
	For patients with no previous mobility impairments who report one or more falls, consider performing the "Get-Up and Go Test": http://www.ncbi.nlm.nih.gov/pubmed/3487300. Patients having difficulty with this test should be referred to a physical/occupational therapist for a full fall evaluation.		
	If the patient has had an increase in falls or a decline in function, a medical evaluation of the cause is warranted.		
HIV	For ages 13–64 screen with at least one HIV test in their lifetime.		
	Test periodically for patients at-risk (sexually active without barrier protection, multiple partners, men who have sex with men, all pregnant women, history of sexually transmitted diseases).[6,22]		

(continues)

TABLE 38-1 Healthcare Maintenance Guidelines for Adults with Developmental Disabilities *(continued)*

NOTE: Health problems that are seen more frequently in this population and require additional attention by healthcare providers are highlighted in the shaded area.

Health Problem	19 – 40 Years	40 – 65 Years	65 Years and Older
Hearing	Screen annually subjectively or objectively with office-based testing (Whisper Test).		
	—	Refer to audiology at regular intervals. Refer to patients for hearing assessment every five years after age 50 (every three years throughout life for patients with Down syndrome). Reevaluate hearing if problems are reported or changes in behavior are noted.[17]	
	Comments *Other syndromes associated with hearing impairments include Cornelia de Lange, Noonan, Usher, and Smith-Magenis.*[16] *Methods for testing may include the following:*		

Method	Applicable for Developmental Age (years)
OtoAcoustic Emissions (OAE)	> 0
Auditory Brainstem Responses (ABR)	> 0
Behavioral observation audiometry	> 0
Pure tone audiometry with visual reinforcement	> 1
Whispered speech	> 3
Pure tone (play) audiometry	> 3–4

Health Problem	19 – 40 Years	40 – 65 Years	65 Years and Older
Hypertension	Measure blood pressure annually.[22]		
	Comments *For patients with spasticity/contractures, may need to do a wrist or thigh blood pressure measurement. Document type of measurement used.*		
Immunizations	See Centers for Disease Control Recommended Adult Immunization Schedule: http://www.cdc.gov/mmwr/PDF/wk/mm5901-Immunization.pdf.		
Obesity	Measure height and weight annually.[22]		
	Comments *Consider weight on home scale in more familiar setting. Accommodations for patients unable to stand include using a Lift Team, a wheelchair scale, Hoyer Lift, and/or hospital bed which includes a scale.*		
Osteoporosis	Consider bone mineral density (BMD) screening earlier and at regular intervals for high-risk patients. Check serum vitamin D 25 OH levels at regular intervals.		
	—		Although the age to begin screening is unclear, some authors suggest age 40 for patients residing in institutions and age 45 for patients residing in the community. Multiple sources recommend BMD screening beginning for the general population at age 65 every three to five years if normal baseline test; at age 60 every one to two years if high risk. (AAFP, USPSTF, AACE).[10]

TABLE 38-1 Healthcare Maintenance Guidelines for Adults with Developmental Disabilities (continued)

NOTE: Health problems that are seen more frequently in this population and require additional attention by healthcare providers are highlighted in the shaded area.

Health Problem	19 – 40 Years	40 – 65 Years	65 Years and Older
Osteoporosis (continued)	**Comments** High risk factors in patients with developmental disabilities include: mobility impairments, long term use of antiepileptic drugs or antipsychotics, Down syndrome, Cerebral Palsy, and Prader-Willi syndrome. High risk factors in the general population include: osteopenia on plain films, history of vertebral fractures, early menopause, chronic steroid use, low body weight, cigarette use and positive family history of osteoporosis. See FRAX: WHO Fracture Risk Assessment Tool: www.shef.ac.uk/FRAX/. Note that mobility is not calculated in this assessment tool.		
Prostate Cancer (Men)	—	Insufficient evidence to recommend routine screening in men under age 75.[20]	Screening not recommended for men over age 75.[20]
	Comments Family history is often difficult to obtain with this population. Patients at high-risk include positive family history at an early age and African American men.		
Testicular Cancer (Men)	Routine screening not recommended. Prompt assessment and evaluation of testicular problems when young men present with signs and symptoms of testicular disease.[20]	—	
	Comments Clinical exam is especially important in this population who may not be able to report symptoms and may have difficulty with the self exam technique.		
Thyroid Disease	Perform thyroid stimulating hormone (TSH) test every three years.[16] Thyroid function tests should be performed annually for patients with Down syndrome.[17]		Perform TSH test annually.
	Comments Symptoms of thyroid disease are often not elicited due to cognitive impairment and/or communication difficulties in patients with developmental disabilities. Consider TSH testing if unexplained change in behavior or level of functioning. Increased risk for thyroid disease seen in patients with Down syndrome and the elderly.		
Tuberculosis	Screen routinely based on likelihood of exposure. (CDC 2005, AAFP 2008).		
	Comments Consider PPD skin testing every one to two years for patients who live or work in aggregate settings (board and care homes, intermediate care facilities, day programs).		

(continues)

TABLE 38-1 Healthcare Maintenance Guidelines for Adults with Developmental Disabilities *(continued)*

NOTE: Health problems that are seen more frequently in this population and require additional attention by healthcare providers are highlighted in the shaded area.

Health Problem	19 – 40 Years	40 – 65 Years	65 Years and Older
Vision	Screen annually subjectively or objectively with office-based tests.		
	Refer to ophthalmology for exam and glaucoma screening at least once before age 40 and by age 30 for patients with Down syndrome.[17]	Refer for ophthalmologic exam and glaucoma screening every two to three years or as recommended by ophthalmologist.	
	Comments *Screen more frequently for persons with diabetes, those on long-term psychiatric medication, and those with syndromes associated with vision deficits/ocular abnormalities, such as Cornelia de Lange, Fragile X, Down, Smith-Magenis, Tuberous Sclerosis, and Velocardiofacial.[16]*		

Counseling	19 – 40 Years	40 – 65 Years	65 Years and Older
Lifestyle Modification/ Healthy Quality of Life	Discuss: • Adequate calcium and vitamin D supplementation. • Advanced directive. • Dental hygiene. • Fall risk assessment and prevention. • Nutrition and physical activity. • Tobacco and substance abuse cessation. • Sexual health, including: contraception, sexually transmitted disease prevention, and healthy relationships.		
	Comments *Include caregivers, health advocates, and parents/family members to help reinforce teaching concepts.*		
Medication Review	Review medications at regular intervals with patients and caregivers to assure adherence with regimen and evaluate for side effects and drug interactions.		
	Comments *High rates of polypharmacy exist.*		
Safety	Review safety practices per individual circumstance, such as stranger and street safety for patients who live independently; prevention of head trauma in patients with frequent seizures; and street safety for patients with unpredictable behavior.		

REFERENCES

1. American Academy of Pediatrics Committee on Sports Medicine and Fitness. Atlantoaxial instability in Down syndrome: subject review. *Pediatrics.* 1995 Jul;96:151-4.
2. American Academy of Pediatrics; American Academy of Family Physicians; American College of Physicians-American Society of Internal Medicine. A consensus statement on health care transitions for young adults with special health care needs. *Pediatrics.* 2002 Dec;110(6):1304-6.
3. American College of Obstetricians and Gynecologists (ACOG) Committee on Practice Bulletins—Gynecology. ACOG Practice Bulletin no. 109: Cervical cytology screening. *Obstetrics & Gynecology.* 2009 Dec;114(6):1409-20.
4. American Cancer Society (ACS). ACS guidelines for the early detection of cancer. American Cancer Society Web site. 2008. Available at: www.cancer.org/docroot/PED/content/ped_2_3x _ACS_Cancer_Detection_Guidelines_36.asp. Accessed: February 2, 2010.

TABLE 38-1 Healthcare Maintenance Guidelines for Adults with Developmental Disabilities *(continued)*

REFERENCES *(continued)*

5. Breast Health Access for Women with Disabilities (BHAWD). (2003). *Breast health and beyond for women with disabilities: a provider's guide to the examination and screening of women with disabilities.* Alta Bates Summit Medical Center, Rehabilitation Services Department; Oakland;2003.

6. Centers for Disease Control and Prevention. *Sexually transmitted diseases; treatment guidelines 2006.* Department of Health and Human Services Centers for Disease Control and Prevention Web site. Available at: www.cdc.gov/std/treatment/. Accessed February 22, 2010.

7. Centers for Disease Control. Summary of HPV screening recommendations. Department of Health and Human Services Centers for Disease Control and Prevention Web site. Available at: www.cdc.gov/std/hpv/ScreeningTables.pdf. Accessed February 22, 2010.

8. Centers for Disease Control. Immunization recommendations. Department of Health and Human Services Centers for Disease Control and Prevention Web site. Available at: www.cdc.gov/vaccines/recs/schedules/adult-schedule.htm. Accessed February 22, 2010.

9. Cohen WI, ed. Health care guidelines for individuals with Down syndrome: 1999 revision. (1999) Down Syndrome Research Foundation Web site. 2010. Available at:www.dsrf.org/?section_copy_id=968&section_id=5040. Accessed February 22, 2010.

10. Gonzales R, Kutner JS. *Current Practice Guidelines in Primary Care 2009.* McGraw Hill 2009.

11. Fletcher R, Loschen E, Stavrakaki C, First M, eds. *Diagnostic Manual—Intellectual Disability; A textbook of diagnosis of mental disorders in persons with intellectual disability.* Kingston, NY:NADD Press; 2007. *This was put out by the National Association for Dual Diagnosis and the American Psychiatric Association.*

12. Havercamp SM, Scandlin D, Roth M. Health disparities among adults with developmental disabilities, adults with other disabilities, and adults not reporting disability in North Carolina. *Public Health Reports.* 2004 Jul-Aug;119(4):418-26.

13. Iacono T, Sutherland G. Health screening and developmental disabilities. *Journal of Policy and Practice in Intellectual Disabilities.* 2006 Sept;3(3):155-63.

14. Massachusetts Department of Mental Retardation, University of Massachusetts Medical School's Center for Developmental Disabilities Evaluation and Research. Preventive health recommendations for adults with mental retardation. The Official Web Site of the Commonwealth of Massachusetts. 2010. Available at: www.mass.gov/Eeohhs2/docs/dmr/health_screening_brochure.pdf. Accessed February 22, 2010.

15. National Heart, Lung, and Blood Institute. Risk Assessment Tool for Estimating Your 10-year Risk of Having a Heart Attack. Available at: hp2010.nhlbihin.net/atpiii/calculator.asp. Accessed February 22, 2010.

16. New York State Office of Mental Retardation & Developmental Disabilities. (2009). Preventive Health Care Screening Guidelines for People Aging with Intellectual and Other Developmental Disabilities. Available at: www.omr.state.ny.us/document/image/hp_brochures_preventhealthfinal.pdf. Accessed February 22, 2010.

17. Prasher V, Janicki M, eds. *Physical Health of Adults with Intellectual Disabilities (International Association for the Scientific Study of Intellectual Disabilities).* Blackwell Publishing, Ltd. Osney Mead: Oxford. 2002.

18. Prater CD, Zylstra R. Medical care of adults with mental retardation. *American Family Physician.* 2006 June 15;73(12): 2175-83. Review.

19. Saslow D, Runowicz CD, Solomon D, et al.; American Cancer Society (ACS). American Cancer Society guideline for the early detection of cervical neoplasia and cancer. *A Cancer Journal for Physicians.* 2002 Nov-Dec;52(6):342-62.

20. Sullivan, W. F., Berg, J. M., Bradley, E., Cheetham, T., Denton, R., Heng, J., . . . McMillan, S. (2011). Primary care of adults with developmental disabilities: Canadian consensus guidelines. *Canadian Family Physician, 57,* 541–553.

21. The American Geriatric Society. Breast cancer screening in older women (reviewed and updated in 2005). The American Geriatric Society Web site. 2010. Available at: www.americangeriatrics.org/education/crp_index.shtml. Accessed: February 22, 2010.

22. The U.S. Preventative Services Task Force. Guide to clinical preventative services, 2009. U.S. Department of Health and Human Services Web site. 2009. Available at: www.ahrq.gov/clinic/pocketgd.htm. Accessed: February 22, 2010. *Recommendations of the U.S. Preventative Services Task Force. Pocket guide, abridged version of the recommendations.*

23. U.S. Public Health Service. Closing the gap: A national blueprint for improving the health of individuals with mental retardation. Report of the Surgeon General's Conference on Health Disparities and Mental Retardation. Washington, DC. February 2001. Washington, D.C. Available at: www.surgeongeneral.gov/topics/mentalretardation/. Accessed: February 22, 2010.

24. Wilkinson JE, Cerreto MC. Primary care for women with intellectual disabilities. *Journal of the American Board of Family Medicine.* 2008 May-Jun;21(3)215-22.

25. Wilkinson JE, Culpepper L, Cerreto M. Screening tests for adults with intellectual disabilities. *Journal of the American Board of Family Medicine.* 2007 Jul-Aug;20(4):399-407. *This article takes a more evidence- based approach to recommending screening.*

C. *Patient education*

1. Primary focus should be on developing a trusting relationship with the patient and caregivers (Figure 38-4).

2. Provide lifestyle modification counseling to promote a healthy and happy quality of life (Table 38-1, counseling section).

3. Provide information on community resources to support patients, caregivers, and families.

4. Review safety practices for prevention of accidents and victimization.

V. Self-management resources and tools

A. *Healthcare provider resources*

1. Office of Developmental Primary Care, University of California, Department of Family & Community Medicine (http://developmentalmedicine.ucsf.edu).

2. Developmental Disabilities Division, State of California (www.ddhealthinfo.org).

3. Society for the Study of Behavioural Phenotypes (information on specific genetic syndromes and specific health risks) (http://www.ssbp.co.uk/ssbp/pages/syndrome-sheets.php).

4. Health assessment forms, yearly health checks, and other information (http://www.cddh.monash.org/disability-health-assessment.html).

5. National Women's Health Information Center (women with disabilities website) (http://www.iassid.org/pdf/healthguidelines-2002.pdf).

6. Information and resources for providers, women with disabilities, and families (www.4woman.gov/wwd/).

7. Developmental Disability Nurses Association (resources for healthcare providers and families) (www.ddna.org).

FIGURE 38-4 *Communicating with Patients with Developmental Disabilities*

Person-first language was developed by disability advocates to educate the community-at-large. It emphasizes the individual before the disability. For example, "This is Tom, he has Down syndrome," rather than, "Tom's retarded." Some people, especially those in the Autism and Deaf communities view their disability as an integral part of who they are. They may use other language to identify themselves and members of their community. It is always appropriate to use the language your patient prefers.

Avoid describing people with disabilities as overly courageous, brave, or special merely for having a disability. It is not unusual for them to accomplish significant things. It is always appropriate to celebrate the achievement of personal goals and milestones.

Also, avoid describing people with disabilities as overly pitiful and unfortunate. Most people with disabilities do not consider their lives tragic. They rate their quality of life far higher than many nondisabled people estimate.

Likewise, don't assume that people are unhappy or heroic simply because they are caring for a relative or friend who has a disability. It is helpful to inquire what challenges they face and assistance they need. Most caregivers appreciate empathy and assistance if they struggle with discrimination or lack of respite and accommodation.

Instead of. . .	Use . . .
Afflicted with . . . suffers from . . .	She has Down syndrome
Confined to a wheelchair/wheelchair-bound	Uses a wheelchair
Caretaker	Caregiver, or person who cares for, advocates for, or serves people . . .
Handicapped parking	Accessible parking
Mentally retarded	Person with an intellectual disability
"Normal" or "healthy"	Nondisabled/typical/neurotypical

Used with permission from the Office of Developmental Primary Care, Department of Family & Community Medicine, University of California, San Francisco.

B. Patient and caregiver resources

1. State of California Regional Center System (www.dds.ca.gov/RC/Home.cfm).

2. Support for Families (http://www.suportforfamilies.org).

3. Family Voices (http://www.familyvoices.org).

4. Oral health tips (http://www.nidcr.nih.gov/OralHealth/Topics /DevelopmentalDisabilities/PracticalOralCare PeopleIntellectualDisability.htm).

REFERENCES

American Academy of Pediatrics, American Academy of Family Physicians, & American College of Physicians. (2011). Supporting the health care transition from adolescence to adulthood in the medical home. *Pediatrics, 128*(1), 182–200. Retrieved from http://pediatrics .aapublications.org

American Association on Intellectual and Developmental Disabilities. (2010). Definition of intellectual disability. Retrieved from http ://www.aamr.org/content_100.cfm?navID=21

Centers for Disease Control and Prevention. (2009). Prevalence of autism spectrum disorders: Autism and Developmental Disabilities Monitoring Network, United States, 2006. *Morbidity and Mortality Weekly Report, 58*(SS-10), 1–24.

Cohen, W. I. (1999). Health care guidelines for individuals with Down Syndrome: 1999 revision. Down Syndrome Research Foundation. Retrieved from http://dsrf.org/index.cfm?fuseaction=inform.search Results&requestTimeout=500

Developmental Disabilities Assistance and Bill of Rights Act of 2000. Public Law 106-402. Retrieved from http://frwebpage .access.gpo.gov/cgi-bin/getdoc.cgi?dbname=106_cong_public _laws&docid=f:publ402.106.pdf

Glassman, P., Anderson, M., Jacobsen, P., Schonfeld, S., Weintraub, J., White, A., . . . Young, D. (2003). Practical protocols for the prevention of dental disease in community settings for people with special needs: The protocols. *Special Care Dentistry, 23*(5), 160–164.

Harder and Company Community Research. (2008). *A blind spot in the system: Health care for people with developmental disabilities: Findings from stakeholder interviews (September 2008).* Unpublished manuscript. San Francisco, CA.

Havercamp, S. M., Scandlin, D., & Roth, M. (2004). Health disparities among adults with developmental disabilities, adults with other disabilities and adults not reporting disability in North Carolina. *Public Health Report, 119*(4), 418–426.

Horwitz, S. M., Kerker, B. D., Owens, P. L., & Zigler, E. (2000). The health status and needs of individuals with mental retardation. Department of Epidemiology and Public Health, Yale University School of Medicine; Department of Psychology, Yale University, New Haven, CT. Retrieved from http://info.specialoplympics.org /Special+Olympics+Public+Website/English/Initiatives/Research /Health Research/Health+Status+and+Needs.htm

Johnson, C., & Myers, S. (2007). Identification and evaluation of children with autism spectrum disorders. *Pediatrics, 120*, 1183–1215.

Kozma, C. (2008). Down syndrome and dementia. *Topics in Geriatric Rehabilitation, 24*(1), 41–53.

Krahn, G. L., Hammond, L., & Turner, A. (2006). A cascade of disparities: Health and health care access for people with intellectual disabilities. *Mental Retardation and Developmental Disabilities Research Reviews, 12*:22–27.

Lennox, N., Bain, C., Rey-Conde, T., Purdie, D., Bush, R., & Pandeya, N. (2007). Effects of a comprehensive health assessment programme for Australian adults with intellectual disability: A cluster randomized trial. *International Journal of Epidemiology, 36*, 139–146.

New York State Office of Mental Retardation and Developmental Disabilities (2009). Preventative health care screening guidelines for people aging with intellectual and other developmental disabilities. Retrieved from www.omr.state.ny.us/document/image/hpbrochures preventhealthfinal.pdf

Sobsey, D., & Doe, T. (1991). Patterns of sexual abuse and assault. *Sexuality and Disability, 9*(3), 243–259.

Sullivan, W. F., Berg, J. M., Bradley, E., Cheetham, T., Denton, R., Heng, J. . . . McMillan, S. (2011). Primary care of adults with developmental disabilities: Canadian consensus guidelines. *Canadian Family Physician, 57*, 541–553.

Svien, L. R., Berg, P., & Stephenson, C. (2008). Issues in aging with cerebral palsy. *Topics in Geriatric Rehabilitation, 24*(1), 26–40.

United Cerebral Palsy. (2011). United cerebral palsy organization. Retrieved from http://www.ucp.org

U.S. Public Health Service (USPHS). (2001). *Closing the gap: A national blueprint for improving the health of individuals with mental retardation.* Report of the Surgeon General's conference on health disparities and mental retardation. Washington, DC. Retrieved from http://www .surgeongeneral.gov/topics/mentalretardation/

Yeargin-Allsopp, M. (2010, March 12). *Trends in the Epidemiology of Cerebral Palsy.* Keynote lecture at the Annual Update on Developmental Disabilities Conference at University of California, San Francisco, San Francisco, California.

HEALTHCARE MAINTENANCE FOR TRANSGENDERED INDIVIDUALS

Charles E. Williamson

I. Introduction and general background

Transgender people living in the United States are a marginalized and medically underserved community. Because of social stigmatization and institutional barriers, accessing health care is difficult, if not impossible, for many transgender patients. In fact, 30–40% of transgender persons in the United States rely on urgent care and emergency departments for their immediate healthcare needs (Feldman & Bockting, 2003). Nearly a third of transgender patients surveyed in multiple studies report discrimination, hostility, and outright refusal of medical care, resulting in a reluctance to seek routine and even urgent care (Herbst et al., 2008; Minter & Daley, 2003). As a result, the rates of preventable illnesses, such as HIV, are higher in the transgender community than in any other population. However, it has been demonstrated that routine medical care focusing on healthcare maintenance for transgender individuals can be delivered in the primary care setting safely and compassionately, without the need for specialty or psychiatric referrals (Alpert et al., 2006).

A. Transgender identity

1. Definition and overview

   The term "transgender" is a broadly used term to describe people whose gender identities, expression, and behaviors differ from their birth gender, irrespective of their physical appearance or sexual orientation (Feldman & Bockting, 2003; Kenagy,

2005). The terms "transsexual," "transvestite," and "gender identity disorder" have all been used to describe the same population, but these terms may be offensive to transgender patients. It is important to recognize that gender is seen by many as more than a binary concept. There is a spectrum of gender identity and expression that ranges from cross-dressing for entertainment or erotic purposes to those who consider themselves bi-gendered (Feldman & Goldberg, 2007; Sobralske, 2005). The term "gender identity disorder" is a clinical term listed in the fourth edition of the American Psychiatric Association's *Diagnostic and Statistical Manual of Mental Disorders*, and may be found restrictive or stigmatizing by some transgender people (Lombardi, 2001).

   a. Male-to-female (MTF): a biologic male who identifies as female

   b. Female-to-male (FTM): a biologic female who identifies as male

   c. Gender-variant, bi-gendered, or gender-queer: individuals who may be male, female, or of indeterminate gender who choose to identify as both or neither male or female

II. Database (may include but is not limited to)

A. Subjective

1. Pertinent past medical history, as outlined in Chapter 37, with focus on the following additional data

   a. Previous medical illnesses, with emphasis on a history of blood clots

   b. Sexually transmitted infection history and HIV status, including date of last screening tests

   c. Surgeries, with emphasis on any feminization or masculinization procedures, such as breast augmentation (for MTFs) or mastectomy (for FTMs). Other surgeries include facial feminization and tracheal shaving (MTF) and sexual reassignment surgeries, such as metoidoplasty and phalloplasty (FTM), and vaginoplasty (MTF).

   d. Cosmetic procedures, including those done by nonlicensed laypersons, such as silicone injections

   e. Previous psychiatric hospitalizations

   f. Medications, with emphasis on hormonal therapy, including names of medications, dosage, route, and source (i.e., Internet, Mexico, buying from friends, and so forth)

g. Immunization status, with emphasis on hepatitis A and B vaccines

h. Hepatitis C risk factors and antibody status

i. History of injuries, with emphasis on screening for abuse and domestic violence

2. Family history, with emphasis on cardiovascular disease and cardiac risk factors

3. Occupational history: screen for paid sex work and source of income to appropriately identify risk factors and need for support

4. Personal and social history

a. Legal status of name and gender identity (important for billing and documentation)

b. History of alcohol, tobacco, and drug use

c. History of depression or suicidal ideation or attempts

d. Relationships and social support network

e. Housing status

f. Future goals for feminization or masculinization, such as gender reassignment surgery

g. Successes and failures with gender reassignment, including anything currently bothering the patient about their appearance

B. *Objective*

1. Physical examination may be deferred until strong clinician–patient relationship is established, unless review of symptoms warrants immediate examination. Refer to Chapter 37 for general recommendations on frequency of physical examinations.

2. The patient should be prepared for the need for a physical examination in advance and given an opportunity to discuss their feelings about being examined.

3. Genital and breast examinations may cause particular distress for patients. Discuss with the patient in advance the rationale for the examination and ascertain how the patient would like one to refer to their anatomy (i.e., genitals, instead of penis or vagina).

4. For patients who have not had gender reassignment surgery, care should be taken to examine for cutaneous yeast infections around the breast areas for FTMs (if the patient practices breast binding) and around the genitals for MTFs (if the patient practices genital binding).

5. For patients who have had gender reassignment surgery, the clinician must familiarize themselves with the particular surgical technique used and screen for applicable complications.

6. For patients who have had silicone injections, the clinician should carefully examine the patient for signs of cellulitis or tissue deformity.

III. Assessment

A. *As outlined in Chapter 37, the current risk factors and health status of the patient should be identified, the patient's motivation to change unhealthy habits should be assessed, and the patient's ability to successfully accomplish adult developmental milestones should be determined.*

B. *Identify the patient's gender reassignment goals and barriers to the goals. Assess for benefits of hormonal gender reassignment therapy and undesirable side effects, such as weight gain and increased cardiovascular risk.*

C. *Identify psychosocial needs of the patient.*

IV. Plan

A. *Diagnostics (screening and secondary prevention tests)*

1. Screen for diseases and conditions based on the patient's risk profile. Note that normal laboratory values are often gender specific. There are no established guidelines for determining normal laboratory values for transgender patients, but the general rule is to use the biologic gender normal values until 2 years of hormone therapy have been completed, then use the normal values of the assigned gender (Feldman & Goldberg, 2007).

2. Screen for diseases and conditions specific to the transgender population.

a. MTF: check prolactin levels every 6 months to screen for prolactinoma, and excess use of estrogen for all patients receiving estrogen therapy. If prolactin level is less than 25, continue therapy. If the level is greater than 25, consider decrease in estrogen therapy. If greater than 100, stop estrogen therapy for at least 8 weeks and recheck. Obtain a magnetic resonance image if still elevated (Alpert et al., 2006).

b. MTF: because the prostate gland is not removed during gender reassignment surgery, the current screening guidelines for prostate cancer for the general population should be followed for all MTF patients.

   c. FTM: a complete blood count and liver function tests should be drawn every 6 months for all patients receiving testosterone therapy to screen for polycythemia and transaminitis (Alpert et al., 2006).

3. Screen for high-risk sexual behavior at every clinic visit. Test for sexually transmitted infections and HIV every 6 months for those with risk factors. Consider testing more frequently for patients engaged in paid sex work.

4. Screen for depression and suicidal ideation at every clinic visit.

5. There is no evidence to support the need for mammograms in MTF individuals. MTF patients do not seem to have an increased risk of breast cancer when using hormone replacement therapy (Feldman & Goldberg, 2006).

6. For FTM patients, the screening recommendations for cervical cancer are the same as for the general population (Feldman & Goldberg, 2006). However, special care is required to explain the rationale for cervical cancer screening to the FTM patient and should only be offered after establishing a strong relationship with the patient.

B. Treatment

1. Refer to Chapter 37 for immunization recommendations.

2. For prescribing/furnishing/drug ordering guidelines for hormonal therapy, see Table 39-1. Use the appropriate drug interaction database when prescribing hormone therapy to avoid adverse drug interactions, especially for patients taking HIV antiretroviral, antidepressant, and anticonvulsant medications.

   a. MTF patients: Most MTF patients can be successfully transitioned with the use of estrogen and spironolactone alone. Always limit estrogen to one type and use the lowest effective dose. Consider adding additional antiandrogen drugs if beard growth is not adequately suppressed or if patient becomes hypotensive on spironolactone. Patients who have had an orchiectomy or gender reassignment surgery require only estrogen to maintain a feminine appearance.

   b. FTM patients: Most FTM patients can be successfully transitioned with the use of testosterone alone. Testosterone dose should not necessarily be reduced after hysterectomy or

sex reassignment surgery. All patients should have a complete blood count, complete metabolic profile, and for MTF patients a baseline prolactin level. Recheck laboratory values after 1 month of therapy and then at least every 6 months. Patients should be educated that it takes approximately 2 years to transition regardless of the dosage of hormones. Increasing the dose of hormone therapy will not hasten the transitioning process. Note that the use of hormones for gender reassignment is off label and the provider should obtain informed consent before initiating therapy.

3. Particular emphasis should be placed on smoking cessation strategies for patients receiving estrogen therapy because of the increase risk of thromboemboli.

4. Consider referring HIV-positive patients for care at a specialty clinic, unless the provider is trained in HIV-AIDS.

5. Consider a psychiatric or mental health referral for patients who have mental illnesses, such as depression. Routine referral for psychiatric care is not otherwise warranted and may alienate patients.

C. Patient education

1. Primary focus should be on developing a trusting relationship with the patient and assisting the patient to overcome previous negative experiences with healthcare providers.

2. Provide health counseling with particular attention to HIV prevention.

3. Provide information on community resources, such as legal and housing assistance.

4. Periodic health counseling as outlined in Chapter 37.

V. Self-management resources and tools

1. Vancouver Coastal Health Clinic has excellent resources for both providers and patients on a variety of topics related to transgender health promotion, mental health, and other topics (www.transhealth.vch.ca)

2. An online textbook produced by Dr. Nick Gorton has evidence-based recommendations and resources for primary care providers caring for transgendered individuals (www.nickgorton.org)

TABLE 39-1 Hormone Guidelines for Sex Reassignment

Name of Drug	Purpose	Dosage	Precautions	Contraindications	Average Cost for 30-Day Generic Supply
Estradiol	Feminization	2–8 mg/d	Deep venous thrombosis, pulmonary embolism, other thromboembolism, thrombophlebitis, hypertension, impotence, prolactinoma, diabetes, nausea or vomiting, migraine or headache, gallbladder disease, abnormal liver function tests, mood disorder or depression, melasma (skin darkening), acne, lipid abnormalities, hypertriglyceridemia, increased risk of heart attack, increased risk of breast cancer, hepatitis, stroke, increased risk of other cancers	Presence of estrogen-dependent cancer; history of thromboembolism or severe thrombophlebitis	$4–$16
Premarin	Feminization	1.25–10 mg/d	Same as estradiol	Same as estradiol	$60–$425
Delestrogen	Feminization	20–80 mg q 2 weeks	Same as estradiol	Same as estradiol	$18–$72 (note that generic form is inconsistently available)
Estradiol patch	Feminization	0.1–0.3 mg/d	Same as estradiol	Same as estradiol	$36–$87
Spironolactone	Antiandrogen	25–200 mg/d	Avoid using concomitantly with digoxin, angiotensin-converting enzyme inhibitors, potassium-sparing diuretics, and AT II receptor antagonists	Renal insufficiency; serum potassium > 5.5 mEq/L	$16–$72
Finasteride	Antiandrogen	5 mg/d	Caution if hepatic insufficiency	No absolute contraindications	$70
Medroxyprogesterone	Antiandrogen	2.5–20 mg/d	Same as estradiol	Same as estradiol	$13–$17
Testosterone cypionate	Masculinization	100–400 mg q 2–4 weeks	May potentiate warfarin; hyperlipidemia, liver disease, cigarette smoking, obesity, family history of coronary artery disease, family history of breast cancer, acne, history of deep venous thrombosis, and erythrocytosis	Active coronary disease, pregnancy	$14–$71
Testosterone transdermal patch	Masculinization	2.5 mg patches: 1–2 per day	Same as testosterone cypionate	Same as testosterone cypionate	$139–$279
Testosterone topical gel	Masculinization	1% gel: 5–10 g/day	Same as testosterone cypionate Caution patients not to apply on genital areas	Same as testosterone cypionate	$291–$582

Source: Adapted from San Francisco Department of Public Health Tom Waddell Health Center Protocols for Hormonal Reassignment of Gender. Retrieved from http://www.sfdph.org/dph /comupg/oservices/medSvs/hlthCtrs/TransGendprotocols122006.pdf

REFERENCES

Alpert, L. M., Bishop, E., Davidson, A., Francivich, J., Freeman, M., Jaye, M. . . . Zevin, B. (2006). *Tom Waddell Health Center protocols for hormonal reassignment of gender.* Retrieved from http://www.sfdph.org/_dph/_comupg/_oservices/_medsvs/_hlthctrs/_transgend protocols122006.pdf

Feldman, J., & Bockting, W. (2003). Transgender health. *Minnesota Medicine, 86*(7), 25–32.

Feldman, J., & Goldberg, J. (2006). *Transgender primary medical care: Suggested guidelines for physicians in British Columbia.* Retrieved from http://www.vch.ca/_transhealth/_resources/_library/_tcpdocs/_guidelines-primcare.pdf

Feldman, J. L., & Goldberg, J. M. (2007). Transgender primary medical care. *International Journal of Transgenderism, 9*(3/4), 3–34.

Herbst, J. H., Jacobs, E. D., Finlayson, T. J., McKleroy, V. S., Neumann, M. S., & Crepaz, N. (2008). Estimating HIV prevalence and risk behaviors of transgender persons in the United States: A systematic review. *AIDS and Behavior, 12*(1), 1–17.

Kenagy, G. P. (2005). Transgender health: Findings from two needs assessment studies in Philadelphia. *Health & Social Work, 30*(1), 19–26.

Lombardi, E. (2001). Enhancing transgender health care. *American Journal of Public Health, 91*(6), 869–872.

Minter, S., & Daley, C. (2003). *Trans Realities: A legal needs assessment of San Francisco's transgender communities.* San Francisco, CA: Transgender Law Center and National Center for Lesbian Rights.

Sobralske, M. (2005). Primary care needs of patients who have undergone gender reassignment. *Journal of the American Academy of Nurse Practitioners, 17*(4), 133–138.

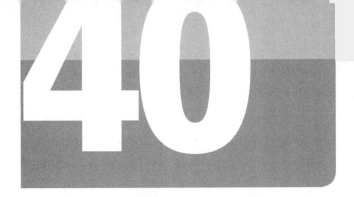

POSTEXPOSURE PROPHYLAXIS FOR HIV INFECTION

Barbara Newlin

I. Definition and overview

The advent of HIV infection in the 1980s brought with it widespread anxiety about the risks of infection in health care and other settings. As soon as antiretroviral medications were approved for use in HIV-infected individuals in the 1990s, the concept of using them in people with known risky exposures arose (postexposure prophylaxis [PEP]). There are an estimated 400,000 occupational exposures to HIV per year in the United States. By 2001, there were 57 confirmed and 138 possible HIV seroconversions caused by occupational exposures (Henderson, 2001).

Antiretrovirals have been used for occupational (PEP) and for nonoccupational exposures (nPEP). Empiric evidence about the effectiveness of PEP, however, is in short supply. The first attempted randomized trial of zidovudine monotherapy for PEP was closed early because of enrollment difficulties. The best evidence for efficacy is a Centers for Disease Control and Prevention case-control study that suggests 81% reduction in risk of HIV infection with use of zidovudine only (Cardo et al., 1997). Randomized controlled trials of PEP are not feasible, but experts agree that the concept of giving antiretroviral medication to arrest infection before it is able to take hold makes sense, and that PEP should be offered to individuals with high-risk exposures to HIV. Indeed, several organizations have developed comprehensive guidelines for the use of PEP (New York State Department of Health AIDS Institute, 2008; Panlilio et al., 2005; World Health Organization, 2005).

A. When should PEP be considered?

Best evidence suggests that the riskiest exposures to HIV occur when large amounts of infectious fluids

(Table 40-1) are injected directly into the body, or contacted by nonintact skin or mucous membranes. Table 40-2 shows the risks of contracting HIV infection through various routes of exposure. Tables 40-3 and 40-4 summarize the 2005 US Public Health Service recommendations for when PEP should be considered for occupational and nonoccupational exposures (sexual, injected drug use, and other exposures). Table 40-5 is an algorithm for considering PEP after nPEP. Table 40-6 summarizes the 2008 New York Health Department (NYHD) guidelines for initiating and following PEP. There are some disagreements in the guidelines as to whether two-drug or three-drug regimens should be used. Generally, two drugs are recommended for lower-risk exposures and three drugs for those of higher risk. The NYHD guidelines recommend three drugs for any exposures risky enough to require PEP (Table 40-6).

The guidelines all agree that the timing of PEP is crucial. It must be started as soon as possible after exposure, with the outside limit of 72 hours. Agreement also exists that PEP should be continued for 28 days to maximize effectiveness (New York State Department of Health AIDS Institute, 2008; Panlilio et al., 2005; World Health Organization, 2005).

B. Weighing the risks and benefits of PEP

The clinician must decide what to recommend to potentially exposed clients. Because of the lack of empiric data, a cost/benefit analysis of PEP is impossible. Factors to weigh include route of exposure; amount of infectious fluid involved; HIV serostatus and stage of disease of the source (including viral load); overall health and pregnancy status of the recipient; mental state of the recipient; and possibility of adverse reactions to the antiretrovirals (Tables 40-3, 40-4, and 40-6). After carefully reviewing all the information, the clinician and the client can together make a decision about whether or not PEP will be initiated, and whether to use a two-drug or three-drug regimen.

II. Database (may include but is not limited to)

A. Subjective

1. History of exposure
   a. When did the exposure occur (exact time and date)
   b. What type of exposure (skin, mucous membrane, percutaneous, or sexual; route of exposure if sexual [vaginal, anal, or oral])
   c. Other details about exposure: trauma involved, deep or shallow, and amount and type of fluid involved

TABLE 40-1 HIV Infectious Fluids

Body fluids infectious for HIV

Blood and plasma

Semen

Amniotic fluid

Vaginal secretions

Cerebrospinal fluid

Synovial fluid

Pleural fluid

Peritoneal fluid

Pericardial fluid

Body fluids noninfectious for HIV

Saliva

Tears

Sweat

Nonbloody urine or feces

Source: Medical Care Criteria Committee. HIV prophylaxis following occupational exposure. New York State Department of Health AIDS Institute, 2008. Available at www.hivguidelnes.org.

TABLE 40-2 Risk of HIV Infection by Routes of Exposure

Exposure Route	Risk Per 10,000 Exposures to an Infected Source	Reference
Blood transfusion	9,000	74
Needle-sharing injection-drug use	67	75
Receptive anal intercourse	50	76, 77
Percutaneous needle stick	30	78
Receptive penile-vaginal intercourse	10	76, 77, 79
Insertive anal intercourse	6.5	76, 77
Insertive penile-vaginal intercourse	5	76, 77
Receptive oral intercourse	1	77†
Insertive oral intercourse	0.5	77†

* Estimate of risk for transmission from sexual exposures assume no condom use.

† Source refers to oral intercourse performed on a man.

Sources: Centers for Disease Control and Prevention. Antiretroviral postexposure prophylaxis after sexual, injection-drug use, or other nonoccupational exposure to HIV in the United States: recommendations from the U.S. Department of Health and Human Services. Morbidity and Mortality Weekly Report 2005; 54 (No. RR-2); Smith et al., 2005.

TABLE 40-3 PEP Recommendations After Percutaneous Injuries (USPHS Guidelines)

Exposure Type	Infection Status of Source				
	HIV-Positive Class 1*	HIV-Positive Class 2*	Source of Unknown HIV Status[†]	Unknown Source[§]	HIV-Negative
Less Severe[¶]	Recommend basic 2-drug PEP	Recommend expanded ≥ 3-drug PEP	Generally, no PEP warranted; however, consider basic 2-drug PEP** for source with HIV risk factors[††]	Generally, no PEP warranted; however, consider basic 2-drug PEP** in settings in which exposure to HIV infected persons is likely	NO PEP warranted
More severe[§§]	Recommend expanded 3-drug PEP	Recommend expanded ≥ 3-drug PEP	Generally, no PEP warranted; however, consider basic 2-drug PEP** for source with HIV risk factors[††]	Generally, no PEP warranted; however, consider basic 2-drug PEP** in settings in which exposure to HIV infected persons is likely	NO PEP warranted

* HIV-positive, class 1 — asymptomatic HIV infection or known low viral load (e.g., <1,500 ribonucleic acid copies/mL). HIV-positive, class 2 — symptomatic HIV infection, acquired immunodeficiency syndrome, acute seroconversion, or known high viral load. If drug resistance is a concern, obtain export consultation. Initiation of PEP should not be delayed pending expert consultation, and, because expert consultation alone cannot substitute for face-to-face counseling, resources should be available to provide immediate evaluation and follow-up care for all exposures.

[†] For example, deceased source person with no samples available for HIV testing.

§ For example, a needle from a sharps disposal container.

¶ For example, solid needle or superficial injury.

** The recommendation "consider PEP" indicate that PEP is optional; a decision to initiate PEP should be based on a discussion between the exposed person and the treating clinician regarding the risks versus benefits of PEP.

[††] If PEP is offered and administered and the source is later determined to be HIV-negative, PEP should be discontinued.

§§ For example, large-bore hollow needle, deep puncture, visible blood on device, or needle used in patient's artery or vein.

Sources: Centers for Disease Control and Prevention. Updated U.S. Public Health Service guidelines for the management of occupational exposures to HIV and recommendations for Postexposure Prophylaxis. Morbidity and Mortality Weekly Report 2005; 54 (No. RR-9); Panlilio et al., 2005.

TABLE 40-4 PEP Recommendations for Skin and Mucous Membrane Exposures (USPHS 2005)

Exposure Type	Infection Status of Source				
	HIV-Positive, Class 1[†]	HIV-Positive, Class 2[†]	Source of Unknown HIV Status[§]	Unknown Source[¶]	HIV-Negative
Small volume**	Consider basic 2-drug PEP[††]	Recommend basic 2-drug PEP	Generally, no PEP warranted[§§]	Generally, no PEP warranted	No PEP warranted
Large volume[¶¶]	Recommend basic 2-drug PEP	Recommend expanded ≥3-drug PEP	Generally, no PEP warranted; however, consider basic 2-drug PEP[††] for source with HIV risk factors[§§]	Generally, no PEP warranted; however, consider basic 2-drug PEP[††] in settings in which exposure to HIV-infected persons is likely	No PEP warranted

* For skin exposures, follow-up is indicated only if evidence exists of compromised skin integrity (e.g., dermatitis, abrasion, or open wound).

[†] HIV-positive, class 1 — asymptomatic HIV infection or known low viral load (e.g., <1,500 ribonucleic acid copies/mL). HIV-positive, class 2 — symptomatic HIV infection, AIDS, acute seroconversion, or known high viral load If drug resistance is a concern, obtain expert consultation. Initiation of PEP should not be delayed pending expert consultation, and because expert consultation alone cannot substitute for face-to-face counseling, resources should be available to provide immediate evaluation and follow-up care for all exposures.

§ For example, deceased source person with no samples available for HIV testing.

¶ For example, splash from inappropriately disposed blood.

** For example, a few drops.

[††] The recommendation "consider PEP" indicates that PEP is optional; a decision to initiate Pep should be based on a discussion between the exposed person and the treating clinician regarding the risks versus benefits of PEP.

§§ If Pep is offered and administered and the source is later determined to be HIV-negative, PEP should be discontinued.

¶¶ For example, a major blood splash.

Sources: Centers for Disease Control and Prevention. Updated U.S. Public Health Service guidelines for the management of occupational exposures to HIV and recommendations for Postexposure Prophylaxis. Morbidity and Mortality Weekly Report 2005; 54 (No. RR-9); Panlilio et al, 2005.

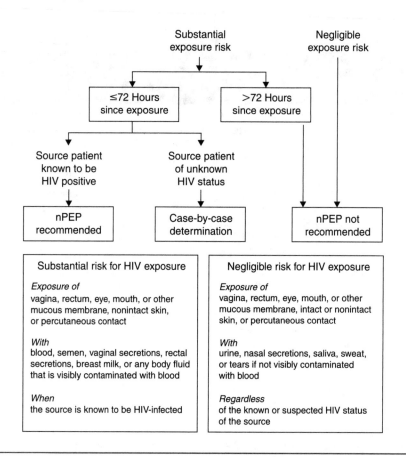

TABLE 40-5 Algorithm for Considering PEP After Non-Occupational HIV Exposures (nPEP)

Sources: Centers for Disease Control and Prevention. Antiretroviral postexposure prophylaxis after sexual, injection-drug use, or other nonoccupational exposure to HIV in the United States: recommendations from the U.S. Department of Health and Human Services. Morbidity and Mortality Weekly Report 2005; 54 (No. 44-2); Smith et al., 2005.

d. Information about the exposure source
   i. Known HIV-positive? Able to document? Stage of illness? Type of antiretrovirals taken now and in the past? Viral load at present time?
   ii. If HIV status is unknown or documented negative, are there risk factors for HIV infection present? Does the source have signs or symptoms of primary HIV infection (fever, rash, or flu-like symptoms) (Table 40-8)? Can the source be located and can a rapid HIV test be obtained?

2. Patient history, including but not limited to
   a. Any history of HIV infection or use of antiretrovirals, previous exposures to HIV, previous PEP, previous HIV testing, other HIV risk factors; liver or kidney disease (especially hepatitis A, B, or C); allergies or adverse reactions to medications; previous sexually transmitted infections; surgeries

   b. General health history: any chronic disease
   c. Social history: sexual history, pregnancy, relationships, social support, living circumstances, and health habits

3. Review of systems

   Complete review of systems is appropriate with emphasis on mouth; skin; liver; gastrointestinal; kidney; genitalia; neurologic (especially headache and peripheral neuropathy history); and psychiatric symptoms.

B. *Objective*

1. Physical examination
   a. Examine area of exposure and assess for trauma, lesions, bruising excoriations, or other breaks in the integrity of skin or mucous membranes, and cleanliness.
   b. Skin: baseline to identify existing lesions or rashes
   c. Head: baseline for headaches or sinus tenderness

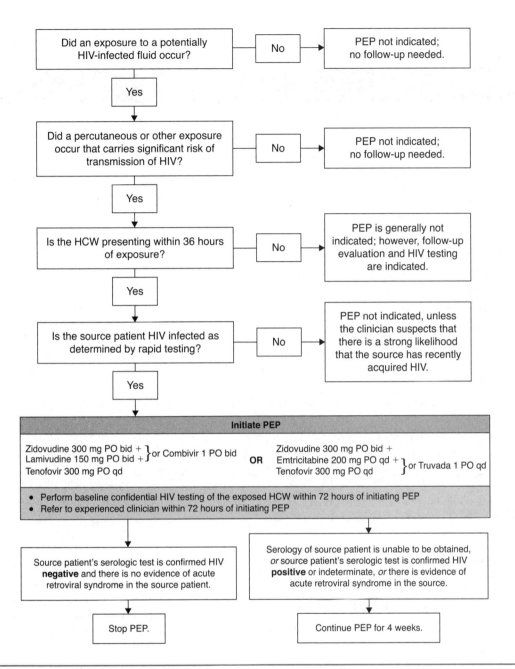

TABLE 40-6 Algorithm for Determining Need to Initiate PEP (New York State Department of Health AIDS Institute, 2008)

Source: Medical Care Criteria Committee. HIV prophylaxis following occupational exposure. New York State Department of Health AIDS Institute, 2008. Available at www.hivguidelines.org.

d. Mouth: baseline for lesions or periodontal disease

e. Abdomen: baseline liver and spleen size and tenderness, general state of abdomen

f. Neurologic: baseline general neurology (especially DTRs and sensory examination)

g. Genital and anal examination for sexual exposures

2. Diagnostic testing

See Table 40-7 for a chart of laboratory examinations recommended before and during PEP and nPEP

TABLE 40-7 Recommended Laboratory Testing and Monitoring for PEP and nPEP (USPHS Guidelines 2005)

Note: STD Screen is recommended for sexual exposures and PRN for others

Test	Baseline	During nPEP*	4–6 Weeks After Exposure	3 Months After Exposure	6 Months After Exposure
HIV antibody testing	E†, S§		E	E	E
Complete blood count with differential	E	E			
Serum liver enzymes	E	E			
Blood urea nitrogen/creatinine	E	E			
Sexually transmitted diseases screen (gonorrhea, chlamydia, syphilis)	E, S	E¶	E¶		
Hepatitis B serology	E, S		E¶	E¶	
Hepatitis C serology	E, S			E	E
Pregnancy test (for women of reproductive age)	E	E¶	E¶		
HIV viral load	S		E**	E**	E**
HIV resistance testing	S		E**	E**	E**
CD4+ T lymphocyte count	S		E**	E**	E**

*Other specific tests might be indicated dependent on the antiretrovirals prescribed. Literature pertaining to individual agents should be consulted.

†E = exposed patient, S = source.

§ HIV antibody testing of the source patient is indicated for sources of unknown serostatus.

¶ Additional testing for pregnancy, sexually transmitted diseases, and hepatitis B should be performed as clinically indicated.

** If determined to be HIV infected on follow-up testing; perform as clinically indicated once diagnosed.

Sources: Centers for Disease Control and Prevention. Antiretroviral postexposure prophylaxis after sexual, injection-drug use, or other nonoccupational exposure to HIV in the United States: recommendations from the U.S. Department of Health and Human Services. Morbidity and Mortality Weekly Report 2005; 54 (No. RR-2); Smith et al., 2005.

III. Assessment

A. Determine the diagnosis and its significance

1. Determine the level of risk for HIV exposure and weigh the benefits of treatment.

2. Determine the significance of possible exposure to the patient and significant others, noting the amount of psychologic distress present.

3. Assess the motivation and ability of the patient to follow through with the treatment plan.

4. Note the amount of social support to help with coping during this stressful time.

IV. Plan

A. Diagnostic tests (Table 40-7)

B. Management

1. The area of exposure should be washed gently with soap and water (for skin) or rinsed liberally with clean water or saline solution (for mucous membranes). Genitals and anal area may be gently bathed with mild soapy water, but douching is not recommended. Any trauma should be appropriately treated. Avoid squeezing, scrubbing, or otherwise traumatizing the area of exposure.

2. PEP recommended

   a. If significant exposure has occurred (Tables 40-2, 40-3, and 40-4), decide on two-drug or three-drug regimen and initiate

      i. Two-drug regimens include AZT/3TC (Combivir; data supports use) or TDF/FTC (Truvada; less toxicity seen). See Table 40-11 for dosing and Table 40-10 for major side effects (Gupta, 2009; Landowitz & Ebrahamzadeh, 2009)

      ii. Three-drug regimens consist of one of the two combinations mentioned previously plus a protease inhibitor, usually LPV/r (lopinavir boosted with ritonavir [Kaletra®]) or another potent

TABLE 40-8 Signs and Symptoms of HIV Primary Infection (Acute Retroviral Syndrome)

Symptom/Sign	%
Fever	96
Lymphadenopathy	74
Pharyngitis	70
Rash Erythematous maculopapular with lesions on face, trunk and sometimes extremities, including palms and soles; mucocutaneous ulceration involving mouth, esophagus or genitals	70
Myalgia or arthralgia	54
Diarrhea	32
Headache	32
Nausea and vomiting	27
Hepatosplenomegaly	14
Weight loss	13
Thrush	12
Neurologic symptoms Meningoencephalitis or aseptic meningitis; peripheral neuropathy or radiculopathy; facial palsy; Guillain-Barré syndrome; brachial neuritis; or cognitive impairment or psychosis	12

Sources: Centers for Disease Control and Prevention. Antiretroviral postexposure prophylaxis after sexual, injection-drug use, or other nonoccupational exposure to HIV in the United States: recommendations from the U.S. Department of Health and Human Services. Morbidity and Mortality Weekly Report 2005; 54 (No. RR-2); Smith et al., 2005.

TABLE 40-9 Counseling for Any Person Having Experienced Exposure to HIV Whether PEP Has Been Recommended or Not

Exposed HCP should be advised to use precautions (e.g., avoid blood or tissue donations, breastfeeding, or pregnancy) to prevent secondary transmission, especially during the first 6–12 weeks postexposure.
For exposures for which PEP is prescribed, HCP should be informed regarding • possible drug toxicities and the need for monitoring, • possible drug interactions, and • the need for adherence to PEP regimens.
Consider reevaluation of exposed HCP 72 hours post-exposure, especially after additional information about the exposure or source person becomes available.

Sources: Centers for Disease Control and Prevention. Updated U.S. Public Health Service guidelines for the management of occupational exposures to HIV and recommendations for Postexposure Prophylaxis. Morbidity and Mortality Weekly Report 2005; 54 (No. RR-9); Panlilio et al., 2005.

protease inhibitor with a low side effect profile (Tables 40-10 and 40-11) (Gupta, 2009; Landowitz & Ebrahamzadeh, 2009; Panlilio et al., 2005). The NYHD guidelines recommend three drugs for any exposure risky enough to warrant PEP, using triple nucleoside reverse transcriptase inhibitors NRTI drug combinations (Table 40-6). Resistance profiles from the source patient may be helpful in choosing PEP drugs. Strict adherence to drug regimens is essential for effectiveness and to avoid drug resistance. An HIV pharmacist should be consulted if feasible.

b. Follow-up should ideally be referred to an HIV specialist. The client should be seen and follow-up at least after the first 3 weeks, or earlier if they are experiencing any problems, especially symptoms of HIV primary infection (Table 40-8).

c. Supportive counseling to ensure adherence to the medication regimen and alleviate anxiety is highly recommended (Table 40-9).

3. PEP not recommended

a. If significant exposure has not occurred, counsel patient on why PEP is not recommended and how to avoid further exposures.

b. Advise patient to follow-up if experiencing any problems, especially symptoms of HIV primary infection (Table 40-8).

C. *Patient education*

Mechanism of HIV infection, possible medication toxicities, strict adherence to medications regimen, mechanism of resistance development, strategies for not infecting others, and signs and symptoms of primary infection (Tables 40-8 and 40-9).

V. Clinician and patient resources

1. HIV Warmline: 1-800-933-3413

2. PEP Line: 1-888-HIV-4911

3. National HIV/AIDS Clinicians' Consulting Center: http://www.nccc.ucsf.edu.
   A comprehensive website including links to many HIV-related guidelines, including PEP. It is advisable to check frequently for updates to these guidelines.

TABLE 40-10 Major Side Effects of Antiretrovirals Which May Be Used for PEP

Class and Agent	Side Effect and Toxicity
Nucleoside reverse transcriptase inhibitors (NRTI)	**Class warning: all NRTIs have the potential to cause lactic acidosis with hepatic steatosis**
Zidovudine (Retrovir®; ZDV, AZT)	Anemia, neutropenia, nausea, headache, insomnia, muscle pain, and weakness
Lamivudine (Epivir®, 3TC)	Abdominal pain, nausea, diarrhea, rash, and pancreatitis
Stavudine (Zerit™; d4T)	Peripheral neuropathy, headache, diarrhea, nausea, insomnia, anorexia, pancreatitis, elevated liver function teats (LFTs), anemia, and neutropenia
Didanosine (Videx®; ddI)	Pancreatitis, lactic acidosis, neuropathy, diarrhea, abdominal pain, and nausea
Emtricitabine (Emtriva, FTC)	Headache, nausea, vomiting, diarrhea, and rash. Skin discoloration (mild hyperpigmentation on palms and soles), primarily among nonwhites
Nucleotide analogue reverse transcriptase inhibitor (NtRTI)	**Class warning: All NtRTIs have the potential to cause lactic acidosis with hepatic steatosis**
Tenofovir (Viread®; TDF)	Nausea, diarrhea, vomiting, flatulence, and headache
Nonnucleoside reverse transcriptase inhibitors (NNRTIs)	
Efavirenz (Sustiva®; EFV)	Rash (including cases of Stevens-Johnson syndrome), insomnia, somnolence, dizziness, trouble concentrating, abnormal dreaming, and teratogenicity
Protease inhibitor	
Indinavir (Crixivan®; IDV)	Nausea, abdominal pain, nephrolithiasis, and indirect hyperbilirubinemia
Nelfinavir (Viracept®; NFV)	Diarrhea, nausea, abdominal pain, weakness, and rash
Ritonavir (Norvir®; RTV)	Weakness, diarrhea, nausea, circumoral paresthesia, taste alteration, and elevated cholesterol and triglycerides
Saquinavir (invirase®; SQV)	Diarrhea, abdominal pain, nausea, hyperglycemia, and elevated LFTs
Fosamprenavir (Lexiva®, FOSAPV)	Nausea, diarrhea, rash, circumoral paresthesia, taste alteration, and depression
Atazanavir (Reyatazr; ATV)	Nausea, headache, rash, abdominal pain, diarrhea, vomiting, and indirect hyperbilirubinemia
Lopinavir/ritonavir (Kaletra®; LPV/RTV)	Diarrhea, fatigue, headache, nausea, and increased cholesterol and triglycerides
Fusion inhibitor	
Enfuvirtide (Fuzeon®; T-20)	Local Injection site reactions, bacterial pneumonia, insomnia, depression, peripheral neuropathy, and cough

Sources: Package inserts; Panel on Clinical Practices for Treatment of HIV Infection. Guidelines for the use of antiretroviral agents in HIV-infected adults and adolescents—April 7, 2005. Washington, DC: National Institutes of Health; 2005. Available at http://aidsinfo.nih.gov/guidelines /default_db2.asp?id=50.

Sources: Centers for Disease Control and Prevention. Updated U.S. Public Health Service guidelines for the management of occupational exposures to HIV and recommendations for Postexposure Prophylaxis. Morbidity and Mortality Weekly Report 2005; 54 (No. RR-9); Panlilio et al., 2005.

TABLE 40-11 The Main Antiretrovirals Recommended for PEP with Dosage and Approximate Cost (adapted from USPHS guidelines 2005)

Medication	Adult Dosage	Cost (In Dollars for 4 Weeks
Combination tablets		
Lopinavir/ritonavir (Kaletra®)	3 tablets twice daily 400 mg lopinavir/100 mg ritonavir	650
Zidovudine/lamivudine (Combirvir®)	1 tablet twice daily 300 mg zidovudine/150 mg lamivudine	640
Zidovudine/lamivudine/ abacavir (Trizivir®)	1 tablet twice daily 300 mg zidovudine/150 mg lamivudine/300 mg abacavir	1,020
Lamivudine/abacavir (Epzicom®)	1 tablet once daily 300 mg lamivudine/600 mg abacavir	760
Emtricitabine/temofovir (Truvada®)	1 tablet once daily 200 mg emtricitabine/300 mg tenofovir	800

Sources: Centers for Disease Control and Prevention. Updated U.S. Public Health Service guidelines for the management of occupational exposures to HIV and recommendations for Postexposure Prophylaxis. Morbidity and Mortality Weekly Report 2005; 54 (No.RR-9).All material in the Morbidity and Mortality Weekly Report Series is in the public domain and may be used and reprinted without permission; Panlilio et al., 2005.

REFERENCES

Cardo, D. M., Culver, D. H., Ciesielski, C. A., Srivastava, P. U., Marcus, R., Abiteboul, D. . . . Bell, D. M. (1997). A case-control study of HIV seroconversion in health care workers after percutaneous exposure. Centers for Disease Control and Prevention Needlestick Surveillance Group. *New England Journal of Medicine, 337*(21), 1485–1490.

Gupta, A. (2009). *Johns Hopkins HIV guide: Post-exposure prophylaxis, 2010.* Retrieved from http://www.hopkins-hivguide.org/managemnet/antiretroviral_therapy/post-exposure_prophylaxis

Henderson, D. K. (2001). HIV postexposure prophylaxis in the 21st century. *Emerging Infectious Diseases, 7*(2), 254–258.

Landowitz, R., & Ebrahamzadeh, P. (2009). *Management of occupational and non-occupational HIV exposure.* Retrieved from http://www.clinicaloptions.com/inPractice/HIV/Epidemiology,%20Testing,%20and%20Prevention/ch5_HIV_Exposure/Pages/Page%201.aspx

New York State Department of Health AIDS Institute. (2008). *HIV prophylaxis following occupational exposure.* Retrieved from http://www.hivguidelines.org/GuidelineDocuments/PEP%201.27.10%20for%20PDF.pdf

Panlilio, A. L., Cardo, D. M., Grohskopf, L. A., Heneine, W., Ross, C. S., & U.S. Public Health Service. (2005). Updated U.S. public health service guidelines for the management of occupational exposures to HIV and recommendations for postexposure prophylaxis. *Morbidity and Mortality Weekly Report 54*(RR-9), 1–17.

Smith, D. K., Grohskopf, L. A., Black, R. J., Auerbach, J. D., Veronese, F., Struble, K. A. . . . Greenberg, A. U. (2005). Antiretroviral postexposure prophylaxis after sexual, injection-drug use, or other nonoccupational exposure to HIV in the United States: Recommendations from the U.S. Department of Health and Human Services. *Morbidity and Mortality Weekly Report, 54*(RR-2), 1–20.

World Health Organization. (2005). *Post-exposure prophylaxis to prevent HIV infection: Joint WHO/ILO guidelines on post-exposure prophylaxis (PEP) to prevent HIV infection.* Retrieved from http://whqlibdoc.who.int/publications/2007/9789241596374_eng.pdf

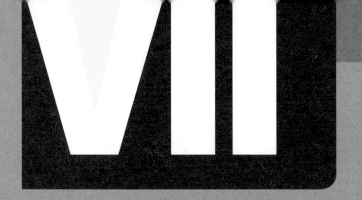

COMMON ADULT PRESENTATIONS

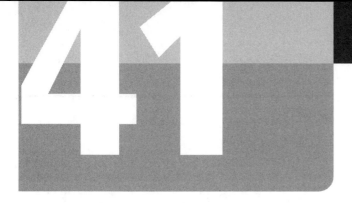

ABSCESS ASSESSMENT AND MANAGEMENT

Rosalie D. Bravo

I. Introduction and general background

Abscesses are inflamed, localized soft tissue masses that are encapsulated collections of pus (Baddour, 2009; Rogers & Perkins, 2006). The etiology is most commonly caused by bacterial infection, of which methicillin-resistant *Staphylococcus aureus* (MRSA) and methicillin-susceptible *S. aureus* are the most common causative organisms (Frazee et al., 2005; Moran et al., 2006). Bacteria enter the dermis and deeper subcutaneous tissues as a result of a break in the integrity of the skin surface. These minor skin traumas may occur from shaving, abrasions, insect bites, splinters, or other foreign bodies. Abscesses may also occur spontaneously in healthy individuals without predisposing conditions. They begin as localized erythema and tenderness on the skin, and as they develop they enlarge and may become firm and indurated. The center of the abscess softens and is filled with purulent exudate or pus consisting of leukocytes, protein, and bacteria. A pustular point or head may develop. This softened area is known as the area of fluctuance. Characteristically, abscesses are painful, warm, well-circumscribed, indurated, and erythematous. They are often located on the buttocks, axillae, or the extremities but they may occur anywhere on the skin. Treatment of an abscess is directed at evacuating the collection of pus by incision and drainage. An abscess may have surrounding cellulitis where the adjacent subcutaneous tissue is inflamed, warm, and tender. The presence of cellulitis in the setting of an abscess presents added complexity and requires antibiotic therapy in addition to incision and drainage (Fitch, Manthey, McGinnis, Nicks, & Pariyadath, 2007; Rogers & Perkins, 2006).

II. Database (may include but is not limited to)

A. Subjective

1. Risk factors for MRSA
   a. Injection drug use
   b. Immunosuppression
   c. Incarceration in prison
   d. Sharing sports equipment
   e. Recent hospitalization or antibiotic therapy
   f. Injection drug use
   g. Men having sex with men (Gorwitz, Jernigan, Powers, & Jernigan, 2006)

2. Precipitating factors
   a. Recent minor skin trauma
   b. Insect stings
   c. Mechanical manipulation of ingrown hairs or comedones (blackheads or whiteheads)
   d. Other foreign bodies, such as splinters or sutures

3. Past health history
   a. Screen for history of abscesses or soft tissue infections
   b. Medical illnesses: immunosuppression, valvular heart disease, diabetes mellitus, or cancer
   c. Medication history: steroid use or recent antibiotic therapy
   d. History of last tetanus vaccination

4. Family or relative history of abscesses or soft tissue infections

5. Personal and social history: health-related behaviors and injection drug use

6. Review of systems
   a. Localized skin symptoms of pain, erythema, warmth, and induration
   b. Systemic symptoms: fevers, chills, regional adenopathy, malaise, nausea, and vomiting

B. Objective

1. General appearance
   a. Age, gender, race, and body habitus
   b. Appearance of chronic illness, such as cachexia or temporal wasting

2. Vital signs: temperature, pulse, respiratory rate, and blood pressure

3. Careful skin examination

   a. Note location and dimensions of erythema; dimensions of induration; visible abrasions or puncture wounds; presence of central fluctuance; and purulent, serous, or sanguinous drainage.

   b. Observe for erythematous streaking from the primary abscess site.

4. Examine lymph nodes for adenopathy.

5. Cardiac: auscultation for murmurs because patients with valvular heart disease or prosthetic valves are at risk for bacteremia (Rogers & Perkins, 2006).

III. Assessment

A. Determine the diagnosis

Diagnosis is a clinical decision based on the history and the physical examination findings. Differentiate between abscesses requiring incision and drainage alone versus incision and drainage with antibiotics. It is important to consider host factors, such as diabetes, immunosuppression, valvular heart disease, or cancer, because comorbid conditions may also change the treatment plan to include antibiotic therapy and hospital admission.

B. Differential diagnosis

1. Simple cutaneous abscess requiring incision and drainage

2. Cutaneous abscess with surrounding cellulitis requiring incision and drainage and antibiotic therapy

3. Cutaneous abscess in the setting of patients at risk for bacteremia

4. Furuncle, an abscess involving a hair follicle and the adjacent soft tissue

5. Carbuncle, a larger abscess involving a group of hair follicles

6. Arteriovenous malformation

7. Hydradinitis suppurativa, abscesses that involve the apocrine sweat glands located in the axillary or groin area

C. Complications

1. Bacteremia

2. Endocarditis

3. Osteomyelitis

4. Tenosynovitis

5. Septic thrombophlebitis

IV. Plan

A. Diagnostics

1. Ultrasound if readily available may determine the presence of a fluid collection and the size and depth of the abscess.

2. Needle aspiration to assess for presence of pus if physical examination alone is indeterminate.

3. Aerobic and anaerobic wound cultures from spontaneous wound drainage or obtained during incision and drainage procedure.

4. Other tests based on the severity of systemic signs and symptoms, such as fevers, rigors, and malaise, may include complete blood count with differential and blood cultures. Blood tests are not necessary for a healthy patient with a simple abscess.

B. Treatment

1. Warm moist compresses if the furuncle or abscess is small and firm.

2. Tetanus prophylaxis if the patient has not had a tetanus vaccination within 10 years.

3. Incision and drainage for fluctuant abscesses and all carbuncles.

4. Antimicrobial therapy in addition to incision and drainage if there is a surrounding cellulitis. Antibiotics are unnecessary for immunocompetent patients who have a simple cutaneous abscess without surrounding cellulitis (Hankin & Everett, 2007; Rajendran et al., 2007). Prescribe antibiotics for patients who have abscesses with surrounding cellulitis and for patients who are diabetic, immunocompromised, have valvular heart disease, or who have other comorbid conditions that increase the risk of bacteremia. Select antibiotics that are effective in treating MRSA and group A streptococcus. Be familiar with regional guidelines for MRSA treatment. Duration of antibiotic therapy should be based on the resolution of symptoms (Baddour, 2009; Hepburn et al., 2004).

   a. Clindamycin, 300–450 mg tid to qid for 7–10 days or

   b. Trimethoprim–sulfamethoxazole, 160 mg/800 mg (one to two tablets based on weight) bid for 7–10 days or

   c. Doxycycline, 100 mg bid for 7–10 days

   d. Antibiotic prophylaxis with a single dose of a cephalosporin. For severe PCN allergies, vancomycin 1 g intravenous single dose. Give antibiotics 60 minutes before incision and drainage for patients with prosthetic heart valves, stents, or implantable cardiac devices (Rogers & Perkins, 2006).

5. Analgesic therapy

C. Incision and drainage procedure

1. Description: incision and drainage is a surgical procedure in which an incision is made into the fluctuant area of an abscess to drain the purulent contents of an abscess. The incision is then left open to promote further drainage.

2. Indication: the presence of a cutaneous abscess measuring 5 mm or greater where there is evidence of a collection of purulent exudate or pus.

3. Contraindications to incision and drainage in the outpatient setting

   a. Cellulitis without an underlying abscess.
   b. The location of the abscess is such that the incision may cause a disfiguring defect.
   c. Abscesses are in locations that pose a risk for complications, such as those located on the hands or plantar surfaces; those located over arteries or large blood vessels, such as those on the neck or over the antecubital fossa; and those on or around the nasolabial folds or orbital region of the face.
   d. For large or deep abscesses that require more pain management than a local anesthetic, provide conscious sedation or general anesthesia for the patient to tolerate the procedure.

4. Procedure

   a. Materials
      i. Gown, gloves, face shield, and one pair of sterile gloves
      ii. One bottle of povidine iodine or chlorhexidine solution
      iii. Eight to 10 packs of sterile 4 × 4s and alcohol wipes
      iv. One #11 or #15 blade scalpel
      v. One small curved hemostat for blunt dissection
      vi. One 10-cc syringe
      vii. One 22-gauge needle for drawing up the local anesthetic
      viii. One 25-gauge needle for infiltrating lidocaine
      ix. Lidocaine 1% or bupivicaine 0.5%
      x. One irrigation kit or a 30- to 60-ml syringe and splash guard
      xi. One 1-L bottle of sterile water or normal saline solution
      xii. Swabs for bacterial culture and sterile basin
      xiii. 0.25- or 0.50-in plain wound packing material, top dressings, and tape
      xiv. Cotton-tip swabs or blunt-edged forceps
   b. Incision and drainage procedure
      i. Wash your hands and observe universal precautions.
      ii. Identify the patient by asking his or her name and assess the patient's allergy history.
      iii. Discuss the risks and benefits of the procedure, such as procedural pain, scar from the incision, reduced pain after abscess is drained, and wound healing.
      iv. Obtain the patient's consent.
      v. Consider premedication with an anxiolytic or analgesic medication.
      vi. Position the patient so that the abscess is easily accessible.
      vii. Put on gloves and a face shield.
      viii. Cleanse the skin in with povidine iodine or chlorhexidine in a circular motion starting from the center of the abscess and working outward. Allow the cleaning solution to dry.
      ix. Cover the surrounding area with sterile drapes so that the abscess is exposed.
      x. Infiltrate the intradermal tissue under the surface of the wound with a local anesthetic agent, such as lidocaine or bupivicaine, using a 22- or 25-gauge needle. The maximum dose of lidocaine 1% solution without epinephrine is 4 mg/kg (Hsu, 2010). Bupivicaine without epinephrine should not exceed a dose of 1–2 mg/kg (Hsu). Bupivicaine or lidocaine with epinephrine is not indicated for the incision and drainage procedure because local vasoconstriction is not necessary and plain bupivicaine and lidocaine both provide a minimum duration of anesthesia for 30 minutes, which is sufficient to complete the procedure. If the patient is allergic to lidocaine, then conscious sedation should be considered. Inject parallel to the skin surface. Do not inject perpendicular to the skin surface (i.e., into the deeper tissues) because this may spread the infection. An alternative method is to inject in a field block pattern where the anesthetic agent is injected around the entire peripheral field surrounding the abscess but not directly over the site to be incised.
      xi. Put on sterile gloves.
      xii. Palpate for the most fluctuant part of the abscess and make a small incision with a #11 blade scalpel over the center.

If possible make the incision along the Langer's lines or skin-tension lines to promote optimal cosmetic results. The depth and length of the incision are variable and should be based on the size and location of the abscess. The incision should not puncture the back wall of the abscess capsule. Extend the incision. The goal of the incision is to provide an opening large enough to allow for drainage of the abscess and insertion of packing material. In addition, the incision should be large enough to insert the curved hemostat into the incision to break up loculations. This is called blunt dissection, which allows for further drainage of pus. Gently compress the outer sides of the abscess to express more drainage. Insert the curved hemostats and explore the abscess cavity, and open the hemostats to break up loculations.

xiii. Collect a culture of the wound using aerobic and anaerobic culture medium. Cultures are beneficial if it is a first abscess, if the abscess worsens after incision and drainage, or if there has been a history of antibiotic treatment failure.

xiv. Irrigate the incised abscess with normal saline solution using the large syringe and splash guard. An 18-gauge angiocatheter may be attached without the needle to the syringe. Irrigate until the drainage is clear or slightly serous.

xv. Insert the 0.25- or 0.50-in packing gauze into the abscess taking care to loosely pack into the entire wound cavity. The goal is to keep the wound open to promote drainage and prevent closure of the wound. Closure of the wound without adequate drainage may lead to reformation of the abscess.

xvi. Cover the wound with a sterile top dressing and paper tape. For additional information and a streaming video of the incision and drainage procedure, visit www.nejm.org (Fitch et al., 2007).

5. Follow-up

a. The patient should return within 48–72 hours for a wound check.

b. Remove the packing and assess the amount of drainage. If the drainage is minimal, then warm soaks should be initiated and continued until the wound is healed. If the wound continues to have purulent drainage, then the wound should be irrigated with normal saline, explored again to assess for any unbroken loculations, and then repacked with new gauze. The patient should return again in 48 hours (Fitch et al., 2007; Kronfol, 2009).

6. Criteria for hospital admission or referral for specialty consultation

a. Patients with signs of systemic toxicity, such as fevers, rigors, or unstable vital signs, should be admitted for parenteral antibiotics.

b. Patients who have failed appropriate initial treatment.

c. The location of the abscess is such that the incision may cause a disfiguring defect. Refer immediately to a dermatologist or plastic surgeon.

d. Abscesses located on the hands or plantar surfaces should be immediately referred to an orthopedic or plastic surgeon.

e. Abscesses located over arteries or large blood vessels on the neck or over the antecubital fossa or inguinal areas should be immediately referred to an otolaryngologist or vascular surgeon.

f. Abscesses on or around the nasolabial folds may pose the risk of septic cavernous venous thrombosis and should be immediately referred to an otolaryngologist.

D. Patient education

Instruct the patient in the signs and symptoms of worsening infection (fevers or chills, increasing pain, redness or swelling, and increasing purulent drainage or recurrent abscess) and inform the patient of expected outcomes: the wound will likely heal in 7–10 days but may take longer. There will likely be a scar from the incision. This may be minimized by limiting direct sun exposure and wearing a sun block if the scar is in an exposed area.

REFERENCES

Baddour, L. M. (2009). Skin abscesses, furuncles, and carbuncles. *UpToDate*. Retrieved from http://www.uptodate.com/online/content/topic.do?topicKey=skin_inf/4615

Fitch, M. T., Manthey, D. E., McGinnis, H. D., Nicks, B. A., & Pariyadath, M. (2007). Videos in clinical medicine: Abscess incision and drainage. *New England Journal of Medicine, 357*, e20. Retrieved from http://content.nejm.org/cgi/video/357/19/e20/

Frazee, B. W., Lynn, J., Chalebois, E. D., Lambert, L., Lowery, D., & Perdreau-Remington, F. (2005). High prevalence of methicillin-resistant *Staphylococcus aureus* in emergency department skin and soft tissue infections. *Annals of Emergency Medicine, 45*(3), 311–320.

Gorwitz, R. J., Jernigan, D. B., Powers, J. H., Jernigan, J. A., and Participants in the CDC-Convened Experts' Meeting on Management of MRSA in the Community. (2006). Strategies for clinical management of MRSA in the community: Summary of an experts' meeting convened by the Centers for Disease Control and Prevention. Retrieved from http://www.cdc.gov/ncidod/dhqp/ar_MRSA_ca_public.html

Hankin, A. & Everett, W. W. (2007). Are antibiotics necessary after incision and drainage of a cutaneous abscess? *Annals of Emergency Medicine, 50*, 48–51.

Hepburn, M. J., Dooley, D. P., Skidmore, P. J., Ellis, M. W., Starnes, W. F., & Hasewinkle, W. C. (2004). Comparison of short-course (5 days) and standard (10 days) treatment for uncomplicated cellulitis. *Archives of Internal Medicine, 164*(15), 1669–1674.

Hsu, D. (2010). Infiltrative anesthetics. *UpToDate.* Retrieved from http://www.uptodate.com/online/content/topic.do?topicKey=ped_proc/5677

Kronfol, R. (2009). Technique of incision and drainage for skin abscess. *UpToDate.* Retrieved from http://www.uptodate.com/online/content/topic.do?topicKey=ped_proc/9189

Moran, G. J., Krishnadasan, A., Gorwitz, R. J., Fosheim, G. E., McDougal, M. S., Carey, R. B. . . . Talan, D. A. (2006). Methicillin-resistant *S. aureus* infections among patients in the emergency department. *New England Journal of Medicine, 355*(7), 666–674.

O'Malley, G. F., Dominici, P., Giraldo, P., Aguilera, E., Verma, M., Lares, C. . . . Williams, E. (2009). Routine packing of simple cutaneous abscesses is painful and probably unnecessary. *Academic Emergency Medicine, 16*(5), 470–474.

Rajendran, P. M., Young, D., Maurer, T., Chambers, H., Perdreau-Remington, F., Ro, P., & Harris, H. (2007). Randomized, double-blind, placebo-controlled trial of cephalexin for treatment of uncomplicated skin abscesses in a population at risk for community-acquired methicillin-resistant *Staphylococcus aureus* infection. *Antimicrobial Agents Chemotherapy, 51*(11), 4044–4048.

Rogers, R. L., Perkins, J., (2006). Skin and soft tissue infections. *Primary Care: Clinics in Office Practice, 33*, 697–710.

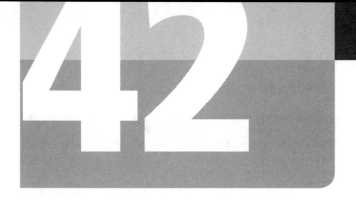

ANEMIA

Michelle M. Marin

I. Introduction and general background

Anemia is defined as a decrease in the red blood cell (RBC) number, hemoglobin concentration, or the volume of packed red blood cells (hematocrit) in the blood. The World Health Organization defines anemia by laboratory definition as hemoglobin of less than 13 g/dl for adults, less than 12 g/dl for menstruating females, and less than 11 g/dl for pregnant females (Beutler & Waalen, 2006). The World Health Organization defines anemia by laboratory definition as hemoglobin of less than 13 g/dl for adults, less than 12 g/dl for menstruating females, and less than 11 g/dl for pregnant females. However, data from the Scripps-Kaiser and NHANES study, recommend that lower limits of hemoglobin be stratified based on gender and race (black men ages 20–59: 12.9 g/dl; black men > 60 years: 12.7 g/dl; black women ages 20–49: 11.5 g/dl; black women > 50 years: 11.5 g/dl; white men ages 20–59: 13.7 g/dl; white men > 60 years: 13.2 g/dl; white women ages 20–49: 12.2 g/dl; white women > 60 years: 12.2 g/dl) (Beutler & Waalen, 2006).

Anemia is a sign and consequence of disease or treatments. Exceptions occur with volume expansion as seen in pregnancy causing a physiologic anemia and with high altitudes causing elevated RBC mass. It can be caused by a variety of systemic disorders and diseases and by a primary hematologic disorder. As a result, most individuals' physical symptoms and signs reflect the underlying illness rather than the anemia itself. Correct identification of the underlying disease is essential for appropriately directed treatment.

Erythropoiesis is the regulated process of RBC production through a series of steps (NAAC, 2002). In adults, this process occurs in the bone marrow of the sternum, ribs, vertebrae, and pelvis. The process begins when pluripotent stem cells are dedicated and the hematopoietic precursor cells mature with growth factors and hormones. The key to erythropoietin production is the availability of oxygen, which is carried to the tissues bound to the hemoglobin. When oxygen is low, then erythropoietin (90% from the kidney) triggers the red cell production to meet tissue demand. This production feedback system can only occur when all the needed substrates are in place: normal renal production of erythropoietin, a functioning bone marrow, and an adequate support of substrates of hemoglobin synthesis (NAAC, 2002).

Anemia classification is based on (1) excessive RBC loss, (2) inadequate or ineffective RBC production, (3) abnormal RBC destruction, or (4) morphologic characteristics. These characteristics of cell size are microcytic, normocytic, and macrocytic (Table 42-1). Common microcytic anemias are iron deficiency, thalassemia, and sideroblastic anemia. The most common causes of normocytic anemias include anemia of chronic disease, hemolytic anemia, bone marrow failure or infiltration, endocrine disorders, and renal disease. Common macrocytic anemias are vitamin B_{12} and folate deficiencies. Multiple etiologies of anemia can coexist together requiring a step-wise diagnostic approach critical to not missing a treatable cause. Outside of the usual categories of anemia lies a unique group of poorly diagnosed anemias that occurs in the geriatric population, accounting for 43% of hypoproliferative anemia (Makipour, Kanapuru, & Ershler, 2008) (Table 42-1).

A. Microcytic anemias

1. Iron deficiency anemia

    a. Definition and overview: Iron deficiency is a microcytic and hypochromic (decrease in hemoglobin concentration) anemia. It occurs when the bone marrow iron stores are less than what is needed to produce RBCs. Common causes of iron deficiency are:

       i. Low-iron diets caused by inadequate intake, increased demand as in pregnancy, or rapid growth in teenage years.

       ii. Poor absorption seen with gastric atrophy, achlorhydria, or gastric surgery; dietary fibers, calcium, and starches that block absorption of iron from nonmeat sources.

       iii. Blood loss caused by menstrual bleeding, large intra-abdominal or joint bleeding, or occult gastrointestinal and genitourinary bleeding. Of note, it takes 20 ml/day of blood for the usual stool hemoccult test to become positive (Umbreit, 2005). One milliliter of blood loss is equivalent to the loss of 0.5 mg of iron (Tables 42-1 and 42-2).

TABLE 42-1 Separating Anemia by MCV

Hypochromic Microcytic MCV < 80 fl	Normochromic/Normocytic MCV 80–100	Macrocytic MCV > 100 fl
Iron deficiency	Acute hemorrhage	Megaloblastic: vitamin B$_{12}$ and folate deficiencies and drug induced
Thalassemia	Acute hemolysis	Reticulocytosis: intense red blood cell stimulation caused by acute hemolysis or hemorrhage (reticulocytes are large, young red blood cells)
Sideroblastic	Early iron deficiency, folate, and vitamin B$_{12}$ deficiency	Chronic liver disease
Hemoglobinopathies	Anemia of chronic disease Chronic inflammation Acute and chronic infections Cancer Chronic kidney disease	Myelodysplastic syndromes: bone marrow failure or infiltration
Lead poisoning	Alcoholic liver disease Endocrinopathies Bone marrow failure or infiltration Pregnancy	Endocrinopathies Postsplenectomy

Source: Collins-Bride, G., & Saxe, J. (Eds.). (1998). *Nurse practitioner/physician collaborative practice: Clinical guidelines for ambulatory care.* San Francisco, CA: UCSF Nursing Press. Used with permission from the UCSF Nursing Press.

b. Prevalence and incidence: Iron deficiency anemia is the most common nutritional deficiency (Umbreit, 2005). It affects more than 3 million people according to the National Heart, Lung and Blood Institute. Iron deficiency results in increased pediatric and maternal mortality; decreased work production; delayed childhood development; and with mild to moderate deficiency, an increased risk for developing infectious diseases. There are estimates that 4% of US women between the ages of 20 and 49 years have iron deficiency anemia. The incidence of anemia increases with age with 10% seen in the 65 years and older age group (Schrier, 2010). This increase is associated with a significant increase in morbidity and mortality, impaired cognition, decrease in exercise tolerance, and decrease in quality of life measures.

2. Thalassemia

a. Definition and overview: Thalassemia syndromes are a group of inherited autosomal-recessive anemias classified by defects in the synthesis of one or more of the hemoglobin globin chain subunits. These defects can occur either in the α or β globin chains of hemoglobin. The combined imbalances of globin and inadequate hemoglobin production result in a variety of clinical manifestations. The former

TABLE 42-2 Differentiating Anemias

	MCV	RDW	Retics	Iron	TIBC	% Sat	Ferritin
Iron deficiency	D	I	D	D	I	D	D
Iron depletion	N	N	N	N	I	D	D
β-Thalassemia	D ↓	D	I	N	N	N	N
Sideroblastic	D	H	I	NII	NID	NII	N
Chronic disease	D or N	N	NID	D	N/D	N/I/D	N
Lead poisoning	D	N	I	N	N	N	N

I, increased; D, decreased; D ↓, decreased greater than expected in iron deficiency;
N, normal; II, increased significantly.

causes hypochromia and microcytosis, the latter leads to ineffective erythropoiesis and hemolytic anemia (Giardina & Forget, 2008). The diagnosis of thalassemia is made by a hemoglobin electrophoresis test (Table 42-3).

   i. α-Thalassemia trait: loss of one α gene, not anemic but mean cell volume (MCV) may be low.

   ii. α-Thalassemia minor: loss of two genes of α globin, hematocrit is low and MCV is 60–75 fl.

   iii. Hemoglobin H: loss of three α genes, moderate microcytic anemia.

   iv. β-Thalassemia minor: mild microcytic anemia, asymptomatic.

   v. β-Thalassemia intermedia: severe anemia often requiring RBC transfusion.

   vi. β-Thalassemia major: condition is life threatening requiring chronic transfusions and possibly hematopoietic cell transplantation.

  b. Prevalence and incidence: Thalassemias are the most common single genetic disorders known. They are encountered in every ethnic group and geographic location, although most common in the Mediterranean basin and tropic and subtropic areas of Asia and Africa. Thalassemia in these regions ranges from 2.5 to 15%. In the United States, 15% of African Americans are silent carriers of α-thalassemia, with 3% carrying the trait; 1–15% of those of Mediterranean origin carry the trait. For β-thalassemia, 10–15% of Mediterranean and 0.8% of African Americans in the United States are affected (Hoffman et al., 2008). Interestingly, thalassemias are most common in areas that are historically known for endemic malaria.

  3. Sideroblastic anemia

  a. Definition and overview: Sideroblastic anemias are a group of disorders with ringed iron-laden sideroblasts in the bone marrow accompanied by moderate to severe microcytic anemia. The classification of sideroblastic anemias is distinguished between diseases of the heme synthesis pathway and those diseases of mitochondrial DNA or those with defects in the nuclear DNA. There are two primary X-linked inherited forms that are recognized early in life. Acquired types are caused by exposures from toxins or drugs (alcohol, lead, or zinc). Once the offending toxin is removed, recovery occurs within 1–2 weeks (Gehrs & Friedberg, 2002). Others are associated with ringed sideroblasts, the myelodysplastic syndrome of refractory anemia.

  b. Prevalence and incidence: The incidence of sideroblastic anemia is low. Acquired types are more prevalent than hereditary types. Many individuals are stable for years but in a subset of patients who belong to the myelodysplastic syndrome category, 5% go on to develop leukemia. Acquired sideroblastic anemias are not fully established because of the multiple triggers and clinical presentations (Schwartz, 2007).

B. Normocytic anemias

  1. Definition and overview: The MCV is within normal limits but hemoglobin and hematocrit are decreased mildly to moderately. Individuals are generally asymptomatic. Nearly all anemias are normocytic in their initial stages (Brill & Baumgardner, 2000).

  2. Anemia of chronic disease and anemia of chronic inflammation (ACD)

  a. Definitions and overview: This is an anemia of underproduction of RBCs often associated with chronic inflammatory disease. A decreased life span of the RBC and inhibition of hematopoiesis, deregulation of iron absorption and transport, and decreased

TABLE 42-3 Thalassemia Percent of Abnormal HGB and Degrees of Anemia

	HgbA	HgbA2	HgbF	Comments
Normal	97–99%	1–3%	<1%	
β-Thalassemia (minor)	80–95%	4–8%	1–5%	MCV 55–75, Hct 28–40%, peripheral smear mildly abnormal, heterozygous trait
β-Thalassemia (intermediate)	0–30%	0–10%	6–100%	Moderate anemia
β-Thalassemia (major)	0%	4–10%	90–96%	Homozygous trait, marked microcytosis with severe anemia
α-Thalassemia trait	Normal	Normal	Normal	Heterozygous trait, 2/4 genes normal, MCV 60–7 fl, Hct 28–40%, diagnosis of exclusion

erythropoietin production defines this anemia (Gardner & Benz, 2008). Hepcidin, an iron regulatory peptide produced by the liver, is thought to be the central regulator in iron metabolism and is controlled by the erythropoietic activity in the bone (Kemna, 2008). ACD is usually seen as normocytic, normochromic, or mildly microcytic with a low reticulocyte count. Iron stores may be normal or increased. The most common causes are usually multifactorial.

  i. Chronic systemic diseases, such as diabetes, congestive heart failure, and chronic obstructive pulmonary disease
  ii. Chronic inflammation, such as rheumatoid arthritis and inflammatory bowel disease
  iii. Neoplasm
  iv. Chronic liver and kidney disease
  v. Chronic infection, such as HIV/AIDS
  vi. Endocrine deficiencies, such as hypothyroidism, diabetes, adrenal or pituitary insufficiencies, and hypogonadism
  vii. Uncompensated blood loss
  viii. Hypersplenism

  b. Prevalence and incidence: This is the second most common form of anemia world-wide, second to iron deficiency. In a review of hospitalized patients, estimated prevalence is 20–40% for ACD (Tefferi, 2007).

3. Hemolytic anemia
  a. Definition and overview: Hemolytic anemia is a normocytic, normochromic anemia where there is a premature destruction of RBCs for which the bone marrow cannot compensate. This occurs when RBC survival is less than normal (120 days) or when the bone marrow is impaired (Linker, 2007). This can be seen congenitally with recognition early in life as in sickle cell disease or later in life when exposed to a stressor, such as G6PD. The acquired type usually occurs in adulthood, in those persons older than 40 years of age and in those with mechanical hemolysis, paroxysmal nocturnal hemolysis, or warm and cold reactive antibodies.
  b. Prevalence and incidence: Hemolytic anemia represents 5% of all anemias (Schick, 2010). Autoimmune hemolytic anemia occurs in 10% of systemic lupus erythematosus, most occurring in women older than 65 years of age (Schwartz, 2007). The underlying disorder and etiology of hemolysis dictates survival.

C. Macrocytic anemias

1. Definition and overview: Megaloblastic anemias are a group of diverse anemias that share the failure in the synthesis and assembly of DNA resulting in ineffective erythropoiesis. Findings of MCV greater than 100 suggest megaloblastic anemia, but with MCV greater than 110 it is much more likely to be present. The most common causes of megaloblastosis are vitamin B_{12} and folate deficiencies. Deficiencies of one of these vitamins can cause malabsorption of the other vitamin. Megaloblastic disease, especially when combined with microcytic anemia, can be present with or without anemia.

2. Vitamin B_{12} deficiency
  a. Definitions and overview: Vitamin B_{12} (cobalamin) deficiency is a problem of either inadequate intake over several years or of inadequate absorption. Lifelong subclinical vitamin B_{12} deficiency, 50% with normal vitamin B_{12} levels, when challenged with abnormal absorption or altered metabolism can tip individuals into symptomatic deficiency. (Oh & Brown, 2003). Low levels of vitamin B_{12} elevates homocysteine, which is associated with cardiovascular disease (Elmadfa & Singer, 2009). Megaloblastic anemia identifies this disorder. Common causes are:
    i. Pernicious anemia associated with autoimmune disorders.
    ii. Gastrectomy, bariatric surgery, and intestinal surgeries.
    iii. Small-bowel disorders, such as inflammatory bowel disease, bacterial overgrowth, tape worms, enteritis, sprue, and celiac disease all affecting the terminal ileum.
    iv. Long-term vegan diets without dairy products or eggs.
    v. Medications inhibiting absorption, such as metformin, proton pump inhibitors, and histamine 2 blockers.
    vi. Food: cobalamin malabsorption syndrome when nutritional intake is adequate and there is no evidence of other causes of malabsorption or pernicious anemia.
  b. Prevalence and incidence: Determining the frequency of vitamin B_{12} deficiency anemia is difficult because the etiologies are diverse. Pernicious anemia is 0.25–0.5 cases per 1,000 in those older than 70 years of age. Although usually seen in adults older than 40 of Scandinavian or Northern European ancestry, it can also be seen in any population. Nutritional deficiency is seen worldwide; however, in affluent countries inadequate absorption is more common. It is estimated that vitamin B_{12} deficiency occurs in 10–15% of those older than 60 years and is

thought to be a result of atrophic gastritis (Baik & Russell, 1999).

3. Folic acid deficiency

a. Definitions and overview: Folic acid is present in most fruits and vegetables. A typical diet of 50 mg/d should be adequate. Folic acid stores of 5–20 mg last about 4 months. Common causes of folic acid deficiency include:
   i. Inadequate diet of fruits and vegetables.
   ii. Inflammatory bowel disease, such as sprue.
   iii. Cultural or ethnic cooking destroying folate, as in prolonged stewing.
   iv. Medications interfering with absorption, such as methotrexate, phenytoin, acyclovir, oral contraceptives, colchicine, and trimethoprim.
   v. Increased demand in pregnancy and lactation; hyperemesis gravidarum; and intrinsic hematologic disease, such as malignancy infiltration in the bone marrow.

b. Prevalence and incidence: The Food and Drug Administration mandated that folic acid be added to enriched grain products in 1998, which resulted in a significant decrease in folate deficiency. In temperate zones, folate deficiency is most common in alcoholics. Tropical sprue, which is endemic near the equator, results in malabsorption of this critical vitamin.

II. Database (may include but is not limited to)

A. Subjective: microcytic

1. Iron deficiency anemia, thalassemia, and sideroblastic anemia

   a. Past health history
      i. Medical illnesses: recurrent iron deficiency anemia, anorexia, gastrointestinal or genitourinary malignancy, celiac disease, atrophic gastritis, *Helicobacter pylori*, helminthic infections, and chronic inflammatory conditions
      ii. Surgical history: partial or total gastroenterostomy, gastric resection, or splenectomy
      iii. Obstetric and gynecological history: heavy menses, multiparty, recent pregnancy, and parturition
      iv. Medication history: nonsteroidal anti-inflammatory drugs, steroids, chemotherapy, iron or multivitamins, salicylates, antacids that block iron absorption, and health food products
      v. Exposure history: toxic exposures, such as lead poisoning and potent marrow toxic agents

   b. Family history
      i. Anemia
      ii. Chronic inflammatory diseases
      iii. Malignancy
      iv. Lead poisoning

   c. Personal and social history
      i. Diet inadequate in iron, dairy, or animal products
      ii. Heavy alcohol use
      iii. Intravenous drug use and sharing needles
      iv. Travel to sub-Sahara Africa exposing the person to schistosoma, such as *Trichuris* infections, and malarial zones.
      v. Regular blood donations

2. Thalassemia

   a. Past health history
      i. Medical illnesses: chronic microcytic anemia and iron overload.
      ii. Surgical history: splenectomy or hematopoietic stem cell transplant.
      iii. Obstetric history: pregnancy or stillborn fetus caused by hydrops fetalis.
      iv. Medication history: chelation therapy and RBC transfusions.

   b. Family history
      i. Thalassemia and hemoglobinopathies
      ii. Ethnicity: Mediterranean, Southeast Asian, Chinese, and African American descent

3. Sideroblastic anemia

   a. Past health history
      i. Medical illness: copper deficiency, vitamin B_6 deficiency, and myelodysplastic syndrome
      ii. Medication history: excessive use of zinc supplements, antibiotics, copper chelating agents, antituberculosis agents, and chemotherapy
      iii. Exposure history: lead poisoning and prolonged exposure to cold

   b. Family history
      i. Sideroblastic anemia
      ii. Mitochondrial disease

   c. Personal and social history
      i. Chronic excessive alcohol intake
      ii. Coin ingestion

4. Review of systems for microcytic anemias

   a. Constitutional: degree of symptoms depends on the degree and rate of anemia development. Marked fatigue and decreased exercise tolerance may be the earliest symptoms along with weakness, postural faintness, headache, and weight loss. Pica, especially eating ice, is common.

b. Skin and nails: pallor; bruising; koilonchia (spoon nails); and brittle nails.

c. Ears, nose, and throat: bleeding, fissures at corners of mouth, and painful mouth.

d. Neck: swollen neck glands.

e. Pulmonary: cough, shortness of breath, and hemoptysis.

f. Cardiac: chest pain, palpitations, and tachycardia

g. Abdomen: tenderness, masses, changes in bowel habits, bleeding hemorrhoids, hematemesis, melena or bright red blood per rectum, distention, and difficulty swallowing.

h. Genitourinary: bloody urine

i. Gynecological: heavy and or irregular menses, pregnancy, and multiple pregnancies

j. Skeletal: bone tenderness

B. *Subjective: normocytic anemias*

1. Anemia of chronic disease
   a. Past health history
      i. Medical illness: anemia; chronic diseases, such as renal disease; inflammatory bowel disease; autoimmune disorders; malignancies; sickle cell disease; and liver disease
      ii. Surgical history: cholecystectomy, prosthetic cardiac valves, and stem cell transplant
      iii. Medication history: penicillin, quinine, and quinidine
      iv. Exposure history: parvovirus 19
   b. Family history
      i. G6PD deficiency
      ii. Sickle cell disease
      iii. Hereditary anemia disorders
      iv. Autoimmune disorders
      v. Renal or liver disease
   c. Personal and social history
      i. Diet including fava beans

2. Hemolytic anemia
   a. Past medical history
      i. Medical illnesses: previous hemolysis, chronic hemolytic anemia, systemic lupus erythematosus, rheumatoid arthritis, chronic lymphocytic leukemia, non-Hodgkin's lymphoma, various carcinomas, idiopathic thrombocytopenic purpura and thrombotic thrombocytopenic purpura,

G6PD deficiency, malaria, and cold agglutinin disease
      ii. Surgical: prosthetic heart valves, patches, and vascular grafts
      iii. Medications: antimalarials, sulfonamides, nitrofurantoin, sulfanyureas, quinine, quinidine, interferon, phenacetin, high-dose penicillin, and blood transfusions
      iv. Exposures: infectious agents, such as parasites; viruses, such as Epstein-Barr or cytomegalovirus; measles; syphilis; enteric bacteria; spider bites and snake venom; copper; and organic compounds
   b. Family history
      i. G6PD deficiency
      ii. Autoimmune hemolytic anemia
      iii. Red cell membrane disorders
   c. Personal and social history
      i. Aggressive exercise causing microvascular trauma

3. Review of symptoms for normocytic anemia and anemia of chronic disease and hemolysis
   a. Constitutional: fatigue, weakness, postural faintness, poor exercise tolerance, and abrupt or gradual onset.
   b. Skin: rash, yellowing color, bruising, petechiae, pale skin, and nails
   c. Neck: swollen lymph nodes.
   d. Pulmonary: shortness of breath
   e. Cardiac: palpitations, tachycardia, and chest pain
   f. Abdominal: right upper quadrant pain, abdominal fullness, and decreased appetite
   g. Extremities: leg ulcers and edema
   h. Joints: swollen painful joints
   i. Bladder: dark or bloody urine

C. *Subjective: macrocytic and megaloblastic*

1. Vitamin B_{12} deficiency
   a. Past health history
      i. Medical history: thyroid disease, diabetes mellitus, Addison's disease, idiopathic hypoparathyroidism, autoimmune hemolytic diseases, tropical sprue, atrophic gastritis, regional enteritis, folate deficiency, or gastric cancer
      ii. Surgical: gastrectomy, bariatric surgery, or intestinal surgery
      iii. Medications: metformin, colchicine, cholestyramine, histamine 2 blockers, proton pump inhibitors, multivitamins, and azidothymidine

iv. Exposures: intestinal tape worm infestation and repeated and prolonged (> 6 hr) nitrous oxide inhalation especially in the elderly (Longo, 2009)

b. Family history
   i. Pernicious anemia
   ii. Autoimmune disorders, such as diabetes mellitus type 1 and thyroid disorders, vitiligo, hypoparathyroidism, and Addison's disease

c. Personal and social history
   i. Vegan diet
   ii. Alcohol use

2. Folate deficiency

   a. Past health history
      i. Medical history: vitamin B_{12} deficiency, chronic hemolytic anemia, sprue, atrophic gastritis, small bowel disease, psoriasis, epilepsy, and chronic hemodialysis
      ii. Obstetric and gynecological history: pregnancy
      iii. Medications: methotrexate, pentamidine, trimethoprim, cancer chemotherapy, triampterene, phenytoin, primadone, phenobarbital, and sulfasalazine

   b. Family history
      i. Hereditary disorders
      ii. Gluten sensitivities

   c. Personal and social history
      i. Alcohol abuse
      ii. Narcotic addiction
      iii. Inadequate diet

3. Review of systems: macrocytic or megaloblastic anemia, vitamin B_{12} or folic acid deficiency.

   a. Constitutional: fatigue, decreased exercise tolerance, weakness, and weight loss
   b. Skin: yellow skin, pallor, vitiligo, and rashes.
   c. Mouth: cheilosis, stomatitis, sore smooth tongue, and atrophic glossitis
   d. Neck: sense of fullness in the thyroid region
   e. Pulmonary: shortness of breath
   f. Cardiac: tachycardia, chest pain, palpitations.
   g Abdominal: diarrhea, pain, anorexia, nausea, constipation, bowel incontinence, and sense of fullness
   h. Bladder: incontinence
   i. Neurologic: paresthesias, balance problems, and difficulty walking
   j. Extremities: edema
   k. Neuropsychiatric: depression, irritability, dementia, and insomnia

III. Physical examination

A. *Evaluate weight and height.*

B. *Complete vital signs: postural blood pressure and pulse, respiratory rate, and temperature.*

C. *See Table 42-4 for physical examination findings seen in anemia.*

IV. Assessment

A. *Determine the diagnosis: after the health history and physical examination. Guide the work-up based on the clues found. Review previous complete blood cell count (CBC) to evaluate what might be the individual's true normal count.*

B. *Differentiate the anemia and assess the severity of the disease.*

   1. Microcytic anemias

      a. Iron deficiency anemia
         i. CBC: white cell and platelet abnormalities give clues about bone marrow malfunction, such as myelodysplastic or myeloproliferative disorder.
         ii. Assess anemia based on the MCV (Table 42-1).
         iii. Order iron studies: ferritin, iron, total iron binding capacity, and reticulocyte count with a peripheral blood smear (Table 42-5).
         iv. Determine the type of microcytic anemia. If iron deficiency, order stool guaiac and urinalysis to rule out blood loss from the gastrointestinal and genitourinary tracts, respectively. It is critical not to miss an occult gastrointestinal lesion, frequently a malignancy. Refer patients older than age 50, or younger than age 50 with a positive family history of colon cancer, to gastroenterology for endoscopy and colonoscopy. Young patients with iron deficiency anemia, weight loss, and persistent abdominal discomfort should also be referred to gastroenterology. Young menstruating women who are asymptomatic and otherwise healthy likely have iron deficiency anemia caused by menses combined with inadequate dietary iron intake.

TABLE 42-4 Physical Examination Findings Seen with Anemia

Location	Finding	Implication
Skin and nails	Pallor	Decreased number of red blood cells
	Petechiae	Thrombocytopenia, leukemia, disseminated intravascular coagulation
	Telangiectasia and spider angiomas	Liver disease
	Jaundice, icterus	Hemolytic and megaloblastic anemia, liver disease
	Decreased elasticity of skin, brittle nails	Long-standing anemia
	Koilonychia (spoon nails) Hair loss	Long-standing anemia, especially iron deficiency
	Rash	Systemic lupus erythematosis
Neck	Thyromegaly or masses	Endocrinopathies
Mucous membranes	Pallor, cheilosis, and stomatitis	Leukemia, pernicious anemia, or severe iron deficiency
	Smooth red tongue and atrophic glossitis	Vitamin B_{12} deficiency
Lymph nodes	Lymphadenopathy	Leukemia, lymphoma, HIV
Heart	Tachycardia, loud murmurs, decreased PMI, congestive heart failure, functional murmurs, hypertension	Severe anemia, pregnancy, renal disease
Pulmonary	Tachypnea	Severe anemia
Abdomen	Splenomegaly, hepatomegaly, or hepatic tenderness	Leukemia, lymphoma, hemolytic anemia, liver disease, autoimmune disease
Central nervous system	Decreased vibratory and position sense/ataxia, and decreased vibration of 256-degree tuning fork	Pernicious anemia Sideroblastic anemia
Skeletal	Bone tenderness, swollen joints	Hematologic disease, rheumatoid arthritis, autoimmune disorders
Rectal	Guiaic-positive stool, or bright red blood per rectum	Gastrointestinal bleeding
Extremities	Edema	Heart failure, renal failure, cirrhosis, hepatitis
	Leg ulcers	Chronic hemolytic anemia, iron deficiency

v. A therapeutic trial of iron reevaluating the results can be helpful because only an iron-deficient state will diminish (see the treatment section).

b. Thalassemia anemia

i. If iron studies are normal and abnormal peripheral smear is reported, consider thalassemia based on the individual's history. Milder forms of thalassemia need to be distinguished from iron deficiency and more severe forms need to be distinguished from other hemoglobinopathies.

ii. Thalassemias are congenital. Compare current CBC to previous CBCs. Microcytosis is usually significant, whereas the RBC count is normal or elevated.

iii. If no diagnosis, order hemoglobin A_2, globin chain synthesis ratio, and hemoglobin electrophoresis (Table 42-3).

c. Sideroblastic anemia

i. Review the CBC and iron studies; iron overload is suggestive of sideroblastosis.

ii. A bone marrow biopsy with appropriate staining ultimately is the gold standard for this diagnosis.

2. Normocytic anemia

a. Anemia of chronic disease. This is a diagnosis of exclusion when CBC and iron stores are normal. Identify potential causes of this anemia.

i. Consider ordering an erythrocyte sedimentation rate and a C-reactive protein to look for chronic inflammatory states. C-reactive protein is most useful to distinguish infectious from noninfectious inflammation.

ii. Rule out liver disease with liver functions tests, thyroid disease with a thyroid-

TABLE 42-5 Red Blood Cell Morphology

Description of Red Blood Cell		Associated with Disease
Anisocytosis	Excessive number of red blood cells of various sizes	Larger size = vitamin B_{12} or folate deficiency, drug effect Smaller size = iron deficiency
Hypochromia (decreased hemoglobin content in the red blood cell)	Central pallor	Iron deficiency
Macro-ovalocytes	Oval red blood cell	Vitamin B_{12} or folate deficiency, liver disease, myelodysplastic syndrome
Polychromasis	Wright's stain: large grayish blue with pink	Reticulocytes Increased levels in a peripheral smear are a result from a variety of anemias or from damage to the bone marrow
Poiklocytosis	Abnormal red blood cell shapes, such as:	(below is not inclusive list)
	Acanthocytes (spur cells)	Severe liver disease
	Echinocytes (burr cells)	Uremia, red blood cell volume loss
	Schistocytes (schizocytes)	Microangiopathic or macroangiopathic hemolytic anemia
	Spherocytes	Autoimmune hemolytic anemia, G6PD deficiency, hereditary spherocytosis
	Target cells	Thalassemia, liver disease, hemoglobin C, sickle cell disease
	Teardrop cells	Myelofibrosis, infiltrative processes of marrow
	Rouleaux formation	Paraproteinemia, such as multiple myeloma
Red blood cell inclusions		(below is not inclusive list)
	Basophilic stippling	Lead poisoning, thalassemia, myelofibrosis
	Pappenheimer (iron) bodies	Sideroblastic anemia, lead poisoning
	Parasites	Malaria, babesiosis
Hypersegmentation	Neutrophil nuclei with more than seven lobes	Vitamin B_{12} or folate deficiency, drug effects

stimulating hormone level, and renal disease with a serum creatinine and urinalysis.

  b. Hemolytic anemia
   i. With a careful health and medication history and physical examination, look at the normocytic anemia MCV for reticulocytosis.
   ii. Order an indirect bilirubin, and lactate dehydrogenase blood test.
   iii. Consider ordering a direct antiglobin test or Coombs to confirm immune-mediated hemolysis. Order a G6PD blood test 1–2 months after acute hemolysis.
   iv. Consider ordering a cold agglutinin titer.
 3. Macrocytic and megaloblastic anemias
  a. Vitamin B_{12} deficiency
   i. CBC with elevated MCV and a peripheral smear with macro-ovalocytes and hypersegmented polymorphonuclear cells are seen with vitamin B_{12} and folate deficiency.
   ii. Order a vitamin B_{12} and a folate level to differentiate the common causes of megaloblastic anemia.
   iii. Consider serum methylmalonic level that has increased sensitivity and specificity for confirming vitamin B_{12} deficiency. Additional serological testing for parietal and intrinsic factor antibiotics has replaced the Schilling test (Oh & Brown, 2003).
   iv. Low cobalamin distinguishes vitamin B_{12} from myelodysplastic syndrome.
  b. Folate deficiency: with normal vitamin B_{12} level, low serum folate level, normal methylmalonic level, and elevated homocysteine, folate deficiency is the probable diagnosis.

V. Goals of clinical management

A. *Choose a cost-effective approach for diagnosing anemia.*

B. *Choose a treatment plan that normalizes RBC level and minimizes the risk of anemia relapse (Table 42-6).*

C. *Select an approach that maximizes the patient's short- and long-term adherence to treatment.*

VI. Plan

A. *Microcytic anemias*

1. Iron deficiency anemia

   a. If medically stable, treat with oral iron on an empty stomach beginning with ferrous sulfate, 325 mg, two to three times a day. After 6 weeks of therapy, may be able to decrease dose to twice per day, depending on the CBC results.

   b. Oral iron can cause nausea, vomiting, abdominal discomfort, diarrhea, and constipation. To

TABLE 42-6 Laboratory Tests with Normal Values

Test	Normal	Comment
Complete blood count	Hemoglobin: F: 12–15.5 g/dl M: 13.6–17.5 g/dl Hematocrit: F: 35–49% M: 39–49%	Physiologic variation because of age, smoking, and altitude
Red blood cell indices		
Red blood count	F: 3.5–5.2 10 × 6th/mcl M: 4.3–6 10 × 6th/mcl	
Mean cell volume	80–100 fl	
Mean cell hemoglobin concentration	31–36 g/dl	Increased with spherocytosis, hemolysis; decreased in other anemias
Mean cell Hgb	26–34 pg	Increased with macrocytosis; decreased with microcytosis
Red cell distribution width	11.5–14.5%	Measures variation of red blood cell size; decreased in iron deficiency
White blood cell count	4.5–11 10 × 3rd/mcl	
Platelets	15,000–450,000 µl	
Reticulocyte count	33–137 10 × 3rd/mcl	Separates hypoproliferative from hemolytic anemia or blood loss; expect increase of two to three times in 10 days after anemia starts if normal erythropoietin and bone marrow
Iron supply studies	50–175 mcg/dl	
Serum iron, total iron binding capacity	250–460 mcg/dl	Is increased in iron deficiency anemia
% transferring saturation	25–50%	Low in iron deficiency < 16%
Ferritin	M: 10–300 µg/ml F: 10–200 µg/ml	Most useful in separating iron deficiency from ACD, thalassemia; lowest levels correlate with depleted bone marrow
Haptoglobin	4–316	Low level helpful in DX of HELLP; high levels helpful in ruling out significant intravascular hemolysis
Folate	165–760 ng/ml	
Vitamin B$_{12}$	140–820 pg/ml	

Sources: Gomella, L., & Haist, S. (2007). *The famous scut monkey handbook: Clinician's pocket reference* (11th ed.). New York, NY: McGraw-Hill; Nicoll, D., McPhee, S., Pignone, M., & Lu, C. (2007). *Pocket guide to diagnostic tests* (5th ed.). New York, NY: McGraw-Hill Medical.

decrease side effects advise the patient to take iron with food, decrease the medication frequency, or use another ferrous product with less iron per dose. Parental iron is a potential option for patients who are unable to absorb oral iron or who cannot or will not adhere to oral iron regimen, and who have continued blood loss in chronic disease. Refer to a hematologist if considering parental iron.

    c. Plan to give iron 1–2 months for anemia correction then an additional 4–5 months to replenish iron stores (ferritin level to 50 mcg/ml). Expect a rise in the reticulocyte count in 1 week.

    d. Although medication nonadherence is the most common cause of response failure, having the incorrect diagnosis has to be considered.

    e. Plan for patient follow-up with laboratory values at 1, 2, 4, and 6 months to ensure full recovery.

2. Thalassemia

    a. Individuals with mild disease should be identified to prevent repeated unnecessary diagnostic anemia evaluations and to prevent patients from taking iron unnecessarily.

    b. For those with hemoglobin H disease, 1 mg of folate daily should be prescribed.

    c. Individuals who have severe anemia and need to be treated with red cell transfusions and chelation therapy should be referred to a hematologist.

3. Sideroblastic anemia

    a. If medically stable, no treatment is needed. Patients often do not respond to erythropoietin therapy.

    b. Occasionally, these patients need RBC transfusions. A hematologist should be managing their anemia.

B. Normocytic anemias

1. Anemia of chronic disease

    a. Treat underlying conditions.

    b. In most cases, correction of anemia is not indicated. However, erythropoietin can be effective for those individuals with renal failure, cancer, and inflammatory disorders.

2. Hemolytic anemias

    a. Treat illness and discontinue drugs that may have triggered this anemia.

    b. Prednisone is the standard initial treatment in autoimmune hemolytic anemia. Symptomatic individuals should receive transfusions. In those who fail remission or cannot sustain remission, a splenectomy is recommended. Immunosuppressive agents are used in those persons who fail to respond with splenectomy.

    c. Instruct patients to take 1 mg of folate daily. In those individuals with G6PD deficiency, avoid giving oxidant medications (e.g., sulfamethoxazole). In those susceptible to hemolysis, avoid giving medications known to trigger hemolytic anemia.

    d. Hematology evaluation and management are indicated.

C. Macrocytic and megaloblastic anemias

1. Vitamin B_{12} deficiency anemia

    a. Administer cobalamin, 1,000 mg, parenterally daily for 1 week, then weekly for 1 month, then monthly lifelong. In severe anemia, serum potassium, and hematocrit may drop with initial treatment with cobalamin.

    b. Oral cobalamin, 1,000–2,000 mcg daily, can be substituted with equal effect (Vidal-Alaball, Butler, Cannings-John, & Goringe, 2009).

    c. It is important to appropriately investigate macrocytosis. All patients with suspected myelodysplastic disease need a hematologic evaluation.

    d. Those individuals who do not respond to vitamin B_{12} treatment, who are medically unstable, or whose vitamin B_{12} and folic acid levels are normal should be referred to a hematologist.

2. Folate deficiency anemia

    a. Avoid treating patients with potential cobalamin deficiency with folate alone unless vitamin B_{12} deficiency anemia has been ruled-out and treated because this may lead to progressively severe neuropsychiatric disease caused by untreated vitamin B_{12} deficiency.

    b. Administer folate, 1 mg daily. In 1 week, the patient should begin to have a sense of improvement with increase in reticulocytes. CBC corrects in 2 months, and then the patient may be tapered to folate, 0.5 mg/d long term.

D. Client education

1. Provide verbal and written information regarding

    a. The disease process, including signs and symptoms and underlying etiologies.

    b. Diagnostic tests that include a discussion about preparation, actual procedures, and follow-up care.

    c. Management plan: rationale, action, use, side effects, and cost of therapeutic interventions, and the need for adhering to the long-term treatment plans.

VII. Self-management resources and tools

1. The American Society of Hematology's website is www .bloodthevitalconnection.org/for. This website provides both an overview of anemia and other links for additional information for patients.

2. The National Institutes of Health (www.nhi.gov) has a collection of patient information sites that discuss anemia with handouts under links on dietary supplementation.

REFERENCES

Baik, H. W., & Russell, R. (1999). Vitamin B12 deficiency in the elderly. *Annual Review of Nutrition, 19*, 357–377.

Brill, J., & Baumgardner, D. (2000). Normocytic anemia. *American Family Physician, 62*(10), 2255.

Beutler, E., & Waalen, J. (2006). The definition of anemia: what *is* the lower limit of normal of the blood hemoglobin concentration? *Blood, 107*(5), 1747–1750.

Elmadfa, I., & Singer, I. (2009). Vitamin B12 and homocysteine status among vegetarians: a global perspective. *American Journal of Clinical Nutrition, 89*(5), 1693S–1698S.

Gardner, L., & Benz, Jr., E. (2008). Anemia of chronic disease. In R. Hoffman, H. Heslop, B. Furie, E. Benz, Jr., P. McGlave, L. Silberstein, & S. Shattil (Eds.), *Hematology: Basic principles and practice* (5th ed., pp. 469–474). Philadelphia, PA: McGraw-Hill.

Gehrs, B., & Friedberg, R. (2002). Autoimmune hemolytic anemia. *American Journal of Hematology, 69*(4), 258–271.

Giardina, P., & Forget, B. (2008). Thalassemia syndromes. In R. Hoffman, H. Heslop, B. Furie, E. Benz, Jr., P. McGlave, L. Silberstein, & S. Shattil. (Eds.), *Hematology: Basic principles and practice* (5th ed.). Philadelphia, PA: McGraw-Hill.

Kemna, E. H. (2008). Hepcidin: from discovery to differential diagnosis. *Haematologia, 9*(3), 90–97.

Linker, C. (2007). Blood. In S. McPhee & M. Papadakis (Eds.), *Current medical diagnosis & treatment* (pp. 493–507). New York, NY: McGraw-Hill.

Longo, D. (2009). Examination of blood smears and bone marrow and red blood cell disorders. In A. Fauci, E. Braunwald, D. Kasper, S. Hauser, D. Longo, J. Jameson, & J. Loscalzo (Eds.), *Harrisons's manual of medicine* (17th ed., pp. 321–328). New York, NY: McGraw-Hill.

Makipour, S., Kanapuru, B., Ershler, W. B. (2008). Unexplained anemia in the elderly. *Seminars in Hematology, 45*(4), 250–254.

Oh, R. C., & Brown, D. L. (2003). Vitamin B12. *American Family Physician, 67*(5), 979–986.

Schick, P. (2010). *Hemolytic anemia, Version 2010*. Retrieved from www .emedicine.medscape.com/article/201066.

Schrier, S. (2010). To be old is to be inflamed? *Blood, 115*(18), 3651–3652.

Schwartz, R. (2007). Autoimmune and intravascular hemolytic anemias. In L. Goldman, D. Ausiello, W. Arend, J. Armitage, D. Clemmons, J. Drazen, . . . J. Newman. (Eds.), *Goldman Cecil medicine: Expert consult* (23rd ed., pp. 1194–1202). Philadelphia, PA: W. B. Saunders.

Tefferi, A. (2007). Nonhemolytic normochromic, normocytic anemias. In L. Goldman, D. Ausiello, W. Arend, J. Armitage, D. Clemmons, J. Drazen, . . . J. Newman. (Eds.), *Goldman Cecil medicine: Expert consult* (23rd ed., pp. 1228–1230). Philadelphia, PA: W. B. Saunders.

Umbreit, J. (2005). Iron deficiency: A concise review. *American Journal of Hematology, 78*, 225–231.

Vidal-Alaball, J., Butler, C., Cannings-John, R., & Goringe, A. (2009). Oral vitamin B$_{12}$ versus intramuscular vitamin B$_{12}$ for vitamin B$_{12}$ deficiency (review). *The Cochrane Collaboration*. Retrieved from www .thecochranelibrary.com

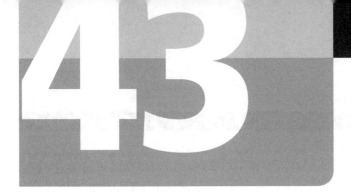

ANTICOAGULATION THERAPY (ORAL)

Fran Dreier and Linda Ray

I. Introduction

Long-term oral anticoagulant therapy (OAT) with warfarin (Coumadin®) is indicated for numerous conditions (Table 43-1). Used for primary and secondary prevention of thromboembolism (TE), OAT requires careful and meticulous management by the clinician to achieve effective and safe outcomes. Although the best practice model for anticoagulation management is a dedicated anticoagulation service, the primary clinician often oversees warfarin therapy. Warfarin management can be complex because the drug possesses what one anticoagulation expert (Ansell, 2009) describes as a "high risk/benefit profile." Warfarin has a narrow therapeutic index and thus requires close and careful follow-up; what may be a therapeutic dose at one point in time may be subtherapeutic or supratherapeutic at other times. The discussion that follows is intended to increase clinician comfort with managing OAT.

The anticoagulants used for OAT are the vitamin K antagonists. Warfarin is the vitamin K antagonist most commonly used; it is an oral agent often referred to by its trade name Coumadin®. Warfarin is often described as a "blood thinner," but in reality it does not make blood more watery. Nonetheless, the term "blood thinner" is an accepted descriptor, particularly when discussing this topic with patients. Blocking vitamin K recycling in the liver hinders synthesis and activation of selected clotting proteins. The net effect is to slow down the clotting cascade in the systemic circulation. At therapeutic doses, warfarin lengthens the time to form a fibrin clot by approximately 10–15 seconds beyond normal clotting speed.

A. Monitoring warfarin therapy

The test for monitoring warfarin therapy is the prothrombin time as measured in seconds. Because of problems of interlaboratory reliability with prothrombin time measurements, a test measure directly related to prothrombin time called the International Normalized Ratio (INR) was developed. INR is a more reliable tool for monitoring warfarin therapy because it allows for standardization of measurement between institutions and laboratories. (Nicoll, McPhee, Pignone, & Lu, 2007). The INR is intended to be used only for warfarin monitoring; it is not a measure of liver function. Although a person not on warfarin likely has an INR between 0.8 and 1.2, after treatment with OAT is started the time until clotting formation extends, the INR rises, and the blood is described as being "thinner."

B. Target population

Indications associated with increased clot risk are shown in Table 43-1, along with the usual target INR for that indication. For the rare patient who develops a clot while therapeutic on warfarin, the target INR range is usually increased by 0.5–1. For the patient whose bleeding risk is heightened, such as a patient at risk for falls, the treatment intensity may be reduced to an INR as low as 1.5. Older patients deserve special consideration. Common barriers to an older patient taking warfarin safely include cognitive impairment, increased fall risk, visual or hearing impairment, or dependency on others for warfarin dosing (Evans-Molina, Henault, Regan, & Hylek, 2003).

In the setting of atrial fibrillation (AF), warfarin is highly effective in preventing complications of TE, particularly stroke, in patients of any age (Wolf, Abbott, & Kannel, 1991). The CHADS2 score is a widely used scheme for evaluating stroke risk in patients with lone or nonvalvular AF (Gage et al., 2001) (Table 43-2). Current research suggests patients with a score of greater than or equal to 1 benefit from warfarin, unless risk for bleeding outweighs the potential for benefit. Patients with AF and a score of 0 are usually treated with aspirin (Fang et al., 2008). AF in the setting of valvular disease or comorbidities confers increased stroke risk.

The clinician should keep in mind that an individual's risk of complications of thrombosis and bleeding may change over time and therefore the indication for treatment, target INR, and treatment duration should be reevaluated from time to time.

C. Associated risks

As reported by the Centers for Medicare and Medicaid Services (2009), those at increased risk of bleeding

TABLE 43-1 Indications with Therapeutic INR Range of 2–3

Indications with Therapeutic INR Range of 2–3	Duration of OAT
Treatment of DVT/PE (collectively known as VTE)	
Provoked by transient risk factor	3–6 months
Unprovoked	> 6 months
Recurrent	Long-term
Stroke/TIA/systemic arterial embolism, secondary prevention	Long-term
Prevention of systemic embolism (ACS, AF, valvular heart disease, severe left ventricular dysfunction [EF < 30%], postsurgical VTE prophylaxis)	Varies with indication
Pulmonary hypertension	Long-term
Mechanical prosthetic valves in the aortic position*	Long-term
Antiphospholipid antibody syndrome (without other risk factors) and other inherited thrombophilias	Long-term
Indications with Therapeutic INR Range of 2.5–3.5	**Duration of OAT**
Recurrent thromboembolism on therapeutic warfarin	Long-term
Mechanical prosthetic valves in the mitral position or ball and cage valves in any position	Long-term

* Goal INR 2.5–3.5 if patients have additional risk factors (e.g., AF)

Source: Adapted from Hirsch, J., Guyatt, G., Albers, G., Harrington, R., & Schünemann, H. J. (2008). Executive summary: American College of Chest Physicians evidence-based clinical practice guidelines (8th ed.). *Chest, 133*, 71S–109S.

while on warfarin are patients with the following: INR greater than 4, labile INR, history of gastrointestinal bleeding, existing cerebrovascular disease, serious heart disease, anemia, malignancy, trauma, renal insufficiency, concomitant drugs, advanced age, and prior stroke. It is axiomatic that the higher the INR, the greater the risk for bleeding complications. However, an elevated INR does not cause spontaneous bleeding; there must be some concomitant tissue trauma or inflammation to initiate the bleeding.

TABLE 43-2 CHADS2 Score for Assessment of Stroke Risk in Patients with Atrial Fibrillation

Congestive Heart Failure*	1 pt
Hypertension	1 pt
Age ≥ 75 years	1 pt
Diabetes	1 pt
Stroke (previous TIA or CVA)	2 pts

*Ejection fraction < 25% or have had a heart failure exacerbation in the last 90 days

Risk of events per year without OAC:
    0 points = 1.9%
    1 point = 2.8%
    2 points = 4%
    3 points = 5.9%
    4 points = 8.5%
    5 points = 12.5%
    6 points = 18.2%

Source: Adapted from Gage, B. F., Waterman, A. D., Shannon, W., Boechler, M., Rich, M. W., & Radford M. J. (2001). Validation of clinical classification schemes for predicting stroke: Results from the National Registry of Atrial Fibrillation. *Journal of the American Medical Association, 285*, 2864–2870.

D. Treatment duration

Patients who are at high risk of TE need life-long OAT (Table 43-1). Long-term therapy is also recommended for patients with saddle or massive pulmonary embolism (i.e., significant clot burden). Short-term therapy, which usually lasts 3–6 months, is appropriate for indications where clot risk is transitory or triggered by a provoking event, such as a single-event deep venous thrombosis after hip replacement. The duration of an individual's treatment is strongly influenced by whether their clot was considered to be provoked or unprovoked. The issue of duration of OAT for various indications is a subject of active research. The American College of Chest Physicians intermittently publishes updated evidence-based clinical guidelines for antithrombotic therapy, including recommendations for treatment duration. These guidelines can be found online at http ://www.chestjounal.org/content/vol133/6_suppl.

E. Variables that affect response to warfarin

1. Diet

The most frequent cause for a change in INR in a patient who has been otherwise stable is a change in oral vitamin K intake (e.g., loss of appetite) or absorption (e.g., acute diarrheal illness). Patients should be encouraged to maintain a consistent amount of vitamin K in their diet from week to week. Vitamin K is present in varying quantities in most food, and deficiency is rare. The daily adequate intake recommended by the US Department of Agriculture is 120 mcg for men and 90 mcg for women (2001). Certain foods are very rich in vitamin K, and far exceed the daily adequate intake in a single serving. It is generally agreed that the foods highest in vitamin K are dark green leafy vegetables, such as kale and spinach. Some of the cruciferous vegetables are moderately high in vitamin K. The nature of the patient's vitamin K intake should be assessed at every visit, and the patient should be reminded periodically of the role of vitamin K in warfarin management. Some common vitamin K–rich foods are listed in Table 43-3. A comprehensive list can be found at www.nal.usda.gov/fnic/foodcomp/Data/SR17/wtrank/sr17w430.pdf. Supplements, both tablet and liquid forms, and multivitamins may contain significant amounts of vitamin K; clinicians should ask about supplement use at each visit.

2. Alcohol intake

Alcohol can affect the INR unpredictably. Paradoxically, chronic alcohol use tends to lower the INR, whereas acute binge drinking tends to increase the INR. Light to moderate drinking (i.e., up to two servings of alcohol [12 oz of wine, 24 oz of beer, 2 oz of hard liquor] at one time) may be less problematic. Alcohol also increases the likelihood of injury if ingested in excess, may cause bleeding by irritating the upper gastrointestinal tract, and may impair platelet function. Abstention from alcohol does simplify warfarin management (Wittkowsky, 2009b).

3. Comorbidities

An acute illness or a worsening of a chronic illness may affect warfarin stability. Changes in liver, cardiac, or thyroid function are likely to alter usual dose requirements. In general, severe illness tends to reduce an individual's warfarin requirement. For reasons not fully understood, fever itself may independently cause an increased response to warfarin (Self, 2000).

4. Medications and nutritional supplements: interactions

a. Drug interactions

Many drug interactions with warfarin have been documented. For most agents, there is

significant individual variability among patients as to timing and extent of the interaction. Drug interactions may vary both among individuals and within a drug class itself (see Table 43-4 for a partial list of interactions). It is important that the clinician very clearly educate patients to report any acute illness, new medicines, or change in medicines. It is critical that clinicians maintain meticulous communication, to ensure that all are aware of new drugs that have been prescribed. If there is no alternative to an agent that interacts, the clinician may choose to preemptively alter warfarin dose or increase the frequency of INR checks to enhance patient safety. This is often done in consultation with an anticoagulation specialist. A comprehensive list of interactions can be found in the article by Holbrook and colleagues (2005). Fortunately, first-generation penicillins are not known to interact with warfarin.

Pain medications represent a special category of consideration because the need for acute or chronic analgesia arises so frequently in the primary care setting. Nonsteroidal anti-inflammatory drugs (NSAIDs), both nonselective and selective (cyclooxygenase-2 inhibitors), should be avoided in patients taking warfarin because they increase the risk of gastrointestinal bleeding (Battistella, Mamdani, Juurlink, Rabeneck, & Laupacis,

TABLE 43-3 Foods Rich in Vitamin K

Beet greens*	Lettuce†
Broccoli	Mustard greens*
Brussel sprouts	Seaweed (nori)
Cauliflower	Soybean oil‡
Collard greens*	Spinach*
Kale*	Turnip greens*

* Extremely high in vitamin K.
† Except iceberg.
‡ In large quantities.

Source: U.S. Department of Agriculture, Agricultural Research Service. (2009). USDA National Nutrient Database for Standard Reference, Release 22. Nutrient Data Laboratory Home Page. Retrieved from http://www.ars.usda.gov/ba/bhnrc/ndl

TABLE 43-4 Warfarin–Drug Interactions

Increase in INR	Decrease in INR
Alcohol	Alcohol
Amiodarone*	Antiretrovirals (some)†
Antiretrovirals (some)†	Carbamazepine
Azoles‡	Phenobarbital*
Cimetidine*	Rifampin/rifabutin*
Erythromycin*	Sucralfate
Fibrates*	Vitamin K (phytonadione)*
Fluoroquinolones (some)*	
Phenytoin	
Statins	

This is not a comprehensive list. INR should be monitored after initiating or modifying any drug therapy.

* Significant interaction.

† The reader is advised to go to literature for specifics of individual drugs of this class.

‡ Azoles include antifungals, metronidazole, and sulfamethazole, a component of Bactrim®/Septra®.

Source: Adapted from UCSF Medical Center, Comprehensive Hemostasis and Antithrombotic Service (CHAS), updated 2/2009.

2005; Cheetham, Levy, Niu, & Bixler, 2009). If a patient must take an NSAID, it is best for the patient to take the shortest acting agent, at the smallest dose, for the briefest time. If a patient must be on chronic NSAID therapy, the clinician should consider monitoring stool guaiacs. Although adding a drug from the class of proton pump inhibitors should theoretically confer some protection to the upper gastrointestinal tract, this does not protect the lower gastrointestinal tract.

The safest alternative for a patient requiring short-term pain relief is acetaminophen. Although it does not relieve inflammation, when the dosage does not exceed 2 g/day, there is very small likelihood that an interaction will occur. However, the INR may increase with the use of 4 g/day (Carrier, Gréoire, & Wells, 2009). Tramadol may increase the INR; narcotics do not by themselves alter the INR or platelet function.

b. Supplements

It has been estimated that 50% of patients are taking some form of nutritional supplement and that up to 60% do not report use of alternative therapies to their healthcare providers (Wittkowsky, 2009a). Although there are relatively few case reports of supplement–warfarin interactions to date, potential interactions do exist, either by diminishing platelet activity or by directly affecting the INR (Table 43-5). The clinician is advised to check Web-based information systems for further information regarding these products (the Natural Pharmacist, www.tnp.com; the Pharmacist's Letter, www .natural pharmacist.com; the National Institutes of Health, http://dietary-supplements.info.nih .gov; and Natural Standards, http://www .naturalstandard.com).

F. Issues of dosing and follow-up in OAT therapy

1. OAT therapy is best managed using a systematic approach of patient assessment, addressing dose adjustment, and scheduling the next follow-up interval. The use of a flow sheet or electronic record is strongly advised to help the clinician interpret the visit data in the context of overall INR trends and usual dose patterns (Garcia et al., 2008).

2. At each visit the clinician should assess the patient's overall health status. The clinician should confirm actual dosing at each visit with direct and specific questions

   a. Based on the 7-day week, tell me what dose you take on what days.
   b. Do you recall having missed any doses recently, particularly in the last 7 days?

   Additional areas to cover at each visit are shown in Table 43-6.

3. Current guidelines indicate that the stable patient with therapeutic readings should undergo testing every 4 weeks (Ansell, 2009), although there is recent evidence suggesting that the stable patient without significant comorbidities might be followed less frequently (Witt et al., 2009). Testing every 1 to 2 weeks is recommended if the INR is not within therapeutic range or if warfarin dose is changed. In certain situations, such as a very high (supratherapeutic) INR, it may be advisable to retest in 1 or 2 days.

TABLE 43-5 Warfarin and Commonly Used Dietary Supplements/Herbal Medicines

Herbs and Dietary Supplements	Impact or Effect
American ginseng	May either potentiate warfarin or inhibit warfarin effect
Chinese herbs and medicines	Impact determined by active ingredients
Coenzyme Q-10	May have a procoagulant effect or increase INR; avoid or monitor closely for 3 months at time of supplement initiation
Echinacea	No case reports of interaction with warfarin
Fish oil and omega-3 fatty acids	Antiplatelet activity; may increase bleeding risk
Garlic	Antiplatelet activity when taken in large quantities
Ginko biloba	Antiplatelet activity; may increase bleeding risk (hemorrhagic stroke case reports)
Glucosamine	May increase INR (based on a few isolated case reports)
Multivitamins containing vitamin K	Inhibits warfarin; choose product with ≤ 30 mcg vitamin K

Source: Adapted from Dennehy, C. (2010, April 9–11). *An evidence based look at popular dietary supplements.* Presented at Clinical Pharmacotherapy 2010, UC Davis.

TABLE 43-6 Warfarin Management: Questions to Ask at Follow-up Visits

Current dose and tablet strength
Any changes in health status?
Any unusual bruising or bleeding?
Any change in diet?
Any new medicines or supplements?
Any change in medicines or supplements?
Any falls?
Any questions?

G. Managing variations in INR

1. One of the challenges of managing OAT is deciding how to respond to INR variations. Small INR variations occur from visit to visit for even the more stable patient, and not all INR variations require new dose adjustment. The trend of a patient's INR readings is more important than any single INR. Precipitous change in dosing should be avoided, because it is responsible for some of the difficulty that can occur in attempting to maintain INRs within target range.

2. When presented with an INR that is out of target range, the clinician should look for variables that affect warfarin stability, determine if these variables are transient or continuing, and review or reinforce topics in patient education that may explain the variation in the INR reading. If a subtherapeutic or supratherapeutic value can be explained by a transient change in a variable, the provider should adjust the dose for 1 or 2 days and then rechallenge the patient with the prior dose, with follow-up in 1 or 2 weeks.

3. Variables affecting warfarin stability (Oertel, 2005) include the following

   a. Changes in other medications, including additions or deletions of routine, over-the-counter and herbal medications, and dose changes of current medications

   b. Intercurrent illness, especially febrile or diarrheal illness

   c. Dietary habits (wide swings in amount of intake or type of foods)

   d. Alcohol intake

   e. Travel, which can alter lifestyle habits and dosing schedules

   f. Issues of patient adherence

4. A patient's response to chronic warfarin treatment may vary over time, and occasionally a previously stable patient requires a new weekly warfarin dose in the absence of any clear influencing variables.

5. The degree of response to an INR out of range should also be based on the patient's risk category. For example, a single low value is more concerning for patients with a mechanical mitral valve than it is for a patient with lone AF. A supratherapeutic value is more concerning when there is a high risk for falls or a past history of gastrointestinal bleeding. Patients at higher risk for complications require closer follow-up than patients at lower risk.

6. Although computer-based programs and warfarin dosing tables are available to aid clinicians in making dose adjustments, these are not likely to address individual patient variables and a clinician's familiarity with a patient's case history. Some guidelines for dose adjustments include

   a. Change the total weekly dose by approximately 10–15%, depending on the magnitude of the INR variation and the stability and risk profile of the patient.

   b. Use a single-strength tablet to propose a schedule of multiples (e.g., two and three tablets alternating) or fractions (e.g., dose reduction from one tablet daily to half a tablet Monday, Wednesday, and Friday, and one tablet the other 4 days). Although dosing with one tablet strength is easier for some patients to manage than using tablets of different strengths, using a combination of 1- and 5-mg tablets can offer good dosing flexibility for most patients.

   c. Before changing to a new dose, evaluate the patient's risk for confusion, dose error, practicality and cost of dose adjustment, and patient preference (Wong, Wilson, & Wittkowsky, 1999).

7. Patients with persistently unstable INRs may benefit from receiving either Coumadin® or a generic from the same manufacturer each time (Wittkowsky, 2009b). Some patients whose INRs are persistently unstable without clear cause may benefit from adding 100 mcg of a vitamin K supplement daily. It may be necessary to adjust the patient's usual dose based on an initial lowering of INR because of the added vitamin K (Hirsch, Guyatt, Albers, Harrington, & Schünemann, 2008).

8. Subtherapeutic INRs

   If an INR is below goal, inquire about a recent change in vitamin K intake, along with the possibility of missed doses or an error in dosing. See Table 43-7 for additional guidelines for evaluating a subtherapeutic INR.

TABLE 43-7 Evaluation of Subtherapeutic INR

Dose error? (particularly missed dose)
Increase in vitamin K intake?
New medication or supplement?
Change in medication or supplement?
Improvement in heart or liver function?
Change in usual manufacturer of tablet?

TABLE 43-8 Possible Causes of Supratherapeutic INR

Dose error
Diet change
Change in medicine or supplement
Acute illness
Decrease in liver function
Decrease in cardiac function
Change in usual manufacturer of tablet
Laboratory error

9. Supratherapeutic INRs

If an INR is above goal, inquire whether the patient has increased bruising or frank bleeding. An INR greater than 4 carries an increased risk of serious bleeding (Beyth, 2005). Inquire about intercurrent illness, acute dose error, recent addition of antibiotics, or reduction in dietary vitamin K intake or in total dietary intake (Table 43-8). See Table 43-9 for specific guidelines for managing supratherapeutic INRs.

II. Patient education and safety

A. Patient education is the cornerstone of safe and effective warfarin management. This requires that the patient have a basic understanding of the purpose and mechanism of anticoagulation. At the beginning of treatment it should be made clear to patients that although warfarin does slow clotting, it does not cause bleeding. Warfarin comes in nine strengths; each strength is consistently coded to a different color, although shape and manufacturer do vary. The coding of color to strength helps to prevent dosing errors and to discover them quickly when they occur.

B. To promote adherence and minimize error, warfarin dosing should be tailored to the individual patient. Some patients achieve their best INR control with one single-strength daily dose, although those less susceptible to confusion or error can manage a variable dose. Equal daily dosing causes less confusion and is associated with lower rates of dose error. However, using the same dose every day may require the patient to have tablets in more than one strength or to split tablets. Although warfarin comes in multiple strengths, many patients need a dose that falls somewhere in between these strengths. In some cases it is not possible to achieve a target INR with 7 days of equal dosing.

TABLE 43-9 Recommendations for the Management of Excessive Oral Anticoagulation or Bleeding

INR supratherapeutic, but < 5 with no significant bleeding	Lower or omit dose, monitor more frequently, resume at lower dose when INR is therapeutic. If only minimally elevated or associated with a transient variable, dose adjustment may not be necessary.
INR > 5 but < 9, no significant bleeding	Omit the next one or two doses, monitor more frequently, resume therapy at adjusted dose when INR is therapeutic. Alternatively, omit dose and give 1–2.5 mg vitamin K orally, particularly for those at increased risk of bleeding. If more rapid reversal is required because the patient needs urgent surgery, give vitamin K ≥ 5 mg orally, expecting INR reduction within 24 hours. If INR remains high, give additional vitamin K of 1–2 mg.
INR > 9, no significant bleeding	Hold warfarin therapy and give a higher dose of vitamin K (2.5–5 mg) orally, expecting INR to reduce significantly within 24–48 hours. Monitor the INR more frequently, give additional vitamin K if needed, and resume therapy at an adjusted dose when the INR is in therapeutic range.
INR therapeutic or elevated with serious or life-threatening bleeding	Hold warfarin therapy and give vitamin K by slow intravenous infusion along with fresh frozen plasma, prothrombin complex concentrate, or recombinant factor VIIa. For life-threatening bleeding, recombinant factor VIIa is supplemented with vitamin K, 10 mg by slow infusion, repeated as necessary.

Source: Adapted from Hirsch, J., Guyatt, G., Albers, G., Harrington, R., & Schünemann, H. J. (2008). Executive summary: American College of Chest Physicians evidence-based clinical practice guidelines (8th ed.). *Chest, 133,* 72S–73S.

C. The fundamentals of safe warfarin therapy should be reinforced frequently:

1. Clarify warfarin tablet strength and dosing schedule at each visit. It should be clear to the patient whether the dosing instructions are given in terms of milligrams or tablets. It is most precise to talk with patients about their weekly dosing schedule in terms of specific milligrams per day rather than number of tablets per day. However, many patients know their warfarin only by its color and prefer instructions given in tablets per day. It is critical to patient safety that the patient, caregiver, and clinician have a clear mutual understanding of what dose is being recommended.

2. Reinforce dietary guidelines and the need to report any significant changes.

3. Report any signs of warfarin complications, which include unusual bruising, epistaxis, bleeding gums, hematuria, hematochezia, or melena.

4. Report if any medicines or supplements have been started, changed, or discontinued. Avoid aspirin, NSAIDs, and all nonprescription medications unless approved by the clinician.

5. Report any acute illness, especially vomiting or diarrhea, or significant change in health status.

6. Avoid activities that increase risk of injury, particularly contact sports.

7. Call the clinic or go to an acute care setting in case of a fall or serious injury, particularly head trauma. Because the most devastating potential complication of warfarin therapy is intracranial bleeding, even minor head trauma should prompt a call to the clinic or an urgent care visit.

D. Special considerations

1. Multiple providers: it is best to identify a single provider for warfarin management and prescription refills. This simple strategy can help to avoid potentially serious errors in dosing.

2. Women and gynecological issues: women who are of childbearing age must be informed about the teratogenic risks of warfarin. They should be advised to use contraception and to tell their clinician about wishes to become pregnant. They should also be counseled that warfarin may augment or prolong menstruation. Because warfarin can unmask an existing gynecological issue in a woman of any age, patients should report unusual, heavy, or intermenstrual bleeding.

3. Combined warfarin and antiplatelet therapy (often referred to as "dual" or "triple" therapy):

some patients, such as those with coronary artery disease, may be taking warfarin along with one or two antiplatelet agents (i.e., aspirin and clopidogrel [Plavix®]). Because the risk of bleeding has been shown to be significantly higher in these patients, the need for antiplatelet therapy should be carefully evaluated (Douketis et al., 2008). If the patient does require dual or triple therapy, one option is to lower the INR target within the limits of safety given the patient's indication for warfarin.

4. Planned interruptions of OAT: the relative risk of bleeding during a procedure versus developing a thrombus without anticoagulation determines whether and when an individual may need to interrupt warfarin. In a case of low risk for thrombosis, the dose may be stopped safely 5 days before the procedure, and resumed when the clinician performing the procedure deems it safe, usually the day of or day after the procedure. More complicated situations require a decision tree as to whether to bridge the patient with low-molecular-weight heparin or lengthen the time off warfarin. A minority of patients may require hospitalization for heparinization preprocedure and postprocedure. The CHADS$_2$ score can help with risk stratification for patients with lone AF who need to interrupt OAT treatment. A patient with a CHADS$_2$ score of 5–6 is considered to be high risk for TE when OAT is suspended (Table 43-10). More detailed guidelines for bridging decisions, developed by the Comprehensive Hemostasis and Anticoagulation Service (CHAS) at the University of California, San Francisco, are in Table 43-11.

5. Oral procedures: some oral procedures can be safely performed at an INR of 2. The decision to alter warfarin dosing is based on how much bleeding the procedure may induce. See Table 43-12 for guidelines for oral procedures.

TABLE 43-10 Risk of Thromboembolism for Patients with AF Interrupting Warfarin

Low risk	CHADS$_2$ score of 0–2
	No history of CVA or TIA
Moderate risk	CHADS$_2$ score of 3 or 4
High risk	CHADS$_2$ score of 5–6
	Recent (i.e., within 3 months) stroke or TIA
	Rheumatic valvular heart disease

Source: Adapted from Douketis, J. D., Berger, P. B., Dunn, A. S., Jaffer, A. K., Spyropoulos, A. C., Becker, R. C., & Ansell, J. (2008). The perioperative management of antithrombotic therapy: American College of Chest Physicians evidence-based clinical practice guidelines (8th ed.). *Chest, 133,* 305S.

TABLE 43-11 A Reference for Perioperative Management of Patients on Long-Term Anticoagulation Therapy

February 2009 University of California San Francisco Medical Center Comprehensive Hemostasis and Antithrombotic Service (CHAS)		
(Note: These recommendations are not intended to replace individual clinician judgment. Decisions should account for patient preferences and provide informed decision making about the risks and benefits of anticoagulation)		

	Low Thromboembolic Risk	Moderate Thromboembolic Risk	High Thromboembolic Risk
	Non-valvular atrial fibrillation (AF) with CHADS$_2$ score (see reverse) of 0–2 (and no prior stroke or TIA) Single VTE occurred > 12 months ago and no other risk factors Mechanical bi-leaflet heart valve in aortic position without AF or other risk factors for stroke	Non-valvular AF with CHADS$_2$ score of 3 or 4 VTE within the past 3–12 months Active cancer treated within 6 months or palliative Bileaflet aortic heart valve with one of the following: AF, prior stroke/TIA, hypertension, diabetes, heart failure, age > 75 yr Known non-severe thrombophilic conditions (heterozygous carrier of factor V Leiden mutation or factor II mutation)	Acute venous or arterial thromboembolic event < 3 months ago (Elective surgery should be delayed for 3 months. If surgery is necessary within 1 month of venous event, a temporary IVC filter may be indicated) Nonvalvular atrial fibrillation *with* a CHADS$_2$ score of 5 or 6, or recent (within 3 months) stroke or TIA Mechanical heart valve in aortic position *and* ≥ 2 risk factors[2] Mechanical heart valve with a recent (within 6 months) stroke or TIA, or AF Mechanical heart valve in mitral position Caged ball or tilting disk aortic heart valve > 1 prosthetic heart valve Rheumatic mitral valve disease Known severe thrombophilia (deficiency of protein C, protein S or antithrombin, antiphospholipid antibodies, or multiple thrombophilic abnormalities)
Low Bleeding Risk Endoscopic procedures w/o biopsy Urologic procedures w/o biopsy Skin biopsy	Perform procedure under *full or reduced* anticoagulation: **Before procedure:** No change in warfarin dose, **OR** Hold 1–2 warfarin doses prior to procedure to allow INR to decline to around 2 or less No bridging necessary	Perform procedure under *full or reduced* anticoagulation: **Before procedure:** No change in warfarin dose, **OR** Hold 1 warfarin dose prior to procedure to allow INR to decline to around 2 or less No bridging necessary	Perform procedure under *full* anticoagulation: **Before procedure:** No change in warfarin dose

TABLE 43-11 A Reference for Perioperative Management of Patients on Long-Term Anticoagulation Therapy *(continued)*

February 2009 University of California San Francisco Medical Center Comprehensive Hemostasis and Antithrombotic Service (CHAS)			
(Note: These recommendations are not intended to replace individual clinician judgment. Decisions should account for patient preferences and provide informed decision making about the risks and benefits of anticoagulation)			
	Low Thromboembolic Risk	**Moderate Thromboembolic Risk**	**High Thromboembolic Risk**
Low Bleeding Risk *(continued)* Potentially bloodless surgery [e.g., cataract] Consider risk of anesthesia administration (e.g., retrobulbar administration with cataract surgery) Dental procedures: cleaning, simple extractions, restorations, endodontics, prosthetics	✓ INR day of procedure **After procedure:** Resume/continue previous warfarin dose on the evening of surgery or when deemed safe and with the approval of the surgeon or proceduralist No bridging necessary	✓ INR day of procedure **After procedure:** Resume/continue previous warfarin dose on the evening of surgery or when deemed safe and with the approval of the surgeon or proceduralist No bridging necessary	✓ INR day of procedure **After procedure:** Continue previous warfarin dose on the evening of surgery or when deemed safe and with the approval of the surgeon or proceduralist
High Bleeding Risk All invasive cardiac procedures (e.g., heart valve replacement, coronary artery bypass graft) Certain Interventional radiologic procedures Endoscopic procedures with biopsy Higher risk urologic procedures: TURP, prostate biopsy, lithotripsy, prostatectomy, bladder surgery Multiple dental extractions, gingival and alveolar surgery Ophthalmic lid, lacrimal, or orbital surgery Neurosurgical procedures Major vascular surgery Major cancer surgery Any major surgery	Perform procedure when INR < 1.5: **Before procedure:** Stop warfarin 5 days prior to procedure (take last dose 6 days prior to procedure) No bridging necessary vs. bridge with low dose SQ enoxaparin 30 mg SQ q12h (note: for mechanical valve, use full dose) If bridged with enoxaparin, last dose should be given no sooner than 24 hours prior to procedure ✓ INR day of procedure **After procedure:** Resume previous warfarin dose on the evening of surgery or when deemed safe and with the approval of the surgeon or proceduralist If the intervention increases the risk of thrombosis, administer prophylactic enoxaparin No bridging necessary vs. bridge with low dose SQ enoxaparin 30 mg SQ q12h (note: for mechanical valve, use full dose)	Perform procedure when INR < 1.5: **Before procedure:** Stop warfarin 5 days prior to procedure (take last dose 6 days prior to procedure) Pre-procedure enoxaparin bridging optional for patients with CHADS$_2$ score of 3 Start enoxaparin 1 mg/kg SC q12h (preferred), or low dose SQ enoxaparin 30 mg SQ q12h (for AF/VTE only) when INR < 2, about 4 days prior to procedure Last dose of enoxaparin should be given no sooner than 24 hours prior to procedure (IV UFH should be stopped 4 hours prior to procedure) ✓ INR day prior to procedure	Perform procedure when INR < 1.5: **Before procedure:** Stop warfarin 5 days prior to procedure (take last dose 6 days prior to procedure) Start bridge therapy with enoxaparin 1 mg/kg SC q12h when INR < 2, about 4 days prior to procedure Last dose of enoxaparin should be given no sooner than 24 hours prior to procedure ✓ INR day prior to procedure

TABLE 43-11 A Reference for Perioperative Management of Patients on Long-Term Anticoagulation Therapy (*continued*)

	February 2009 University of California San Francisco Medical Center Comprehensive Hemostasis and Antithrombotic Service (CHAS)		
(Note: These recommendations are not intended to replace individual clinician judgment. Decisions should account for patient preferences and provide informed decision making about the risks and benefits of anticoagulation)			
	Low Thromboembolic Risk	Moderate Thromboembolic Risk	High Thromboembolic Risk
High Bleeding Risk (*continued*)		**After procedure:** Resume full-dose bridge therapy with enoxaparin 1 mg/kg SC q12h 48–72 hours after surgery when hemostasis achieved and with the approval of the surgeon or proceduralist. Dose may be "stepped up" starting with prophylactic dose within 12 hours of surgery with approval of the surgeon or proceduralist. Continue until INR therapeutic for 2 consecutive days. Resume preoperative or preprocedure warfarin dose on the evening of surgery or when deemed safe and with the approval of the surgeon or proceduralist.	**After procedure:** Resume bridge therapy with enoxaparin 1 mg/kg SC q12h q 12h 48–72 hours after surgery when hemostasis achieved and with the approval of the surgeon or proceduralist. Dose may be "stepped up," starting with prophylactic dose within 12 hours of surgery. Continue until INR therapeutic for 2 consecutive days. Resume previous warfarin dose on the evening of surgery or when deemed safe and with the approval of the surgeon or proceduralist.

For patients with decreased CrCl (<30 mL/min) who may require immediate reversal of anticoagulation, consider the use of unfractionated heparin instead of enoxaparin. Do NOT bolus IVUFH in these patients.

Management of patients on antiplatelet therapy

Management of antiplatelet therapy must be individualized.

Bare metal stents, Dual antiplatelet therapy with aspirin and clopidogrel *should not* be interrupted for a minimum of four weeks and any elective procedures should be delayed until six weeks following implantation.

Drug eluting stents, (e.g., Cypher® or Taxus® stent), dual antiplatelet therapy with aspirin and clopidogrel *should not* be interrupted for a minimum of 12 months and any elective procedure should be delayed until two weeks following completion of the ideal course (at least 12 months) of dual antiplatelet therapy.

Patients with either type of stent should remain on aspirin for an extended period of time.

Discontinuation of **NSAIDs** (e.g., ibuprofen, naproxen) should be considered for patients undergoing invasive procedures.

Aspirin: Should not be discontinued for routine procedures

CHADS$_2$ score for assessment of stroke risk in atrial fibrillation patients

Recent or current heart failure*	1 point
Diagnosis of hypertension+	1 point
Age ≥ 75 years	1 point
Diagnosis of diabetes	1 point
History of previous CVA or TIA	2 points

* Ejection fraction < 25% or have had a heart failure exacerbation in last 90 days

+Score as yes in patients with this diagnosis even if currently controlled

Dental procedures: Specific guidelines are available for dental procedures. See *Guidelines for the management of anticoagulation during oral surgery.*

TABLE 43-12 Guidelines for the Management of Anticoagulation During Oral Surgery

Patients who require interventional or surgical procedures while they are taking anticoagulants can pose a therapeutic dilemma for clinicians. The need for alteration of anticoagulant therapy in patients undergoing general dentistry, periodontal, and oral surgical procedures is dependent on several factors including the intensity of anticoagulation, the type of procedure, and the likelihood of thrombosis versus bleeding. Because of the risk for thromboembolism, patients undergoing invasive procedures who require interruption of their anticoagulant therapy should have it interrupted for the shortest possible time period. The trend to lower intensity of anticoagulation allows many procedures to be performed without interruption of therapy while maintaining the INR at approximately 2.0.

All patients undergoing any procedure associated with a risk for bleeding should have the **INR evaluated within 24 hours before the procedure**. If interruption of therapy is necessary, it must be individualized. When therapy is interrupted, it should usually be resumed the evening of the procedure if hemostasis has been achieved.

Low-Risk or Routine Procedures can usually be performed with an INR of 2–3 and include

   a. Routine hygiene and light scaling.

   b. Routine restorative procedures including fillings performed under local infiltrative anesthesia.

   c. Simple, single extractions. Multiple and surgical extractions may require modification of anticoagulant therapy.

   d. Sockets should be sutured and packed with a local hemostatic agent, such as Gelfoam or Surgicel®.

Moderate-Risk Procedures can be performed with an INR of approximately 1.5.

   a. Procedures requiring mandibular blocks to accomplish adequate local anesthesia.

   b. Deep scaling.

   c. Multiple extractions or other extensive periodontal surgery.

   d. Sockets should be sutured and packed with a local hemostatic agent, such as Gelfoam or Surgicel®.

High-Risk Procedures should only be performed when the INR is normalized. Periprocedural heparinization in the hospital setting may be necessary for some patients, for example those with mechanical heart valves who are at a high risk of both bleeding and development of thrombosis.

   a. Multiple extractions or extraction of impacted teeth.

   b. Major reconstructive procedures.

General Guidelines

A. Aspirin and other nonsteroidal anti-inflammatory drugs should not routinely be used in most patients for postoperative analgesia because of their antiplatelet effect. An exception is once daily aspirin, 81–325 mg, when prescribed for patients with a cardiovascular or cerebrovascular indication. This therapy should not be interrupted at any time and should be continued before and after the dental procedure. In addition, therapy with clopidogrel (Plavix®) should not be interrupted when it is used in patients with drug-eluting stents.

B. A thorough medication history should be obtained before the planned procedure. Keep in mind that herbal medications may also influence hemostasis.

C. Prophylactic antibiotics are required for patients at risk of bacterial endocarditis. See the AHA guidelines for recommendations.

D. Patients should be instructed to avoid chewing hard foods, to avoid hot liquids, and to perform vigorous mouth washing for 24–48 hours after procedures. They should use external ice packs and biting pressure on gauze pads to control localized bleeding.

E. Tranexamic acid mouthwashes have been suggested as an intervention to minimize bleeding after oral surgical procedures. In a well-designed 2003 study, a 5% solution of tranexamic acid used immediately after surgery and four times a day for 2 days was as effective as a 5-day course to reduce bleeding (Carter, G., & Goss, A., 2003).

F. Patients undergoing major procedures who have had anticoagulant therapy interrupted should be scheduled for a follow-up anticoagulation clinic appointment within 7–14 days. Patients who have required bridging with low-molecular-weight heparin need earlier follow-up.

References

Dalen, J. E., & Hirsh, J. (Eds.). (2008). Eighth ACCP Consensus Conference on Antithrombotic Therapy. *Chest, 133*, 67S–887S.

Douketis, J. D., et al. (2008). The perioperative management of antithrombotic therapy: American College of Chest Physicians evidence-based clinical practice guidelines (8th edition). *Chest Supplement, 133*, 299S–339S.

(continues)

TABLE 43-12 Guidelines for the Management of Anticoagulation During Oral Surgery *(continued)*

References

Ferrieri, G. B., et al. (2007). Oral surgery in patients on anticoagulant treatment without therapy interruption. *Journal of Oral and Maxillofacial Surgery, 65,* 1149–1154.

Douketis, J. D. (2003). Perioperative anticoagulation management in patients who are receiving oral anticoagulant therapy: A practical guide for clinicians. *Thrombosis Research, 108,* 3–13.

Carter, G., et al. (2003). Tranexamic acid mouthwash versus autologous fibrin glue in patients taking warfarin undergoing dental extractions: A randomized prospective clinical study. *Journal of Oral and Maxillofacial Surgery, 61,* 1432–1435.

Carter, G., & Goss, A. (2003). Tranexamic acid mouthwash: A prospective randomized study of a 2-day regimen vs 5-day regimen to prevent post-operative bleeding in anticoagulated patients requiring dental extractions. *International Journal of Oral and Maxillofacial Surgery, 32,* 504–507.

Dunn, A. S., & Turpie, A. G. G. (2003). Perioperative management of patients receiving oral anticoagulants. *Archives of Internal Medicine, 163,* 901–908.

Wilson, W., et al. (2007). Prevention of endocarditis. Guidelines from the American Heart Association. (The Council on Scientific Affairs of the American Dental Association has approved the guideline as it relates to dentistry.) *Circulation, 116,* 1736–1754.

Nishimura, R. A., et al. (2008). ACC/AHA 2008 Guideline update on valvular heart disease: Focused update on infective endocarditis. A report of the American College of Cardiology/American Heart Association Task Force on Practice Guidelines. *Circulation, 118,* 887–896.

Addendum: preparation of 5% tranexamic acid mouthwash

Tranexamic acid is freely soluble in water. A 500-mg tablet of tranexamic acid can be crushed and dispersed in 10 ml of water immediately before administration. Alternatively, a liquid can be prepared by mixing crushed tablets with water and then filtering out the insoluble excipients to give a clear solution. A maximum expiry date of 5 days is suggested for this preparation, which has not been formally tested.

Source: Adapted from Kayser, S. R., Kearns, G., & Smith, R. (2009). The Anticoagulation Clinic, Division of Oral Surgery, University of California San Francisco.

6. Travel: diets often change significantly when patients travel. Counsel patients to maintain their intake of vitamin K–rich food at its usual level and to maintain the usual 24-hour dosing interval across changing time zones.

7. Discontinuing warfarin: if a patient is at high risk of falls or of dose error (as may occur in dementia), or if the patient is unable or unwilling to adhere to monitoring schedules, the clinician should reevaluate if the risk of bleeding outweighs the possible benefits of treatment. Chronic warfarin treatment should prompt periodic review of the risk/benefit ratio for each individual patient.

8. Self-management: patients on lifelong anticoagulation sometimes ask about the possibility of self-testing at home with their own fingerstick point-of-care device. This is a viable option for some, and many insurance companies now pay for the machine and supplies. Before a patient begins self-testing it is wise to confirm that the patient's fingerstick values are concordant with venipuncture values. Some patients demonstrate a persistent discordance and in that case are not candidates for self-testing.

9. Specialty referral: patients at higher risk for bleeding (e.g., INR goal of 3–3.5) or thrombosis (an example of the latter is a patient who has had an arterial clot) may do best with services offering specialty management, such as a hematology or dedicated anticoagulation clinic.

REFERENCES

Ansell, J. E. (2009). The value of an anticoagulation management service. In J. Ansell, L. Oertel, & A. Wittkowsky (Eds.), *Managing oral anticoagulation therapy* (3rd ed., pp. 1–8). St. Louis, MO: Wolters Kluwer Health.

Battistella, M., Mamdani, M. M., Juurlink, D. N., Rabeneck, L., & Laupacis, A. (2005). Risk of upper gastrointestinal hemorrhage in warfarin users treated with nonselective NSAIDs or COX-2 inhibitors. *Archives of Internal Medicine, 165,* 189–192.

Beyth, R. (2005). Assessing risk factors for bleeding. In J. Ansell, L. Oertel, & A. Wittkowsky (Eds.), *Managing oral anticoagulation therapy* (2nd ed., pp. 1–6). St. Louis, MO: Wolters Kluwer Health.

Carrier, M., Gréoire, L. G., & Wells, P. S. (2009). Factors that influence warfarin effect. In J. Ansell, L. Oertel, & A. Wittowsky (Eds.), *Managing oral anticoagulation therapy* (3rd ed., pp. 183–191). St. Louis, MO: Wolters Kluwer Health.

Centers for Medicare and Medicaid Services. (2009). *Decision memo for prothrombin time (INR) monitor for home anticoagulation management.* Retrieved from www.cms.hhs.gov

Cheetham, C. T., Levy, G., Niu, F., & Bixler, F. (2009). Gastrointestinal safety of nonsteroidal antiinflammatory drugs and selective cyclooxygenase-2 inhibitors in patients on warfarin. *Annals of Pharmacotherapy, 43,* 1765–1773.

Douketis, J. D., Berger, P. B., Dunn, A. S., Jaffer, A. K., Spyropoulos, A. C., Becker, R. C., & Ansell, J. (2008). The perioperative management of antithrombotic therapy: American College of Chest Physicians evidence-based clinical practice guidelines (8th ed). *Chest Supplement, 133,* 299S–339S.

Evans-Molina, C., Henault, L. E., Regan, S., & Hylek, E. M. (2003). Nurse assessment of warfarin candidacy among geriatric patients with atrial fibrillation referred to an anticoagulation clinic. *Journal of Thrombosis and Thrombolysis, 16*(1 & 2), E310S.

Fang, M. C., Go, A. S., Chang, Y., Borowsky, L., Pomernacki, N. K., & Singer, D. E. (2008). Comparison of risk stratification schemes to predict thromboembolism in people with nonvalvular atrial fibrillation. *Journal of the American College of Cardiology, 51*, 810–815.

Gage, B. F., Waterman, A. D., Shannon, W., Boechler, M., Rich, M. W., & Radford, M. J. (2001). Validation of clinical classification schemes for predicting stroke: Results from the National Registry of Atrial Fibrillation. *Journal of the American Medical Association, 285*, 2864–2870.

Garcia, D. A., Witt, D. M., Hylek, E., Wittkowsky, A. K., Nutescu, E. A., Jacobson, A., . . . Ansell, J. (2008). Delivery of optimized anticoagulant therapy: Consensus statement from the Anticoagulation Forum. *Annals of Pharmacotherapy, 42*, 979–988.

Hirsch, J., Guyatt, G., Albers, G., Harrington, R., & Schünemann, H. J. (2008). Executive summary: American College of Chest Physicians evidence-based clinical practice guidelines (8th ed). *Chest Supplement, 133*, 71S–109S.

Holbrook, A. M., Pereira, J. A., Labiris, R., McDonald, H., Douketis, J. D., Crowther, M., & Wells, P. S. (2005). Systemic overview of warfarin and its drug and food interactions. *Archives of Internal Medicine, 165*, 1095–1106.

Nicoll, D., McPhee, S., Pignone, M., Lu, C. M. (2007). *Pocket guide to diagnostic tests*, 5e. Retrieved from http://www.accesspharmacy.com/pocketDiagnostic.aspx

Oertel, L. (2005). Managing maintenance therapy. In J. Ansell, L. Oertel, & A. Wittkosky (Eds.), *Managing oral anticoagulation therapy* (2nd ed., pp. 1–40). St. Louis, MO: Wolters Kluwer Health.

Self, T. H. (2000). *Warfarin and other oral anticoagulants*. Retrieved from http://www.medscape.com/viewarticle/410539

Witt, D. M., Delate, T., Clark, N. P., Martell, C., Tran, T., & Crowther, M. A. Warfarin Associated Research Projects and other EnDeavors (WARPED) Consortium (2009). Outcome and predictors of very stable INR control during chronic anticoagulation therapy. *Blood, 114*, 952–956.

Wittkowsky, A. K. (2009a). Initiation and maintenance dosing of warfarin and monitoring the INR. In J. Ansell, L. Oertel, & A. Wittkowsky (Eds.), *Managing oral anticoagulation therapy* (3rd ed., pp. 173–182). St. Louis, MO: Wolters Kluwer Health.

Wittkowsky, A. K. (2009b). Pharmacology of warfarin and related anticoagulants. In J. Ansell, L. Oertel, & A. Wittkowsky (Eds.), *Managing oral anticoagulation therapy* (3rd ed., pp. 149–160). St. Louis, MO: Wolters Kluwer Health.

Wolf, P. A., Abbott, R. D., & Kannel, W. B. (1991). Atrial fibrillation as an independent risk factor for stroke: The Framingham Study. *Stroke, 22*, 983–988.

Wong, W., Wilson, N. J., & Wittkowsky, A. K. (1999). Influence of warfarin regimen type on clinical and monitoring outcomes in stable patients on an anticoagulation management service. *Pharmacotherapy, 19*, 1385–1391.

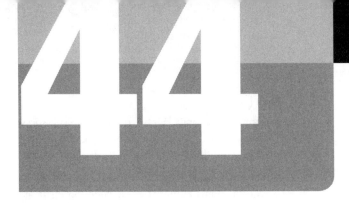

ANXIETY

Esker-D Ligon and Donald E. Tarver II

I. Introduction and general background

Anxiety disorders are commonly encountered, yet not adequately addressed, in the primary care setting. It is estimated that 8% of patients presenting for primary care services have a form of anxiety disorder, and presence of such disorders may increase the disability of existing chronic medical conditions (Kroenke, Spitzer, Williams, Monahan, & Lowe, 2007). Despite increased awareness of the prevalence of these disorders, less than 40% of patients with anxiety are diagnosed and treated in the primary care setting (Kroenke et al., 2007). Although some providers hold the sentiment that treatment of mental health disorders in the primary care setting is too time consuming, the reality exists that lack of treatment prevents one from being able to adequately address physical health issues.

Anxiety disorders contribute to functional impairments, disability, decreased health outcomes, comorbidity, and high use of health services. Given the impact of these disorders and the emerging trend toward the provision of integrated services, primary care providers should be equipped to properly screen and treat patients presenting with anxiety symptoms.

The etiology of anxiety disorders involves the interaction of environmental, biochemical, psychosocial, and genetic factors. Many types of anxiety disorders exist; however, this guideline focuses on the identification and treatment of the four most common: (1) generalized anxiety disorder, (2) social anxiety disorder, (3) panic disorder with or without agoraphobia, and (4) posttraumatic stress disorder (PTSD). Primarily found is generalized anxiety disorder; secondarily panic disorder; and thirdly social phobia (Kroenke et al., 2007). With improved screening by

primary care providers, PTSD may be found to have higher rates than previously known, especially for persons who are homeless or of low socioeconomic status who may be chronically exposed to violence and other forms of trauma (Bobo, Warner, & Warner, 2007; Meredith et al., 2009).

Diagnosis of anxiety disorders in the primary care setting is often influenced by a variety of factors. Many patients present with a variety of somatic complaints, or problems with sleep. Some patients use substances to self-medicate symptoms; substance use, although a separate problem, is often a symptom of an underlying disorder. It is imperative that providers adequately assess for such disorders. Cultural factors may also confound the diagnosis of anxiety disorders (Brenes et al., 2008). Each culture or demographic group has a set of norms for addressing mental health disorders, which may be influenced by stigma. Cultural identity involves not only ethnicity, acculturation and biculturalism, and language but also age, gender, socioeconomic status, sexual orientation, religious and spiritual beliefs, disabilities, political orientation, and health literacy, among other factors (American Psychiatric Association [APA], 2000).

Anxiety disorders across a spectrum of intensity and clinical relevance may present at anytime during the course of primary care examination. It is normal for patients to have situational nervousness on first meeting with a stranger, including a new primary care provider. This must not be overinterpreted as a sign of a significant or enduring psychiatric condition for which treatment is indicated. Similarly, the sometimes stressful nature or unfamiliarity of treatment center settings may cause a patient to present as anxious or agitated. If there are actual or perceived sociocultural differences between the provider and the patient there may be a greater chance of initial anxiety. The provider should acknowledge any known cause for concern, and then further engage the patient in understanding any extrinsic or intrinsic cause of observed anxiety. Sometimes a sincere apology for inconvenience that the patient may have encountered for any reason goes far to help situational anxiety subside.

As for the clinically significant anxiety disorder that may require treatment, signs and symptoms of such disorders may be gleaned through the means that follow. A provider should endeavor to honestly be aware of personal biases, prejudices, or lack of knowledge pertaining to particular personal issues or cultural standards of a given patient. Be sure that privacy is ensured and that the provider assumes a nonjudgmental tone toward anything that the patient may be encouraged to reveal. Despite inquiring in a warm, nonjudgmental manner, some topics are inherently difficult for some patients to discuss. They may feel embarrassed and guarded, and the interviewer may need to phrase questions in different ways and repeatedly. Throughout any clinical encounter the provider needs to be alert for signs of increased agitation, such as increased restlessness or pacing, clenched fists, verbal threats, or increasing verbal volume. When one detects such agitation, it is advisable to refrain from further discussion of distressing topics that are not germane to the patient's current presentation (Lange, Lange, & Cabaltica, 2000).

II. Database (may include but is not limited to)

A. Subjective

1. Symptomatology and relevant supporting data

   Patients may present with a variety of complaints related to anxiety disorders. Providers should inquire about the duration of symptoms, effect of symptoms on patient's functioning, and relationships between symptoms and contributory factors.

   a. Feelings of nervousness, anxiety, panic, excessive worry, or feeling generally stressed and overwhelmed

   b. Negative thoughts, ruminative or obsessive thinking; unrelenting pessimism, feelings of foreboding, and excessive guilt

   c. Adrenergic effects: irregular heartbeat, tachycardia, and palpitations; shortness of breath, diaphoresis, lightheadedness, paresthesias, and tremors

   d. Sleep disturbance: insomnia, hypersomnia, nightmares, and restless sleep

   e. Marked avoidance of specific situations and social withdrawal

   f. Restlessness, irritability, agitation, and excessive anger

   g. Appetite disturbance

   h. Difficulty with memory or concentration

   i. Persistent sense of fear, foreboding, apprehensiveness, and hypervigilance

   j. Suicidality: ideation, thoughts of being better off dead or that life is not worth living, and planned or attempted suicidal acts

   k. Somatic complaints: headaches, gastrointestinal complaints, back and neck pain, chest pain, and excessive concern with physical health

   l. Precipitating stressors, events, and losses (include community violence and vicarious trauma)

   m. Substance use: changes in types, frequency, and quantity of alcohol or drugs, including street drugs or prescribed medications

   n. Past health history: history of other mental health disorders and medical illnesses causing or exacerbating signs and symptoms of anxiety (e.g., hyperthyroidism)

B. Objective

1. Appearance and kinetic behavior: restlessness, writhing hands, biting nails, shaking legs or feet, rocking, sitting unusually still, appearing tense, and altered grooming and hygiene

2. Mental status examination: include mood, affect, speech, thought content, thought process, memory and concentration, and assessment of insight and judgment

3. Evidence-based screening tools: it is advisable that primary care practice settings adopt a screening tool for early identification of comorbid anxiety disorders.

   a. Refer to the following link for an example of an anxiety screening tool (an adaptation of the General Anxiety Disorder-7 screening tool [Marcus, 2008]): http://www.aafplearninglink.org/Resources/Upload/File/Anxiety%20Screen.pdf. The anxiety screening tool should be used to screen for the emergence of anxiety disorder symptoms. Screening should be repeated periodically to objectively measure changes after behavioral or psychotherapeutic intervention.

   b. DREAMS mnemonic is a useful interview tool to screen for PTSD (Lange et al., 2000).

      i. *Detachment* (alexithymia) or feeling emotionally numb

      ii. *Reexperiencing* the event via nightmares, flashbacks

      iii. *Event* with emotional effects, such as distress, feeling unsafe, fear

      iv. *Avoidance* of reminder places, activities, or people

      v. *Month* duration of symptoms or longer

      vi. *Sympathetic* hyperactivity (e.g., insomnia, irritability)

4. Diagnostic studies: include laboratory testing for metabolic syndromes, thyroid disorders, hormonal imbalances, or substance intoxication or occult use.

5. Collateral data: include information from members of a multidisciplinary treatment team when possible. With the permission of the patient a brief discussion with family members or friends may yield corroborating or missing information about manifestations of the patient's anxiety, or provide perspective on the causes, duration, intensity, and possible remedies of the patient's condition. Collateral contacts may also yield immensely helpful information regarding suicidal statements, failure to eat or function normally, or use of substances.

III. Assessment

A. *Determining a diagnosis*

Refer to the decision trees for anxiety in the *Diagnostic and Statistical Manual of Mental Disorders, 4th Edition, Text Revised* (DSM-IV-TR) published by the American Psychiatric Association (2000), or the *DSM-IV Primary Care Version* (American Psychiatric Association, 1995). The DSM-IV-TR classification and the specific diagnostic criteria are meant to serve as guidelines to be informed by clinical judgment in the categorization of the patient's conditions and are not meant to be applied in a rote fashion. The following are summarized criteria for the four anxiety disorders common to primary care settings. As a general rule, symptoms cannot be attributable to the effects of a substance, nor another medical or psychiatric condition.

1. Panic attack (not a codable disorder): a feature of many anxiety disorders characterized by the following:
   a. Palpitations or rapid heart rate
   b. Sweating
   c. Trembling or shaking
   d. Shortness of breath
   e. Feeling of choking
   f. Chest pain or discomfort
   g. Nausea or stomach upset
   h. Dizziness or lightheadedness
   i. Feelings of unreality or self-detachment
   j. Fear of dying
   k. Numbness or tingling of extremities
   l. Chills or hot flushes

2. Generalized anxiety disorder: excessive anxiety and worry about a variety of situations. Patient reports difficulty controlling the anxiety, and it interferes with their ability to function. Anxiety is associated with at least three of six symptoms as noted previously.

3. Social anxiety disorder: fear of being embarrassed or humiliated in social or performance situations when exposed to unfamiliar people or possible scrutiny by others. Exposure to feared situation provokes anxiety, and in some cases a panic attack. In most cases, the patient recognizes fear is excessive or unreasonable. The feared situation is avoided or experienced with intense anxiety; avoidance may interfere with normal functioning or cause marked distress.

4. Panic disorder with or without agoraphobia: recurrent unexpected panic attacks and at least one of the attacks has been followed by at least a month of one of the following symptoms: persistent worry about having another attack, worry about the consequences of the attack, or significant change in behavior related to attacks.

5. Agoraphobia (not a separate codable disorder)
   a. Fear about being in situations that would be difficult to escape or in which help would not be available if a panic attack was experienced
   b. Significant avoidance of such situations, enduring situations in distress, or requiring a companion to function

6. PTSD
   a. Condition may be acute (lasting < 3 months) or chronic (lasting > 3 months).
   b. Person has been exposed to an event in which they witnessed or experienced something that threatened life, serious injury, or damage to personal integrity; their response included intense fear, helplessness, or horror and lasts for longer than 1 month. The traumatic event is reexperienced in one of four ways:
      i. Intrusive distressing recollections of the event.
      ii. Distressing dreams or nightmares of the event.
      iii. Having a sense of reliving the event, including flashbacks and hallucinations.
      iv. Intense psychologic or physiologic response to triggers and cues reminiscent of the event
   c. Persistent avoidance of stimuli associated with the trauma including avoidance of triggers associated with trauma, inability to remember important details of trauma, anhedonia, isolation, restricted emotions, and sense of shortened lifespan.
   d. Increased state of arousal evidenced by sleep disturbance, irritability, poor concentration, hypervigilance, or becoming easily startled.

B. *Functional assessment and severity of illness*

1. When determining the severity of illness, consider the following factors: patient's current clinical status; psychosocial factors affecting the clinical situation; the patient's highest level of past functioning; and the patient's quality of life.

2. A functional assessment may be useful at assessing strengths and disease severity, and should focus on the patient's ability to perform essential activities of daily living. Information gathered may also facilitate the monitoring of treatment by assessing important beneficial and adverse effects of treatment.

IV. Plan

Anxiety disorders are a common and often disabling mental disorder. Treatment is indicated when symptoms of the disorder interfere with functioning or cause significant distress. Effective treatment for anxiety disorders should lead not only to reduction in frequency and intensity of symptoms, but should optimally yield full remission of symptoms and return to a premorbid level of functioning. A range of evidence-based psychosocial and pharmacologic interventions exist for treatment of anxiety disorders and should be instituted for all patients requiring treatment.

The treatment plan is ideally collaboration between the patient, the provider, and other members of the treatment team. It should include a variety of biologic and sociocultural interventions to create an integrated treatment plan. Optimally, interventions should encourage recovery from illness through community integration and empower patients to make choices that improve their quality of life. Considerations that guide the choice of an initial treatment modality include patient preference, the risks and benefits of treatment, past treatment history, presence of co-occurring conditions, cost, and treatment availability.

A. Medication selection

When making the decision to use pharmacologic treatments, providers must consider a patient's ability to remain compliant with treatment. Before selecting a specific medication one must balance the risks associated with the medication against the benefits of treatment and consider the following: potential side effects, potential drug interactions or contraindications, pharmacologic properties, co-occurring medical and psychiatric conditions, and the strength of the evidence for the particular medication in treatment of anxiety disorders.

Please refer to Table 52-3 on antidepressant medications in Chapter 52 for a list of treatment options. The use of benzodiazepines is often a controversial issue. Additionally, the treatment of PTSD is often complex and may require a specialty referral.

Benzodiazepines are appropriate as monotherapy only in the absence of a co-occurring mood disorder, and may be preferred (as monotherapy or in combination with antidepressants) for patients with very distressing or impairing symptoms in whom rapid symptom control is critical. The benefit of rapid response must be balanced against the potential for depressive and sedative side effects, and physiologic dependence that may lead to difficulty discontinuing the medication. Addition of benzodiazepines to a selective serotonin reuptake inhibitor (SSRI) or serotonin-norepinephrine reuptake inhibitor is a common augmentation strategy to target residual symptoms. They are also commonly used to treat severe presentations initially with another agent, followed by a gradual taper of the benzodiazepine.

When the goal is to prevent panic attacks rather than reduction of symptoms after an attack has occurred, a regular dosing schedule rather than an "as needed" schedule is preferred. In such instances, agents with a longer half-life, such as clonazepam, may provide better coverage than short half-life agents, such as lorazepam.

PTSD may manifest with a variety of physical and psychiatric symptoms, which must be addressed to successfully treat this disorder. Treatment often requires a multidisciplinary approach, including polypharmacy in some cases (Bobo et al., 2007). Severe cases should be referred to a psychiatric or mental health clinician. Refer to Table 44-1 for possible pharmacotherapeutic options to treat PTSD.

B. Medication management

1. Educate patients about the likely time course of treatment associated with a particular medication. Pharmacotherapy should generally be continued for 1 year or more after acute response to promote further symptom reduction and decrease risk of recurrence.

2. Patients with anxiety disorders can be sensitive to medication side effects; thus, low starting doses of medications are recommended with a gradual increase to a full therapeutic dose over several days and as tolerated by the patient. Underdosing of antidepressants is common in treatment of anxiety disorders, and is a frequent source of partial response or nonresponse.

3. Medication monitoring involves assessment of the change in symptoms, such as frequency and intensity of panic attacks, level of anticipatory anxiety, degree of agoraphobic avoidance, quality of sleep, persistence of somatic symptoms, and severity of interference and distress related to anxiety disorders.

   a. Patients typically require monitoring every 1–2 weeks when first starting a new medication, then every 2–4 weeks until the dose is stabilized.

   b. Less frequent monitoring is required after stabilization and reduction of symptoms.

4. Discontinuation of medication should be performed in a gradual and collaborative manner. This allows for continual assessment of the effects of the taper, the patient's response to any changes that emerge and, if required, treatment may be reinitiated at a previously effective dose. However, medications can be discontinued much more quickly in urgent conditions, such as pregnancy. Before advising a taper of effective pharmacotherapy, one should consider the duration of symptom remission, the presence

TABLE 44-1 Pharmacotherapeutic Options for Treating PTSD

Medication	Starting Dose (mg)	Effective Dose (mg)	Maximum Dose/Day
First line			
Fluoxetine (Prozac)	20 mg/day	20–40 mg/day	200 mg/day
Paroxetine (Paxil)	20 mg/day	20–50 mg/day	50 mg/day
Sertraline (Zoloft)	50 mg/day	50–200 mg/day	80 mg/day
Citalopram (Celexa)	20 mg/day	20–40 mg/day	60 mg/day
Escitalopram (Lexapro)	10 mg/day	10–20 mg/day	20 mg/day
Fluvoxamine (Luvox)	50 mg/day	50–300 mg/day	300 mg/day
Non-SSRI antidepressants			
Venlafaxine (Effexor)	37.5–75 mg b.i.d.	50–250 mg b.i.d.	300 mg/day
Mirtazapine (Remeron)	15 mg q.h.s.	15–45 mg q.h.s.	45 mg/day
Trazodone (Desyrel)	25–50 mg q.h.s.	25–150 mg q.h.s.	175 mg/day
Amitriptyline (Elavil, Amitid, Amitril) – TCA	25–100 mg q.h.s.	50–300 mg/day	300 mg/day
Clomipramine (Anafranil) – TCA	25 mg q.h.s.	25–250 mg q.h.s.	250 mg/day
Desipramine (Norpramine) – TCA	25 mg/day	100–300 mg/day	300 mg/day
Doxepin (Adapin, Sinequen) – TCA	25 mg q.h.s.	75–300 mg q.h.s.	300 mg/day
Imipramine (Tofranil, Presamine, Janimine) – TCA	25 mg q.h.s.	50–300 mg q.h.s.	300 mg/day
Nortriptyline (Pamelor, Avetyl) – TCA	25 mg q.h.s.	50–150 mg q.h.s.	150 mg/day
Phenelzine (Nardil) – MAOI	15 mg t.i.d.	15–30 mg t.i.d.	90 mg/day
Augmenting agents			
Antiadrenergic agents			
Prazosin	1 mg b.i.d.	5–20 mg/day	40 mg/day
Clonidine	0.1 mg b.i.d.	0.2–1.2 mg/day	2.4 mg/day
Guanfacine	1 mg q.h.s.	1–2 mg/day	3 mg/day
Propranolol (Inderal®)	20–40 mg b.i.d.	160–480 mg/day	640 mg/day
Mood stabilizers/anticonvulsants			
Valproate (Depakote)	300–600 mg b.i.d.	Blood levels of 50–100 mcg/mL.	Blood levels of greater than 100 mcg/mL.
Carbamazepine (Tegretol)	200 mg/day	Blood levels of 4–12 mcg/mL.	Blood levels of greater than 12 mcg/mL
Lamotrigine (Lamictal)	25–50 mg/day	50–250 mg b.i.d.	500 mg/day
Topiramate (Topamax)	25–50 mg/day	100–400 mg/day	400 mg/day
Gabapentin (Neurontin)	300 mg q.h.s.	300–600 mg t.i.d.	3600 mg/day
Lithium	300–600 mg b.i.d.	300–600 mg t.i.d.	Blood levels of greater than 1.2 mEq/L
Atypical antipsychotics			
Risperidone (Risperdal)	1 mg/day	1–3 mg b.i.d.	6 mg/day
Olanzapine (Zyprexa)	25–5 mg/day	5–20 mg/day	20 mg/day
Quetiapine (Seroquel)	25 mg/day	150–750 mg/day divided b.i.d.–t.i.d.	800 mg/day
Miscellaneous agents			
Zolpidem (Ambien)	5 mg q.h.s.	5–10 mg q.h.s.	10 mg/day
Zaleplon (Sonata)	5 mg q.h.s.	5–10 mg q.h.s.	20 mg/day
Diphenhydramine (Benadryl)	25 mg q.h.s.	25–50 mg q.h.s.	50 mg/day
Buspirone (BuSpar)	7.5 mg b.i.d.	30 mg/day	60 mg/day

Source: Bobo, W., Warner, C., & Warner, C. (2007). The management of post traumatic stress disorder (PTSD) in the primary care setting. *Southern Medical Journal, 100*(8), 797–801. Reprinted with permission.

of current or impending psychosocial stressors in the patient's life, and the extent to which the patient is motivated to discontinue the medication. This discussion should also include the possible outcomes of taper, including discontinuation symptoms and recurrence of panic symptoms.

C. Psychosocial interventions

Psychosocial treatment is recommended for pregnant women and other patients who prefer nonpharmacologic treatment and can invest the time and effort required to attend weekly sessions. Psychosocial treatments for anxiety disorders should be conducted by professionals with an appropriate level of training and experience in the relevant approach.

1. Cognitive-behavioral therapy (CBT): CBT is a time-limited treatment, generally 10–15 weekly sessions, which yields durable effects. It can be successfully administered individually or in a group format. CBT and other psychosocial treatments are not readily available in some geographic areas. Self-directed forms of CBT may be useful for patients who do not have ready access to a trained CBT therapist. CBT for anxiety disorders generally includes psychoeducation, self-monitoring, countering anxious beliefs, exposure to fear cues, modification of anxiety-maintaining behaviors, and relapse prevention.

2. Combined treatment should be considered for patients who have failed to respond to monotherapy, and may also be used under certain clinical circumstances (e.g., using pharmacotherapy for temporary control of severe symptoms that are impeding the patient's ability to engage in psychosocial treatment). Such treatment may also enhance long-term outcomes by reducing the likelihood of relapse when pharmacologic treatment is stopped.

3. Other group therapies: patient support groups are not recommended as monotherapy, although they may be useful adjuncts to other effective treatments for some patients.

4. Couples or family therapy may be helpful in addressing co-occurring relationship dysfunction. When initiating treatments for anxiety disorders, educate significant others about the nature of the disorder, enlisting their assistance to improve treatment adherence.

5. Complementary and alternative medicine methods, such as Tai Chi and meditation, and regular exercise

regimens have been proven to be helpful at addressing anxiety in some cases (van der Watt, Laugharne, & Janca, 2008).

D. Referral to specialty care

As a primary care provider, it is important to have the ability to differentiate cases that can be managed in one's own setting from more severe cases that require consultation or referral to dedicated psychiatric care. If response to an adequate trial of a first-line treatment (e.g., CBT, SSRI, or serotonin-norepinephrine reuptake inhibitor) is unsatisfactory, it is appropriate for the provider and the patient to consider a change to another treatment. Decisions about whether and how to make changes depends on the level of response or lack thereof to the initial treatment, the feasibility of other treatment options, and the severity of remaining symptoms and impairment. After first- and second-line treatments and augmentation strategies have been exhausted, either because of lack of efficacy or patient intolerance, providers are encouraged to consult with experienced colleagues or refer the patient to dedicated psychiatric services.

V. Special populations

A. Dually diagnosed patients

There is a high prevalence of self-medication with alcohol and other substances by persons with anxiety disorders (Arch, Craske, Stein, Sherbourne, & Roy-Byrne, 2006). It is often advantageous for patients to receive integrated treatment of both conditions (Mueser, Noordsy, Drake, & Fox, 2003). Patients often decrease their use of substances once the underlying anxiety is effectively addressed (Denning, 2000). Providers should exercise caution when prescribing medications because of potential interactions with substances of abuse. Extreme caution should be used when using benzodiazepines to treat patients using alcohol or opiates. Patients should be educated about the additive effects of the previously mentioned substances.

B. Pregnant women

For women with anxiety disorders who are pregnant, nursing, or planning to become pregnant, psychosocial interventions should be implemented. Pharmacotherapy may be indicated but requires discussion of the potential benefits and risks with the patient and, when possible, her obstetrician. Such discussions should also consider the potential risks to the patient and the child of untreated psychiatric illness, including anxiety disorders and any co-occurring psychiatric conditions.

C. Older adults

There are important safety considerations for SSRIs, tricyclic antidepressants, and benzodiazepines, which include increased risk of falls and osteoporotic fractures in patients age 50 and older. Caution and careful monitoring are indicated when prescribing medications to elderly patients, because they may produce sedation, fatigue, ataxia, slurred speech, memory impairment, and weakness.

D. Children and adolescents

Children and adolescents may present with different symptoms than adults. Please refer to the DSM-IV-TR for further information. There is also a higher risk of suicidality as a potential adverse effect of SSRIs and other antidepressants in this population.

VI. Self-management resources and tools

A. Patient and client educational handouts and resources

1. Educational handouts for patients and families can be found at www.nimh.nih.gov. Many handouts are available in multiple languages, and are updated periodically.

2. The Anxiety and Phobia Workbook (Bourne, 2005).

3. National Alliance for the Mentally Ill (NAMI).

4. National Center for PTSD website (www.ncptsd.va.gov) has factsheets and resources for patients and providers.

5. Anxiety Disorders Association of America website (www.adaa.org) has resources for patients and providers.

REFERENCES

American Psychiatric Association (APA). (1995). *Diagnostic and statistical manual of mental health disorders* (4th ed.): *Primary care version.* Arlington, VA: APA.

American Psychiatric Association (APA). (2000). *Diagnostic and statistical manual of mental health disorders* (4th ed.), *text revision.* Washington, DC: APA.

Arch, J., Craske, M., Stein, M., Sherbourne, C., & Roy-Byrne, P. (2006). Correlates of alcohol use among anxious and depressed primary care patients. *General Hospital Psychiatry, 28,* 37–42.

Bobo, W., Warner, C., & Warner, C. (2007). The management of post traumatic stress disorder (PTSD) in the primary care setting. *Southern Medical Journal, 100*(8), 797–801.

Bourne, E. (2005). *The anxiety and phobia workbook* (4th ed.). Oakland, CA: New Harbinger.

Brenes, G., Knudson, M., McCall, W., Williamson, J., Miller, M., & Stanley, M. (2008). Age and racial differences in the presentation and treatment of generalized anxiety disorder in primary care. *Journal of Anxiety Disorders, 22,* 1128–1136.

Denning, P. (2000). *Practicing harm reduction psychotherapy: An alternative approach to addictions.* New York, NY: Guilford.

Kroenke, K., Spitzer, R., Williams, J., Monahan, P., & Lowe, B. (2007). Anxiety disorders in primary care: Prevalence, impairment, comorbidity, and detection. *Annals of Internal Medicine, 146*(5), 317–325.

Lange, J., Lange, C., & Cabaltica, R. (2000). Primary care treatment of post-traumatic stress disorder. *American Family Physician, 62*(5), 1035–1040, 1046.

Marcus, D. A. (2008). Chronic pain. *A primary care guide to practical management* (2nd ed.). Totowa, NJ: Humana Press.

Meredith, L., Eisenman, D., Green, B., Basurto-Davila, R., Cassells, A., & Tobin, J. (2009). System factors affect the recognition and management of posttraumatic stress disorder by primary care clinicians. *Medical Care, 47*(6), 686–694.

Mueser, T., Noordsy, D., Drake, R., & Fox, L. (2003). Integrated treatment for dual disorders: A guide to effective practice. New York, NY: Guilford.

van der Watt, G., Laugharne, J., & Janca, A. (2008). Complementary and alternative medicine in the treatment of anxiety and depression. *Current Opinion in Psychiatry, 21*(1), 37–42.

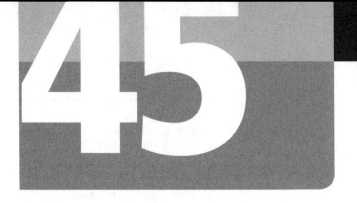

ASTHMA IN ADOLESCENTS AND ADULTS

Susan L. Janson

I. Introduction and general background

Asthma is an inflammatory disease of the airways characterized by airflow obstruction that is reversible (at least partially) either spontaneously or with treatment. Airway inflammation and bronchospasm causes recurring symptoms of wheezing, coughing, breathlessness, and the sensation of chest tightness that occurs particularly at night or early morning. The obstruction to airflow in the airways is the result of mucosal inflammation caused by inflammatory cell infiltration with neutrophils, eosinophils, and lymphocytes, in addition to mast cell activation and epithelial cell injury. Airway inflammation contributes to hyperresponsiveness of the airway and airway narrowing caused by bronchoconstriction of airway smooth muscle. In some patients, persistent changes in airway structure occur resulting in airway remodeling.

A. Pathogenesis

The etiology of asthma is unknown but the strongest predictor for developing asthma is atopy, the genetic predisposition for development of an immunoglobulin (Ig) E–mediated response to common aeroallergens. Viral respiratory infections may also contribute and are the most important cause of asthma exacerbations. There is considerable variability in the pattern of airway inflammation indicating phenotypic differences of expression that may influence response to treatment. Onset of asthma for most people begins early in life

with recurrent wheezing, atopic disease, and a history of parental asthma.

Understanding of the pathogenesis of asthma is evolving as genetic and phenotypic variations are identified. Research has focused on an imbalance of Th1 and Th2 cytokines in allergic diseases including asthma that result in either overexpression of Th2 or underexpression of Th1 cells. Th2 cells mediate inflammation, whereas Th1 cells respond to infection. The "hygiene hypothesis" illustrates how this imbalance may occur, as in westernized civilizations, where exposure to infections is limited resulting in persistence of Th2 dominance in genetically susceptible children (Busse & Lemanske, 2001).

B. Prevalence

Asthma affects 21 million people in the United States and more than 300 million worldwide. Early in life the prevalence of asthma is higher in boys, but at puberty the gender ratio shifts toward girls and asthma is seen predominantly in women after puberty. Asthma exacerbations are responsible for more than $37 billion in direct costs annually in the United States (Kamble & Bharmal, 2009).

C. Factors that precipitate or aggravate asthma

1. Allergens: Exposure to aerosolized allergens (aeroallergens) for people who are sensitized to them is an important precipitant of asthma. Outdoor allergens are primarily pollens from trees and plants that occur in seasonal waves. Patients with these sensitivities have more frequent exacerbations during the time of heavy pollination if they are sensitized. Even more important are the perennial indoor allergens (molds, house dust mites, cockroaches, and animal dander) because of the length of time people stay indoors.

2. Irritants: The most important airway irritant exposure is environmental tobacco smoke. Other irritants include bleach, perfume, strong odors (paint fumes, cooking gas, and wood smoke) and air pollution, with increased exposure in closed, poorly ventilated areas.

3. Medication and drugs: Some medications are known to trigger airway constriction through neural or metabolic pathways. These include β-blockers, aspirin, nonsteroidal anti-inflammatory drugs, and sulfites.

4. Comorbid conditions that exacerbate asthma: Among the chronic conditions that make asthma

harder to control are gastroesophageal reflux (GERD), rhinitis and sinusitis, obesity, and chronic stress and depression. Evidence is stronger for the first two but efforts should be made to treat and control all of these conditions when present.

II. Database (may include but is not limited to)

A. Subjective

1. Past health history
   a. Age of onset of disease
   b. History of emergency department visits, hospitalizations, need for intubation, and mechanical ventilation
   c. Need for systemic or oral corticosteroids and frequency of use
   d. Symptoms: recurrent wheezing, shortness of breath, chest tightness, cough that is worse at night, and sputum production
   e. Pattern of symptoms
      i. Perennial, seasonal, or both
      ii. Continual, episodic, or both
      iii. Onset, duration, and frequency (number of days or nights per week or month)
      iv. Diurnal variations, especially nocturnal and on awakening in early morning
   f. Precipitating or aggravating factors
      i. Viral respiratory infections
      ii. Environmental allergens, indoor (e.g., mold, house dust mite, cockroach, and animal dander or secretions) and outdoor (e.g., pollen)
      iii. Home characteristics (age, location, heating and cooling system, wood-burning stove, humidifier, carpeting over concrete, molds or mildew, floor coverings, and stuffed or upholstered furniture)
      iv. Smoking (patient or others in home or work)
      v. Exercise
      vi. Occupational chemicals or allergens
      vii. Environmental change (relocation or remodeling)
      viii. Irritants (second-hand tobacco smoke, strong odors, air pollutants, dusts, particulates, vapors, gases, and aerosols)
      ix. Emotions or stress
      x. Medications (e.g., aspirin, other nonsteroidal anti-inflammatory drugs, β-blockers)
      xi. Food, food additives, and preservatives (e.g., sulfites)
      xii. Changes in weather and exposure to cold air
      xiii. Endocrine factors (e.g., menses, pregnancy, and thyroid disease)
      xiv. Comorbid conditions (e.g., sinusitis, allergic rhinitis, GERD, and allergic responses to specific foods or alcohol).
   g. History of exacerbations
      i. Prodromal signs and symptoms
      ii. Rapidity of onset and duration and frequency
      iii. Severity (need for urgent care, hospitalization, or intensive care unit care)
      iv. Impact (number of days missed from work or school, limitation of activities, nocturnal awakening, and economic impact)

2. Family history: Allergies, atopy, or asthma

3. Occupational and environmental history: Work-related exposures, such as vapors, gas, dusts, fumes, isocyanates, or cedar

4. Personal and social history: Tobacco smoking and second-hand tobacco exposure

5. Review of systems
   a. Constitutional signs and symptoms: fatigue caused by sleep disruption.
   b. Ear, nose, and throat: congestion, sneezing, runny nose, sinus headache, and postnasal drip.
   c. Respiratory: recurrent wheezing, cough, breathlessness, chest tightness, and increased mucus production.
   d. Cardiac: palpitations during times of severe breathlessness.
   e. Gastrointestinal: heartburn or dyspepsia.
   f. Psychiatric: anxiety or depression.

B. Objective

1. Physical findings
   a. General appearance: anxious; labored breathing; hyperexpansion of the chest (especially in children); use of accessory muscles; hunched shoulders; and deformed chest
   b. Ear, nose, and throat: pale and boggy nasal mucosa; thin and watery nasal secretions; red or streaked posterior pharynx; and thrush (associated with inhaled corticosteroid use [ICS])
   c. Lungs: diffuse or scattered expiratory wheezes, prolonged expiration, wheezing with forced exhalation, and decrease in air entry and movement
   d. Cardiac: tachycardia (if hypoxic)
   e. Skin: atopic dermatitis or eczema; pallor or cyanosis (if hypoxic)

2. Supporting data from relevant diagnostic tests and assessment of severity and control (Tables 45-1 and 45-2)

TABLE 45-1 Classifying Asthma Severity and Initiating Treatment in Adolescents ≥ 12 Years of Age and Adults

Components of Severity		Intermittent	Persistent		
			Mild	Moderate	Severe
Impairment Normal FEV₁/FVC: 8–19 yr 85% 20–39 yr 80% 40–59 yr 75% 60–80 yr 70%	Symptoms	≤ 2 d/wk	≥ 2 d/wk but not daily	Daily	Throughout the day
	Nighttime awakenings	≤ 2 times per month	3–4 times per month	> 1 per week but not nightly	Often 7 times per week
	Short-acting β₂-agonist use for symptom control (not prevention of EIB)	≤ 2 d/wk	> 2 d/wk but not daily, and not more than one time on any day	Daily	Several times per day
	Interference with normal activity	None	Minor limitation	Some limitation	Extremely limited
	Lung function	Normal FEV₁ between exacerbations FEV₁ > 80% predicted FEV₁/FVC normal	FEV₁ > 80% predicted FEV₁/FVC normal	FEV₁ > 60% but < 80% predicted FEV₁/FVC reduced 5%	FEV₁ < 60% predicted FEV₁/FVC reduced > 5%
Risk	Exacerbations requiring oral systemic corticosteroids	0–1/yr (see note)	≥ 2/yr (see note) →		
		← Consider severity and interval since last exacerbation. → Frequency and severity may fluctuate over time for patients in any severity category. Relative annual risk of exacerbation may be related to FEV₁.			
Recommended step for initiating treatment		Step 1	Step 2	Step 3	Step 4 or 5
				and consider short course of oral systemic corticosteroids	
		In 2–6 weeks, evaluate level of asthma control that is achieved and adjust therapy accordingly.			

Abbreviations: EIB, exercise-induced bronchospasm; FEV₁, forced expiratory volume in 1 second; FVC, forced vital capacity; ICU, intensive care unit.

The stepwise approach is meant to assist, not replace, the clinical decision making required to meet individual patient needs.

Level of severity is determined by assessment of both impairment and risk. Assess impairment domain by patient's and caregiver's recall of previous 2–4 weeks and spirometry. Assign severity to the most severe category in which any feature occurs.

At present, there are inadequate data to correspond frequencies of exacerbations with different levels of asthma severity. In general, more frequent and intense exacerbations (e.g., requiring urgent, unscheduled care, hospitalization, or ICU admission) indicate greater underlying disease severity. For treatment purposes, patients who had ≥ 2 exacerbations requiring oral systemic corticosteroids in the past year may be considered the same as patients who have persistent asthma, even in the absence of impairment levels consistent with persistent asthma.

Source: National Heart, Lung and Blood Institute, National Asthma Education and Prevention Program, & National Institutes of Health. (2007). *Expert panel report: Guidelines for the diagnosis and management of asthma* (Publication No. 97-4051). Bethesda, MD: Author.

III. Assessment

A. Differential diagnosis

1. Asthma

2. Emphysema and chronic bronchitis

3. Upper airway disease: allergic rhinitis and sinusitis

4. Vocal cord dysfunction

5. Obstructions of large airways (foreign body, tumor, and lymph nodes)

6. Obstructions of small airways (cystic fibrosis, bronchiolitis, and bronchopulmonary dysplasia)

7. Recurrent cough not caused by asthma

8. Aspiration

9. Heart disease (congestive heart failure)

TABLE 45-2 Assessing Asthma Control and Adjusting Therapy in Adolescents ≥ 12 Years of Age and Adults

		Classifying of Asthma Control		
		Well Controlled	**Not Well Controlled**	**Very Poorly Controlled**
Impairment	Symptoms	≤ 2 d/wk	> 2 d/wk	Throughout the day
	Nighttime awakenings	≤ 2 times per month	1–3 times per week	≥ 4 times per week
	Interference with normal activity	None	Some limitation	Extremely limited
	Short-acting β₂-agonist use for symptom control (not prevention of EIB)	≤ 2 d/wk	> 2 d/wk	Several times per day
	FEV_1 or peak flow	> 80% predicted/ personal best	60–80% predicted/ personal best	< 60% predicted/ personal best
	Validated questionnaire ATAQ	0	1–2	3–4
	ACQ	≤ 0.75*	≥ 1.5	N/A
	ACT	≥ 20	16–19	≤ 15
Risk	Exacerbations requiring oral systemic corticosteroids	0–1/yr	≥ 2/yr (see note) →	
		Consider severity and interval since last exacerbation		
	Progressive loss of lung function	Evaluation requires long-term follow-up care		
	Treatment-related adverse effects	Medication side effects can vary in intensity from none to very troublesome and worrisome. The level of intensity does not correlate to specific levels of control but should be considered in the overall assessment of risk.		
Recommended action for treatment		Maintain current step. Regular follow-ups every 1–6 months to maintain control. Consider step down if well controlled for at least 3 months.	Step up 1 step and Reevaluate in 2–6 weeks. For side effects, consider alternative treatment options.	Consider short course of oral systemic corticosteroids. Step up 1–2 steps, and Reevaluate in 2 weeks. For side effects, consider alternative treatment options.

Abbreviations: EIB, exercise-induced bronchospasm; ICU, intensive care unit.

*ACQ values of 0.76–1.4 are indeterminate regarding well-controlled asthma.

The stepwise approach is meant to assist, not replace, the clinical decision making required to meet individual patient needs.

The level of control is based on the most severe impairment of risk category. Assess impairment domain by patient's recall of previous 2–4 weeks and by spirometry or peak flow measures. Symptom assessment for longer periods should reflect a global assessment, such as inquiring whether the patient's asthma is better or worse since the last visit.

At present, there are inadequate data to correspond frequencies of exacerbations with different levels of asthma control. In general, more frequent and intense exacerbations (e.g., requiring urgent unscheduled care, hospitalization, or ICU admission) indicate poorer disease control. For treatment purposes, patients who had ≥ 2 exacerbations requiring oral systemic corticosteroids in the past year may be considered the same as patients who have not-well-controlled asthma, even in the absence of impairment levels consistent with not-well-controlled asthma.

Validated questionnaires for the impairment domain (the questionnaires do not assess lung function or the risk domain)

ATAQ = Asthma Therapy Assessment Questionnaire© (see sample in "Component 1: Measures of Asthma Assessment and Monitoring.")

ACQ = Asthma Control Questionnaire© (user package may be obtained at www.qoltech.co.uk or juniper@qoltech.co.uk)

ACT = Asthma Control Test™ (see sample in "Component 1: Measure of Asthma Assessment and Monitoring.")

Minimal important difference: 1.0 for the ATAQ; 0.5 for the ACQ; not determined for the ACT.

Before step up in therapy:

Review adherence to medication, inhaler technique, environmental control, and comorbid conditions.

If an alternative treatment option was used in a step, discontinue and use preferred treatment for that step.

Source: National Heart, Lung and Blood Institute, National Asthma Education and Prevention Program, & National Institutes of Health. (2007). *Expert panel report: Guidelines for the diagnosis and management of asthma* (Publication No. 97-4051). Bethesda, MD: author.

B. *Severity, control, and response to treatment (Tables 45-1 and 45-2)*

1. Classify severity: Intermittent, mild persistent, moderate persistent, or severe persistent. Severity of asthma is the intrinsic intensity of the disease and is most easily determined when the patient is not on long-term treatment. Severity is measured in two domains: impairment and risk. Impairment is assessed by history of activity limitation and by spirometry to assess airway caliber. Risk is assessed by the likelihood of frequent exacerbations, also assessed by history and by forced expiratory volume in 1 second (FEV_1). Predictors of asthma exacerbation include severe airflow obstruction; two or more emergency department visits or hospitalizations in the last year; intubation or intensive care unit admission for asthma in the last 5 years; patient report of feeling in danger from asthma; depression; and certain demographic characteristics (female, nonwhite, not using corticosteroid medication, and current smoking).

2. Classify asthma control: Asthma can be classified as well controlled, not well controlled, or very poorly controlled. Asthma control is classified when the patient is currently on a controller medication, considering domains of impairment and risk. Control is the degree to which the symptoms, impairments, and risk are minimized and the goals of therapy are met. Control is assessed by symptoms, night-time awakenings, need for a short-acting β-agonist for relief of symptoms, and ability to engage in usual activities. Several standardized questionnaires have been developed for the assessment of asthma control as reported by patients.

3. Assess responsiveness to therapy: Responsiveness is the ease with which asthma control is achieved by therapy.

C. *Significance and motivation*

Assess the significance of asthma to the patient and family, including how much asthma interferes with quality of life, work, and play. Determine willingness and ability to follow the treatment plan and properly inhale medications.

IV. Goals of clinical management to control asthma

A. *Reduce impairment*

1. Prevent chronic symptoms and night-time awakenings

2. Require only infrequent use of short-acting β-agonist (infrequent use is ≤ 2 d/wk) for quick relief of symptoms

3. Maintain normal (or near normal) lung function

4. Maintain normal activity levels: exercise and attendance at work and school

B. *Reduce risk*

1. Prevent recurrent exacerbations and minimize need for urgent care

2. Prevent progressive loss of lung function; for youth, prevent reduced lung growth

3. Provide optimal pharmacotherapy with minimal or no adverse effects

V. Plan

A. *Diagnostic tests*

1. Pulmonary function testing (spirometry) (Figure 45-1): Spirometry is needed to diagnose asthma because medical history and physical examination are not reliable ways to exclude other causes of respiratory impairment. The key measures are FEV_1, forced vital capacity (FVC), and FEV_1/FVC ratio. For those who cannot sustain expiration for the length of time necessary to measure FVC, FEV in

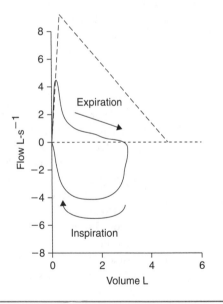

FIGURE 45-1 Flow-Volume Loop Generated by Spirometry

R. Pellegrino, G. Viegi, V. Brusasco, R. O. Crapo, F. Burgos, R. Casaburi, A. Coates, C. P. M. van der Grinten, P. Gustafsson, J. Hankinson, R. Jensen, D. C. Johnson, N. MacIntyre, R. McKay, M. R. Miller, D. Navajas, O. F. Pedersen, and J. Wanger. Interpretative strategies for lung function tests, *European Respiratory Journal*, Nov 2005; 26:948–968. Reprinted with permission from the European Respiratory Society.

6 seconds is used as a substitute for FVC. Significant reversibility is demonstrated by an increase in FEV_1 or FVC of 200 ml and greater than or equal to 12% change from baseline after inhaling two puffs of albuterol at 90 mcg/puff (Pellegrino et al., 2005). Some patients with the symptoms of asthma do not demonstrate reversibility until they have a 2-week trial of oral corticosteroids.

2. Chest radiograph to exclude other causes of airway obstruction

3. Allergy testing by skin tests or in vitro tests

4. Exhaled nitrous oxide testing to detect inflammation

5. Additional testing
   a. Flow–volume loops
   b. Bronchoprovocation challenge testing with methacholine or cold air.

B. Management

1. Medications: A stepwise approach to pharmacologic therapy is recommended (Table 45-3)

   a. Quick relief "rescue" medications are short-acting β_2-agonists. These include albuterol-HFA, levalbuterol-HFA, and pirbuterol, which are prescribed for any severity of asthma. Patients should be instructed to inhale two puffs every 4–6 hours as needed for symptoms of asthma. They also may be used 20–30 minutes before exercise to prevent exercise-induced bronchospasm.

   b. Long-acting "controller" medications
      i. ICS are the most effective to reduce airway inflammation and control persistent asthma. It is essential to step-down therapy to identify the minimum medication necessary to maintain control.
      ii. Long-acting β_2-agonists (LABA) added if asthma is not controlled with ICS alone. Do not use LABA as monotherapy. Consider discontinuing LABA when control is achieved.
      iii. Consider combined ICS and LABA in one inhaler if asthma is not controlled by ICS alone.
      iv. When initiating therapy monitor at 2- to 4-week intervals to ensure that asthma control is achieved.
      v. Consider adding a leukotriene receptor antagonist (e.g., montelukast (sold as Singulair®) if allergies are a strong component of the asthma.

   c. Anti-IgE therapy: Omalizumab (Xolair®)
      i. Consider for adolescents older than 12 years and adults with severe uncontrolled asthma, skin test positive to perennial allergens, and elevated IgE. Skin testing is given subcutaneously under direct observation.
      ii. Be alert to the possibility of anaphylaxis if giving this medication.

2. Environmental control

   a. Reduce exposure to allergens to which the patient is sensitized and exposed (dust mites, animal dander, mold, cockroach, and pollens).

   b. Effective allergen avoidance requires a multifaceted, comprehensive approach (e.g., carpets harbor dust mites so remove or vacuum often; use allergen-proof mattress and pillow covers to protect against dust mites; wash all bed linens in hot water at least every 2 weeks; eliminate any cockroach infestation and do not leave food or garbage out or exposed; remove mold and mildew; and repair leaks).

   c. Avoid exposure to environmental tobacco smoke and other respiratory irritants (wood smoke, perfume, strong odors and fumes, bleach, and cleaning products).

   d. Avoid exertion outside when air pollution levels are high.

   e. Avoid use of nonselective β-blockers.

   f. Avoid sulfite-containing food and foods to which the patient is sensitive.

3. Treat and control comorbid diseases that aggravate asthma

   a. Allergic rhinitis or sinusitis (consider leukotriene receptor antagonist, antihistamine, nasal corticosteroid spray, and nasal saline washes).

   b. GERD: consider use of a proton pump inhibitor; elevate head of bed at night; no food at bedtime; and decrease use of alcohol and caffeine. See Chapter 56 for further suggestions.

   c. Other conditions that make asthma harder to control include obesity, depression, family barriers to self-management, and vocal cord dysfunction.

4. Consider specialty consultation for uncontrolled asthma that has not responded to maximal therapy, when allergy immunotherapy or omalizumab is being considered, or when exacerbations require hospitalizations.

5. Follow-up should be at frequent intervals until control is achieved and then at 3- to 6-month intervals to maintain control. More frequent follow-up is determined by individual characteristics, past history, and psychosocial factors that increase risk.

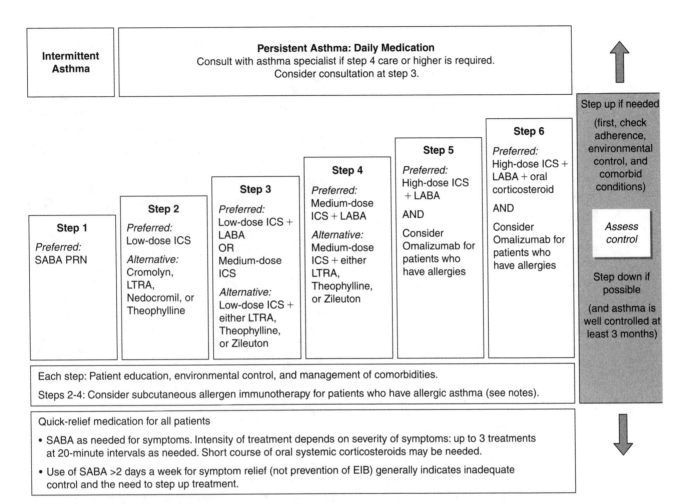

TABLE 45-3 Stepwise Approach for Managing Asthma in Adolescents ≥12 Years of Age and Adults

Key: **Alphabetical order is used when more than one treatment option is listed within either preferred or alternative therapy.** EIB, exercise-induced bronchospasm; ICS, inhaled corticosteroid; LABA, long-acting inhaled beta$_2$-agonist, LTRA, leukotriene receptor antagonist; SABA, inhaled short-acting beta$_2$-agonist.

Notes:

The stepwise approach is meant to assist, not replace, the clinical decision making required to meet individual patient needs.

If alternative treatment is used and response is inadequate, discontinue it and use the preferred treatment before stepping up.

Zileuton is a less desirable alternative due to limited studies as adjunctive therapy and the need to monitor liver function. Theophylline requires monitoring of serum concentration levels.

In step 6, before oral corticosteroids are introduced, a trial of high-dose ICS + LABA + either LTRA, theophylline, or zileuton may be considered, although this approach has not been studied in clinical trials.

Step 1, 2, and 3 preferred therapies are based on Evidence A; step 3 alternative therapy is based on Evidence A for LTRA, Evidence B for theophylline, and Evidence D for zileuton. Step 4 preferred therapy is based on Evidence B, and alternative therapy is based on Evidence B for LTRA and theophylline and Evidence D zileuton. Step 5 preferred therapy is based on Evidence B. Step 6 preferred therapy is based on (EPR—2 1997) and Evidence B for omalizumab.

Immunotherapy for steps 2–4 is based on Evidence B for house-dust mites, animal danders, and pollens; evidence is weak or lacking for molds and cockroaches. Evidence is strongest for immunotherapy with single allergens. The role of allergy in asthma is greater in children than in adults.

Clinicians who administer immunotherapy or omalizumab should be prepared and equipped to identify and treat anaphylaxis that may occur.

Source: National Heart, Lung and Blood Institute, National Asthma Education and Prevention Program, & National Institutes of Health. (2007). *Expert panel report: Guidelines for the diagnosis and management of asthma* (Publication No. 97-4051). Bethesda, MD: Author.

C. Patient education and training in self-management of asthma

1. Elicit the patient's concerns and questions regarding asthma.

2. Describe airway inflammation and bronchospasm.

3. Teach the patient how to recognize and avoid individual triggers: explain the cumulative effect of precipitating factors.

4. Instruct the patient not to smoke and to avoid second-hand smoke.

5. Review all of the patient's medications, including the purpose, actions, dosage, side effects, and interactions. Explain how each medication works to relieve, control, or prevent asthma signs and symptoms.

6. Demonstrate the proper use of the metered-dose inhaler or dry powder inhaler and also spacer device for metered-dose inhaler containing corticosteroid medication (Boxes 45-1 through 45-3). Have the patient demonstrate proper use periodically or at each follow-up visit.

7. For patients who meet the criteria for moderate-persistent or severe-persistent asthma, demonstrate the use and rationale of peak flow meters (for use at home or in the office) before the initiation of therapy. See the Patient Education Supplement: Peak Expiratory Flow Rate Monitoring (Box 45-4 Supplement). Recommend daily morning measurements on awakening before inhaling medications. Teach the patient how to measure and interpret

---

BOX 45-1 Instructions for Using a Metered-Dose Inhaler With or Without a Spacer

1. To begin, shake the inhaler five or six times.

2. Remove the mouthpiece cover. If using a spacer, place the spacer over the mouthpiece at the end of the inhaler.

3. Put your lips and teeth over the inhaler mouthpiece or the spacer mouthpiece and breathe in slowly. As you do so, squeeze the top of the canister once. Keep inhaling even after you finish the squeeze. Continue inhaling slowly and deeply.

4. After inhaling, remove the inhaler or spacer from your mouth and hold your breath for up to 10 seconds.

If you need another dose of medication, repeat the previous steps.

BOX 45-2 Patient Instructions for Using a Dry Powder Disk Inhaler

1. Hold the disk level in one hand. With the other hand, put your thumb in the appropriate notch and push it away from you as far as it goes. The mouthpiece will appear and snap into place.

2. Keep the disk horizontal. Again with your thumb, slide the lever away from you until it clicks. The disk is now ready to deliver medication.

3. Put your lips around the mouthpiece. Breathe in quickly and deeply through your mouth—not your nose.

4. After inhaling, remove the disk from your mouth and hold your breath for up to 10 seconds.

5. To close the disk, put your thumb in the notch and slide it back toward you as far as it goes. The disk will click shut, and the lever will automatically return to its original position. The disk is now ready for your next dose.

Ask your pharmacist for a demonstration when you pick up the medication from the pharmacy.

BOX 45-3 Instructions for Using a Dry Powder Tube Inhaler

1. To begin, twist the cover off and set it down.

2. Next, load the dose of medication. Twist the base grip to the right as far as it will go. Twist it back to the left. You will hear a click, which means it is ready to go.

3. You do not need to shake the inhaler.

4. Bring the inhaler to your lips in a horizontal position. Put your lips over the tube and take a fast and powerful deep breath. Continue inhaling quickly and deeply.

5. Hold your breath for up to 10 seconds.

6. If you need another dose of medication, repeat the previous steps. The tube inhaler is designed to deliver one dose at a time.

7. Do not blow into your inhaler after loading a dose because the medication will become saturated with condensation and difficult to dispense.

8. When you are finished, place the cover back on the inhaler and twist shut. Keep your inhaler dry and store it at room temperature.

the peak flow rate readings (Box 45-5). Provide written guidelines for what the patient should do when the readings fall below a specified level.

8. Have a written action plan directing the patient what to do during an exacerbation. Include when the patient should call his or her provider, increase or add medications, or go to the emergency department (Figure 45-2).

9. Encourage adequate hydration, proper nutrition, and adequate rest.

10. Encourage the patient to keep regular appointments for follow-up and evaluation, even if the symptoms of asthma are not present.

D. Asthma education resources

1. American Academy of Allergy, Asthma and Immunology: www.aaaai.org

2. American Lung Association: www.lungusa.org

3. Association of Asthma Educators: www.asthma educators.org

4. National Heart, Lung and Blood Institute Information Center: www.nhlbinih.gov

5. U.S. Environmental Protection Agency: www .airnow.gov

BOX 45-4 Supplement
Patient Education Supplement: Peak Expiratory Flow Rate Monitoring

What is a peak expiratory flow rate?

Peak expiratory flow rate is a measurement of the highest speed at which you can blow out air when you exhale as hard and as fast as you can. This measurement tells us how much impediment, or obstruction, there is in your airways. Flow rates decrease when asthma obstructs, or narrows, your airways. Flow rates are normal when there is no, or minimal, obstruction of your airways.

What are the steps to measuring a peak expiratory flow rate?

1. Place the indicator at the base of the numbered scale.
2. Stand up or sit up straight with head erect.
3. Take a deep breath.
4. Place the meter in your mouth and close your lips around the mouthpiece.
5. Blow out as hard and as fast as possible.
6. Write down the achieved measurement. This is where the indicator stops.
7. Repeat this process two more times.
8. Record the highest of the 3 measurements.

When and how often should you measure and record peak flow rates?

You and your provider will plan this during your visits.

Source: NHLBI National Asthma Education and Prevention Program: "Expert Panel Report II: Guidelines for the Diagnosis and Management of Asthma." National Institutes of Health Publication No. 97-4051, Bethesda, MD, 1977.

BOX 45-5 Instructions for Using a Peak Flow Meter

The peak flow meter helps you to monitor your asthma by measuring the maximum airflow you can blow out of your lungs.

Ask your clinician about where to set the color-coded indicators. They can help determine the status of your airflow.

1. To begin, hold the meter by the handgrip. Slide the measurement arrow to the bottom of the scale, next to the mouthpiece. (One device requires you to shake the arrow to the bottom of the device).

2. Raise the meter horizontally, inhale deeply from room air, then place your mouth over the mouthpiece and blow forcefully. Make sure your lips act as a seal over the mouthpiece so that no air escapes. Make sure your tongue is not in the mouthpiece.

3. The measurement arrow will slide up the scale. The number that it stops on is your peak flow reading.

4. Repeat the test two more times. Each time, remember to slide the measurement arrow back to its start position near the mouthpiece. Remember the highest reading of your three blows.

5. Record the highest reading, with the date and time. Your clinician will help determine a personalized scale to use with your meter, dependent on your age, height, and gender.

Asthma Action Plan

PROVIDER INSTRUCTIONS

At initial presentation, determine the level of asthma severity
- Level of severity is determined by both impairment and risk and is assigned to the most severe category in which any feature occurs.

At subsequent visits, assess control to adjust therapy
- Level of control is determined by both impairment and risk and is assigned to the most severe category in which any feature occurs.
- Address adherence to medication, inhaler technique, and environmental control measures.
- Sample patient self-assessment tools for asthma control can be found at http://www.asthmacontrol.com/index.html http://www.asthmacontrolcheck.com

Stepwise approach for managing asthma:
- Therapy is increased (stepped up) if necessary and decreased (stepped down) when possible as determined by the level of asthma severity or asthma control.

Asthma severity and asthma control include the domains of current impairment and future risk.

Impairment: frequency and intensity of symptoms and functional limitations the patient is currently experiencing or has recently experienced.

Risk: the likelihood of either asthma exacerbations, progressive decline in lung function (or, for children, reduced lung growth), or risk of adverse effects from medication.

ASTHMA MANAGEMENT RECOMMENDATIONS:

— Ensure that patient/family receive education about asthma and how to use spacers and other medication delivery devices.

— Assess asthma control at every visit by self-administered standardized test or verbal history.

— Perform spirometry at baseline and at least every 1 to 2 years for patients ≥ 5 years of age.

— Update or review the Asthma Action Plan every 6 to 12 months.

— Perform skin or blood allergy tests for all patients with persistent asthma.

— Encourage patient/family to continue follow-up with their clinician every 1 to 6 months even if asthma is well controlled.

— Refer patient to a specialist if:
- there are difficulties achieving or maintaining control OR
- step 4 care or higher is required (step 3 care or higher for children 0-4 years of age) OR
- immunotherapy or omalizumab is considered OR
- additional testing is indicated OR
- if the patient required 2 bursts of oral systemic corticosteroids in the past year or a hospitalization.

HOW TO USE THE ASTHMA ACTION PLAN:

Top copy (for patient):
- Enter specific medication information and review the instructions with the patient and/or family.
- Educate patient and/or family about factors that make asthma worse and the remediation steps on the back of this form.
- **Complete and sign the bottom of the form and give this copy of the form to the patient.**

Middle copy (for school, childcare, work, etc):
- Educate the parent/guardian on the need for their signature on the back of the form in order to authorize student self-carry and self-administration of asthma medications at school and also to authorize sharing student health information with school staff.
- **Provide this copy of the form to the school/childcare center/work/caretaker or other involved third party. (This copy may also be faxed to the school, etc.)**

Bottom copy (for chart):
- **File this copy in the patient's medical chart.**

FOR MORE INFORMATION:

To access the August 2007 full version of the NHLBI Guidelines for the Diagnosis and Treatment of Asthma (EPR-3) or the October 2007 Summary Report, visit **http://www.nhlbi.nih.gov/guidelines/asthma/index.htm.**

©2008, Public Health Institute (RAMP)

FIGURE 45-2 Asthma Action Plan

Source: Reprinted with permission from Regional Asthma Management and Prevention (RAMP), a program of the Public Health Institute. The RAMP Asthma Action Plan was supported by Cooperative Agreement Number 1U58DP001016-01 from the Centers for Disease Control and Prevention. The contents of the RAMP Asthma Action Plan are solely the responsibility of the authors and do not necessarily represent the official views of the CDC.

My Asthma Plan ENGLISH

Patient Name: _____

Medical Record #: _____

Provider's Name: _____   DOB: _____

Provider's Phone #: _____   Completed by: _____   Date: _____

Controller Medicines	How Much to Take	How Often	Other Instructions
		_____ times per day **EVERY DAY!**	❑ Gargle or rinse mouth after use
		_____ times per day **EVERY DAY!**	
		_____ times per day **EVERY DAY!**	
		_____ times per day **EVERY DAY!**	

Quick-Relief Medicines	How Much to Take	How Often	Other Instructions
❑ Albuterol (ProAir, Ventolin, Proventil) ❑ Levalbuterol (Xopenex)	❑ 2 puffs ❑ 4 puffs ❑ 1 nebulizer treatment	Take ONLY as needed (see below — starting in Yellow Zone or before excercise)	NOTE: If you need this medicine more than two days a week, call physician to consider increasing controller medications and discuss your treatment plan.

Special instructions when I am ⬤ *doing well,* ⬤ *getting worse,* ⬤ *having a medical alert.*

GREEN ZONE

Doing *well.*

⊙

- No cough, wheeze, chest tightness, or shortness of breath during the day or night.
- Can do usual activities.

Peak Flow (for ages 5 and up):
is _____ or more. (80% or more of personal best)

Personal Best Peak Flow (for ages 5 and up): _____

PREVENT asthma symptoms every day:

☐ Take my controller medicines (above) every day.

☐ Before exercise, take _____ puff(s) of _____

☐ Avoid things that make my asthma worse. (See back of form.)

YELLOW ZONE

Getting *worse.*

⊙

- Cough, wheeze, chest tightness, shortness of breath, or
- Waking at night due to asthma symptoms, or
- Can do some, but not all, usual activities.

Peak Flow (for ages 5 and up):
_____ to _____ (50 to 79% of personal best)

CAUTION. Continue taking every day controller medicines, AND:

☐ Take _____ puffs or _____ one nebulizer treatment of quick relief medicine. If I am not back in the *Green Zone* within 20-30 minutes take _____ more puffs or nebulizer treatments. If I am not back in the *Green Zone* within one hour, then I should:

☐ Increase _____

☐ Add _____

☐ Call _____

☐ Continue using quick relief medicine every 4 hours as needed. Call provider if not improving in _____ days.

RED ZONE

Medical Alert

☹

- Very short of breath, or
- Quick-relief medicines have not helped, or
- Cannot do usual activities, or
- Symptoms are same or get worse after 24 hours in Yellow Zone.

Peak Flow (for ages 5 and up):
less than _____ (50% of personal best)

MEDICAL ALERT! Get help!

☐ Take quick relief medicine: _____ puffs every _____ minutes and get help immediately.

☐ Take _____

☐ Call _____

Danger! Get help immediately! Call 911 if trouble walking or talking due to shortness of breath or if lips or fingernails are gray or blue. For child, call 911 if skin is sucked in around neck and ribs during breaths or child doesn't respond normally.

Health Care Provider: My signature provides authorization for the above written orders. I understand that all procedures will be implemented in accordance with state laws and regulations. Student may self carry asthma medications: ❑ Yes ❑ No   self administer asthma medications: ❑ Yes ❑ No (This authorization is for a maximum of one year from signature date.)

_____   _____
Healthcare Provider Signature   Date

ORIGINAL (Patient) / CANARY (School/Child Care/Work/Other Support Systems) / PINK (Chart)

©2008, Public Health Institute (RAMP)

FIGURE 45-2 Asthma Action Plan *(continued)*

Source: Reprinted with permission from Regional Asthma Management and Prevention (RAMP), a program of the Public Health Institute. The RAMP Asthma Action Plan was supported by Cooperative Agreement Number 1U58DP001016-01 from the Centers for Disease Control and Prevention. The contents of the RAMP Asthma Action Plan are solely the responsibility of the authors and do not necessarily represent the official views of the CDC.

Controlling Things That Make Asthma Worse

❏ **SMOKE**
- Do not smoke. Attend classes to help stop smoking.
- Do not allow smoking in the home or car. Remaining smoke smell can trigger asthma.
- Stay away from people who are smoking.
- If you smoke, smoke outside.

❏ **DUST**
- Vacuum weekly with a vacuum with a high efficiency filter or a central vacuum. Try to make sure people with asthma are not home during vacuuming.
- Remove carpet if possible. Wet carpet before removing and then dry floor completely.
- Damp mop floors weekly.
- Wash bedding and stuffed toys in hot water every 1-2 weeks. Freeze stuffed toys that aren't washable for 24 hours.
- Cover mattresses and pillows in dust-mite proof zippered covers.
- Reduce clutter and remove stuffed animals, especially around the bed.
- Replace heating system filters regularly.

❏ **PESTS**
- Do not leave food or garbage out. Store food in airtight containers.
- Try using traps and poison baits, such as boric acid for cockroaches. Instead of sprays/bombs, use baits placed away from children, such as behind refrigerator.
- Vacuum up cockroach bodies and fill holes in with caulking or copper wool.
- Fix leaky plumbing, roof, and other sources of water.

❏ **MOLD**
- Use exhaust fans or open windows for cross ventilation when showering or cooking.
- Clean mold off hard surfaces with detergent in hot water and scrub with stiff brush or cleaning pad, then rinse clean with water. Absorbent materials with mold may need to be replaced.
- Make sure people with asthma are not in the room when cleaning.
- Fix leaky plumbing or other sources of water or moisture.

❏ **ANIMALS**
- Consider not having pets. Avoid pets with fur or feathers.
- Keep pets out of the bedroom of the person with asthma.
- Wash your hands and the hands of the person with asthma after petting animals.

❏ **ODORS/SPRAYS**
- Avoid using strongly scented products, such as home deodorizers and incense, and perfumed laundry products and personal care products.
- Do not use oven/stove for heating.
- When cleaning, keep person with asthma away and don't use strong smelling cleaning products.
- Avoid aerosol products.
- Avoid strong or extra strength cleaning products.
- Avoid ammonia, bleach, and disinfectants.

❏ **POLLEN AND OUTDOOR MOLDS**
- Try to stay indoors when pollen and mold counts are high.
- Keep windows closed during pollen season.
- Avoid using fans; use air conditioners.

❏ **COLDS/FLU**
- Keep your body healthy with enough exercise and sleep.
- Avoid close contact with people who have colds.
- Wash your hands frequently and avoid touching your hands to your face.
- Get an annual flu shot.

❏ **WEATHER AND AIR POLLUTION**
- If cold air is a problem, try breathing through your nose rather than your mouth and covering up with a scarf.
- Check for Spare the Air days and nights and avoid strenuous exercise at those times.
- On very bad pollution days, stay indoors with windows closed.

❏ **EXERCISE**
- Warm up before exercising.
- Plan alternate indoor activities on high pollen or pollution days.
- If directed by physician, take medication before exercise. (See Green Zone of Asthma Action Plan.)

©2008, Public Health Institute (RAMP)

FIGURE 45-2 Asthma Action Plan *(continued)*

Source: Reprinted with permission from Regional Asthma Management and Prevention (RAMP), a program of the Public Health Institute. The RAMP Asthma Action Plan was supported by Cooperative Agreement Number 1U58DP001016-01 from the Centers for Disease Control and Prevention. The contents of the RAMP Asthma Action Plan are solely the responsibility of the authors and do not necessarily represent the official views of the CDC.

SCHOOL AUTHORIZATION FORM
To be completed by Parent/Guardian and turned in to the school

AUTHORIZATION AND DISCLAIMER FROM PARENT/GUARDIAN: I request that the school assist my child with the asthma medications listed on this form, and the Asthma Action Plan, in accordance with state laws and regulations.
❑ Yes ❑ No.

My child may carry and self-administer asthma medications and I agree to release the school district and school personnel from all claims of liability if my child suffers any adverse reactions from self-administration of asthma medications:
❑ Yes ❑ No.

_____   _____
Parent/Guardian Signature   Date

AUTHORIZATION FOR USE OR DISCLOSURE OF HEALTH INFORMATION TO SCHOOL DISTRICTS

Completion of this document authorizes the disclosure and/or use of individually identifiable health information, as set forth below, consistent with Federal laws (including HIPAA) concerning the privacy of such information. Failure to provide all information requested may invalidate this authorization.

USE AND DISCLOSURE INFORMATION:

Patient/Student Name: _____ / _____
　　　　　　　　　　　　　Last　　　　　　　First　　　　　MI　　　Date of Birth
I, the undersigned, do hereby authorize (name of agency and/or health care providers):

(1)_____ (2)_____ to provide
health information from the above-named child's medical record to and from:

_____   _____
School or school district to which disclosure is made   Address / City and State / Zip Code

_____   _____
Contact person at school or school district   Area Code and Telephone Number

The disclosure of health information is required for the following purpose:
_____

Requested information shall be limited to the following: ❑ All health information; or ❑ Disease-specific information as described:
_____

DURATION:
This authorization shall become effective immediately and shall remain in effect until _____(enter date) or for one year from the date of signature, if no date entered.
RESTRICTIONS:
Law prohibits the Requestor from making further disclosure of my health information unless the Requestor obtains another authorization form from me or unless such disclosure is specifically required or permitted by law.
YOUR RIGHTS:
I understand that I have the following rights with respect to this Authorization: I may revoke this Authorization at any time. My revocation must be in writing, signed by me or on my behalf, and delivered to the health care agencies/persons listed above. My revocation will be effective upon receipt, but will not be effective to the extent that the Requestor or others have acted in reliance to this Authorization.
RE-DISCLOSURE:
I understand that the Requestor (School District) will protect this information as prescribed by the Family Equal Rights Protection Act (FERPA) and that the information becomes part of the student's educational record. The information will be shared with individuals working at or with the School District for the purpose of providing safe, appropriate, and least restrictive educational settings and school health services and programs.

I have a right to receive a copy of this Authorization. Signing this Authorization may be required in order for this student to obtain appropriate services in the educational setting.

APPROVAL: _____ _____ _____
　　　　　　　Printed Name　　　　　　　　　Signature　　　　　　　　Date

_____ _____
Relationship to Patient/Student   Area Code and Telephone Number

---

FIGURE 45-2 Asthma Action Plan *(continued)*

Source: Reprinted with permission from Regional Asthma Management and Prevention (RAMP), a program of the Public Health Institute. The RAMP Asthma Action Plan was supported by Cooperative Agreement Number 1U58DP001016-01 from the Centers for Disease Control and Prevention. The contents of the RAMP Asthma Action Plan are solely the responsibility of the authors and do not necessarily represent the official views of the CDC.

This Asthma Plan was developed by a committee facilitated by the Regional Asthma Management and Prevention (RAMP) Initiative, a program of the Public Health Institute. This publication was supported by Cooperative Agreement Number 1U58DP001016-01 from the Centers for Disease Control and Prevention. Its contents are solely the responsibility of the authors and do not necessarily represent the official views of CDC. This plan is based on the recommendations from the National Heart, Lung, and Blood Institute's, "Guidelines for the Diagnosis and Management of Asthma," NIH Publication No. 07-4051 (August 2007). The information contained herein is intended for the use and convenience of physicians and other medical personnel and may not be appropriate for use in all circumstances. Decisions to adopt any particular recommendation must be made by qualified medical personnel in light of available resources and the circumstances presented by individual patients. No entity or individual involved in the funding or development of this plan makes any warranty or guarantee, express or implied, of the quality, fitness, performance or results of use of the information or products described in the plan or the Guidelines. For additional information, please contact RAMP at (510) 302-3365, http://www.rampasthma.org.

FIGURE 45-2 Asthma Action Plan *(continued)*

Source: Reprinted with permission from Regional Asthma Management and Prevention (RAMP), a program of the Public Health Institute. The RAMP Asthma Action Plan was supported by Cooperative Agreement Number 1U58DP001016-01 from the Centers for Disease Control and Prevention. The contents of the RAMP Asthma Action Plan are solely the responsibility of the authors and do not necessarily represent the official views of the CDC.

REFERENCES

Busse, W. W., & Lemanske, Jr., R. F. (2001). Asthma. *New England Journal of Medicine, 344*(5), 350–362.

Kamble, S., &. Bharmal, M. (2009). Incremental direct expenditure of treating asthma in the United States. *Journal of Asthma, 46*(1), 73–80.

Pellegrino, R., Viegi, G., Brusasco, V., Crapo, R. O., Burgos, F., Casaburi, R., . . . Wagner, J. (2005). Interpretive strategies for lung function tests. *European Respiratory Journal, 26*, 948–968.

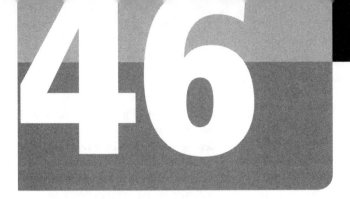

BENIGN PROSTATIC HYPERPLASIA

Jean N. Taylor-Woodbury

I. Introduction and general background

The prostate is a muscular gland roughly triangular in shape and located in the lower abdomen between a man's bladder and rectum. According to some anatomic descriptions it has a median lobe and two lateral lobes and physically surrounds the neck of the bladder and the urethra (Venes, 2009). Other sources, such as the classification system of Lowsley, attribute five lobes to the prostate: (1) anterior, (2) posterior, (3) media, (4) right lateral, and (5) left lateral (Tanagho, 2008). Partly muscular and partly glandular, the prostate has ducts opening into the prostatic portion of the urethra. Normally the prostate is roughly 2 × 4 × 3 cm and weighs approximately 20 g; it is enclosed in a fibrous capsule containing smooth muscle fibers in its inner layer. Muscle fibers also separate the glandular tissue and encircle the urethra. The gland secretes a thin, opalescent, slightly alkaline fluid that forms part of the seminal fluid (Venes, 2009). The gland is responsible for secreting liquid that then mixes with additional fluids secreted by the seminal vesicles, and with the sperm produced by the testicles.

A. Benign prostatic hyperplasia

1. Definition and overview: Benign prostatic hyperplasia (BPH) is generally considered to be a progressive disease and is considered to be the most common benign tumor in men (Meng, Stoller, & Walsh, 2010). The etiology of BPH is not known, but it is believed to be multifactorial with testicular androgens being the most probable controlling factor for the prostatic enlargement (Barry, 2009; Meng et al., 2010).

Hyperplasia of the prostate occurs in a nodular pattern, increasing the cell numbers and occurring to varying amounts in the stroma or epithelium and glandular tissue of the prostate (Barry, 2009; Meng et al., 2010). The hyperplasia begins in the area around the urethra and gradually increases in nodules over a period of years. As BPH progresses, the affected individual may or may not develop lower urinary tract symptoms (LUTS), which may include urinary frequency, hesitancy, urgency, nocturia, decreased force of stream, intermittent stream, incomplete bladder emptying, and incontinence or dribbling.

Prostatic enlargement may cause obstruction of the bladder outlet and compression of the urethra. If this occurs, compromised urinary flow and deterioration of the upper urinary tract and renal failure can result (Emberton et al., 2008).

Does BPH increase the risk for development of prostatic carcinoma? Most current clinical research suggests that although BPH may not result in prostatic carcinoma, pathologic changes that are associated with BPH may be associated with prostatic carcinoma (Bushman, 2009). An extensive study by Negri et al. (2005) concluded that the development of BPH seemed to be increased in those with a family history of bladder cancer, but not with those having a family history of prostatic carcinoma. Some studies have indicated an association between chronic inflammation and both BPH and prostatic carcinoma (Abdel-Meguid, Mosli, & Al-Maghrabi, 2009) and have found that prostatic cancer develops in 83% of prostate glands where BPH is also found (Bostwick et al., 1992). A study conducted by Hammarsten and Högstedt (2002) suggests that fast-growing BPH is a factor that increases the risk of developing clinical prostate cancer. The authors note that these findings support the hypothesis of an association between the development of BPH and clinical prostate cancer. The association between BPH and prostate cancer is complicated and controversial. To date, no clear-cut answers exist as to the actual association and risk.

2. Prevalence and incidence: BPH is very common, beginning around age 45 with development of accompanying symptoms by the age of 65 in whites and 60 in blacks (Fauci et al., 2009). It affects up to 80% of men 80 years or older (Barnard & Aronson, 2009). Not all men, however, who have histologic BPH are symptomatic with lower urinary tract symptoms (LUTS). Twenty-five percent of men age 55 and 50% age 75 report signs and symptoms

(Meng et al., 2010). Up to 80% of men 80 years of age and older report being affected by BPH (Barnard & Aronson, 2009).

It is difficult to predict who will develop BPH because the risk factors are poorly understood, although some studies have indicated racial differences and some have indicated a genetic link. Age is considered a correlate to likelihood of BPH and its progression. For those who progress early, findings have suggested that approximately half of all men younger than age 60 who require surgical intervention for BPH may have an inherited form of BPH that is an autosomal-dominant trait. According to Meng et al. (2010), the first-degree male relatives of those with the heritable form of BPH have a fourfold increased relative risk of developing BPH.

More recent studies have also indicated that diabetes and obesity increase the risk of BPH and BPH symptom progression, whereas exercise and moderate alcohol consumption seem to decrease the risk of BPH and BPH progression (Parsons, 2007; Platz et al., 1998; Sea, Poon, & McVary, 2009).

II. Database (may include but is not limited to)

A. Subjective

1. BPH
   a. Current symptoms and severity: The American Urological Association (McVary et al., 2010) offers effective tools for screening symptoms and severity (Appendices 46-1 and 46-2).
   b. Past health history
      i. Medical illnesses: any prostatic disease, renal disease, renal infection, or renal calculi; and any bladder disease, dysfunction, or recurrent infections.
      ii. Sexual history to include practices and any history of infection.
      iii. History of diabetes mellitus and obesity.
      iv. History of physical trauma to the bladder or the urethra.
      v. History of neurologic disease or injury.
      vi. Any history of cancer.
      vii. Surgical history: bladder surgery, urethral surgery, or penile surgery.
      viii. Trauma history: brain trauma including infarct or hemorrhagic stroke; trauma to bladder, urethra, or penis
      ix. Exposure history: any prior chemical or radioactive exposures to the lower genitourinary tract or perineal area.
      x. Medication history: medications and supplements that may impact on urinary flow or retention (e.g., antihistamine and decongestant use). Note any history of use of medications or supplements for treatment of existing or prior genitourinary disorders or disease, or prostatic disease.
      xi. A history of eye disease or cataracts should also be evaluated. Boehringer, Ingelheim and the Food and Drug Administration notified healthcare professionals of revisions to precautions and adverse reactions sections of the prescribing information for tamsulosin (Flomax®), indicated for the treatment of the signs and symptoms of BPH. A surgical condition termed "intraoperative floppy iris syndrome" (IFIS) has been observed during phacoemulsification cataract surgery in some patients treated with α_1 blockers including Flomax®. Most of these reports were in patients taking the α_1 blocker when IFIS occurred, but in some cases the α_1 blocker had been stopped before surgery. It is recommended that male patients being considered for cataract surgery, as part of their medical history, be specifically questioned to ascertain whether they have taken Flomax® or other α_1 blockers. If so, the patient's ophthalmologist should be prepared for possible modifications to their surgical technique that may be warranted should IFIS be observed during the procedure (United States Food and Drug Administration, 2005).
   c. Family history
      i. Prostatic disease, particularly in first-degree relatives, includes age of onset of disease
      ii. Diabetes
      iii. Neurologic disorders
      iv. Cancer
   d. Occupational and environmental history
      i. Work-related exposures, such as chemical or radiation exposures
      ii. Degree of access to appropriate facilities for voiding
   e. Personal and social history
      i. Recreational drug use, including methamphetamines, and tobacco
      ii. Dietary intake and caffeine
   f. Review of systems
      i. Abdomen: suprapubic pain (suggestive of acute urinary retention) and flank pain.
      ii. Genitourinary: urethral discharge; dysuria; irritative symptoms (urgency, frequency, or

nocturia); or obstructive symptoms (hesitancy, decreased or intermittent stream flow, sensation of incomplete void, and dribbling incontinence).

   iii. Neurologic: focal neurologic findings suggestive of neurologic etiology of the presenting urinary symptoms, such as lower extremity weakness, radiculopathic or neuropathic symptoms (e.g., saddle anesthesia).

B. Objective

1. Physical examination findings

   a. An abdominal examination may demonstrate a palpable, distended bladder, which may be asymptomatic if LUTS are otherwise mild or absent.

   b. Absence of costovertebral angle pain

   c. Absence of urethral discharge or other genital findings suggestive of infection or sexually transmitted infection as a source of the LUTS

   d. A digital rectal examination should be done and may reveal an enlarged prostate, which may be focal or diffuse. However, the size of the prostate correlates poorly with either the symptoms or the signs of BPH.

   e. A focused neurologic examination should be accomplished to rule out a neurogenic bladder.

2. Supporting data from relevant diagnostic tests

   a. Urinalysis by either dipstick or microscopic examination to evaluate for hematuria or urinary tract infection.

   b. Measurement of the serum prostate-specific antigen (PSA) should be considered for those patients with at least a 10-year life expectancy and for whom the knowledge of prostate cancer would change symptom or disease management, and for those whom the PSA level might change the management of their LUTS (McVary et al., 2010).

III. Assessment

A. Determine the diagnosis

Ready access to International Classification of Diseases-9 codes related to urologic disorders is available at the American Urologic Association's website at http://www.auanet.org/content/practice-resources /coding-tips/basics.cfm, or on-line at any number of websites specializing in International Classification of Diseases-9 codes, such as http://www.icd9data .com/2009/Volume1/580-629/600-608/600/default .htm.

1. BPH

2. Prostatitis

3. Prostatic neoplasms (benign or malignant)

4. Other conditions that may explain the patient's presentation

   a. Diabetes mellitus
   b. Urethral stricture
   c. Bladder neck contracture
   d. Bladder stone
   e. Neurogenic bladder

B. Assess the severity of the disease.

C. Assess the significance of the problem to the patient and significant others

IV. Goals of clinical management

A. Choose a cost-effective approach for screening or diagnosing BPH.

B. Select a treatment plan that returns the client to a symptom-free state in a safe and effective manner.

C. Select an approach that maximizes client adherence.

V. Plan

A. Screening: There are no screening tests for BPH. Examination is usually done in response to complaints of symptoms, although prostatic hyperplasia may be detected during a routine digital rectal examination.

B. Diagnostic tests (see Box 46-1 for a description of relevant diagnostic studies and Figure 46-1 for the suggested approach for BPH diagnosis and treatment)

C. Management (includes treatment, consultation, referral, and follow-up care)

1. BPH

   a. If symptoms are mild (American Urological Association Symptom Scale of less than or equal to 7 or no bothersome symptoms), then watchful waiting is indicated.

   b. If symptoms are moderate to severe, then discuss treatment options with the patient.

BOX 46-1 *Description of Relevant Diagnostic Studies*

Common prostate studies may include, but are not limited to the following:

1. Urinalysis (may be done by dipstick testing or microanalysis). According to the American Urological Association, routinely measuring the serum creatinine levels in the initial assessment of men with lower urinary tract symptoms is not indicated (McVary et al., 2003, being revised).

2. Prostate-specific antigen should be offered as an option to men with at least a 10-year life expectancy and for whom knowledge of the presence of prostate cancer would change health management or for men in whom the prostate-specific antigen measurement may change the management of their voiding symptoms (McVary et al., 2003, being revised).

3. Urine cytology may be considered if there is a predominance of irritative (versus obstructive) symptoms and if the patient has a history of smoking or other significant risk factors for bladder carcinoma.

4. Optional tests for men with moderate to severe urinary symptoms include test of postvoid residual and urinary flow. If there is significant postvoid residual volume, transabdominal kidney ultrasound or intravenous urography by radiograph may be helpful in evaluating for hydronephrosis (American College of Radiology, 1995 revised 2007).

Source: Adapted from McVary, K. T., Roehrborn, C. G., Avins, A. L., Barr, M. J., Bruskewitz, R., . . . Wei. T. (2010). *Management of BPH.* American Urological Association Education and Research, Inc. Retrieved from http://www.auanet.org/content/guidelines-and-quality-care/clinical-guidelines.cfm?sub=bph and American College of Radiology. (1995, last reviewed 2008). *ACR appropriateness criteria®: obstructive voiding symptoms secondary to prostate disease.* Retrieved from http://www.acr.org/SecondaryMainMenuCategories/quality_safety/app_criteria/pdf/ExpertPanelonUrologicImaging/ObstructiveVoidingSymptomsSecondarytoProstateDisease Doc9.aspx.

c. If patient chooses noninvasive therapy, may choose watchful waiting or the following medical therapy.
  i. Phenoxybenzamine, 5–10 mg orally twice daily
  ii. Prazosin, 1–5 mg orally twice daily (according to the current American Urological Association guideline for the management of BPH [2003, being revised], there is insufficient evidence to support the use of either phenoxybenzamine or Prazosin for the treatment of LUTS with BPH)
  iii. Alfuzosin, 10 mg orally daily
  iv. Doxazosin, 1–8 mg orally daily
  v. Tamsulosin, 0.4 or 0.8 mg orally daily
  vi. Terazosin, 1–10 mg orally daily
  vii. In using α-blockers, a gradual upward titration is recommended to minimize the risk of orthostatic hypotension that may occur with the use of this class of medications
  viii. 5α-Reductase inhibitors (used for individuals with prostates > 40 mL by ultrasonographic examination (Meng, Stoller, & Walsh, 2010)
    a. Dutasteride, 0.5 mg orally daily
    b. Finasteride, 5 mg orally daily
  ix. Combination therapy: α-blocker and 5α-reductase inhibitor
  x. Based on expert panel recommendations, and noted in the American Urological Association guideline for the Management of Benign Prostatic Hyperplasia (McVary et al., 2010), phytotherapeutics and other dietary supplements are not currently recommended for the treatment of LUTS with BPH. It is noted that Saw Palmetto (Serenoa repens) has shown some promise in treating BPH, but no sound studies support the efficacy of other phytotherapeutics, such as African prune tree (Pygeum africanum) and Rye pollen (Secale cereale) (Dedhia & McVary, 2008). Until adequate and sound methodologic studies (i.e., randomized, placebo-controlled) are done that support the efficacy and safety of phytotherapeutics, they are not recommended for the treatment of LUTS and BPH (Dedhia & McVary, 2008; Dreikorn, 2002).

d. If the patient desires invasive therapy, refer to the urology service.
  i. The specialist may consider additional optional diagnostic tests, such as pressure flow, urethrocystoscopy, or prostate ultrasound.
  ii. Minimally invasive surgical options include transurethral laser-induced prostatectomy, transurethral needle ablation of the prostate, transurethral electrovaporization of the prostate, and hyperthermia.
  iii. Conventional surgical therapy includes transurethral resection of the prostate,

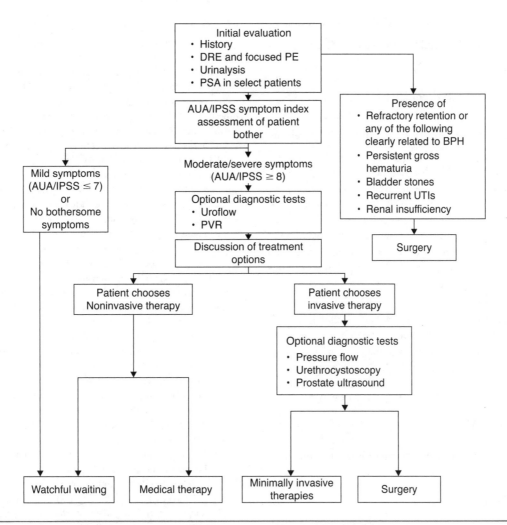

FIGURE 46-1 Benign Prostatic Hyperplasia (BPH) Diagnosis and Treatment

Source: Benign Prostatic Hyperplasia (2003) (being revised) Roehrborn, C. G., McConnell, J. D., Barry, M. J., Benaim, E., Bruskewitz, R. C., Blute, M. L., Holtgrewe, H. L., Kaplan, S. A., Lange, J. L., Lowe, F. C., Roberts, R. G., Stein, B. S.: AUA Guideline on the Management of Benign Prostatic Hyperplasia: Diagnosis and Treatment Recommendations. American Urological Association Education and Research, Inc., ©2003. Used with permission. http://www.auanet.org/content /guidelines-and-quality-care/clinicalguidelines.cfm?sub=bph

transurethral incision of the prostate, and open simple prostatectomy.

2. Adverse effects of treatment

Regardless of treatment approach, patient education around both desired and the potential for undesired or adverse effects of the treatment should be thorough. The adverse effects depend on the treatment course and may range from no adverse effects, to either asymptomatic or symptomatic hypotension with the use of α-blockers, to more severe side effects with surgical intervention. For example, beyond the risk of immediate surgical complications, transurethral resection of the prostate has the potential to result in retrograde ejaculation, erectile dysfunction, urinary incontinence, inability to void, and infection (DuBeau, 2009).

D. *Client education*

1. Assist the patient and significant others in expressing and coping with concerns and feelings related to the respective prostate disease process and disease management.

2. Provide verbal and, preferably, written information regarding

   a. The disease process, including signs and symptoms and underlying etiologies.

   b. Diagnostic tests, including a discussion about preparation, cost, the actual procedures, and after-care.

   c. Management (rationale, action, use, side effects, and cost of therapeutic interventions; and the need for adhering to long-term treatment plans).

VI. Self-management resources and tools

A. Patient and client education brochures or frequently asked question documents:

1. The National Institutes of Health's (2010) website (http://www.nlm.nih.gov/medlineplus/prostate diseases.html): has patient and client education brochures and frequently asked question documents in English and Spanish. The documents include visual resources and include a link to a number of other resources, including to the American Urological Association Foundation Urologyhealth.com website (http://www.urology health.org/adult/).

2. The Merck Source Resource Library (Krames, 2002–2009): provides a superb and accessible section on BPH, which includes a high-quality interactive human atlas. For more information go to http://www.merckengage.com/common/ms_transition.aspx?WT.mc_id=MESOURCE and http://visn12.kramesonline.com/Medications/3,S,83023

3. Johns Hopkins Medical School: offers a Health Alerts electronic subscription service for BPH, which provides regular updates on BPH and treatments.

REFERENCES

Abdel-Meguid, T., Mosli, H., & Al-Maghrabi, J. (2009). Prostate inflammation. Association with benign prostatic hyperplasia and prostate cancer. *Saudi Medical Journal, 30*(12), 1563–1567.

American College of Radiology. (1995, last reviewed 2008). *ACR appropriateness criteria®: obstructive voiding symptoms secondary to prostate disease.* Retrieved from http://www.acr.org/SecondaryMainMenuCategories/quality_safety/app_criteria/pdf/ExpertPanelonUrologicImaging/ObstructiveVoidingSymptomsSecondarytoProstateDiseaseDoc9.aspx.

American Urological Association Foundation. (2010). *UrologyHealth.org.* Retrieved from http://www.urologyhealth.org/adult/

Barnard, R. J., & Aronson, W. J. (2009). Benign prostatic hyperplasia: Does lifestyle play a role? *The Physician and Sports Medicine, 37*(4), 141–146.

Barry, M. J. (2009). Approach to benign prostatic hyperplasia. In A. H. Goroll & A. G. Mulley, *Primary care medicine: Office evaluation and management of the adult patient* (6th ed.) (pp. 974–979). Philadelphia: Wolters Kluwer/Lippincott, Williams & Wilkins.

Bostwick, D., Cooner, W., Denis, L., Jones, G. W., Scardino, P. T., & Murphy, G. P. (1992). The association of benign prostatic hyperplasia and cancer of the prostate. *Cancer, 70*(Suppl 1), 291–301.

Bushman, W. (2009). Etiology, epidemiology, and natural history of benign prostatic hyperplasia. *Urologic Clinics of North America, 36*(4), 403–415.

Dedhia, R. C., & McVary, K. T. (2008). Phytotherapy for lower urinary tract symptoms secondary to benign prostatic hyperplasia. *The Journal of Urology, 179*(6), 2119–2125.

Dreikorn, K. (2002). The role of phytotherapy in treating lower urinary tract symptoms and benign prostatic hyperplasia. *World Journal of Urology, 19*(6), 426–435.

DuBeau, C. (2009). Benign prostate disorders. In J. Halter, J. Ouslander, M. Tinneti, S. Studenski, K. High, & S. Asthana (Eds.), *Hazzard's geriatric medicine and gerontology* (6th ed., pp. 348–374). New York, NY: McGraw-Hill Professional. Retrieved from http://www.accessmedicine.com/content.aspx?aID=5118484

Emberton, M., Cornel, E. B., Bassi, P. F., Fourcade, R. O., Gómez, J. M., & Castro, R. (2008). Benign prostatic hyperplasia as a progressive disease: A guide to the risk factors and options for medical management. *International Journal of Clinical Practice, 62*(7), 1076–1086.

Fauci, A., Braunwald, E., Kasper, D., Hauser, S., Longo, D., Jameson, J., & Loscalzo, J. (2009). *Harrison's manual of medicine* (17th ed.). New York, NY: McGraw-Hill. Professional.

Hammarsten, J., & Högstedt, B. (2002). Calculated fast-growing benign prostatic hyperplasia—a risk factor for developing clinical prostate cancer. *Scandinavian Journal of Urology and Nephrology, 36*(5), 330–338.

McVary, K. T., Roehrborn, C. G., Avins, A. L., Barr, M. J., Bruskewitz, R., . . . Wei. T. (2010). *Management of BPH.* American Urological Association Education and Research, Inc. Retrieved from http://www.auanet.org/content/guidelines-and-quality-care/clinical-guidelines.cfm?sub=bph

Meng, M., Stoller, M., & Walsh, T. (2010). Urologic disorders. In S. McPhee & M. Papadakis (Eds.), *Current medical diagnosis & treatment 2010* (49th ed., pp. 850–871). Retrieved from http://www.accessmedicine.com/content.aspx?aID=11857

Negri, E., Pelucchi, C., Talamini, R., Montella, M., Gallus, S., Bosetti, C., . . . La Vecchia, C. (2005). Family history of cancer and the risk of prostate cancer and benign prostatic hyperplasia. *International Journal of Cancer, 114*(4), 648–652.

Parsons, J. (2007). Modifiable risk factors for benign prostatic hyperplasia and lower urinary tract symptoms: New approaches to old problems. *The Journal of Urology, 178*, 395–401.

Platz, F., Kawachi, I., Rimm, E., Colditz, G., Stampfer, M., Willett, W., & Giovannucci, E. (1998). Physical activity and benign prostatic hyperplasia. *Archives of Internal Medicine, 158*(21), 2349–2356.

Sea, J., Poon, K., & McVary, K. (2009). Review of exercise and the risk of benign prostatic hyperplasia. *The Physician and Sports Medicine, 37*(4), 75–83.

Tanagho, E. (2008). Anatomy of the genitourinary tract. In E. Tanagho & J. McAninch (Eds.), *Smith's general urology* (17th ed., pp. 1–16). New York, NY: McGraw-Hill. Retrieved from http://www.accessmedicine.com/content.aspx?aID=3125000

U.S. Food and Drug Administration. (2005). *Tamsulosin: Safety warning/recommendation statement.* Retrieved from http://www.fda.gov/Safety/MedWatch/SafetyInformation/SafetyAlertsforHumanMedicalProducts/ucm151211.htm

Venes, D. (Ed.). (2009). *Taber's cyclopedic medical dictionary.* Philadelphia, PA: F.A. Davis Company. Retrieved from http://online.statref.com/document.aspx?fxid=57&docid=48018

APPENDIX 46-1:
THE AMERICAN UROLOGICAL ASSOCIATION (AUA) SYMPTOM INDEX FOR BENIGN PROSTATIC HYPERPLASIA (BPH) AND THE DISEASE SPECIFIC QUALITY OF LIFE QUESTION

Patient Name: _____ Date of birth: _____ Date completed _____

	Not at All	Less than 1 in 5 Times	Less than Half the Time	About Half the Time	More than Half the Time	Almost Always	Your score
1. Over the past month, how often have you had a sensation of not emptying your bladder completely after you finished urinating?	0	1	2	3	4	5	
2. Over the past month, how often have you had to urinate again less than two hours after you finished urinating?	0	1	2	3	4	5	
3. Over the past month, how often have you stopped and started again several times when you urinated?	0	1	2	3	4	5	
4. Over the past month, how often have you found it difficult to postpone urination?	0	1	2	3	4	5	
5. Over the past month, how often have you had a weak urinary stream?	0	1	2	3	4	5	
6. Over the past month, how often have you had to push or strain to begin urination?	0	1	2	3	4	5	
	None	**1 Time**	**2 Times**	**3 Times**	**4 Times**	**5 or More**	
7. Over the past month, how many times did you most typically get up to urinate from the time you went to bed at night until the time you got up in the morning?	0	1	2	3	4	5+	

Total Symptom Score

Score: 1-7: *Mild* 8-19: *Moderate* 20-35: *Severe*

The possible total runs from 0 to 35 points with higher scores indicating more severe symptoms. Scores less than seven are considered mild and generally do not warrant treatment.

The International Prostate Symptom Score uses the same 7 questions as the AUA Symptom

Index (presented above) with the addition of the following Disease Specific Quality of Life

Question (bother score) scored on a scale from 0 to 6 points (delighted to terrible):

"If you were to spend the rest of your life with your urinary condition just the way it is now, how would you feel about that?"

Source: McVary, K. T., Roehrborn, C. G., Avins, A. L., Barr, M. J., Bruskewitz, R., . . . Wei. T. (2010). *Management of BPH*. American Urological Association Education and Research, Inc. Retrieved from http://www.auanet.org/content/guidelines-and-quality-care/clinical-guidelines. cfm?sub=bph. Used with permission.

APPENDIX 46-2:
BENIGN PROSTATIC HYPERPLASIA (BPH) IMPACT INDEX ("BOTHER" SCORE)

Patient Name: _____ DOB: _____ ID: _____ **Date of assessment** _____

Initial Assessment ❑ Monitor during: _____ Therapy ❑ after: _____ Therapy/surgery ❑ _____

BPH Impact Index

1. Over the past month how much physical discomfort did any urinary problems cause you?	None ❑ Only a little ❑ Some ❑ A lot ❑
2. Over the past month, how much did you worry about your health because of any urinary problems?	None ❑ Only a little ❑ Some ❑ A lot ❑
3. Overall, how bothersome has any trouble with urination been during the past month?	Not at all bothersome ❑ Bothers me some ❑ Bothers me a little ❑ Bothers me a lot ❑
4. Over the past month, how much of the time has any urinary problem kept you from doing the kind of things you would usually do?	None of the time ❑ Most of the time ❑ A little of the time ❑ All of the time ❑ Some of the time ❑
	Total Score: (Scoring based on 0-4 point scale)

Source: Benign Prostatic Hyperplasia (2003) (being revised) Roehrborn, C. G., McConnell, J. D., Barry, M. J., Benaim, E., Bruskewitz, R. C., Blute, M. L., Holtgrewe, H. L., Kaplan, S. A., Lange, J. L., Lowe, F. C., Roberts, R. G., Stein, B. S.: AUA Guideline on the Management of Benign Prostatic Hyperplasia: Diagnosis and Treatment Recommendations. American Urological Association Education and Research, Inc., © 2003. Used with permission. http://www.auanet.org/content/guidelines_and_quality_care/clinicalguidelines.cfm?sub=bph

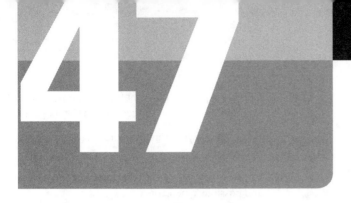

CHRONIC OBSTRUCTIVE PULMONARY DISEASE

Lynda A. Mackin

I. Introduction and general background

Chronic obstructive pulmonary disease (COPD) is an umbrella name for two major pulmonary obstructive disorders: chronic bronchitis and emphysema. Although each disorder has its own distinctive pathophysiology, many COPD patients have a combination of chronic bronchitis and emphysema.

A. COPD

1. Definition and overview

   COPD is defined as follows: "the physiological finding of nonreversible pulmonary function impairment" (Mannino, Homa, Akinbami, Ford, & Redd, 2002). The main pathophysiologic problem in COPD is expiratory airflow obstruction. In the case of chronic bronchitis, loss of structural integrity and bronchospasm in the larger airways, plus excess mucous production, are the cause of obstruction. In emphysema, smaller, more distal airways and alveoli are damaged, resulting in loss of structural integrity during expiration and destruction of the alveolar–capillary membrane. The small airway changes result in early collapse during expiration; the loss of surface area at the alveoli–capillary level impairs gas exchange.

   Smoking is recognized to be the most common cause of COPD, but environmental exposures and toxins can also be the cause. Additionally, COPD is now increasingly being described as a systemic disease evidenced by nutritional depletion and skeletal muscle dysfunction (Decramer, De Benedetto, Del Ponte, & Marinari, 2005).

2. Prevalence and incidence

   In 2007, it was estimated that 12 million people living in the United States were physician-diagnosed with COPD (National Institutes of Health/National Heart, Lung and Blood Institute [NIH/NHLBI], 2009) and an additional 12 million had COPD but have not been diagnosed (Mannino et al., 2002; National Health Interview Survey, 2007; NIH/NHLBI, 2009). Currently, COPD is the fourth leading cause of death in the United States (NIH/NHLBI, 2009). Per 2007 data, the prevalence of COPD was reported to be higher in females than males, with the exception of the 65 years and older age group, where there is no gender difference (NIH/NHLBI, 2009). COPD accounted for 53.6% of all deaths caused by lung disease in the United States in 2006 (NIH/NHLBI, 2009). In terms of ethnicity, COPD prevalence is higher in whites compared to blacks in males aged 45–64 years and in both males and females ages 65 years and older (NIH/NHLBI, 2009).

II. Database (may include but is not limited to)

A. Subjective

1. COPD

   a. Past health history
      i. Medical illnesses: asthma, allergies, nasal polyps, sinusitis, childhood respiratory infections, and other respiratory diseases
      ii. Surgical history: chest or lung
      iii. Exposure history: environmental tobacco smoke exposure, occupational dusts and fume exposures toxins; indoor and outdoor air pollution (Global Initiative for Chronic Obstructive Lung Disease [GOLD], 2009)
      iv. Medication history: medications taken to relieve symptoms currently and in the past (oral or inhaled bronchodilators and oral or inhaled steroids)
   b. Family history: obstructive pulmonary disease
   c. Occupational and environmental history
      i. Work-related exposures: toxins and fumes
      ii. Exposure to home cooking or heating fuels

    d. Personal and social history: smoking
    e. Review of systems
        i.   Constitutional signs and symptoms: fatigue, activity intolerance, weight change, and fevers; impact of symptoms on activities of daily living and occupational and recreational pursuits
        ii. Ear, nose, and throat: allergic rhinitis, sinus symptoms, and postnasal drip
        iii. Respiratory: chronic cough (with or without sputum production; may be intermittent); chronic sputum production; and progressive, persistent dyspnea (worsens with activity or on exertion)
        iv. Cardiac: chest pain, fluid retention and peripheral edema, and dysrhythmias

B. *Objective*
    1. Physical examination findings (Table 47-1)
    2. Spirometry: See Table 47-2 (GOLD, 2008, updated 2009).
        a. A key component of the COPD diagnosis is spirometric testing. Key spirometric values are the forced vital capacity (FVC) and the forced expiratory volume in one second (FEV_1), percentage predicted. If the FEV_1 is less than 80% predicted value, this is considered indicative of airway obstruction. Additionally, if the FVC/FEV_1 ratio is less than 0.7, this is also indicative of airway obstruction.
        b. Spirometry determines the severity of airflow obstruction and is performed before and after inhaled bronchodilator administration; this allows for determination of reversibility of airflow obstruction (if present).
    3. Chest radiograph: may demonstrate hyperinflation and flattened diaphragms.

    4. Check complete blood count (may see polycythemia in chronic hypoxemia) and complete metabolic panel.
    5. Pulse oximetry: Saturation is reduced in cases of hypoxemia.
    6. Consider arterial blood gases: reflects hypoxemia and possible hypercapnia.
    7. Consider α_1-antitrypsin deficiency screen (in cases of younger onset of symptoms and more extensive disease).
    8. To assess systemic effect of disease, the BODE Index may be useful (Celli et al., 2004): the BODE Index is a multidimensional mortality prediction that incorporates body mass index, severity of airflow obstruction, dyspnea, and exercise capacity as measured by 6-minute walk performance.

III. Goals of clinical management

A. *Relieve symptoms*

B. *Prevent disease progression*

C. *Increase exercise tolerance*

D. *Improve health status*

E. *Prevent and treat complications and exacerbations*

F. *Reduce mortality*

G. *Prevent or minimize side effects of treatments*

TABLE 47-1 Classic Physical Examination Findings in Chronic Bronchitis and Emphysema

Chronic Bronchitis	Emphysema
Overweight	Thin
Cyanotic but breathing comfortably at rest	Not cyanotic, breathing looks comfortable
Noisy breath sounds, rhonchi, wheezing	Quiet, distant breath sounds
Peripheral edema	No peripheral edema

Most chronic obstructive pulmonary disease patients have clinical characteristics of both chronic bronchitis and emphysema to varying degrees.

TABLE 47-2 Spirometric Classification of COPD Severity Based on Post-Bronchodilator FEV_1

Stage I: Mild FEV_1/FVC < 0.70
$FEV_1 \geq 80\%$ predicted
Stage II: Moderate FEV_1/FVC < 0.70
$50\% \leq FEV_1 < 80\%$ predicted
Stage III: Severe FEV_1/FVC < 0.70
$30\% \leq FEV_1 < 50\%$ predicted
Stage IV: Very Severe FEV_1/FVC < 0.70
$FEV_1 < 30\%$ predicted or $FEV_1 < 50\%$ predicted plus chronic respiratory failure

FEV_1: forced expiratory volume in one second; FVC: forced vital capacity; respiratory failure: arterial partial pressure of oxygen (PaO_2) less than 8.0 kPa (60 mm Hg) with or without arterial partial pressure of CO_2 ($PaCO_2$) greater than 6.7 kPa (50 mm Hg) while breathing air at sea level.

IV. Components of COPD management (GOLD, 2009)

A. Assess and monitor disease

1. Detailed history: past medical history, comorbidities, review of current treatments and responses including use of steroids, family history, exposures, and impact on life and social activities

2. Spirometry: assess severity; for stages II–IV include bronchodilator reversibility testing.

B. Reduce risk factors

1. Smoking cessation or prevention

   a. Single most important intervention

   b. Studies demonstrate that repeated recommendations to quit from primary care provider are effective.

   c. Success rates improve if both group support and nicotine replacement or adjuncts are used.

2. Eliminate or reduce occupational exposures, and indoor and outdoor pollution.

C. Manage stable COPD

1. Determine severity through spirometry and symptom review.

2. Stepwise treatments (Table 47-3).

3. Treatments per national and cultural preferences, patient's skills, and medication availability

   a. Short-acting β-agonists (SABA) inhalers: may be used on a scheduled or as-needed basis. Albuterol, levoalbuterol, pirbuterol, and others; promotes bronchodilation, thus improving airflow.

   b. Anticholinergic bronchodilator inhalers: may be used on a scheduled or as-needed basis. Ipratropium (Atrovent®), tiotropium (Spriva®), and anticholinergics promote bronchodilation and also decrease mucus hypersecretion, thus improving airflow and decreased dyspnea.

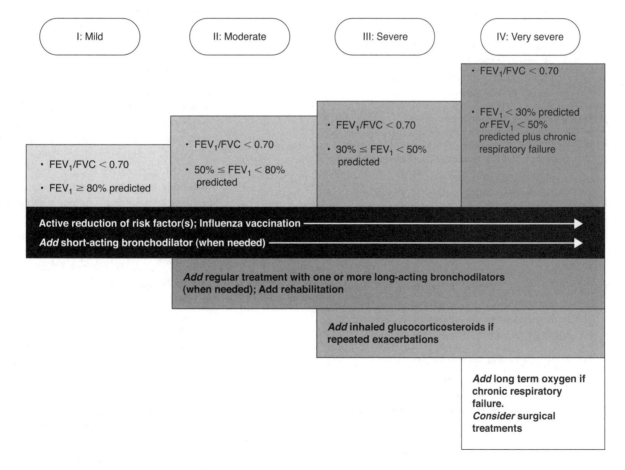

TABLE 47-3 Therapy at Each Stage of COPD

Source: Citation used with permission. From the Global Strategy for the Diagnosis, Management, and Prevention of Chronic Obstructive Pulmonary Disease, Global Initiative for Chronic Obstructive Lung Disease (GOLD) 2009. Available from: http://www.goldcopd.org.

c. Combination SABA and anticholinergic: albuterol and ipratropium (Combivent®); provides synergy especially for chronic bronchitis.

d. Long-acting β-agonist (LABA): salmeterol xinafoate (Serevent Discus®); formoterol fumarate (Foradil Aerolizer®); longer-lasting bronchodilator effect than SABA agents; should not be used for quick relief.

e. Long-acting oral bronchodilator: not first-line treatment; theophylline (oral tablets)

f. Inhaled corticosteroid and long-acting bronchodilator combinations: fluticasone propionate and salmeterol (Advair®); approved for use in COPD in 250 (fluticasone propionate)/50 (salmeterol) strength, one inhalation twice a day; budesonide and formoterol fumerate (Symbicort®)160/4.5 mcg, two inhalations twice day

g. Oral corticosteroids: for exacerbations, or in selected cases, chronic therapy; dosages, burst, and taper schedules vary

h. Vaccines: pneumococcal and seasonal influenza

i. Nonpharmacologic treatments: pulmonary rehabilitation; supplemental oxygen therapy (when hypoxemia is present); and referral for surgery (in selected cases)

j. See Table 47-4 for complete listing of medications (GOLD, 2009)

D. Manage exacerbations

1. Definition: "An exacerbation of COPD is defined as an event in natural course of disease characterized by change in the patient's baseline dyspnea, cough, and/or sputum that is beyond normal day-to-day variation, is acute in onset and may warrant a change in regular medication..." (GOLD, 2009, p. 62). The discussion that follows here only applies to mild exacerbations that can be safely treated as an outpatient. The reader is directed to the GOLD (2009) Guidelines for complete information regarding management of exacerbations in moderate and severe cases and recommendations for emergency department and hospital treatment.

2. Etiology and clinical presentation

a. Most exacerbations are caused by lower respiratory tract infection or air pollution.

b. Can be viral or bacterial. Most common bacterial etiologies are *Streptococcus pneumoniae*, *Moraxella catarrhalis*, and *Haemophilus influenza*.

c. Key history: severity of obstruction (FEV$_1$), current medication regimen, duration of new or worsening symptoms, and prior exacerbations (quantity and frequency and need for antibiotics, particularly in the last 3 months).

d. Cardinal symptoms: increased dyspnea, increased sputum production, and increased sputum volume.

3. Clinical evaluation

a. Physical examination: tachypnea; tachycardia; altered mental status (serious sign); increased work of breathing; poor air entry; wheezing; rhonchi; and complaints of increased shortness of breath

b. Arterial blood gas: PaO$_2$ less than 60 or Spo$_2$ less than 90%; moderate to severe acidosis (pH < 7.36) plus hypercapnia (PaCO$_2$ 45–60) in the patient with respiratory failure indicates the need for mechanical ventilation

c. Chest radiograph: identify alternative diagnosis (pneumonia or congestive heart failure).

d. Electrocardiogram: look for right ventricular hypertrophy, arrhythmias, and ischemia. Others: sputum culture; metabolic panel; and complete blood count (may not be necessary for outpatient treatment, but should be considered). Spirometry or peak expiratory flow measurements are not considered helpful in the midst of exacerbation.

4. Exacerbation treatment

a. Determine treatment site. Strongly consider hospitalization for the following: changes in mental status; inability to care for oneself; inadequate home care; uncertain diagnosis; inadequate outpatient response to treatment; inability to eat or sleep because of symptoms; worsening hypoxemia and hypercapnia; and high-risk comorbidity (pneumonia, dysrhythmias, congestive heart failure, diabetes mellitus, or renal or liver failure) (GOLD, 2009)

b. Outpatient treatment of exacerbation: summary of GOLD Guidelines Component 4: Manage Exacerbations (2009).

   i. Increase bronchodilator dose and frequency.

   ii. Oral corticosteroids (if baseline FEV$_1$ is less than 50% predicted, prednisone 30–40 mg orally daily for 7–10 days); consider inhaled corticosteroid (if not already on).

   iii. Antibiotic treatment: reserved for cases presenting with all three cardinal symptoms or that have two cardinal symptoms, of which one is increased sputum purulence.

      a. First line: β-lactam (penicillin or ampicillin–amoxicillin); tetracycline; and trimethoprim–sulfamethoxazole (in areas where there are high levels

TABLE 47-4 Commonly Used Formulations of Drugs used in COPD

Drug	Inhaler (μg)	Solution for Nebulizer (mg/ml)	Oral	Vials for Injection (mg)	Duration of Action (hours)
β₂-agonists					
Short-acting					
Fenoterol	100–200 (MDI)	1	0.05% (Syrup)		4–6
Levalbuterol	45–90 (MDI)	0.21, 0.42			6–8
Salbutamol (albuterol)	100, 200 (MDI & DPI)	5	5 mg (Pill), Syrup 0.024%	0.1, 0.5	4–6
Terbutaline	400, 500 (DPI)		2.5, 5 (Pill)	0.2, 0.25	4–6
Long-acting					
Formoterol	4.5–12 (MDI & DPI)	0.01*			12+
Arformoterol		0.0075			12+
Salmeterol	25–50 (MDI & DPI)				12+
Anticholinergics					
Short-acting					
Ipratropium bromide	20, 40 (MDI)	0.25–0.5			6–8
Oxitropium bromide	100 (MDI)	1.5			7–9
Long-acting					
Tiotropium	18 (DPI), 5 (SMI)				24+
Combination short-acting β₂-agonists plus anticholinergic in one inhaler					
Fenoterol/ Ipratropium	200/80 (MDI)	1.25/0.5			6–8
Salbutamol/ Ipratropium	75/15 (MDI)	0.75/4.5			6–8
Methylxanthines					
Aminophylline			200–600 mg (Pill)	240 mg	Variable up to 24
Theophylline (SR)			100–600 mg (Pill)		Variable up to 24
Inhaled glucocorticosteroids					
Beclomethasone	50–400 (MDI & DPI)	0.2–0.4			
Budesonide	100, 200, 400 (DPI)	0.20, 0.25, 0.5			
Fluticasone	50–500 (MDI & DPI)				
Triamcinolone	100 (MDI)	40		40	
Combination long-acting β₂-agonists plus glucocorticosteroids in one inhaler					
Formoterol/ Budesonide	4.5/160, 9/320 (DPI)				
Salmeterol/ Fluticasone	50/100, 250, 500 (DPI) 25/50, 125, 250 (MDI)				
Systemic glucocorticosteroids					
Prednisone			5–60 mg (Pill)		
Methyl-prednisolone			4, 8, 16 mg (Pill)		

*Formoterol nebulized solution is based on the unit dose vial containing 20 μgm in a volume of 2.0 ml.

of resistance to β-lactamase–producing strains of *S. pneumoniae, M. catarrhalis,* or *H. influenza,* β-lactam agents are not recommended).

    b.   Second line: β-lactam/β-lactamase inhibitor (amoxicillin–clavulanate); macrolides (azithromycin and clarithromycin); and second- or third-generation cephalosporins and ketolides (telithromycin)

    iv.   Patient education on medications, side effects, dosing, when to expect symptoms to improve, signs and symptoms of worsening, and when to call the provider or seek emergency evaluation. Provide an action plan or written instructions for the patient. The patient should be reappointed to see the provider again in 2–3 days, or sooner as needed.

    c.   The reader is referred to GOLD Guidelines (2009). Global strategy for the diagnosis, management, and prevention of COPD for more detailed information about home management of late stage COPD exacerbations, and hospital and end-of-life management.

V. Care from a population health perspective

A. Smoking cessation is by far the most important preventative strategy; smokers should be counseled and supported in achieving cessation at all clinical encounters.

B. Access to quality-controlled spirometry for diagnosis and monitoring.

C. Reduce risks by working for clean air and environment issues at a public health level.

D. Manage comorbidities in addition to COPD symptoms, especially in older adults.

REFERENCES

Celli, B. R., Cote, C. G., Marin, J. M., Casanova, C., Montes de Oca, M., Mendez, R. A., . . . Cabral, H. J. (2004). The body-mass index, airflow obstruction, dyspnea and exercise capacity index in chronic obstructive pulmonary disease. *New England Journal of Medicine, 350,* 1005–1012.

Decramer, M., De Benedetto, F., Del Ponte, A., & Marinari, S. (2005). Systemic effects of COPD. *Respiratory Medicine, 99,* S3–S10.

Global Initiative for Chronic Obstructive Lung Disease (GOLD). (2009). *Global strategy for the diagnosis, management, and prevention of chronic obstructive pulmonary disease.* Retrieved from http://www.goldcopd.com/Guidelineitem.asp?l1=2&l2=1&intId=2003

Mannino, D. M., Homa, D. M., Akinbami, L. J., Ford, E. S., & Redd, S. C. (2002). Chronic obstructive pulmonary disease surveillance—United States, 1971–2000. *Morbidity and Mortality Weekly Review, 51*(SS06), 1–16. Retrieved from http://www.cdc.gov/mmwr/preview/mmwrhtml/ss5106a1.htm

National Health Interview Survey. (2007). Hyattsville, MD: National Center for Health Statistics. Unpublished data tabulated by National Heart, Lung and Blood Institute, 2009.

National Institutes of Health/National Heart, Lung and Blood Institute. (2009). *Morbidity & Mortality. 2009 Chart book on cardiovascular, lung and blood diseases.* Retrieved from http://www.nhlbi.nih.gov/resources/docs/2009_ChartBook.pdf

CHRONIC NONMALIGNANT PAIN MANAGEMENT

Kellie McNerney, JoAnne M. Saxe, and Kelly Pfeifer

I. Introduction and general background

This chapter examines nonpharmacologic treatments, non-opioid medications and the use of chronic opioid medication for the management of chronic nonmalignant pain (CNP). If nonpharmacologic agents and nonopiates fail to relieve pain, the subsequent use of opioids may be indicated. According to the 2009 American Pain Society Guidelines, "evidence is limited, but chronic pain can be effectively treated with chronic opioid therapy" (Chou et al., 2009, p. 1).

Also discussed are patient selection and risk evaluation, a strategy to initiate and monitor chronic opioid therapy, and informed consent and safety issues. One difficulty of managing opioid therapy for CNP patients is that clients may present with a history of risk behaviors, or a potential for or history of substance abuse (Passik & Weinreb, 2000). Definitions of substance use, including dependence, addiction, pseudo-addiction, substance abuse, physical dependence, and tolerance, are important for review and are included in Figure 48-1 (Federation of State Medical Boards of the United States, 2004). Patients with substance abuse history do have chronic pain, perhaps at a higher prevalence than the general population, but there are few studies that document this (Rosenblum et al., 2003). This chapter provides guidelines based on the American Pain Society recommendations for chronic opioid therapy, so that patients in higher-risk populations, including those with histories of substance abuse, can be safely treated (Chou et al., 2009).

The goal of therapy for the clinician is to provide adequate management of CNP in a timely, safe, and effective manner for the patient. The goal of therapy for the patient includes maximizing self-care strategies for pain management and control, optimizing function, and preventing untoward outcomes related to chronic pain (Caudill, 2009; Saxe et al., 2009).

A. Definition and overview

The International Association for the Study of Pain (IASP) defines pain as "an unpleasant sensory and emotional experience associated with actual or potential tissue damage, or described in terms of such damage. Pain is always subjective. Each individual learns the application of the word through experiences related to injury in early life . . ." (IASP, 2009). IASP further describes the subjective nature of pain as "Many people report[ing] pain in the absence of tissue damage or any likely pathophysiological cause; usually this happens for psychological reasons" (IASP). "If they regard their experience as pain and if they report it in the same ways as pain caused by tissue damage, it should be accepted as pain. This definition avoids tying pain to the stimulus" (IASP).

Chronic pain is defined as "pain that persists beyond the normal tissue healing time which is assumed to be three months" (IASP, 2009). Some authors use 6 months as the duration needed to meet the definition of chronic pain (Bedard, 1997; Barclay & Nghiem, 2008; Chou et al., 2009). Chronic pain may occur in the context of numerous diseases and syndromes. For the purpose of this guideline, all chronic pain disorders outside of cancer pain are referred to as CNP.

Chronic pain syndrome is a condition in which a client's pain "consumes and incapacitates his/her life to the point that the pain and suffering becomes his/her main focus" (Saxe et al., 2009, p. 1). Anxiety and depression are common comorbidities, and the client often has difficulty with their work and personal life (Pfeifer, 2006; Saxe et al.). Examples of CNP include but are not limited to osteoarthritis and rheumatoid arthritis; trigeminal and postherpetic neuralgia; fibromyalgia; myofascial pain; low back pain; peripheral neuropathy; phantom limb pain; reflex sympathetic dystrophy; sickle cell disease; temporomandibular joint dysfunction; chronic abdominal pain from such conditions as Crohn's disease or chronic pancreatitis; and headaches, including cluster, tension, and migraine.

B. Prevalence and costs

The prevalence of chronic pain in the general population of the United States has been estimated at between 10% and 35% or 70–105 million people (Rosenblum et al., 2003; Turk, 2006). An international survey of chronic pain revealed an overall prevalence of chronic pain as 22% of the population (Rosenblum et al.). Significant financial burden is attributed to this diagnosis because of loss of productivity and disability and the direct cost of physician visits and medication treatment (Turk, 2006). Costs associated with chronic pain have been estimated to be over $86 billion per year (Turk, 2002).

FIGURE 48-1 Definition of Terms

Addiction is often used interchangeably with substance abuse/dependence and is defined as: "A behavioral pattern of compulsive substance use for non-medical purposes despite the harmful effects. Individuals with addictions compulsively use drugs, are obsessive about securing their supply and have a high tendency to relapse after withdrawal. Compulsive use of controlled substances results in physical, psychological and social harm to the user. This individual seeks continued use despite that harm."

Pseudo-Addiction is the "iatrogenic syndrome resulting from the misinterpretation of relief seeking behaviors as though they are drug-seeking behaviors that are commonly seen with substance use disorders. The relief seeking behaviors resolve upon institution of effective analgesic therapy."

Physical Dependence and Tolerance may be normal physiologic consequences of extended opioid therapy and are not the same as addiction.

Signs of substance abuse and dependence may include some or all of following: Manipulative or abusive behavior directed at caregivers, including intimidation or coercion and aimed at acquisition and continuance of the substance abuse.

- Evidence of compulsive drug use, such as unsanctioned dose increases or unapproved uses, despite side effects.
- Chaotic psychosocial history
- Involvement with the law
- Diversion for sale or misuse of controlled substances
- Signs of poor personal habits, activities of independent living or social dysfunction.
- Physical or emotional deterioration and de-conditioning.

Source: Federation of State Medical Boards of the United States, 2004.

II. Database (may include but is not limited to)

A. Subjective

1. History of the presenting complaint
   The history of the presenting symptom should include the identification of pain: its source onset, location, radiation, duration, characteristics, alleviating factors, aggravating factors, treatments tried, and the response to treatments. The significance of pain (i.e., impact on work, relationships, and activities of daily living) should also be assessed. Pain and functional scales can be helpful in measuring the subjective report of pain (Figure 48-2).

2. Past health history
   a. Medical and psychiatric illnesses, surgical history, hospitalizations, and trauma in relation to the pain syndrome
   b. Medications: current and history of medications
   c. Medication allergies and drug interactions

3. Family history of chronic pain and mental health disorders

4. Occupational history: if pain occurred as a result of a job injury, note any related litigation issues, present ability to work, and goals for work in the future

5. Psychosocial history: to include substance abuse screening. A tool, such as the Cage-Aid (Brown & Rounds, 1995) or equivalent tool, may be used. The Cage-Aid can be downloaded from http://www.aafplearninglink.org/Resources/Upload/CAGE-AID.pdf

6. Review of systems
   a. Constitutional signs and symptoms: fatigue or weight gain
   b. Skin: scar tissue including trauma or surgical scars
   c. Cardiac: chest pain or arrhythmias (assessing risk for side effects or contraindication to medications including opiates)
   d. Respiratory: shortness of breath and sleep apnea (assessing risk for side effects or contraindications to opiates)
   e. Gastrointestinal: constipation
   f. Musculoskeletal: joint swelling or warmth, pain, arthralgias, myalgias, stiffness, and muscle wasting
   g. Neurologic: paresthesias, dysthesias, abnormal gait, muscle strength, symmetry, mood disorders, depression, and anxiety

B. Objective

1. The physical examination: focused on the areas affected, which typically includes the completion of musculoskeletal and neurologic examinations. The initial examination should also include a baseline cardiopulmonary examination, especially if opioids will be considered in the future.

2. Diagnostics

   a. Review pain and functional assessment tools, Patient Health Questionnaire–9 (Spitzer, Kroenke, & Williams, 1999) or equivalent (Figure 48-3), and substance use and abuse risk.

   b. Obtain baseline electrocardiogram for QTc interval measurement before methadone administration (Cohen & Mao, 2009; Krantz et al., 2009).

   c. Review pertinent laboratory studies and imaging or other radiologic examinations.

   d. Review any other relevant past medical documents or diagnostic tests.

III. Assessment

A. Determine the diagnosis (e.g., chronic right upper extremity pain x > 5 years) with appropriate International Classification of Diseases-9 codes (http://www.icd9cm.chrisendres.com)

B. Severity

Assess severity of symptoms (e.g., "moderate pain with frequent episodes of severe pain related to activity interfering with sleep and ability to work").

C. Significance and motivation

Assess significance of diagnosis in relation to functional capacity and mood, and support systems. Determine the

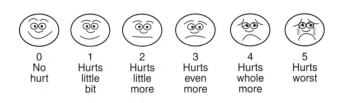

| 0 | 1 | 2 | 3 | 4 | 5 |
| No hurt | Hurts little bit | Hurts little more | Hurts even more | Hurts whole more | Hurts worst |

FIGURE 48-2 CNP Client Pain Questionnaire

Source: From Hockenberry, M. J., Wilson, D.: *Wong's essentials of pediatric nursing*, ed. 8, St. Louis, 2009, Mosby. Used with permission. Copyright Mosby.

client's strengths, ability to follow the treatment plan, and risk for nonadherence.

IV. Goals of clinical management

A. To minimize pain and pain-related distress and disability

B. To decrease related depression and anxiety

C. To improve and maximize patient functioning in relationships, at work, or at home

V. Plan (interventions and ongoing approach to care)

A. Nonmedication strategies include but are not limited to:

1. Cognitive behavioral therapy

   a. Stress reduction
   b. Relaxation techniques
   c. Attention diversion
   d. Goal setting
   e. Pain and symptom diary

2. Physical activity and physical therapy

3. Transcutaneous electrical nerve stimulation unit

4. Heat and cold therapies

5. Pain support group

6. Acupuncture

7. Massage

8. Guided imagery techniques

9. Laugh therapy and laugh yoga (American Pain Society, 2005; Barclay & Nghiem, 2008; Caudill, 2009; Keefe, Somers, & Kothadia, 2009)

B. Nonopiate medication strategies (Barclay, 2008; Caudill, 2009)

1. Acetaminophen: for mild to moderate pain 325–500 mg, one to two tablets, four times daily, not to exceed 4 g/day. Caution with liver disease, alcohol use, hepatitis, and use of other medications metabolized by the liver.

2. Nonsteroidal anti-inflammatory medication (NSAIDs): for mild to moderate pain, may use in conjunction with acetaminophen. Review specific

FIGURE 48-3 Patient Health Questionnaire-9

Client Name: _____ Chart No. _____ Date: _____

Over the last 2 weeks, how often have you been bothered by any of the following problems?	Not at All	Several Days	More than Half the Days	Nearly Every Day
1. Little interest or pleasure in doing things	0	1	2	3
2. Feeling down, depressed, or hopeless	0	1	2	3
3. Trouble falling or staying asleep, or sleeping too much	0	1	2	3
4. Feeling tired or having little energy	0	1	2	3
5. Poor appetite or overeating	0	1	2	3
6. Feeling bad about yourself — or that you are a failure or have let yourself or your family down	0	1	2	3
7. Trouble concentrating on things, such as reading the newspaper or watching television	0	1	2	3
8. Moving or speaking so slowly that other people could have noticed? Or the opposite — being so fidgety or restless that you have been moving around a lot more than usual	0	1	2	3
9. Thoughts that you would be better off dead or of hurting yourself in some way	0	1	2	3

For office coding

0 + _____ + _____ + _____

= Total Score: _____

If you checked off *any* problems, how *difficult* have these problems made it for you to do your work, take care of things at home, or get along with other people?

❏ Not difficult at all   ❏ Somewhat difficult   ❏ Very difficult   ❏ Extremely difficult

PHQ-9 Scoring
For health care professional use

Total Score	Depression Severity
1-4	Minimal Depression
5-9*	Mild Depression
10-14*	Moderate Depression
15-19*	Moderately Severe Depression
20-27*	Severe Depression

* For any score 5 and above offer referral for Behavioral Health Services

medication because dose and timing vary depending on medication. Note precautions associated with hypertension, diabetes, benign prostatic hypertrophy, and individuals older than 50 years of age. NSAIDs are contraindicated in gastrointestinal ulcer disease and chronic kidney disease. Examples include ibuprofen, 400–800 mg every 6–8 hours yet not to exceed a total of 2,400 mg per 24 hours; diflunisal, 500–1,000 mg twice daily; or naproxen, 250–500 mg twice daily. If one class fails, consider switching to another class of NSAIDs (e.g., switching from a nonselective cyclooxygenase inhibitor (e.g., ibuprofen) to a salicylic acid derivative (e.g., trilisate propionic acids) or a selective cyclooxygenase inhibitor (e.g., celecoxib).

3. Topical analgesic creams and patches: for mild to moderate pain, may be used in conjunction with acetaminophen and NSAIDs. Dose varies and is dependent on analgesia desired and individual patient response. Examples include lidocaine 5% patches, up to three patches to the affected area at once for 12 hours within a 24-hour period; lidocaine 4% cream; or capsaicin cream 0.025–0.075%, applied to the affected area up to three to four times daily.

4. Antidepressants: chronic pain can cause depression or may worsen depression. Additionally, depression can worsen with chronic pain. As such, antidepressants may be a useful adjunctive therapy. The specific class of tricyclic antidepressants is helpful for neuropathic pain disorders and sleep disturbance. A baseline electrocardiogram is indicated before initiating this classification of medication to assess for any conduction abnormalities because they may cause arrhythmias. Start with a low dose and titrate up over several weeks. Some antidepressants can change the potency of opiates. Be certain to check for medication interactions.

5. Anticonvulsants: have been used for neuropathic pain, such as diabetic neuropathy and postherpetic neuralgias. Examples include gabapentin, 300–600 mg three times a day. Start at 300 mg at bedtime, titrate up 300 mg weekly. Use with caution in renal insufficiency. Pregabalin (Lyrica®), start 50–150 mg dependent on severity of pain; postherpetic neuralgia may require 150 mg to start, diabetic neuropathy only 50 mg to start. May titrate up to three times a day.

6. Other adjunctive medications: muscle relaxants. Avoid carisoprodol because of abuse potential and availability of other muscle relaxants. Examples include baclofen, 5–20 mg three times daily, or cyclobenzeprine, 5–10 mg three times daily.

C. Opiates

1. Standards for prescribing controlled substances

    The clinician follows the accepted standards for prescribing controlled substances. For example, in the State of California, nurse practitioners and nurse midwives are expected to follow Standardized Procedures for Controlled Substances (Figure 48-4).

2. Starting opiates

    The following recommendations for starting opiates, if indicated, are based on CNP protocols from the Petaluma Health Center (Pfeifer, 2006, adapted with permission from Brian Williams' protocols from Hamakua Health Center) and a San Francisco Community Clinic Consortium Pain Clinic consultant (Berman, 2008) as adapted by Glide Health Services (Saxe et al., 2009) and the American Pain Society, chronic opioid treatment guidelines (2009).

    a. New clients require sufficient visits to complete a full history and physical and to review all prior medical records, pain and functioning questionnaires, depression and substance abuse screenings with appropriate laboratory studies, imaging, and urine drug screen.

    b. A mental health evaluation visit is recommended during this establishment of care. Opiates are not prescribed until these procedures are complete and 30 days have passed. Exceptions can be made if the provider has access to the patient's previous records and, ideally, have been approved by a chronic pain treatment team.

    c. Existing patients receiving primary care may be given a trial of opioid therapy before enrolling in CNP protocol if the primary care provider deems the patient is a candidate for opioid therapy. If the provider believes therapy will be chronic, the provider obtains and completes the same pain questionnaire and depression and substance abuse screening required for adherence to the protocol (e.g., Cage-Aid [Brown & Rounds, 1995], which can be accessed at http://www.aafplearninglink.org/Resources/Upload/CAGE-AID.pdf).

    d. Enrollment in a CNP protocol is indicated if the clinician deems that opioid therapy is appropriate for care. The following matters are discussed with the patient and family in depth, including a signed CNP treatment agreement plan (Figure 48-5):

        i. The prescribed treatment plan, which includes a discussion about associated risks and benefits of opioid treatment, medications to be used, nonopioid

FIGURE 48-4 Furnishing and Ordering Controlled Substances from Schedule II–V at the UCSF DCHS Faculty Practices

I. **POLICY:**

    A. Only nurse practitioners with current furnishing licenses and DEA registration for ordering schedule II–V CS (see Addendum) may furnish these drugs and devices.

    B. The qualified nurse practitioner may initiate, alter, discontinue, and renew category II–V CS included in the UCSF DCHS Faculty Practices Formulary.

    C. As described in the Policies and in the "Furnishing/Ordering Drugs and Devices by Nurse Practitioners" Standardized Procedure.

II. **PROTOCOL**

    A. Definition: This protocol covers the management of Schedule II–V CS for all adults and children seen in the UCSF DCHS Faculty Practices with the following conditions, illnesses, diseases:

        1. Acute traumatic injuries,

        2. Acute infections (e.g., pyelonephritis),

        3. Acute and chronic musculoskeletal disorders,

        4. Acute and chronic neurological disorders (e.g., migraines),

        5. Chronic psychological disorders (e.g., ADHD),

        6. Acute urological conditions (e.g., renal calculi), and/or

        7. Post-surgical pain.

    B. Subjective Data: Subjective information will include but is not limited to:

        1. Relevant health history to warrant the use of the drug or device.

        2. No allergic history to the drug or device.

        3. No past health, family and/or personal-social history, which are an absolute and/or potential for contraindication to the use of the drug or device.

    C. Objective: Objective information will include but is not limited to:

        1. A physical examination to indicate/contraindicate the use of the drug and/or device.

        2. Diagnostics: Laboratory tests or procedures to determine the underlying etiology of pain and/or to indicate/contraindicate use of the drug and/or device, if needed.

    D. Assessment: Subjective and objective data supports the use of the drug and/or device. Contraindications, safety issues, and/or cost concerns have been adequately assessed and documented.

    E. Management:

        1. Diagnostics: Ordering relevant laboratory/diagnostic studies.

        2. Treatment:

            a. The following medications may be used:

                1. Opioid agonists (For example but not limited to: Morphine, morphine controlled–release, hydromorphone, levorphanol, meperidine, methadone, oxymorphone, codeine (with or without aspirin or acetaminophen), hydrocodone, oxycodone or oxycodone controlled-release): Use the guidelines noted in the current UCSF DCHS FP Formulary Guidelines for drug dosage, frequency, route of administration. Schedule II opioid agonist analgesics should be reserved for severe, incapacitating pain. Schedule III opioid agonists should be used for moderate to severe pain.

                2. Stimulants (For example but not limited to: Mixed salts of dextroamphetamine and amphetamines, dextroamphetamine sulfate, atomoxetine, methylphenidate, and pemoline): Use the guidelines noted in the current UCSF DCHS Faculty Practices Formulary Guidelines on page 27.

            b. Drug/device order: Write a separate drug order for each Schedule II–V CS on anti-fraud prescription form. (Note: Telephone orders are acceptable for Schedule III through V CS.) Each order needs to include:

                1. Name, age, telephone number, and the medical record number of the client,

                2. Name of the medication/device,

FIGURE 48-4 Furnishing and Ordering Controlled Substances from Schedule II–V at the UCSF DCHS Faculty Practices (continued)

3. Dosage, frequency, route, duration of the use, amount; and number of refills of the drug/device (Note: CS II may not be refilled. Schedule III CS may only be filled 5 times in a 6 month period),

4. Brief statement regarding the reason for using the drug/device,

5. Printed name, furnishing number, DEA number and signature of the nurse practitioner; and

6. Printed name of the supervising physician.

  c. Supportive/Adjunctive Therapy:

1. Consider using tricyclic antidepressants, sustained-release bupropion, or anticonvulsants for neuropathic pain since these medications may be more effective in managing the pain as compared to opioids.

2. Recommend non-pharmacologic therapies (e.g., thermal therapy, massage, physical therapy, chiropractic, acupuncture, and meditation) as indicated since these modalities may be useful in pain management.

3. Client Education:

  a. Provide the client and/or the client's caregiver with the information and counseling in regards to the action and use of the drug/device. Caution the client and/or the client's caregiver on the pertinent side effects and complications with the chosen drug/device. Advise on how to communicate with the Clinic staff should s/he have any questions/concerns/side effects/complications.

4. Physician Consultation/Referral:

Consult or refer to physician if the client is:

  a. Unresponsive to the drug/device therapy,

  b. Demonstrating unusual or unexpected side effects,

  c. Known to have a history of CS and/or alcohol abuse; and as indicated in the general policy section.

5. Follow-up: In accordance with standard practice or with consulting physician's recommendation.

6. Record keeping: As described in General Policies.

Addendum

Federal Narcotics Law

Federal Narcotics Law: The Federal Controlled Substances Act of 1970 recognized five schedules of drugs based upon their relative abuse potential (Note: California State regulatory requirements have been added.):

Class I: Drugs with no current medical application and maximum abuse potential. Examples: Heroin, lysergic acid diethylamide (LSD), marijuana, 3, 4 methylenedioxymethamphetamine (MDMA [Ecstasy]).

Class II: Includes opioid analgesics (e.g., morphine, methadone, oxycodone, hydrocodone), stimulants (e.g., dextroamphetamine, cocaine, methylphenidate), and depressants (e.g., pentobarbital).Facsimile of Schedule II CS permitted under certain circumstances (e.g., hospice care). Facsimile for emergency dispensing must be followed up with a written and signed transmittal order within 7 days. Refills are prohibited.

Class III: Codeine, hydrocodone, and other opioids in lower doses, in combination products such as Vicodin®, Norco®, and Tylenol #3®. May communicate to pharmacist Schedule III-V CS prescriptions/transmittal orders either orally, in writing, or by facsimile.

Class IV: benzodiazepines (e.g., Valium®, Ativan®, Xanax®, Klonopin®), stimulants such as phentermine. Written prescription required, up to 5 refills allowed within 6 months of issuance for this class.

Class V: Cough medicines with codeine in low dose (Robitussin-AC®). May refill Schedule III-IV's 5 times in 6 months; and refills of Schedule V's as noted by the practitioner.

IMPORTANT: Refills for schedule II medications or future dated prescriptions are not allowed by the Drug Enforcement Agency.

Source: State of California Board of Registered Nursing, 1998, 2004a, 2004b; University of California San Francisco [UCSF], Department of Community Health Systems [DCHS], 2010.

FIGURE 48-5 Pain Management Agreement

Glide Health Services
330 Ellis Street
San Francisco, CA 94102

The purpose of this agreement is to prevent misunderstandings about certain medicines you will be taking for pain management or other medical conditions. This agreement will help both you and your provider comply with laws regarding controlled pharmaceuticals.

I, _____ and _____ have decided together to use a
             Client Name   *Provider Name*

controlled substance for management of pain or other medical condition.

MEDICATION	INSTRUCTIONS	AMOUNT PER WEEK/MONTH

✓ I agree that this medication will only be used by myself and as it is prescribed.

✓ I will not share, sell or trade my medication with anyone.

✓ I will safeguard my medication from loss or theft. Lost or stolen medicine may not be replaced.

✓ If I run out of the medication, Glide Health Services may not refill the prescription early.

✓ I will not seek controlled substances from other medical providers.

✓ I understand that there will be no refills on my medications without a provider visit at Glide.

✓ I agree to share my complete medications history in order to avoid adverse drug interactions.

✓ I will attend all my scheduled appointments, including any referral appointments my clinician has made for me, and follow up as designated in my plan of care.

✓ I agree to bring all unused pain medication to every office visit.

✓ I understand pharmacy records may be reviewed to confirm prescriptions.

✓ I understand I may be required to have random urine or blood testing completed. I agree to this testing, and understand that if I fail to do so, I will be safely tapered off the medication(s).

✓ **I understand if I break this agreement, my provider may stop prescribing these pain medicines.**

✓ **I understand that many pain medicines may cause drowsiness and impair my ability to drive and operate machinery and may impair my thinking and judgment.**

✓ **I understand that misuse of these drugs or use of these drugs in combination with alcohol, unauthorized prescription medications, or illicit drugs may have serious effects including death.**

The prescribing provider has explained that the above medications have possible side effects and may be addictive.

Comments:

_____

_____

_____

_____   _____
Client's Signature   *Date*

_____   _____
Provider Signature   *Date*

therapies to be pursued, and the follow-up interval.

ii. Patient expectations and responsibilities including keeping appointments, adherence to treatment plans, obtaining medications from a single provider, single pharmacy, feedback to provider, and legal issues including diversion.

iii. How to take the medication and importance of dosing and timing of dose and interaction with other medications.

iv. Potential adverse effects of treatment with opioid medication including safety and not driving, and not operating equipment until the patient is tolerant of the medication regime. Other adverse effects include the potential for altered mentation, respiratory depression, and arrhythmias, and the risk of death if used incorrectly or in conjunction with other substances.

v. A review and provision of prophylactic treatment for constipation caused by opiates, because untreated constipation can worsen back and abdominal pain.

vi. Random urine testing is required for all patients on opioid therapy. Because the interpretation of urine tests is frequently misunderstood, providing interpretation guides and training for all providers is strongly recommended. Gourlay, Heit, and Caplan (2010) have noted important de-tails related to this matter at http://issuu.com/cafp.sc/docs/udtmonograph6.3

vii. The procedure for CNP protocol treatment agreement, and minor and major contract breaks, is reviewed including consequences of breaks.

3. Subsequent evaluations

   Subsequent visits are determined by the clinician but initially may be monthly. More frequent visits may be required at the provider's discretion. Exceptions may be made for low-risk clients with stable housing situations. These low-risk patients should be seen every 2–3 months at a minimum. The provider makes this determination after at least 2 months of contact and assessment.

   a. All patients leave a urine sample on monthly or routine follow-up visits but it is up to the provider to determine if urine toxicology screens are done randomly on that visit (Chou et al., 2009; Saxe et al., 2009).

   b. Clinical encounters include an assessment of:

      i. Pain: intensity and response to treatment plan (Figure 48-2)

      ii. Adverse events and side effects of therapy

      iii. Activity and functioning level to evaluate efficacy of treatment plan

      iv. Adherence to essential components of treatment agreement is documented with nonadherence to plan of care and documentation of minor or major contract break on the problem list. Specific plans for addressing contract breaks should be discussed and documented. For example, a setting may consider adopting the following approach: any client with more than two major contract breaks or three minor breaks will be referred for evaluation to a CNP team to determine appropriate action to follow.

   c. Refills of medications are documented in the electronic health record or paper chart to include date, name of opiate, dose, instructions for use, quantity prescribed, and number of refills. The patient brings all pain medication bottles to each and every visit at the request of the provider.

   d. One primary provider writes prescriptions. In their absence, an alternate or covering provider is determined. This arrangement is reviewed with the patient.

   e. Refills on controlled substances should be done during the visit with only enough medication to last until the next visit.

   f. Refills are not completed without an appointment or over the telephone.

   g. Lost medications or stolen medications should not be replaced and recorded as a major contract break. With rare exceptions, providers do not routinely refill lost or stolen medications. Exceptions by provider discretion require documentation of the rationale, and the incident must be recorded as a minor contract break.

   h. A treatment plan for addressing adverse effects is discussed and documented.

4. Medication considerations

   a. Note contraindications to opioid therapy

      i. Absolute contraindications

         a. Allergy to opiate agents

         b. Coadministration of drug capable of inducing life-threatening drug–drug interaction

         c. Active diversion of controlled substances

         d. Unwillingness or inability to comply with treatment plan

         e. Unwillingness to adjust to at-risk activities resulting in serious reinjury

ii. Relative contraindications (prescribe with caution, and more intensive monitoring)

a. Meets criteria for current substance use disorder (e.g., as noted by the *Diagnostic and Statistical Manual of Mental Disorders* [American Psychological Association, 2000])

b. Acute psychiatric instability or high suicide risk

c. History of intolerance, serious adverse effects, or lack of efficacy of opioid therapy

d. Inability to manage opioid therapy responsibly (i.e., cognitive impairment)

e. Severe social instability or inability to manage medications safely

f. Client with sleep apnea not on continuous positive airway pressure machine

g. Elderly clients

b. Assess and address common adverse affects of opioid therapy: constipation, nausea and vomiting, itching, sweating, peripheral edema, urinary retention, myoclonus, hyperalgesia, dyspepsia, changes in cognition, perceptual or affective adverse effects, or sexual dysfunction

c. Short-acting opiates: short-acting medications should not be the mainstay of chronic pain treatment; consider not prescribing short-acting medications, or limiting to one dose at most per day. Short-acting medications for CNP are appropriate in the following situations

i. To manage breakthrough pain during dose adjustments for long-acting medications (starting new medications or transitioning from one to another)

ii. To manage predictable pain flares (long travel or before exercise, dental appointments, and so forth)

iii. To manage chronic pain in patients who do not need high doses of medications (e.g., elderly patients may do well with hydrocodone/acetaminophen, 5/500 mg half a tablet four times daily on a schedule, plus half a tablet as needed for additional pain)

iv. Potency varies considerably; see analgesic comparison tables at http://www.global rph.com/narcoticonv.htm for assistance with converting from one opiate to another, and converting short-acting to long-acting opiates (McAuley, 2009). Cost varies considerably; many are now available as a generic.

v. Short-acting medications are not recommended for chronic pain because of high-risk metabolites (e.g., meperidine/Demerol®); low efficacy (e.g., propoxyphene/Darvocet®); or risk of rebound headaches (e.g., butalbital/Fioricet®).

vi. Types of short-acting opiates (Table 48-1)

d. Long-acting opiates: Long-acting medications should be the primary therapy for patients using opiates for chronic pain. For all patients (especially the elderly), start with low doses and build up slowly, because sedation and respiratory depression can occur with too-rapid dose escalation. Short-acting medications can be used as a "bridge" to manage pain

TABLE 48-1 Short-Acting Opiates

Medication	Strengths	Comments
Hydrocodone combined with acetaminophen or ibuprofen	5-, 7.5-, and 10-mg tablets	Caution: keep acetaminophen dose under 4,000 mg daily, or 2,000 mg in the elderly (e.g., write "max 8 in 24 hours" if 500-mg acetaminophen per tablet).
Oxycodone combined with acetaminophen or aspirin	2.5-, 5-, 7.5-, and 10-mg	Also available in extended release. Caution: keep acetaminophen dose under 4,000 mg daily, or 2,000 mg in the elderly. Approximately 10% of patients do not metabolize oxycodone well and will not get effective pain relief; consider changing opiates if there is a poor response (Chou et al., 2009).
Codeine combined with acetaminophen	30/300 or 60/300	Caution: keep acetaminophen dose under 4,000 mg daily, or 2,000 mg in the elderly.
Morphine	15 and 30 mg	Also available in long-acting form.
Hydromorphone	2, 4, and 8 mg	
Fentanyl transmucosal lozenge	100-, 200-, 400-, 600-, and 800-mcg buccal tablets	Typically used for cancer pain because of rapid action, occasionally used for chronic pain. It is expensive.
Oxymorphone	5 and 10 mg	Also available as extended release

until the correct dose of long-acting medications is determined, and then the short-acting medications can be discontinued. Types of long-acting opiates are provided in Table 48-2.

e. Changing from short-acting to long-acting medications: Changing from short-acting to long-acting medications is the standard of care for chronic pain, because short-acting medications have increased dependence and addiction potential and increased street value, with an increased risk of diversion. Short-acting opiates also may not control baseline pain and require a greater total dose of medications to control pain (Chou et al., 2009; Pfeifer, 2006).

TABLE 48-2 Long-Acting Opiates

Medication	Strengths	Comments
Morphine sulfate (sustained/extended release): examples include Kadian® and MS Contin®	Kadian® (sustained-release pellets in capsules): 10-, 20-, 30-, 50-, 60-, 80-, 100-, and 200-mm capsules MS Contin® (sustained-release tablets): 15-, 30-, 60-, 100-, and 200-mm tablets	Dose varies by product, generally daily to twice a day. Often preferred by providers because diversion potential is lower.
Methadone	5- and 10-mg tablets	Methadone is an appropriate medication for severe pain for patients with CNP, even in opioid-tolerant patients. Titrate up very slowly because methadone has a very long and "highly variable" half-life (Chou et al., 2009). Get a baseline ECG to measure QTc interval, recommend a repeat in 30 days and an ECG early or more frequently at doses over 100 mg daily, because fatal arrhythmias can occur if patients develop long QTc intervals (Krantz et al., 2009). Safe starting dose for opioid-naive patient is 2.5 mg every 8 hours. Increase medication weekly, not more frequently. Use cautious titration and dosing (e.g., consider starting with half-tablets) in the elderly or patients with renal or hepatic dysfunction (Chou et al., 2009). Although withdrawal symptoms are prevented in daily dosing (for methadone clinics), and the half-life is long, the pain relief is at most 8 hours; dosing must be at least every 8–12 hours when prescribing methadone for pain.
Oxycodone controlled release	10-, 15-, 20-, 30-, 40-, 60-, and 80-mm controlled-release tablets	10% of people do not metabolize this drug well, so they do not feel effective relief (Chou et al., 2009). Consider transition to another opiate for patients who request escalation of dose because of inadequate pain control. Considered to have a high street value.
Fentanyl patch	12, 25, 50, 75, and 100 mcg/h patch	The fentanyl patch is not indicated for opiate-naive patients. Change the patch every 48–72 hours (some patients report difficulty with adherence and pain relief after 48 hours). Start at lower doses and start cautiously because of the long half-life. Initial fentanyl transdermal doses are based on daily total morphine requirements for individuals already on opiates. The total daily dosing is then moderately reduced, usually 25–50% (Chou et al., 2009). Considered to have a high street value.
Hydromorphone	Has numerous strengths with short-acting and extended release formulations	It is not commonly used in some community clinics.
Buprenorphine	2- and 8-mg sublingual tablets	This opiate agonist–antagonist is not approved by the Food and Drug Administration for pain, yet some patients with mixed addiction and chronic pain do well on this option. Although prescribed for addiction, they can get some pain relief. Requires special Food and Drug Administration license and training.

Equianalgesic tables provide helpful guidelines with the conversion of dosing between different types of opiates, yet they do not factor in individual patient factors that influence safe dosing (Vissers, Besse, Hans, Devulder, & Morlion, 2010). As such, it has been recommended by notable authorities to reduce dosing on these tables by one-third to two-thirds of the stated dosing (Vissers et al.). A well-referenced web-based opiate conversion chart can be found at http://www.globalrph.com/narcoticonv.htm (McAuley, 2009).

f. Indications to stop opiate therapy: Medication use agreement noncompliance or contract breaks

    i. Institutions differ on the definition of contract breaks and the consequences. At the authors' institution, the number of minor and major contract breaks that require action is defined (Saxe et al., 2009). Examples of minor contract breaks include missed appointments, early refill requests, seeking medications from another provider or different pharmacy, and not adhering to treatment agreement plans.

    ii. Major contract breaks include refusal of urine toxicology screen; lost or stolen medications; drug screening (with high-sensitivity confirmation, such as gas chromatography) indicating that the prescribed medication is absent despite client statements of recent ingestion; client is abusive to staff; pill count discrepancy; or request for pill count is refused.

    iii. Institution has in place consequences of contract breaks; for example, two major contract breaks may be grounds for review by a CNP team and consideration for addiction referral and discontinuation of opioid therapy. Unless there has been fraud or multiple prescribers, consider a standard policy of weaning as opposed to abrupt discontinuation. This increases the chance that the patient will continue to work with the team on other options (complementary treatments, behavioral therapy, and addiction treatment) as opposed to just seeking another provider, and it decreases the likelihood of emergency department visits for withdrawal symptoms. Pharmacies can be instructed to dispense small supplies at a time (a 1-, 3-, or 7-day supply) to assist the weaning

plan (Berman, 2008; Pfeifer, 2006; Saxe et al., 2009).

    iv. Inappropriate use of alcohol or illicit drugs may be considered a major contract break or cause for termination. Some institutional flexibility may be spelled out per chronic pain team. For example, rather than termination, the client must agree to a mental health evaluation and commit to a drug treatment cessation program to continue treatment.

    v. Opioid therapy may be discontinued for patients with multiple minor contract breaks or at the provider's discretion. Otherwise the patient is evaluated by the primary provider frequently until adherence problems have resolved. Final determination to address repetitive contract breaks is made by a CNP team or medical director (Berman, 2008; Pfeifer, 2006; Saxe et al., 2009).

    vi. Opioid therapy is discontinued when the therapy or side effects of the therapy are a greater detriment than benefit as determined by consultation with the client, family, and CNP team.

    vii. Opioid therapy is discontinued if evaluation demonstrates lack of efficacy, the client desires to discontinue therapy, or the cause of pain has resolved.

    viii. Opioid therapy is discontinued when there are serious safety issues as a result of treatment.

    ix. When opioid therapy is discontinued, opioid is tapered and weaned off, unless there is dangerous or illegal behavior. Opioid therapy should be immediately discontinued for unsafe use of medications, diversion of prescription of medication, or alteration or forgery of prescriptions. Provider should treat withdrawal symptoms with noncontrolled medications or refer for addiction counseling (Chou et al., 2009; Saxe et al., 2009).

    x. Clients that have been dismissed from opiate treatment for contract breaks may not receive prescriptions for controlled substances from other providers at the same institution unless that client is first reviewed by a CNP team and approved for renewal of treatment, with a plan in place to address the previous cause of dismissal (Saxe et al., 2009).

5. Referral to mental health and substance abuse

Referral to mental health and substance abuse services for further management is recommended for the following indications:
   a. Patients with a past or current history of behaviors suggestive of substance abuse disorder. It is recommended to include this statement in the patient's treatment agreement.
   b. Patients with psychosocial problems that hinder treatment of pain.
   c. Patients with a diagnosis of depression, anxiety, or other mental health disorders.
   d. Provider's discretion: all patients may benefit from learning cognitive behavioral techniques to improve self-care and function.

6. Consultation with pain specialist or addiction specialist:

Consultation with pain specialist or addiction specialist is indicated when:
   a. Patients who have significant chronic, substantiated pain that develops addiction behaviors in the context of chronic opioid therapy (IASP, 2009; Saxe et al., 2009).
   b. The patient is not well-controlled on current pain treatment plan.
   c. The provider determines the need for consultation.
   d. All consultation is documented as part of the patient record. Not all patients have access to pain management specialists because of financial, insurance, location, availability, and transportation barriers. In these circumstances, review of the case with a CNP team or review of the case with pain specialists by email or telephone consult may be appropriate (Saxe et al., 2009).

VI. Patient education

A. *Assist the patient and family in understanding and coping with chronic pain, and steps of care in terms of CNP protocol*
   1. Provide verbal and written information regarding chronic pain and nonpharmacologic and pharmacologic treatments.
   2. Assist the patient and family in obtaining all prior medical records and diagnostics, and facilitate the request for prior medical records.

B. *Provide self-care strategies as mentioned in nonpharmacologic management of chronic pain*

C. *Discuss management rationale for:*
   1. Nonpharmacologic and nonopiate strategies as first-line treatment and progression to opiates if indicated
   2. CNP team rationale and CNP protocol

D. *Review the individual treatment agreement If the patient proceeds to the CNP protocol*
   1. Discuss medication(s): dose; schedule of dosing; side effects of medications; and safety of activity on medication (e.g., driving or swimming), including risk of death if medications are used incorrectly or combined with substances or dangerous activity.
   2. Provide an explanation that one provider prescribes and one pharmacy dispenses, patient responsibility for managing medications safely, keeping appointments, and random urine screening.
   3. Provide an overview of and the need for signing the individual treatment plan or pain agreement (Figure 48-5).
   4. Discuss the need for documenting the consequences of nonadherence to the treatment plan including discontinuation

E. *Encourage chronic pain support groups*

F. *Encourage mental health provider evaluation for ongoing support*

VII. Chronic pain support resources and tools

A. *American Pain Society: www.ampainsoc.org*

B. *International Association for Study of Pain: www.iasp.org*

C. *Laughter Yoga International: www.laughteryoga.org*

D. *Self-help book, Managing pain before it manages you (Caudill, 2009)*

E. *Kaiser Permanente Chronic Pain Program and Support Group*

REFERENCES

American Pain Society. (2005). Guideline for management of fibromyalgia pain syndrome in adults and children. *APS Clinical Practice Guideline Series, 4.* Retrieved from www.ampainsoc.org/bu/fibromyalgia.htm

American Pain Society (2009). *Guideline for the use of chronic opioid therapy in chronic noncancer pain: Evidence review.* Retrieved at http://www.ampainsoc.org/library/pdf/Opioid_Final_Evidence_Report.pdf

American Psychological Association. (2000). *Diagnostic and statistical manual of mental disorders* (4th ed.). Arlington, VA: American Psychological Association.

Barclay, L., & Nghiem, H. T. (2008). Primary care management of nonmalignant pain reviewed. *Medscape Medical News, Continuing Medical Education.* Retrieved from http://cme.medscape.com/viewarticles/584508

Bedard, M. E. (1997). *Fact sheet on chronic non-malignant pain (CNP).* American Society for Action on Pain. Retrieved from http://www.druglibrary.org/schaeffer/asap/factsheet.html

Berman, P. (2008). *South of Market Health Center chronic non-malignant pain management protocol* (unpublished protocol). San Francisco, CA: South of Market Health Center.

Brown, R. L., & Rounds, L. A. (1995). Conjoint screening questionnaires for alcohol and other drug abuse: Criterion validity in a primary care practice. *Wisconsin Medical Journal, 94*(3), 135–140.

Caudill, M. A. (2009). *Managing pain before it manages you* (3rd ed.). New York, NY: Guilford Press.

Chou, R., Fanciullo, G., Fine, P., Adler, J. A., Ballantyne, J. C., Davies, P., . . . Miaskowski, C. (2009). Clinical guidelines for the use of chronic opioid therapy in chronic noncancer pain. *The Journal of Pain, 10*(2), 113–130.

Cohen, S. P., & Mao, J. (2009). Concerns about consensus guidelines for QTc interval screening in methadone treatment, letters. *Annals of Internal Medicine, 151*(3), 216–217. Retrieved from http://www.annals.org/content/151/3/216.2.full

Federation of State Medical Boards of the United States, Inc. (2004). *Model policy for the use of controlled substances for the treatment of pain.* Retrieved from http://www.fsmb.org/pdf/2004_grpol_controlled_substances.pdf

Gourlay, D., Heit, H. A., & Caplan (2010). Urine drug testing in clinical practice (4th cd.). Retrieved at http://issuu.com/cafp.sc/docs/udtmonograph6.3

IASP. (2009). Recommendations for pain treatment services. Retrieved from http://www.iasp-pain.org

Keefe, F. J., Somers, T. J., & Kothadia, S. M. (2009). Coping with pain. *Pain Clinical Update, 17*(5), 1–6. Retrieved from http://www.iasp-pain.org/AM/Template.cfm?Section=Home&Template=/CM/ContentDisplay.cfm&ContentID=9596

Krantz, M. J., Martin, J., Stimmel, B., Metha, D., & Haigney, M. C. P. (2009). QTc interval screening in methadone treatment. *Annals of Internal Medicine, 150*(6), 387–399. Retrieved from http://www.annals.org/content/150/6/387.full?sid=c75d1581-ab55-4a55-999c-5632ebd20b92

McAuley, D. F. (2009). Opioid (narcotic) analgesic converter. Retrieved from http://www.globalrph.com/narcoticonv.htm

Passik, S. D., & Weinreb, H. J. (2000). Managing chronic non-malignant pain: Overcoming obstacles to the use of opioids. *Advances in Therapy, 17*(2), 70–80.

Pfeifer, K. (2006). *Petaluma Health Center chronic nonmalignant pain management protocol* (unpublished protocol). Petaluma, CA: Petaluma Health Center.

Rosenblum, A., Joseph, H., Fong, C., Kipnis, S., Cleland, C., & Portenoy, R. K. (2003). Prevalence and characteristics of chronic pain among chemically dependent patients in methadone maintenance and residential treatment facilities. *Journal of the American Medical Association, 289*(18), 2370–2378. Retrieved from http://jama.ama-assn.org/content/289/18/2370.full

Saxe, J. M., Smith, V., Ligon, E. D., McNerney, K., Hill, K., & Nierman, J. (2009). *Glide Health Services chronic nonmalignant pain management protocol* (unpublished protocol). San Francisco, CA: Glide Health Services.

Spitzer, R. L., Kroenke, K., & Williams, J. B. W. (1999). Validation and utility of a self-report version of PRIME-MD: The PHQ primary care study. *Journal of the American Medical Association, 282*(18), 1737–1744.

State of California Board of Registered Nursing. (1998). *An explanation of standardized procedure requirements for nurse practitioner practice.* Retrieved from http://www.rn.ca.gov/pdfs/regulations/npr-b-20.pdf

State of California Board of Registered Nursing. (2004a). *Nurse practitioner expanded furnishing authority for schedule II controlled substances, BPC 2836.1.* Retrieved from http://www.rn.ca.gov/pdfs/regulations/npr-b-51.pdf

State of California Board of Registered Nursing. (2004b). *Criteria for furnishing number utilization by nurse practitioners.* Retrieved from http://www.rn.ca.gov/pdfs/regulations/npr-i-16.pdf

Turk, D. C. (2002). Clinical effectiveness and cost-effectiveness of treatments for patients with chronic pain. *Clinical Journal of Pain, 18*, 355–365.

Turk, D. (2006). Pain hurts-individual, significant others and society! *American Pain Society Bulletin, 16*(1). Retrieved from http://www.ampainsoc.org/pub/bulletinwin06/pres1./html

Vissers, K. C., Besse, K., Hans, G., Devulder, J., & Morlion, B. (2010). Opioid rotation in the management of chronic pain: Where is the evidence? *Pain Practice, 10*(2), 85–93.

CHRONIC VIRAL HEPATITIS

Miranda Surjadi

I. Introduction and general background

The liver is one of the largest organs in the body, weighing approximately 1–1.5 kg. Most cells in the liver consist of hepatocytes. Hepatocytes are responsible for the synthesis of serum proteins (albumin, coagulation factors, and many hormonal and growth factors); the production of bile; the regulation of nutrients; and metabolism and conjugation of lipophilic compounds for excretion in the bile or urine. Although there are many causes of liver diseases, one of the most common is viral infections. Chronic viral hepatitis implies persistence of viral infection for 6 months or more after initial exposure. The primary causes of chronic viral hepatitis are hepatitis B and C. Long-term complications of chronic viral hepatitis include hepatocellular carcinoma (HCC), cirrhosis, and complications of hepatic synthetic function failure and portal hypertension (Ghany & Hoofnagle, 2005).

A. Chronic hepatitis B

1. Definition and overview

   Chronic hepatitis B is defined as persons positive for hepatitis B surface antigen for more than 6 months. Worldwide, there are 350 million individuals infected with chronic hepatitis B. In the United States, there are approximately 1.25 million people infected with chronic hepatitis B. The hepatitis B virus (HBV) is a DNA virus from the hepadnavirus family. It replicates by forming an RNA intermediate, which is copied using reverse transcriptase to generate DNA strands (Lavanchy, 2004; McQuillan et al., 1999).

2. Prevalence and incidence

   In the United States, the prevalence is approximately 1% of the population. The prevalence is greatest in Alaskan natives, first-generation immigrants from Southeast Asia, injection drug users, and men who have sex with men. Risk of HBV chronicity varies with age. In an adult, the risk for developing chronic HBV is approximately 10%. In a newborn, the risk for chronicity is 90% (without HBV vaccine and hepatitis B immunoglobulin). People who have chronic hepatitis B are at high risk to develop HCC. The risk increases by 10-fold and can happen in the absence of cirrhosis (Lok & McMahon, 2009).

B. Chronic hepatitis C

1. Definition and overview

   a. The hepatitis C virus (HCV) is a single-stranded, enveloped RNA virus from the flaviviridae family. Exposure to HCV results in chronic infection in 75–80% of the cases. Persistence of HCV RNA in the serum for 6 months or more after exposure results in chronic hepatitis C infection. HCV replicates with a high mutation rate, thereby resulting in heterogeneity within the HCV genome.

   b. Hepatitis C has six major genotypes with quasi-species within the genotypes. Genotype 1 is the most common genotype in the United States, accounting for approximately 70% of the population. Genotypes 2 and 3 account for 25% of the United States population. Genotypes 4, 5, and 6 are rare and account for the remainder. Genotypes do not influence progression of liver disease, but it does predict the success of HCV treatment. Genotype 1 needs 48 weeks of HCV therapy and is successful in 40–50% of patients. Genotypes 2 and 3 only require 24 weeks of HCV therapy and the success rates are 75–80%.

   c. Chronic HCV infection results in cirrhosis in 20% of the cases. Cirrhosis usually takes 20–30 years to develop in immunocompetent adults. Alcohol, HIV, and coinfection with other hepatitis viruses increase the likelihood of developing cirrhosis (Ghany, Strader, Thomas, & Seeff, 2009).

2. Prevalence and incidence

   It is estimated that 180 million people are infected with hepatitis C worldwide. In the United States, there are approximately 4–5 million individuals infected with HCV. The prevalence is greatest in people who have injected drugs, had blood transfusions before 1987, engage in high-risk sexual activity, and who were born from HCV-positive mothers. The risk for HCC is 1–5% per year in persons with chronic HCV and cirrhosis (Ghany et al., 2009).

II. **Database** (may include but is not limited to)

A. Subjective

1. Chronic hepatitis B
   a. Past health history
      i. Medical illnesses: HIV, coinfection with hepatitis C or D, hepatitis A, nonalcoholic fatty liver disease, diabetes mellitus, hyperlipidemia, obesity, other illnesses that may affect liver enzymes or liver function
      ii. Obstetric and gynecological history: recent pregnancy may flare HBV; risk of transmission to fetus and efficacy of hepatitis B immunoglobulin and HBV vaccine depends on the level of maternal HBV DNA
      iii. Exposure history: born in endemic area, parents born in endemic area, healthcare worker, sexual exposure, or injection drug use (IDU)
      iv. Medication history
         a. Medications that can cause flare of HBV, such as steroids, chemotherapy, and biologic agents (tumor necrosis factor-α inhibitors)
         b. Hepatotoxic medications, such as tuberculosis medications, methotrexate, and statins
   b. Family history
      i. Chronic hepatitis B
      ii. HCC
   c. Occupational and environmental history: work-related exposures: healthcare worker
   d. Personal and social history
      i. Sexual history, illicit drug use, and alcohol use
      ii. Household contacts
   e. Review of systems
      i. Constitutional signs and symptoms: fatigue, weight loss, fevers and chills (acute HBV)
      ii. Skin, hair, and nails: itching and bruising
      iii. Ear, nose, and throat: jaundice
      iv. Chest: gynecomastia
      v. Cardiac: shortness of breath, chest pain, and palpitations
      vi. Abdomen: abdominal pain, nausea, vomiting, and clay-colored stools
      vii. Genitourinary: dark urine
      viii. Musculoskeletal: joint pains
      ix. Extremities: pedal edema
      x. Neurologic: confusion, tremors, and sleep–wake cycle disturbance

2. Chronic hepatitis C
   a. Past health history
      i. Medical illnesses: HIV, coinfected with hepatitis B, nonalcoholic fatty liver disease, other illnesses that may affect liver function and enzymes
      ii. Obstetric and gynecological history: mother-to-child transmission is less than 5% (except with HIV coinfection, then the risk is 20%).
         a. Breastfeeding in an HCV-infected mother is safe for the baby.
      iii. Exposure history: IDU, blood transfusions, sexual exposure, and needlestick exposure
      iv. Medication history: hepatotoxic medications, such as tuberculosis medications, methotrexate, and statins
   b. Family history
      i. Other viral hepatitis
      ii. HCC
   c. Personal and social history
      i. IDU, other illicit drugs, and alcohol intake
      ii. Housing, access to telephone, and refrigerator
      iii. Mental health and psychiatric history: suicidal and homicidal ideation
   d. Review of systems
      i. Constitutional signs and symptoms: fatigue, fevers, and chills (acute HCV)
      ii. Skin: jaundiced, itchy, and bruising
      iii. Ear, nose, and throat: jaundiced
      iv. Cardiac: shortness of breath, chest pain, and palpitations
      v. Abdomen: abdominal pain, nausea, vomiting, and clay-colored stools
      vi. Genitourinary: dark urine
      vii. Musculoskeletal: joint pains
      viii. Extremities: pedal edema
      ix. Neurologic: confusion, tremors, and sleep–wake cycle disturbances

B. Objective

1. Physical examination findings (Table 49-1)

2. Supporting data from relevant diagnostic tests (Tables 49-2 through 49-5)

TABLE 49-1 Physical Examination Findings

Condition	Associated Findings (may or may not include)
Chronic hepatitis B and C	Assess:
	1. Vital signs: temperature, heart rate
	2. General appearance: lethargy (hepatic encephalopathy)
	3. Skin and hair: jaundiced, pruritus, bruising (cirrhosis)
	4. Eyes: icteric sclerae (cirrhosis)
	5. Chest and lungs: spider nevi, gynecomastia, crackles (from right heart failure caused by portal hypertension)
	6. Cardiovascular: increased jugular venous pressure (caused by right heart failure from portal hypertension)
	7. Abdomen: ascites, fluid wave, caput medusae, hepatomegaly, splenomegaly (cirrhosis)
	8. Extremities: palmar erythema, pedal edema (cirrhosis)
	9. Neurologic: asterixis, tremors, behavioral changes (hepatic encephalopathy)
	10. Genitourinary: testicular atrophy, dark urine (cirrhosis)

TABLE 49-2 HBV Serologic Tests

Test	Clinical Implications	Comments
Hepatitis B surface antigen (HBsAg)	If positive for ≥ 6 months, denotes chronic infection	
Hepatitis B core antibody IgG (IgG anti-HBc)	Past exposure to HBV	
Hepatitis B core antibody IgM (IgM anti-HBc)	Acute exposure to HBV Reactivation of chronic infection	
Hepatitis B surface antibody (HBsAb)	Immunity to HBV	Vaccine-induced immunity will not have positive anti-HBc
Hepatitis B DNA (HBV DNA)	Active viral replication	May be present in inactive disease state, but usually < 2,000 IU/ml
Hepatitis B E antigen (HBeAg)	Active viral replication	May be negative in those with a precore mutant HBV
Hepatitis B E antibody (HBeAb)	Low replicative state	
Hepatitis D virus	RNA virus that needs HBsAg to replicate	Consider ordering if coinfection of HDV is suspected
Hepatitis B genotype and resistance	Quasispecies of HBV (genotype A responds well to pegylated interferon) Resistance to antiviral medications based on mutations of HBV	Consider ordering if past resistance to antiviral therapy is suspected or when considering pegylated interferon therapy

TABLE 49-3 Common Liver Tests

Function	Test	Definition	Clinical Implications	Comments
Marker of hepatocellular injury	Aspartate aminotransferase (AST)	Found mainly in hepatocytes. Released into bloodstream when there is liver injury	Increased in viral hepatitis AST:ALT ratio 2:1 in alcoholic hepatitis	Found in liver, heart, skeletal muscle, brain
Marker of hepatocellular injury	Alanine aminotransferase (ALT)	Found mainly in hepatocytes. Released into bloodstream when there is liver injury	Increased in viral hepatitis ALT > AST in chronic viral hepatitis	Found in liver
Marker of cholestatic injury	Alkaline phosphatase	Canicular enzyme that plays a role in bile production	Increased in hepatobiliary disease, bone disease, pregnancy, hyperparathyroidism	Found in liver, bone, intestine, and placenta
Marker of cholestatic injury	Bilirubin	Breakdown product of hemolysis. Taken up by liver cells and conjugated to water-soluble product. Excreted in bile.	Elevations may indicate hepatic or extrahepatic disorder	Hepatitis and cirrhosis causes conjugated hyperbilirubinemia
Marker of liver function	Albumin	Major component of plasma proteins. Liver synthesizes albumin.	Decreased in cirrhosis from chronic liver disease Also decreased in nephrotic syndrome, malabsorption, protein-losing enteropathy	Indication of severity of liver disease
Marker of liver function	Prothrombin time	Liver produces clotting factors I, II, V, VII, and X. Prothrombin time depends on the activity of these clotting factors.	Increased in cirrhosis from chronic liver disease Also increased with warfarin, vitamin K deficiency	Vitamin K is needed to activate some of the clotting factors

TABLE 49-4 HCV Serologic Tests

Test	Definition	Clinical Implications	Comments
Hepatitis C antibody (HCV Ab)	Detects antibodies to hepatitis C virus	Positive in patients who have been exposed to hepatitis C.	Will stay positive even if HCV treatment is successful.
Hepatitis C viral load (HCV RNA)	Quantifies viral load by PCR	Positive in patients with chronic hepatitis C. Useful in monitoring response to HCV therapy.	HCV RNA values will wax and wane. Values do not correlate with liver disease progression.
Hepatitis C genotype	Quasispecies of HCV (genotypes 1–6)	Useful in determining how successful HCV treatment will be and how long treatment duration will be.	Genotype 1: 40–50% SVR with 48 weeks of pegylated interferon and ribavirin. Genotypes 2 and 3: 75–80% SVR with 24 weeks of pegylated interferon and ribavirin. Other genotypes: SVR variable, treatment is individually based.

TABLE 49-5 Interpretation of Chronic HBV Serologies

	Replicative Phase	Nonreplicative Phase
HBsAg	+	+
HBsAb	–	–
HBcAb (total)	+	+
HBeAg	±	–
HBeAb	–	±
ALT	Normal or elevated	Normal
HBV DNA	≥ 2,000 IU/ml	< 2,000 IU/ml

III. Assessment

A. *Determine the diagnosis*

1. Chronic hepatitis B (Tables 49-2 and 49-5)

2. Chronic hepatitis C (Tables 49-4 and 49-7)

3. Other conditions that may explain the patient's elevated liver function tests

   a. Autoimmune hepatitis: antinuclear antibody (ANA)/anti–smooth muscle antibody positive; chronic necroinflammatory liver disease of unknown etiology

   b. Nonalcoholic steatohepatitis and fatty liver disease: associated with diabetes mellitus, hyperlipidemia, and obesity

   c. Primary biliary cirrhosis: antimitochondrial antibody (AMA) positive in 95%; chronic cholestatic liver disease

   d. Hemachromotosis: most common genetic disorder in the white population; the extent of liver injury is associated with the accumulation of hepatic iron

   e. Wilson's disease: autosomal-recessive defect of cellular copper export; decreased ceruloplasmin

   f. α_1-Antitrypsin deficiency: genetic disorder that affects lungs and liver

   g. Primary sclerosing cholangitis: chronic biliary duct inflammation; associated with inflammatory bowel disease

B. *Severity: assess the severity of the disease; cirrhotic patient or intact liver function.*

C. *Significance: assess the significance of the problem to the patient and significant others.*

D. *Motivation and ability: determine the patient's willingness and ability to follow the treatment plan.*

IV. Goals of clinical management

A. *HCC screening and surveillance: choose a cost-effective approach for screening.*

B. *Treatment goals*

1. Chronic HBV (Table 49-6)

   a. Convert hepatitis B surface antigen positive to negative (very rare)

   b. Convert hepatitis B E antigen positive to negative with the development of hepatitis E antibodies

   c. HBV DNA undetectable

   d. Normalization of liver enzymes

2. Chronic HCV

   a. Goal is sustained viral response (SVR): HCV RNA undetectable 6 months after termination of HCV therapy

TABLE 49-6 Treatment for Chronic HBV Patients

Generic Name	Dose	Resistance Rate
Lamivudine	100 mg daily	14–32% in 1 yr
Adefovir	10 mg daily	29% in 5 yrs
Entecavir	0.5, 1 mg daily	1.2% in 5 yrs
Telbivudine	600 mg daily	25% in 2 yrs
Tenofovir	300 mg daily	None
Pegylated interferon	1 SQ q wk × 48 wks	None

TABLE 49-7 Side Effects of HCV Therapy: Pegylated Interferon and Ribavirin

Drug	Side Effects
Pegylated interferon	Flu-like symptoms
	Depression, anxiety, irritability
	Complete blood count abnormalities: neutropenia, thrombocytopenia
	Anorexia, nausea, diarrhea, vomiting (rare)
	Alopecia
	Skin irritation around shot
	Thyroid abnormalities (rare)
	Retinal disorders (rare)
Ribavirin	Anemia
	Insomnia
	Birth defects (need double contraception)
	Rash, pruritus
	Numbness, tingling in extremities

b. Genotype 1: SVR in 40–50% of patients with 48 weeks of HCV therapy.

c. Genotypes 2 and 3: SVR in 75–80% of patients with 24 weeks of HCV therapy.

d. Genotypes 4, 5, and 6: these genotypes are rare and HCV treatment is individualized.

e. Cirrhosis, HIV coinfection: African-American men tend to have a decreased response to HCV therapy.

C. *Patient adherence: select an approach that maximizes patient adherence.*

V. Plan

A. *HCC screening and surveillance*

The American Association for the Study of Liver Diseases recommends screening with abdominal ultrasound with or without alpha fetoprotein (AFP) every 6–12 months. AFP alone is not recommended as a screening tool, unless in rare cases where imaging is not available.

B. *Who to screen*

1. All cirrhotics

2. All patients with family history of HCC

3. In chronic hepatitis B patients
   a. All Asian men 40 years and older
   b. All Asian women 50 years and older
   c. All Africans 20 years and older

C. *Diagnostic tests*

1. Chronic hepatitis B: if hepatitis B surface antigen is positive for more than 6 months, then chronic HBV infection

   a. Complete blood count; complete metabolic panel; coagulation tests (prothrombin time and international normalized ration [INR], activated partial thromboplastin time, and thrombin time)

   b. HBV DNA, hepatitis B E antigen, hepatitis B E antibody

   c. HIV

   d. AFP

   e. Hepatitis serologies: hepatitis C Ab, hepatitis A total Ab

   f. Other tests to rule out other types of liver diseases if etiology is not certain: ANA, iron studies, AMA, anti–smooth muscle antibody, ceruloplasmin, lipids, glucose (gastrointestinal [GI]–hepatology specialist may order these tests)

   g. Imaging: see special populations who need HCC surveillance

   h. Liver biopsy: for staging of liver disease if indicated to start treatment (usually this is ordered by the GI–hepatology specialist). If cirrhosis is present, then liver biopsy is not needed.

2. Chronic hepatitis C: if HCV antibody is positive, then confirm chronic HCV infection with an HCV RNA (qualitative or quantitative).

   a. If HCV RNA negative, then recheck in 6 months to confirm resolved hepatitis C. Two negative HCV RNA tests 6 or more months apart confirms resolved hepatitis C.

   b. If HCV RNA is positive, then this is chronic HCV. There is no need to use HCV RNA as a monitoring tool for liver disease progression. HCV RNA, both qualitative and quantitative, is used primarily in the setting of HCV therapy.

      i. Complete blood count, complete metabolic panel, and coagulation studies

      ii. HCV genotype, HIV, and AFP

      iii. Hepatitis serologies: HepBsAg, HepBsAb, HepBcAb, HepA total Ab (vaccinate for hepatitis A and B if not immune)

      iv. Other tests to rule out other types of liver diseases if etiology is uncertain: ANA, iron studies, AMA, anti–smooth muscle antibody, ceruloplasmin, lipids, glucose (GI–hepatology specialist may order these)

      v. Baseline imaging to look for cirrhosis

      vi. Liver biopsy: for staging of liver disease if indicated to start treatment (usually this is ordered by the GI–hepatology specialist). If cirrhosis is already present, liver biopsy is not needed.

D. Management

1. Chronic hepatitis B: Refer chronic HBV patients to specialists when they are in chronic active phase (Table 49-5). If hepatitis B surface antigen is positive, note if:
   a. Hepatitis B E antigen positive
      i. Alanine aminotransferase (ALT) elevated
      ii. HBV DNA greater than or equal to 20,000 IU/ml
      iii. Refer to specialist for treatment
   b. Hepatitis B E antigen negative
      i. ALT elevated
      ii. HBV DNA greater than or equal to 2,000 IU/ml
      iii. Refer to specialist for treatment
   c. Cirrhotics: refer all to specialist for treatment despite ALT or HBV DNA level
   d. Inactive chronic hepatitis B
      i. ALT normal
      ii. HBV DNA less than 2,000 IU/ml
      iii. Followed by primary care provider every 6 months: ALT, HBV DNA
         a. Refer to specialist when ALT becomes abnormal or if HBV DNA is persistently greater than 2,000 IU/ml for 6 months or more
         b. Follow HCC surveillance guidelines for all chronic hepatitis B patients (both active and inactive)
         c. Vaccinate for hepatitis A if not immune

2. Chronic hepatitis C
   a. Who to refer to specialist for HCV treatment
      i. Patients who are willing to undergo 6–12 months of HCV treatment
      ii. Compensated liver disease and stable laboratory values:
         a. Hemoglobin greater than 12 for women, hemoglobin greater than 13 for men
         b. WBC greater than 3,000, neutrophil count greater than 1,500, platelets greater than 80,000
         c. Prothrombin time and INR normal
         d. Direct bilirubin normal
         e. Indirect bilirubin normal (unless Gilbert's dz)
         f. Albumin normal
         g. Creatinine normal
         h. Thyroid-stimulating hormone normal
      iii. Social history: no drugs, no tobacco, and housing stable
      iv. Psychiatric history: not active depression or anxiety; no recent suicidal or homicidal ideations or intent (< 5 years)
      v. Willingness to use double contraception throughout HCV therapy and for 6 months afterward
   b. Who not to refer to specialist for HCV therapy
      i. Decompensated liver disease as manifested by history of ascites, pedal edema, encephalopathy, and variceal bleeding. If these patients are appropriate candidates, they should be referred to a liver transplant center for evaluation. Calculate the model for end-stage liver disease (MELD) score. If the score is 10 or greater, refer to a liver transplant center (http://www.unos.org/resources/meldpeldcalculator.asp?index=98)
      ii. Autoimmune conditions that worsen on HCV therapy: autoimmune hepatitis, ulcerative colitis, Crohn's disease, systemic lupus erythematosus, rheumatoid arthritis, and so forth
      iii. Any current or recent history of malignancy (within 5 years, except for basal cell or squamous cell cancer)
      iv. Social history: current drug and alcohol use, housing is not stable, no access to telephone or refrigerator
      v. Psychiatric history: uncontrolled depression or anxiety or recent suicidal or homicidal ideation or intent within 5 years
      vi. Pregnant or trying to get pregnant
      vii. Severe chronic obstructive pulmonary disease, cardiac history (recent myocardial infarction or poorly controlled congestive heart failure), or retinal abnormalities on ophthalmology examination
   c. Chronic HCV patients who are being followed by primary care providers (those who do not want treatment or are not good candidates for treatment).
      i. Cirrhotic patients
         a. HCC surveillance
         b. Monitor liver function and liver enzymes every 3–6 months as needed: INR, total bilirubin, albumin, aspartate aminotransferase (AST) and ALT
            i. HCV RNA is not useful in monitoring of liver disease and does not predict progression of liver disease
               a. Refer to liver transplant when appropriate
               b. Vaccinate for hepatitis A and B
               c. Patient education: low-salt diet; avoid alcohol, raw fish, and shellfish

d. Chronic HCV: not cirrhotic
   i. Monitor ALT and AST every 6–12 months as needed
   ii. HCV RNA is not useful in monitoring of liver disease and does not predict progression of liver disease
   iii. Vaccinate for hepatitis A and B
   iv. Patient education: avoid alcohol, support groups
   v. Update patients on future HCV therapies (specifically targeted antiviral therapy [STAT-C] agents) that are coming in 2011, which may increase sustained viral response to HCV therapy

E. **Client education**

1. Discuss transmission and vaccinate appropriately

2. Chronic hepatitis C treatment side effects
   a. Table 49-7
   b. Advice for patients currently undergoing treatment with pegylated interferon and ribavirin
      i. Drink plenty of clear liquids. Try to drink between 8 and 10 glasses of water or another clear liquid every day. Increase this amount if you are vomiting.
      ii. Avoid drinks that have alcohol; caffeine (coffee, cola, and strong tea); or lots of sugar (most soft drinks).
      iii. Try to get plenty of sleep at night. Take short naps during the day.
      iv. Eat small, nutritious meals. Crackers, clear sodas, and ginger ale can help settle your stomach. Greasy, high-fat foods (including most "fast food") can make you feel worse. Try to eat even if you are not very hungry.
      v. Exercise lightly. Walking and lifting light weights are good exercises.
      vi. Take your medicine at bedtime, so that you can sleep through the side effects.
      vii. Take any pain relievers recommended by your doctor. A pain reliever about a half hour before your pegylated interferon injection can help make the side effects less severe. Do not take any pain reliever, however, unless your doctor says it is okay.
      viii. Avoid situations or "triggers" that make you feel worse, such as loud noises, bright lights, strong odors, or skipped meals.
      ix. Do not color or perm your hair until after your treatment is finished.
      x. Do not use harsh detergents or soaps that might irritate your skin.
      xi. Simple, unscented lotions can help dry, itchy skin. If taking ribavirin gives you a rash, Benadryl lotion might help.
   c. For patients who are having mood symptoms on pegylated interferon and ribavirin therapy
      i. Talk about your feelings with a family member, friend, or someone else that you trust. Join a support group.
      ii. Tell people close to you when you are taking your HCV treatment. Tell them that it can affect your moods.
      iii. Avoid things that can make you feel stressed, such as too much caffeine, sugar, or nicotine.
      iv. Learn ways to relax. Meditate or breathe quietly. Walk or do light exercise.
      v. Take care of your body. Eat healthy meals, get lots of sleep, and drink plenty of water.
      vi. If you are taking medicine because you are depressed, be sure not to skip a dose. Keep all of your appointments with your psychiatrist or therapist.

VI. Self-management resources and tools

1. American Association for the Study of Liver Diseases: www.aasld.org

2. National Institute of Diabetes and Digestive and Kidney Diseases: http://www2.niddk.nih.gov/

3. American Liver Foundation: http://www.liverfoundation.org/

REFERENCES

Ghany, M., & Hoofnagle, J. H. (2005). Approach to the patient with liver disease. In D. L. Kasper, A. S. Fauci, D. L. Longo, E. Braunwald, S. L. Hauser, & J. L. Jameson (Eds.), *Harrison's principles of internal medicine* (pp. 1808–1813). New York, NY: McGraw Hill.

Ghany, M. G., Strader, D. B., Thomas, D. L., & Seeff, L. B. (2009). Diagnosis, management, and treatment of hepatitis C: An update. *Hepatology, 49*(4), 1335–1374.

Lavanchy, D. (2004). Hepatitis B virus epidemiology, disease burden, treatment, and current and emerging prevention and control measures. *Journal of Viral Hepatitis, 11*(2), 97–107.

Lok, A. S., & McMahon, B. J. (2009). Chronic hepatitis B: Update 2009. *Hepatology, 50*(3), 1–36.

McQuillan, G. M., Coleman, P. J., Kurszon-Moran, D., Moyer, L. A., Lambert, S. B., & Margolis, H. S. (1999). Prevalence of hepatitis B virus infection in the United States: The National Health and Nutrition Examination Surveys. *American Journal of Public Health, 89*(1), 14–18.

CONGESTIVE HEART FAILURE

Barbara Boland

I. Introduction and general background

Heart failure is a common condition seen in the primary care setting. It is a complex syndrome that can result from the alteration in any one of a number of cardiac determinants.

A. Definition and overview

Congestive heart failure is a clinical syndrome caused by decreased cardiac filling or output, which results in an increase in pulmonary and systemic venous pressures and fluid retention. Heart failure occurs when the ventricle is unable to fill with or eject sufficient blood to meet the body's needs. It is characterized by specific symptoms and is largely diagnosed through history and physical examination.

Heart failure can be left- or right-sided. Left-sided heart failure occurs when the left ventricle is not able to pump sufficiently to meet the body's demands. Patients with left-sided heart failure have symptoms of dyspnea and fatigue. Right-sided heart failure is often a result of left-sided failure. When the left ventricle fails, fluid backs up in the lungs and ultimately into the venous system causing edema and hepatic congestion. Patients frequently have symptoms of both types of heart failure.

There are two major clinical subsets that cause decreased cardiac output and heart failure: systolic dysfunction and diastolic dysfunction. Systolic dysfunction occurs when the heart loses its ability to contract normally. Common causes are ischemic and nonischemic dilated cardiomyopathy. Diastolic dysfunction is abnormal filling of the left or right ventricle, caused by impaired myocardial relaxation or stiffness of the heart muscle. Common causes are chronic hypertension with left ventricular hypertrophy and hypertrophic or restrictive cardiomyopathies.

There are also classifications of heart failure. Functional classification generally relies on the New York Heart Association Functional Classification. The classes (I–IV) are

1. Class I: no symptoms with or limitations in ordinary activities

2. Class II: slight, mild limitation of activity; the patient is comfortable at rest or with mild exertion

3. Class III: marked limitation of any activity; the patient is comfortable only at rest

4. Class IV: severe limitations; any physical activity causes discomfort and symptoms occur at rest (American Heart Association, 2009; The Criteria Committee of the New York Heart Association, 1994)

In the 2009 guidelines, the American College of Cardiology Foundation/American Heart Association working group reviewed the four stages of heart failure, developed in 2001

1. Stage A: Patients at high risk for developing heart failure but without structural heart disease or symptoms of heart failure

2. Stage B: Structural heart disease but without signs or symptoms of heart failure

3. Stage C: Structural heart disease with prior or current symptoms of heart failure

4. Stage D: Refractory heart failure requiring specialized interventions (end stage)

This system emphasizes both the development and the progression of the disease (Jessup et al., 2009).

B. Prevalence and incidence

The estimated prevalence of heart failure in adults age 20 and older is 5,800,000 (3,200,000 males and 2,500,000 females). Heart failure is primarily a disease of the elderly. After age 65, the incidence of heart failure approaches 10 per 1,000 population. Seventy-five percent of heart failure cases have antecedent hypertension, which highlights the need for better hypertension control (Lloyd-Jones et al., 2010).

The significance of this is underscored by the mortality associated with heart failure. People diagnosed with heart failure have sudden cardiac death at six to nine times the rate of the general population. Mortality from heart failure is higher for African American males and females than for their white counterparts. Follow-up of Framingham Heart Study participants (original and offspring) from the 1950s to 1990s, aged 65–74 with heart failure, revealed a 1-year mortality of one in five dying (Lloyd-Jones et al., 2010).

II. Database (may include but is not limited to)

A. Subjective

1. Past medical history

   a. Medical illnesses: hypertension; coronary artery disease (history of myocardial infarction [MI]); arrhythmia; cardiomyopathy; valvular heart disease including aortic or pulmonic stenosis, mitral or tricuspid stenosis, or mitral or aortic regurgitation; rheumatic fever; congenital heart disease including left to right shunt or A-V fistula; myocarditis; hyperlipidemia; peripheral vascular disease; anemia; thyroid disease; infections including HIV; diabetes; systemic lupus erythematosus; obstructive sleep apnea; and alcohol or cocaine abuse

   b. Surgical history: cardiac surgeries, including valve replacements

   c. Medication history: drugs that may worsen heart failure, such as nonsteroidal anti-inflammatory drugs, antiarrhythmic drugs (ibutilide [Corvert®] and sotalol), calcium channel blockers, thiazolidinediones, and metformin; chemotherapy, such as anthracyclines, cyclophosphamide, trastuzumab, bevacizumab; herbal medications and natural supplements, such as ephedra (also called Ma huang)

2. Family history: history of atherosclerosis; MI; CVA; peripheral arterial disease; sudden cardiac death; arrhythmias; conduction disease (often requiring pacemakers); heart failure; or cardiomyopathy

3. Occupational and educational history

   a. Level of education

   b. Exposures to chemicals

   c. Days missed from work or school

4. Personal and social history

   a. Tobacco, alcohol, and drug use (cocaine and stimulants)

   b. Diet

   c. Exercise

   d. Culture

   e. Living situation

5. Review of symptoms

   a. Constitutional signs and symptoms: fatigue, weight gain or loss

   b. Skin, hair, and nails

   c. Eye, ear, nose, and throat

   d. Respiratory: wheezing, shortness of breath, orthopnea, dyspnea with or without exertion, paroxysmal nocturnal dyspnea, and cough

   e. Cardiac: chest pain, palpitations, edema, syncope, and presyncope

   f. Gastrointestinal: increasing abdominal girth; abdominal pain, especially right-upper quadrant; anorexia; and nausea

   g. Genitourinary: sexually transmitted disease exposure

   h. Neurologic: lightheadedness or dizziness

   i. Psychiatric: anxiety or depression

   j. Functional capacity: ability to dress, bathe, climb stairs, exercise, and perform activities of daily living

   k. Practitioners can also group symptoms according to left- or right-sided heart failure

      i. Left-sided: orthopnea, dyspnea on exertion, paroxysmal nocturnal dyspnea, cough, and fatigue.

      ii. Right-sided: anorexia, nausea, right-upper quadrant abdominal pain, edema, and nocturia.

B. Objective

1. Physical examination findings

   a. Height, weight, and body mass index

   b. Vital signs: narrow pulse pressure; orthostatic blood pressures

   c. Pulsus alterans

   d. Skin: diaphoresis, pallor or cyanosis, and cool temperature

   e. HEENT

   f. Thyroid

   g. Lungs: rales, wheezing

   h. Cardiac: tachycardia; elevated jugular venous pressure; S3; laterally displaced PMI; murmur; and edema (peripheral or sacral)

   i. Abdomen: increased abdominal girth; abdominal tenderness (particularly in the right-upper quadrant); hepatomegaly; and hepatojugular reflux

   j. Vascular: pulses

2. Supporting data from relevant diagnostic tests

   Heart failure is a diagnosis that is based primarily on history and physical examination. The following findings may support one's diagnosis

   a. Laboratory studies: often used to rule out or evaluate other causes of symptoms (e.g., anemia and thyroid disease); complete blood count (CBC), electrolytes, calcium, magnesium, creatinine, liver-function tests, fasting glucose, urinalysis, lipid panel, and thyroid-stimulating hormone.

b. B-type natriuretic peptide (BNP) and NT pro-BNP can be useful in diagnosis and disease management. "It is recommended that they be assessed in all patients suspected of having heart failure, especially when the diagnosis is not certain" (Heart Failure Society of America, 2010, p. 482); however, using them to screen asymptomatic patients is not recommended (Heart Failure Society of America, 2010).

c. Normal ranges are: BNP less than 100 pg/ml and NT pro-BNP less than or equal to 60 pg/ml for males and 12–150 for females, which may vary by age (Quest Diagnostics, 2009).

d. Chest radiograph: cardiomegaly, pulmonary edema

e. Electrocardiogram: left ventricular hypertrophy, evidence of prior MI, arrhythmia, and conduction problems

f. Echocardiogram: abnormalities in ventricular size, systolic or diastolic function, wall motion, and valvular functioning

III. Assessment

A. Determine the diagnosis

1. Congestive heart failure

2. Other conditions that may explain the patient's presentation

   a. Chronic obstructive pulmonary disease
   b. Anemia
   c. Angina or myocardial ischemia
   d. Cardiac tamponade
   e. Valvular heart disease
   f. Atrial fibrillation or other arrhythmia
   g. Pericarditis
   h. Venous insufficiency
   i. Cirrhosis
   j. Pulmonary embolism
   k. Chronic fatigue
   l. Deconditioning
   m. Pneumonia
   n. Sleep apnea
   o. Depression
   p. Obesity
   q. Renal disease or failure

B. Severity: assess the severity of the disease.

C. Significance: assess the significance of the problem to the patient and their significant others.

D. Motivation and ability: determine the patient's willingness and ability to follow the treatment plan.

IV. Goals of clinical management

A. Screening or diagnosis: choose a cost-effective approach for screening and diagnosing congestive heart failure.

B. Treatment: select a treatment plan that controls heart failure in a safe and effective manner.

C. Patient adherence: select an approach that maximizes patient adherence. Identify barriers to adherence and compliance.

D. Prevention of complications.

V. Plan

A. Screening

Screening is usually only done when the patient has symptoms. Patients with the following conditions have higher risk for left ventricular dysfunction and heart failure and should be periodically evaluated with routine history, physical examination, and echocardiography as indicated for this risk.

1. Hypertension

2. Diabetes

3. Obesity

4. Coronary artery disease (e.g., after MI, revascularization)

5. Peripheral arterial disease or cerebrovascular disease

6. Valvular heart disease

7. Family history of cardiomyopathy in a first-degree relative

8. History of exposure to cardiac toxins

9. Sleep-disordered breathing

10. Test findings: sustained arrhythmias

11. Abnormal electrocardiogram (e.g., left ventricular hypertrophy, left bundle branch block, pathologic Q waves); cardiomegaly on chest radiograph (Heart Failure Society of America, 2010)

B. Diagnostic tests

1. Laboratory studies: BNP; NT pro-BNP; those used to rule out or evaluate other causes of symptoms, such as CBC, electrolytes, calcium, magnesium, creatinine, liver-function tests, fasting glucose, urinalysis, lipid panel, and thyroid-stimulating hormone.

2. Chest radiograph: cardiomegaly, pulmonary edema.

3. Electrocardiogram: Left ventricular hypertrophy, evidence of prior MI, arrhythmia, and conduction problems.

4. Echocardiogram: abnormal ventricular size and systolic or diastolic function; wall motion abnormalities; valvular abnormalities (Hunt et al., 2009; Jessup et al., 2009).

C. Management (includes treatment, consultation, referral, and follow-up care)

1. Acute heart failure: immediate intervention of oxygen, stat chest radiograph, echocardiogram, laboratory studies, diuresis; arrange hospital admission.

2. Acute or chronic heart failure

   a. Treatment of systemic illness or underlying condition that may be contributing: thyroid disease, uncontrolled diabetes mellitus, or infection.

   b. Eliminate drugs (cocaine) and medications: nonsteroidal anti-inflammatory drugs, calcium channel blockers, thiazolidinediones, antiarrhythmic drugs, ephedra, or toxins that may be contributing to heart failure.

   c. Lifestyle
      i. Smoking cessation
      ii. Alcohol cessation or restriction (1–2 glasses per day)
      iii. Illicit drug use cessation
      iv. Activity: temporary restriction if very symptomatic; otherwise, encourage regular exercise 20–30 minutes three to five times per week.
      v. Diet: sodium restriction of 2–3 g/day; less than 2 g/day in moderate to severe heart failure.
      vi. Fluids: restrict daily intake to less than 2 L in patients with serum sodium less than 130 mEq/L or difficult to control fluid retention.

   d. Weight loss if needed

   e. Weight monitoring: document weight daily; have plan of how to respond to evidence of volume overload

   f. Aggressive blood pressure management

   g. Lipid management

   h. Pharmacologic therapy (Table 50-1)
      i. Loop diuretics: thiazide diuretics may be used in hypertensive patients; however, loop diuretics are the class of choice. Care must be taken not to over-diurese patients with diastolic dysfunction.
      ii. Angiotensin-converting enzyme inhibitors (ACEI) or angiotensin receptor blockers (ARBs) if unable to tolerate (ACEI) for symptomatic and asymptomatic patients with ejection fraction less than 40%
      iii. β-Blockers
      iv. Hydralazine
      v. Nitrates
      vi. Aldosterone antagonist (spironolactone)
      vii. Digoxin (Heart Failure Society of America, 2010): biventricular pacing, implantable defibrillators, and cardiac transplant are considerations for advanced cases (Bashore & Granger, 2007).

   i. Health maintenance
      i. Annual flu vaccine
      ii. Pneumococcal vaccine
      iii. Medic alert information

   j. Referral to heart failure disease management program
      i. Patients recently hospitalized for heart failure and those at high risk
      ii. High-risk patients include those with
         a. Renal insufficiency
         b. Diabetes
         c. Depression
         d. Persistent New York Heart Association Class III or IV symptoms
         e. Chronic obstructive pulmonary disease
         f. Active comorbidities
         g. Frequent hospitalization
         h. Inadequate social supports
         i. Persistent nonadherence to therapeutic regimen
         j. Cognitive impairment or poor health literacy (Heart Failure Society of America, 2010)

   k. End of life and palliative care
      i. Consider for patients who have: advanced persistent symptoms at rest despite pharmacologic therapy

TABLE 50-1 Medications

Agent	Initial Dose	Maximum Daily Dose
Loop diuretics		
Furosemide	20–40 qd or bid	600 mg
Bumetanide	0.5–1 mg qd or bid	10 mg
Torsemide	10–20 mg qd	200 mg
Ethacrynic acid	25–50 mg qd or bid	200 mg
Angiotensin-converting enzyme inhibitors		
Enalapril	2.5 mg bid	20 mg bid
Captopril	6.25 mg tid	50 mg tid
Lisinopril	2.5–5 mg qd	40 mg qd
β-Blockers		**Target Dose**
Bisoprolol	1.25 mg qd	10 mg qd
Metoprolol succinate CR/XL	12.5–25 mg qd	200 mg qd
Carvedilol	3.125 mg bid	6.25–25 mg bid

Sources: Heart Failure Society of America. (2010). Executive summary: HFSA 2010 comprehensive heart failure practice guideline. *Journal of Cardiac Failure, 16*(6), 475–539, e1–e193; Hunt, S. A., Abraham, W. T., Chin, M. H., Feldman, A. M., Francis, G. S., Ganiats, T. G., . . . Yancy, C. W. (2009). 2009 focused update incorporated into the ACC/AHA 2005 guidelines for the diagnosis and management of heart failure in adults: A report of the American College of Cardiology Foundation/American Heart Association Task Force on Practice Guidelines: Developed in collaboration with the International Society for Heart and Lung Transplantation. *Circulation, 119*(14), e391–e479.

ii. Hospitalization for heart failure
iii. Poor quality of life, including little or no ability to conduct activities of daily living
iv. Need for continuous intravenous inotropic support
v. Consider hospice referral (Heart Failure Society of America, 2010).
vi. Advanced directives and durable power of attorney should be in place

D. *Client education*

1. Concerns and feelings
   Assist the patient and significant others in expressing and coping with concerns and feelings related to the diagnosis of congestive heart failure, its potential complications, and the management of this disease.

2. Information
   Provide verbal and written information regarding
   a. The disease process, including symptoms, cause, and treatment of patient's heart failure and prognosis and disease progression

b. Diagnostic tests, including what the test measures, normal results, frequency, and importance of testing

c. Management: much of the responsibility for management of this illness lies with the patient and their family. Family members should be encouraged to participate in the patient's care. A good relationship with the primary care provider and a plan detailing how and when to call the provider must be in place. Patients and their families should be educated about
   i. Symptom recognition; weight monitoring; and medication effects, side effects, dosing and titration, and cost
   ii. Diet, including sodium and fluid restrictions
   iii. Tobacco cessation; alcohol limitations or abstinence
   iv. Physical activity: limitations or ways to maintain and increase activity level
   v. Travel restrictions (e.g., high altitude, humid destinations)
   vi. Health maintenance (Dickstein et al., 2008; Heart Failure Society of America, 2010)

VI. Self-management resources and tools

A. Patient and client education

1. The American Heart Association (http://www.heart.org/HEARTORG/Conditions/HeartFailure/Heart-Failure_UCM_002019_SubHomePage.jsp and http://www.hearthub.org/hc-heart-failure.htm): The American Heart Association has print and online education materials and online videos. Websites are available in Spanish, Chinese, Vietnamese, and English.

2. Heart Failure Matters (http://www.heartfailurematters.org/EN/Pages/index.aspx): This is an interactive, multilingual, educational website containing animations, videos, and tools for patients with heart failure. It is available in English, French, German, and Spanish. It has a family and caregiver section and links to a variety of other related websites.

3. National Heart, Lung and Blood Institute (http://www.nhlbi.nih.gov/health/dci/Diseases/Hf/HF_WhatIs.html): The National Heart, Lung and Blood Institute website contains educational information on line and for purchase and has websites tailored to selected ethnic audiences. It also has links to recipes, health assessment tools, events, and clinical trial information.

B. Community support groups

1. The American Heart Association offers a variety of community events and support groups for individuals with heart disease.

2. Mended Hearts (http://www.mendedhearts.org/) is an organization for individuals with heart disease. Patients must pay to join. They have group meetings, hospital visiting programs, an annual convention, educational resources, and various events. Patients can join a local chapter.

REFERENCES

American Heart Association. (2009). *Classification of functional capacity and objective assessment.* Retrieved from http://www.americanheart.org/presenter.jhtml?identifier=4569

Bashore, T. M., & Granger, C. B. (2007). Congestive heart failure. In M. A. Papadakis & S. J. McPhee (Eds.), *2007 current consult medicine* (pp. 746–747). New York, NY: McGraw Hill.

Dickstein, K., Cohen-Solal, A., Filippatos, G., McMurray, J. J., Ponikowski, P., Poole-Wilson, P. A., . . . Zamorano, J. L. (2008). ESC guidelines for the diagnosis and treatment of acute and chronic heart failure 2008: The Task Force for the Diagnosis and Treatment of Acute and Chronic Heart Failure 2008 of the European Society of Cardiology. *European Heart Journal, 29*(19), 2388–2442.

Heart Failure Society of America. (2010). Executive summary: HFSA 2010 comprehensive heart failure practice guideline. *Journal of Cardiac Failure, 16*(6), 475–539, e1–e193.

Hunt, S. A., Abraham, W. T., Chin, M. H., Feldman, A. M., Francis, G. S., Ganiats, T. G., . . . Yancy, C. W. (2009). 2009 focused update incorporated into the ACC/AHA 2005 guidelines for the diagnosis and management of heart failure in adults: A report of the American College of Cardiology Foundation/American Heart Association Task Force on Practice Guidelines: Developed in collaboration with the International Society for Heart and Lung Transplantation. *Circulation, 119*(14), e391–e479.

Jessup, M., Abraham, W. T., Casey, D. E., Feldman, A. M., Francis, G. S., Ganiats, T. G., . . . Yancy, C. W. (2009). 2009 focused update: ACCF/AHA guidelines for the diagnosis and management of heart failure in adults. A report of the American College of Cardiology Foundation/American Heart Association Task Force on Practice Guidelines. *Circulation, 119*(14), 1977–2016.

Lloyd-Jones, D., Adams, R., Brown, T. M., Carnethon, M., Dai, S., DeSimone, G., . . . Wylie-Roserr, J. (2010). Heart disease and stroke statistics. 2010 Update. A report from the American Heart Association. *Circulation, 121*:e84-e88.

Quest Diagnostics. (2009). Congestive heart Failure (CHF) risk testing: BNP (B-type natriuretic peptide) and proBNP. Retrieved from http://www.questdiagnostics.com/hcp/topics/bnp/bnp.html

The Criteria Committee of the New York Heart Association. (1994). *Nomenclature and criteria for diagnosis of diseases of the heart and great vessels* (9th ed., pp. 253–256). Boston, MA: Little, Brown & Co.

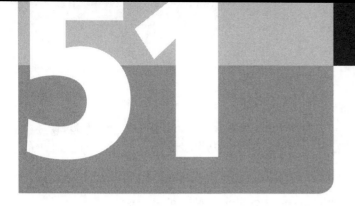

DEMENTIA

Jennifer Merrilees

I. Introduction and general background

Dementia is a syndrome of decline in two or more cognitive domains (e.g., memory, language, visuospatial, or executive function) that results in deficits of functional capacity (American Psychiatric Association, 1994). It is usually a chronic and progressive neurodegenerative disease. Common causes of dementia include Alzheimer's disease (AD), vascular dementia, frontotemporal dementia (FTD), and dementia with Lewy bodies (DLB). Other disorders that may be associated with dementia are Huntington's disease, HIV-AIDS, Parkinson's disease, alcoholism, and head trauma. Rapidly progressive dementias are rare and may include Creutzfeldt-Jakob disease. At this time there is no cure for dementia, although current research aimed at the reversal or prevention of dementia is underway.

Given the aging population, the prevalence of AD is expected to rise, making this a critical public health problem, not only for patients with the disease, but for the people and health systems that care for them (2009 Alzheimer's disease facts and figures, 2009). Neurologists and geriatricians with expertise in dementia can assist with the evaluation, diagnosis, and management. Referrals may be considered as part of a thorough work-up, but should be done when symptoms are less typical (Santacruz & Swagerty, 2001).

There is no single test for dementia and the evaluation is directed at clarifying the nature of the impairment and identification of possible causes (Table 51-1). There is evidence that approximately 9% of patients have a potentially treatable cause for dementia (e.g., an electrolyte abnormality), yet less than 1% show a reversal of symptoms with treatment (Clarfield, 2003). Despite this, a comprehensive evaluation is considered critical to correctly identify and diagnose patients with dementia and to initiate appropriate management.

A. Alzheimer's disease

1. Definition

   AD is the most common cause of dementia. Although the sites of earliest damage in AD are the hippocampus and entorhinal cortex (areas that are important in memory function), the disease eventually affects multiple regions of the brain. Neuronal death is caused by the over-accumulation of amyloid plaques and neurofibrillary tangles. The strongest risk factor for AD is advanced age, although prior head injury, family history of AD, and cardiovascular factors, such as hypertension, pose increased risk for development of AD. When AD occurs in a person younger than age 65, it has been referred to as pre-senile, early age onset, younger-onset, or early onset AD. Most cases are not familial, although genetic risk increases in early age of onset AD, when a first-degree relative has AD, and in the presence of certain genetic mutations (U.S. Preventative Services Task Force, 2003).

2. Prevalence

   AD is the cause in 60–80% of people with a dementia (2009 Alzheimer's disease facts and figures, 2009). The incidence of AD increases with advanced age (approximately 5% of people between ages 65 and 74 have AD; this incidence rises to 25–47% in people older than age 85 [Boustani, Peterson, Hanson, Harris, & Lohr, 2003]).

B. Vascular dementia

1. Definition

   Vascular dementia (also referred to as multi-infarct dementia) is caused by cerebrovascular ischemia and lacunar infarcts in the brain (also called white matter disease). Symptoms are similar to AD, although the onset may be more easily identified and the progression of symptoms can be characterized by "stepwise" changes, reflecting the occurrence of strokes. Risk factors include strokes, hypertension, hypercholesteremia, and diabetes. Vascular dementia may coexist with AD or DLB (referred to as mixed dementia).

2. Prevalence

   Vascular dementia is considered the second most common cause for dementia, occurring in approximately 20–30% of people with dementia.

TABLE 51-1 Possible Causes of Dementia (Partial List)

Neurodegenerative	Alzheimer's disease, Down syndrome, Parkinson's disease, dementia with Lewy bodies, frontotemporal dementia, multisystem atrophy, Huntington disease
Cerebrovascular	Vascular dementia, vasculitis
Prion-associated	Creutzfeldt-Jakob disease, Gerstmann-Sträussler-Scheinker syndrome, fatal familial insomnia
Neurogenetic	Spinocerebellar ataxias, mitochondrial encephalopathies, Wilson's disease
Infectious	Meningitis, encephalitis, leukoencephalopathy, neurosyphilis, Whipple's disease, HIV
Toxic or metabolic	Systemic: thyroid, parathyroid, adrenal, liver, kidney, sarcoidosis, vitamin deficiencies, hypoxia/ischemia, drugs, alcohol, heavy metals
Miscellaneous	Multiple sclerosis, neoplastic, hydrocephalus

C. Dementia with Lewy bodies

1. Definition and overview

The symptoms of DLB can be similar to AD with several important distinctions. Diagnostic criteria for DLB include the presence of visual hallucinations; parkinsonian signs (stiffness, slowness of movement, shuffling gait); and fluctuations in alertness and attention (McKeith, 2006). DLB is caused by the accumulation of Lewy bodies containing α-synuclein, which deposit within neurons and affect multiple brain regions.

2. Prevalence

DLB is considered the third most common cause for dementia. It is thought to occur in approximately 18–20% of cases of dementia.

D. Frontotemporal dementia

1. Definition and overview

There are multiple variants of FTD with terminology and diagnostic criteria under refinement. FTD is caused by focal damage to the frontal and anterior temporal lobes of the brain. Behavioral variant FTD is the most common clinical subtype characterized by an array of behavior, personality, emotional, and cognitive changes. Average age at onset is 56 years (Miller et al., 1998). Because of related biology, amyotrophic lateral sclerosis may occur in conjunction with FTD. There are two aphasic subtypes of FTD. The first is called semantic dementia, in which the patient exhibits a loss of word and object meaning. The second aphasic variant, termed progressive nonfluent aphasia, is characterized by halting speech and difficulty with speech expression (Boxer & Miller, 2005). Other related movement disorders include corticobasal degeneration, progressive supranuclear palsy (Sha, Hou, Viskontas, & Miller, 2006), and motor neuron disease. Tauopathy and nontauopathy proteins have been identified as cellular mechanisms for FTD.

2. Prevalence

FTD is recognized as the most common presenile dementia, typically occurring between 50 and 60 years of age. FTD represents approximately 10–20% of dementia cases.

II. Database (may include but is not limited to)

A. Subjective

One of the most important steps in the evaluation of a person with suspected dementia is a discussion of the symptoms and associated features with the patient and an informant (someone who knows the patient well). It is critical to involve an informant to verify information: patients with dementia may have limited insight and may mask their deficits with good social graces. The focus of the interview is aimed at onset and duration of symptoms and whether they represent a change from the patient's baseline abilities. Taking a careful history is critical to determine how the symptoms have progressed and potential temporal relationships of related factors (e.g., medical conditions, medications, stroke events, and so forth). It is important to understand the pattern and character of the deficits. Patients and families can be encouraged to maintain a log or journal to help in the evaluation of the person with suspected cognitive deficits. It can be helpful to start with general questions: "What are you concerned about?" moving to more specific questions, such as "What was the very first thing that was different or caused you concern?" and "How have the symptoms progressed: have they worsened, stayed the same, or improved?"

A careful review of medications (prescription and over-the-counter) should be conducted. Request that the patient bring all medications to the evaluation to clarify dosages, expiration dates, and the patient's understanding of the purpose and administration for the medications.

1. Alzheimer's disease

    a. Patient or family reports of deficits in short-term memory; finding the right word; visual–spatial; or executive function (organization and planning). Statements may include: "She seems more forgetful," "she takes longer to get things done," "she is getting lost in familiar places," "she repeats the same question multiple times," "she cannot multitask as well as before," "she cannot come up with the right word to use," or "she is having trouble learning new things, such as the computer."

    b. Report of personality or behavioral changes: apathy, depression, or irritability. Common complaints may include: "she is quieter," "she doesn't engage in activities as in the past," or "she easily angers."

    c. Report of patient's functional decline: paying bills late; forgetting appointments; misplacing personal items; diminished standards in personal hygiene and grooming (e.g., not showering as often, appearance that is unkempt, or wearing the same clothes over again); and problems with driving (e.g., running through stop signs, driving too fast or slow, getting lost, new traffic violations, or car accidents).

    d. Report of risk factors for AD. For example, a family history of AD or a history of head injury with or without a loss of consciousness may increase the risk for development of the disease.

2. Vascular dementia

    a. Patient or family reports of deficits in short-term memory; finding the right word; navigation; or executive function (organization and planning).

    b. Report of personality or behavioral changes: apathy, depression, irritability, or anxiety.

    c. Report of patient's functional decline: paying bills late, forgetting appointments, misplacing personal items, diminished standards in personal hygiene and grooming.

    d. Report of a stroke-like event that coincides with the previously mentioned cognitive, behavioral, and functional changes. It may be possible to identify a specific time-point that symptoms presented. Medical review that reveals the presence of vascular risk factors (hypertension, hypercholesteremia, or diabetes)

3. Dementia with Lewy bodies (DLB)

    a. Patient or family reports of deficits in visual-spatial abilities; navigation; executive function (organization and planning); short-term memory; or finding the right word.

    b. Report of personality or behavioral changes. Visual hallucinations that may or may not be distressing to the patient. Common complaints may include a sense that someone is looking over their shoulder; vague movement in their peripheral vision or a report of seeing small people or animals when nothing is there; and misperceiving objects (e.g., mistaking a tree for the figure of a person). Other examples of behavioral changes may include anxiety, apathy, and depression.

    c. Report of functional decline. Examples include misplacing personal items; trouble with driving or navigation (getting lost, driving in the wrong portion of the lane, and new dents and scrapes on the car); paying bills late; and forgetting appointments.

    d. Report of motor symptoms suggestive of parkinsonism (shuffling gait or dragging feet more while walking, bradykinesia, stiffness, and falls caused by tripping).

    e. Report of sleep changes suggestive of rapid eye movement behavior disorder. Symptoms may include new onset of thrashing and moving while sleeping, arm and leg movements as if warding off an attack, hitting the bed partner during sleep, or falling out of bed during sleep.

4. Frontotemporal dementia

    a. Report of executive dysfunction, poor judgment, speech and language changes that may include loss of object and word meaning, or dysarthria. Common complaints may include: "she has been making risky decisions," "she cannot seem to organize tasks," "she doesn't know what certain words mean anymore," and "her speech is halting and it is hard to get words out."

    b. Report of personality and behavioral changes: apathy, disinhibition, impulsivity, social or personal misconduct, unusual eating behaviors, compulsions, and diminished empathy. Common complaints: "she has become a different person," "she has been yelling at people," "she doesn't care about things, doesn't care about me," "she says she will do things, but doesn't," "she makes suggestive comments to others," "she talks to strangers more readily," "she has become self-centered," "her eating behavior has changed (eats more, carbohydrate cravings, or exhibits food fads)."

    c. Report of functional decline: trouble with task completion; trouble maintaining a job; diminished abilities in managing financial and legal matters (not getting tasks completed or showing poor judgment, such as making risky investments, unusual purchases, giving away money); and diminished standards in hygiene and grooming.

    d. Report of motor symptoms suggestive of amyotrophic lateral sclerosis; corticobasal degeneration; or progressive supranuclear palsy (falls, weakness, or diminished ability to control limb movements).

    e. Report of a family history suggestive of FTD that may include dementia, behavioral disorders, or psychiatric disorders (Table 51-2).

B. Objective

1. Mental status screening and evaluation

    a. Use a reliable and valid instrument. The Mini-Mental Status Examination (Folstein, Folstein, & McHugh, 1975) and the Montreal Cognitive Assessment are tools that provide brief screening of memory, language, executive function, and visual–spatial abilities. The Mini-Mental Status Examination has a sensitivity of 71–92% and specificity of 56–96% (Costa, Williams, & Somerfield, 1996). Population-based normative data for age and education level are available (Crum, Anthony, Bassett, & Folstein, 1993). The Montreal Cognitive Assessment is available in multiple languages and is free of charge: the test and administration instructions are available through the website (http://www.mocatest .org). The Montreal Cognitive Assessment has a sensitivity of 90% in identifying mild cognitive impairment and a specificity of 87% (Nasreddine et al., 2005).

    b. Full neuropsychologic testing by a neuropsychologist may be necessary to accurately demonstrate the presence and character of deficits.

2. Functional assessment

    a. A reliable and valid instrument that assists in comparing present with past performance in functional domains can be used in conjunction with the clinical interview.

    b. Functional abilities can be assessed in multiple domains including occupational performance; finances; driving; use of computer; household tasks (e.g., housekeeping and cooking); and personal hygiene.

    c. Examples of functional assessment instruments include the Functional Activities Questionnaire (Pfeffer, Kurosaki, Harrah, Chance, & Filos, 1982) and the Instrumental Activities of Daily Living Scale (Lawton &

Brody, 1969). Both tools are easy to administer and have good reliability and validity (Costa et al., 1996; Graf, 2007). A disadvantage of both tools is the reliance on self- or informant-report rather than direct observation of functional abilities.

    d. An instrumental activities of daily living scale is available at http://consultgerirn.org

3. Assessment of mood

    a. Evaluation should include an assessment for depression because mood disorders share similar features with neurodegenerative conditions.

    b. A commonly used screen is the Geriatric Depression Scale. Using a yes/no format, patients answer questions about their mood over the past week. A long version (30 items) and a short version (15 items) are available. Scoring guidelines are provided to rate the severity of depression. The Geriatric Depression Scale has 92% sensitivity and 89% specificity (Yesavage et al., 1983).

    c. The Geriatric Depression Scale is available at http://consultgerirn.org

4. Physical and neurologic examination

    a. The routine physical examination should be completed to identify the presence of any medical problems (e.g., hypertension or atrial fibrillation)

    b. The neurologic examination should include an assessment of motor abilities, reflexes, coordination, gait and balance, and an assessment for focal neurologic signs.

5. Relevant diagnostic tests

    a. Laboratory screening routinely includes complete blood count (to rule out anemia and infection); serum chemistries; thyroid and liver function; vitamin B_{12} (to rule out metabolic conditions); and urinalysis (to rule out infection). Rapid plasma reagent test (RPR), folate acid level or homocysteine, and methylmalonic acid may be warranted depending on clinical findings and history. See Table 51-3 for a summary of routine laboratory screening.

    b. Other tests may be indicated based on the history or physical examination (e.g., electrocardiography or electroencephalography).

    c. Brain imaging: optional, although recommended by most specialists. Brain imaging can help detect the degree and pattern of atrophy and may identify other causes for cognitive deficits (e.g., stroke, white matter ischemia, or tumors). The most common

TABLE 51-2 Features of Dementia

Syndrome	Symptoms	Onset	Areas of Brain Affected	Biochemical	Possible Associated Symptoms	Progression
Alzheimer's disease	Short-term memory loss, word-finding difficulty, visual–spatial difficulties (getting lost or disoriented)	Gradual; more common after age 65, but can occur earlier	Multiple areas; global atrophy on imaging	Deficits in acetylcholine	Apathy, depression, diminished insight over time	Slowly progressive over 7–10 yrs (or longer)
Dementia with Lewy bodies	Recurrent and well-formed visual hallucinations, fluctuating cognition, parkinsonian symptoms, visual–spatial deficits, short-term memory loss	Gradual	Multiple areas; global atrophy on imaging	Deficits in acetylcholine and dopamine	Rapid eye movement sleep behavior disorder, falls, anxiety	Slowly progressive
Vascular dementia	Dependent on the location of ischemia	May be sudden with identifiable onset	Cortical or subcortical changes on imaging		Irritability, apathy	Dependent on management of stroke risk factors
Frontotemporal dementia	Behavior and personality change: apathy, disinhibition, poor judgment, social misconduct, executive dysfunction	Gradual; before age 60	Frontal and anterior temporal lobes (anterior sections of the brain)	Deficits in serotonin	Speech and language changes occur in the aphasic variant. Motor deficits occur in progressive supranuclear palsy and corticobasal degeneration, and amyotrophic lateral sclerosis (related disorders), diminished insight early in disease (behavioral variant frontotemporal dementia)	Progressive over 6–8 yrs

TABLE 51-3 Common Laboratory Screening in Assessment of Dementia

Laboratory tests
Complete blood cell count
Serum electrolytes, including magnesium
Serum chemistry panel, including liver function
Thyroid function
Vitamin B$_{12}$
Folate acid level or homocysteine
Methylmalonic acid
Urinalysis
Serologic tests for syphilis*
Toxicology screening*
Human immunodeficiency virus*

* Based on clinical relevance.

imaging technique used is magnetic resonance imaging.

    d. Genetic testing: may be pursued if there is a strong family history and a desire for confirmation.

        i. Apolipoprotein E4 allele is found approximately three times more frequently in those with AD than in those without. Yet, many people with AD do not have the APOE4 allele and many with the allele do not develop AD. Thus, the presence may denote a general risk for AD but there is no definitive link (Boustani et al., 2003).

        ii. Referral to a genetic counselor is often indicated to clarify the presence of genetic risk and to discuss the implications of genetic testing.

III. Assessment

A. Determine the diagnosis

1. *Diagnostic and Statistical Manual of Mental Disorders-IV* criteria requires the presence of cognitive impairments to the degree that functional abilities are reduced and represent a decline from the patient's normal abilities (American Psychiatric Association, 1994).

2. Criteria exists for the different causes for dementia.

    a. Alzheimer's disease: insidious onset and progressive cognitive impairment (McKhann et al., 1984).

    b. Vascular dementia: two or more strokes by history, examination, or imaging of single stroke temporally related to onset of dementia (Chui et al., 1992).

    c. Dementia with Lewy bodies: fluctuating cognition, attention, and alertness; recurrent visual hallucinations; and parkinsonism. Suggestive features include rapid eye movement sleep behavior disorder and neuroleptic sensitivity (McKeith, 2006).

    d. Frontotemporal dementia: early decline in social and interpersonal conduct, loss of insight, and emotional blunting. Supportive features include decline in personal hygiene and grooming; mental rigidity and inflexibility; distractibility; hyperorality and dietary changes; perseverative and stereotyped behavior; and press of speech, economy, and stereotyped (Neary et al., 1998).

3. If cognitive impairment is present, and there is no decline in functional abilities, consider a diagnosis of mild cognitive impairment.

    a. Mild cognitive impairment is used to describe a condition that may or may not precede the development of dementia (Petersen et al., 1999).

    b. Schedule follow-up testing within 6 months to a year or as needed.

B. Determine the significance of the diagnosis for the patient and family.

IV. Goals of clinical management

A. Desired outcomes for the patient with dementia is that he or she remains as independent as possible in an environment that matches his or her functional abilities and that the dementia and comorbid conditions are well managed.

V. Plan

A. Conduct further work-up or referral to specialist as needed.

Referrals are indicated when symptoms are atypical, occurring in a younger patient, are suggestive of a rapidly progressive dementia, or confounded by difficult psychiatric or behavioral disturbances (Santacruz & Swagerty, 2001). Referrals may also be helpful when a second opinion is desired.

B. Medication treatment

1. There are several classes of medications used to treat disease symptoms or improve cognitive function. Currently, there are no agents available to cure dementia. Medications can be used for monotherapy and as combination therapy.

2. Table 51-4 outlines commonly used medications.

3. Dietary supplements and other medications: ginkgo biloba, vitamin E, and estrogen have been considered as treatment for AD, although research has not provided compelling evidence in favor of these medications (Andrade & Radhakrishnan, 2009; Boustani et al., 2003).

4. If the patient has vascular disease or mixed dementia, then he or she should receive stroke prophylaxis and education regarding modification of cardiovascular risk factors.

C. Safety management

1. Make referrals as needed: for example, if wandering or getting lost is a concern, discuss strategies for maintaining safety and refer the patient and family to the Safe Return program operated through the Alzheimer's Association.

2. Driving
   a. Depending on cognitive and motor findings, the patient can be requested to not drive, complete test of driving abilities through the department of motor vehicles, or be referred to a driver's safety course that will assess driving ability.
   b. Reporting to the department of motor vehicles of the diagnosis of dementia should be consistent with state laws: some states have mandatory reporting requirements.
   c. Referral to adult protective services if there is concern for the well-being of the patient or the caregiver.

D. Management of behavioral symptoms

Behavioral changes occur commonly in dementia and contribute to caregiver distress (Craig, Mirakhur, Hart, McIlroy, & Passmore, 2005; de Vugt et al., 2006). The changes may be caused by structural changes in the brain, a result of neurotransmitter depletion, by changes in how the patient perceives and responds to environmental stimuli, or a combination of all of the above.

1. The first step in managing these symptoms is to discuss the character, frequency, and severity of the symptoms with the patient and caregiver. Describe the behavior specifically (e.g., not just "sundowning," but agitation in the evening that includes pacing, repetitive statements that this is not their house, pushes caregiver away, and tries to open front door to leave the house).

2. Identify whether the symptoms are hazardous, annoying, or tolerable. It should be noted that not all behaviors are problematic. For example, wandering is a beneficial form of exercise as long as the patient can engage in the activity safely. Other behaviors are hazardous, such as agitation and aggression that may be physically dangerous to the patient or the caregiver.

TABLE 51-4 Medications Used in the Treatment of Dementia

Drug	Indications	Possible Side Effects	Other Considerations
Cholinesterase inhibitors Donepezil (Aricept®); Galantamine (Razadyne®, Reminyl®); Rivastigmine (Exelon®)	Used primarily in AD and DLB to slow the breakdown of acetylcholine, a neurotransmitter important for memory. May be helpful in managing the hallucinations and fluctuating cognition of DLB.	Gastrointestinal (nausea, vomiting, diarrhea). Contraindicated in patients with bradycardia.	Obtain baseline electrocardiogram before initiation in patients with cardiovascular conditions. Rivastigmine available in patch form. Galantamine is available in generic form.
N-methyl-D-aspartate antagonist Memantine (Namenda®)	Used to reduce glutamate-mediated excitotoxicity. Approved for treatment of advanced AD (Mini-Mental Status Examination scores ≤ 15).	Constipation, dizziness, and headache.	Large clinical studies are underway to evaluate effectiveness in FTD.
Selective serotonin reuptake inhibitors	Used to treat the serotonin deficits that may contribute to behavioral symptoms that occur in FTD.	Gastrointestinal (nausea and diarrhea), agitation.	

a. Develop an individualized plan of care for managing behavioral symptoms.

b. Strategies for managing behavioral symptoms fall into five categories. In many cases, using a combination of interventions is necessary.

i. Environmental (e.g., modifying the patient's environment). Examples include: to decrease agitation it can be helpful to provide activities that are enjoyable for the patient and match their functional level, or use of communication techniques that are simpler, easier to understand, and that do not provoke an argument. For patients vulnerable to sweepstake offers in the mail, have mail diverted to a post office box where it can be screened before reaching the patient. If the patient is having disturbing visual illusions, remove the stimuli from their environment.

ii. Behavioral (substitution for a behavior that is more tolerable or safer). Examples include substitution of sugar-free candy or nonalcoholic beverages for patients with food cravings.

iii. Pharmacologic (using a medication targeted specifically for the behavior). Examples include a selective serotonin reuptake inhibitor to treat agitation. Antipsychotics are associated with increased risk of death (Gill et al., 2007) and should be used only in cases of severe agitation, aggression, or psychosis, and in conjunction with an assessment for potential medical reasons for the behavior.

iv. Physical (a physical restraint or barrier to prevent patient's movement). These strategies should only be considered as a last resort. It may be necessary to move the patient to a more protected and supportive environment.

v. Internal to the caregiver (gain acceptance for the behavior). Counseling and education regarding expected disease symptoms, identification of strategies for effective behavior management, and obtaining respite and support from caregiving duties are examples of helpful interventions.

E. Conduct patient and family education

1. Discuss implications of diagnosis as it pertains to the patient's occupation and other responsibilities.

2. Provide education regarding dementia diagnosis, progression, and goals of care in a manner that is consistent with their values, culture, education, and abilities.

3. Review of medication indications and side effects with a discussion of expected and realistic goals of treatment (e.g., treatment is for symptomatic improvement and not a cure or reversal of disease). Expected benefits may be mild improvement in memory function and other disease symptoms. It is recommended that 6–12 months of therapy is needed to adequately assess the benefit of therapy (California Workgroup on Guidelines for Alzheimer's Disease Management, 2008).

4. Discuss common side effects of the acetylcholinesterase inhibitors including gastrointestinal upset and vivid dreams. Slow titration of medication, use of the patch, or administration of medication in the morning and not bedtime are common strategies to prevent these side effects. These medications are not indicated for patients with bradycardia: it may be necessary to obtain an electrocardiogram before initiation of therapy.

5. Educate regarding the importance of exercise: physical exercise has been linked to improvement of mood, maintenance of mobility, and decrease in the risk for falls, and may improve cognition (Vogel et al., 2009; Williams & Tappen, 2007).

6. Provide information regarding educational and supportive resources available in the community.

7. Provide information about advance directives and durable power of attorney while the patient is in the early stages of disease and able to articulate his or her wishes. Make referrals for legal and financial advice, especially if there are concerns about the patient's judgment, decision-making, or vulnerability.

8. Discuss that the need for a formal evaluation for capacity may be warranted if a surrogate decision-maker is needed. Psychiatrists typically conduct such evaluations.

9. Discuss possible participation in research on dementia. The National Institutes of Health maintains a listing of all clinical trials at www.clinicaltrials.gov.

10. Discuss strategies for ensuring safety concerns (e.g., door alarms and medical alert tags).

11. Discuss end-of-life care.

a. Assess the patient's and family's cultural values and preferences (per advance directives if available).

b. Discuss goals for managing patient care, regarding dementia and any comorbid conditions.

c. Emphasize comfort measures (e.g., simplify medication regimen, maximize comfort for patient, and initiate referral for hospice care as indicated).

F. Follow-up care

1. Follow-up assessment of the person with dementia is typically every 6 months to a year or sooner if needed and should include:

   a. An assessment of daily function to assess progression of disease and to identify concerns of the patient or family.

   b. Cognitive status testing to assess progression of disease.

   c. Review for comorbid physical or neuropsychiatric conditions.

   d. Review of current medications to assess for therapeutic effectiveness and potential negative side effects.

   e. Physical examination as appropriate.

   f. Continuation of patient and family education as needed and referrals for education and support as needed.

VI. Assessment and management of concomitant conditions

There are factors that may negatively impact the status of the patient with dementia and their caregiver. For example, depression has been shown to contribute to excess disability of the patient with dementia. The selective serotonin reuptake inhibitors are the ideal medication for treating depression (Swartz, Barak, Mirecki, Naor, & Weizman, 2000). Sudden changes in the patient's behavior may not be caused by advancing disease, but may be a result of physical illness (e.g., pneumonia or urinary tract infection). Sudden changes warrant both a medical evaluation and a review of the patient's medications.

VII. Assessment of the status of the family and caregiver

Caregiving responsibilities may include a variety of tasks ranging from management of medications and appointments; decision-making, money management, and guarding the safety of the patient; and assistance with walking, dressing, and other aspects of physical care. Dementia family caregiving is associated with negative physical and emotional outcomes for the caregiver (Schulz & Martire, 2004), although many express satisfaction with their roles. Race, ethnicity, financial resources, supportive resources, and preparation are only a few of the factors that impact the caregiver's experience with this role. Caregiver outcomes

include evidence of the use of effective skills in caregiving with minimal stress reported.

A. Assess the caregiver's physical and emotional health concerns

1. Assess their level of strain.

   a. The Modified Caregiver Strain Index is a 13-item survey designed to measure strain for certain aspects of caregiving with higher scores indicative of greater strain (Travis, Bernard, McAuley, Thornton, & Kole, 2003). The Caregiver Strain Index has good reliability and is easy to administer and score (Thornton & Travis, 2003).

   b. The Caregiver Strain Index is available at http://consultgerirn.org

   c. Assess the caregiver's coping strategies for managing the strain of caregiving and promote positive strategies (e.g., exercise, counseling, and so forth).

2. Assist the caregiver in identifying activities that are pleasurable for them and methods for incorporating these activities into their lifestyle.

3. Refer to caregiver support groups, counseling, respite care, or other services

VIII. General resources

A. The Alzheimer's Association

(http://www.alz.org; or 1-800-272-3900) is a national organization with local offices and can be a resource for all types of dementia.

B. Alzheimer's Disease Education and Referral Center

(www.alzheimers.org; or 1-800-438-4380), a sponsored service by the National Institute on Aging.

C. Guideline for Alzheimer's Disease Management:

California Workgroup on Guidelines for Alzheimer's Disease Management (http://www.alz.org/national /documents/2008_Guidelines_Final_Report.pdf)

D. The Hartford Institute for Geriatric Nursing, College of Nursing, New York University

Contains best practice information on the care of older adults and multiple assessment tools with administration and scoring instructions (http://consultgerirn .org/ or www.hartfordign.org)

REFERENCES

2009 Alzheimer's disease facts and figures. (2009). *Alzheimers Dementia and Geriatric Cognitive Disorders, 5*(3), 234–270.

American Psychiatric Association. (1994). *Diagnostic and statistical manual of mental disorders, 4th Ed. Rev.* Washington, DC: Author.

Andrade, C., & Radhakrishnan, R. (2009). The prevention and treatment of cognitive decline and dementia: An overview of recent research on experimental treatments. *Indian Journal of Psychiatry, 51*(1), 12–25.

Boustani, M., Peterson, B., Hanson, L., Harris, R., & Lohr, K. N. (2003). Screening for dementia in primary care: A summary of the evidence for the U.S. Preventive Services Task Force. *Annals of Internal Medicine, 138*(11), 927–937.

Boxer, A. L., & Miller, B. L. (2005). Clinical features of frontotemporal dementia. *Alzheimer Disease and Associated Disorders, 19*(Suppl. 1), S3–S6.

California Workgroup on Guidelines for Alzheimer's Disease Management. (2008). *Guideline for Alzheimer's disease management.* Unpublished manuscript.

Chui, H. C., Victoroff, J. I., Margolin, D., Jagust, W., Shankle, R., & Katzman, R. (1992). Criteria for the diagnosis of ischemic vascular dementia proposed by the State of California Alzheimer's Disease Diagnostic and Treatment Centers. *Neurology, 42*(3 Pt. 1), 473–480.

Clarfield, A. M. (2003). The decreasing prevalence of reversible dementias: An updated meta-analysis. *Archives of Internal Medicine, 163*(18), 2219–2229.

Costa, P., Williams, T., & Somerfield, M. (1996). Early identification of Alzheimer's disease and related dementias. Clinical Practice Guideline, Quick Reference Guide for Clinicians. *AHCPR Publication No. 97-0703:* Rockville, MD, *19,* 1–28.

Craig, D., Mirakhur, A., Hart, D. J., McIlroy, S. P., & Passmore, A. P. (2005). A cross-sectional study of neuropsychiatric symptoms in 435 patients with Alzheimer's disease. *American Journal of Geriatric Psychiatry, 13*(6), 460–468.

Crum, R. M., Anthony, J. C., Bassett, S. S., & Folstein, M. F. (1993). Population-based norms for the Mini-Mental State Examination by age and educational level. *Journal of the American Medical Association, 269*(18), 2386–2391.

de Vugt, M. E., Riedijk, S. R., Aalten, P., Tibben, A., van Swieten, J. C., & Verhey, F. R. (2006). Impact of behavioural problems on spousal caregivers: A comparison between Alzheimer's disease and frontotemporal dementia. *Dementia and Geriatric Cognitive Disorders, 22*(1), 35–41.

Folstein, M. F., Folstein, S. E., & McHugh, P. R. (1975). "Mini-mental state". A practical method for grading the cognitive state of patients for the clinician. *Journal of Psychiatric Research, 12*(3), 189–198.

Gill, S. S., Bronskill, S. E., Normand, S. L., Anderson, G. M., Sykora, K., Lam, K., . . . Rochon, P. A. (2007). Antipsychotic drug use and mortality in older adults with dementia. *Annals of Internal Medicine, 146*(11), 775–786.

Graf, C. (2007). The Lawton Instrumental Activities of Daily Living (IADL) Scale. *Annals of Long-Term Care, 15*(7).

Lawton, M., & Brody, E. (1969). Assessment of older people: Self-maintaining and instrumental activity of daily living. *Gerontologist, 15,* 179–186.

McKeith, I. G. (2006). Consensus guidelines for the clinical and pathologic diagnosis of dementia with Lewy bodies (DLB): Report of the consortium on DLB International Workshop. *Journal of Alzheimer's Disease, 9*(Suppl. 3), 417–423.

McKhann, G., Drachman, D., Folstein, M., Katzman, R., Price, D., & Stadlan, E. M. (1984). Clinical diagnosis of Alzheimer's disease: Report of the NINCDS-ADRDA Work Group under the auspices of Department of Health and Human Services Task Force on Alzheimer's Disease. *Neurology, 34*(7), 939–944.

Miller, B. L., Boone, K., Mishkin, F., Swartz, J., Koras, N., & Kushii, J. (1998). Clinical and neuropsychological features of FTD. In A. Kertesz & D. Munoz (Eds.), *Pick's disease and Pick complex* (pp. 23–33). New York, NY: Wiley-Liss.

Nasreddine, Z. S., Phillips, N. A., Bedirian, V., Charbonneau, S., Whitehead, V., Collin, I., . . . Chertkow, H. (2005). The Montreal Cognitive Assessment, MoCA: A brief screening tool for mild cognitive impairment. *Journal of the American Geriatrics Society, 53*(4), 695–699.

Neary, D., Snowden, J. S., Gustafson, L., Passant, U., Stuss, D., Black, S., . . . Benson, D. F. (1998). Frontotemporal lobar degeneration: A consensus on clinical diagnostic criteria. *Neurology, 51*(6), 1546–1554.

Petersen, R. C., Smith, G. E., Waring, S. C., Ivnik, R. J., Tangalos, E. G., & Kokmen, E. (1999). Mild cognitive impairment: Clinical characterization and outcome. *Archives of Neurology, 56*(3), 303–308.

Pfeffer, R. I., Kurosaki, T. T., Harrah, C. H., Jr., Chance, J. M., & Filos, S. (1982). Measurement of functional activities in older adults in the community. *The Journals of Gerontology, 37*(3), 323–329.

Santacruz, K. S., & Swagerty, D. (2001). Early diagnosis of dementia. *American Family Physician, 63*(4), 703–713, 717–718.

Schulz, R., & Martire, L. M. (2004). Family caregiving of persons with dementia: Prevalence, health effects, and support strategies. *American Journal of Geriatric Psychiatry, 12*(3), 240–249.

Sha, S., Hou, C., Viskontas, I. V., & Miller, B. L. (2006). Are frontotemporal lobar degeneration, progressive supranuclear palsy and corticobasal degeneration distinct diseases? *Nature Clinical Practice Neurology, 2*(12), 658–665.

Swartz, M., Barak, Y., Mirecki, I., Naor, S., & Weizman, A. (2000). Treating depression in Alzheimer's disease: integration of differing guidelines. *International Psychogeriatrics, 12*(3), 353–358.

Thornton, M., & Travis, S. S. (2003). Analysis of the reliability of the modified caregiver strain index. *The Journals of Gerontology Series B: Psychological Sciences and Social Sciences, 58*(2), S127–S132.

Travis, S. S., Bernard, M. A., McAuley, W. J., Thornton, M., & Kole, T. (2003). Development of the family caregiver medication administration hassles scale. *Gerontologist, 43*(3), 360–368.

U.S. Preventative Services Task Force. (2003). Screening for dementia: Recommendations and rationale. *Annals of Internal Medicine, 138*(11), 925–926.

Vogel, T., Brechat, P. H., Lepretre, P. M., Kaltenbach, G., Berthel, M., & Lonsdorfer, J. (2009). Health benefits of physical activity in older patients: A review. *International Journal of Clinical Practice, 63*(2), 303–320.

Williams, C. L., & Tappen, R. M. (2007). Effect of exercise on mood in nursing home residents with Alzheimer's disease. *American Journal of Alzheimer's Disease & Other Dementias, 22*(5), 389–397.

Yesavage, J., Brink, T., Rose, T., Lum, O., Huang, V., Adey, M., . . . Leirer, V. O. (1983). Development and validation of a geriatric depression screening scale: A preliminary report. *Journal of Psychiatric Research, 17,* 37–49.

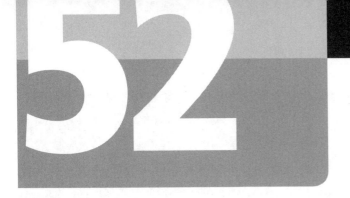

DEPRESSION

Matt Tierney and Beth Phoenix

I. Introduction and general background

A. Definition, overview, and epidemiology

Depression is a distinct mood disorder defined by the presence of numerous symptoms of specified duration (Figure 52-1). Depression can be expressed as major depressive disorder or as dysthymic disorder, also called "minor depression." It can also occur as part of a bipolar mood disorder in which depressive episodes alternate with manic or hypomanic episodes, or where both manic–hypomanic and depressive symptoms are manifested during the same period of time (mixed episode). Depression can appear similar to, or accompany, other psychiatric disorders, such as anxiety disorders, thought disorders, and substance abuse disorders. Thus, clinicians should be familiar with the current version of the *Diagnostic and Statistical Manual of Mental Disorders* (DSM) to distinguish depression from other psychiatric illnesses. As with all psychiatric illness, medical causes of depressive symptoms must be ruled out before determining a diagnosis of depression. Therefore, clinical evaluation should involve the assessment of biologic, psychologic and social factors.

The 12-month prevalence of major depressive disorder has been estimated at 6.7%, with over 80% of that group having moderate to severe depression, and lifetime prevalence of major depressive disorder has been estimated at 16.6% (Kessler, Chiu, Demier, Merikangas, & Walters, 2005). The prevalence of depression in primary care settings is estimated between 5% and 9% among adults (U.S. Department of Health and Human Services, Depression Guideline Panel, 1993), so it is important for the primary care provider to screen for, assess, and treat depression. Although depression is comparable in prevalence to other disorders commonly seen in primary care, it remains underrecognized by primary care providers (Wittkampf et al., 2009). Depression is not only underdiagnosed, it is also undertreated; it is estimated that only about 20% of Americans with depression receive care consistent with treatment guidelines (Gonzalez et al., 2010). Fortunately, initiatives to improve quality of depression care in primary care settings have resulted in the development of a number of diagnostic and treatment planning tools (MacArthur Initiative on Depression & Primary Care, 2009).

Depression is a significant public health problem; the World Health Organization rates depression as the leading cause of years of health lost to disability worldwide (Daly, 2009). Depression has a significant impact on public health for multiple reasons: it is common and interferes with many aspects of functioning; the typical age of onset is in the teenage or young adult years; and the disorder can easily become chronic, particularly if treatment is not prompt and adequate. If depressive episodes are not adequately treated, the brain becomes sensitized to being in a depressed state, which is then more likely to recur in the future. This phenomenon, called "kindling," may lead to depressive episodes that are more frequent, more severe, and of longer duration, with incomplete recovery between episodes. For this reason, it is important to prevent long-term morbidity through early diagnosis and aggressive treatment with the goal of complete remission.

In addition to the significant burden of depression-related disability, depression is also a significant cause of premature mortality from suicide. Many adults who died by suicide visited their primary care provider within 1 month of their deaths; thus, familiarity with suicide risk factors is strongly recommended (Luoma, Pearson, & Martin, 2002). The SAD PERSONS mnemonic (Table 52-1) summarizes major risk factors for suicide. The combination of severe depression and excessive alcohol consumption is implicated in a substantial majority of completed suicides in the United States, making substance use assessment a critical part of depression screening.

The U.S. Preventive Services Task Force (USPSTF) recommends depression screening for adults when support services are in place to accurately diagnose and treat depression, including the ability to provide follow-up. USPSTF does not recommend a specific screening instrument. The following two questions, sometimes referred to as the PHQ-2, are effective in identifying most cases of depression (Löwe, Kroenke, & Gräfe, 2005): "Over the past 2 weeks, have you felt down,

FIGURE 52-1 Patient Health Questionnaire-9 (PHQ-9)

Client Name: _____ Chart No. _____ Date: _____

Over the last 2 weeks, how often have you been bothered by any of the following problems?	Not at all	Several days	More than half the days	Nearly every day
1. Little interest or pleasure in doing things	0	1	2	3
2. Feeling down, depressed, or hopeless	0	1	2	3
3. Trouble falling or staying asleep, or sleeping too much	0	1	2	3
4. Feeling tired or having little energy	0	1	2	3
5. Poor appetite or overeating	0	1	2	3
6. Feeling bad about yourself — or that you are a failure or have let yourself or your family down	0	1	2	3
7. Trouble concentrating on things, such as reading the newspaper or watching television	0	1	2	3
8. Moving or speaking so slowly that other people could have noticed? Or the opposite — being so fidgety or restless that you have been moving around a lot more than usual	0	1	2	3
9. Thoughts that you would be better off dead or of hurting yourself in some way	0	1	2	3

For office coding

0 + _____ + _____ + _____

= Total Score: _____

If you checked off *any* problems, how *difficult* have these problems made it for you to do your work, take care of things at home, or get along with other people?

❏ Not difficult at all ❏ Somewhat difficult ❏ Very difficult ❏ Extremely difficult

PHQ-9 Scoring
For health care professional use

Total Score	Depression Severity
1-4	Minimal Depression
5-9*	Mild Depression
10-14*	Moderate Depression
15-19*	Moderately Severe Depression
20-27*	Severe Depression

* For any score 5 and above offer referral for Behavioral Health Services

TABLE 52-1 SAD PERSONS Mnemonic for Suicide Risk Factors

S ex (male)
A ge (elderly or adolescent)
D epression
P revious suicide attempts
E thanol abuse
R ational thinking loss (psychosis)
S ocial supports lacking
O rganized plan to commit suicide
N o spouse (divorced > widowed > single)
S ickness (physical illness)

Source: Adapted from Patterson, W. M., Dohn, H. H., Bird, J., & Patterson, G. A. (1983). Evaluation of suicidal patients: The SAD PERSONS scale. *Psychosomatics, 24*(4), 343–349.

TABLE 52-2 Depression Risk Factors

Other serious physical and mental health problems
Concurrent substance abuse or dependence
Family history of depression or suicide
Childhood depression; physical, emotional, or sexual abuse
Long-term use of certain medications
Personality traits, such as having low self-esteem and being overly dependent, self-critical, or pessimistic
Having recently given birth
Unemployment or low socioeconomic group
Female gender
Poor social support
Negative life events, such as bereavement, new onset of illness, institutionalization, financial strain, work-related distress, or experience of discrimination

depressed, or hopeless?" and "'Over the past 2 weeks, have you felt little interest or pleasure in doing things?"

A positive response to either of these questions warrants a more thorough screening for depression using diagnostic criteria from the DSM (Figure 52-1). The Geriatric Depression Scale may be used to screen for and monitor depressive symptoms in older adults (Kurlowicz & Greenberg, 2007).

II. **Database** (Table 52-2)

A. Subjective

1. Past health history: depression; anxiety; other psychiatric illness; trauma history including head trauma; chronic medical illnesses (e.g., HIV-AIDS, hepatitis C); physical disability; new serious health diagnosis; obstetric history; medication history, including current medications, medications or supplements taken in the past and effect on depression

2. Family history: depression, including death by suicide; other psychiatric illness; alcoholism or other substance abuse

3. Occupational history: presence or absence of rewarding and meaningful work

4. Personal and social history: support systems; substance use, including alcohol, nicotine, narcotics, and illicit drugs; relationship status; precipitating factors (stressors and losses)

5. Review of systems: somatic complaints without focal findings, including headaches and other

pain; anhedonia, depressed mood, hypersomnia or insomnia, psychomotor agitation or slowing; indecisiveness or decrease in concentration; fatigue or loss of energy; changes in appetite or weight; feeling guilty or poor self-esteem; suicidal thoughts or plans; irritability; pressured speech or thoughts; increase in goal-directed behaviors or risk-taking behaviors or in activities that have a high potential for negative consequences (e.g., buying sprees or sexual indiscretions); expansive or euphoric mood; psychosis including paranoia and auditory or visual hallucinations; and inability to care for activities of daily living.

B. Objective

1. Physical examination findings

    a. Vital signs, including weight

    b. Thyroid examination

    c. Neurologic examination if indicated. Clinical assessment sometimes reveals that suspected depression is actually another illness, often an organic brain illness (Cassem & Bernstein, 1997). Many discrete neurologic disorders (e.g., Parkinson's disease, Alzheimer's disease, cerebral vascular accidents, multiple sclerosis, traumatic brain and spinal cord injuries, dementias, and epilepsy) are associated with increased risk of depression (Fann & Tucker, 1995; Schneck & Buzan, 2000). Thus, a neurologic examination is often indicated in the physical assessment of depression.

d. Mental status examination

   i. Appearance and behavior: patient may demonstrate poor hygiene, poor eye contact, and inability to engage with interviewer.

   ii. Motor function: may demonstrate motor slowing or agitation.

   iii. Affect: can vary from anxious or irritable, to depressed with constricted affect.

   iv. Mood: use the patient's own description of mood.

   v. Language: assess flow and volume. Speech may be quiet with few words and slow; or may exhibit some nervous pressure.

   vi. Thought process: may be slow, evidenced by increased latency of response.

   vii. Thought content: what are the patient's main concerns? Patient may have suicidal or homicidal thoughts with or without a plan to carry these out (these are medical emergencies). Depressive symptoms may include obsessions, perseverations, paranoid ideas, feelings of depersonalization or unreality, and morbid thoughts. Psychotic depression may include auditory or visual hallucinations, or delusions.

   viii. Cognition: assess possible changes in all areas, including orientation, concentration, or memory; visuospatial skills or ability to abstract; and executive functioning.

   ix. Insight: rated good, fair, or poor based on the patient's awareness of their depressive symptoms. Patients who are unsure or unaware that symptoms may be caused by depression are rated fair or poor.

   x. Judgment: rated good, fair, or poor based on the patient's ability to gather and organize information to make plans and function well.

2. Data from diagnostic tests. No single test is associated with a definitive diagnosis of depression; however, the following should be considered as part of a basic work-up of depressive symptoms from other causes or of medical problems associated with depression

   a. Complete blood count to rule out anemia

   b. Metabolic panel to rule out possible medical causes of depressive symptoms

   c. Thyroid-stimulating hormone and free T4 to rule out thyroid dysregulation

   d. Serum vitamin B_{12} and folic acid levels to rule out vitamin deficiencies

   e. Drug of abuse screen to rule out co-occurring substance use disorders

   f. Hormone levels (gender specific) to rule out endocrine dysregulation

III. Assessment

A. Determine the diagnosis (DSM-IV-TR)

1. Major depressive disorder: presence of five out of nine depressive symptoms, with one of the symptoms being depressed mood or anhedonia, occurring daily for at least 2 weeks.

2. Dysthymia (minor depression): presence of three depressive symptoms (including depressed mood) for a duration of at least 2 years, with symptoms present more days than not.

3. Major depressive disorder and dysthymia ("double depression"): persistent low-grade depression with periods of more severe depressive symptoms.

4. Other psychiatric conditions that may explain the patient's presentation

   a. Bipolar disorder: if patient currently meets criteria for a depressive episode but also has a history of sustained expansive, euphoric, or irritable mood with pressured speech or thoughts, with increase in goal-directed behaviors or risk-taking activities, or with reduced need for sleep without feeling fatigue.

   b. Thought disorder: presence of psychosis, disorganized thinking, or paranoia.

   c. Anxiety disorder: when patient does not meet all criteria for a depressive disorder, but may have some of the symptoms accompanied by disabling worry about things that are out of the patient's control.

   d. Substance abuse disorder: if depressive symptoms are better accounted for by substance intoxication or withdrawal.

   e. Other medical conditions that explain symptoms, including but not limited to thyroid or other endocrine disorders, dementia, anemia, and malnutrition.

   f. Medication side effects (Table 52-3)

5. Specifiers may be used if appropriate

   a. Severity: mild, moderate, or severe, based on the presence of suicidal thoughts and the impact depression has on the patient's functional ability

   b. Chronicity: single episode, recurrent, or chronic

   c. With or without psychotic features

   d. With atypical features: presence of weight gain and hypersomnia. Although "typical

TABLE 52-3 Medications That May Cause Depression

Acyclovir	Clonidine	Metoclopramide
Alcohol	Cocaine (withdrawal)	Metrizamide
Amantadine	Contraceptives	Metronidazole
α methyldopa	Corticosteroids	NSAIDs
Amphetamines (withdrawal)	Cycloserine	Opiates
Anabolic steroids	Dapsone	Pentazocine
Anticonvulsants	Digitalis	Pergolide
Antihistamines	Disopyramide	Phenylpropanolamine
Antineoplastic agents	Disulfiram	Physostigmine
Antipsychotic medications	Estrogens	Prazosin
Baclofen	Ethambutol	Progestins, implanted
Barbiturates	Fluoroquinolone antibiotics	Reserpine
Benzodiazepines	Guanethidine	Statins
β-adrenergic blockers	Interferon alfa	Sulfonamides
Bromocriptine	Isotretinoin	Thiazide diuretics
Calcium channel blockers	Levodopa	
Cimetidine	Mefloquine	

Note. NSAIDs = nonsteroidal anti-inflammatory drugs.

Source: Schatzberg, A., & Nemeroff, C. (2009). *The American Psychiatric Publishing Textbook of Psychopharmacology* (4th Ed.). Washington, D.C.: APA. Reprinted with permission from the *American Psychiatric Publishing Textbook of Psychopharmacology*, (Copyright 2009). American Psychiatric Publishing, Inc.

depression" is characterized by insomnia and weight loss, "atypical depression" is characterized by hypersomnia and weight gain. This specifier can be misleading, because both types of depression are commonly seen in the primary care setting.

e. In remission: partial (alleviation of some but not all symptoms) or full (complete alleviation of symptoms); early (< 6 months) or sustained (> 6 months)

B. *Significance and motivation*

Assess the significance of depression to the patient and significant others, including impact on work, relationships, and activities. Determine the patient's willingness and ability to follow the treatment plan. Assess for presence of social supports and other patient strengths that may influence the ability to recover from depression.

IV. **Goals of clinical management**

A. *Screening and diagnosing depression*

Although there is no consensus on screening for depression, the USPSTF notes that "recurrent screening may be most productive in patients with a history of depression, unexplained somatic symptoms, comorbid psychological conditions (e.g., panic disorder or generalized anxiety), substance abuse, or chronic pain. The optimal interval for screening is unknown" (U.S. Department of Health and Human Services, 2009, p. 125).

B. *Treatment*

Select a treatment plan that leads to sustained full remission of depressive symptoms. Approximately one-third of depressed patients achieve remission with their initial treatment regimen, and approximately another one-third require several treatment regimens. Another one-third fail to respond to two or more adequate trials of antidepressant monotherapy, which is considered treatment-resistant depression (Gaynes et al., 2009). Treatment resistance is associated with a range of comorbid physical and mental disorders, including substance abuse.

1. Treatment phases

a. Acute phase: 0–16 weeks. Plan: initiate treatment and monitor weekly for first month and at least once a month thereafter.

b. Continuation phase: 16–20 weeks after symptom remission. Plan: continue treatment, monitor every 2–3 months.

c. Maintenance phase: 6 months symptom-free. Plan: continue monitoring and treatment every 2–3 months.

d. Discontinuation: consider treatment discontinuation only after patient has been symptom-free for 6–12 months. Patients with a history of depression should continue to be monitored for several months after the completion of a course of treatment, and patient education should include a review of the early signs of depression and a review of the importance of immediately resuming previously successful treatment in the event of a symptom relapse (American Psychiatric Association, 2000).

C. Patient adherence

Select an approach that maximizes patient adherence, including but not limited to cost, frequency of treatment, tolerability of treatment, and patient health beliefs.

V. Plan

A. Diagnostic tests to rule out other causes of depressive symptoms

Complete blood count with differential; complete metabolic panel, vitamin B_{12}, folate, thyroid-stimulating hormone, free T4; Gamma-glutamyl transferase (GGT) or breathalyzer if alcohol use suspected; consider a drug of abuse screen and a more thorough toxicology screen (e.g., heavy metal screen) if indicated by history. HIV testing if indicated by history.

B. Management (includes treatment, consultation, referral, and follow-up care)

1. Medication management (Figure 52-2). Medication treatment should always include consideration of the following: patient history of medication treatment for depression; cost and insurance coverage; past or anticipated side effects; and concurrent patient medications (Table 52-4 and Table 52-5).

2. Psychotherapy: for mild to moderate depression, psychotherapy has generally been found to be equal in efficacy to pharmacologic treatment (Wolf & Hopko, 2008), and the combination of medication and psychotherapy is more effective than either modality alone. Circumstances under which referral for psychotherapy should be considered as a first-line treatment option include patient preference and pregnancy and lactation.

3. Combined treatment with antidepressants and psychologic treatment is recommended for
   a. Partial response to either treatment alone
   b. Patients with personality disorders or complex psychosocial problems
   c. Patients with a history of chronic or severe depression

4. Consultation with physician: concurrent medical illness or suspicion of same and polypharmacy treatment.

5. Referral to mental health or psychiatric specialty for evaluation or management: psychotic symptoms, suspicion of bipolar disorder or thought disorder, prior treatment-resistant depression, active suicidal ideation or plan, and concurrent psychiatric or neurologic disorder.

C. Client education

1. Information: provide verbal and written information regarding
   a. The disease process, including but not limited to signs and symptoms and possible causes and risks, including self-harm
   b. The importance of treatment, including non-pharmacologic treatment, with the goal of complete and sustained remission of depression; expected treatment duration; and community resources to manage psychiatric crises
   c. Selection of written educational materials should consider
      i. Patient educational and reading level
      ii. Availability of materials in patient's preferred language
      iii. Accuracy of information and freedom from commercial bias

2. Counseling
   a. Supportive counseling, focusing on problem-solving and use of coping strategies (MacArthur Initiative on Depression & Primary Care, 2009)
   b. Behavioral recommendations: regular exercise, especially aerobic exercise; balanced diet; presence of supportive relationships; and sleep hygiene

VI. Self-management resources and tools

Brief educational or self-management interventions, such as manualized or book-based therapies and the use of interactive web-based or other computer programs based on cognitive-behavioral approaches, have been shown to improve depression outcomes for patients treated in primary care settings (McNaughton, 2009).

A. Educational resources (books and websites)

1. Patient education brochures about depression in English and Spanish can be downloaded or ordered from the National Institutes for Mental Health (http://www.nimh.nih.gov/health/publications /depression/complete-index.shtml). The National

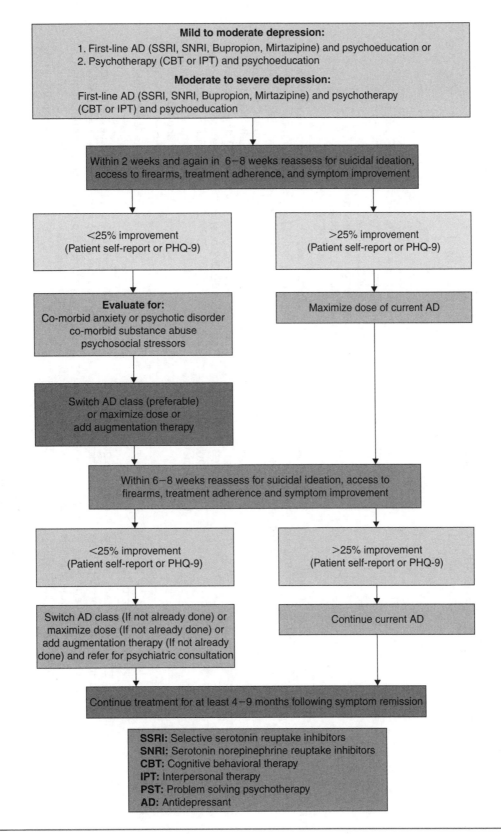

FIGURE 52-2 Primary Care Treatment Algorithm for Depression

Source: Reprinted with permission from Wolters Kluwer. From Fancher, T., McCarron, R. M., Kukoyi, O., & Bourgeois, J. A. (2009). Chapter 2: Mood disorders—Depression. In R. M. McCarron, G. L. Xiong, & J. A. Bourgeois (Eds.), Lippincott's Primary Care Psychiatry, p. 31.

TABLE 52-4 Section II—Information Guide To Antidepressants Revised—March 2009

Antidepressant*	Therapeutic Dose Range (mg/day)	Initial Suggested Dose**	Titration Schedule	Advantages	Disadvantages
Selective Serotonin Reuptake Inhibitors (SSRIs)					
Citalopram (Celexa)	20–40	20 mg in morning with food (10 mg in elderly or those with panic disorder)	Maintain initial dose for 4 weeks before dose increase. If no response, increase in 10 mg increments every 7 days as tolerated.	Helpful for anxiety disorders. Few drug interactions. Generic available.	
Escitalopram (Lexapro)	10–30 mg	10 mg for escitalopram	Increase to 20 mg if partial response after 4 weeks	More potent s-enantiomer of citalopram, 10 mg dose effective for most. FDA labeling for general anxiety disorder. Reduces all three symptom groups of PTSD.	More expensive than citalopram.
Fluoxetine (Prozac)	10–80	20 mg in the morning with food (10 mg in elderly and those with comorbid panic disorder)	Maintain 20 mg for 4–6 weeks and 30 mg for 2–4 weeks before additional dose increases. Increase in 10 mg increments at 7-day intervals. If significant side effects occur within 7 days, lower dose or change medication.	Helpful for anxiety disorders. Long half-life good for poor adherence, missed doses; less frequent discontinuation symptoms. Reduces all three symptom groups of PTSD. Generic available.	Slower to reach steady state and eliminate when discontinued. Sometimes too stimulating. Active metabolite has half-life ~10 days and renal elimination. Inhibitor of cytochrome P450 2D6 and 3A4. Use cautiously in the elderly and others taking multiple medications.
Fluoxetine Weekly (Prozac Weekly)	90	Initiate only after patient stable on 20 mg daily	Start 7 days after last dose of 20 mg.		No generic available.
Paroxetine (Paxil)	10–50 (40 in elderly)	20 mg once daily, usually in the morning with food (10 mg in elderly and those with comorbid panic disorder)	Maintain 20 mg for 4 weeks before dose increase. Increase in 10 mg increments at intervals of approximately 7 days up to maximum dose of 50 mg/day (40 elderly)	FDA labeling for most anxiety disorders. Reduces all three symptom groups of PTSD. Generic available.	Sometimes sedating. Anticholinergic effects can be troublesome. Inhibitor of CYP2D6 (drug interactions) Discontinuation/withdrawal symptoms.
(Paxil CR)	25–62.5 (50 in elderly)	25 mg daily (12.5 mg in elderly and those with panic disorder)	Increase by 12.5 mg at weekly intervals, maintain 25 mg for 4 weeks before dose increase	May cause less nausea and GI distress.	Generic not available

TABLE 52-4 Section II—Information Guide To Antidepressants *(continued)*
Revised—March 2009

Antidepressant*	Therapeutic Dose Range (mg/day)	Initial Suggested Dose**	Titration Schedule	Advantages	Disadvantages
Selective Serotonin Reuptake Inhibitors (SSRIs) *(continued)*					
Sertraline (Zoloft)	25–200	50 mg once daily, usually in the morning with food (25 mg for elderly)	Maintain 50 mg for 4 weeks. Increase in 25–50 mg increments at 7-day intervals as tolerated. Maintain 100 mg for 4 weeks before next dose increase.	FDA labeling for anxiety disorders including PTSD. Safety shown post MI. Generic available.	Weak inhibitor of CYP2D6–drug interactions less likely.
Serotonin and Norepinephrine Antagonist					
Mirtazapine (Remeron)	15–45	15 mg at bedtime	Increase in 15 mg increments (7.5 mg in elderly) as tolerated. Maintain 30 mg for 4 weeks before further dose increase.	Few drug interactions. Less or no sexual dysfunction. Less sedation as dose increases. May stimulate appetite. Generic available.	Sedation at low doses only (≤ 15 mg). Weight gain due to appetite stimulation.
Norepinephrine and Dopamine Reuptake Inhibitor					
Bupropion † (Wellbutrin)	200–450	100 mg twice a day (once a day in elderly)	Increase to 100 mg three times a day after 7 days (slower titration for elderly). After 4 weeks, increase to maximum 150 mg three times a day if necessary. Hepatic impairment: 75 mg/day	Can be stimulating. Less or no sexual dysfunction. Generic available.	At higher doses may induce seizures. Contra-indicated in persons with seizure disorders or eating disorders. Stimulating effect can increase anxiety or insomnia.
Bupropion SR† (Wellbutrin SR)	200–400 mg	150 mg once a day (100 mg in elderly)	Increase to 150 mg twice a day after 7 days (100 bid elderly). Increase to 200 mg twice a day after 4 weeks (150 bid elderly) if insufficient response. Hepatic impairment: 100 mg daily.	Also indicated for smoking cessation (Zyban). Generic available.	Do not split or crush SR or XL products. CYP2B6 inhibitor
Bupropion XL† (Wellbutrin XL)	300–450 mg	150 mg once daily (in the morning)	Increase to 300 mg daily after 7 days. Increase to 450 mg per day after 4 weeks if necessary. Hepatic impairment: 150 mg		Generic XL not available.

(continues)

TABLE 52-4 Section II—Information Guide To Antidepressants *(continued)* Revised—March 2009

Antidepressant*	Therapeutic Dose Range (mg/day)	Initial Suggested Dose**	Titration Schedule	Advantages	Disadvantages
Serotonin and Norepinephrine Reuptake Inhibitors					
Venlafaxine (Effexor, Effexor XR)	75–375	75 mg with food; 37.5 mg if anxious, elderly or debilitated	Immediate release (IR) dose should be divided two or three times a day. For extended release (XR) give 37.5 mg in a.m., then increase to 75 mg in a.m. after 1 week, 150 mg in the a.m. after 2 weeks. If partial response after 4 weeks increase to 225 mg in the a.m. Norepinephrine effect only occurs above 150 mg.	Helpful for anxiety disorders, neuropathic pain, and vasomotor symptoms. XR version should be taken once a day. May reduce all three symptom groups of PTSD. Generic available (IR and XR)	May increase blood pressure at higher doses. Risk for drug interactions similar to fluoxetine. Discontinuation/ withdrawal symptoms. Sexual dysfunction.
Desvenlafaxine (Pristiq)	50–400	50 mg once daily	No evidence that higher doses are associated with greater effect.	Active metabolite of venlafaxine.	Dose adjustment if CrCl < 30 ml/min. Gradually increase dosing interval when discontinuing when taken for ≥ 6 weeks (taper dose if dose > %50 mg/ day).Sexual dysfunction. Generic not available.
Duloxetine	40–60	40 or 60 mg as a single or divided dose (20 or 40 mg elderly)	Dose can be increased after 1 week. Maximum dose 120 mg/d although doses > 60 mg/d have not been shown to be more effective.	Also approved for general anxiety disorder and pain associated with diabetic neuropathy and fibromyalgia.	Dose adjustment if CrCl < 30 ml/min. Urinary hesitancy. Sexual dysfunction. Generic not available.
Tricyclic Antidepressants: Secondary Amines					
Desipramine‡ (Norpramin)	100–300 (25–100 in elderly)	50 mg in the morning (10 or 25 mg elderly)	Increase by 25 to 50 mg every 3 to 7 days to initial target dose of 150 mg (75 or 100 mg elderly) for 4 weeks. Target serum concentration: > 115 ng/ml.	More effect on Norepinephrine than serotonin. Effective for diabetic neuropathy and neuropathic pain. Compliance and effective dose can be verified by serum concentration. Generic available.	Can be stimulating, but sedating to some patients. Anticholinergic, cardiac, and hypotensive (less than tertiary amines); caution in patients with BPH or cardiac conduction disorder or CHF

TABLE 52-4 Section II—Information Guide To Antidepressants (continued) Revised—March 2009

Antidepressant*	Therapeutic Dose Range (mg/day)	Initial Suggested Dose**	Titration Schedule	Advantages	Disadvantages
Tricyclic Antidepressants: Secondary Amines (continued)					
Nortriptyline ‡ (Pamelor)	25–100	25 mg (10 mg in elderly) in the evening	Increase in 10–25 mg increments every 5–7 days as tolerated to 75 mg/day. Obtain serum concentration after 4 weeks; target range: 50–150 ng/mL.	Less orthostatic hypotension than other tricyclics. Compliance and effective dose can be verified by serum concentration. Generic available.	Anticholinergic, cardiac, and hypotensive (less than tertiary amines); caution in patients with BPH or cardiac conduction disorder or CHF.

*There are more antidepressants than those listed in this table. However, this list provides a reasonable variety of drugs that have different side effects and act by different neurotransmitter mechanisms. The January 29, 2009, issue of *The Lancet* includes a meta-analysis and an editorial concluding that sertraline offers the best balance among efficacy, acceptability, and costs compared to 11 other agents. [1,2,3]

Treatment of Parkinson's disease may include selegiline (Eldepryl), which is a selective monoamine oxidase inhibitor (MAOI) at low doses only. Because the use of many antidepressants is contraindicated in conjunction with a nonselective MAOI, caution with or discontinuation of Eldepryl may be in order. Selegiline is also available as a higher dose and nonselective, transdermal patch (Emsam) approved for the treatment of major depressive disorder.

**For SSRIs, venlafaxine, and the tricyclic antidepressants, start at the beginning of the therapeutic dosing range. If side effects are bothersome, reduce the dose and increase slower. In the elderly, the debilitated or those sensitive to medications, start lower. For all antidepressants, allow four weeks at a therapeutic dose, then assess for response. If only partial or slight response but well tolerated, then increase the dose. If no response, worse symptoms, or intolerable side effects, switch antidepressants.

For treatment of depression in pregnancy, TCAs and SSRIs (particularly fluoxetine) are generally the agents of choice. However, the SSRIs have been associated with persistent newborn pulmonary hypertension with maternal use and 20 weeks of gestation, a slight decrease in gestational age, lower birth weight, and neonatal withdrawal or adaptation syndrome. Paroxetine has been associated with first-trimester cardiovascular malformations (ventricular and atrial septal defects); hence the use of paroxetine should be avoided during the first trimester. TCAs have been associated with neonatal withdrawal symptoms and anticholinergic adverse effects. There are insufficient data about other newer antidepressants, although there may be a link between bupropion and spontaneous abortion.

[2]Parikh SV. Antidepressants are not all created equal. *The Lancet.* Early Online Publication, Jan 29, 2009. DOI:10.1016/S0140-6736(09)60047-7

[3]Cipriani A. Furukawa TA, Salanti G, Geddes JR, Higgins JPT, Churchill R, Watanabe N, Nakagawa A, Omori IM, McGuire H, Tansella M, Barbui C. Comparative efficacy and acceptability of 12 new-generation antidepressants: a multiple-treatments meta-analysis. *The Lancet,* Early Online Publication, 29 January 2009. DOI:10-1016/S0140-6736(09)60046-5

[3] Qaseem A, Snow V, Denberg TD, Forciea MA, Owens DK. Using second-generation antidepressants to treat depressive disorders: a clinical practice guideline from the American College of Physicians. *Annals of Internal Medicine,* 2008 Nov 18;149(10):725–733.

For women planning to breast feed, an antidepressant with the lowest excretion into breast milk, i.e., lowest infant serum concentrations and fewer adverse reactions, should be considered. These include sertraline, paroxetine and nortriptyline. Citalopram and fluoxetine have the highest concentrations in breast milk and more reports of infant adverse effects. A 40% decrease in breast milk concentration can be achieved by switching to escitalopram at 25% of the citalopram dose. Venlafaxine is detectable in the serum and associated with less weight gain in breast-fed infants. Less information is available about bupropion, mirtazepine and trazodone, although the concentrations in breast milk infant serum are low. The TCAs are nearly undetectable in infant plasma concentrations and low concentrations are found in breast milk but have less advantageous side effect profiles.

†Avoid bupropion in patients with a history of seizures, eating disorders, significant central nervous system lesions, or recent head trauma.

‡Tricyclic antidepressants (TCAs) have lower costs but somewhat higher discontinuation rates compared to SSRIs and second generation antidepressants due to side effects. The TCA are more lethal in overdose than SSRIs. TCAs may be contraindicated in patients with certain physical comorbidities such as recent myocardial infarction, cardiac conduction defects, urinary retention, narrow angle glaucoma, orthostatic hypotension, and cognitive impairment.

Source: Courtesy of MacArthur Foundation Initiative on Depression and Primary Care. MacArthur Toolkit—Copyright April 2006 3 CM LLC. Used with permission. Also available at http://www.depression-primarycare.org/

TABLE 52-5 Section III. Clinician Antidepressant Fact Sheet
Page 2 of 2

Antidepressant Side Effects

Side effects account for as many as two-thirds of all premature discontinuations of antidepressants. Most side effects are early onset and time limited (e.g., SSRI decreased appetite, nausea, diarrhea, agitation, anxiety, headache). These can be managed by temporary aids to tolerance. Some side effects are early-onset and persistent or late onset (e.g., SSRI apathy, fatigue, weight gain, sexual dysfunction) and may require additional medications or a switch in antidepressant.

Strategies for Managing Antidepressant Side Effects:

1. Allow patient to verbalize his/her complaint about side effects.
2. Wait and support. Some side effects (i.e., GI distress) will subside over 1–2 weeks.
3. Lower the dose temporarily.
4. Treat the side effects (see table).
5. Change to a different antidepressant.
6. Discontinue medications and start psychological counseling.

Side Effect	SSRIs & Efflexor	Tricyclics (nortriptyline, amitriptyline, imipramine)	Bupropion	Mirtazapine	Management Strategy
Sedation	±	++	–	+	Give medication at bedtime. *Increase* Remeron dose. Try caffeine.
Anticholinergic-like symptoms: Dry mouth/eyes, Constipation, Urinary retention, Tachycardia	±	+++	–	±	Increase hydration. Sugarless gum/candy Dietary fiber. Artificial tears. Consider switching medication.
GI distress Nausea	++	–	+	±	Often improves in 1–2 weeks. Take with meals. Consider antacids or H2 blockers.
Restlessness Jitters/Tremors	+	±	++	–	Start with small doses, especially with anxiety disorder. Reduce dose temporarily. Add beta-blocker (propranolol 10–20 mg bid/tid). Consider short trial of benzodiazepine.
Headache	+	–	+	–	Lower dose. Acetaminophen.
Insomnia	+	–	+	–	Trazodone 25–100 mg po qhs (can cause orthostatic hypotension and priapism). Take medication in A.M.
Sexual Dysfunction	++	–	–	–	May be part of depression or medical disorders. Decrease dose. Consider a trial of Viagra. Try adding bupropion 100 mg qhs or bid. Try adding buspirone 10–20 mg bid/tid. Try adding cyproheptadine 4 mg 1–2 hrs. before sex.

TABLE 52-5 Section III. Clinician Antidepressant Fact Sheet *(continued)*
Page 2 of 2

Side Effect	SSRIs & Efflexor	Tricyclics (nortriptyline, amitriptyline, imipramine)	Bupropion	Mirtazapine	Management Strategy
Seizures	–	–	+	±	Discontinue antidepressant.
Weight gain	±	±	±	++	Exercise Diet Consider changing medications
Agranulocytosis	–	–	–	±	Monitor for signs of infection, flu-like symptoms Stop drug, check WBC

Key: – Very unlikely   ± Uncommon   +Mild   ++ Moderate

Source: Courtesy of MacArthur Foundation Initiative on Depression and Primary Care. MacArthur Toolkit—Copyright April 2006 3 CM LLC. Used with permission. Also available at http://www.depression-primarycare.org/

Institutes for Mental Health also produced a brief video about depression (http://www.youtube.com/watch?v=GB5DSmdyutI).

2. The MacArthur Initiative on Depression and Primary Care (www.depression-primarycare.org) includes patient education materials as part of its Depression Management Tool Kit (2009).

3. Beyond Blue (www.beyondblue.org.au), an organization to address issues related to depression in Australia, has information about depression in multiple languages including Spanish, Chinese, and Vietnamese.

4. The Antidepressant Skills Workbook, a self-management manual for adults with depression, can be downloaded free from www.comh.ca/antidepressant-skills/adult/.

5. Feeling Good: The New Mood Therapy (Burns, 1980) describes a cognitive therapy approach to depression management. It is commonly used as self-guided treatment and in depression treatment programs.

6. A free interactive skills program based on cognitive-behavioral and interpersonal psychotherapy approaches can be found at http://moodgym.anu.edu.au.

B. Community support groups

1. National Alliance on Mental Illness website (www.nami.org). This support, education, and advocacy organization offers a variety of educational materials about depression including fact sheets, podcasts, and video clips.

2. The Depression and Bipolar Support Alliance (www.dbsalliance.org) offers educational brochures about depression and other mood disorders and conducts in-person and online support groups and educational events.

REFERENCES

American Psychiatric Association. (2000, April). *Practice guideline for the treatment of patients with major depressive disorder.* Retrieved from http://www.psychiatryonline.com/pracGuide/PracticePDFs/MDD2e_Inactivated_04-16-09.pdf

Burns, D. D. (1980). *Feeling good: The new mood therapy.* New York, NY: William Morrow.

Cassem, N. H., & Bernstein, J. G. (1997). Depressed patients. In N. H. Kassem, T. A. Stern, J. F. Rosenbaum, & M. S. Jellinek (Eds.), *Massachusetts General Hospital: Handbook of general psychiatry* (4th ed., pp. 35–68). St. Louis, MO: Mosby.

Daly, R. (2009, January 2). Depression biggest contributor to global disease burden. *Psychiatric News, 44*(1), 7.

Fann, J. R., & Tucker, G. J. (1995). Mood disorders with general medical condition. *Current Opinion in Psychiatry, 8,* 13–18.

Gaynes, B. N., Warden, D., Trivedi, M. H., Wisniewski, S. R., Fava, M., & Rush, A. J. (2009). What did STAR*D teach us? Results from a large-scale, practical, clinical trial for patients with depression. *Psychiatric Services, 60*(11), 1439–1445.

Gonzalez, H. M., Vega, W. A., Williams, D. R., Taraf, W., West, B. T., & Neighbors, H. W. (2010). Depression care in the United States: Too little for too few. *Archives of General Psychiatry, 67*(1), 37–46.

Kessler, R. C., Chiu, W. T., Demier, O., Merikangas, K. R., & Walters, E. E. (2005). Prevalence, severity, and comorbidity of 12-month DSM-IV disorders in the National Comorbidity Survey Replication. *Archives of General Psychiatry, 62*(6), 617–627.

Kurlowicz, L., & Greenberg, S. A. (2007). The Geriatric Depression Scale (GDS). In *Try this: Best practices in nursing care to older adults, issue 4.* Retrieved from http://consultgerirn.org/uploads/File/trythis/issue04.pdf

Löwe, B., Kroenke, K., & Gräfe, K. (2005). Detecting and monitoring depression with a two-item questionnaire (PHQ-2). *Journal of Psychosomatic Research, 58*(2), 163–171.

Luoma, J. B., Pearson, J. L., & Martin, C. E. (2002). Contact with mental health and primary care prior to suicide: A review of the evidence. *American Journal of Psychiatry, 159,* 909–916.

MacArthur Initiative on Depression & Primary Care. (2009). *Depression management toolkit.* Retrieved from http://www.depression-primarycare.org/

McNaughton, J. L. (2009). Brief interventions for depression in primary care: A systematic review. *Canadian Family Physician, 55*(8), 789–796.

Schneck, C. D., & Buzan, R. D. (2000). Mood disorders in neurologic illness. *Current Treatment Options in Neurology, 2,* 151–168.

U.S. Department of Health and Human Services, Depression Guideline Panel. (1993). *Clinical practice guideline No. 5, depression in primary care: Volume 1. Detection and diagnosis.* (AHCPR Publication No. 93-0550). Rockville, MD: Author.

U.S. Department of Health and Human Services. (2009). *Guide to clinical preventative services, 2009 recommendations of the U.S. Preventive Services Task Force (pocket guide, Abridged version of the recommendations).* Retrieved from http://www.ahrq.gov/clinic/uspstf

Wittkampf, K., van Ravesteijn, H., Baas, K., van de Hoogen, H., Schene, A., Bindels, P., Van Weert, H. (2009). The accuracy of Patient Health Questionnaire-9 in detecting depression and measuring depression severity in high-risk groups in primary care. *General Hospital Psychiatry, 31*(5), 451–459.

Wolf, N. J., & Hopko, D. R. (2008). Psychosocial and pharmacological interventions for depressed adults in primary care: A critical review. *Clinical Psychology Review, 28,* 131–161.

Zuithoff, N. P., Vergouwe, Y., King, M., Nazareth, I., Hak, E., Moons, K. G., & Geerlings, M. I. (2009). A clinical prediction rule for detecting major depressive disorder in primary care: The PREDICT-NL study. *Family Practice, 26*(4), 241–250.

DIABETES MELLITUS

Barbara A. Boland

I. Introduction, general background, prevalence, and incidence

Diabetes mellitus is a metabolic disorder characterized by hyperglycemia that results from decreased insulin secretion, insulin resistance, or both. There are several types of diabetes. The most common types are type 1, type 2, and gestational diabetes.

Approximately 23.6 million children and adults in the United States (7.8% of the population) have diabetes. Of these, 17.9 million are diagnosed, 5.7 million are undiagnosed, and 57 million have prediabetes. Type 1 diabetes accounts for approximately 5–10% of diagnosed diabetes cases, whereas type 2 makes up the other 90–95% (American Diabetes Association, 2009a). This number is predicted to increase from 23.6 million in 2009 to 44.1 million in 2034 (Huang, Basu, O'Grady, & Capretta, 2009).

A. Type 1 diabetes

1. Definition and overview

   Type 1 diabetes is caused by an autoimmune process that destroys the β cells in the pancreas, thereby resulting in little or no insulin production. Individuals with type 1 diabetes cannot live without administration of exogenous insulin. Type 1 diabetes is usually diagnosed early in life (before age 30) and often presents acutely with symptoms and high blood sugars.

B. Type 2 diabetes

1. Definition and overview

   Type 2 diabetes is usually the result of insulin resistance, although it can also be caused by decreased insulin production. Individuals with type 2 diabetes are often obese. Risk factors for type 2 include age older than 45 years; obesity; sedentary lifestyle; family history of diabetes; history of gestational diabetes; delivery of a baby over 9 lb; race or ethnicity (African Americans, Latinos, Native Americans, and Asian Americans/Pacific Islanders); and the aged population. Type 2 diabetes is becoming more common in children and adolescents.

C. Gestational diabetes

1. Definition and overview

   Gestational diabetes occurs in 3–12% of pregnancies. Pregnancy is an insulin-resistant state. Women with a history of gestational diabetes have a 40–60% chance of developing type 2 diabetes in the next 5–10 years after their pregnancy; therefore, they should have their blood sugar monitored periodically. For more indepth information see Chapter 32 on Gestational Diabetes.

II. Database (may include but is not limited to)

A. Subjective

1. Past medical history

   a. Medical illnesses: pancreatitis, pancreatic cancer, cystic fibrosis, hemachromatosis (can damage the pancreas), Cushing's syndrome, glucagonoma, and pheochromocytoma; history of cerebral vascular accident, myocardial infarction, hypertension, hyperlipidemia, and peripheral arterial disease

   b. Surgical history: pancreatic surgery and liver surgery

   c. Trauma history: pancreatic trauma

   d. Obstetric and gynecological history: history of gestational diabetes or delivery of baby weighing greater than 9 lb; contraception method

   e. Medication history: medications that increase blood glucose levels or interfere with the release of insulin (e.g., glucocorticoids, pentamidine, nicotinic acid, thyroid hormone, phenytoin, and thiazides). Any over-the-counter or herbal medication (e.g., sweetened cough preparations).

2. Family history

   a. Diabetes mellitus

   b. Other endocrine disorders

3. Occupational and educational history

   a. Education level

   b. Occupation

   c. Days missed from school or work

4. Personal and social history

   a. Tobacco, alcohol, and drug use

   b. Diet history and recall

   c. Exercise

   d. Cultural history, living arrangements, housing, and psychosocial supports and problems

5. Review of symptoms

   a. Constitutional signs and symptoms: fatigue, weight loss, and polydipsia

   b. Skin, hair, and nails; slowed wound healing

   c. Eye, ear, nose, and throat; blurry vision; and gum infections or dental disease

   d. Respiratory: shortness of breath

   e. Cardiac: chest pain

   f. Gastrointestinal: polyphagia and symptoms of gastroparesis

   g. Genitourinary: polyuria, recurrent vaginal yeast infections, and sexual or erectile dysfunction

   h. Neurologic: decreased sensation or tingling and numbness in extremities

   i. Psychiatric: history of stress

B. Objective

   1. Physical examination findings

      a. Height, weight, body mass index (note body mass index > 25)

      b. Vital signs, including orthostatic blood pressure measurements

      c. Skin: acanthosis nigricans; fungal infections of feet or toenails; and cracks in skin or wounds, especially hands and feet

      d. HEENT: eyes for retinopathy, vision test for blurry vision, teeth or gum inflammation, and poor dentition

      e. Thyroid: thyromegaly

   f. Lungs: crackles consistent with cardiovascular sequela.

   g. Cardiac: irregular heartbeat, cardiomegaly, and murmurs

   h. Abdomen: hepatomegaly

   i. Vascular: peripheral pulses, bruits, and edema

   j. Neurologic: sensory; motor strength; and deep tendon reflexes (patellar and Achilles)

   k. Foot examination: inspection; pulses in dorsalis pedis and posterior tibial, determination of proprioception, vibration, and monofilament sensation

   2. Psychiatric: note symptoms of anxiety or depression

   3. Supporting data from relevant diagnostic tests (Table 53-1)

III. Assessment

A. Determine the diagnosis (International Classification of Diseases-9 codes related to diabetes are available online from a variety of sites).

   1. Type 1 diabetes: latent autoimmune diabetes in adults

   2. Type 2 diabetes

   3. Gestational diabetes

   4. Maturity onset diabetes of the young

   5. Diseases of the pancreas

      a. Pancreatitis

      b. Pancreatic malignancy

   6. Liver disease

      a. Cirrhosis

      b. Hemochromatosis

   7. Endocrinopathies

      a. Cushing's disease

      b. Acromegaly

      c. Glucagonoma

TABLE 53-1 Criteria for the Diagnosis of Diabetes

1. $HgbA_{1C} \geq 6.5\%$. The test should be performed in a laboratory using a method that is NGSP certified and standardized to the DCCT assay.
   or

2. Fasting plasma glucose concentration $\geq$ 126 mg/dl (fasting is defined as no caloric intake for at least 8 hours).
   or

3. 2-hour plasma glucose $\geq$ 200 mg/dl during a 75-g oral glucose tolerance test.
   or

4. Symptoms of hyperglycemia or hyperglycemic crisis plus a random plasma glucose $\geq$ 200 mg/dl.

5. In the absence of unequivocal hyperglycemia, criteria 1–3 should be confirmed by repeat testing.

Source: American Diabetes Association. (2010). Standards of medical care in diabetes—2010. *Diabetes Care, 33*(1), S11–S61.

d. Pheochromocytoma

e. Hyperthyroidism

8. Medication induced

a. Glucocorticoids

b. Phenytoin

c. Thyroid hormone

d. Pentamidine

e. Nicotinic acid

f. Thiazide diuretics

B. *Severity: assess the severity of the disease*

C. *Significance: assess the significance of the problem to the patient and significant others*

D. *Motivation and ability: determine the patient's willingness and ability to follow the treatment plan*

IV. Goals of clinical management

A. *Screening or diagnosing diabetes: choose a cost effective approach for screening and diagnosing diabetes*

B. *Treatment: Select a treatment plan that controls glucose in a safe and effective manner, without causing hypoglycemia*

C. *Patient adherence: select an approach that maximizes patient adherence*

D. *Prevention of complications: glycemic control*

V. Plan

A. *Screening*

1. High-risk groups

a. Family history: first- or second-degree relatives

b. Symptoms of hyperglycemia

c. Age 45 and older; if normal, check every 3 years

d. Obesity; body mass index greater than 25

e. Patients in high-risk ethnic groups: African Americans, Hispanic Americans, Native Americans, and Asian Americans/Pacific Islanders. The American Diabetes Association recommends screening the following groups who have signs of insulin resistance or conditions associated with insulin resistance:

i. History of impaired fasting glucose or impaired glucose tolerance

ii. History of hypertension or vascular disease

iii. Hyperlipidemia

iv. History of gestational diabetes or delivery of baby weighing over 9 lb

v. History of polycystic ovary syndrome

vi. Sedentary lifestyle

vii. Acanthosis nigricans (American Diabetes Association, 2010c)

B. *Primary prevention of diabetes*

Individuals at high risk for developing type 2 diabetes (those with impaired glucose tolerance, impaired fasting glucose, or an $HgbA_{1C}$ of 5.7–6.4%), should be referred to structured programs that emphasize lifestyle changes, including moderate weight loss (7% body weight) and regular physical activity (150 min/wk). They should be encouraged to adopt dietary strategies including reduced calories, reduced intake of dietary fat, and the inclusion of foods containing whole grains and fiber (14 g fiber per 1,000 kcal).

In addition, patients at very high risk for developing diabetes (combined impaired fasting glucose and impaired glucose tolerance plus other factors, such as $HgbA_{1C}$ greater than 6, hypertension, low high-density lipoprotein, elevated triglycerides, and family medical history of diabetes in a first-degree relative) and who are obese and less than 60 years of age, should be considered for treatment with metformin.

Those with prediabetes should be monitored for the development of diabetes annually (American Diabetes Association, 2010a). Prediabetes, also known as impaired fasting glucose, is defined by fasting glucose levels of 100–125 or glucose levels of 140–199 at 2 hours post challenge glucose load (American Association of Clinical Endocrinologists Diabetes Mellitus Clinical Practice Guidelines Task Force, 2007).

C. *Diagnostic tests and diagnostic criteria (Tables 53-1 and 53-2)*

1. Fasting serum glucose (no caloric intake for at least 8 hr): greater than or equal to 126

2. Random serum glucose greater than or equal to 200 with symptoms of hyperglycemia

3. Two-hour plasma glucose greater than or equal to 200 during an oral glucose tolerance test, using glucose load containing the equivalent of 75 g anhydrous glucose dissolved in water.

4. $HgbA_{1C}$ greater than or equal to 6.5%. The test should be performed in a laboratory using a method that is certified by the National Glycohemoglobin Standardization Program and standardized to the Diabetes Control and Complications Trial assay (American Diabetes Association, 2010c).

D. Management (includes treatment, consultation, referral, and follow-up care)

Many aspects of management are similar for both type 1 and type 2 diabetes.

Providers must first investigate the cause of the diabetes, especially if it is related to infection or medication use, and treat the patient accordingly. Patients initially presenting with type 1 diabetes may be hospitalized, depending on their symptoms and degree of illness (e.g., diabetic ketoacidosis).

Both type 1 and type 2 diabetes require meal planning and consideration of the amount of carbohydrates and fats ingested.

1. Diet
    a. Goals: normal blood glucose levels, attain and maintain reasonable body weight, and normalize lipids
    b. Calories: individuals with type 2 diabetes often need caloric reduction
    c. Protein: 15–20% of daily calories
    d. Fat: saturated less than 7% of daily calories; minimize transfats
    e. Cholesterol: less than 300 mg/day
    f. Carbohydrates: 45–60% of daily calories (American Association of Clinical Endocrinologists Diabetes Mellitus Clinical Practice Guidelines Task Force, 2007; American Diabetes Association, 2010c). Monitoring carbohydrates, whether by carbohydrate counting, exchanges, or experience-based estimation, remains a key strategy in achieving glycemic control.

2. Exercise
    a. At least 150 min/wk of moderate-intensity aerobic physical activity (50–70% of maximum heart rate) (Table 53-3)
    b. Patients with type 2 diabetes without complications should perform resistance training three times per week (American Diabetes Association, 2010c)

3. Medications
    a. For type 1 diabetes management, the mainstay of the treatment plan is insulin, either the basal or bolus regimen via injection or insulin pump.
    b. Dosing of insulin for type 1 is often 0.2–0.8 units per kg of body weight per day (The Merck Manuals Online Medical Library, 2009). Based on the findings of the Diabetes Control and Complications Trial and Epidemiology of Diabetes Interventions and Complications (National Diabetes Information Clearinghouse, 2009), and the risk for hypoglycemia, it is imperative that patients with type 1 diabetes check their blood glucose level and base insulin dosing on the amount of carbohydrates eaten and the corresponding blood glucose correction. Patients with type 1 diabetes usually require several injections throughout the day to control their blood glucose and

TABLE 53-2 Clinical Interpretations of Plasma Glucose Concentrations

Glucose Concentration (mg/dl)	Clinical Interpretation
Fasting	
< 100	Within the reference range
100–125	Impaired fasting glucose/prediabetes mellitus
≥ 126	Overt diabetes mellitus
2-hr postchallenge load (75-g oral glucose tolerance test)	
< 140	Within the reference range
140–199	Impaired fasting glucose/prediabetes mellitus
≥ 200	Overt diabetes mellitus

Source: American Association of Clinical Endocrinologists Diabetes Mellitus Clinical Practice Guidelines Task Force. (2007). American Association of Clinical Endocrinologists medical guidelines for clinical practice for the management of diabetes. *Endocrine Practice, 13*(Suppl. 1), 1–68.

TABLE 53-3 Exercise Rules and Precautions

Type 1
Avoid vigorous exercise in the presence of ketosis
Wear properly fitted footwear
Before starting, screen for vascular or neurologic complications
Caution in patients with retinopathy, neuropathy, and peripheral vascular disease
High-risk patients should start slowly
Precautions
Carry identification that includes diagnosis and medication list
If taking sulfonylureas, meglitinides, or insulin, check glucose before starting and carry carbohydrates
Check glucose before and after exercise
Avoid exercise in extreme temperatures and humidity
Proper equipment
Proper warm-up and stretching
Adequate hydration
Stop for any pain, lightheadedness, or shortness of breath

Source: American Diabetes Association. (2010). Standards of medical care in diabetes—2010. *Diabetes Care, 33*(1), S11–S61.

prevent complications; therefore, some prefer using an insulin pump that can be programmed for basal and bolus delivery.

c. For type 2 diabetes management, treatment usually begins with lifestyle modification, exercise, and then oral agents. This treatment plan is, however, usually guided by the patient's HgbA$_{1C}$ level, blood glucose levels, and their comorbidities. There are several algorithms for the treatment of type 2 diabetes (American Diabetes Association, 2007; Joslin Diabetes Center & Joslin Clinic, 2009a; Rodbard et al., 2009) (Figure 53-1).

　i. Oral agents (Table 53-4a and b)

　ii. Injectable (other than insulin)

　　a. Exenatide (Byetta): class-incretin mimetic; dose 5–10 mcg taken 60 minutes before a meal (type 2 only)

　　b. Pramlintide (Symlin): class-synthetic hormone; dose for type 1 is 15–60 mcg and for type 2 is 60–120 mcg taken before meals

　　　i. Insulins (Table 53-5a and b)

　　　ii. Self glucose monitoring

　iii. According to the Joslin Diabetes Center & Joslin Clinic (2009b), "The frequency of self glucose monitoring is highly individualized and should be based on such factors as glucose goals, exercise, medication changes and patient motivation. Patients with type 1 diabetes should monitor at least three times a day. In patients with type 2 diabetes, the frequency of monitoring is dependent upon such factors as mode of treatment and level of glycemic control" (p. 2).

4. Clinical goals (Table 53-6)

5. Complications: patients should be educated about potential complications from diabetes and how to prevent them. With this in mind, all diabetic patients should have the following

　a. Dilated eye examination by an ophthalmologist annually

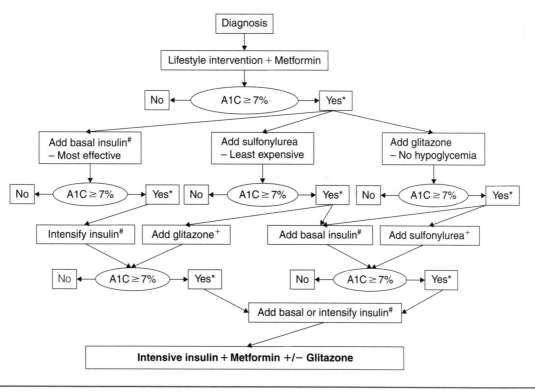

FIGURE 53-1 Algorithm for Management of Type 2 Diabetes Mellitus

Source: Copyright 2007 American Diabetes Association. From *Diabetes Care*, Vol. 30, 2007; S4–S41. Reprinted with permission from the American Diabetes Association.

TABLE 53-4a Oral Agents

Generic	Brand Name	Daily Dose (Min-Max)	Dosing
Sulfonylureas			
Glipizide	Glucotrol®	2.5–40 mg	QD-BID
Glipizide controlled release	Glucotrol XL®	2.5–20 mg	QD
Glimepiride	Amaryl®	1–8 mg	QD
Glyburide	Micronase®, Diabeta®	1.25–20 mg	QD-BID
Micronized glyburide	Glynase®	0.75–12 mg	QD-BID
Meglitinide analogs			
Repaglinide	Prandin®	0.5–16 mg	BID before meals
D-Phenylalanine derivative			
Nateglinide	Starlix®	120–360 mg	TID before meals
Biguanides			
Metformin	Glucophage®	500–2,550 mg	QD-TID with meals
Metformin extended release	Glucophage XR® Glumetza®	500–2,000 mg	QD with a meal
Metformin	Riomet® (oral solution)	(5 cc = 500 mg) 500–550 mg	QD-TID with meals
Thiazolidinediones			
Pioglitzaone	Actos®	15–45 mg	QD
Rosiglitazone	Avandia®	4–8 mg	QD-BID
Alpha-glucosidase inhibitors			
Acarbose	Precose®	25–300 mg	TID with meals
Miglitol	Glyset®	25–300 mg	TID with meals
DPP-4 inhibitors			
Sitagliptin	Januvia®	100 mg	QD
Saxagliptin	Onglyza®	2.5–5 mg	QD

TABLE 53-4b Oral Agents

Combinations	Brand Name
Glyburide/metformin	Glucovance®
Glipizide/metformin	Metaglip®
Rosiglitazone/metformin	Actosplus Met
	Avandamet®
Rosiglitazone/glimepiride	Avandaryl®
Pioglitazone/glimepiride	Duetact®
Sitagliptin/metformin	Janumet®

TABLE 53-5a Insulins

Generic Name	Brand Name	Type	Onset	Peak	Duration
Aspart	NovoLog®	Rapid	10–20 min	1–3 hr	3–5 hr
Lispro	Humalog®	Rapid	5–15 min	30–75 min	2–4 hr
Glulisine	Apidra®	Rapid	5–15 min	30–75 min	2–4 hr
Regular insulin	Novolin® R	Short acting	30–60 min	2–4 hr	5–8 hr
	Humulin® R	Same	Same	Same	Same
NPH	Novolin® N	Intermediate	1–3 hr	6–10 hr	16–24 hr
	Humulin® N	Same	Same	Same	Same
Glargine	Lantus®	Long acting	45 min–4 hr	None	24 hr
Detemir	Levemir®	Long acting	45 min–4 hr	None	24 hr

TABLE 53-5b Insulins

Premixed	Brand Name
NPH/Regular	Novolin® 70/30
	Humulin® 70/30
	Humulin® 50/50
Lispro protamine/lispro	Humalog® Mix 75/25
Lispro protamine/lispro	Humalog® Mix 50/50
Aspart protamine/aspart	Novolog® Mix 70/30

TABLE 53-6 Clinical Goals

	American Diabetes Association	American Association of Clinical Endocrinologists
Preprandial glucose	70–130	< 110
2-hour postprandial glucose	< 180	< 140
HgbA$_{1c}$	< 7	≤ 6.5
Blood pressure	< 130/80	< 130/80
Lipids	Low-density lipoprotein: < 100 mg/dl	Same
	High-density lipoprotein: men > 40 mg/dl, women > 50 mg/dl	Same
	Triglycerides: < 150 mg/dl	
Urine microalbumin	< 30 mg albumin/g creatinine	

Sources: American Association of Clinical Endocrinologists Diabetes Mellitus Clinical Practice Guidelines Task Force. (2007). American Association of Clinical Endocrinologists medical guidelines for clinical practice for the management of diabetes. *Endocrine Practice, 13*(Suppl. 1), 1–68; American Diabetes Association. (2010). Standards of medical care in diabetes—2010. *Diabetes Care, 33*(1), S11–S61.

b. Foot examination at every primary care provider visit (with monofilament) and by a podiatrist every 12 months (for patients without complications)

c. Foot care education

d. Dental examination every 6 months

e. Annual influenza vaccine

f. Pneumococcal vaccine

g. Blood pressure at every visit

h. Smoking cessation counseling at every visit

i. Review self-management goals at every visit

j. Laboratory studies: HgbA$_{1C}$ every 3–6 months (depending on control)

k. Urine microalbuminuria yearly

l. Creatinine every 3 months

m. Annual lipid panel

n. Liver function tests if on thiazolidinedione medications

o. Medications: Aspirin, 75–162 mg/day for patients with type 1 or type 2 diabetes at increased cardiovascular risk (most men > 50 years of age or women > 60 years of age who have at least one additional major risk factor [i.e., family medical history of cardiovascular disease, hypertension, smoking, dyslipidemia, or albuminuria]) (American Diabetes Association, 2010a).

p. Angiotensin-converting enzyme inhibitors or angiotensin receptor blockers for patients with hypertension or microalbuminuria (American Diabetes Association, 2010a; Joslin Diabetes Center & Joslin Clinic, 2009b).

6. Sick-day guidelines

a. Prevent dehydration and ketosis

b. Adequate fluid and calorie intake

c. Alert patient to signs and symptoms of hypoglycemia and hyperglycemia

d. Include patient's family and significant others in the plan

7. Referral

a. Patients with diabetes should be referred to an endocrinologist for the following reasons:

i. Starting an insulin pump

ii. Recurrent diabetic ketoacidosis

iii. Recurrent hypoglycemia

iv. Unable to adequately control glucose or erratic blood glucose readings

v. Patient request or provider discomfort

b. Women of childbearing age should be referred for preconception care.

c. Mental health referrals should be made as needed: screen for depression, diabetes-related stress, anxiety, eating disorders, and cognitive impairment when self-management is poor.

d. All patients with diabetes mellitus should be referred for diabetes self-management education classes.

E. *Client education: diabetes self-management education*

1. Concerns and feelings

Assist the patient and significant others in expressing and coping with concerns and feelings related to the diagnosis of diabetes, its potential complications, and the management of this disease. Assist the patient to develop strategies to promote behavior change.

2. Information: provide verbal and written information regarding:

a. The diabetes disease process, including signs and symptoms of hyperglycemia and hypoglycemia; pathophysiology of type 1 and type 2 diabetes; and complications of diabetes.

b. Diagnostic tests, including what they mean, normal results, frequency, and importance of testing.

c. Management

i. Meal planning and exercise: how to incorporate these into the patient's lifestyle

ii. Rationale, action, use, side effects, and cost of therapeutic interventions, including medications

iii. Self glucose monitoring: what the parameters are and how to interpret the results for self-management decision making (American Diabetes Association, 2010b)

iv. Adherence to long-term treatment plans

v. Prevention of complication, self-management strategies

vi. Travel instructions, medical alert identification, sick-day guidelines, and health maintenance.

VI. Self-management resources and tools

A. *Patient and client education*

There are numerous educational opportunities for individuals with diabetes, either online, by mail, or by telephone.

1. National Diabetes Education Program

The National Diabetes Education Program has publications available by mail or online that are geared toward different age groups (from teenagers to older adults) and ethnic backgrounds and are written in a variety of languages (www.YourDiabetesInfo.gov)

2. American Diabetes Association

The American Diabetes Association's (2009a) website has extensive patient information on line, brochures for purchase, and a hotline number for patients who want to speak with someone directly (www.diabetes.org)

3. Joslin Diabetes Center

The Joslin Diabetes Center has patient education on line, brochures, and cookbooks for purchase, including some for children and teenagers, and has Spanish and Asian American websites (www.joslin.org)

4. Juvenile Diabetes Research Foundation International

The Juvenile Diabetes Research Foundation International provides online or printed information for adults, teenagers, and children and has links to Facebook, Twitter, and You Tube. In addition, it has links to community events, local chapters, and affiliates around the globe (www.jdrf.org)

B. Community support groups

There are numerous support groups for individuals with diabetes, in addition to those listed previously.

1. Defeat Diabetes Foundation, Inc

Click for state and see local support groups (http://www.defeatdiabetes.org/)

2. American Diabetes Association

Website has a link to community events and programs, including those geared for specific ethnic groups (http://www.diabetes.org/)

3. Diabetes Health

Website links to multiple community events (http://www.diabeteshealth.com/)

REFERENCES

American Association of Clinical Endocrinologists Diabetes Mellitus Clinical Practice Guidelines Task Force. (2007). American Association of Clinical Endocrinologists medical guidelines for clinical practice for the management of diabetes. *Endocrine Practice, 13*(Suppl. 1), 1–68.

American Diabetes Association. (2007). Standards of medical care in diabetes—2007. *Diabetes Care, 30*(1), S11.

American Diabetes Association. (2009). *Community events.* Retrieved from http://www.diabetes.org/community-events/

American Diabetes Association. (2009a). *Diabetes statistics.* Retrieved from http://www.diabetes.org/diabetes-basics/diabetes-statistics/

American Diabetes Association. (2010a). Executive summary: Standards of medical care in Diabetes—2010. *Diabetes Care, 33*(1), S4–S10.

American Diabetes Association. (2010b). National standards for diabetes self-management education—2010. *Diabetes Care, 33*(1), S89–S96.

American Diabetes Association. (2010c). Standards of medical care in diabetes—2010. *Diabetes Care, 33*(1), S11–S61.

Huang, E. S., Basu, A., O'Grady, A., & Capretta, J. C. (2009). Projecting the future diabetes population size and related costs for the U.S. *Diabetes Care, 32*(12), 2225–2229.

Joslin Diabetes Center & Joslin Clinic. (2009a). *Clinical guideline for pharmacological management of type 2 diabetes.* Retrieved from http://www.joslin.org/joslin_clinical_guidelines.html

Joslin Diabetes Center & Joslin Clinic. (2009b). *Clinical guidelines for adults with diabetes.* Retrieved from http://www.joslin.org/joslin_clinical_guidelines.html

National Diabetes Information Clearinghouse. (2009). *DCCT and EDIC: The diabetes control and complications trial and follow-up study.* Retrieved from http://diabetes.niddk.nih.gov/dm/pubs/control/

Rodbard, H. W., Jellinger, P. S., Davidson, J. A., Einhorn, D., Garber, A. J., Grunberger, G., ... Schwartz, S. S. (2009). Statement by an American Association of Clinical Endocrinologists/American College of Endocrinology consensus panel on type 2 diabetes mellitus: An algorithm for glycemic control. *Endocrine Practice, 15*(6), 540–559.

The Merck Manuals Online Medical Library. (2009). *Diabetes mellitus.* Retrieved from http://www.merck.com/mmpe/sec12/ch158/ch158b.html#sec12-ch158-ch158b-1183

EPILEPSY

M. Robin Taylor and Paul Garcia

I. Definition and description

This chapter helps the primary care provider evaluate the patient with previously diagnosed epilepsy. Epilepsy refers to a group of conditions that are characterized by the recurrent disturbance of cerebral function (seizures) because of excessive neuronal discharges in the brain occurring in a paroxysmal manner. An epileptic seizure occurs when the cerebral cortex is rendered hyperexcitable (because of an increase in excitatory neurotransmission, a decrease in inhibitory neurotransmission, or a disturbance in brain circuitry) by any of a number of causes including metabolic disturbances, injuries, strokes, tumors, and developmental abnormalities (Lowenstein, 2008). Depending on the site in the brain that is affected, the disturbance of function may consist of a loss or impairment of consciousness, a disturbance of behavior, or an abnormality of motor or sensory function. When the cause is easily reversible (e.g., hyponatremia, hypoglycemia, alcohol withdrawal, medication toxicity, or fever), the seizure is said to be "provoked" and the patient's condition is not considered epilepsy. When the cause is not readily reversible and seizures have occurred on more than one occasion, the chance for further seizures is high and the patient is said to have epilepsy (Marks & Garcia, 1998).

Epilepsy is a common condition in all medical practices and almost all practitioners are called on to care for patients with epilepsy. At any point in time, 0.5–1% of the population will have epilepsy (Marks & Garcia, 1998). Because a person may develop epilepsy or have epilepsy remit at various stages in their life, the lifetime risk for developing epilepsy is considerably higher, approximately 3% (Marks & Garcia). The lifetime risk for having an epileptic seizure (including provoked seizures) is approximately 10% (Marks & Garcia). People of all ages, genders, and ethnicities are affected by epilepsy. As a group, people with epilepsy face both medical and psychosocial challenges (including employment and educational barriers). The lifetime risk for dying from a seizure-related death is estimated to be as high as 25% (Hauser & Hesdorffer, 1990). Recent studies suggest that successful treatment of epilepsy both prolongs life and improves quality of life (Choi et al., 2008; Wiebe, Blume, Girvin, & Eliasziw, 2001).

II. Database (may include, but is not limited to)

A. Subjective

1. Seizure history

   a. Description of seizures from patient and witnesses

   b. Most recent seizures: characteristics and frequency

   c. Any changes in seizure pattern (including characteristics and frequency)

   d. Triggering events (stress, fatigue, alcohol, and menstruation)

   e. Impairment of consciousness

   f. Any recent intervention including paramedics, emergency department visits, or benzodiazepines

   g. Any previous intervention, including surgery

   h. Previous diagnostic work-up, including electroencephalogram (EEG) and magnetic resonance imaging (MRI); last visit with Neurology.

2. Antiepileptic drugs (AEDs) and medications

   a. Name, formulation, strength, and dosing schedule. Recent change from brand to generic or between different generics? Adherence to medication.

   b. Dose changes: drugs tried in the past and responses (therapeutic and toxic)

   c. Signs and symptoms of AED toxicity including blurred vision, diplopia, ataxia, somnolence or fatigue, confusion or mental slowing, and gastrointestinal upset

   d. Concomitant treatment for other conditions that may interact with AEDs (e.g., nonsteroidal anti-inflammatory drugs, antibiotics, oral contraceptives, and anticoagulants)

   e. Use of rescue medications, such as sublingual lorazepam, buccal midazolam, or rectal diazepam

3. Past medical history

   a. Head trauma, developmental and genetic disorders, and neurologic and psychiatric disorders

   b. Recent minor illnesses, especially gastrointestinal disorders with vomiting or fever

   c. Chronic illnesses (e.g., HIV-AIDS, cerebrovascular disease, and cancer)

4. Family history: epilepsy, Alzheimer's disease, neurodegenerative disorders, malignancy, and psychiatric disorders

5. Personal and social history

   a. Occupational history

   b. Habits: alcohol or illicit drug use

   c. Sleep patterns (change in sleep patterns may provoke seizures)

   d. Stress and coping: recent stressors (can provoke seizures), coping strategies, and social support

   e. Recreational activities and safety: driving, swimming, climbing, other risky activities for patients with ongoing seizures, and use of helmets or other protective devices

6. Review of systems

   a. Skin: rash or jaundice

   b. Gastrointestinal: signs and symptoms of chemical hepatitis (e.g., nausea, vomiting, anorexia, abdominal pain, or malaise)

   c. Neurologic: full review of systems

   d. Psychiatric: note affect, and symptoms of active psychiatric disease

B. **Objective**

1. Physical examination

   a. Temperature and blood pressure

   b. Cardiac (rule out cardiac origin)

   c. Neurologic examination

      i. Cranial nerves (special emphasis on nystagmus)

      ii. Cerebellar (special emphasis on gait disturbances and Romberg)

      iii. Focal motor signs and mental status

   d. Skin: rashes

2. Diagnostic testing and work-up

   a. Source (should be neurologist or epileptologist)

   b. Supporting documentation

      i. Abnormal electrocardiogram (not always present)

      ii. Abnormal MRI (not always present). MRI should define the etiology of seizures or be of adequate quality to exclude causes that may progress in the future (e.g., small tumors or vascular malformations).

III. Assessment

A. *Determine the diagnosis*

The following diagnoses should be considered for all patients presenting with seizures

1. Epilepsy (Table 54-1)

2. Cerebrovascular disease

3. Cardiac arrhythmias with resulting cerebral hypoperfusion

4. Syncope

5. Nonepileptic (i.e., psychogenic) seizure

6. Transient ischemic attack

7. Migraine

8. Alzheimer's and other neurodegenerative disorders (can cause seizures in the geriatric population)

9. Infection, may exacerbate seizures

B. *Severity*

1. Determine if seizures are fully controlled.

2. If seizures are not fully controlled, determine if the patient is at the maximum clinically tolerated dose of medication (regardless of serum levels)

3. Assess for AED toxicity (Table 54-2)

C. *Significance*

Assess the significance of the symptoms and chronic nature of this disorder to the patient and significant others.

D. *Patient adherence*

Assess if the patient is able to adhere to the treatment plan.

IV. Goals of clinical management

A. *Achieve seizure-free status with the smallest possible dosage and lowest side effect profile of AED therapy*

B. *Attempt to arrive at AED monotherapy if possible*

C. *Assist the patient to achieve optimal level of functioning with daily activities and quality of life while living with a chronic, often unpredictably relapsing disorder*

V. Plan

A. *Screening: There are no screening tests or preventive strategies for epilepsy.*

TABLE 54-1 Epilepsy Syndromes

	Generalized	Localization-Related (Partial or Focal)
	Seizures begin diffusely throughout the cerebral cortex	Seizures arise from a discrete focus in cerebral cortex or limbic structures (hippocampus or amygdala)
Idiopathic (primary, without clear cause)	**Seizure types:** absence, myoclonic, tonic–clonic **Neurologic examination:** normal **Neuroimaging:** normal **EEG:** normal background with fast (3–6 Hz) generalized spike-and-wave discharges **Common examples:** childhood absence epilepsy, juvenile myoclonic epilepsy, epilepsy with generalized tonic–clonic seizures on awakening **Treatment:** valproate, ethosuximide (effective for absence seizures only), topiramate, lamotrigine, felbamate, levetiracetam, or zonisamide	**Seizure types:** simple partial (awareness unimpaired), complex partial (awareness impaired), or secondarily generalized tonic clonic **Neurologic examination:** normal **Neuroimaging:** normal **EEG:** normal background with focal epileptiform discharges. **Common examples:** benign childhood epilepsy with centro–temporal spikes (Rolandic epilepsy); benign epilepsy with occipital paroxysms **Treatment:** often no medical treatment; all AEDs may be effective except ethosuximide
Symptomatic (secondary; caused by an apparent or assumed brain lesion)	**Seizure types:** atypical absence, myoclonic, tonic, atonic, tonic–clonic **Neurologic examination:** diffuse or multifocal abnormalities **Neuroimaging:** diffuse or multifocal abnormalities common **EEG:** abnormal background with slow (< 3 Hz) generalized or multifocal epileptiform discharges **Common examples:** Lennox-Gastaut syndrome, progressive myoclonus epilepsies **Treatment:** valproate, lamotrigine, levetiracetam, felbamate, rufinamide, tomiramate, zonisamide, ketogenic diet, or corpus callosotomy	**Seizure types:** simple partial (awareness unimpaired), complex partial (awareness impaired), secondarily generalized tonic–clonic **Neurologic examination:** focal abnormalities or normal **Neuroimaging:** focal abnormalities common **EEG:** normal or abnormal background with focal or multifocal epileptiform discharges **Common examples:** temporal lobe epilepsy, frontal lobe epilepsy **Treatment:** carbamazepine, phenytoin, valproate, gabapentin, lacosamide, lamotrigine, leviteracetam, oxcarbazepine, topiramate, zonisamide), or resective surgery

Sources: Adapted with permission from "Management of seizures and epilepsy," 1998, American Family Physician. Copyright © 1998 American Academy of Family Physicians. All Rights Reserved; Adapted from Marks, W. J., Jr., & Garcia, P. A. (1998). Seizures and epilepsy: Current management. *American Family Physician, 57*(7), 1589–1600.

B. Diagnostic tests

1. Blood levels of AEDs: to assess for adherence or possible toxicity. Not all AEDs have defined "therapeutic ranges" (e.g., benzodiazepines and all AEDs released subsequent to valproic acid). Note that AED levels are only a rough guide; many patients require levels in the "toxic" range to achieve complete seizure control and tolerate these levels without significant clinical toxicity. Routine blood level monitoring is not useful.

2. Complete blood count: thrombocytopenia, anemia, and leukopenia secondary to AEDs. Obtain a baseline before initiating a new AED and in early phase of treatment or if patient is symptomatic.

3. Liver function tests: obtain a baseline before initiating a new AED and in early phase of treatment or if patient is symptomatic. Most AEDs can cause elevated liver enzymes, but this is uncommonly clinically significant and usually does not require discontinuation of the AED.

4. Consider other tests if diagnosis is in question (electrolytes, glucose, creatinine, rapid plasma reagin [RPR])

C. Medication management (Tables 54-2 and 54-3)

TABLE 54-2 Oral Antiepileptic Medications

Generic Name	Brand Name	Strengths Available[1] (mg)	Typical Adult Starting Dose[2]	Typical Increment and Rate of Ascension[3]	Most Common Dose-Related Adverse Effects	Non-Dose-Related and Idiosyncratic Reactions
Carbamazepine	Tegretol® Tegretol-XR® Carbatol®	100, 200 100, 200, 400 100, 200, 300	200 mg BID 200 mg BID 200 mg BID	200 mg/wk (dose TID-QID) 200 mg/wk 200 mg/wk	Dizziness, somnolence, ataxia, nausea, vomiting, diplopia, blurred vision	Hyponatremia, rash, Stevens-Johnson syndrome, leucopenia, aplastic anemia, agranulocytosis, transaminitis, hepatic failure
Ethosuximide	Zarontin®	250	250 mg QD to 250 mg BID	250 mg/wk	Anorexia, nausea, vomiting, drowsiness, headache, dizziness	Rash, Stevens-Johnson syndrome, hemopoietic complications
Gabapentin	Neurontin®	100, 300, 400, 600, 800	300 mg TID	300 mg/wk	Somnolence, dizziness, ataxia, fatigue	Rash, weight gain, behavioral changes, extremity edema
Lacosamide	Vimpat®	50, 100, 150, 200	50 mg BID	100 mg/wk to max 400 mg/d	Dizziness, ataxia, vomiting, diplopia, nausea, vertigo	PR interval lengthening
Lamotrigine	Lamictal® Lamictal-XR®	25, 100, 150, 200 25, 50, 100, 200	25 mg QOD to 25 mg BID	25–50 mg/2 wk only for monotherapy (special considerations for polytherapy not addressed here)	Dizziness, ataxia, somnolence, headache, diplopia, blurred vision, nausea, vomiting, rash	Rash, Stevens-Johnson syndrome, transaminitis
Levetiracetam	Keppra® Keppra-XR®	250, 500, 750 500, 750	500 mg BID	1,000 mg/d/2 wk to max 3,000 mg	Somnolence, asthenia, infection, dizziness	Depression, irritability
Oxcarbazepine	Trileptal®	150, 300, 600	300 mg BID	600 mg/d/wk to max 2,400 mg	Dizziness, somnolence, diplopia, fatigue, nausea, vomiting, ataxia, abnormal vision, abdominal pain, tremor, dyspepsia, abnormal gait	Stevens-Johnson syndrome, bone marrow suppression, hyponatremia
Phenobarbital		15, 30, 60, 100	100 mg QD	15–30 mg/wk	Somnolence, cognitive and behavioral effects	Rash, Stevens-Johnson syndrome, hematopoietic complications, transaminitis, hepatic failure

TABLE 54-2 Oral Antiepileptic Medications (continued)

Generic Name	Brand Name	Strengths Available[1] (mg)	Typical Adult Starting Dose[2]	Typical Increment and Rate of Ascension[3]	Most Common Dose-Related Adverse Effects	Non–Dose-Related and Idiosyncratic Reactions
Phenytoin	Dilantin I®	30, 50, 100	300 mg QD	25–30 mg/wk	Ataxia, diplopia, slurred speech, confusion	Rash, Stevens-Johnson syndrome, hematopoietic complications, gingival hyperplasia, coarsening of facial features, transaminitis, hepatic failure
Pregabalin	Lyrica®	25, 50, 75, 100, 150, 200, 225, 300	75 mg BID or 50 mg TID	To max 600 mg/d	Dizziness, somnolence, dry mouth, peripheral edema, ataxia, confusion, asthenia, abnormal thinking, blurred vision, incoordination, weight gain	Weight gain
Rufinamide	Banzel®	200, 400	400–800 mg/d (BID doses)	400–800 mg/d every 2 d to max 3,200 mg/d	Somnolence, dizziness, ataxia, headache, fatigue, nausea	Multiorgan hypersensitivity, QT interval shortening
Tiagabine	Gabitril®	4, 6, 8, 10, 12, 16	4 mg QD	4 mg/wk (dose BID-QID)	Dizziness, nervousness, asthenia, confusion, tremor	
Topiramate	Topamax 1®	25, 50, 100, 200	25 mg BID	50 mg/wk	Somnolence, dizziness, ataxia, slurred speech, psychomotor slowing, cognitive problems, word-finding difficulty	Weight loss, transaminitis, nephrolithiasis
Valproate	Depakote® Depakote-ER®	125, 250, 500 250, 500	250 mg TID	250 mg/wk	Nausea, vomiting, tremor, thrombocytopenia, weight gain	Transaminitis, hepatic failure, pancreatitis, rash, Stevens-Johnson syndrome, hair damage or loss,
Zonisamide	Zonegran®	25, 50, 100	100 mg/d	200 mg/d for 2 wk to max 400 mg/d	Somnolence, anorexia, dizziness, headache, nausea, agitation/ irritability	Stevens-Johnson syndrome, oligohydrosis/hyperthermia, nephrolithiasis

[1]Strengths listed are for tablet or capsule formulations of the brand name agents.

[2]Initiation doses for some agents vary, depending on concomitant medications, body weight, age of patient, and other factors; consult prescribing information for each drug. Doses are for non-urgent initiation of medication; clinical circumstances may necessitate increased doses and accelerated titration. See prescribing information for pediatric doses, which are based on body weight and often must be administered more frequently than in adults.

[3]Rate of ascension may need modification, depending on seizure frequency and occurrence of adverse effects. Note that phenytoin may be increased in 25-mg increments by using a halved 50-mg Dilantin® Infatab® tablet or by 30 mg using a 30-mg Dilantin Kapseal® capsule.

Sources: Prepared by Robin Taylor, NP, and Paul Garcia, MD. Reviewed by Brian Alldredge, PharmD. Adapted with permission from "Management of seizures and epilepsy," 1998, American Family Physician. Copyright © 1998 American Academy of Family Physicians. All Rights Reserved; Adapted from Marks, W. J., Jr., & Garcia, P. A. (1998). Seizures and epilepsy: Current management. American Family Physician, 57(7), 1589–1600.

TABLE 54-3 Medication Treatment Strategies for Patients with Epilepsy

Establish an epilepsy syndrome diagnosis for each patient (**Table 54-1**).
Select medications appropriate for that epilepsy syndrome (**Table 54-1**).
Among the syndrome-appropriate medications, choose the agent best suited for the particular patient, based on patient and medication characteristics (**Table 54-2**).
Initiate and titrate the medication at doses, increments, and rates appropriate for that medication to enhance tolerability (**Table 54-2**).
Ascend the medication, regardless of serum levels, until complete seizure control is achieved, or until persistent, unacceptable side effects occur.
If satisfactory seizure control is not achieved, transition the patient to another agent appropriate for the epilepsy syndrome being treated. Attempt to arrive at antiepileptic drug monotherapy for each patient.
If trials with one or two agents fail to achieve acceptable results, refer the patient to an epilepsy specialist for consultation.

Sources: Adapted with permission from "Management of seizures and epilepsy," 1998, American Family Physician. Copyright © 1998 American Academy of Family Physicians. All Rights Reserved; Adapted from Marks, W. J., Jr., & Garcia, P. A. (1998). Seizures and epilepsy: Current management. *American Family Physician, 57*(7), 1589–1600.

D. Referral guidelines

Refer to neurology or epileptology when

1. Diagnosis of epilepsy is in question
2. Seizures are uncontrolled on one AED at maximum tolerated dose
3. Complete seizure control, but with bothersome or intolerable AED side effects
4. AED withdrawal if patient desires, after 2–3 years of seizure control
5. Pregnant woman with a seizure disorder

E. Client education

1. Provide verbal and written information about the etiology and treatment of epilepsy.
2. Discuss the importance of adherence to medication regimes, emphasizing that the maximum tolerated dose is one increment below the dose at which the patient experiences side effects.
3. Review the importance of lifestyle issues on seizure control: regular sleep–wake schedule and minimal or no alcohol

VI. Self-management resources

A. An excellent resource for patient and families can be found at: http://www.epilepsy.com/

This site is sponsored by the Epilepsy Therapy Project. The individuals involved with this site are among the top epilepsy experts in the country. A wide variety of resources are available on diagnosis, treatment, clinical trials, and support for family and caregivers.

The site has a function called "My Epilepsy Diary," which allows patients and families to enter seizures, medications, side effects, healthcare appointments, and so forth. It can be used to set alerts so that patients remember to take their medications at the proper times. The site also has a section for healthcare professionals, with more sophisticated information that tends to be highly accurate and carefully reviewed: http://professionals.epilepsy .com/homepage/index.html

B. Seizure Tracker

Seizure Tracker is a web-based site that allows patients to enter data on medication dosages, seizure frequencies, use of rescue medications, and so forth and then share this information with healthcare providers of their choosing: https://www.seizuretracker.com/

C. Epilepsy Foundation

Another useful site is the Epilepsy Foundation site (previously, "Epilepsy Foundation of America"): http://www .epilepsyfoundation.org/. A good resource for patients and families, it can be used to identify local Epilepsy Foundation affiliates throughout the country: http://www .epilepsyfoundation.org/aboutus/affiliatelookup .cfm. The local affiliates can help direct patients and families to local resources (advocacy, job training, support groups, and so forth).

REFERENCES

Choi, H., Sell, R. L., Lenert, L., Muennig, P., Goodman, R. R., Gilliam, F. G., & Wong, J. B. (2008). Epilepsy surgery for pharmacoresistant temporal lobe epilepsy: A decision analysis. *Journal of the American Medical Association, 300*(21), 2497–2505.

Hauser, W. A., & Hesdorffer, D. C. (1990). *Epilepsy: Frequency, causes and consequences.* New York, NY: Demos Publications.

Lowenstein, D. H. (2008). Seizures and epilepsy. In A. S. Fauci, E. Braunwald, D. L. Kasper, S. L. Hauser, D. L. Longo, J. L. Jameson, & J. Loscalzo (Eds.), *Harrison's Principles of Internal Medicine Online, 17e:.* http://www.accessmedicine.com/content.aspx?aID=2901171

Marks, W. J., Jr., & Garcia, P. A. (1998). Seizures and epilepsy: Current management. *American Family Physician, 57*(7), 1589–1600.

Wiebe, S., Blume, W. T., Girvin, J. P., & Eliasziw, M. (2001). Effectiveness and efficiency of surgery for temporal lobe epilepsy study group: A randomized, controlled trial of surgery for temporal-lobe epilepsy. *New England Journal of Medicine, 345*(5), 311–318.

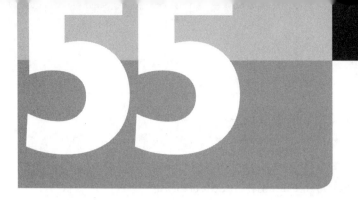

LOW BACK PAIN

H. Kate Lawlor

I. Introduction and general background

Up to 60% of the American population experience low back pain (LBP) at some time during their adult life (Atlas & Deyo, 2001). After upper respiratory infections, back pain is the next most common reason to seek nonemergent care (Atlas & Deyo, 2001). The differential diagnosis is lengthy, and a precise diagnosis cannot be made in more than 80% of cases (Chou et al., 2007); yet, most patients with LBP in a primary care setting spontaneously improve in 1–4 weeks and need no evaluation beyond the initial history and physical (Atlas & Deyo, 2001). The diagnostic challenge is to identify those patients who require a more extensive or urgent evaluation.

The differential diagnosis includes both muscular and focal spine disorders (i.e., disc herniation and spinal stenosis); regional nonspinal disorders (i.e., pelvic inflammatory disease and prostatitis); and systemic diseases (i.e., ankylosing spondylitis and metastatic cancer). Even if anatomic defects like narrowed disc space or the vertebral osteophytes of degenerative arthritis are found on radiographs, causality cannot be absolutely assumed, because these defects are also common in asymptomatic patients and increase in frequency with age (Ehrlich, 2003). More than one-third of asymptomatic individuals older than age 60 have evidence of disc herniation or spinal stenosis on specialized imaging (Ehrlich, 2003).

Table 55-1 lists the potential causes of LBP grouped by category. The most common causes are pain from mechanical or degenerative processes. The most frequent sources of pain in these categories are spinal stenosis and symptomatic herniated disc (Chou et al., 2007). The obligation for the clinician is to promptly identify those patients whose pain may be caused by select, urgent conditions, such as, in order of frequency, ankylosing spondylitis, cord compression,

a compression fracture, spondylolisthesis, cancer, cauda equine syndrome, or referred pain from abdominal or genitourinary sources (Chou et al., 2007).

These guidelines review the history and physical examination necessary to differentiate functional LBP from more urgent causes. The treatment and patient education for functional or nonspecific causes of LBP that are appropriately managed by primary care providers are included. For most patients, the history and physical examination is sufficient to exclude the "red flags" that suggest more serious disorders (Ehrlich, 2003) (Table 55-2).

II. Database (may include but is not limited to)

A. Subjective

1. History of present illness

   a. Onset and duration (intermittent versus constant)
   b. Circumstances when first occurred (e.g., trauma or work-related)
   c. Location and radiation of pain
   d. Quality and severity of pain (use specific descriptors and pain severity scale)
   e. Progression of symptoms over time
   f. Aggravating and alleviating factors
   g. Worse with bending, lifting, prolonged standing, or sitting (most common with mechanical back pain)
   h. Worse in morning or afternoon and evening hours (pain on waking or shifting positions, suggests vertebral instability [e.g., spondylolisthesis])
   i. Relief with activity; worse with rest (typical of ankylosing spondylitis)
   j. Relief with sitting (suggestive of spinal stenosis)
   k. Worse with cough, bowel movement, or sneezing (suggests nerve entrapment)
   l. Interventions attempted to relieve pain; results
      i. Medications (aspirin, nonsteroidal anti-inflammatory drugs [NSAIDs], others)
      ii. Herbal products
      iii. Chiropractic care
      iv. Physical therapy or massage
      v. Acupuncture
      vi. Heat or cold application
   m. Associated signs and symptoms
      i. Constitutional symptoms: fever, malaise, fatigue, weight loss (each suggests a more serious concern)

TABLE 55-1 Most Common Causes of Low Back Pain

1. Mechanical
   A. Poor back or core abdominal muscle tone (may be secondary to obesity, pregnancy, or deconditioning)
   B. Chronic postural or lumbar-sacral strain

2. Structural or degenerative
   A. Degenerative joint disease (osteoarthritis, degenerative disc disease, or facet arthrosis)
   B. Sacroiliitis
   C. Scoliosis or kyphosis
   D. Disc protrusion or herniation
   E. Spinal stenosis (narrowing of spinal canal)
   F. Osteoporosis
   G. Cauda equina syndrome (characterized by lower-extremity weakness and sensory loss, saddle anesthesia, fecal incontinence, urinary retention, or incontinence)

3. Trauma
   A. Fall
   B. Work-related injury
   C. Compression fracture caused by fall, osteoporosis, or chronic steroid use
   D. Subluxation of facet joint (spondylolisthesis)

4. Inflammatory
   A. Ankylosing spondylitis (or other spondyloarthropathies)
   B. Rheumatoid arthritis

5. Infection
   A. Osteomyelitis
   B. Referred pain from pelvic inflammatory disease or prostatitis
   C. Tuberculosis

6. Cancer
   A. Multiple myeloma
   B. Metastatic cancer of prostate, breast, and lung
   C. Spinal cord tumors

7. Vascular
   A. Dissecting abdominal aneurysm (usually history of hypertension)

8. Psychogenic
   A. Tension or stress related
   B. Malingering (often in setting of workers compensation suit)

Source: Adapted from Atlas, S., & Deyo, R. (2001). Evaluating and managing acute low back pain in the primary care setting. *Journal of General Internal Medicine, 16,* 120–131.

ii. Ocular: painful, inflamed, or gritty eye (uveitis is associated with ankylosing spondylitis)

iii. Neurologic
   a. Burning pain that radiates down anterior, posterior, or lateral aspect of one or both legs ("sciatica", 95% sensitive for nerve root irritation [Atlas & Deyo, 2001]). Sciatica occurs with herniated disc and spinal stenosis. Pain location helps to identify which nerves are affected (Table 55-3).
   b. Sharp back pain with coughing or sneezing (indicative of disc compression)
   c. Leg pain with standing or walking; relief with sitting (suggests spinal stenosis)
   d. Leg or foot weakness; gait disturbance; urinary retention or urinary incontinence; bowel incontinence (these symptoms in the aggregate suggest cauda equina syndrome resulting from cord compression, a surgical emergency)

iv. Abdominal: pain or diarrhea (inflammatory bowel disease can be associated with ankylosing spondylitis)

v. Genitourinary: dysuria; urinary frequency or urgency; recent indwelling catheter use (suggests urinary tract infection). Vaginal

TABLE 55-2 History and Physical Examination Findings Associated with Increased Likelihood of Serious Spinal Condition ("Red Flags")

Disorder	History	Physical Examination and Studies for Diagnosis
All	Failure to improve > 1 month No relief with bed rest	Unpredictable physical examination; see specific disorders below
Cancer	Age > 50 years Previous history of cancer (especially multiple myeloma) Unexplained weight loss of > 10 lb in 6 months Failure to improve after 1 month Multiple risk factors present	Lymphadenopathy Plain lumbosacral spine films Magnetic resonance imagining (MRI) Elevated erythrocyte sedimentation rate (ESR)
Fracture	Age > 50 years; especially > 70 years Weight < 57 kg History of smoking (increased risk of osteoporosis) History of significant trauma (fall from height, motor vehicle accident, or a direct blow) History of osteoporosis Prior or current steroid use Substance abuse (increased risk of falls; alcohol use causes decreased bone density)	Vertebral point tenderness Plain lumbosacral spine film
Bone infection	Fever or chills Pain increased at rest Recent skin or genitourinary infection Recreational injection drug use	Fever > 100°F Tenderness over a spinous process MRI Elevated ESR, positive C-reactive protein
Ankylosing spondylitis	Male sex, < 45 years old Positive family history of irritable bowel disease, ankylosing spondylitis Pain > 3 months, especially buttock pain Pain in latter part of night, morning stiffness Pain improved with exercise May be associated with irritable bowel disease, psoriasis, uveitis, plantar fasciitis, or Achilles tendinitis	May have decreased chest expansion Decreased spinal flexibility in sideway, frontal, and backward motions May have sacroiliac joint tenderness May have radiologic evidence of sacroiliitis on anteroposterior pelvic plain films Elevated ESR, positive C-reactive protein 90% + histocompatibility complex (HLA)-B27
Cauda equina syndrome	Urinary retention or incontinence Bowel incontinence Progressive leg or foot weakness Sensory loss in lower extremities	Saddle anesthesia Diminished anal sphincter tone Severe unilateral or bilateral leg or foot weakness Bladder distention MRI

Source: Adapted from Atlas, S., & Deyo, R. (2001). Evaluating and managing acute low back pain in the primary care setting. *Journal of General Internal Medicine, 16*, 120–131; and Chou, R., Qaseem, A., Snow, V., Casey, D., Cross, J. T. Jr., Shekelle, P., . . . American Pain Society Low Back Pain Guidelines Panel. (2007). Diagnosis and treatment of low back pain: A joint clinical practice guideline from the American College of Physicians and the American Pain Society. *Annals of Internal Medicine, 147*(7), 478–491.

discharge or pelvic pain (suggests pelvic infection)

    vi. Vascular: chest pain or abdominal pain (LBP with these symptoms may signal an abdominal aortic aneurysm)

    vii. Skin: history of psoriasis (associated with ankylosing spondylitis) or recent skin infection (may cause spinal infection)

    viii. Psychologic: recent sleep disturbances; depressed or anxious mood; diminished participation in social events (may signal depression)

  n. Patient's concern or theory about the source of symptoms

2. Past health history

  a. Prior spinal diagnoses, fractures, or surgery

  b. Previous radiologic or imaging studies of spine. Prior bone density testing.

  c. Medications

    i. Used for back pain (especially opiates; dosage and frequency)

    ii. Prescription (steroid use can be a risk factor for osteoporosis and compression fractures)

    iii. Over the counter

    iv. Herbal or alternative

3. Family history

  a. Disc disease

  b. Osteoporosis

  c. Rheumatoid arthritis or ankylosing spondylitis

  d. Coronary vascular disease

  e. Scoliosis

  f. Osteoarthritis

4. Occupational

  a. Physical requirements of job

  b. How many hours worked per week

  c. Recent job injury

  d. Prior ergonomic assessments performed and results

  e. Current worker's compensation claim or permanent disability

  f. Job satisfaction

5. Personal and social (factors that may predict poorer or delayed resolution)

  a. Other pending litigation: occupational or trauma

  b. Impact of pain on activities of daily living or current relationships

  c. History of depression

  d. Outstanding disability claims

  e. Habits

    i. Smoking (risk factor for osteoporosis)

    ii. Injectable drug use (risk factor for spinal infection)

    iii. Alcohol use (be alert to increased use for self-medicating for pain)

    iv. Recreational drug use

B. *Objective: physical examination (patient should be undressed; examination should include but is not limited to)*

1. Height (loss of height suggests kyphosis or compression fracture)

2. Weight (unexplained weight loss suggests cancer; low body weight is risk factor for osteoporosis; and obesity is risk factor for osteoarthritis)

3. Age (> 50 years at greater risk for cancer; > 75 years at greater risk for osteoporosis)

4. Gender (males at greater risk for ankylosing spondylitis)

5. Vital signs, including temperature (fever > 100°F suggests infection)

6. Spine (performed with patient unclothed in gown and underwear)

In the absence of a history suggestive of a serious condition, systemic disease or illness not localized to the back region (Table 55-1), a focused spine and neurologic examination as described previously should be an adequate screening examination to rule out serious or urgent causes of LBP, unless any "red flags" (Table 55-2) are identified (Ehrlich, 2003).

  a. Inspection: look for changes in normal spine curvature that may occur if muscle spasm, scoliosis, kyphosis, or ankylosing spondylitis

  b. Standing: assess symmetry and posture

  c. Palpation: assess for bone tenderness versus muscle spasm. With patient forward flexed, assess for abnormal curvature of spine; may suggest kyphosis or scoliosis.

  d. Range of motion: assess flexibility and complaints of pain. Ask which movement causes the most pain. Flexion causes increased pressure on the disc; extension narrows the diameter of the spinal canal; lateral bending causes increased pain if disc is herniated.

  e. Gait; check heel and toe walking separately (heel walk involves the anterior tibialis and L4 innervation; toe walk uses the gastrocsoleus and S1 innervation)

7. Focused neurologic examination

Straight leg raises: screens for nerve root irritation, most commonly caused by a herniated disc. While supine, the affected leg should be elevated with the ankle dorsiflexed and the knee fully extended. A positive response ("sciatica") reproduces sharp or burning pain when the limb is raised to 30–70 degrees: pain in the buttocks, posterior leg, or contralateral leg is 95% sensitive for nerve root irritation caused by herniated disc (Chou et al., 2007). Sciatica caused by spinal stenosis is more common in older patients, and pain is often bilateral (Table 55-3 for examination findings associated with impingement of specific nerve roots). If positive straight leg raises or a "red flag" are present, proceed with a more detailed neurologic examination of the lower extremities as described next. If the straight leg raise test is negative, further neurologic examination is not needed (Atlas & Deyo, 2001).

8. Expanded neurologic examination

    a. Comparative muscle strength testing of upper and lower extremities: quadriceps, knee, great toe, and foot dorsiflexion
    b. Sensation testing of lower extremities and feet
    c. Reflex testing of patellae and Achilles tendon
    d. Measure leg length: difference of more than 2 cm can cause significant postural alterations that can result in LBP
    e. Measure muscle mass of thighs and calves: difference of more than 2 cm may indicate neurologic involvement of limb with smaller muscle mass
    f. If symptoms and examination findings are consistent with cauda equina syndrome (severe unilateral or bilateral leg weakness, urinary retention and distended bladder or fecal incontinence), check for saddle anesthesia and diminished anal sphincter tone.

9. Systemic examination

    a. Eye examination: if complaints of eye pain or irritation. Anterior uveitis can be associated with ankylosing spondylitis.
    b. Pulmonary examination (chest expansion decreased in ankylosing spondylitis)
    c. Cardiac examination: note evidence of aortic valve incompetence (ankylosing spondylitis) including testing for aortic bruits to assess if aortic aneurysm.
    d. Urinary examination: assess for distended bladder (saddle anesthesia or diminished anal sphincter tone with fecal incontinence and urinary retention suggests cauda equina syndrome, a surgical emergency)
    e. Genitourinary examination: note any pelvic tenderness or masses, or cervical motion tenderness or discharge (suggests pelvic inflammatory disease in females); urethral discharge or dysuria (can be associated with ankylosing spondylitis); and prostate enlargement or tenderness or masses (can signal infection or prostate cancer in males).
    f. Rectal examination: check for saddle anesthesia or diminished anal sphincter tone

C. **Diagnostic tests** (might include, but not limited to)

    1. Radiographs: basic imaging findings are poorly correlated with specific symptoms and are not sensitive for important abnormalities (Chou et al., 2007). In addition, in several studies of

TABLE 55-3 Specific Nerve Root Impingements Associated with Particular Physical Examination Findings

Strength	Unilateral Altered Sensation	Reflex	Nerve Root
Iliapsoas: have the patient seated with legs dangling over the edge of the examination table. Then stabilize their pelvis by placing your hand over their iliac crest while the patient actively raises their thigh from the table. Secondly, place your other hand over the distal femoral portion of their knee, and ask the patient to attempt to raise their thigh further from the table while you resist this motion. Compare resistance results testing on the other, uninvolved side (Hoppenfeld, 1976, p. 250).	Anterior thigh/groin	—	L2
Quadriceps: squatting then rising, or strengthening a bent knee against resistance while seated	Anterolateral thigh	Patellar	L3
Quadriceps; ankle dorsiflexion (heel walking)	Medial ankle/foot	Patellar	L4
First toe dorsiflexion	Dorsum of foot	—	L5
Ankle plantar flexion (toe walking)	Lateral plantar foot	Achilles	S1

Note: Over 95% of herniated discs involve the L4-5 or L5–S1 interspaces (Chou et al., 2007).

Sources: Atlas, S., & Deyo, R. (2001). Evaluating and managing acute low back pain in the primary care setting. *Journal of General Internal Medicine, 16,* 120–131; Hoppenfeld, S. (1976). *Physical exam of the spine and the extremities.* East Norwalk, CT: Appleton-Century-Crofts/Prentice-Hall.

asymptomatic individuals, disc degeneration was a common finding that increased with age (Atlas & Deyo, 2001). Therefore, plain radiographs of the spine have a very low sensitivity and specificity in most cases and should not be obtained in patients with nonspecific LBP.

   a. Only consider plain radiograph of the lumbosacral spine when
      i. There are "red flags" in the patient's history or physical examination (Table 55-2).
      ii. If the patient has not improved after a 1-month course of conservative therapy, especially if the patient is older than 50 years and has a history of unexplained weight loss.
   b. Consider additional pelvic radiograph to look for sacroiliitis if suspicion of ankylosing spondylitis based on patient's history or examination (Chou et al., 2007).
   c. Consider chest radiographs if findings suggestive of abdominal aortic aneurysm.
   d. Advanced radiographic studies (computerized tomography, magnetic resonance imaging [MRI]) are appropriate to consider in the situations discussed next. In general, MRI, if available, is preferable over CT because it does not use ionizing radiation and provides better visualization of soft tissue, vertebral marrow, and the spinal canal (Jarvik & Deyo, 2002).
      i. If severe or progressive neurologic deficits
      ii. If suspicion of infection, tumor, or cauda equina syndrome, early study is warranted
      iii. If sciatic symptoms suggest disc herniation or spinal stenosis, but
         a. Treat with course of conservative care first (discussed later), which may be sufficient (Atlas & Deyo, 2001)
         b. If surgery is likely to be needed for unimproved symptoms of disc herniation or spinal stenosis, consider referral to orthopedist or surgical specialist before advanced studies are ordered, because they may have a particular preferred test.

2. Routine blood and urine testing is unnecessary. Select tests may be helpful if particular pathology is suspected
   a. Erythrocyte sedimentation rate: if question of malignancy, ankylosing spondylitis, or consideration of infection
   b. Complete blood count: may be used as screening test for neoplasms, infections, or inflammatory processes

   c. Prostate-specific antigen: if suspicion of metastatic prostate cancer
   d. Urinalysis: if question of urinary tract disease
   e. C-reactive protein: as screen for vertebral infection or ankylosing spondylitis
   f. HLA-B27: as screen for ankylosing spondylitis (rate of reliability as a screen differs markedly among ethnic populations; strongest association with ankylosing spondylitis is in whites) (Khan, 2002).
   g. Serum calcium and vitamin D level if concern of osteoporosis
   h. Alkaline phosphatase

3. Electromyography and nerve conduction studies should be reserved for use by specialists in recalcitrant or complex cases.

III. Assessment

More than 85% of cases of acute LBP presenting to a primary provider cannot reliably be attributed to a specific disease or spinal abnormality (Chou et al., 2007), and patients recover within 4 weeks of conservative therapy as described (Atlas & Deyo, 2001).

A. *Determine if evidence of nerve impingement caused by disc herniation or spinal stenosis (Tables 55-2 and 55-3).*

B. *Determine if presence of "red flags" suggests more serious pathology (cancer, infection, or inflammatory condition; Table 55-2).*

C. *If no red flags are present, even if evidence of simple nerve impingement (i.e., no evidence of cauda equina), treat as functional musculoskeletal back pain and follow the plan outlined next.*

D. *Determine if medicolegal issues concerning possible worker's compensation or disability claim are present. If there are medicolegal issues, refer to a specialist.*

IV. Plan

A. *Acute LBP (< 2–4 weeks; may include sciatica, but no "red flags")*
   1. Physical measures: in a synthesis of 17 randomized and controlled trials of nonpharmacologic therapies

for LBP (Chou & Huffman, 2007a), only the following interventions showed evidence of efficacy.

a. Bed rest only if sciatic or muscle symptoms make walking or sitting difficult. Limit use of bed rest for only severe pain; bed rest for more than 48 hours is not only of no value, it is detrimental (Ehrlich, 2003).

b. Avoid prolonged sitting or standing; get up at regular intervals (every 30 minutes) to walk and stretch the back.

c. Activity modification as warranted by pain level and location. Avoid heavy lifting or extreme spinal flexion.

d. Local application of moist heat or cold.

e. Spinal manipulation by physical therapist (PT) or osteopathic doctor (DO) may be helpful.

f. Massage may relieve pain.

g. Other nonpharmacologic therapies, such as acupuncture, back schools, low-level laser, lumbar supports, traction, transcutaneous electrical nerve stimulation units, and ultrasonography, lack reliable evidence of effectiveness in managing acute LBP. There have been no studies that evaluate the effect of different mattresses or pillows on pain intensity.

2. Medications. A review of 51 controlled trials for the treatment of LBP from the Cochrane Central Registry of Controlled Trials found the following (Chou & Huffman, 2007b)

a. NSAIDs were superior to placebo for global improvement of back pain with or without sciatica. No one agent was found to be superior to any other drug in the same class.

b. Acetaminophen at dosages up to 4 g/day produced relief equivalent to NSAIDs for patients who could not tolerate NSAIDs.

c. There was insufficient evidence to judge the independent benefit of aspirin.

d. Opioid analgesics offered moderate benefits in relieving pain not controlled by NSAIDs or acetaminophen. Their use should be limited to less than 2 weeks, reserved for patients whose pain cannot be controlled by agents in (a) or (b), or who should not use medications listed in (a) or (b).

e. Muscle relaxants (e.g., diazepam, tizanidine, cyclobenzaprine, and baclofen): use for less than 2 weeks; reserved for patients whose pain cannot be controlled alone by agents in (a) because of severe muscle spasm. Most effective when combined with NSAID or acetaminophen. Use associated with a higher incidence of adverse events.

f. Antidepressants, antiepileptic drugs, and systemic corticosteroids (including epidural steroid injections for patients with sciatica) were not shown to offer any independent pain relief.

3. File a "Physician's First Report of Injury" if symptoms are caused by a work-related injury

4. Follow-up care after symptoms have resolved.

a. Exercises and activities per PT or DO to improve muscle strength and reduce likelihood of recurrence; exercising in warm water can be an effective analgesic. Do not do any exercises that increase the pain.

b. Encourage return to work and activities of daily living as tolerated.

c. Begin program of daily walking and low-stress aerobic activities once pain has resolved.

d. Consider encouraging patient to attend community-based exercise program or gym program to support performance of exercises to strengthen core musculature and reduce likelihood of recurrence.

5. Consult or refer for evaluation by an orthopedic spine surgeon or neurosurgeon if

a. Symptoms consistent with cauda equina syndrome-immediate surgical referral

b. Lower limb weakness or sensory losses

c. Progressive neurologic deficit

d. Presence of "red flags" (symptoms suggestive of cancer, bone infection, or ankylosing spondylitis require referral to other appropriate specialists)

e. Abnormal findings on CT or MRI

f. Failure to secure relief of symptoms, or worsening of symptoms after 1 month of conservative measures described previously

6. Patient education (sample in Figure 55-1)

a. Provide written information that includes

i. Most common cause of symptoms

ii. Difference in symptoms caused by musculoskeletal strain versus nerve root impingement

iii. Reassurance that testing is rarely helpful initially, and spontaneous resolution is most common

iv. Physical recommendations

v. Analgesic recommendations

vi. Exercise and activity precautions

vii. Call or see provider if

    a. No improvement after 2 weeks of sciatic symptoms

    b. No improvement after 1 month of nonspecific LBP

c. Symptoms progress in severity

d. "Red flags" occur

viii. Conditioning or prevention recommendations once acute phase subsides

B. Subacute LBP (1–3 months)

1. Physical measures (Chou & Huffman, 2007a)

   a. Intermittent bed rest (of no more than 48 hours at a time) only if radicular symptoms persist

   b. Modify activity as needed to control symptoms

   c. Low-stress aerobic exercise (walking or swimming) as tolerated; avoid heavy lifting, prolonged sitting, or standing

   d. Treatment by PT or DO

   e. Local heat and cold if patient finds this helpful

   f. Acupuncture and massage therapy demonstrate short-term symptom relief

   g. Cognitive-behavioral therapy to promote relaxation shows good evidence of benefit in comparative trials

   h. Lumbar corsets, traction, transcutaneous electrical nerve stimulation unit use, and ultrasonography have failed to demonstrate benefit in numerous controlled trials

2. Medications (Chou & Huffman, 2007b)

   a. Nonnarcotic analgesics only (e.g., acetaminophen, NSAIDs) unless contraindicated

   b. Consider course of tricyclic antidepressants (e.g., amitriptyline) if radicular pain is present (when used for nerve pain, start at 10 mg qhs, then increase to 25 mg qhs after 1 week, then up to 50 mg qhs as maintenance dose). This is a subtherapeutic dose for depression. Caution with use in patients with history of bipolar disease, mood swings, glaucoma, or history of palpitations.

   c. Short-term use of benzodiazepines may offer some benefit if skeletal muscle spasm persists; other skeletal muscle relaxants did not demonstrate benefits in controlled trials (Chou and Huffman, 2007b).

   d. Opioids should be avoided because of risk of dependency or abuse, unless brief course needed for severe pain (1–2 weeks).

3. Conditioning (after initial pain has subsided; unlikely to be covered by insurance)

   a. Biofeedback

   b. "Back school"

   c. Conditioning training by PT or DO or other health professional to improve core muscle strength. More rigorous conditioning regimens are associated with the best outcomes (Chou et al., 2007).

   d. Ergonomic evaluation of workplace if symptoms suggest aggravation by work activities.

4. Referral for specialty evaluation (Atlas & Deyo, 2001)

   a. Refer for surgical evaluation if patient with sciatica has no improvement after 4–6 weeks of conservative therapy, or imaging with CT or MRI shows lesion in area that corresponds to symptoms.

   b. Refer for diagnostic or specialty evaluation if new "red flag" symptoms appear while patient is being treated with conservative therapy.

   c. Refer for evaluation by specialist if symptoms are caused by a workplace injury or the patient plans to file a disability claim.

5. Patient education (see sample patient education handout in Figure 55-1)

   Provide written information that includes all the teaching points detailed in requirements described in the management of acute episode of LBP

6. Career counseling: consider referral for vocational evaluation if patient's work repeatedly produces back pain despite conditioning, and is not amenable to surgical correction.

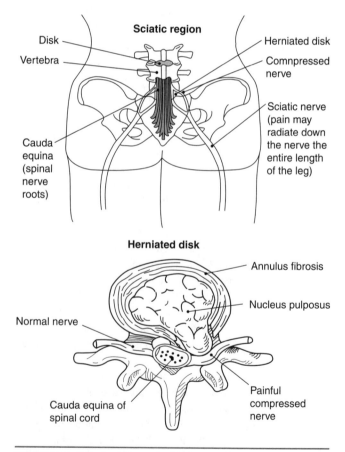

FIGURE 55-1a Sample Patient Education Handout
Adapted with permission from Low Back Pain, April 15, 2007, *American Family Physician*. Copyright © 2007 American Academy of Family Physicians. All rights reserved.

FIGURE 55-1b Sample Patient Education Handout

What is low back pain?
Low back pain is when you feel sore or uncomfortable in your lower back or buttocks.

What causes low back pain?
It is usually caused by muscle strain in your lower back. If you strain a muscle in your back, it can hurt to move it.

Another cause of low back pain is a bulging disc. Discs in your spine give cushioning and support. When a disc bulges, or "herniates," it may irritate a nerve (see drawings). This can cause pain that travels down your thigh or leg. Pain caused by nerve irritation is called sciatica (sigh-AT-tic-ah).

In rare cases, back pain may be caused by an infection, cancer, or other diseases.

Who gets low back pain and why?
Three out of four people have low back pain at some time in their lives. You can get low back pain from straining to lift heavy objects or by twisting your back. People often hurt their backs when they are moving furniture, playing sports, or gardening.

How long will it last?
Most people slowly start to feel better over a few weeks. Nearly all people are completely better within six to eight weeks.

How will my health care provider find the cause of the pain?
Your provider will ask you questions about your pain and will give you a physical examination.

Will I need to have an x-ray or scan?
Most people don't need to have these tests. Your provider will decide if you should have one after he or she examines you.

Will bed rest help?
You may need to rest in bed for a day or two, but too much bed rest can stop you from getting better. Some people worry that staying active will hurt their backs more. Getting back to your normal activities may hurt or be uncomfortable, but it shouldn't cause any damage.

What can I do to help with the pain?
- Try not to do things that make the pain worse, like sitting for a long time, lifting heavy objects, or bending or twisting.
- Stick to your normal activities as much as you can. Gentle exercise like walking helps you get better more quickly.
- Some over-the-counter medicines can help pain or swelling. These include ibuprofen (brand name: Advil or Motrin), naproxen (brand name: Aleve or Naprosyn), and acetaminophen (brand name: Tylenol). Your healthcare provider may give you medicine to help with pain or muscle spasms.
- Try using heating pads or taking a warm bath or shower.
- Your provider can show you some gentle exercises to help stretch your back and make the muscles stronger.
- A physical therapist, massage therapist, or chiropractor may help with your pain and make you feel better.

When should I return to work?
Your healthcare provider can tell you when it's okay for you to return to work. It is important to try to keep active. But, if you have to sit for many hours or do a lot of physical activity at work, you may need to make some changes for a while.

How can I prevent low back pain?
You can prevent low back pain with physical therapy, exercises, and stretching. Supports and back belts do not prevent low back pain.

Keep in shape, lose weight if you are overweight, and exercise regularly. Being inactive can lead to low back pain. Regular exercise like walking, swimming, or biking is good for your back. These activities put less stress on your back than sitting and standing.

Don't lift heavy objects by bending over at the waist. Bend your hips and knees and then squat to pick up the object. Keep your back straight and hold the object close to your body. Don't twist your body while you are lifting.

If you have to sit at your desk or drive for a long time, take breaks to stretch.

How can I tell if my back pain is serious?
You should get medical care right away if:
- You are older than 50
- The pain was caused by an injury such as a fall or car crash
- You have trouble sleeping because of the pain
- You lose weight without trying or have a fever, chills, or a history of cancer
- You have trouble urinating or controlling your bowels

Tell your healthcare provider if the pain goes down your leg below your knee, or if your leg, foot, or groin feels numb. See your doctor if your pain doesn't get better after two or three weeks of treatment.

(continues)

C. Recurrent or chronic LBP (> 3 months)

1. Appropriate to do radiologic or imaging studies, or blood tests if not resolved yet, especially if pain is arising from work setting

2. Refer to specialist for further evaluation and management, especially if work-related or a disability claim was filed

3. Physical measures (Chou et al., 2007)
   a. Modify activity to control symptoms; avoid heavy lifting and prolonged sitting and standing
   b. Low-stress aerobic exercise
   c. Massage
   d. Medium firm mattress for sleep
   e. Yoga as long as no radicular (sciatic) symptoms
   f. Manipulation by PT or DO
   g. Acupuncture may offer additive short-term pain relief
   h. Cognitive-behavioral therapy for short-term pain relief. Not effective in improving functional status (Chou & Huffman, 2007a)

4. Medications (Chou & Huffman, 2007b)
   a. Nonnarcotic analgesics only (acetaminophen or NSAIDs)
   b. Consider a course of low-dose tricyclic antidepressant if it has not been tried for back pain (see previous discussion).

5. Refer to pain management specialist or physiatrist who specializes in the spine if insufficient relief with previously mentioned measures and no evidence of structural disorder or other cause of pain.

6. Conditioning (can use if not previously attempted, or if had good relief with prior use)
   a. Biofeedback
   b. "Back school": interdisciplinary rehabilitation most effective when presented at patient's work-site (Chou & Huffman, 2007a)
   c. Conditioning training by PT or DO
   d. Ergonomic evaluation of workplace if symptoms suggest aggravation by work activities and evaluation was not already conducted

7. Patient education (Figure 55-1)

V. Self-management resources and tools

A. Patient and client education

The Internet has volumes of information available on the causes, evaluation, and treatment of LBP. The following are suggested because the vocabulary is appropriate for a lay audience, they do not focus exclusively on surgical remedies, and they are not overly long. This list is not exclusive; other websites may be found to be valuable.

1. American Academy of Rheumatology (http://www.rheumatology.org/patients/factsheet/backpain)

2. Annals of Internal Medicine, Low Back Pain (http://www.medicinenet.com/low_back_pain/page4.htm)

3. Family Doctor, An Overview of Low Back Pain (http://www.familydoctor.org/online/famdocen/home/common/pain/treatment)

4. Handout on Health: Back Pain (NIH Publication No. 09-5282), National Institute of Arthritis and Musculoskeletal and Skin Diseases Information Clearinghouse, National Institutes of Health.

REFERENCES

Atlas, S., & Deyo, R. (2001). Evaluating and managing acute low back pain in the primary care setting. *Journal of General Internal Medicine, 16,* 120–131.

Chou, R., & Huffman, L. (2007a). Nonpharmacologic therapies for acute and chronic low back pain: A review of the evidence for an American Pain Society/American College of Physicians Clinical Practice Guideline. *Annals of Internal Medicine, 147*(7), 492–504.

Chou, R., & Huffman, L. (2007b). Medications for acute and chronic low back pain: A review of the evidence for an American Pain Society/American College of Physicians Clinical Practice Guideline. *Annals of Internal Medicine, 147*(7), 505–514.

Chou, R., Qaseem, A., Snow, V., Casey, D., Cross, J. T., Jr., Shekelle, P., . . . American Pain Society Low Back Pain Guidelines Panel. (2007). Diagnosis and treatment of low back pain: A joint clinical practice guideline from the American College of Physicians and the American Pain Society. *Annals of Internal Medicine, 147*(7), 478–491.

Ehrlich, G. (2003). Back pain. *The Journal of Rheumatology, 30*(67), 26–31.

Jarvik, J. G., & Deyo, R. (2002). Diagnostic evaluation of low back pain with emphasis on imaging. *Annals of Internal Medicine, 137,* 586–597.

Khan, M. A. (2002). Update on spondyloarthropathies. *Annals of Internal Medicine, 136*(12), 896–907.

GASTROESOPHAGEAL REFLUX DISEASE

Karen C. Bagatelos, Geraldine Collins-Bride, and Fran Dreier

I. Definition and overview

Gastroesophageal reflux disease (GERD) is defined as chronic symptoms or mucosal damage produced by the abnormal reflux of stomach acid to the esophagus (Kahrilias, 2008). It is the most common gastrointestinal (GI) diagnosis recorded during outpatient clinic visits in the United States (Kahrilias, 2008). GERD affects 19 million adults, accounting for 4,590,000 outpatient visits and 96,000 hospitalizations annually (The Practice Parameters Committee of the American College of Gastroenterology, Wang, & Sampliner, 2008). Prevalence is estimated at 20–25% of adults (Talley & Vakil, 2005; The Practice Parameters Committee of the American College of Gastroenterology et al., 2008.).

A. Significance and complications

Recognizing and treating GERD is important, not only to relieve bothersome symptoms but also to avoid the complication of Barrett's esophagus and esophageal carcinoma, the incidence of which is rising (Kahrilias, 2008). Barrett's esophagus involves the replacement of normal squamous epithelium with columnar epithelium, which can occur when normal esophageal mucosa is exposed to stomach acid. The columnar epithelium can then develop dysplasia, a precursor to cancer, and subsequently cancer. The worldwide incidence of esophageal cancer is 4 cases per 100,000 (Hauser, Pardi, & Poterucha, 2008). The mortality rate is high in this population, with a low survival rate.

Additional complications associated with GERD include esophagitis, esophageal ulceration, and esophageal strictures. Respiratory manifestations, such as chronic cough, shortness of breath, and exacerbation of asthma, are also commonly seen. It is important to always consider GERD in patients with respiratory symptoms to prevent more severe respiratory complications (Galmiche, Zerbib, & Des Varannes, 2008). The reflux of acid seen with GERD can also cause sore throats and tooth decay. Antisecretory therapy and other treatment modalities for GERD produce a huge economic burden.

B. Pathophysiology and etiology of GERD

Several factors can contribute to the development of GERD. In normal individuals (i.e., those who do not have GERD), four mechanisms protect the esophageal epithelium from being damaged by reflux of gastric contents (Hauser et al., 2008)

1. A competent lower esophageal sphincter (LES), which acts as a barrier to reflux

2. Effective movement of contents through the esophagus

3. Secondary peristalsis, which sweeps refluxed material back into the stomach and closes the LES

4. The acid-neutralizing effect of swallowed saliva and mucous present in the upper GI (UGI) tract

From a broad perspective, the final common path in the development of GERD is altered gastric motility or injury to the UGI tract. Esophageal dysmotility is associated with a great many illnesses, including rheumatologic and endocrine disorders. Altered gastric motility may be associated with a weak LES or transient LES relaxation, weak or disordered esophageal peristalsis, or delayed gastric emptying. Local esophageal damage can be caused by increased gastric acid secretion or the retrograde passage of bile and pancreatic juice. Mucosal injury further decreases the rate of passage of the bolus of food through the UGI tract. Additional factors that decrease the flow of acid and food through the UGI tract include reduced saliva, increased hydrochloric acid, and decreased mucosal blood flow. Specific structural or physiologic conditions, such as a hiatal hernia or obstructive sleep apnea (Hauser et al., 2008), also decrease the rate of passage of food through the UGI tract. Motility is also affected by factors that increase abdominal pressure (pregnancy, weight gain, obesity, and tight clothing) and by hormonal influences (progesterone, cholecystokinin, secretin, and low gastrin). Hormonal influences can cause transient LES relaxation, excess acid production, and decreased UGI tract motility (Table 56-1).

TABLE 56-1 GERD Common Etiologies

Causative Factor	Clinical Examples
Motility disorders	Esophageal dysmotility caused by diminished peristalsis: rheumatologic and endocrine disorders, such as Sjögren syndrome and scleroderma
	Altered gastric motility including a weak lower esophageal sphincter or transient lower esophageal sphincter relaxation, weak or disordered esophageal peristalsis, and delayed gastric emptying seen with gastroparesis or gastric outlet obstruction
Local damage	Increased gastric acid secretion or the retrograde passage of bile and pancreatic juices that cause damage to the esophageal mucosa
Change in resistance to gastric acid	Factors that decrease the flow of acid and food through the upper gastrointestinal tract, such as reduced saliva (Sjögren syndrome, anticholinergic medications), increased hydrochloric acid (stress response or gastrinoma), or decreased mucosal blood flow (radiation therapy or ischemia)
Structural and physiologic changes	Associated with the following conditions: hiatal hernia, obstructive sleep apnea, weight gain, obesity, pregnancy, or wearing tight clothing
Hormonal influences	Progesterone, cholecystokinin, secretin, and low gastrin

II. Database (may include but is not limited to)

A. Subjective

1. Past medical history

   a. Peptic ulcer disease (associated with a hypersecretory state)

   b. Obesity (body mass index > 29) causes increased pressure on the stomach and lower esophagus causing more acid to reflux

   c. Gallbladder disease may cause symptoms similar to GERD

   d. Pregnancy in the later trimesters can exacerbate reflux because of increased pressure on the upper digestive tract

   e. Neurologic disease, such as a stroke or brain tumor, or any condition that affects neural pathways, including neurologic medications

   f. Diabetes can cause gastroparesis, which in turn causes increased reflux

   g. Collagen-vascular disease (scleroderma, mixed connective tissue disease, and systemic lupus erythematosis) can cause changes in the mucosa or the circulation in the UGI tract

   h. Recurrent pulmonary infections (possible aspiration) and asthma

   i. Cerebral palsy and other neurodevelopmental disabilities

   j. Medications: aspirin, nonsteroidal anti-inflammatory drugs, hormones, vitamins, adrenergics, and anticholinergics)

2. Family history

   a. Peptic ulcer disease, GI cancer, gallbladder disease

   b. Diabetes, rheumatologic, and other endocrine disorders

3. Personal and social

   a. Current life stressors: stress can reduce the esophageal perception thresholds for pain (Mizyad, Fass, & Fass, 2009).

   b. Habits

      i. Alcohol, tobacco, caffeine (coffee, colas, and tea)

      ii. Diet: fatty or low-protein diet, spiced foods, citrus, carbonated beverages, chocolate, mints and mint tea, eating large meals, or late night eating

4. Review of systems

   a. Gastrointestinal

      i. Pain: the typical symptom is heartburn, retrosternal burning sensation originating in the subxyphoid region and spreading upward into the chest occurring 30–60 minutes after meals. In severe episodes there are esophageal spasms or noncardiac chest pain. The pain can radiate into the neck, shoulders, and back.

      ii. Dysphagia, episodes of choking

      iii. Regurgitation of gastric contents into the mouth

      iv. Nausea and vomiting (can be seen with GERD, although not a common associated symptom)

v. Aggravating factors for these symptoms
a. Position (laying down, especially postprandial reclining; bending over and lifting heavy objects)
b. Wearing tight clothing or belts
c. Tobacco, alcohol, and caffeine
d. Diet as noted previously
b. Ear, nose, and throat: chronic sore throat, early morning hoarseness
c. Mouth: complaint of bad breath (halitosis)
d. Cardiac: full cardiac review of systems is indicated
e. Pulmonary: cough (especially nocturnal cough), wheezing, shortness of breath not typically seen with GERD

B. Objective

1. Physical examination
a. General: appearance, development, nourishment; note tight clothing if present
b. Weight
c. Ear, nose, and throat: dentition changes, tooth decay, and pharyngeal erythema
d. Cardiac examination: should be normal in a patient with GERD
e. Chest examination: wheezing, adventitious sounds
f. Abdominal examination: obesity, epigastric tenderness, distention, and tympanic bowel sounds
g. Rectal examination: stool hemoccult

III. Assessment

A. Determine the diagnosis

GERD is most commonly diagnosed by history and presenting symptoms. The following diagnoses should be considered for all patients presenting with symptoms of GERD

1. Cardiac disease or angina
2. Esophageal stricture or mass
3. Esophageal motility disorder
4. Esophageal spasm
5. *Helicobacter pylori* infection
6. Gastroparesis
7. Peptic ulcer disease
8. Zollinger-Ellison syndrome

B. Severity

Assess the severity of the disease, including duration of symptoms (diagnosed or undiagnosed) and risk for complications of untreated or poorly treated GERD.

C. Significance and motivation

Assess the significance of the symptoms and often chronic nature of this disorder to the patient. Determine the motivation and ability of the patient to follow through with the treatment plan; that often involves significant lifestyle modification of habits, food choices, and timing of meals.

IV. Goals of clinical management

A. Screening

Although the American College of Gastroenterology recommends screening endoscopy for patients with reflux lasting greater than 12 months, especially those older than 50 years, there are no long-term studies demonstrating that screening contributes to the prevention of cancer or to increased life expectancy (Shaheen & Ransohoff, 2002).

B. Treatment

1. Medical management is designed to promote gastric emptying, augment the resting tone of the LES, and favorably alter the nature of refluxed material through nonpharmacologic and pharmacologic means.

2. Treatment aims to assist the patient in the management of GERD symptoms and enhance lifestyle modification to prevent recurrence of symptoms and disease.

C. Prevention of complications

These include Barrett's esophagus, adenocarcinoma, esophagitis, dysphagia caused by esophageal strictures, narrowing or spasm, ulcers, persistent pain, and bleeding.

V. Plan

A. Screening

There are no screening tests available for the early detection or prevention of GERD. However, there are preventive measures that can be taken. These include maintaining normal body weight; reducing stress; and avoiding tobacco, excess alcohol, and caustic foods.

B. Diagnostic tests

1. Laboratory tests: complete blood count, stool for occult blood, *H. pylori* serum antibody or *H. pylori* stool antigen (*H. pylori* stool antigen is highly

sensitive and specific for determining if current infection exists). In unrelenting cases, check serum gastrin to evaluate for Zollinger-Ellison syndrome.

2. Electrocardiogram if chest pain is present. Consider additional cardiology diagnostic studies if angina is suspected.

3. UGI series: if dysphagia is present, consider UGI series to rule out a stricture or mass.

4. Endoscopy is indicated in the following circumstances, from the American Society for Gastrointestinal Endoscopy practice guideline (2007)

   a. Alarming signs or symptoms, including persistent vomiting, hematemesis, evidence of GI blood loss, involuntary weight loss, progressive dysphagia, anemia, evidence of GI bleeding, chest pain proven to be of noncardiac etiology; or a mass, stricture, or ulcer found on imaging studies.

   b. Wheezing, orthopnea, or atypical respiratory symptoms

   c. Unrelenting symptoms despite therapy, or family history of esophageal cancer (The Practice Parameters Committee of the American College of Gastroenterology et al., 2008).

   d. Patients who have reflux of many years' duration should receive an endoscopy to screen for Barrett's esophagus. If Barrett's esophagus is confirmed then surveillance endoscopy should be done every 6 months to 3 years, depending on pathologic findings and the endoscopist's recommendations (The Practice Parameters Committee of the American College of Gastroenterology et al., 2008).

   e. Recurrent symptoms after antireflux surgery.

5. Special studies

   Additional evaluation includes tests to measure reflux and more precisely evaluate the motility of the esophagus and stomach (gastric emptying study, manometry with a 24-hour pH study, and endoscopy with biopsy). A gastric emptying study may reveal decreased gastric emptying, which can cause functional dyspepsia. A manometry with pH study can quantify the amount of reflux that a patient has in 24 hours, and also measures the pressure in the upper and lower esophageal sphincter. These tests provide evidence for determining if the patient is an appropriate surgical candidate.

C. Management

Most patients (80–95%) with GERD respond to management with weight reduction, antacids or other medication, habit changes, elevation of the head of the bed, stress reduction, and other nonsurgical measures. For those who cannot be managed successfully with these measures but do respond to proton-pump inhibitors (PPIs), and who do not want to take medication indefinitely, surgery is a viable option.

1. Nonpharmacologic measures

   a. Mechanical measures: raise the head of the bed 8–10 inches, and maintain an upright posture for a minimum of 30–60 minutes after eating.

   b. Dietary measures
      i. Decrease or discontinue alcohol, coffee, tea, and carbonated beverages
      ii. Eat several small meals per day
      iii. Do not eat within 3 hours of bedtime
      iv. Avoid fatty foods, acidic foods, caffeine, mint, and any other aggravating foods

   c. Smoking cessation

   d. Weight loss when body mass index is greater than 29

   e. Habits: stress management

2. Pharmacologic measures

   a. For mild symptoms: patients with infrequent symptoms often respond well to antacids. Liquid preparations can be used, 15 ml (double-strength preparations) and 30 ml (single-strength preparations) 1 and 3 hours after meals and at bedtime until symptoms resolve.

   b. For mild to moderate symptoms: histamine H_2 antagonists (H_2 blockers) can be effective. H_2 blockers work best when given as a divided dose twice daily. Dosage must be adjusted for patients with renal impairment (crcl < 50). If symptoms respond to these, do not progress to the next treatment modality.

   c. For moderate to severe symptoms or when symptoms do not respond to H_2 blockers, consider treatment with PPIs. PPIs are potent inhibitors of gastric acid secretion. PPIs can be used intermittently as needed, although H_2 blockers have a more rapid onset of action and are a better choice for prn use than PPIs. For severe symptoms, the PPI of choice (often determined by insurance company formularies) can be given twice daily, once daily, or in conjunction with an H_2 blocker. These regimens should achieve resolution of symptoms and complete healing of the esophagus in 8 weeks. If symptoms recur within 6 months, chronic therapy may be needed with either daily or twice-daily dosing of a PPI (Table 56-2).

TABLE 56-2 Commonly Used GERD Medications*

Medication Category with Examples	Initial Dose	Maintenance Dose	Precautions
Antacids			Use with caution in renal impairment
			Many drug interactions, especially with higher doses (e.g., antipsychotics, anticonvulsants, and calcium channel blockers)
Aluminum hydroxide and magnesium hydroxide (Alamag OTC, Maalox®)	5–10 ml or 2–4 tablets 1–3 hours after meals and HS	PRN according to symptoms	
Calcium carbonate and magnesium hydroxide (Mylanta® Gelcaps, Mylanta® Supreme or Rolaids® Extra Strength)	Same as above	Same as above	Constipation is a frequent side effect
Histamine H$_2$ antagonists			Many adverse reactions including cardiac arrhythmias, reversible confusional states, and increased prolactin levels.
			Use with caution in renal impairment (crcl < 50)
			Monitor for vitamin B$_{12}$ deficiency with long-term use
Ranitidine (Zantac®)	150 mg BID or 300 mg QD (taken in the evening or at HS if single dose)	150 mg HS	
Famotidine (Pepcid®)	20 mg BID, take second dose in the evening or at HS	20 mg HS	
Nizatidine (Axid®)	150 mg BID or 300 mg QD (taken in the evening or at HS if single dose)	150 mg QD	
Proton pump inhibitors (PPIs)	Usually prescribed for 6–8 weeks for initial treatment		Check for drug interactions
			Good safety profile. Long-term safety use best studied with omeprazole, the first PPI on the market
			Long-term use of PPIs: adjust to the lowest dose for symptom control (Kahrilias, Shaheen, & Vaezi, 2008)
			Take before breakfast. If BID dosing, take second dose before evening meal.
			No dose adjustment required for renal impairment
Omeprazole (Prilosec®)	20–40 mg QD	20–40 mg QD	Take 30 minutes before a meal
Lansoprazole (Prevacid®)	15–30 mg QD	15–30 mg QD	Take 30 minutes before a meal
Pantoprazole (Protonix®)	20–40 mg QD	20–40 mg QD	Take at least 1 hour before a meal
Rabeprazole (Aciphex®)	20 mg QD	20 mg QD	
Esomeprazole (Nexium®)	40 mg QD	40 mg QD	

* Reflects suggested dosages for GERD. Dosages for erosive esophagitis and other esophageal disorders may vary.

d. For patients with slow gastric emptying, consider using

    i. Metoclopramide (Reglan®), 10 mg tid to qid. This agent increases the rate of gastric and esophageal emptying by stimulating the smooth muscle of the intestine. The potential side effects of metoclopramide should be reviewed with the patient before initiating treatment. The most serious, although infrequent, side effects include tardive dyskinesia, agranulocytosis, supraventicular tachycardia, hyperaldosteronism, and neuroleptic malignant syndrome.

    ii. Cisapride (Propulsid®), 10 mg qid ac and hs. This agent is very effective in enhancing gastric emptying. Cisapride has fewer side effects than metoclopramide; however, given its risk for potentially life-threatening arrhythmias, it is only available for limited access protocol use by gastroenterologists.

    iii. For nausea one can use ondansetron (Zofran®) or promethazine (although the latter often produces drowsiness).

    iv. Domperidone has been found to be effective but is not approved by the US Food and Drug Administration.

e. For patients with gastroparesis who do not respond to medications, consider a referral to a tertiary medical center for a gastric stimulator.

3. Surgical options

The most common surgical procedure performed for GERD is the Nissen fundoplication. This surgery may be indicated in a small number of patients with severe reflux who do not have successful resolution of symptoms with PPIs. Surgical therapy for the appropriate group has been found to be more effective than medical treatment in two controlled randomized studies during a 36-month period, although long-term effectiveness is controversial (De Vault & Castell, 2005). The patient must undergo detailed evaluation by a gastroenterologist before surgery can be considered. Presurgical evaluation includes endoscopy, UGI series, and esophageal manometry with a 24-hour pH study.

It is important for both clinician and patient to understand that even in the hands of an experienced surgeon, the Nissen fundoplication will most likely fail after some years and need a revision. One study suggests that deterioration in both the LES pressure and endoscopic histology back to the presurgical level occurs 5–6 years postoperatively (De Vault & Castell, 2005). The same authors also reviewed another study of 55 postoperative subjects, interviewed 2.9 years after surgery. Of these subjects, 67% reported heartburn, 33% reported regurgitation, and 33% reported regular use of prescription GERD medications.

D. *Follow-up*

1. Follow-up in approximately 4–6 weeks after initiating treatment or sooner if symptoms increase in severity. Assess adherence to treatment plan.

2. Gastroenterology consult if symptoms worsen or complications occur. If no response to treatment, consider EGD, UGI series, or Cine-esophagram.

3. Assess for side effects of medications. There is some controversy regarding the possible association of PPIs with osteoporosis and decreased bone mineral density. A recent study suggests that the apparent association between PPI use and decreased bone mineral density may be related to factors independent of PPI use (Targownik & Leung, 2010).

E. *Patient education*

1. Assist the patient and family in verbalizing their concerns and coping strategies with respect to the disease process and its management.

2. Provide verbal and written information about the pathophysiology of GERD and its treatment. The National Institutes of Health has a very good handout that is available for distribution. See the website below.

3. Discuss what the patient can expect with diagnostic testing, including preparation and after-care.

4. Explain the therapeutic benefit and side effects of any prescribed treatment.

5. Stress that follow-up is recommended in person or by telephone to monitor treatment response and make appropriate treatment regimen changes.

VI. Self-management resources

A. *The National Institutes of Health*

The National Institutes of Health has multiple brochures for patients. Refer to their website at http://digestive.niddk.nih.gov/ddiseases/pubs/gerd/ for their publication on GERD.

B. *The Mayo Clinic*

The Mayo Clinic also has excellent resources at http://www.mayoclinic.com/health/gerd/DS00967

REFERENCES

American Society for Gastrointestinal Endoscopy, Standards of Practice Committee. (2007). Role of endoscopy in management of GERD. *Gastrointestinal Endoscopy, 66*(2), 219–224.

De Vault, K. R., & Castell, D. O. (2005). Guidelines for the diagnosis and treatment of gastroesophageal reflux disease. *American Journal of Gastroenterology, 100*(1), 190–200.

Galmiche, J. P., Zerbib, F., & Des Varannes, S. B. (2008). Review article: Respiratory manifestations of gastro-esophageal reflux disease. *Alimentary Pharmacology & Therapeutics, 27*(8), 449–464.

Hauser, S. C., Pardi, D. S., & Poterucha, J. J. (2008). *Mayo Clinic Gastroenterology and Hepatology Board Review*. Rochester, Minnesota: Mayo Clinic Scientific Press.

Kahrilias, P. J. (2008). Gastroesophageal reflux disease. *The New England Journal of Medicine, 359*(16), 1700–1707.

Kahrilias, P. J., Shaheen, N. J., & Vaezi, M. F. (2008). American Gastroenterological Association medical position statement on management of gastroesophageal reflux disease. *Gastroenterology, 135*(4), 1383–1391.

Mizyad, I., Fass, S. S., & Fass, R. (2009). Gastro-Oesophageal reflux disease and psychological comorbidity. *Alimentary Pharmacology & Therapeutics, 29*(4), 351–358.

Shaheen, N., & Ransohoff, D. (2002). Gastroesophageal reflux, Barrett esophagus and esophageal cancer. *Journal of the American Medical Association, 287*(15), 1982–1986.

Talley, N. J., & Vakil, N. (2005). Guidelines for the management of dyspepsia. *American Journal of Gastroenterology, 100*, 2324–2337.

Targownik, L. E., & Leung, S. L. (2010). Proton-pump inhibitor use is not associated with osteoporosis or accelerated bone mineral density loss. *Gastroenterology, 138*(3), 896–904.

The Practice Parameters Committee of the American College of Gastroenterology, Wang, K. K., & Sampliner, R. (2008). Updated guidelines 2008 for the diagnosis, surveillance and therapy of Barrett's esophagus. *American Journal of Gastroenterology, 103*, 788–797.

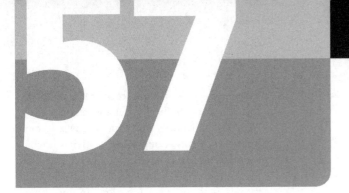

HERPES SIMPLEX INFECTIONS

Hattie C. Grundland and Geraldine Collins-Bride

I. Introduction and general background

Herpes simplex is a DNA virus belonging to the herpes virus group. The virus causes a reoccurring vesicular eruption to the skin or mucus membrane surfaces that have a prior contact exposure. Similar to other herpes viruses, after initial infection a latent state is established that can be followed by reactivation of the virus and recurrent local disease. Herpes simplex virus (HSV) infection is life-long. The course of disease, however, varies among individuals from asymptomatic to recurrent clinical presentations.

A. Types of HSV

1. HSV-1

   HSV-1 is responsible for most of the infections in the face and upper body. Oral and perioral lesions often referred to by the public as "cold sores" or "fever blisters" are common presentations. HSV-1 can infect mucus membranes or abraded skin at any site including the eye, the genitals, and nongenital skin. Serious manifestations of HSV disease, such as encephalitis and meningitis, are rare in the immunocompetent patient. HSV is a common infection worldwide. Each year in the United States there are approximately 500,000 primary infections (Scott, Coulter, & Lamey, 1997). HSV-1 is commonly transmitted in childhood with 90% of individuals seropositive for HSV-1 by the fourth decade of life (Buddingh, Schrum, & Lanier, 1953; Corey, 1986).

2. HSV-2

   HSV-2 is responsible for most of the infections in the genitalia. Most cases of recurrent genital herpes are caused by HSV-2, although seroprevalence trends show genital herpes caused by HSV-1 may be increasing (Langenberg, Corey, Ashley, Leong, & Straus, 1999; Xu et al., 2006). A total of 20–25% of the adult population has serologic evidence of HSV-2 infection (Fleming et al., 1997). Subclinical viral shedding is common and genital infections acquired in this manner are unrecognized in 80–90% of cases. In addition, the individual may not attribute such symptoms as vulvar rashes, irritation, or fissures with genital herpes ulcers. Thus, subclinical viral shedding is a key factor in both horizontal (to a partner) and vertical (mother to newborn) transmission (Schillinger et al., 2008).

   HSV-2 infection is an important risk factor in HIV acquisition (Todd et al., 2006). In persons with HIV infection, the HIV virus can be detected consistently in genital ulcers caused by HSV-2, offering an explanation for the increased risk of HIV acquisition in individuals with HSV-2 (Schacker et al., 1998).

   Neonatal infection with HSV is associated with high neonatal morbidity and mortality. Most pregnant women with a history of recurrent genital herpes can deliver their infants vaginally with a risk of neonatal transmission of less than 8% (Prober et al., 1987). The risk of neonatal transmission is greatest in women who have their first outbreak of genital herpes in pregnancy, especially near the time of delivery. In women with active genital lesions at the time of delivery a cesarean section delivery is recommended. There is limited evidence that the use of routine serologic screening for HSV-2 or prophylactic antiviral therapy in women with a history of recurrent HSV decreases neonatal herpes infection, and therefore neither intervention is recommended by the U.S. Preventative Services Task Force (U.S. Department of Health & Human Services [USDHHS], 2009).

B. Clinical presentations: primary, nonprimary first-episode, and recurrent HSV

1. Primary infection

   This is the first clinical episode in an individual without antibodies to HSV-1 or HSV-2. Primary infection can be severe with painful genital ulcers and systemic symptoms, such as fever, myalgias, malaise, and tender inguinal lymphadenopathy. Lesions classically appear as vesicles or pustules that open to form shallow ulcers. Symptoms usually occur within a few weeks after infection and resolve within 2 weeks (Figure 57-1). Complications of HSV infection are more likely in primary infection and can include aseptic meningitis, sacral autonomic nervous system dysfunction, and disseminated lesions (Corey et al., 1983).

2. Nonprimary first-episode infection

This is the first clinical episode of herpes in an individual with serologic evidence of prior infection with either HSV-1 or HSV-2. The clinical presentation usually is less severe compared to primary infection with fewer local lesions, mild to no systemic symptoms, and shorter duration of symptoms (Corey et al., 1983; Kimberlin & Rouse, 2004).

3. Recurrent infection

Recurrent clinical episodes of herpes typically are less severe than primary and nonprimary first episodes. Systemic symptoms are uncommon. Time of healing of local ulcers and duration of viral shedding is shorter (Wald, Zeh, Selke, Ashley, & Corey, 1995). Triggers that may cause recurrent disease include acute illness, stress, sunlight, fatigue, and menstrual periods. Fifty percent of patients with recurrent episodes experience prodromal symptoms, such as sensitivity to touch (hyperesthesia), local tingling or itching, and peripheral nerve pain (Kimberlin & Rouse, 2004). Most patients experience fewer recurrences over time, from 25% of days in the first year after infection to 4% of days in later years. A smaller number of patients

develop frequent recurrence of HSV outbreaks that can cause both physical and emotional distress. For individuals who experience six or more outbreaks yearly, suppressive antiviral therapy should be offered (Centers for Disease Control and Prevention, 2010). Although the medical complications from recurrent infection are uncommon, the psychosocial and psychosexual impact can cause significant distress for patients.

II. Database

A. Subjective

1. Past medical history and situational factors (may include but is not limited to)

   a. History of similar ulcer eruption (i.e., location of lesion and duration of the outbreaks). Note results of culture if done previously.

   b. History of contact exposure to individual with known HSV infection

   c. History of stimulus known to trigger eruption: sunlight, menses, fever, other illnesses, stress, and increased sexual activity

   d. History of rash, eczema, and erythema-multiforme

   e. History of immunocompromise: HIV-AIDS, leukemia, and lymphoma

   f. History of sexual practices, including oral–genital contact

   g. Currently pregnant

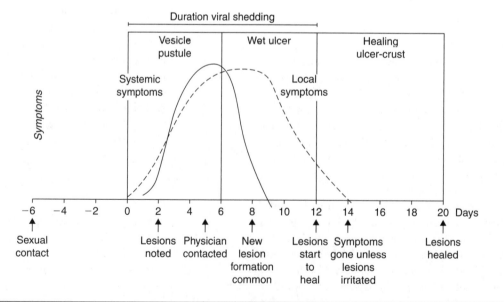

FIGURE 57-1 Clinical Course of Primary Genital Herpes Simplex Virus Infection

Source: Corey, L., Adams, H. G., Brown, Z. A., & Holmes, K. K. (1983). Genital herpes simplex virus infections: Clinical manifestations, course, and complications. *Annals of Internal Medicine, 98*(6), 958–972. Reprinted with permission.

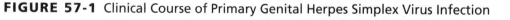

2. Occupational history
   a. Exposure history
   b. Type of profession (e.g., healthcare worker and dentist [herpetic whitlow])
   c. Contacts and personal protection
3. Symptomatology
   a. Fever, headache, malaise, myalgias, and tender lymph nodes
   b. Burning pain, tingling, hyperesthesia, or itching of involved skin and mucus membranes defines the prodromal symptoms of recurrent infection preceding outbreak of lesions by up to 2 days.
   c. Depending on the site of infection
      i. Genital lesions: dysuria, urinary retention, sacral or genital paresthesias, rectal tenesmus, and constipation
      ii. Oral lesions: facial paresthesias, mouth pain (gingivastomatitis), difficulty eating, and visual disturbances or pain
   d. No symptoms

B. *Objective*
1. Vital signs: fever infrequent, most common in primary infection or with secondary complications, such as aseptic meningitis
2. Skin: tender, single, or clustered vesicles, pustules, or ulcers on a clean erythematous base. Ulcers may appear crusted over in the period before resolution. Most frequently occurs in or around the mouth, on the vulva, on penile glans or shaft, or perianally. May occur on distal fingers (herpetic whitlow), especially of healthcare workers.
3. Eye: unilateral conjunctivitis, blepharitis with vesicles on the lid margin, keratitis with dendretic lesions, or with punctuate opacities on ophthalmic examination
4. Mouth: small ulcers located on the soft palate, buccal mucosa, tongue, or floor of the mouth
5. Lymph: may have tender, nonfluctuant regional lymphadenopathy, especially in primary outbreaks.
6. Genitourinary: may see urethral, vaginal, or rectal discharge depending on severity of involvement. If rectal involvement, may see only swollen inflamed mucosa on anoscopy, not distinct lesions.

III. Assessment

A. *Determine the diagnosis*
1. Primary
2. Nonprimary first-episode

3. Recurrent
4. Other conditions that may explain the patient's presentation
   a. Infectious genital ulcer diseases: syphilis, chancroid, lymphogranuloma venereum, or granuloma inguinale
   b. Noninfectious genital ulcers: Behçet syndrome, Crohn's disease, or fixed drug eruption
   c. Mucopurulent cervical discharge: *Chlamydia*, gonorrhea, or mycoplasmas
   d. Vulvar rashes: contact dermatitis or impetigo
   e. Orolabial ulcers: aphthous stomatitis
   f. Herpes zoster
   g. Other etiologies of proctitis

B. *Severity*

Assess the severity of the infection including diagnosis of complications
1. Urine retention resulting from bladder neck spasm.
2. Proctitis particularly in men who have sex with men (Klausner, Kohn, & Kent, 2003).
3. Constipation
4. Difficulty eating solid foods
5. Secondary bacterial infections caused by streptococci or staphylococci
6. Erythema multiforme
7. Herpes keratitis
8. Disseminated herpes
9. Aseptic meningitis
10. Neonatal herpes
11. Emotional stress and psychologic morbidity especially seen with recurrent genital HSV.

IV. Goals of clinical management

A. *Choose a cost-effective approach for diagnosing HSV infection*

B. *Select a treatment plan that addresses the patient's symptom severity, frequency of recurrence, transmission risk to uninfected partner, and cost*

C. *Select an approach that maximizes patient adherence*

D. *Provide an education plan that empowers patients to cope with a recurrent sexually transmitted disease through self-management resources*

V. Plan

A. Screening

The American Academy of Family Physicians and the United States Preventive Services Task Force recommend against routine serologic screening for the general population and for pregnant women to prevent neonatal HSV infections. Counseling around the risks and benefits of serologic screening should be discussed and offered to select groups of patients including patients who may have HSV-infected sex partners and HIV-positive patients (American Academy of Family Physicians, 2009; USDHHS, 2009).

B. Diagnostic tests

1. HSV viral culture if active lesions are present.

   The sensitivity of viral culture is highest when lesion vesicles are unroofed and the base of an ulcer can be sampled. As lesions start to heal, the culture sensitivity decreases rapidly (Corey et al., 1983). Determination of the HSV-type of infection predicts recurrence risk (50% with HSV-2, 10% with HSV-1) but otherwise is not necessary or helpful.

2. HSV polymerase chain reaction.

   Improved sensitivity over culture but at increased cost. In many laboratories this test is performed only on cerebral spinal fluid.

3. Pap smear taken from active lesion to check for presence of multinucleated giant cells.

   Limited use because of low sensitivity, but specificity is good. It is most useful for lesions late in the course of an outbreak.

4. Type specific herpes virus serology.

   Used primarily to rule out HSV diagnosis if the serology is negative at least 6 weeks after the onset of the outbreak. May also be used to determine primary herpes infection if patient is seronegative during initial symptoms then converts to seropositive after 6 weeks from the onset of the outbreak.

5. Diagnostic tests as necessary to rule out etiologies other than HSV infection include syphilis serology to rule out primary or secondary syphilis.

6. HIV screening should be offered to all patients.

C. Management

1. Preventive

   a. Avoid contact with persons with a known or suspected active herpes lesion.

   b. Use of condoms, gloves, or other barrier methods.

   c. Avoid or decrease exposure to known recurrence triggers.

   d. Antiviral medications used to treat or suppress recurrent outbreaks or prophylactic therapy of an infected person to prevent horizontal transmission to an uninfected partner (Table 57-1).

2. Symptomatic

   a. Sitz bath or cool compresses

   b. Topical anesthetic or viscous lidocaine as needed

   c. Anticonstipating diet or stool softeners as needed

   d. Nonsteroidal anti-inflammatory medications to reduce pain

   e. Antiviral medications for primary or recurrent outbreaks (Table 57-1)

3. Criteria for consultation or specialty referral

   a. Generalized involvement

   b. Any complications present

   c. Pregnancy

4. Follow-up

   a. As medically indicated for patients with primary herpes, depending on the severity of the infection.

   b. Not medically necessary for follow-up with infrequent recurrent outbreaks, although some patients may require follow-up visits to focus on counseling and education.

   c. Patients on suppressive therapy should be reevaluated every 12 months.

D. Patient education

1. Goal: educate on the clinical course of the disease, emphasizing risk factors for HSV transmission. Address concerns and feelings to help patients cope with herpes.

   a. Discuss the natural history of HSV infection including outbreak recurrence and risk of transmission during symptomatic and asymptomatic disease.

   b. Advise patients to inform current and future sex partners of exposure risks, including the avoidance of contact with a herpes lesion from onset of prodrome until complete healing of the lesion.

   c. Review appropriate use of prescribed medications.

   d. Consider suppressive therapy as a strategy to decrease transmission to uninfected partners for those patients with frequent outbreaks (Corey et al., 2004).

   e. Review the use of condoms and other barrier methods to help decrease transmission.

TABLE 57-1 Drug Treatment of Herpes Simplex Infections

HSV Type	Drug	Dosage	Notes
Oral HSV primary	Acyclovir*	200 mg orally five times daily or 400 mg orally three times daily for 7–10 days	Begin treatment early in infection
Oral HSV recurrent	Acyclovir or Penciclovir	200 mg orally five times daily for 10 days or 1% cream every 2 hours while awake for 4 days	Treatment for recurrent oral herpes offers mild benefit Although the evidence does not support topical treatment, some patients report successful use
Genital HSV primary	Acyclovir or Famciclovir or Valacyclovir	400 mg orally three times a day for 7–10 days or 200 mg orally five times a day for 7–10 days 250 mg orally three times a day for 7–10 days 1 g orally twice a day for 7–10 days	Extending treatment is an option if healing is incomplete after 10 days of therapy
Genital HSV recurrent	Acyclovir or Famciclovir or Valacyclovir	400 mg orally three times a day for 5 days or 800 mg orally twice a day for 5 days or 800 mg orally three times a day for 2 days 125 mg orally twice daily for 5 days or 1,000 mg orally twice daily for 1 day 500 mg orally twice a day for 3 days or 1 g orally once a day for 5 days	Begin treatment at first sign of infection; an option for patients with mild or infrequent recurrent symptoms (< 6 outbreaks per year)
Genital HSV suppressive	Acyclovir or Famciclovir or Valacyclovir	400 mg orally twice a day 250 mg orally twice a day 500 mg orally once a day or 1 g orally once a day	An option for patients with more frequent or severe symptoms (> 6 outbreaks per year) Shown to decrease transmission in discordant couples with HSV-2
HSV treatment in patients with HIV			See Chapter 64, Primary Care of HIV-infected Adults*

*Intravenous acyclovir therapy should be provided for patients who have severe primary HSV disease or complications that necessitate hospitalization (e.g., disseminated infection, pneumonitis, or hepatitis) or central nervous system complications (e.g., meningitis or encephalitis). The recommended regimen is acyclovir, 5–10 mg/kg body weight intravenously every 8 hours for 2–7 days or until clinical improvement is observed, followed by oral antiviral therapy to complete at least 10 days of total therapy.

Source: Centers for Disease Control and Prevention. (2010). *Sexually transmitted diseases: Treatment Guidelines 2006*. Retrieved from http://www.cdc.gov/std/treatment/2006/genital-ulcers.htm#genulc3

f. Inform current and prospective sex partners of exposure risks.

g. Advise women who are pregnant or become pregnant to tell their clinician or obstetrician about their history of HSV infection.

h. Understand that HSV infection is associated with increased HIV transmission

i. Address concerns and psychologic impact of HSV infection and provide printed, web-related and telephone resources to assist patients in their understanding and coping.

VI. Self-management resources and tools

A. Patient education

1. Herpes Resource Center
   American Social Health Association
   (1-800-230-6039; http://ashatd.org)

2. National Institute of Allergy and Infectious Disease (http://niaid.nih.gov)

3. Centers for Disease Control and Prevention (http://cdc.gov)

B. Community support groups

1. The Herpes Resource Center has an affiliated network of local support (HELP) groups for people concerned about herpes simplex virus. The network of support groups can be accessed on the American Social Health Association website (http://ashatd.org)

REFERENCES

American Academy of Family Physicians. (2009). *Summary of AAFP recommendations for clinical preventive services.* Retrieved from http://www.aafp.org/online/en/home/clinical/clinicalrecs.html

Buddingh, G. J., Schrum, D. I., & Lanier, J. C. (1953). Studies of the natural history of herpes simplex infections. *Pediatrics, 11*(6), 595–610.

Centers for Disease Control and Prevention. (2010). *Sexually transmitted diseases: Treatment Guidelines 2006.* Retrieved from http://www.cdc.gov/std/treatment/2006/genital-ulcers.htm#genulc3

Corey, L., Adams, H. G., Brown, Z. A., & Holmes, K. K. (1983). Genital herpes simplex virus infections: Clinical manifestations, course and complications. *Annals of Internal Medicine, 98*(6), 958–972.

Corey, L. (1986). Genital herpes. In A. Nahmias & B. Roizman (Eds.), *The Herpes viruses* (pp. 1–35). New York, NY: Plenum Press.

Corey, L., Wald, A., Patel, R., Sacks, S. L., Tyring, S. K., Warren, T., . . . Valacyclovir Transmission Study Group. (2004). Once-daily valacyclovir to reduce the risk of transmission of genital herpes. *New England Journal of Medicine, 350*(1), 11–20.

Fleming, D. T., McQuillan, G. M., Johnson, R. E., Nahmias, A. J., Aral, S. O., . . . St. Louis, M. E. (1997). Herpes simplex virus type 2 in the United States, 1976 to 1994. *New England Journal of Medicine, 337*(16), 1105–1111.

Kimberlin, D. W., & Rouse, D. J. (2004). Clinical practice. Genital herpes. *New England Journal of Medicine, 350*(19), 1970–1977.

Klausner, J. D., Kohn, R., & Kent, C. (2003). Etiology of clinical proctitis among men who have sex with men. *Clinical Infectious Disease, 38*(2), 300–302.

Langenberg, A. G., Corey, L., Ashley, R. L., Leong, W. P., & Straus, S. E. (1999). A prospective study of new infections with herpes simplex virus type 1 and type 2. Chiron HSV Vaccine Study Group. *New England Journal of Medicine, 341*(19), 1432–1438.

Prober, C. G., Sullender, W. M., Yasukawa, L. L., Au, D. S., Yeager, A. S., & Arvin, A. M. (1987). Low risk of herpes simplex virus infections in neonates exposed to the virus at the time of vaginal delivery to mothers with recurrent genital herpes simplex virus infections. *New England Journal of Medicine, 316*, 240–244.

Schacker, T., Ryncarz, A. J., Goddard, J., Diem, K., Shaughnessy, M., & Corey, L. (1998). Frequent recovery of HIV-1 from genital herpes simplex virus lesions in HIV-1-infected men. *Journal of the American Medical Association, 280*(1), 61–66.

Schillinger, J. A., McKinney, C. M., Garg, R., Gwynn, R. C., White, K., Lee, F., . . . Frieden, T. (2008). Seroprevalence of herpes simplex virus type 2 and characteristics associated with undiagnosed infection. *Sexually Transmitted Disease, 35*(6), 599–606.

Scott, D. A., Coulter, W. A., Lamey, P. J. (1997). Oral shedding of herpes simplex virus type 1: A review. *Journal of Oral Pathology Medicine, 26*(10), 441–447.

Todd, J., Grosskurth, H., Changalucha, J., Obasi, A., Mosha, F., & Balira, R. (2006). Risk factors influencing HIV infection incidence in a rural African population: A nested case-control study. *Journal of Infectious Disease, 193*(3), 458–466.

U.S. Department of Health & Human Services. (2009). *Guide to clinical preventive services, 2009 recommendations of the U.S. Preventative Services Task Force (USPSTF)* (pocket guide, abridged version of the recommendations). Rockville, MD: Agency for Healthcare Research and Quality.

Wald, A., Zeh, J., Selke, S., Ashley, R. L., & Corey, L. (1995). Virologic characteristics of subclinical and symptomatic genital herpes infections. *New England Journal of Medicine, 333*(12), 770–775.

Xu, F., Sternberg, M. R., Kottiri, B. J., McQuillan, G. M., Lee, F. K., & Nahmias, A. J. (2006). Trends in herpes simplex virus type 1 and type 2 seroprevalence in the United States. *Journal of the American Medical Association, 296*(8), 964–973.

HYPERTENSION

Judith Sweet

I. Introduction and definition

Hypertension (HTN) is an elevation in arterial blood pressure (BP) confirmed when the average of two or more (seated) readings done at two or more office visits is greater than 140 systolic or 90 diastolic. Hypertension (HTN) is a continuous and independent risk factor for cardiovascular disease, and the presence of additional risk factors (elevated total cholesterol, high-density lipoprotein cholesterol < 35, smoking, diabetes, and left ventricular hypertrophy as the most important) compounds the risk from HTN.

Elevated systolic BP (SBP) is now considered to be as important a risk factor as diastolic HTN. Diastolic HTN is a stronger cardiovascular risk factor, and more common before the age of 50 than systolic HTN, whereas systolic HTN is more common after the age of 50 than diastolic HTN (Seventh Report of the Joint National Committee on Prevention, Detection, Evaluation, and Treatment of High Blood Pressure [JNC 7], 2004).

A. Prevalence

The National Health and Nutrition Examination Survey (NHANES) (Burt et al., 1995) reported a decade ago that more than 50 million Americans have elevated BP. Based on 1999–2000 NHANES data, there was an estimated 65 million Americans with hypertension (Cutler et al., 2008). Suboptimal BP (> 115 mm Hg SBP) has been estimated by the World Health Organization (2002) to be responsible for 62% of cerebrovascular disease and 49% of ischemic heart disease, with possibly as many as 1 billion people at risk. The World Health Organization considers HTN to be the main attributable risk factor for death worldwide (JNC 7, 2004).

1. Classification of BP (adults)

   The JNC 7 (2004) report simplifies the categorization of BP into four categories: (1) normal, (2) pre-HTN, (3) HTN stage 1, and (4) HTN stage 2 (Table 58-1). The designation of "pre-HTN" is meant to identify those individuals at high risk of developing frank HTN who may benefit from adapting lifestyle modifications that either lower BP or slow the rate of progression (JNC 7, 2004). This stage should not be viewed as a disease category, but rather as a warning and an incentive for care providers to strongly counsel these individuals regarding lifestyle modifications. These individuals are not candidates for medication treatment unless they also have diabetes or kidney disease (JNC 7, 2004).

   The treatment goal recommended by JNC 7 (2004) for both stage 1 and stage 2 HTN, regardless of the presence or absence of risk factors or target organ damage, is less than 140/90. If there are other "compelling conditions" present (heart failure, diabetes, renal disease, post–myocardial infarction, history of stroke or high risk of cardiovascular disease), different standards apply (which are not covered in this chapter) (JNC 7, 2004, p. 33).

II. Database

A. Subjective

1. Most patients are asymptomatic.

   Although most patients are asymptomatic, some may experience headaches, dizziness, blurred vision, tinnitus, chest pain, shortness of breath, nausea, vomiting, extremity swelling, or anxiety, which may be unrelated to secondary causes of end organ damage.

2. The following symptoms suggest secondary HTN

   a. Muscle cramps, polyuria, weakness, and excessive thirst: primary aldosteronism

TABLE 58-1 Classification of Blood Pressure for Adults (18 years and Older)

BP Classification	SBP mm Hg	DBP mm Hg
Normal	< 120	and < 80
Prehypertension	120–139	or 80–89
Stage 1 hypertension	140–159	or 90–99
Stage 2 hypertension	≥ 160	or ≥ 100

b. Headache, pallor, palpitations, sweating, and flushing: pheochromocytoma

c. Hirsutism, easy bruising, and symptoms of diabetes mellitus: Cushing's syndrome

d. Severe chest pain radiating to back: aortic dissection or aneurysm

e. Claudication: coarctation of aorta

f. Snoring and daytime fatigue: sleep apnea

g. Palpitations, insomnia, anxiety, and weight loss: hyperthyroidism (see Chapter 66 on thyroid disorders)

3. Symptoms suggestive of target organ damage

a. Exertional chest pain, shortness of breath, orthopnea, peripheral edema, and paroxysmal nocturnal dyspnea: coronary artery disease or congestive heart failure

b. Fatigue, pruritus, or peripheral edema: renal failure

c. Syncopal episodes or dizziness, memory loss, motor weakness, speech difficulties, or other focal neurologic findings: cerebrovascular disease

d. Claudication and sudden loss of vision: peripheral arterial disease

4. Past medical history

a. History and work-up of HTN (When was patient first told he or she has high BP?); course of treatment and complications including medications tried and failed or with adverse effects.

b. Diabetes, lipid abnormalities, gout, cardiovascular and cerebrovascular disease, and renal disease.

c. Use of prescribed or over-the-counter drugs that may influence BP or interfere with the effectiveness of an antihypertensive drug (e.g., hormonal contraceptives, steroids, nonsteroidal anti-inflammatory drugs, alcohol, cocaine, amphetamines, appetite suppressants or other "diet" supplements, tricyclic antidepressants, monoamine oxidase inhibitors, or decongestants [pseudoephedrine and phenylpropanolomines or analogues]) (Table 58-2).

d. Dietary supplement use including products containing "herbal ecstasy," Ma Huang/ephedra, ergot-containing products, and St. John's Wort.

e. If overweight, note history of weight gain.

5. Family history: History of HTN, stroke, sudden cardiac death, diabetes, congestive heart failure, renal disease, or other cardiovascular disease.

6. Personal and social history: habits

a. Alcohol use: chronic use and withdrawal elevates BP

b. Recreational or street drug use, especially cocaine, crack, and amphetamines; anabolic steroids; recent withdrawal from narcotics

c. Diet: this includes sodium intake, use of canned or prepared foods, vegetable and fruit intake, fat and cholesterol intake

d. Exercise: type, frequency, and level of exercise

e. Tobacco use: not a cause of HTN but is an additional risk factor for cardiovascular disease, and withdrawal may be associated with elevated BP

7. Ethnic or racial background

May affect responsiveness to certain medications (e.g., overall improved BP control with diuretics for African Americans), and a factor in lifestyle modifications (e.g., dietary choices) (JNC 7, 2004).

8. Other factors influencing BP control

Emotional stress including social support system (if any), family and living situation, employment and working situation and stress, ability to obtain and pay for healthcare services, and educational level.

B. Objective

1. Physical examination

a. Vital signs including BP taken after patient has been sitting quietly for at least 5 minutes with arm resting on a flat surface with feet on the floor, and the patient should not have used caffeine, tobacco, or alcohol and should not have exercised for at least 30 minutes before the BP measurement. Initial evaluation should include BP measurement in both arms. At least two measurements should be obtained and the average of the two recorded. Periodic standing BP measurements are recommended for those at risk for postural BP changes or with such symptoms, and when adding or changing medications. The preferred method of BP measurement is the auscultatory (not digital) method, and the proper sized cuff is essential; the cuff bladder should encircle at least 80% of the arm (JNC 7, 2004).

b. Fundoscopic evaluation for arteriovenous nicking, arteriolar narrowing, papilloedema, hemorrhages, or exudates.

c. Assess neck for carotid bruits, distended veins, and enlarged thyroid.

d. Evaluate the heart for precordial heave, thrills, rate, murmurs, or other extra sounds, such as S3 and S4.

e. Auscultate the lungs for adventitious sounds (e.g., wheezing).

f. Evaluate the abdomen for bruits, enlarged kidneys, or striae.

g. Assess the extremities for diminished or absent peripheral arterial pulses, edema, or femoral artery bruits.

h. Neurologic assessment as baseline and for evaluation of abnormal sensory, motor, and cognitive findings suggestive of end-stage disease.

2. Diagnostic tests
a. Laboratory: urinalysis, blood glucose, hematocrit, serum potassium, creatinine and estimated glomerular filtration rate, calcium, and fasting lipid profile
b. Twelve-lead electrocardiogram

TABLE 58-2 Common Substances Associated with Hypertension in Humans

Prescription Drugs	Street Drugs and Other "Natural Products"	Food Substances	Chemical Elements and Other Industrial Chemicals
Cortisone and other steroids: (both corticosteroids and mineralosteroids), adrenocorticotropic hormone (ACTH)	Cocaine and cocaine withdrawal	Sodium chloride	Lead
Estrogens (usually just oral contraceptive agents with high estrogenic activity)	Ma Huang, "herbal ecstasy," and other phenyl propanolamine analogues	Ethanol	Mercury
Nonsteroidal anti-inflammatory drugs	Nicotine and withdrawal	Licorice	Thallium and other heavy metals
Phenylpropanolamines and analogues	Anabolic steroids	Tyramine-containing foods (with monoamine oxidase inhibitors)	Lithium salts, especially the chloride
Cyclosporine and tacrolimus	Narcotic withdrawal	Caffeine	
Erythropoietin	Methylphenidate		
Sibutramine	Phencyclidine		
Ketamine	Ketamine		
Desflurane	Ergotamine and other ergot-containing herbal preparations		
Carbamazepine	St. John's Wort		
Bromocryptine			
Metoclopramide			
Antidepressants (especially venlafaxine)			
Buspirone			
Clonidine (abrupt withdrawal) with or without the simultaneous initiation of beta-adrenergic blocking agents			
Pheochromocytoma: beta-adrenergic blocking agent without alpha blocker first; glucagon			
Clozapine			
Weight loss drugs			

Source: Adapted from Seventh Report of the Joint National Committee on Prevention, Detection, Evaluation, and Treatment of High Blood Pressure (JNC 7). (2004, p. 59). U.S. Department of Health and Human Services, NIH Publication no. 0405230. Retrieved from http://www.nhlbi.nih.gov/guidelines/hypertension/jnc7full.htm

c. If secondary HTN is suspected based on the patient's presentation, other tests should be included (Table 58-3)

III. Assessment

A. *Determine the diagnosis*

1. Pre-HTN

2. Primary HTN, stages 1 or 2

3. Secondary HTN

B. *Severity*

Assess severity based on level of BP and presence or absence of other risk factors or other compelling diseases.

C. *Significance and patient's motivation and ability*

Assess the significance of this diagnosis to the patient and to significant others. Additionally, assess patient's understanding of the disorder and willingness and ability to follow a treatment plan, including lifestyle modifications.

IV. Goals of clinical management

A. *Public health goal*

Reduce the cardiovascular; and renal morbidity and mortality.

B. *Individual's goal related to self-management and patient adherence*

Choose a plan including medications, lifestyle modifications, and follow-up that is tailored to the patient.

C. *BP goal*

Primary focus should be on attaining an SBP below 140, because most persons reach the diastolic BP goal once the SBP goal is reached. In persons with renal disease or diabetes, the goal is less than 130/80 (JNC 7, 2004).

V. Plan and management (Figure 58-1)

A. *Lifestyle modification (Table 58-4)*

This is the first step in counseling and treating patients with pre-HTN and stage 1 HTN, and is an essential component of treatment in treating stage 2 HTN. In some patients, lifestyle modifications are definitive therapy, and in others may reduce the number and doses of antihypertensives required to reach goal BP.

1. Weight

Weight loss of as little as 10 lb (4.5 kg) reduces BP or prevents HTN in many overweight individuals (JNC 7, 2004).

2. Diet

Adoption of the DASH (Dietary Approaches to Stop Hypertension) dietary plan (Sacks et al., 2001)

a. Dietary sodium of less than 2.4 g of sodium daily.

b. Four to five servings of fruits and vegetables to increase potassium and other nutrients.

c. Daily low-fat dairy for adequate calcium intake.

d. Low-fat and low cholesterol dietary choices.

3. Alcohol

Alcohol intake should be limited to 1 oz or less daily of ethanol (two drinks in men) and no more than 0.5 oz (one drink in women).

TABLE 58-3 Screening Tests for Identifiable Causes of Hypertension

Diagnosis	Diagnostic Test
Chronic kidney disease	Estimated glomerular filtration rate
Coarctation of the aorta	Computerized tomography angiography
Cushing's syndrome and other glucocorticoid excess states including chronic steroid therapy	History; dexamethasone suppression test
Drug induced or related	History and drug screening
Pheochromocytoma	24-hours metanephrine and normetanephrine
Primary aldosteronism and other mineralocorticoid excess states	24-hour urinary aldosterone level or specific measurements of other mineralocorticoids
Renovascular hypertension	Doppler flow study; magnetic resonance angiography
Sleep apnea	Sleep study with O_2 saturation
Thyroid or parathyroid disease	Thyroid-stimulating hormone, serum parathyroid hormone

Source: Seventh Report of the Joint National Committee on Prevention, Detection, Evaluation, and Treatment of High Blood Pressure (JNC 7). (2004). U.S. Department of Health and Human Services, NIH Publication no. 0405230. Retrieved from http://www.nhlbi.nih.gov/guidelines /hypertension/jnc7full.htm

4. Exercise

   Regular aerobic activity, such as brisk walking, is recommended most days of the week.

5. Tobacco abstinence

   For overall cardiovascular risk reduction, smoking cessation is essential and should be a major focus of counseling for providers.

6. Stress management

   For hypertensive patients in whom stress seems to be an important factor, whether consciously perceived by the individual or not, stress management

should be considered as a recommendation or intervention. Stress management techniques that have been found to be successful in clinical trials include cognitive-behavioral interventions, biofeedback with focus on breathing regulation, Transcendental Meditation™, and self-regulated slow breathing using a Food and Drug Administration approved device that regulates breathing rate (e.g., RESPeRATE™) (Elliott & Izzo, 2006; Mann, 2000; Linden, Lenz, & Con, 2001; Rainforth et al., 2007; Spence, Barnett, Linden, Ransden, & Taenzer, 1999).

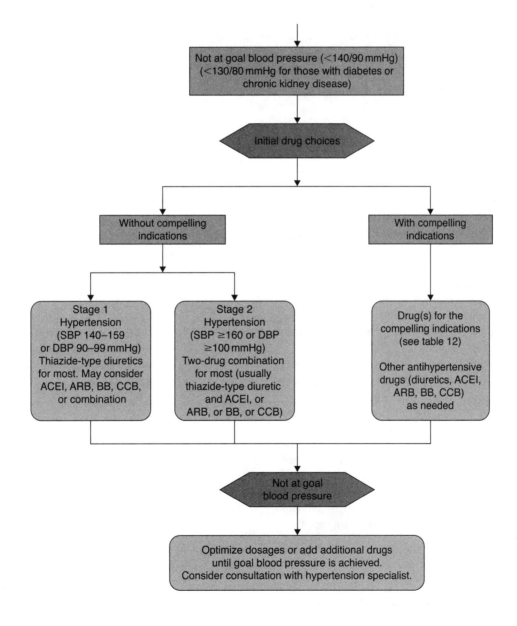

FIGURE 58-1 Algorithm for Treatment of Hypertension
Source: JNC 7, p. 31.

TABLE 58-4 Lifestyle Modifications to Prevent and Manage Hypertension

Modification	Recommendation	Approximate SBP Reduction
Weight reduction	Maintain normal body weight (body mass index 18.5–24.9 kg/m²)	5–20 mm Hg/10 kg of weight loss
Adopt DASH eating plan	Consume a diet rich in fruits, vegetables, and low-fat dairy products with a reduced content of saturated and total fat	8–14 mm Hg
Dietary sodium reduction	Reduce dietary sodium intake to no more than 100 mmol per day (2.4 g sodium or 6 g sodium chloride)	2–8 mm Hg
Moderation of alcohol consumption	No more than two drinks (e.g., 24 oz beer, 10 oz wine, or 3 oz 80-proof whiskey) per day in most men, and to no more than one drink per day in women and lighter weight persons	4–9 mm Hg
Physical activity	Engage in regular aerobic physical activity, such as brisk walking (at least 30 minutes per day, most days of the week).	2–4 mm Hg
Stress management	Consider if this seems to be a factor: relaxation and breathing exercises, cognitive behavioral approaches, meditation, device-guided slow breathing	Variable

Source: Adapted from Seventh Report of the Joint National Committee on Prevention, Detection, Evaluation, and Treatment of High Blood Pressure (JNC 7). (2004, p. 26). U.S. Department of Health and Human Services, NIH Publication no. 0405230. Retrieved from http://www.nhlbi .nih.gov/guidelines/hypertension/jnc7full.htm

B. Pharmacologic treatment (Table 58-5)

Reducing elevated BP with medications has been shown in numerous studies to decrease the incidence of cardiovascular mortality and morbidity.

1. Factors to be considered in the selection of therapy are

   a. Cost of medication
   b. Metabolic and subjective side effects
   c. Potential drug–drug interactions
   d. Concomitant diseases that may be beneficially or adversely affected by the antihypertensive agent chosen
   e. Ethnicity and race: there is a great variance in HTN-related morbidity and mortality among various ethnic groups in the United States, because of many factors including physiologic differences in response to some drugs; socioeconomic conditions; access to healthcare services; attitudes and beliefs related to health information; and differences in lifestyle practices, such as diet (JNC 7, 2004)
      i. African Americans may respond to a low-sodium diet and diuretics with greater BP reductions than other demographic subgroups (JNC 7, 2004).
      ii. Mexican Americans and Native Americans tend to have lower control rates of HTN than non-Hispanic whites and African Americans (JNC 7, 2004).
      iii. African Americans and Asians have a three to four times higher risk of developing angioedema and more cough associated with the use of angiotensin-converting enzyme inhibitors than whites (JNC 7, 2004).

2. General treatment guidelines

   a. The preferred initial agent is a thiazide-type diuretic, because agents from this drug class have been shown in numerous studies to be superior to all other agents in preventing the cardiovascular complications of HTN (JNC 7, 2004).
   b. Most hypertensive patients require two or more antihypertensives from different drug classes to reach goal BP range (JNC 7, 2004).
   c. However, simplify the regimen to once-daily dosing if possible for greater adherence.
   d. In some patients on once-daily dosing, there may be a trough effect: waning of effectiveness of medications at the end of dosing interval. Therefore, it is best to measure the BP just before the next dose to determine the need for dosage adjustment (JNC 7, 2004).
   e. In stage 2 HTN, consider starting therapy with two drugs, either as separate prescriptions or in fixed-dose combinations, because this increases the likelihood of reaching BP goal more promptly than with one agent (JNC 7, 2004).

C. Patient education

It is essential that this be done in the language in which the patient is fluent (verbal and written) and at a reading level appropriate to patient's education. When in doubt, aim at a sixth grade or lower level of reading.

1. Provide verbal and written information on cardiovascular risk factors associated with HTN and long-term prognosis of HTN if untreated.

TABLE 58-5 Pharmacological Therapy* (JNC 7, 2004; Sutters, 2011)

Class of Drug	Drug Name	Usual Dose Range/mg/day	Usual Daily Frequency	Mechanism	Comments
Thiazide diuretics	Chlorthalidone	12.5–25	1	Decreased plasma volume and extracellular fluid volume, decreased cardiac output initially, followed by decreased total peripheral resistance with normalization of cardiac output. Long-term effects include slight decreases in extracellular fluid volume.	For thiazide and loop diuretics, lower doses and dietary counseling should be used to avoid metabolic changes (e.g., potassium, sodium losses). Check electrolytes 1–2 weeks after initiating these medications.
	Chlorthiazide	125–500	1–2		
	Hydrochlorathiazide	12.5–50	1		
	Indapamide	1.25–2.5	1		
	Polythiazide	2–4	1		
	Metolazone (Mykrox)	0.5–1.0	1		
	Metolazone (Zaroxolyn)	2.5–5.0	1		
Loop diuretics	Bumetanide	0.5–2	2	See thiazides.	Higher doses may be needed for patients with renal impairment or congestive heart failure. Ethacrynic acid is the only alternative for patients with allergy to thiazide and sulfur-containing diuretics.
	Ethacrynic acid	50–100	1–2		
	Furosemide	10–80	2		
	Torsemide	2.5–10	1		
Potassium-sparing diuretics	Amiloride	5–10	1–2	Promotes excretion of water and sodium while retaining potassium through disruption of sodium and potassium exchange in the distal nephrons.	Weak diuretics, used mainly in combination with other diuretics to avoid or reverse hypokalemia from the diuretics. Avoid when serum creatinine ≥ 2.5. May cause hyperkalemia, especially if concomitant angiotensin-converting enzyme inhibitors or potassium supplements.
	Triamterene	50–100	1–2		
Aldosterone receptor blockers	Eplerenone	50–100	1	Promotes excretion of water and sodium while retaining potassium by blocking aldosterone receptors	May cause hyperkalemia especially if concomitant angiotensin-converting enzyme inhibitors or potassium supplements. Spironalactone may cause gynecomastia and menstrual irregularities.
	Spironalactone	25–50	1		

(continues)

TABLE 58-5 Pharmacological Therapy* (JNC 7, 2004; Sutters, 2011) *(continued)*

Class of Drug	Drug Name	Usual Dose Range/mg/day	Usual Daily Frequency	Mechanism	Comments
β-Blockers	Atenolol	25–100	1	Decreased cardiac output and increased total peripheral resistance; decreased plasma renin activity; atenolol, betaxolol, bisoprolol, and metroprolol are cardioselective.	Selective agents also inhibit in higher doses (e.g., all may aggravate asthma).
	Betaxolol	5–20	1		
	Bisoprolol	2.5–10	1		
	Metoprolol	25–100	1–2		
	Metoprolol extended release	25–100	1		
	Nadolol	40–120	1		
	Propranolol	40–160	2		
	Propranolol long-acting	60–180	1		
	Timolol	10–40	2		
β-Blockers with intrinsic sympathomimetic activity	Acebutolol	200–800	2	See β-blockers Acebutolol is cardioselective.	Use intrinsic sympathomimetic activity agents for those with bradycardia who must receive β-blockers.
	Penbutolol	10–40	1		
	Pindolol	10–40	2		
Combined α- and β-blockers	Carvedilol	12.5–50	2	Same as β-blockers, plus $_1$-blockade.	Possibly more effective in blacks than other blockers; May cause postural effects: titration should be based on standing blood pressure.
	Labetolol	200–800	2		
α-1 Receptor blockers	Doxasozin	1–16	1	Block postsynaptic$_1$-receptor blockade and cause vasodilation.	All may cause postural effects: titration should be based on standing blood pressure.
	Prazosin	2–20	2–3		
	Terazosin	1–20	1–2		
Angiotensin-converting enzyme inhibitors	Benzapril	10–40	1	Block formation of angiotensin II by cleaving angiotensin I thereafter promoting vasodilation and reducing the circulation of aldosterone that results in decreased sodium and water retention. They also increase bradykinin and vasodilatory prostaglandins.	Diuretic doses should be reduced or discontinued before starting angiotensin-converting enzyme inhibitors whenever possible to prevent excessive hypotension. May cause hyperkalemia in patients with renal impairment or in those receiving potassium-sparing agents. Can cause acute renal failure in patients with severe bilateral renal artery stenosis or severe stenosis in artery in a solitary kidney.
	Captopril	25–100	2		
	Enalapril	5–40	1–2		
	Fosinopril	10–40	1		
	Lisinopril	10–40	1		
	Moexiprol	7.5–30	1		
	Perindopril	4–8	1		
	Quinapril	10–80	1		
	Rampiril	2.5–2.0	1		
	Trandolopril	1–4	1		

TABLE 58-5 Pharmacological Therapy* (JNC 7, 2004; Sutters, 2011) (continued)

Class of Drug	Drug Name	Usual Dose Range/mg/day	Usual Daily Frequency	Mechanism	Comments
Angiotensin II receptor blockers	Candesartan	8–32	1	Blocks the angiotensin II receptor thus inhibiting the action of angiotensin II as noted previously. Bradykinin levels are not altered so there is lower incidence of an associated dry cough than with angiotensin-converting enzyme inhibitors.	See angiotensin-converting enzyme inhibitors.
	Eprosartan	400–800	1–2		
	Irbesartan	150–300	1		
	Losartan	25–100	1–2		
	Olmesartan	20–40	1		
	Telmisartan	20–80	1		
	Valsartan	80–320	1–2		
Calcium channel blockers	Amlodipine	2.5–10	1	Block inward movement of calcium ion across cell membranes and cause smooth muscle relaxation.	Dihydropyridines—more potent peripheral vasodilators than other calcium channel blockers and, as such, may cause more dizziness, headache, flushing, peripheral edema, and tachycardia.
	Diltiazem (Sutters, M, 2011)				
	• Cardizem SR®	180–360	2		All can reduce sinus rate and produce heart block, especially in combination with other antihypertensives.
	• Cardizem CD®	180–240	1		
	• Dilacor XR®	180–480	1		
	• Tiazac SA®	180–540	1		
	Felodipine	2.5–2.0	1		
	Isradipine	2.5–10	2		
	Nicardipine	20–40	3		
	Nicardipine sustained release	60–120	2		
	Nifedipine long-acting	30–60	1		
	Nisoldipine	10–40	1		
	Verapamil (long acting and sustained release) (Sutters, 2011)	180–480	1–2		
Central α₂-agonists	Clonidine	0.1–0.8	2	Stimulate central₂-receptors that inhibit efferent sympathetic activity.	Do not withdraw abruptly because the person may develop rebound hypertension.
	Clonidine patch	0.1–0.3	1 per week		
	Guanabenz	4–64	2		
	Guanfacine	0.5–2	1		
	Methyldopa	250–1,000	2		
Peripheral adrenergic antagonists	Reserpine	0.1–0.25	1	Inhibits catecholamine release from neuronal storage sites. Depletion of tissue stores from catecholamines.	May cause serious orthostatic and exercise-induced hypotension.
Direct vasodilators	Hydralazine	25–100	2	Direct smooth muscle vasodilation (primary arteriolar).	Individuals taking hydralazine may develop a lupus-like syndrome that usually resolves when the medication is stopped.
	Minoxidil	2.5–40	1–2		

*"In some patients treated once daily, the antihypertensive effect may diminish toward the end of the dosing interval (trough effect). Blood pressure (BP) should be measured just prior to dosing to determine if satisfactory BP control is obtained" (JNC 7, 2004, p. 11).

2. Elicit the patient's concerns regarding the diagnosis, including his or her acceptance of the diagnosis.

3. Provide the patient with a written copy of his or her BP reading at each visit. If possible provide a wallet card that contains multiple readings.

4. Come to a mutual agreement with the patient on BP goal.

5. Provide specific, preferably written, information on lifestyle modifications that you are recommending for this patient.

6. Be sure to underscore the importance of the need to continue treatment, most likely for their lifetime. Emphasize "control does not mean cure" (JNC 7, 2004, p. 62)

7. Include in the education that most individuals with HTN are usually asymptomatic, so the patient will not usually be able to tell if the BP is elevated or not based on his or her symptoms.

8. Have the patient repeat his or her understanding of treatment regimen before the end of the visit.

9. Include in the patient education cautions regarding use of cold preparations and over-the-counter analgesics (e.g., pseudoephedrine, nonsteroidal anti-inflammatory drugs, respectively).

10. Encourage the use of validated home BP-monitoring devices for interested and able patients, especially those with refractory HTN.

D. Follow-up and monitoring

1. If treating initially with lifestyle modifications alone, have the patient follow-up in 3 months to assess both effectiveness on BP and the patient's ability to carry through lifestyle changes.

2. After initiating antihypertensive drug therapy, have the patient return in 1 month for a BP check and review of adverse or other effects of medications.

3. Continue follow-up visits at 1- to 3-month intervals until BP goal is achieved.

4. If stage 2 HTN or with the presence of other comorbid conditions, such as diabetes or chronic kidney disease, more frequent visits may be warranted.

5. Once the BP is stable schedule visits at 3- to 6-month intervals.

6. Laboratory follow-up

   a. Check serum electrolytes 2–4 weeks after starting a diuretic.

   b. Check serum potassium and creatinine 2–4 weeks after starting an angiotensin-converting enzyme inhibitor.

   c. Check serum electrolytes and creatinine at least annually for all patients on antihypertensive medications.

7. Have the patient bring in all medications to each follow-up visit.

8. Failure to reach target BP goal

   a. Consider nonadherence to medication or lifestyle recommendations, including excessive sodium intake or increased alcohol intake.

   b. Consider use of over-the-counter medications or street drugs.

   c. Evaluate for high levels of stress or psychiatric conditions that can affect BP, such as anxiety disorders and panic disorder.

   d. Reconsider secondary causes for HTN.
   Always maintain an attitude of empathetic concern and genuine interest in developing the best possible, workable plan for the patient, as a partner in treatment.

REFERENCES

Burt, V. L., Whelton, P., Roccella, E. J., Brown, C., Cutler, J. A., Higgins, M., . . . LaBarthe, D. (1995). Prevalence of hypertension in the US adult population. Results from the Third National Health and Nutrition Examination Survey, 1988–1991. *Hypertension, 25*, 305–313.

Cutler, J. F., Sorlie, P. D., Wolz, M., Thom, T., Fields, L. E., & Roccella, E. J. (2008). Trends in hypertension prevalence, awareness, treatment, and control rates in United States adults between 1988–1994 and 1999–2004. *Hypertension, 52*, 818–827. doi: 10.1161/_HYPERTENSIONAHA.108.113357

Elliott, W. J., & Izzo, J. L. (2006). Device-guided breathing to lower BP: Case report and clinical overview. *Medscape General Medicine, 8*(3), 23. Retrieved from http://www.ncbi.nlm.nih.gov/pmc/articles/PMC1781326/

Linden, W., Lenz, J. W., & Con, A. H. (2001). Individualized stress management for primary hypertension, a randomized trial. *Archives of Internal Medicine, 161*, 1071–1080.

Mann, S. J. (2000). The mind/body link in essential hypertension: Time for a new paradigm. *Alternative Therapies in Health and Medicine, 6*(2), 39–45.

Rainforth, M. V., Schneider, R. H., Nidich, S. I., Gaylord-King, C., Salerno, J. W., & Anderson, J. W. (2007). Stress reduction programs in patients with elevated blood pressure: A systematic review and meta-analysis. *Current Hypertension Reports, 9*, 520–528. Retrieved from http://www.springerlink.com/content/68148x30475t6562/fulltext.pdf

Sacks, F. M., Svetkey, L. P., Vollmer, W. M., Appel, L. J., Bray, G. A., Harsha, D., . . . DASH-Sodium Research Collaborative Research Group (2001). Effects on blood pressure of reduced dietary sodium and the Dietary Approaches to Stop Hypertension (DASH) diet. DASH-Sodium Collaborative Research Group. *New England Journal of Medicine, 344,* 3–10.

Seventh Report of the Joint National Committee on Prevention, Detection, Evaluation, and Treatment of High Blood Pressure (JNC 7). (2004). U.S. Department of Health and Human Services, NIH Publication no. 0405230. Retrieved from http://www.nhlbi.nih.gov /guidelines/hypertension/jnc7full.htm

Spence, J. D., Barnett, P. A., Linden, W., Ransden, V., & Taenzer, P. (1999). Lifestyle modification to prevent and control hypertension: Recommendations on stress management. Canadian Hypertension Society, Canadian Coalition for High Blood Pressure Preventions and Control, Laboratory Centre for Disease Control at Health Canada, Heart and Stroke Foundation of Canada. *Canadian Medical Association Journal, 160*(9), S46–S50. Retrieved from http://www .ncbi.nlm.nih.gov/pmc/articles/PMC1230339/

Sutters, M. (2011). Chapter 11. Systemic hypertension. In S. McPhee, Maxine A. Papadakis, & M. W. Rabow (Eds.), *Current medical diagnosis & treatment,* 50th ed., AccessMedicine, New York: McGraw-Hill.

World Health Organization. (2002). *World Health Report: Reducing risks, promoting healthy life.* Geneva, Switzerland: World Health Organization. Retrieved from http://www.who.int/whr/2002/

INTIMATE PARTNER VIOLENCE (DOMESTIC VIOLENCE)

Cecily Cosby, JoAnne M. Saxe, and Janice Humphreys

I. Introduction

Violence in the United States, in particular intimate partner violence (IPV) (also commonly referred to as domestic violence), continues to be a significant public health concern (Bureau of Justice Statistics, 2009). Although there are many stereotypes about victims of IPV, abuse can occur between members of heterosexual or homosexual couples and does not require sexual intimacy, legal ties, or even cohabitation. The intention is to intimidate and control the other person and instill fear in the victim. Victims, survivors for those who withstand the violence, can be men or women, educated or illiterate, wealthy or poor, and any age (U.S. Department of Justice; National Center for Victims of Crime, 2008a).

According to the 2009 California Penal Code Handbook (Section 1M.6, 137W, 242, 243, 273.5), acts of partner abuse include those that intentionally or recklessly cause, or attempt to cause, bodily injury, or that place another person in reasonable apprehension of imminent serious bodily injury. IPV is considered by many as a prelude to murder (Ferguson, 2007).

A. Definition and overview

There are three general categories of IPV that often occur together: (1) physical abuse or battering, (2) sexual abuse, and (3) psychological abuse. Included within these categories can be such actions as isolating the victim, birth-control sabotage, employment sabotage, and economic abuse. Although all states have legislation that defines IPV, those definitions vary across states. IPV constitutes the willful intimidation, assault, battery,

sexual assault, or other abusive behavior perpetrated by one family member, household member, or intimate partner against another (National Center for Victims of Crime, 2008a). In most state laws addressing IPV, the relationship necessary for a charge of domestic assault or abuse generally includes a spouse, former spouse, persons currently residing together or those that have within the previous year, or persons who share a common child. In addition, as of 2007, most states provide some level of statutory protection for victims of dating violence (National Center for Victims of Crime, 2008b & 2008c). Dating violence is defined as violence committed by a person who is or has been in a social relationship of a romantic or intimate nature with the victim (U.S. Department of Health & Human Services, 2009).

B. Prevalence and incidence

IPV, a source of traumatic stress, affects between 25% and 30% of women of all ages (Tjaden, Thoennes, National Institute of Justice, & Centers for Disease Control and Prevention, 1998). Nonlethal IPV is highest among women aged 16–24 and women residing in low-income households (Greenfeld et al., 1998). A recent analysis of the Behavioral Risk Factor Surveillance System Survey in 16 states and two territories reported the following estimates of lifetime physical or sexual IPV: 20.5% for Hispanic women, 9.7% for Asian women, 29.2% for black women, and 26.8% for white women (Black & Breiding, 2008). Among African American women between the ages of 15 and 24 years, IPV is the leading cause of premature death from homicide and injury (Rennison & Welchans, 2002). Although several population-based surveys have found that IPV is significantly more common among women of color, particularly African American and Native American women, when differences attributable to race, income, education, and employment are considered, the differences attributable to race decrease (Caetano & Cunradi, 2003; Tjaden & Thoennes, 2000).

IPV can occur in all kinds of intimate relationships, including marriage, committed same-sex or opposite-sex relationships, and dating relationships of adults and adolescents. However, IPV most often is committed by men against women (Briere, 1992). Although the severity of IPV can vary, the type of IPV that is repetitive and prolonged has been most closely associated with negative health sequelae (Humphreys & Campbell, 2010). This violence results in nearly 2 million injuries and nearly 1,300 deaths. Of the IPV injuries, more than 555,000 require attention by a healthcare provider, and more than 145,000 are serious enough to warrant hospitalization for 1 or more nights. In 2004, nearly 33% of female homicide victims were killed by intimate partners (Bureau of Justice Statistics, 2009).

C. Consequences

Research suggests that the risk of suffering from six or more chronic physical symptoms increases with the number of forms of violence experienced, even when the last episode was over 30 years ago (Nicolaidis et al., 2004). IPV costs in the United States are estimated at $12.6 billion on an annual basis, 0.1% of the gross domestic product (Waters et al., 2004). IPV also results in more than 18.5 million mental health care visits each year and 13.6 million days of lost productivity from paid work and household chores among IPV survivors and the value of IPV murder victims' expected lifetime earnings (Centers for Disease Control and Prevention, 2003).

In addition to the injuries inflicted on women during violent episodes, physical and psychologic abuses are linked to a number of adverse health effects. These include arthritis; chronic neck or back pain; migraine or other types of headache; sexually transmitted infections (including HIV); chronic pelvic pain; peptic ulcers; irritable bowel syndrome; and frequent indigestion, diarrhea, or constipation (Coker, Smith, Bethea, King, & McKeown, 2000). Psychologic consequences include posttraumatic stress disorder, depression, substance abuse, and suicidal behaviors (Ellsberg, Jansen, Heise, Watts, & Garcia-Moreno, 2008). Six percent of all pregnant women are battered. Pregnancy complications, including low weight gain, anemia, infections, and first- and second-trimester bleeding, are significantly higher for abused women, as are maternal rates of depression, suicide attempts, and substance abuse (Parker, McFarlane, & Soeken, 1994).

D. Risk factors

Factors that should heighten the clinician's index of suspicion regarding the possibility of IPV include medical records indicating repeated visits or previous injuries, a history of IPV or a history with inconsistent descriptions of injuries, and a past history of suicide attempts. Vague and nonspecific responses to questions with a history of anxiety, depression, sleeplessness, fatigue, or chronic somatic complaints may indicate intrafamilial crisis. Abuse is a frequent precipitant of suicide attempts, and those who attempt suicide are likely to have a history of IPV (Ellsberg et al., 2008).

E. Special populations

Special populations at increased risk of IPV include the poor or homeless; teenagers; pregnant or immigrant women; those with chronic illnesses (HIV) or disabilities; lesbian, gay, bisexual, and transgender individuals; and older victims (Table 59-1).

F. Screening

Whether IPV screening reduces violence or improves health outcomes for women is unknown. Although the US Preventive Services Task Force (USPSTF, 2004) could not determine the balance between the benefits and harms of screening for family and IPV among children, women,

or older adults (Chamberlain, 2005; Nelson, Nygren, McInerney, & Klein, 2004), the physical and psychological sequelae of IPV are considered sufficiently prevalent by other organizations to justify routine screening. Some suggest the USPSTF has only considered interventions based in health care and has ignored extensive literature from psychologists, sociologists, and criminologists. Furthermore, there is clear evidence from recent studies that IPV screening is not associated with harm (Koziol-Mclain & Campbell, 2001; MacMillan et al., 2009).

Grounds for screening can be made based on the high prevalence of undetected abuse among women patients (only 1 in 10 victims of IPV is appropriately identified in the healthcare setting), the potential value of this information in helping such patients, and the low cost and low risk of screening (Punukollu, 2003). Although there are some variations in recommendations, most suggest the screening of all women, and should include men who are in partner relationships with other men (American Academy of Family Physicians, 2009; American College of Obstetricians and Gynecologists, 2002; American Medical Association Council on Scientific Affairs, 1992; Substance Abuse and Mental Health Services Administration, 2009) (Table 59-2).

Evidence-based approaches in the primary care setting for preventing IPV are seriously lacking. Only two studies of interventions to decrease IPV in women that recruited only pregnant women showed a trend (not statistically significant) in women reporting decreased violence after brief counseling or outreach interventions (McFarlane, Soeken, & Wiist, 2000; Parker, McFarlane, Soeken, Silva, & Reel, 1999). There are no studies of interventions with health outcomes for older children, women who are not pregnant, or older adults. No study has examined, in a comparative design, the effectiveness of screening when the end point is improved outcomes for women, as opposed to identification of abuse (Wathen & MacMillan, 2003). The safety and effectiveness of such interventions as advocacy, career counseling plus critical consciousness awareness, cognitive behavioral counseling, cognitive trauma therapy, nurse support and guidance, peer support groups, safety planning, and shelters are included in a review by Sandowski (2009).

II. Database (may include but is not limited to)

A. Subjective

Although many individuals may not bring up the subject of abuse on their own, many will discuss it in a private, confidential setting when asked simple, direct, nonjudgmental questions. See Table 59-3 for approaches to phrasing questions. A variety of tools can be used to

TABLE 59-1 Special IPV Risk Populations

Risk	Data	Sources
Chronic illness (HIV)	The IPV risk for women with HIV may be as high as 67%, a rate three to four times greater than among HIV-negative women. HIV-positive women seem to experience IPV at rates comparable to HIV-negative women from the same underlying populations; however, their abuse seems to be more frequent and more severe.	Brief, Vielhauer, & Keane, 2006; Gielen et al., 2007; Cobb, 2008
Individuals with disabilities	Those with disabilities and deaf women have an increased risk of both typical and unique forms of violence. The greater the degree of cognitive impairment, the greater the risk for victimization and abuse.	Curry, Powers, Oschwald, & Saxton, 2004
Immigrant women	More difficult for these women to seek or obtain help because of abusive partners using immigration status against her, threatening deportation. Language barriers, isolation, and a lack of familiarity with the United States social system. Fear that if she reports violence she will be treated with insensitivity, hostility, or discrimination by authorities. Low level of awareness about IPV among immigrants or refugees. Not seen as a problem in their community. May be recognized, but only as a family or private issue. Community members may condone IPV or do not consider various abusive or controlling acts to be IPV.	Kulwicki & Miller, 1999; Murdaugh et al., 2004; Moracco et al., 2005; Shiu-Thornton, Senturia, & Sullivan, 2005; Yoshihama, 2008
Lesbian, gay, bisexual, or transgender individuals	A multicity study on urban men who have sex with men found that one in five men had been physically battered by a partner; 1 in 20 had been sexually battered during the previous 5 years. Lifetime prevalence of IPV was 39.2% and 22% of men reported physical abuse in the last 5 years. Lesbian, gay, bisexual, or transgender individuals who are incarcerated are sexually assaulted at a rate 15 times higher than that of the general inmate population. From 2001 to 2005, about 3% of females experiencing nonfatal IPV reported that the offender was another female. In 2003, lesbian, gay, bisexual, or transgender individuals experienced 6,523 incidents of domestic violence; 44% were men, 36% women, and 2% were transgender. In 2007, 3% of male victims of violent crime were hurt by an intimate partner.	Relf et al., 2004; Greenwood et al., 2002; Jenness et al., 2007; National Coalition of Anti-Violence Programs, 2008; Barber, 2008
Poor or homeless	Women living in disadvantaged neighborhoods are more than twice as likely to be the victims of IPV as women in more affluent neighborhoods. Between 25% and 50% of homeless families have lost their homes as a result of intimate partner abuse.	Benson & Fox, 2004
Pregnant women	In one study, homicide was the leading cause of pregnancy-related death. Abused women were twice as likely to begin prenatal care during the third trimester and more likely to abuse substances before and during pregnancy.	McFarlane, Parker, Soeken, & Bullock, 1992; Martin, English, Clark, Cilenti, & Kupper, 1996; Horton & Cheng, 2001; Frye, 2001
Teenagers	As many as 12% of youth in grades 7 through 12 have been victims of physical dating violence, and 20% of youth have suffered from psychologic dating violence. African American and Hispanic teenagers, teenagers receiving lower grades in school, and those with mental illness have been found to be at higher risk for being victims. Approximately 25% of adolescents report verbal, physical, emotional, or sexual abuse from a dating partner each year. One in five high school girls have been physically or sexually abused by a dating partner. 22% of battered teenagers began prenatal care in the third trimester of pregnancy, compared to 7.5% of nonbattered teenagers.	CDC, 2003, 2008; Silverman, Raj, Mucci, & Hathaway, 2001

TABLE 59-2 IPV Screening Recommendations

Organization	Recommendation	Sources
American Academy of Family Physicians	Screen during routine office visits for early intervention.	American Academy of Family Physicians, 2009
American College of Obstetricians and Gynecologists	Screen all patients at routine obstetric and gynecological visits, family planning visits, and preconception visits. Suggested questions: 1. Within the past year—or since you have been pregnant—have you been hit, slapped, kicked or otherwise physically hurt by someone? 2. Are you in a relationship with a person who threatens or physically hurts you? 3. Has anyone forced you to have sexual activities that made you feel uncomfortable?	American College of Obstetricians and Gynecologists, 2002
American Medical Association	Screen in primary care settings and provide a structured approach to documentation and referral to appropriate community resources.	American Medical Association, 1992.
American Nurses Association	Universal screening, routine assessment, and documentation in any healthcare setting.	American Nurses Association, 2000.
Canadian Task Force on Preventive Health Care	Suggested questions: 1. Have you ever been in a relationship with someone who has hit you, kicked you, slapped you, punched you, or threatened to hurt you? 2. Currently? 3. When you were pregnant did anyone ever physically hurt you? 4. Are you in a relationship with someone who yells at you, calls you names, or puts you down?	MacMillan & Wathan, 2001
National Consensus Guidelines on Identifying and Responding to Domestic Violence Victimization in Health Care Settings	APPENDIX D: Suggested Assessment Questions and Strategies APPENDIX E: Validated Abuse Assessment Tools APPENDIX F: Expanded Assessment APPENDIX G: Indicators of Abuse APPENDIX H: Safety Plan and Discharge APPENDIX I: Interventions with Current or Past Victims of Domestic Violence	National Advisory Committee, Family Violence Prevention Fund, 2004.
Substance Abuse and Mental Health Services Administration	Includes recommended questions for mental health providers to screen both a client who might be an abuser, or a victim of abuse.	SAMHSA Treatment Improvement Protocols, Appendix C, 2009.
United States Preventive Services Task Force	Insufficient evidence to recommend for or against the use of specific screening tools, although suggest clinicians be alert to signs of abuse and use selective screening questions if indicated. Appropriate actions include document the abuse, provide treatment for injuries and psychologic injuries, and give protective services information.	United States Preventive Services Task Force, 1996, 2004; Nelson, Nygren, McInerney, & Klein, 2004.

TABLE 59-3 Screening History Questions

Phrasing Questions: The Use of One of the Victimization Scales, Physical–Sexual, Psychologic–Emotional, Stalking.
1. "Are you in a relationship in which you have been physically hurt or threatened by your partner? Have you ever been in such a relationship?"
2. "Has your partner ever destroyed things that you cared about? Ever threatened or abused your children? Ever forced you to have sex when you didn't want to?"
3. "What happens when you and your partner disagree or fight? Do you ever feel afraid of your partner?"
4. "Has your partner ever prevented you from leaving the house, seeking friends, getting a job, or continuing your education?"
5. "If your partner uses alcohol or drugs is s/he ever physically or verbally abusive to you when using?"
6. "Do you have guns or other weapons in your home? If so, has your partner ever threatened to use them?"

TABLE 59-4 Physical Examination

Components of the Physical Examination
Assess general appearance: Level of distress
Vital signs
Other physical examination data:
1. Look carefully for multiple abrasions and contusions to different anatomic sites and multiple injuries in various stages of healing.
2. Most accidents involve the extremities, whereas IPV injuries often involve the face, neck, chest, breasts, abdomen, genitalia, or anus.
Mental status examination: Evaluate mood, orientation, thought processes, and judgment.

Additional components of the physical examination are listed in Table 59-4.

accurately measure victimization and offer the clinician specific scales in the areas of physical, sexual, psychological, and emotional victimization, and stalking to guide their inquiries (Basile, Hertz, & Back, 2007; Centers for Disease Control and Prevention, 2006).

1. When IPV is identified,
   a. It is important to determine the identity of the person allegedly inflicting the injuries and document the circumstances surrounding the event, any past history of abuse, the nature of the injuries, and use of any threats or weapons. Whenever possible, use the patient's exact words and quotation marks.
   b. Additional history related to other health-risk behaviors (e.g., alcohol or drug use, tobacco) and chronic conditions, such as sleep problems, depression, and eating disorders, should be elicited. These conditions, along with currently being the victim of IPV, are predictors of the women's physical and psychologic health (Svavarsdottir & Orlygsdottir, 2009).

B. *Objective*

Perform a complete head-to-toe examination or focused evaluation as indicated by history or report of injuries. Document the character and extent of all physical injuries, including areas of pain and tenderness, even if there is as yet no obvious bruising or injury. It is recommended to use photos or drawings whenever possible.

III. Assessment

Evaluate the extent of any injuries and the need for immediate medical intervention. See Table 59-5 for additional components of the assessment. Assess the need for mandatory reporting as cited in the respective state's penal codes. Mandatory reporting, the legal requirement in less than 10 states requiring health professionals to report suspected instances of IPV to the police, is a somewhat controversial legal intervention. Although mandatory reporting may result in some escalation in partner violence as a result of angering the abuser, it is thought by some authorities that the benefits of helping the victim and perpetrator to receive treatment outweighs this risk. Another concern related to mandatory reporting includes the violation of provider–patient confidentiality that is important for effective treatment to occur (American College of Emergency Physicians, 2011; Rodriguez, 2001; Sachs, 2007).

A summary of the reporting requirements of all states can be found at http://www.ndaa.org/apri/programs/vawa/dv_reporting_requirements.html (National District Attorneys Association, 2008).

IV. Goals of clinical management

The goals in managing victims of IPV include consistent screening through thoughtful inquiry in a safe and confidential environment, identifying immediate injury and safety risks, appropriate reporting and referral, and the provision of information and support. Being aware of immigration concerns and cultural or ethnic differences is an important element in patient care. The acronym 'RADAR' summarizes

TABLE 59-5 Assessment

Components of the Assessment

Determine the diagnosis (not mutually exclusive).
1. History of prior IPV.
2. Recent IPV without observable injury.
3. Current history of IPV with observable injury.
   a. Report as required by state regulations.

Determine the ICD9 codes for IPV, which are divided into four categories (Rudman, 2000).
1. Adult maltreatment and abuse (995-81).
2. The primary diagnosis (underlying reason for admittance).
3. Modifier codes that provide details (E-codes).
4. History codes that provide information on previous incidents (V-codes).

Assess for suicidal or homicidal ideation.

Evaluate the safety of the patient and family members and children.

Identify any immediate risk and need for emergency housing, legal, or social service consultations.

Assess social support systems.

Determine ongoing risk of IPV.

Physical abuse ranking scale. Greater than 5 indicates high danger (Wadman & Foral, 2007).
1. Throwing things, punching the wall—lower risk
2. Pushing, shoving, grabbing, throwing things
3. Slapping with an open hand
4. Kicking, biting
5. Hitting with closed fists
6. Attempted strangulation
7. Beating up, pinning to the wall or floor, repeated
8. Threatening with a weapon
9. Assault with a weapon—higher risk

action steps that the clinician can use to recognize and treat victims of IPV (Alpert, 2004).

R emember to routinely inquire about partner violence

A sk directly about violence (see questions in Table 59-3), always in a private area

D ocument suspected or reported partner violence in the patient's chart

A ssess patient safety (lethality or abuse scales)

R eview patient options

V. Plan

A. Diagnostic testing
Obtain radiographs, computed tomography, or magnetic resonance imaging based on the extent of injury.

B. Management
Interventions designed to decrease health-risk behaviors, treat chronic health conditions or illnesses, and offer best practice first response to women who are victims of IPV can be offered to reduce the short- and long-term effects of violence on their physical and psychologic health (Svavarsdottir & Orlygsdottir, 2009).

Patient management includes treatment, consultation, referral, and follow-up care. In the event there is a history of recent sexual assault (within 72 hours), it is important to refer the patient to the sexual assault response team or emergency department. In most instances law enforcement involvement is necessary to authorize a forensic examination and a report is filed both via telecommunications and in writing to the respective authorities. The clinician will follow the reporting guidelines as cited in the respective State's penal codes.

C. Client and patient education
Priority educational areas include the nature of IPV and the identification of emergency strategies. A personalized safety plan for patients can be found at http://www.domesticviolence.org/personalized-safety-plan/

VI. Self-management resources and tools

The clinician can provide patient education brochures or frequently asked question documents and Community Support Groups and the National Domestic Violence Hotline: (1-800-799-SAFE) (1-800-799-7233).

REFERENCES

Alpert, E. J. (2004). *Partner violence: How to recognize and treat victims of abuse* (4th ed.). Waltham, MA: Massachusetts Medical Society.

American College of Emergency Physicians. (2011). *Domestic family violence.* Retrieved from http://www.acep.org/Content.aspx?id=29184

American Academy of Family Physicians. (n.d.). *Family and intimate partner violence and abuse.* Retrieved from http://www.aafp.org/online/en/home/policy/policies/f/familyandintimatepartner-violenceand abuse.html

American College of Obstetricians and Gynecologists. (2002). *Violence against women.* Retrieved from http://www.acog.org/departments/dept_notice.cfm?recno=17&bulletin=585

American Medical Association Council on Scientific Affairs. (1992). *Diagnostic and treatment guidelines on elder abuse and neglect.* Chicago, IL: American Medical Association.

American Nurses Association. (2000). *Position statement on violence against women.* Retrieved from http://www.nursingworld.org/Social CausesHealthCare

Barber, C. F. (2008). Domestic violence against men. *Nursing Standard, 22*(51), 35–39.

Basile, K. C., Hertz, M. F., & Back, S. E. (2007). *Intimate partner violence and sexual violence victimization assessment instruments for use in health-care settings.* Version 1. Atlanta, GA: Centers for Disease Control and Prevention, National Center for Injury Prevention and Control.

Benson, M., & Fox, G. (2004). When violence hits home: How economics and neighborhood play a role. Washington, DC: National Institutes of Justice.

Black, M. C., & Breiding, M. J. (2008). Adverse health conditions and health risk behaviors associated with intimate partner violence—United States, 2005. *Morbidity and Mortality Weekly Report, 57,* 113–118.

Brief, D., Vielhauer, M., & Keane, T. (2006). University of California, San Francisco, AIDS Health Project. The interface of HIV, trauma, and posttraumatic stress disorder. *Focus, 21*(4), 1–4.

Briere, J. (1992). Medical symptoms, health risk, and history of childhood sexual abuse. *Mayo Clinic Proceedings, 67*(6), 603–604.

Bureau of Justice Statistics. (2009). *Domestic violence and sexual assault data resource center.* Retrieved from http://bjs.ojp.usdoj.gov/

Bureau of Justice Statistics. (2009). *Intimate homicide.* Retrieved from http://bjs.ojp.usdoj.gov/content/homicide/intimates.cfm

Caetano, R., & Cunradi, C. (2003). Intimate partner violence and depression among whites, blacks, and hispanics. *Annals of Epidemiology, 13*(10), 661–665.

California Penal Code Handbook 2009. (2008). Matthew Bender & Company LexisNexis.

Centers for Disease Control and Prevention. (2003). *National Center for Injury Prevention and Control. Costs of intimate partner violence against women in the United States.* Retrieved from http://www.cdc .gov/violenceprevention/pdf/IPVBook-a.pdf

Centers for Disease Control and Prevention. (2006). *Measuring intimate partner violence victimization and perpetration: A compendium of assessment tools.* Retrieved from http://www.cdc.gov/ncipc/dvp/Compendium/IPV%20Compendium.pdf

Centers for Disease Control and Prevention. (2008). *Understanding teen dating violence fact sheet 2008.* Retrieved from http://www.cdc.gov/violenceprevention/pdf/DatingAbuseFactSheet-a.pdf

Chamberlain, L. (2005). The USPSTF recommendation on intimate partner violence: What we can learn from it and what we can do about it. *Family Violence Prevention and Health Practice, 1,* 1–24.

Cobb, A. J. (2008, August 25–28). *The intersection: HIV/AIDS and intimate partner violence.* Paper presented at the Ryan White All-Grantee Meeting, Washington, DC.

Coker, A., Smith, P., Bethea, L., King, M., & McKeown, R. (2000). Physical health consequences of physical and psychological intimate partner violence. *Archives of Family Medicine, 9,* 451–457.

Curry, M. A., Powers, L. E., Oschwald, M., & Saxton, M. (2004). Development and testing of an abuse screening tool for women with disabilities. *Journal of Aggression, Maltreatment and Trauma, 8*(4), 123–141.

Ellsberg, M., Jansen, H. A., Heise, L., Watts, C. H., & Garcia-Moreno, C. (2008). Intimate partner violence and women's physical and mental health in the WHO multi-country study on women's health and domestic violence: An observational study. *Lancet, 371*(9619), 1165–1172.

Ferguson, E. E. (2007). Domestic violence by another name: Crimes of passion in Fin-de-Siecle Paris. *Journal of Women's History, 19*(4), 12–34.

Frye, V. (2001). Examining homicide's contribution to pregnancy-associated deaths. *Journal of the American Medical Association, 285*(11), 1510–1511.

Gielen, A. C., Ghandour, R. M., Burke, J. G., Mahoney, P., McDonnell, K. A., & O'Campo, P. (2007). HIV/AIDS and intimate partner violence: Intersecting women's health issues in the United States. *Trauma, Violence, & Abuse, 8*(2), 178–198.

Greenfeld, L. A., Rand, M. R., Craven, P. A., Klaus, C. A., Perkins, C. A., Ringel, C., . . . Fox, J. A. (1998). *Violence by intimates: Analysis of data on crimes by current or former spouses, boyfriends, and girlfriends* (No. NCJ 167237). Rockville, MD: U.S. Dept of Justice, Bureau of Justice Statistics.

Greenwood, G. L., Relf, M. V., Huang, B., Pollack, L. M., Canchola, J. M., & Cantania, J. A. (2002). Battering victimization among a probability-based sample of men who have sex with men. *American Journal of Public Health, 92*(12).

Horton, I. L., & Cheng, D. (2001). Enhanced surveillance for pregnancy-associated mortality-Maryland, 1993–1998. *Journal of the American Medical Association, 285,* 1455–1459.

Humphreys, J., & Campbell, J. C. (Eds.). (2010). *Family violence and nursing practice* (2nd ed. in press). Philadelphia, PA: Lippincott Williams & Wilkins.

Jenness, V., Maxsom, C., Matsuda, K. N., & Sumner, J. M. (2007). Violence in California correctional facilities: An empirical examination of sexual assault. Center for Evidence-Based Corrections, University of California, Irvine. Retrieved from http://ucicorrections.seweb.uci.edu/pdf/PREA_Presentation_PREA_Report_UCI_Jenness_et_al.pdf

Koziol-Mclain, J., & Campbell, J. C. (2001). Universal screening and mandatory reporting: An update on two important issues for victims/survivors of intimate partner violence. *Journal of Emergency Nursing: JEN: Official Publication of the Emergency Department Nurses Association, 27*(6), 602–606.

Kulwicki, A. D., & Miller, J. (1999). Domestic violence in the Arab American population: Transforming environmental conditions through community education. *Issues in Mental Health Nursing, 20,* 199–215.

MacMillan, H. L., & Wathan, C. N. (2001). Prevention and treatment of violence against women: systematic review & recommendations. London, Ontario: Canadian Task Force.

MacMillan, H. L., Wathen, C. N., Jamieson, E., Boyle, M. H., Shannon, H. S., Ford-Gilboe, M., ... McMaster Violence Against Women Research Group 2009). Screening for intimate partner violence in health care settings: A randomized trial. *Journal of the American Medical Association, 302*(5), 493–501.

Martin, S. L., English, K. T., Clark, K. A., Cilenti, D., & Kupper, L. L. (1996). Violence and substance use among North Carolina pregnant women. *American Journal of Public Health, 86*(7), 991–998.

McFarlane, J., Parker, B., Soeken, K., & Bullock, L. (1992). Assessing for abuse during pregnancy: Severity and frequency of injuries and associated entry into prenatal care. *Journal of the American Medical Association, 267*(23), 3176–3178.

McFarlane, J., Soeken, K., & Wiist, W. (2000). An evaluation of interventions to decrease intimate partner violence to pregnant women. *Public Health Nursing, 17*(6), 443–451.

Moracco, K. E., Hilton, A., Hodges, K. G., & Frasier, P. Y. (2005). Knowledge and attitudes about intimate partner violence among immigrant Latinos in rural North Carolina. *Violence Against Women, 11*, 337–352.

Murdaugh, C., Hunt, S., Sowell, R., & Santana, I. (2004). Domestic violence in Hispanics in the southeastern United States: A survey and needs analysis. *Journal of Family Violence, 19*, 107–116.

National Advisory Committee. (2004 update). *National consensus guidelines on identifying and responding to domestic violence victimization in health care settings.* Retrieved from http://endabuse.org/userfiles/file/Consensus.pdf

National Center for Victims of Crime. (2008a). *Domestic violence.* Retrieved from http://www.ncvc.org/ncvc/main.aspx?dbName=DocumentViewer&DocumentID=32347

National Center for Victims of Crime. (2008b). *Dating violence resource center.* Retrieved from http://www.ncvc.org/ncvc/main.aspx?dbID=DB_DatingViolenceResourceCenter101

National Center for Victims of Crime. (2008c). *Teen dating violence fact sheet.* Retrieved from http://www.ncvc.org/ncvc/AGP.Net/Components/documentViewer/Download.aspxnz?DocumentID=42307

National Coalition of Anti-Violence Programs. (2008). *Lesbian, gay, bisexual and transgender domestic violence in the United States in 2007.* Retrieved from http://www.avp.org/publications/reports/documents/2007NCAVPDVREPORT.pdf

National District Attorneys Association. (2008). *State domestic violence reporting requirements.* Retrieved from http://www.ndaa.org/apri/programs/vawa/dv_reporting_requirements.html

Nelson, H. D., Nygren, P., McInerney, Y., & Klein, J. (2004). Screening women and elderly adults for family and intimate partner violence: a review of the evidence for the U.S. preventive services task force. *Annals of Internal Medicine, 140*(5), 387–396.

Nicolaidis, C., Curry, M., McFarland, B., & Gerrity, M. (2004). Violence, mental health and physical symptoms in an academic internal medicine practice. *Journal of General Internal Medicine, 19*(8), 819–827.

Parker, B., McFarlane, J., & Soeken, K. (1994). Abuse during pregnancy: Effects on maternal complications and infant birth weight in adult and teen women. *Obstetrics & Gynecology, 841*, 323–328.

Parker, B., McFarlane, J., Soeken, K., Silva, C., & Reel, S. (1999). Testing an intervention to prevent further abuse to pregnant women. *Research Nursing Health, 22*(1), 59–66.

Punukollu, M. (2003). Domestic violence: Screening made practical. *Journal of Family Practice, 52*(7), 537–543.

Relf, M., Huang, B., Campbell, J., & Cantania, J. (2004). Gay identity, interpersonal violence, and HIV risk behaviors: An empirical test of theoretical relationships among a probability-based sample of urban men who have sex with men. *Journal of the Association of Nurses in AIDS Care, 15*(2), 14–26.

Rennison, C. M., & Welchans, S. (2002). Intimate partner violence. *Bureau of Justice Statistics Special Report,* (NCJ 178247). Washington, DC: US Department of Justice, Bureau of Justice Statistics.

Rodriguez, M. A. (2001). Mandatory reporting of domestic violence injuries to the police. *Journal of the American Medical Association, 286*(5), 580–583.

Rudman, W. J. (2000). *Coding and documentation of domestic violence.* San Francisco: Family Violence Prevention Fund; 2000; endabuse.org/userfiles/file/HealthCare/codingpaper.pdf

Sachs, C. J. (2007). Mandatory reporting of injuries inflicted by intimate partner violence. *American Medical Association Journal of Ethics, Virtual Mentor, 9*(12), 842–845.

SAMHSA/CSAT. (n.d.). *Treatment improvement protocol 39: Guidelines for assessing violence.* Retrieved from http://www.ncbi.nlm.nih.gov/bookshelf/br.fcgi?book=hssamhsatip&part=A71687#A71688.

Sandowski, L. (2009). Intimate partner violence towards women. *Clinical Evidence (Online),* Feb. 13;2009. pii: 1013.

Shiu-Thornton, S., Senturia, K., & Sullivan, M. (2005). Like a bird in a cage: Vietnamese women survivors talk about domestic violence. *Journal of Interpersonal Violence, 20*, 959–976.

Silverman, J. G., Raj, A., Mucci, L., & Hathaway, J. (2001). Dating violence against adolescent girls and associated substance use, unhealthy weight control, sexual risk behavior, pregnancy, and suicidality. *Journal of the American Medical Association, 286*(5), 572–579.

Svavarsdottir, E. K., & Orlygsdottir, B. (2009). Intimate partner abuse factors associated with women's health: A general population study. *Journal of Advanced Nursing, 65*(7), 1452–1462.

Tjaden, P., Thoennes, N., National Institute of Justice, & Centers for Disease Control and Prevention. (1998, November). *Prevalence, incidence, and consequences of violence against women: Findings from the national violence against women survey.* Washington, DC: National Institute of Justice and Centers for Disease Control and Prevention.

Tjaden, P., & Thoennes, N. (2000). *Extent, nature and consequences of intimate partner violence: Findings from the national violence against women survey* (No. NCJ 181867). Washington, DC: U.S. Department of Justice.

U.S. Department of Health and Human Services (USDHHS). National Women's Health Information Center (2009). *Violence Against Women: Dating Violence.* Retrieved from http://www.womenshealth.gov/violence/types/dating.cfm

U.S. Department of Justice. (n.d.). *Domestic violence.* Retrieved from http://www.ovw.usdoj.gov/domviolence.htm

U.S. Preventive Services Task Force. (1996). Screening for family violence. In *Guide to clinical preventive services* (2nd ed., pp. 556–565). Baltimore, MD: Williams & Wilkins.

U.S. Preventive Services Task Force. (2004). *Screening for family and intimate partner violence: Recommendation statement.* Agency for

Healthcare Research and Quality, Rockville, MD. Retrieved from http://www.ahrq.gov/clinic/3rduspstf/famviolence/famviolrs.htm

Wadman, M. C., & Foral, J. (2007). *Domestic violence, determining risk.* Emedicinehealth. Retrieved from http://www.emedicinehealth.com/domestic_violence/page7_em.htm

Waters, H., Hyder, A., Rajkotia, Y., Basu, S., Rehwinkel, J. A., & Butchart, A. (2004). *The economic dimensions of interpersonal violence.* Department of Injuries and Violence Prevention, World Health Organization, Geneva. Retrieved from http://whqlibdoc.who.int/publications/2004/9241591609.pdf

Wathen, C. N., & MacMillan, H. L. (2003). Interventions for violence against women: Scientific review. *Journal of the American Medical Association, 289*(5), 589–600.

Yoshihama, M. (2008). *Literature on intimate partner violence in immigrant and refugee communities: Review and recommendations.* In Family Violence Prevention Fund for The Robert Wood Johnson Foundation. *Intimate partner violence in immigrant and refugee communities: Challenges, promising practices and recommendations.* Retrieved from https://folio.iupui.edu/bitstream/handle/10244/788/ipvreport20090331.pdf

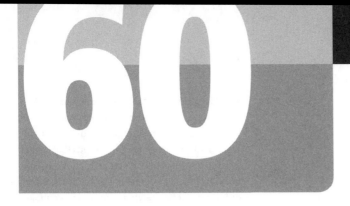

IRRITABLE BOWEL SYNDROME

Karen C. Bagatelos and Geraldine Collins-Bride

I. Definition and overview

Irritable bowel syndrome (IBS) is a "functional bowel disorder," a disorder of intestinal motility and visceral sensory perception. There are no structural or biochemical causes associated with IBS. Although often associated primarily with the lower intestinal tract, IBS can actually be seen along the entire gastrointestinal tract. The main symptoms of IBS are abdominal pain and discomfort associated with a change in the consistency or frequency of stool, and relief of the pain with defecation (Ringel, Sperber, & Drossman, 2001). This constellation of symptoms led to the development of the Rome Criteria, which was done in conjunction with the World College of Gastroenterology in Rome, Italy, in 1998 (Rome I), again in 1999 (Rome II), and subsequently in 2006 (Rome III). The Rome criteria are used to aid in the diagnosis of IBS.

The following is a list of the Rome III criteria for IBS diagnosis: recurrent abdominal pain or discomfort at least 3 days per month in the last 3 months associated with two of the following features

1. Improvement with defecation
2. Onset associated with change in frequency of stool
3. Onset associated with a change in the form of stools (Drossman, 2006)

Other features that are included in the diagnosis are

1. Abnormal stool frequency (more than three bowel movements per day or less than three per week)
2. Abnormal stool form, abnormal stool passage, passage of mucus, and abdominal bloating or

distention (Drossman, Camilleri, Mayer, & Whitehead, 2002)

3. Exacerbation triggered by stressful life events

Diagnosis can be made if all other diagnoses, structural or metabolic, have been eliminated. One must keep in mind that symptom expression differs among patients and may be any combination of the above.

A. Epidemiology

1. The prevalence of IBS is 1–2 in 10 or 10–20% of the population.

   Studies have also shown a prevalence of 8–22 per 100 adults (Ringel et al., 2001). These numbers are difficult to assess because in many patients symptoms resolve or medical attention and treatment is not sought. Approximately 10–20% of patients with IBS actually seek care (Lehrer & Lichenstein, 2009). The costs of healthcare use and absenteeism from work are substantial. It is estimated that approximately 8 billion dollars is spent per year in the United States on the care of patients with IBS (Hauser, Pardi, & Poterucha, 2008).

2. Risk factors

   Female gender confers greater risk with a ratio of 2:1. These numbers may be somewhat inflated because females seek medical care more frequently than males, thus the number of men with IBS may not be accurately reported. The prevalence of IBS decreases with age; however, there have been rare cases of new-onset IBS in the elderly. There are no consistent racial or ethnic differences in individuals with and without IBS (Hauser et al., 2008). Although IBS seems to have a "familial component," a confirmed genetic risk has not been clearly established. IBS has been associated with psychiatric illness and can also be exacerbated by stress, anxiety, and depression. Studies have shown that physical and sexual abuse may have a role in the development of IBS (Lehrer & Lichenstein, 2009). In some cases the onset of symptoms can occur after acute inflammatory conditions of the gastrointestinal tract. Food sensitivities and allergies may also have a role.

B. Pathophysiology

The etiology of IBS is not completely understood. There are many possible mechanisms and causative factors. In some patients, IBS seems to be associated with visceral hypersensitivity as demonstrated by balloon distention studies (Yuan et al., 2003). These studies have shown that IBS patients have lower thresholds for pain. Balloon inflation in the sigmoid colon causes increased pain in

IBS patients as opposed to normal controls (Horwitz & Fisher, 2001). Patients with IBS can have hypersensitivity throughout the entire digestive tract.

IBS is also associated with altered bowel motility. Signals from the central nervous system are either exaggerated or diminished, which causes an increase or decrease in bowel motility (Horwitz & Fisher, 2001), thus explaining why some patients have diarrhea-predominant and others have constipation-predominant IBS. It has been postulated that serotonin or other neurotransmitters can play a role. There can be underexpression or overexpression of some neurotransmitters or increased amounts of receptors in the central and enteric (intestinal) nervous system transmitting signals at abnormal rates. This etiology remains under investigation.

The possible role of bacterial overgrowth and inflammation is also being investigated. Bacterial overgrowth may be the primary cause of IBS symptomatology in some patients because some improve significantly with antibiotic treatment. In some patients, the flora of the digestive tract becomes imbalanced, with "bad" bacteria overcoming "good" bacteria. Psychosocial factors, such as stress and anxiety, and dietary factors can also play a role in the expression of this syndrome (Drossman et al., 2002).

II. Database (may include but is not limited to)

A. Subjective findings

1. Past medical history

   a. Multiple abdominal surgeries: can cause adhesions
   b. Surgery that has damaged the vagus nerve: any upper abdominal surgery, in particular gastric and esophageal surgeries, can cause diarrhea (Ukleja, Woodward, & Achem, 2002).
   c. Psychiatric illness, including trauma and abuse
   d. Substance abuse (including laxatives)
   e. Thyroid disease
   f. Food allergies, especially lactose intolerance
   g. Carcinoid syndrome: causes profound diarrhea
   h. Gastroesophageal reflux disease: frequently seen in patients with slow overall motility

2. Medications prone to altering gastrointestinal motility, such as opiates or laxatives

3. Family history: IBS, inflammatory bowel disease, colon cancer, diabetes, and thyroid disease

4. Psychosocial history

   a. Habits: alcohol, tobacco, or illicit drug use
   b. Situational stressors, coping mechanisms, and social support systems

   c. Exercise and physical activity: sedentary lifestyle is commonly seen in patients with constipation and other bowel motility disorders
   d. Diet history: note typical diet, foods that trigger symptoms, amount of water and caffeine intake, use of artificial sweeteners (sorbitol, saccharin, or NutraSweet), chewing gum, and fiber intake

5. Review of systems

   a. Fever, chills, weight gain or loss, and fatigue
   b. Changes in skin, hair, nails, and other symptoms suggestive of thyroid disease
   c. Lower abdominal pain relieved with defecation, particularly in the left lower quadrant
   d. Constipation, diarrhea, or alternating diarrhea and constipation
   e. Bloating (upper and lower intestinal tract) and gas
   f. Frequency of stools and presence of mucus or blood in the stool (patients with IBS typically do not have blood in the stool)
   g. Anxiety, depression, other psychiatric symptoms
   h. Nausea, vomiting, dyspepsia, and other upper gastrointestinal symptoms

B. Objective findings

1. Physical examination: a full physical examination is recommended with particular attention to

   a. Vital signs (note any orthostatic changes), weight, and body mass index
   b. Thyroid examination
   c. Abdominal examination noting bowel sounds, any masses, and tenderness (especially in the left lower quadrant)
   d. Pelvic examination noting any uterine or adnexal enlargement
   e. Mental status examination noting appearance, behavior, mood, affect, and thought content

III. Assessment

A. Determine the diagnosis

IBS is a diagnosis of exclusion. That being said, many patients with IBS undergo expensive and unnecessary testing and continue to pursue diagnostic work-ups in search of the answer to "what is wrong with me?" The diagnostic and management approaches to patients with IBS rest with careful history and physical examination skills in additional to building a strong therapeutic alliance with the patient to help understand the underlying disorder and symptom-based treatment. The following diagnoses should be considered for all patients presenting with suspected IBS.

1. Bacterial infections

2. Colon cancer

3. Diverticulosis and diverticulitis

4. Eating disorders

5. Adhesions

6. Fecal incontinence

7. In females: ovarian tumors, endometriosis, and adnexal cysts

8. Inflammatory bowel disease

9. Atypical colitis, microscopic colitis, or lymphocytic colitis

10. Thyroid disease, diabetes, and other endocrinologic disorders

11. Celiac disease

12. Depression, anxiety, and other mental health disorders

13. Pelvic floor dysfunction caused by pelvic floor damage

14. Arteriovenous malformations with bleeding

15. Large polypoid mass (can cause constipation) or a malignant tumor

16. Trauma to the rectum

B. *Severity: assess the severity of the disease.*

C. *Significance: assess the significance of the symptoms and chronic nature of the disorder to the patient and significant others.*

IV. Goals of clinical management

A. *Assist the patient with medications, stress management, and psychosocial support.*

B. *Prevent pain by performing adequate pain assessments and referring to pain management for assistance if needed.*

C. *Assist the patient to achieve optimal level of functioning with daily activities and quality of life while living with a chronic, often relapsing disorder.*

V. Plan

A. *Screening: there are no screening tests available for early detection or prevention of IBS.*

B. *Diagnostic studies: based on symptoms and history*

1. Diet diary. The diet diary is an essential initial diagnostic tool for IBS management. The diary helps both the patient and the clinician to make associations between symptoms and foods. It also engages the patient in a meaningful way as a partner in both the diagnostic and treatment processes. The diary should note time of meals and snacks, type of foods eaten, and associated gastrointestinal symptoms before or after food consumption, noting the time frame of symptom development.

2. For recommended first- and second-line symptom-based diagnostic testing see Tables 60-1 and 60-2.

3. Alarm symptoms warranting a gastroenterology referral include unrelenting symptoms despite treatment, rectal bleeding, abnormal stool studies, anemia, anorexia, blood in stools, severe unrelenting diarrhea or constipation, nocturnal symptoms, onset in patients older than 50 years, or a palpable abdominal or rectal mass (Kolfenbach, 2007; World Gastroenterology Organization Global Guideline, 2009).

C. *Management*

The mainstay of any treatment regimen for patients with suspected or confirmed IBS is first and foremost to build a therapeutic alliance with the patient. The underpinnings of this alliance include careful listening, validation of symptoms, and compassion for the distress that symptoms may cause for the patient. Once such an alliance is built, it provides a platform for working with the patient through the symptom-based diagnostic and treatment process.

There are few studies that offer convincing evidence of effectiveness in curing the IBS symptom complex (Akehurst & Kaltenthaler, 2001). Current treatment guidelines focus on symptom-based treatment (World Gastroenterology Organization Global Guideline, 2009).

1. For diarrhea-predominant symptoms

   a. Diet: all patients should be on a restrictive diet that includes no dairy, carbonated beverage, caffeine, alcohol, red meat, artificial fats, and artificial sweeteners (sorbitol-containing products). Limit gas-producing vegetables, such as onions, garlic, beans, broccoli, cabbage, brussel sprouts, asparagus, and cauliflower.

   b. Concentrated fiber to help form stools (i.e., one heaping tablespoon of psyllium fiber or other similar fiber in 4 oz of water one to three times per day). Patients should try insoluble fiber, incorporated into their diet, such as whole grain foods, fresh fruits, fresh

TABLE 60-1 Initial Symptom-Based Diagnostic Work-Up for Irritable Bowel Syndrome

Diarrhea-Predominant Symptoms	Constipation-Predominant Symptoms	Upper Gastrointestinal-Predominant Symptoms
Stool sample: culture and sensitivity, ova and parasites, and *Clostridium difficile* • To rule out bacterial and parasitic infections	Complete blood count with differential • To look for evidence of anemia seen with malignancies, IBD, and other systemic disease • To look for leukocytosis seen with IBD and infections	Upper gastrointestinal series with a small bowel follow through • To rule out structural abnormality or adhesions; also to evaluate transit time with constipation and diarrhea
Stool sample for *Giardia* • To rule out *Giardia lamblia* infection. Increased risk in individuals with immunocompromise and those with a recent travel history	Thyroid-stimulating hormone • To rule out hyperthyroid and hypothyroid disorders	Abdominal sonogram • To rule out gallstones
Stool sample for fecal occult blood • To rule out malignancy, IBD, and other systemic causes of intestinal bleeding	Plain abdominal film (also called a "flat plate of the abdomen") • To look for a bowel obstruction or ileus, adhesions, and pseudo-obstruction	Serum liver function tests • To evaluate liver health and rule out hepatitis, cirrhosis, and other liver diseases
Stool sample for fecal fat • Seen with malabsorption	Stool sample for fecal occult blood • To rule out malignancy, IBD, and other systemic causes of intestinal bleeding	Serum lipase and amylase • To rule out pancreatitis
Complete blood count with differential • To look for evidence of anemia seen with malignancies, IBD, and other systemic disease • To look for leukocytosis seen with IBD and infections	Serum potassium and calcium • To rule out hypokalemia and hypercalcemia, both associated with constipation	
Erythrocyte sedimentation rate • Nonspecific marker of inflammatory bowel disease (IBD) and malignancy		
Fasting blood sugar • To rule out diabetes mellitus, which can present with diarrhea because of diabetic gastroenteropathy		
Thyroid-stimulating hormone • To rule out hyperthyroid and hypothyroid disorders		
Electrolytes (depending on severity of symptoms) • To look for electrolyte disturbances seen with severe diarrhea and malabsorption		

TABLE 60-2 Second-Line Symptom-Based Diagnostic Work-Up for Irritable Bowel Syndrome

Diarrhea-Predominant Symptoms	Constipation-Predominant Symptoms	Upper Gastrointestinal-Predominant Symptoms
Celiac serologies (tissue transglutaminase IgA most sensitive) • To rule out celiac sprue disease	Colonoscopy or flexible sigmoidoscopy with a barium enema • To rule out mucosal (atypical colitis) or structural abnormalities	Endoscopy • To rule out celiac disease, gastric or duodenal ulcer, and gastroesophageal reflux disease with esophageal spasm
Repeat stool sample for ova and parasites and *Clostridium difficile* • To rule out a recurrent bacterial infection or *C. difficile*, commonly seen with recent history of antibiotic use	Abdominal and pelvic computerized tomography scan • To rule out cancer and other pathologic conditions	
Allergy testing • To look for food allergies		
Endoscopy • To rule out celiac disease by taking small bowel biopsies looking for villous blunting with diarrhea, bloating, and pain		

vegetables, wheat bran, and beans. Insoluble fiber absorbs water from the intestinal tract and helps to decrease diarrhea.

c. Loperamide, 4 mg two to four times daily, as needed to reduce stool frequency.

d. Empiric antibiotic trial (see options below) followed by a probiotic to treat bacterial overgrowth and repopulate the intestines with beneficial flora. Probiotics have been found to be beneficial in some patients. A recent systematic review from the American College of Gastroenterology Task Force on the treatment of IBS concluded that lactobacillus alone does not seem to be effective in single-organism studies and combinations of probiotic studies. However, bifidobacterium does demonstrate some efficacy (American College of Gastroenterology Task Force on Irritable Bowel Syndrome, 2009). Future studies are needed to determine the efficacy of specific strains of probiotics in the treatment of IBS (Aragon, Graham, Borum, & Doman, 2010). With further study, it may be possible to target symptoms with specific strains of bacteria that facilitate better targeting of treatment and enhanced efficacy (Spiller, 2008). At this time, it is not possible to make recommendations as to a specific brand or bacterial strain because no documented studies exist. There is also no

standardization of these products. One of the following antibiotics regimens may be used

i. Rifaximan, 400 mg po tid for 7 days
ii. Levofloxacin, 500 mg po daily for 7 days
iii. Ciproflaxacin, 500 mg po bid for 7 days
iv. Metronidazole, 500 mg po tid for 7 days

2. For constipation-predominant symptoms

a. High-fiber diet with the addition of dietary fiber, psyllium, or Benifiber® (i.e., one heaping tablespoon in 8 oz of fluids one to two times per day with plenty of water). Also add insoluble fiber (see list mentioned previously). This helps the stool absorb water to facilitate passage and prevent constipation.

b. Laxatives: polyethylene glycol (Miralax®), 18 g mixed in 8 oz of liquid one to two times per day; Bisacodyl (Dulcolax®) tablets as directed. Senna or Cascara tablets should be avoided long term secondary to melaosis coli, which worsens constipation in the long term.

c. Empiric antibiotic followed by a probiotic as mentioned previously

d. Chloride channel activator that acts to increase intestinal fluid secretion and intestinal motility: lubiprostone (Amitiza®), 24 mcg twice daily.

e. Increase oral fluids: water is best, followed by low-sugar-content fluids.

f. Exercise: assist the patient in developing a regular daily exercise and activity plan. Physical activity has been shown to promote healthier bowel motility.

3. For abdominal pain–predominant IBS

    a. Antispasmodic agents

        i. Dicyclomine (Bentyl®), 20 mg four times per day. Can titrate up to a maximum of 160 mg per day.

        ii. Hyoscyamine, 0.125–0.25 mg every 4 hours prn pain. Take before food. Maximum dosage is 1.5 mg in 24 hours. Because of anticholinergic properties, use these medications with caution in the geriatric population.

    b. Low-dose tricyclic antidepressants (help to reduce visceral sensation): amitriptyline, 25 mg at bedtime, may titrate up to 100 mg at bedtime.

    c. Serotonin reuptake inhibitor or other antidepressant if depression is suspected

    d. Pain management: suggest nonpharmacologic measures first, such as relaxation, acupuncture, and meditation. Avoid the use of narcotic analgesics because of their highly addicting potential. See Chapter 48 on chronic pain for further suggestions.

4. For alternating diarrhea and constipation

    a. High-fiber diet (insoluble fiber) examples include whole grain foods; fresh fruits; fresh vegetables; wheat bran; beans; or a fiber supplement, such as psyllium husk, methylcellulose (Citrucel®), or Benifiber. The dose for constipation is one tablespoon in 8 oz of fluid one to two times per day and the dose for diarrhea is one tablespoon in 4 oz of water one to three times per day.

    b. Antidiarrheal medications during diarrhea phase (loperamide, 4 mg bid to qid) and laxative during constipation phase (polyethylene glycol, 18 g in 8 oz of liquid)

    c. Empiric antibiotic followed by a probiotic.

5. For abdominal bloating–predominant symptoms

    a. Empiric antibiotic followed by a probiotic.

    b. Food diary to correlate any aggravating foods.

    c. Diet: avoid cruciferous vegetables (cauliflower, broccoli, cabbage, and so forth) and dairy products (Table 60-3).

Incorporate stress management strategies, if needed, refer for psychiatric treatment. In the event of refractory pain, a referral to gastroenterology is warranted.

D. Follow-up

Reevaluate the patient in 3–6 weeks after initial treatment program and evaluation are done. If symptoms persist consider changing treatment regimen or obtaining further diagnostic testing as indicated based on predominant symptoms. The following are recommendations for further testing after the initial evaluation, which are often done by a gastroenterologist

1. Refractory constipation: evaluate colonic transit time, pelvic floor function, and adhesions by considering the following additional tests

    a. Colonic transit test

    b. Anorectal manometry

    c. Rectal sensation testing and emptying study

2. Refractory diarrhea: evaluate for bacterial overgrowth, laxative abuse, atypical colitis, carcinoid syndrome, and increased colonic transit

    a. Stool chemistry for surreptitious laxative abuse

    b. Duodenal aspirate for bacterial overgrowth

    c. Colonic biopsies for microscopic or collagenous colitis

    d. Urinary 5-hydroxy indolacetic acid for carcinoid syndrome

    e. Small bowel transit study for increased transit

TABLE 60-3 Diet Strategies for the Management of Constipation and Diarrhea: AVOID THE FOLLOWING FOODS

Constipation	Diarrhea
Prepared protein-laden foods: cooked, fried, baked, steamed, or canned	Caffeine: found in coffee, tea, cola, and chocolate
Wheat products: bread, pasta, cookies, pastries, and so forth	Nicotine from cigarettes or chewing tobacco
Supplementary iron	Gas-producing foods, such as beans, broccoli, cabbage, and apples
Dairy products: all dairy	Dairy products that contain lactose
Supplementary calcium	High sugar foods, such as juices, soda, candy, cookies, and other packaged sweets
All processed foods	Foods high in fat, such as bacon, sausage, butter, oils, and deep fried foods
	Sorbitol and xylitol, and other artificial sweeteners

3. Pain: evaluate small or large intestine for obstruction, intermediate obstruction, cancer, or adhesions

    a. Plain abdominal radiograph for obstruction and intermediate-obstruction

    b. CT scan of the abdomen for cancer and obstruction

    c. CT enterography for cancer, obstruction, and colitis

    d. Upper gastrointestinal series with a small bowel follow through for adhesions; can also evaluate transit time

E. **Client education**

1. Assist the patient and family in verbalizing their concerns and coping strategies with respect to the disease process and management.

2. Provide verbal and written information about the pathophysiology of IBS and treatment.

3. Discuss what the patient can expect with diagnostic testing, preparation, and after-care.

4. Explain the therapeutic benefits and side effects of any prescribed treatment.

5. Reassure the patient that assistance is available when needed.

6. Emphasize the importance of stress management and good mental health in coping with this disorder

VI. Self-management eResources

A. *The National Institutes of Health has multiple brochures for IBS patients*
(http://digestive.niddk.nih.gov/ddiseases/pubs/ibs/)

B. *Irritable Bowel Syndrome Association*
(http://www.ibsgrouporg/ibsassociation)

REFERENCES

Akehurst, R., & Kaltenthaler, E. (2001). Treatment of irritable bowel syndrome: A review of randomized controlled trials. *Gut, 48*, 272–282.

American College of Gastroenterology Task Force on Irritable Bowel Syndrome, Brandt, L. J., Chey, W. D., Foxx-Orenstein, A. E., Schiller, L. R., Schoenfeld, P., Talley, N. J., . . . Quigley, E. M. (2009). An evidence-based systematic review on the management of irritable bowel syndrome. *American Journal of Gastroenterology, 104*(Suppl. 1), S1–S35.

Aragon, G., Graham, D. B., Borum, M., & Doman, D. B. (2010). Probiotic therapy for irritable bowel syndrome. *Gastroenterology and Hepatology, 6*(1), 39–44.

Drossman, D. A. (2006). The functional GI disorders and the Rome III process. *Gastroenterology, 130*(5), 1377–1390.

Drossman, D. A., Camilleri, M., Mayer, E. A., & Whitehead, W. E. (2002). AGA technical review on irritable bowel syndrome. *Gastroenterology, 123*(6), 2108–2131.

Hauser, S. C., Pardi, D. S., & Poterucha, J. J. (2008). *Mayo Clinic gastroenterology and hepatology board review*. Rochester, Minnesota: Mayo Clinic Scientific Press.

Horwitz, B. J., & Fisher, R. S. (2001). The irritable bowel syndrome. *The New England Journal of Medicine, 344*, 1846–1850.

Kolfenbach, L. (2007). The pathophysiology, diagnosis, and treatment of IBS. *Journal of the American Academy of Physician Assistants, 20*(1), 16–20.

Lehrer, J. K., & Lichenstein, G. R. (2009). *Emedicine web by Jennifer Lehrer & Gary Lichenstein*. Retrieved from http://emedicine.medscape.com/article/180389-overview

Ringel, Y., Sperber, A. D., & Drossman, D. A. (2001). Irritable bowel syndrome. *Annual Review of Medicine, 52*, 319–338.

Spiller, R. (2008). Review article: Probiotics and prebiotics in irritable bowel syndrome. *Alimentary Pharmacologic Therapy, 28*(4), 385–396.

Ukleja, A., Woodward, T. A., & Achem, S. R. (2002). Vagus nerve injury with severe diarrhea after laparoscopic antireflux surgery. *Digestive Diseases and Sciences, 47*(7), 1590–1593.

World Gastroenterology Organization Global Guideline. (2009). *Irritable Bowel Syndrome: A global perspective*, 1–20. Retrieved from http://www.worldgastroenterology.org/irritable-bowel-syndrome.html

Yuan, Y. Z., Tao, R. J., Xu, B., Sun, J., Chen, K. M., Miao, F., . . . Xu, J. Y. (2003). Functional brain imaging in irritable bowel syndrome with rectal balloon-distention by using fMRI. *World Journal of Gastroenterology, 9*(6), 1356–1360.

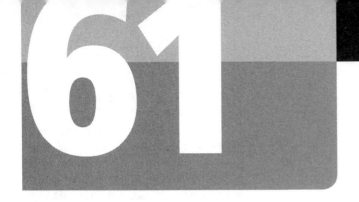

NECK PAIN

Rossana Segovia-Bain

I. Introduction and general background

The cervical (C) spine is a complex structure comprised of vertebrae, intervertebral discs, joints, the spinal cord, nerve roots, blood vessels, muscles, and ligaments. The atlanto-occipital joints (C0–C1) are the two uppermost joints, which are responsible for flexion, extension, and side flexion. The atlantoaxial joint (C1–C2) is the most mobile joint of the spine, rotation being its primary movement. The facet joints, also known as apophyseal joints, allow flexion and extension. This mobility can cause degeneration, most often seen at the C4–C7 levels.

About 25% of the height of the cervical spine is from the intervertebral discs, responsible for the spine's lordotic shape. The nucleus pulposus of the disc acts as a cushion to axial compression; the disc's annulus fibrosus withstands tension within the disc. The cervical vertebrae support the weight of the head and neck (approximately 15 lb). The vertebral arch protects the spinal cord. Cervical nerve roots are named for the vertebra below each root (e.g., the C5 nerve root is between C4 and C5 vertebrae). In the rest of the spine, the nerve root is named for the vertebra above (Magee, 2002).

Given the cervical spine's complex structure, it is vulnerable to injuries and disorders that produce pain and restrict mobility. Neck pain is generally perceived as originating from the inferior aspect of the occiput and the superior aspect of the last cervical vertebra. This forms an imaginary line that is called the "nuchal line" (Bogduk, 2003). The causes of neck pain are various and can be classified as acute, (duration ≤ 3 months) or chronic (lasting ≥ 3 months).

The most common cause of neck pain is mechanical injury, often caused by everyday activities, such as poor posture, repetitive movements, or nonergonomic work stations.

More serious injuries, such as acute trauma or injury, can occur during sports or motor vehicle accidents (MVAs).

Nonmechanical causes of pain are less common and often of an inflammatory or infectious nature, often presenting with "red flags" that should be considered in any differential of neck pain. Other causes of neck pain that should not be overlooked include referred pain and other visceral conditions that can present acutely. Women seem to have an increased incidence of spinal conditions, such as scoliosis in adolescence, osteoporosis with vertebral body fractures, and increased kyphosis after menopause. Men, however, have an increased incidence of kyphosis in adolescence and ankylosing spondylitis in adulthood (Green, 2001).

A. Mechanical spine disease (acute)

1. Definition and overview

   Cervical spine problems that provoke pain account for thousands of primary care evaluations each year. Most patients suffer from acute cervical strains or osteoarthritis (OA). Neck pain can be caused by muscle strains, ligament sprains, arthritis, or nerve impingement. Most strains and sprains recover in 2–4 weeks with conservative treatment. Arthritis neck pain also often responds to medication and physical therapy in the acute-phase period.

2. Prevalence and incidence

   Acute musculoskeletal neck pain is a common problem in the general

   a. population, frequently seen in emergency departments. About 71% of Americans remember at least one episode of neck pain or stiffness during their lifetimes (McReynolds & Sheridan, 2005). Musculoskeletal strains and sprains (sports- or work-related) occur when the cervical muscles are acutely injured, causing spasms of neck and upper back muscles. This can be related to acute sports injury, muscle tension from psychologic stress, poor sleeping habits, poor posture, ergonomics, or habits at work and home environments.

   b. Hyperextension and hyperflexion or "whiplash" occurs when there is a traumatic event that causes the neck to abruptly move forward and backward (e.g., a MVA). This causes severe pain, muscle spasms, and reduced range of motion of the cervical spine.

   c. Herniated nucleus pulposus (HNP) is also commonly known as a "herniated disc" or a "bulging disc." This occurs when the disc extends beyond the margins of the vertebral body. Most herniations are caused by injury to the annulus fibrosus. Disc herniation is classified as disc bulge, protrusion, extrusion, or sequestration.

d. Acute disc herniation causes radicular pain. The most common cause (70–75%) of cervical radiculopathy is foraminal encroachment. During the acute phase, it is possible that the HNP is reabsorbed, thus the reason for initially implementing conservative treatments. HNP in the cervical spine accounts for only 20–25% of radiculopathies. A total of 10% of asymptomatic adults younger than 40 years and 5% of adults older than 40 have been found to have HNP on magnetic resonance imaging (Furman & Simon, 2009; Isaac & Dec, 2009; Steinberg, Akins, & Baran, 1999).

e. Vertebral compression fractures are cervical spine injuries that are classified by the mechanism of the injury, such as flexion, flexion–rotation, extension, extension–rotation, vertical compression, lateral flexion, and idiopathic mechanisms that result in fractures of the ondontoid and atlantooccipital dislocation.

f. MVAs account for 50% of cervical spine injuries; falls account for approximately 20%. About 15% of the injuries occur during sports-related activities. The sports activities with highest incidence of associated cervical spine injuries (and that are considered high risk) include diving, equestrian activities, football, gymnastics, skiing, and hang gliding (Furman & Simon, 2009; Isaac & Dec, 2009; Steinberg et al., 1999).

B. *Mechanical spine disease (chronic)*

"Chronic mechanical cervical spine pain" implies that the condition has been present for 3 or more months. The patient's age is important because spondylosis is generally seen in people older than 25 years of age. About 60% of patients older than 45 years and 85% of patients older than 65 years of age present with spondylosis. Symptoms of OA, however, are not usually found in patients under 60 (Magee, 2002).

1. Definition and overview

   a. OA (also called degenerative joint disease or osteoarthrosis) is the most common form of arthritis and occurs when cartilage in the joints wears down over time. There is no cure but treatment can relieve pain and help patients maintain their activities of daily living.

   b. Spondylosis and spondylolisthesis is degeneration of the discs and vertebrae causing compression of the spinal cord in the neck. OA is the most common cause, most often affecting middle-aged and older people. This is the most common cause of spinal cord

dysfunction in the older than 55 population (Steinberg et al., 1999).

c. Myofascial pain syndrome is a chronic form of muscle pain that centers itself around trigger point areas that are tender on palpation. The pain can radiate to the entire affected muscle. Most people experience muscle pain occasionally and it generally resolves in a few days. However, trigger point myofascial pain has been linked to other pain, such as headaches, jaw pain, arm and leg pain.

d. Musculoskeletal strains and sprains (sports- or work-related) occur when there is an injury to the muscles of the neck caused by prolonged or repetitive neck extension or flexion. This is often related to poor posture at work, such as repetitive leaning or bending of the neck, and nonergonomic work stations, or during hobbies, such as knitting or crocheting. Repetition of the motion causes constant insult to the affected area and prevents healing (Steinberg et al., 1999).

C. *Nonmechanical spine disease*

1. Definition and overview

   Although infections and inflammatory type cervical spine pain are less common, it is important to identify the systemic symptoms, and not delay the diagnosis. Cervical spine diseases can cause secondary mechanical disruption of the nerve root or compression of the cord. It is important to assess systemic symptoms during the history-taking known as "red flags" (Table 61-1) (Glass & Harris, 2004).

   a. Infectious (e.g., osteomyelitis, abscess, or meningitis)

   b. Inflammatory (e.g., rheumatoid arthritis [RA] or Reiter syndrome)

   c. Malignancy (e.g., multiple myeloma, metastatic disease, locally invasive cancer, or primary bone tumor)

   d. Paget disease

   e. Multiple sclerosis with acute myelitis

D. *Referred neck pain*

1. Definition and overview

   This pain generates in an area other than the neck and is also known as trigger point or myofascial pain. In most instances the actual location of the pain or injury is in the proximal structural anatomic area. It seems to be more common in women, although it is also common in older individuals and those with highly stressful or demanding jobs. Referred pain in older patients may be related to cardiac events. Sources of referred neck pain include

   a. Thoracic outlet syndrome

   b. Shoulder or arm joint disease

TABLE 61-1 Red Flags

Possible Cauda Equina Syndrome	Possible Tumor or Infection	Possible Fracture
Saddle anesthesia	Age > 50 or < 20	Major trauma, such as MVA or fall from height
Recent onset of bladder dysfunction, such as urinary retention, increased frequency, or overflow incontinence	History of cancer	Minor trauma or even strenuous lifting (in older or potentially osteoporotic patient)
Severe or progressive neurologic deficit in the lower extremity	Constitutional symptoms, such as recent fever or chills or unexplained weight loss	
On physical examination: • Unexpected laxity of the anal sphincter • Perianal or perineal sensory loss • Major motor weakness: quadriceps (knee extension weakness), ankle plantar flexors, evertors, and dorsiflexors (foot drop)	Risk factors for spinal infection: recent bacterial infection (e.g., urinary tract infection); intravenous drug abuse; or immune suppression (from steroids, transplant, or HIV)	
	Pain that worsens when supine; severe nighttime pain	

Source: Quick Reference Guide for Clinicians Clinical Practice Guideline #14. U.S. Agency for Health Care Policy and Research (1994).

    c. Nerve compression syndrome or brachial plexus disorder
    d. Cardiac ischemia
    e. Lung cancer
    f. Thyroiditis
    g. Tracheal or esophageal disorder
    h. Temporomandibular joint syndrome
    i. Functional or psychiatric illness

II. Database (may include but is not limited to)

Because neck pain is usually multifactorial, it is important to determine if the pain is caused by spinal or extraspinal (soft tissue) injury, or a serious infectious or inflammatory disorder.

A. Subjective

1. Description of the pain including onset; location; duration; radiation; character, quality, and timing; and aggravating and alleviating factors. Determine modifying factors, such as rest, activity, changes in position, course of symptoms, and accompanying symptoms, such as numbness, tingling, weakness, paresthesias, and incontinence. If a traumatic injury, determine the exact mechanism of the injury.

    a. Past health history
        i. Medical illnesses: cancer, osteoporosis, RA, scoliosis, OA, prior neck or low back disorders (work-related or not), MVA, risk factors for aneurysm, infection, immunosuppressive disorder, injection drug use, or trauma
        ii. Surgical history (prior surgery to cervical or lumbar spine, recent surgery)
        iii. Exposure history (e.g., recent exposure to meningitis)
        iv. Medication history: medications for the symptoms or any other disorders
        v. Allergic reactions: to medications or food
    b. Family history: history of any musculoskeletal disorders (e.g., RA or OA)
    c. Occupational and environmental history: a work history is important to establish work-relatedness. If working, type of work, specific tasks, frequency of task, length of time performing same task, and length of time doing the same jobs. Note ergonomics of work station, prior jobs, prior work-related injuries, and job satisfaction.
    d. Personal and social history and health-related behaviors: housing situation (alone or accompanied), support system, smoking, drinking, substance use, and sexual lifestyle
    e. Review of systems
        i. Constitutional signs and symptoms: fever, chills, weight loss, and poor appetite (infectious or malignancy)

ii. Ear, nose, and throat: worsening of neck pain when swallowing (esophageal disorders), headache, visual changes, nuchal rigidity (infectious or malignancy)

iii. Cardiac and pulmonary: cough, dyspnea, worsening with inspiration, chest pressure, pain, arm pain, anxiety, or diaphoresis (myocardial infarction, angina, or lung cancer)

iv. Abdomen: anorexia, nausea, vomiting, and change in bowel function or stool function (gastrointestinal disorders)

v. Genitourinary: flank pain, urinary incontinence, retention, hesitancy, pain, irritation, and itchiness (urinary tract disorders)

vi. Musculoskeletal: active range of motion, activities of daily living, pain with or without movement, swelling, redness, warmth, clicking, or locking.

vii. Neurologic: depressive symptoms, fatigue, headaches (multifactorial mechanical pain), numbness, tingling, weakness, vertigo, or balance disturbances.

B. **Objective**

1. Physical examination findings (Table 61-2)

2. Special tests (Table 61-3)

TABLE 61-2 Physical Examination Findings

Inspection	Loss of cervical lordosis is present with painful acute sprains, fractures, and infectious or neoplastic processes.
Palpation	Palpate the spinous process to define the alignment of the spine. C7 is the most prominent spinous process. Top of thyroid cartilage is parallel to C4, and the cricoids cartilage is parallel to C6. Paraspinous muscle, trapezii, the medial border of the scapula, and sternocleidomastoid muscles palpation may provoke tenderness.
Range of motion *Stabilize the trunk so motion does not occur in the thoracic spine but in the neck only.*	Flexion and extension are estimated visually in degrees. Flexion limitation can also be measured as the distance the chin lacks in touching the sternum. Rotation and lateral bending of neck: the degree of motion is the angle between the vertical axis and midaxis of the face. Rotation is estimated in degrees. Limited range of motion of the neck is usually common and may present with rotation, lateral bending, and flexion and extension.
Neurologic and motor	**Assess:** **C5 Level** Deltoid—C5 axillary nerve (abduct the shoulder to 90 degrees. Push down on the arm to resist activity of the deltoid. True weakness of this muscle should be a uniformed giving way motion). Biceps—C5–C6 musculocutaneous nerve (ask patient to flex the elbow in the supinated position against resistance). Biceps reflex. Sensation —lateral arm: axillary nerve. **C6 Level** Wrist extensor group—C6 radial nerve. Biceps—C6 musculocutaneous nerve. Brachioradialis reflex. Sensation—lateral forearm: musculocutaneous nerve. **C7 Level** Triceps—C7 radial nerve (patient supine and the shoulder flexed about 90 degrees, ask the patient to extend the elbow against resistance). Wrist flexor group—C7 median and ulnar nerves. Finger extensor—C7 radial nerve. Triceps reflex. Sensation—middle finger. **C8 Level** No reflex. Examination is limited to muscle strength and sensation tests. Finger flexors (stabilize the long, index, and little fingers in extension and ask the patient to flex the fingers as you apply resistance). Sensation—ring and little fingers of the hands and distal half of the forearm ulnar side. Neurologic examination is usually normal in cervical strain.

TABLE 61-3 Special Tests

Spurling test	Have patient extend the neck while tilting the head to the side. This narrows the neural foramen and increases or reproduces radicular arm pain that is associated with disc herniation or cervical spondylosis (Green, 2001).
Axial loading test (compression test)	Push down on the patient's head. This provokes neck pain in some patients with disc problems; however, increased low back pain indicates nonorganic finding (Green, 2001).
Hoffmann test	With the patient relaxed in supine position and the hand cradled in the clinician's hand, flick the third fingernail and look for index finger and thumb flexion. If present, it is a sign of long-tract spinal cord involvement in the neck (Green, 2001).
Distraction test	Place one hand with palm open under the patient's chin, the other hand on the occiput, gradually lift the head to remove its weight from the neck. If the patient experiences a relief in symptom, it demonstrates the effect of neck traction, by widening the neural foramen (Hoppenfeld, 1976).
Adson test	Take the patient's radial pulse, abduct, extend, and externally rotate the patient's arm. Ask the patient to take a deep breath and to turn his or her head toward the arm being tested. If there is compression of the subclavian artery, you will feel a marked diminution or absence of the radial pulse (Hoppenfeld, 1976).

III. Assessment

A. Determine the cause of the neck pain, if acute or chronic.

B. Determine if the patient needs immediate referral for consultation (e.g., progressive neurologic symptoms or fracture).

C. Determine if the condition is work-related.

D. Assess the patient's ability to perform his or her usual activities.

E. Assess the patient's pain control and coping abilities.

IV. Goals of clinical management

A. Evidence-based management of the patient's cervical pain presentation.

B. Cost effective plan of treatment.

C. Appropriate management of the patient's condition if work-related.

D. Selection of management approach that maximizes the patient's adherence to the plan of care.

V. Plan

A. Diagnostic criteria non–red flag conditions (Table 61-4)

B. Other diagnostic tests that may be included

1. Blood tests: erythrocyte sedimentation rate, rheumatoid factor, antinuclear antibody if suspecting systemic, infectious, and inflammatory conditions; cardiac enzymes, if indicated.

2. Tuberculosis screening (tuberculin skin test or QuantiFERON®) test, if indicated.

3. Imaging: cervical spine radiograph series, shoulder radiograph series, chest radiograph if indicated based on clinical pulmonary presentation, computerized axial tomography, or magnetic resonance imaging if patient presents with soft tissue, disc signs and symptoms, and not responding to standard treatment within expected time period.

4. Electromyelogram or nerve conduction study to rule out other structures causing the neurologic symptoms when the diagnosis is unclear.

C. Treatment (Table 61-5)

D. Patient education

1. Discuss nature of condition and expected time of recovery.

   a. In acute cases with absent red flags, healing of the soft tissue is expected within a few weeks. Most patients can return to work immediately or within 6 weeks. Some symptoms may still be present in 20–40% of patients 6 months after injury, but the prognosis is good and their symptoms eventually resolve (Petropoulos, 2004).

   b. In chronic cases, explain that periods of acute flare-ups are possible. It is important to focus on the patient's ability to tolerate the pain and aim for the highest possible level of personal function as a goal.

TABLE 61-4 Diagnostic Criteria Non–Red Flag Conditions

Probable Diagnosis	Mechanism	Common Symptoms	Common Signs	Tests and Results
Regional neck pain	Unknown	Diffuse pain	None	None indicated
Cervical strain	Flexion–extension or rotation force, blow to the head or neck	Neck pain, difficult or decreased motion	Limited range of motion because of pain	None indicated
Cervical nerve root compression with radiculopathy	Degenerative condition, trauma	Dermatomal sensory changes, motor weakness	Specific motor, sensory, and reflex changes	None indicated for 4–6 weeks, unless progressive motor weakness
Spinal stenosis	Older patients: degenerative disc disease Younger patients: congenital stenosis	Neck, shoulder, and posterior arm pain, paresthesias in the same distribution as the pain	Weakness of the shoulder girdle and upper arms Signs worse with extension, improved with flexion of the neck	Computed tomography or magnetic resonance imaging shows spinal stenosis

Source: Glass, L. S., & Harris, J. S. (2004). *Occupational medicine practice guidelines: Evaluation and management of common health problems and functional recovery in workers* (2nd ed.). Beverly Farms, MA: OEM Press.

TABLE 61-5 Clinical Characteristics and Management of Cervical Spine Pain

Condition	Clinical Characteristics	Management
Cervical strain and sprain	Most patients can report specific mechanism of injury. May not notice pain immediately but after several hours may have tightness in the neck. Some may report nausea. Physical examination may only show mild abnormalities. May have tenderness or decreased range of motion. After several hours or days, may find more significant soft tissue tenderness, edema, spasms, headaches, and dizziness. With moderate injuries may present with radicular symptoms.	Diagnostic work-up: cervical radiograph to rule out fracture or dislocation if suspected. Treatment: rest in comfortable position, soft cervical collar is appropriate for 1 or 2 days if in the acute phase. Cold packs applied for 15 minutes four to six times a day for the first 2 days, then heat. May also alternate cold and heat if combination promotes better relief. Gentle stretches of the neck and shoulders, (early movements of the stable cervical spine promote recovery). Analgesics according to symptoms especially for nighttime pain. Muscle relaxants are appropriate in the acute phase to relieve spasms and aid with nighttime sleep. Physical therapy that includes cervical traction, massage, and ultrasound can be helpful especially in the first 4 weeks. Encourage early return to normal activities, including work if appropriate.
Acute disc herniation	Pain is usually aggravated by cough, sneeze, straining, and other activities that prolong static position of the neck, especially in flexion–extension and rotation. Lifting, pushing, and pulling may also aggravate the pain. Usually, there is tenderness to palpation of the spinous process. Distraction test relieves the pain, compression test increases the pain. Usually there are associated muscle spasms and trigger point tenderness.	Diagnostic work-up: radiograph may be normal or show degenerative disc disease. May need magnetic resonance imaging, computed tomography, electromyelogram, or nerve conduction study if indicated based on presenting symptoms. Treatment: conservative treatment in the acute phase, absent major progressing symptoms. Rest by limiting activities, soft pillows, elevation of the head of the bed, and soft collar. Physical therapy for traction treatment, home traction for 20 minutes, four times a day; and functional range of motion and strength. Heat or cold compress to the neck for 15 minutes as tolerated. Nonsteroidal anti-inflammatory drugs (NSAIDs) and muscle relaxants used in the acute phase. Patients should be reassured that most disc herniations resolve without residual problems. If symptoms do not resolve within 3–6 weeks, epidural injection may be appropriate depending on presentation of symptoms and degree of limitation on activities of daily living.

TABLE 61-5 Clinical Characteristics and Management of Cervical Spine Pain *(continued)*

Condition	Clinical Characteristics	Management
Chronic disc degeneration (spondylosis or osteoarthritis)	Most common presentations are stiffness and chronic pain that worsens with upright activity. Some patients may report grinding or popping in the neck region. Referred pain to shoulder and arm, and paraspinous process spasms, headaches, fatigue, and sleep disturbances. Difficulty with basic activities of daily living.	Diagnostic tests: anteroposterior and lateral radiograph shows sclerosis in the intervertebral disc area with osteophytes (bone spurs) projecting anteriorly. Osteophytes may also project posteriorly causing stenosis of the cervical canal. Anterior subluxation of one vertebra over the other may also be appreciated on radiographs. Degenerative findings usually at the C5–6 and C6–7 levels. Treatment: usually responsive to traction. NSAIDs and muscle relaxants are helpful especially at nighttime. Cervical pillow, cervical roll, and physical therapy. Epidural injection may also be appropriate. In chronic cases without resolution of major symptoms and with radicular involvement, decompression and fusion surgery may be appropriate.
Cervical radiculopathy	Patients present with neck pain along with radicular pain associated with numbness and paresthesias in the upper extremity along the distribution of the nerve root involved. Muscle spasms or fasciculations may also be present in the myotomes involved. Other symptoms may be weakness, lack of coordination, difficulty with handwriting and performing fine manipulative tasks, dropping objects, and decreased strength. If stenosis of the cervical canal, patient may present with lower extremities symptoms and bowel or bladder dysfunction.	Diagnostic tests: plain radiographs may identify spondylosis or degeneration of the disc and the facet. Magnetic resonance imaging or computed tomography with intrathecal contrast confirms the diagnosis. However, this is not routine care unless progressive symptoms. Electromyelogram or nerve conduction study helps determine the location of the neurologic dysfunction and is commonly used presurgically. Treatment: in most cases, it resolves spontaneously within 6–12 weeks. Nonnarcotic analgesic is usually helpful. May also use short course of oral steroids if appropriate. Physical therapy for traction is useful in the first 2–4 weeks.
Myofascial pain syndrome	Patient may present with multiple localized sites of deep tenderness in the trapezius, rhomboids, and levator scapulae muscles. These are trigger points. Usually diffuse aching-type pain that lasts longer than 3 months along with sleep difficulties. Patients presenting with these symptoms are usually younger than 50 years old.	Diagnostics: radiographs are usually normal. Electroencephalogram if done usually shows abnormalities and indication of sleep disturbances. Treatment: reassurance, psychotherapy, and physical therapy are indicated. Vacation and rest are also recommended to relieve stress. NSAIDs, local trigger point injections with lidocaine with or without corticosteroids may be helpful.
Rheumatoid arthritis	Patient may present with pain in the occiput and radiculopathy of the lower extremity, crepitus, and cervical myelopathy.	Diagnostic tests: laboratory abnormalities are significant for elevated erythrocyte sedimentation rate and rheumatoid factors. Radiographs show osteopenia, joint space narrowing, soft tissue swelling around the involved joints, bone erosions near the capsular attachments of the involved joints, and both malalignment and subluxation of the joints. Treatment: rest, gentle massage, soft cervical collar, isometric exercises, and intermittent heat. Salicylates may give enough pain relief. NSAIDs and epidural injection may be useful. Referral for consultation is advised for further treatment and management.
Cervical fracture	Patient may present with severe neck pain, paraspinous muscle spasms, and point tenderness to the area of fracture. Pain radiates to the shoulder or arm and may be associated with radicular symptoms if nerve root involvement is present.	Diagnostic tests: Anteroposterior, lateral, and odontoid views are the standard. Lateral radiograph should include the occiput superiorly and the top of T1 inferiorly. Swimmer's view may also be indicated to visualize the cervicothoracic junction. If no fracture is seen, it should be evaluated for instability. Treatment: immobilization of cervical spine during transportation to emergency department. Patients whose initial radiograph was negative for fracture, but continues to have pain, may use cervical collar. Repeat radiograph if symptoms persist past 7–10 days. NSAIDs and analgesics are also appropriate.

Sources: Green, W. B. (2001). *Essentials of musculoskeletal care* (2nd ed.). Rosemont, IL: American Academy of Orthopaedic Surgeons; Steinberg, G., Akins, C., & Baran, D. (1999). *Orthopaedics in primary care* (3rd ed.). Hagerstown, MD: Lippincott Williams & Williams.

2. Discuss proper posture and body mechanics.

3. Explain proper use of supportive devices, such as neck pillows and soft collar.

4. Discuss need for a life-long stretching and conditioning exercise program for maintenance and prevention of further disability.

5. Discuss stress reduction techniques.

6. Discuss medication use and compliance and other symptom relief modalities.

7. If determined to be work-related, discuss process of reporting the injury to the employer and assuming care with the employer's occupational health system.

E. Follow-up (acute and chronic)

Follow-up time frame is based on the plan of care and acuity, and severity of the patient's presentation. If imaging or laboratory values have been ordered, follow-up should be prompt to communicate the results to the patient. If patient is taken off work, appropriate follow-up is necessary to determine if the patient is ready to return to work and at what capacity.

VI. Self-management resources and tools

A. Patient and client education Internet-based materials

1. Neck Injuries and Disorders (U.S. National Library of Medicine, 2010): http://www.nlm.nih.gov/medline plus/neckinjuriesanddisorders.html

2. Spine and neck http://orthoinfo.aaos.org/menus/spine.cfm

B. Community support groups

1. Web MD® Health Community: http://exchanges.webmd.com

2. Back Pain Support Group: www.backpainsupportgroup.com

3. Healia Health Communities and Support Groups: http://communities.healia.com

4. eHealth Forum: http://ehealthforum.com

REFERENCES

Bogduk, N. (2003). The anatomy and pathophysiology of neck pain. *Physical Medicine and Rehabilitation Clinics of North America, 14*(3), 455–472.

Furman, M., & Simon, J. (2009). *Cervical disc disease.* Retrieved from http://emedicine.medscape.com/article/305720-print

Glass, L. S., & Harris, J. S. (2004). *Occupational medicine practice guidelines: Evaluation and management of common health problems and functional recovery in workers* (2nd ed.). Beverly Farms, MA: OEM Press.

Green, W. B. (2001). *Essentials of musculoskeletal care* (2nd ed.). Rosemont, IL: American Academy of Orthopaedic Surgeons.

Hoppenfeld, S. (1976). *Physical examination of the spine and extremities.* East Norwalk, CT: Appleton-Century-Crofts.

Isaac, Z., & Dec, K. (2009). *Patient information: Neck pain.* Retrieved from http://www.uptodate.com/online/content/topic.do?topicKey=bone_joi /8884

Magee, D. J. (2002). *Orthopedic physical assessment* (4th ed.). Philadelphia, PA: W.B. Saunders.

McReynolds, T. M., & Sheridan, B. J. (2005). Intramuscular ketorolac versus osteopathic manipulative treatment in the management of acute neck pain in the emergency department: A randomized clinical trial. *Journal of the American Osteopathic Association, 105*(2), 57–68.

Petropoulos, P. (2004). Whiplash injury (PTG). In F. Ferri (Eds.), *Ferri's clinical advisor: Instant diagnosis and treatment.* St. Louis, MO: Mosby.

Steinberg, G., Akins, C., & Baran, D. (1999). *Orthopaedics in primary care* (3rd ed.). Hagerstown, MD: Lippincott Williams & Williams.

U.S. National Library of Medicine. (2010). Neck injuries and disorders. Retrieved from http://www.nlm.nih.gov/medlineplus/neckinjuries anddisorders.html

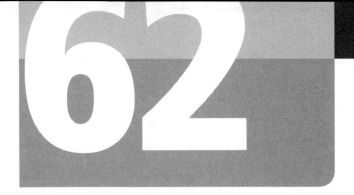

OBESITY

Sherri Borden, David Besio, and Geraldine Collins-Bride

I. Introduction and general background

In a data collection from 2007 to 2008 the Centers for Disease Control and Prevention (CDC) found that approximately 34% of adults in the United States are overweight, and 34% are obese (CDC, 2009d). This documents an increase by the CDC in government databases from 1988 to 1994 where approximately 23% of the population met criteria for obesity (CDC, 2009d).

Obesity trends are more prevalent in minority groups, lower socioeconomic groups, and less educated individuals and contribute to a number of significant chronic healthcare issues. In addition, an overweight and obese population contributes to substantial economic costs, $99.2 billion in 1995 (National Institutes of Health National Heart, Lung and Blood Institute [NIH-NHLBI], 1998).

Clinically, overweight is defined as a body mass index (BMI) of 25–29.9 kg/m^2 and obesity as greater than or equal to 30 kg/m^2. Overweight and obesity for those 18 years and older substantially increases the risks of morbidity for hypertension (HTN), dyslipidemia, type 2 diabetes, coronary artery disease, stroke, gallbladder disease, osteoarthritis, sleep apnea, and respiratory problems. Additional health risks include higher rates of endometrial, breast, prostate, and colon cancer. Overweight individuals also endure social stigmatization and discrimination (NIH-NHLBI, 1998; CDC, 2009b; CDC, 2009c).

The goal of Healthy People 2010 was to promote health and reduce chronic disease associated with diet and weight by reducing the number of adults 20 years or older with a BMI over 30 to 15% of the population. The 2009 draft objectives of Healthy People 2020, discussed later, have been expanded and modified to include changes in State policies, expectations for primary care visits, and nutrition and weight management counseling for individuals older than 2. Although the goals are ambitious, weight-related diseases are a major preventable cause of death, pose an important public health challenge, and should not be overlooked (Healthy People 2010; NIH-NHLBI, 1998).

A. *Healthy People 2020, summarized* (U.S. Department of Health and Human Services, 2009)

1. Objectives retained from 2010
   a. Increase the proportion of adults who are at a healthy weight.
   b. Reduce the proportion of adults who are obese.

2. Objective retained but modified
   a. Reduce the number of children and adolescents who are obese.
   b. For individuals age 2 and older: increase the consumption of fruits, vegetables, whole grains, and calcium. Reduce the consumption of saturated fat and sodium.
   c. Increase the number of healthcare visits that include counseling or education for weight management.
   d. Eliminate very low food security among children in United States households.

3. Objectives new to Healthy People 2020
   a. Prevent inappropriate weight gain in youth and adults.
   b. Increase the number of primary care providers who regularly calculate the BMI of their patients.
   c. Reduce the consumption of calories from solid fats and sugars, increase the number of States with food standards for children, and increase the percentage of schools that offer nutritious food and beverages outside of school meals.
   d. Changes in State level policies for food outlets.

4. Measuring overweight and obesity: BMI provides a reasonable indicator for body fatness and weight categories that may lead to significant health problems. BMI categories are defined as
   a. 18.5–24.9 (normal);
   b. 25–29.9 (overweight)
   c. 30–34.9 (Class I obesity)
   d. 35–39.9 (Class II obesity)
   e. greater than or equal to 40 (Class III obesity).

B. Obesity in adults

1. Most common causes of obesity are the result of energy imbalances

   a. Excessive caloric intake from food, beverages, or alcohol

   b. Lack of activity and exercise and sedentary lifestyle

2. Many medical problems may also contribute to the etiology of obesity

   a. Hypothyroidism

   b. Cushing syndrome

   c. Hypogonadism

   d. Hypothalamic injuries

   e. Polycystic ovary (Stein-Leventhal syndrome)

   f. Pseudo-hypoparathyroidism

   g. Insulinoma

   h. Medications may also contribute to overweight and obesity: corticosteroids; anticonvulsants and psychotropic medications, in particular atypical antipsychotics, such as clozaril and olanzapine; insulin; and select oral hypoglycemic agents

3. Consequences of obesity: as weight increases to the categories of overweight and obesity, risks for chronic health problems increase. These health problems include

   a. Coronary artery disease

   b. Type 2 diabetes

   c. Cancers (endometrial, breast, and colon)

   d. HTN

   e. Dyslipidemia

   f. Stroke

   g. Liver and gallbladder disease

   h. Sleep apnea and respiratory problems

   i. Osteoarthritis

   j. Gynecological problems (abnormal menses and fertility problems)

   k. Metabolic syndrome (Kanaya, 2010). Also known as syndrome X, insulin resistance syndrome, and the dysmetabolic syndrome, metabolic syndrome is a group of risk factors that confers higher risk for stroke, coronary artery disease, and type 2 diabetes. The syndrome includes three or more of the following criteria

      i. Waist circumference according to population-specific criteria:

         a. White, European: men greater than or equal to 102 cm, women greater than or equal to 88 cm

         b. Asian: men greater than or equal to 90 cm, women greater than or equal to 80

         c. Middle East, Mediterranean: men greater than or equal to 94 cm, women greater than or equal to 80 cm

         d. Sub-Saharan Africa: men greater than or equal to 94 cm, women greater than or equal to 80 cm

         e. Central and South American: men greater than or equal to 90, women greater than or equal to 80

      ii. High-density lipoprotein (HDL): men less than 40, women less than 50 or niacin or fibrate use

      iii. Triglycerides: greater than or equal to 150 mg/dl, or niacin or fibrate use

      iv. Blood pressure greater than or equal to 130/85 or taking blood pressure medications

      v. Fasting glucose greater than or equal to 100 mg/dl or using diabetes medications

C. Obesity in children

Obesity among children and adolescents remains a significant problem. The United States has made little progress in this area despite the Healthy People 2010 goal for a reduction in the proportion of children and adolescents who are overweight or obese. Progress toward national prevalence goals to reduce overweight and obesity is monitored by the National Health and Nutrition Examination Survey. The most recent data collection period from 1998 to 2008 used the Pediatric Nutrition Surveillance System, a source of nationally compiled obesity surveillance information obtained from the state and local level for low income, preschool-aged children participating in federally funded nutritional programs. The findings indicate that obesity prevalence increased steadily among preschool-age children from 12.4% in 1998 to 14.5% in 2003 and has remained much the same in 2008 at 14.6% (CDC, 2009a). Obesity is a serious health issue for children and adolescents for numerous reasons including risk of obesity in adolescence and adulthood; increased risk for cardiovascular disease (CVD), such as high blood pressure, high cholesterol, and type 2 diabetes; and alterations in body image with subsequent social stigmatization.

D. Obesity in individuals with mental illness

As in other populations, individuals with mental illness who are overweight or obese are at increased risk for developing chronic diseases, such as CVD and type 2 diabetes. Excessive weight gain is not always addressed by clinicians, such as psychiatrists, primary care physicians, and advanced practice nurses, who feel poorly equipped to deal with this problem and fear patient treatment noncompliance or psychiatric decompensation.

There are no clear interventions to prevent and treat overweight and obesity in this population. According to Boyd (2002), when compared to an individual who maintains their weight, individuals with mental illness who gain more than 11 lbs in adulthood have approximately twice the rate of type 2 diabetes. Excessive weight gain and obesity is two to three times more prevalent than in the general population (Aquila, 2002). This increased occurrence has been strongly associated with several important factors including diet, exercise, environmental factors, and psychotropic medications. Individuals with mental illness tend to eat a diet higher in saturated fat and calories; consume greater amounts of high carbohydrate beverages; and eat a diet lower in fiber, fresh fruits, and vegetables. They also tend to exercise less, living a more sedentary lifestyle as a result of institutionalization and other factors (Greenberg, Chan, & Blackburn, 1999).

Weight gain has also been reported during treatment with many medications, such as conventional antipsychotic agents phenothiazines and thioxanthenes, and was more recently reported in novel antipsychotic agents, such as clozapine, risperidone, and olanzapine (Basson et al., 2001). Although novel antipsychotic medications improve psychiatric outcomes, estimates for associated weight gain range from virtually zero weight gain, as seen in ziprasidone, to an average gain of 4–4.5 kg after 10 weeks of treatment with both olanzapine and clozapine, to nearly 12 kg at 1 year with olanzapine (Fontaine et al., 2001; Allison et al., 1999). The variability of novel antipsychotic weight gain experienced by patients suggests that several factors are involved. Weight gain is often rapid in the first few weeks of treatment and then reaches a plateau. Weight gain with novel antipsychotic treatment has been correlated with an excessive appetite, thought to be directly related to the atypical antipsychotics affinity for histamine H1 receptors of blockade of the hypothalamic sites regulating satiety (Rummel-Kluge et al., 2010).

II. Database

A. Subjective

1. Developmental patterns and past medical history

    a. Infant and childhood obesity: no correlation found in infancy; however, there seem to be links to intrauterine imprinting (Bray & Champagne, 2005). Obesity beginning at age range of 5–6 years has a documented correlation to adult obesity secondary to genetic and environmental factors, such as overfeeding, poor food choices, and sedentary lifestyle.

    b. Adolescent obesity: adolescents with obesity are at an increase risk of CVD, type 2 diabetes, and respiratory and sleep problems. According to the American Academy of Child and Adolescent Psychiatry, adolescent obesity is also associated with lower self-esteem, depression, anxiety, and obsessive–compulsive disorder.

    c. Obesity of early adulthood (postpartum)

    d. Middle-age obesity: decrease in metabolic rate, decrease in activity level, increase in body weight increases the risk of developing CVD and type 2 diabetes.

    e. Past medical history of obesity-related medical problems: arthritis, gallbladder disease, HTN, CVD, diabetes, depression, and obstructive sleep apnea.

2. Family history: note history of obesity; CVD; HTN; genetic syndromes; and thyroid, diabetes, and other endocrine disorders

3. Dietary history

    a. 24-hour recall of current usual intake: type and quantity of food, meal times, and variability of intake

    b. Intake of high caloric foods: sugar; fats; and beverages (alcohol, soda, and fruit juices)

    c. Meal preparation: cooking techniques and use of fats and oils

    d. Emotional and behavioral cues to eating

        i. Internal and emotional reaction to self or others, and sabotaging thoughts, such as "I deserve a treat"

        ii. External sight or smell of food; associations of food with time, place, or activity; and celebration or parties

    e. Availability: cost of food, cooking facilities, and food insecurity

    f. Cultural orientation to food and weight

4. Exercise and activity: note type and amount of daily activity, including assets and barriers to exercise (affordability, access, level of priority, and seasonality)

5. Self-image, self-esteem, and self-confidence: effect on relationships, jobs, and daily life

6. Motivation and interest in weight control.

7. Weight loss and dieting history, including use of over-the-counter (OTC) medications, supplements, and herbal treatments; diuretics and laxatives; diet pills; and prescription drugs. Note history of binge and purge behavior or self-starvation.

8. Review of systems: in general, the mild to moderately obese individual is asymptomatic. In cases of Class III obesity (BMI ≥ 40), the following symptoms can be manifestations of mechanical difficulties or medical consequences

    a. Easy fatigability and dyspnea on exertion
    b. Somnolence
    c. Malaise and weakness
    d. Abdominal bloating and dyspepsia
    e. Ankle swelling
    f. Joint pains, especially weight-bearing joints: low back, hips, knees, and ankles
    g. Skin rashes: acne and chronic candidiasis in skin folds
    h. Menstrual irregularities
    i. Symptoms of depression (see Chapter 52 on Depression)
    j. To rule out endocrine disorders, consider the following history
        i. Lethargy, ankle swelling, somnolence, heat or cold intolerance, hair loss, dry skin, constipation and menstrual irregularities: consider hypothyroidism.
        ii. Acne, increase in hair growth, change in facial appearance, easy bruising, and skin rashes: consider Cushing syndrome.
        iii. Delayed puberty, decreased or absent libido: consider hypogonadism.
        iv. Amenorrhea or menstrual irregularities and hirsutism: consider polycystic ovary syndrome.
        v. Arthralgias, muscle cramps, weakness, numbness or tingling, seizures, and emotional lability: consider pseudo-hypoparathyroidism.

B. **Objective**

1. Physical examination

    a. Most individuals who are obese require general observation; height, weight, and BMI measurement; and a complete set of vital signs. However, a complete physical examination is generally preferred to rule out secondary causes and evidence of obesity-related health risks. The examination should focus in particular on the thyroid, cardiovascular, pulmonary, musculoskeletal, and neurologic examination in all patients.
    b. Measuring abdominal circumference helps assess distribution of fat. Waist circumference provides a clinically acceptable measurement of abdominal fat before and during weight loss. Waist circumference in men should be less than 102 cm (40 in) and in women less

than 88 cm (35 in). Cut-offs can be used to identify increased relative risk for the development of obesity-associated risk factors in most adults with a BMI from 25–34.9.

    c. The following complexes of physical signs may provide clues to underlying endocrine disorders
        i. Cool, dry skin; hoarse voice and facial edema; thick tongue; delayed or absent deep tendon reflexes: consider hypothyroidism.
        ii. Round, "moon face"; hirsutism; truncal obesity; purple striae; ecchymosis: consider Cushing syndrome.
        iii. Small stature; lack of secondary sex characteristics; poor muscular development: consider hypogonadism.
        iv. Short, stocky stature; round face; mental retardation; joint deformities; cataracts; papilledema: consider pseudo-hypoparathyroidism

2. Diagnostic testing: depends on the severity of obesity, potential for secondary cause, and evaluation of obesity-related health risks. Consider the following tests

    a. *Electrolytes, blood-urea-nitrogen, creatinine, and fasting glucose
    b. *Thyroid-stimulating hormone
    c. *Fasting low-density lipoprotein (LDL) and HDL cholesterol, and serum triglycerides
    d. Pulmonary function tests and arterial blood gas
    e. Steroid studies: cortisol level and dexamethasone suppression test
    f. Hemoglobin A_{1C}
    g. Growth hormones
    h. Testosterone
    i. Follicle-stimulating hormone, luteinizing hormone, and prolactin levels

*most commonly ordered as initial screening tests

III. Assessment

A. *Determine the diagnosis: distinguish between secondary and primary obesity. Rule out endocrine disorders as described previously.*

B. *Severity: assess the severity of obesity, including current and future health risks.*

C. *Significance: assess the significance of obesity to the patient and significant others including impact on daily functioning, work, relationships, and self esteem.*

D. Motivation and ability:

1. Assess the motivation of the patient, including reasons for weight reduction, previous history of weight loss, understanding of the causes of obesity, ability to engage in action plan, and financial considerations.

2. Assess stage of change (Prochaska & DiClemente, 1982) to help identify possible interventions and develop patient-specific process goals and cognitive and behavioral therapy strategies (Fabricatore, 2007).

   a. Precontemplation: provide weight and health education, and health benefits of exercise.

   b. Contemplation
      i. Identify and list advantages and disadvantages of weight loss (Brownell, 2000)
      ii. Make a list of potential exercises and activities

   c. Preparation
      i. Positive goal setting (specific, measurable, attainable, reasonable, and time limited)
      ii. Environmental control: stocking the refrigerator with fresh vegetables and fruits, removing easy access to sweets and treats, eating slowly without distractions, using smaller plates and bowls, shopping from a list, menu planning, buying prepackaged healthy calorie-controlled meals to eat as "Plan B," identifying possible alternative exercises, and keeping a food record and exercise log
      iii. Identify potential diet intervention (Figures 62-1 and 62-2)

   d. Action: implement goals of dietary and lifestyle change; reevaluate goals regularly to encourage additional progress.

   e. Maintenance: develop coping strategies for diet and exercise lapses.

   f. Relapse: encourage patient regarding positive accomplishments, reevaluate advantages and disadvantages, and reinitiate preparation strategies.

IV. Goals of clinical management

A. Risk reduction

Although being overweight or obese clearly increases morbidity and mortality, strong evidence suggests that weight loss reduces risk factors for CVD and diabetes. Weight loss reduces blood pressure in both overweight hypertensive and nonhypertensive individuals, lowers serum triglycerides, increases HDL cholesterol, and generally produces reductions in LDL and total serum cholesterol. Additionally, modest weight loss of 5–10% reduces blood glucose levels and HbA$_{1C}$ in some patients with type 2 diabetes (NIH-NHLBI, 1998).

B. Prevention of obesity

Although the physical consequences of obesity are a significant problem, the impact on self-esteem and body image is also an important factor to consider. Physical health is closely linked to mental health and physical problems may negatively impact a patient's body image. Clinicians can play an integral role in helping a patient understand the health risks associated with obesity. Therefore, one of the primary goals should be to initiate healthcare maintenance measures early to prevent or intervene in weight gain. It is important to take into account a variety of factors when choosing treatment plans to provide comprehensive holistic care including the patient's personal, cultural, and family history; knowledge of the development of chronic health conditions; and impact of overweight and obesity on body image.

V. Plan

A. Management

Treatment requires a fundamental change in lifestyle. Weight loss depends on adherence to an agreement outlining lifestyle changes which factor in individual motivation, support systems, and underlying medical or psychologic conditions. The management plan should consist of the following considerations:

1. Treat the underlying cause, if secondary obesity.

2. Establish a patient agreement: determine short- and long-range goals and outcomes, using healthy body weight range based on BMI, patient's desired weight, and practitioner's assessment of desired weight.

3. Diets: although in the short-term lower carbohydrate diets seem to result in weight loss without adverse health consequences (Gardner et al., 2007; Baron, 2010), using a variety of dietary interventions (including low calorie meal replacements) is reasonable because there does not seem to be an advantage of one macronutrient distribution versus another (Sacks et al., 2009). Induce a 500- to 1,000-calorie deficit to promote 1- to 2-lb weight loss per week resulting in approximately an 8–10% total weight loss outcome. Refer to a nutritionist or behaviorist or weight management group (Figure 62-3).

4. Exercise: discuss the health benefits of exercise, even if weight loss is not accomplished. Assist the individual in developing an exercise regimen,

FIGURE 62-1 One Week Food Record

	Day 1	Calories	Day 2	Calories	Day 3	Calories	Day 4	Calories
Breakfast								
Time								
Place								
Hunger level*								
Lunch								
Time								
Place								
Hunger level*								
Dinner								
Time								
Place								
Hunger level*								
Snack (please note all snacks)								
Exercise								

FIGURE 62-1 *One Week Food Record (continued)*

	Day 5	Calories	Day 6	Calories	Day 7	Calories	To Document Intake:
Breakfast							Record everything you eat or drink during the day (as soon as possible after intake). List the food and amount eaten and calories to the best of your ability.
							For example:
							2 slices w/w Light bread 120
Time							8 oz non-fat milk 90
Place							1 hard-boiled egg 80
Hunger level							**Total** **335**
Lunch							
							Goal 1:
Time							
Place							
Hunger level							
Dinner							
							Goal 2:
Time							
Place							
Hunger level							
Snack (please note all snacks)							**Feelings/Comments/Concerns**
Exercise							

* Hunger Level:1 = Starving 10 = Stuffed

Source: Produced by UCSF Nutrition and Food Services. Used with permission by UCSF Medical Center.

FIGURE 62-2 *Wellness Contract*

❑ A goal should be realistic and measurable

- Unrealistic goal: I will eat lots of vegetables every day

- More realistic goal: I will eat two servings of vegetables at dinner three nights this week

- Work towards bigger goals over time

❑ Reward yourself for accomplishing your goal. Examples: take a bubble bath, rent a favorite movie, get a massage, sleep in late, or just pat yourself on the back!

❑ Create no more than 3 goals per week

❑ Check in with a supportive friend, family member, or health professional to help keep you on track.

	Goal	Reward
Food		
Exercise		
Stress Management		

I will focus on these wellness goals for the week.

_____ Signature _____ Date

Source: Produced by UCSF Nutrition and Food Services. Used with permission by UCSF Medical Center.

FIGURE 62-3 *Instructions for Use of the Plate Method*

STEP 1: Fill Half (1/2) of Your Plate with Non-Starchy Vegetables.

- ❑ Non-starchy vegetables are low in calories, low in carbohydrate, and high in fiber. This means non-starchy vegetables can help you feel full and more satisfied with your meal, but not lead to weight gain and high blood sugar.
- ❑ Aim for 1 to 2 cups of any vegetable (EXCEPT starchy vegetables listed in Step 3).
- ❑ Vegetables can be raw or cooked.

STEP 2: Limit Protein to a Quarter (1/4) of Your Plate.

- ❑ Choose lean meat, poultry, or fish. Your portion should not be bigger than the palm of your hand. Try 1 to 2 whole eggs, or just the egg whites for lower cholesterol.
- ❑ Choose tofu, nuts, or seeds. Aim for about 2 tablespoons of nuts and seeds or 1/2 cup of tofu.

STEP 3: Limit Starch to a Quarter (1/4) of Your Plate.

- ❑ Starch is a source of carbohydrate. Carbohydrate turns into an important fuel, called glucose, and limiting the portion size of starch helps control body weight and blood sugar.
- ❑ Choose a bun, tortilla, bread, bagel, rice, grains, cereal, pasta, or a starchy vegetable.
  - If you choose bread, limit to 2 slices or 1/2 bagel.
  - If you choose a hamburger/hotdog bun, limit to 1 bun.
  - If you choose a tortilla, limit to 2 small tortillas or 1 large tortilla.
  - If you choose rice, grains, pasta, cereal, or a starchy vegetable, limit the portion to no more than 1 cup—this is about the size of a woman's fist. Starchy vegetables include beans, potatoes, corn, yams, peas, and winter squash.
- ❑ Choose most of your starches from whole grains, such as whole wheat bread or tortillas, brown rice, whole wheat pasta, whole grain and bran cereals, or beans.

STEP 4: If Desired, Add 1 Portion of Fruit or Milk to Your Meal.

- ❑ Fruit, milk, and yogurt are also sources of carbohydrate. To best control body weight and blood sugar, limit yourself to either fruit or milk at your meal. You may choose to save the fruit or milk as a snack.
- ❑ Because high carbohydrate liquids can quickly raise blood sugar, avoid drinking fruit juice.
- ❑ Examples of fruit portion sizes are:
  - 1 small apple, orange, peach, pear, banana, or nectarine (or half of a larger-size fruit)
  - 3/4 cup fresh pineapple chunks, blueberries, or blackberries
  - 17 grapes
  - 1 and 1/4 cups strawberries or watermelon
  - 1 cup cantaloupe, honeydew, or papaya
- ❑ Choose low fat or nonfat dairy products for heart health and weight control.
- ❑ Examples of milk and yogurt portion sizes are:
  - 1 cup (8 ounces) of non-fat, 1%, or soy milk
  - 2/3 to 1 cup plain non-fat or aspartame-sweetened fruit yogurt

STEP 5: Limit Added Fats.

- ❑ Avoid adding fats to your foods like butter, margarine, shortening, mayonnaise, gravies, cream sauces, salad dressing, and sour cream. Instead, season foods with herbs and spices.
- ❑ Cook using low fat methods such as baking, steaming, broiling, or grilling. Avoid frying foods.

Source: Produced by UCSF Nutrition and Food Services. Used with permission by UCSF Medical Center

(continues)

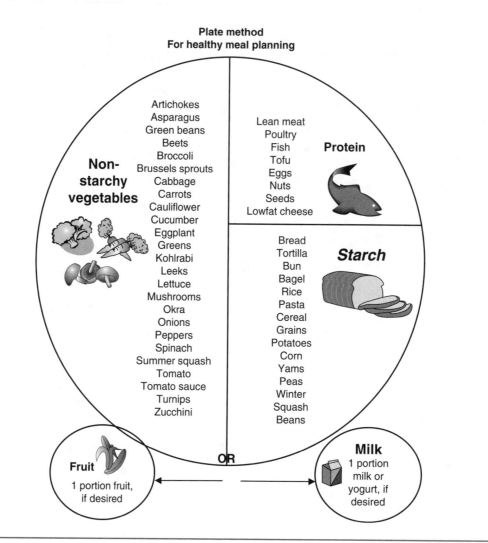

FIGURE 62-3 Instructions for Use of the Plate Method *(continued)*

setting reasonable short-term goals to increase to a long-term goal of six times per week for 60 minutes per session According to the National Weight Control Registry only 9% of participants in the registry reported keeping weight off without engaging in some physical activity. Walking seemed to be the most popular form of physical activity. Half of the participants also combined walking with another form of planned exercise, such as aerobics, bicycling, or swimming (Hill & Wing, 2003).

5. Medications: OTC appetite suppressants are not helpful with long-term management of obesity. Although they do reduce appetite, tolerance and dependence are potentially dangerous side effects.

    a. Pharmacologic therapy

        i. Sibutramine: an appetite suppressant that has been used for long-term use, up to 1 year, and seems to enhance weight loss modestly when used with diet and lifestyle changes. It also may help promote weight control. However, in 2010, the U.S. Food and Drug Administration (FDA) removed sibutramine from the market because of clinical trial data indicating an increased risk of cardiovascular adverse events, including heart attack and stroke, in the studied population (Food and Drug Administration, 2010a).

        ii. Orlistat: a gastric lipase inhibitor, which reduces fat absorption by approximately 30%, is also approved for longer-term use, up to 1 year, and results in modest additional weight loss with diet and lifestyle change (Fabricatore & Wadden, 2003). The recommended dose is 120 mg three times daily. It is currently sold in lower doses (60 mg) OTC as Alli®. Typical side effects from Orlistat are primarily gastrointestinal including flatus, abdominal cramping, fecal incontinence and oily fecal staining. Absorption of fat soluble vitamins may be reduced with Orlistat use. Patients with a history of kidney stones should not be prescribed this medication. There have been rare reports of severe liver injury, including liver failure in patients taking Orlistat (FDA, 2010b). Clinicians should educate all patients taking Orlistat about the signs and symptoms of liver disease (FDA, 2010b).

    iii. Phentermine: the most commonly prescribed appetite suppressant because of low cost, phentermine is approved for only short-term use (≤ 12 weeks) due to potential for abuse. Side effects include increased blood pressure (Snow et al., 2005).

  b. Psychotropic medications, such as bupropion, fluoxetine, and sertraline, also have a short-term anorexic effect and can be helpful in treatment of individuals with coexisting depression. However, these medications are not approved for weight loss by the U.S. Food and Drug Administration (Snow et al., 2005).

  c. Investigational products (Nkansah, 2010)

    i. Bupropion/zonisamide (Empatic®): increases metabolism and suppresses appetite.

    ii. Bupropion/naltrexone (Contrave®): increases metabolism and counteracts body "starvation effect."

    iii. Phentermine/Topiramate (Qnexa®): increases metabolism and satiety.

    iv. Locaserin (no brand yet): selective serotonin 2C receptor agonist. Binds to receptors that regulate appetite.

6. Support groups, including family, friends, work-site support, and structured programs.

7. Cognitive–behavioral therapy for lifestyle modification can be a beneficial addition to a weight loss program.

B. *Follow-up is a critical aspect of success in a weight management program either individual or group-based with frequent visits in the beginning, then negotiated with the patient and their support system. Follow-up should include the following:*

1. Reinforcement of successes and review of difficulties and barriers to change

2. Reevaluation of motivation and degree of adherence

3. Reevaluation of the individual agreement or contract

C. *Bariatric surgery*

This type of treatment is known to be the most effective and intensive treatment for morbid obesity, with improvement noted of medical comorbidities, such as HTN, diabetes mellitus, dyslipidemia, sleep apnea, and gastroesophageal reflux disease. It is recommended for those who meet the surgical criteria and who have not been able to lose weight despite repeated attempts, or maintain weight loss with diet and exercise (Snow et al., 2005). Surgery may be appropriate for those who meet the medical screening criteria: BMI of greater than or equal to 40 or a BMI of 35–39.9 with serious health-related problems, such as diabetes or high blood pressure.

For patients considering weight loss surgery, the practitioner should perform a complete physical and thorough examination of the thyroid as part of the pretreatment evaluation. During this assessment, practitioners should focus on assessing the causes and complications of obesity, including family history of polycystic ovarian disease, hypothyroidism, and medications. The practitioner should screen for existing complications, such as type 2 diabetes, HTN, hyperlipidemia, atherosclerotic CVD, gallbladder disease, gout, cancers, osteoarthritis of the lower extremities, and sleep apnea. Baseline and diagnostic assessments should include electrolytes, liver function tests, complete blood count, total cholesterol, HDL and LDL cholesterol, triglycerides, thyroid function tests, and an electrocardiogram if a recent one is not available (NIH-NHLBI, 1998).

1. Other considerations

  a. Medical conditions that are contraindicated for bariatric surgery include end-stage lung disease, unstable CVD, multiorgan failure, and gastric varices.

  b. Psychiatric conditions with contraindications for weight loss surgery include current drug use, current heavy alcohol intake, active schizophrenia, severe intellectual disability, lack of knowledge regarding surgeries, and medical nonadherence (Bauchowitz et al., 2005).

2. Types of bariatric surgeries

  a. Roux-en-Y gastric bypass (RYGBP) is the most popular procedure in the United States (Baron, 2010). Performed both open and laparoscopically, RYGBP is restrictive and malabsorptive in nature. It provides changes in physiology that seem to effect and reset energy equilibrium. There is strong evidence to suggest that secretion of gastrointestinal hormones, such as grehlin, peptide tyrosine-tyrosine, and glucagon-like peptide-1, are altered by RYGBP helping to promote weight loss (Beckman, Beckman, & Earthman, 2010). Excess body weight loss is anticipated to be approximately 60–70%.

    b. Adjustable gastric banding is primarily restrictive in nature. Placement of a foreign body-band around the upper portion of the stomach creates a small stomach pouch. Based on weight loss and tolerance, this is then adjusted with "fills" to decrease the flow rate of food into the larger portion of stomach to provide a longer feeling of fullness. Anticipated excess body weight loss is approximately 50%.

    c. The biliopancreatic diversion with duodenal switch is primarily malabsorptive. Although expected excess body weight loss is anticipated at approximately 70%, the higher rates of severe side effects, such as diarrhea and nutritional deficiencies, make this surgery less frequently performed (Buchwald, 2005).

    d. Vertical sleeve gastrectomy is restrictive. It limits the volume of food in the stomach by creating a small pouch larger than that created by the lap band procedure. The procedure keeps the pylorus intact, and removes the remainder of the stomach.

3. Preoperative and postoperative care

    a. Diet and lifestyle modifications need to be reinforced.

    b. Medications must be evaluated at the time of surgery. With rapid weight loss, diabetes and antihypertensive medications need to be reduced or eliminated as needed (Pi-Sunyer & Nonas, 2004).

    c. All time-released medications (for RYGBP) and nonsteroidal anti-inflammatory drugs need to be evaluated for appropriateness. Typically to prevent bile sludge and stones, patients who still have a gallbladder are started on Ursodiol®.

    d. Discussion with the surgeon should include medication evaluation for change in delivery (e.g., crushed, liquid, or quartered).

    e. Referral should be made to a registered dietitian experienced with bariatric surgical patients for evaluation of diet and multivitamin and mineral requirement needs.

    f. In addition to surgical complications, multiple early complications need to be monitored for including dehydration, dumping syndrome, nausea and vomiting, and lactose intolerance. Late complications, depending on the type of surgery, may include a variety of vitamin and mineral deficiencies (thiamine, folate, vitamin D, vitamin B_{12}, other fat-soluble vitamins for biliopancreatic diversion with duodenal switch, calcium, and iron); gallstones; weight regain; and other surgical complications.

D. *Patient and family education: patient education and instruction should revolve around the following issues and topics:*

1. Multifactorial etiology of obesity and associated health risks

2. Diet and nutrition counseling with provision of specific caloric and portion information, including sample menus

3. Importance of exercise and physical activity scheduled into daily routine

4. Family involvement and participation and support

5. Patient expectation geared to slow weight loss over months.

VI. Self-management resources

A. *For on-line food record keeping, see the websites www.fitday.com and www.sparklepeople.com*

B. *For healthy nutrition and weight loss diets, see*

1. American Heart Association: www.americanheart.org. See the section "heart hub" for patients for healthy recipes, heart healthy tips, and risk calculators for heart disease

2. United States Department of Agriculture: www.mypyramid.gov. This site has resources on the food pyramid, healthy eating tips, and other nutrition information.

C. *For physical activity and exercise resources*

1. American College of Sports Medicine: www.acsm.org

2. American Heart Association: www.startmoving.org

3. Active at Any Size: http://win.niddk.nih.gov/publications/active.htm#activeat

4. NIA & NASA Exercise Guidelines: http://weboflife.ksc.nasa.gov/exerciseandaging/home.html

REFERENCES

Allison, D. B., Mentor, J. L., Heo, M., Chandler, L. P., Cappelleri, J. C., Infante, M. C., . . . Weiden, P. J. (1999). Antipsychotic-induced weight gain: A comprehensive research synthesis. *American Journal of Psychiatry, 156*(11), 1686–1696.

American Academy of Child and Adolescent Psychiatry. (2006). *Facts for families: Obesity in children and teens. No. 79, updated May 2008.* Retrieved from http://www.aacap.org/galleries/FactsForFamilies/79_obesity_in_children_and_teens.pdf

Aquila, R. (2002). Management of weight gain in patients with schizophrenia. *Journal of Clinical Psychiatry, 63* (Suppl. 4), 33–36.

Baron, R. (2010). Nutritional Disorders. In S. McPhee & M. Papadakis (Eds.), *2010 current medical diagnosis & treatment* (pp. 1136–1138). New York, NY: McGraw-Hill Companies.

Basson, B. R., Kinon, B. J., Taylor, C. C., Szymanski, K. A., Gilmore, J. A., & Tollefson, G. D. (2001). Factors influencing acute weight change in patients with schizophrenia treated with olanzapine, haloperidol, or risperidone. *Journal of Clinical Psychiatry, 62*, 231–238.

Bauchowitz, A. U., Gonder-Frederick, L. A., Olbrisch, M. E., Azarbad, L., Ryee, M. Y., Woodson, M., . . . Schirmer, B. (2005). Psychosocial evaluation of bariatric surgery candidates: A survey of present practices. *Psychosomatic Medicine, 67*(5), 825–832.

Beckman, L. M., Beckman, T. R., & Earthman, C. P. (2010). Changes in gastrointestinal hormones and leptin after roux-en-Y gastric bypass procedure: A review. *Journal of the American Dietetic Association, 110*, 571–584.

Boyd, M. A. (2002). Atypical antipsychotics: Impact on overall health and quality of life. *Journal of the American Psychiatric Nurses Association, 8*(4), 9–17.

Bray, G. A., & Champagne, C. M. (2005). Beyond Energy Balance: There Is More to Obesity than Kilocalories. *Journal of the American Dietetic Association, 105*:S17–S23.

Brownell, K. D. (2000). *The Learn Program for Weight Management 2000.* Dallas, TX: American Health Publishing Company.

Buchwald, H. (2005). Consensus Conference Statement Bariatric Surgery for Morbid Obesity: Health implication for patients, health professionals and third-party payers. *Journal of American College Surgery, 200*, 593–604.

Centers for Disease Control and Prevention. (2009a). Obesity prevalence among preschool aged children—United States, 1998–2008. *Morbidity and Mortality Weekly Review, 58*(28), 769–773. Retrieved from http://www.cdc.gov/mmwr/preview/mmwrhtml/mm5828a1.htm

Centers for Disease Control and Prevention. (Dec. 8, 2009b). Defining overweight and obesity. Retrieved from http://www.cdc.gov/obesity/defining.html

Centers for Disease Control and Prevention. (August 19, 2009c). Overweight and obesity: Health consequences. Retrieved from http://www.cdc.gov/obesity/causes/health.html

Centers for Disease Control and Prevention. (December 23, 2009d). Prevalence of overweight, obesity, and extreme obesity among adults: United States trends, 1960–1962 through 2005 and 2006. Retrieved from http://www.cdc.gov/nchs/data/hestat/overweight/overweight_adult.htm#table1

Fabricatore, A. N. (2007). Behavior therapy and cognitive-behavioral therapy of obesity: Is there a difference? *Journal of the American Dietetic Association, 107*, 92–99.

Fabricatore, A. N., & Wadden, T. A. (2003). Treatment of obesity: An overview. *Clinical Diabetes, 21*(2), 67–72.

Fontaine, K. R., Heo, M., Harrigan, E. P., Shear, C. L., Lakshminarayanon, M., Casey, D. E., . . . Allison, D. B. (2001). Estimating the consequences of anti-psychotic induced weight gain on health and mortality rates. *Psychiatry Research, 101*, 277–288.

Food and Drug Administration. (2010a). Retrieved from http://www.fda.gov/Drugs/DrugSafety/ucm228746.

Food and Drug Administration. (2010b). Retrieved from http://www.fda.gov/Drugs/DrugSafetyPostmarketDrugSafetyInformationforPatientsandProviders/ucm213038.htm

Gardner, C. D., Kiazand, A., Alhassan, S., Kim, S., Stafford, R. S., Balise, R. R., Kraemer, H. C., . . . King, A. C. (2007). Comparison of the Atkins, Zone, Ornish and LEARN diets for change in weight and related risk factors among overweight premenopausal women. The A to Z Weight Loss Study: A randomized trial. *Journal of the American Medical Association, 297*, 969–977.

Greenberg, I., Chan, S., & Blackburn, G. L. (1999). Nonpharmacologic and pharmacologic management of weight gain. *Journal of Clinical Psychiatry, 60*(Suppl. 21), 31–36.

Hill, J., & Wing, R. (2003). The National Weight Control Registry. *The Permanente Journal, Summer, 7*(3), 34–37.

Kanaya, A. M. (2010, February 26). Obesity, metabolic syndrome, and diabetes: Making the connections. Presented at the Obesity Summit 2010, University of California, San Francisco, California.

Mayo Foundation of Medical Education and Research. (1998–2011). *Gastric bypass surgery: Who is it for?* Retrieved from http://www.mayoclinic.com/health/gastric-bypass-surgery/WT00031

National Institutes of Health National Heart, Lung and Blood Institute. (1998). *The clinical guidelines on the identification, evaluations, and treatment of overweight and obesity in adult: The Evidence Report.* Retrieved from http://www.nhlgi.nin.gov/guidelines/obesity/e_txtbk/index.htm

Nkansah, N. (2010, February 26). Medications for obesity: Why no magic bullets? Presented at the Obesity Summit 2010, University of California, San Francisco, California.

Pi-Sunyer, F. X., & Nonas, C. A. (2004). Clinical monitoring. In G. D. Foster & C. A. Nonas (Eds.), *Managing obesity: A clinical guide* (Chapter 3, pp. 43–64). Chicago, IL: American Dietetic Association.

Prochaska, J., & DiClemente, C. C. (1982). Transtheoretical approach: Toward a more integrative model of change. *Psychotherapy: Theory, Research and Practice, 20*, 161.

Rummel-Kluge, C., Komossa, K., Schwarz, S., Hunger, H., Schmid, F., Lobos, C. A., . . . Leucht, S. (2010). Head-to-head comparisons of metabolic side effects of second generation antipsychotics in the treatment of schizophrenia: A systematic review and meta-analysis. *Schizophrenia Research, 123*, 225–233.

Sacks, F. M., Bray, G. A., Carey, V. J., Smith, S. R., Ryan, D. H., Anton, S. D, ... Williamson, D.A. (2009). Comparison of weight-loss diets with different compositions of fat, protein, and carbohydrates. *The New England Journal of Medicine, 360*, 859–873.

Snow, V., Barry, P., Fitterman, N., Qaseem, A., Weiss, K. & Clinical Efficacy Assessment Subcommittee of the American College of Physicians. (2005). Pharmacologic and surgical management of obesity in primary care: a clinical practice guideline from the American College of Physicians. *Annals of Internal Medicine, 142*(7), 525–531.

U.S. Department of Health and Human Services. (2000). *Healthy People 2010.* Objectives. Retrieved from http://www.healthypeople.gov/2010/?visit=1

U.S. Department of Health and Human Services. (2009). *Healthy People 2020 proposed objectives.* Retrieved from http://www.health.gov/healthypeople/

OSTEOARTHRITIS

Diane Putney and JoAnne M. Saxe

I. Introduction and general background

Universally, osteoarthritis (OA) is the most prevalent form of arthritis, with an estimated 800 million persons affected (Guermazi, 2009). In the United States alone, the range has been reported to be from 20–50 million, including over half of all adults older than age 65 (Lozada & Steigelfest, 2009). The economic burden imposed by the debilitating and functional sequelae of OA annually exceeds $120 million in the United States (Guermazi, 2009).

OA is a disease that affects the synovial joints, and ultimately results in the failure of a specific joint (Hunter, 2009a). The etiology of OA is multifactorial, the common denominator being any existing phenomena that contributes to pathologic intra-articular stress. Risk factors include female gender; obesity; increased age; congenital abnormalities in which skeletal misalignment predominates; the preexistence of inflammatory arthropathies (e.g., gout and rheumatoid arthritis [RA]); and in some instances race.

The pathophysiology of OA involves aberrant joint loading, and can also be caused by activity-related risk factors, such as previous isolated joint trauma; surgery; repetitive work-related trauma, such as prolonged kneeling on rigid surfaces; sport activities, particularly those involving running and cutting activities, such as soccer and tennis; and regular wearing of shoes with more than 1-in heels (Chambers, 2005; Iowa State University, 2010; Maly, 2008; Markenson, 2009).

The combination of these biomechanical stressors on the joint can lead to abnormal stress on joint physiology. This abnormal load can cause stress and damage to the structures of the entire joint. Chondrocytes, or cartilage cells, are especially vulnerable to damage over time. Cartilage is a four layer structure comprised of water and connective tissue. Focal ulcerations that form within the cartilage over time can accelerate cartilage loss and herald the formation of sclerosis, or thickening of the ends of bones; osteophyte (bone spur) formation; joint space narrowing; and the appearance of degenerative bone cysts. This series of events, all of which are thought to represent the body's physiologic attempts to mitigate joint damage, instead inevitably result in failure of the affected joint, and attendant pain and disability.

OA is conceptually divided into primary OA that has no known cause and secondary OA, which occurs as a result of specifically identifiable factors.

A. Primary osteoarthritis

1. Definition, overview, prevalence, and incidence: OA is considered to be primary when no clear predisposition or precipitating factors can be associated with its onset (Felson, 2007; Suszynski, 2009).

   Primary OA is associated with aging. The incidence of OA increases from 5% to 40% after the age of 65 (Quellette & Makowski, 2006). With advancing age, cartilage becomes stiffer and the gradual wear and tear on the soft tissue structures and subchondral bone leads to the release of the inflammatory proteins, cytokines and metalloproteinases into the joints (Rutgers, Saris, Dhert, & Creemers, 2010).

   The precise role that gender plays in the pathogenesis of OA remains unclear. The prevalence of OA is significantly greater in women over the age of 65 (Felson, 2007; Quellette & Makowski, 2006). Additionally, data from the Framingham Study noted an increased severity of disease and a greater number of affected joints in women (Harrington & Schneider, 2006; Quellette & Makowski, 2006). There is evidence that women are at significant risk for developing hand, knee, and hip OA with increasing severity after menopause (Mahajan, Tandon, Verma, & Sharma, 2005).

   The incidence of primary OA in certain joints, and specific locations within a joint, can vary with the race of the individual. Whites have the highest rates of OA, regardless of the involved joint (Felson, 2007).

   The extent to which heredity factors into the onset of OA has been rigorously studied in large populations of monozygotic and dizygotic twins, and nontwin groups of siblings (Doherty, 2004; Spector et al., 2006). Findings of these studies conclude that, if OA of the hand or knee is diagnosed in one sibling, the likelihood of their sibling acquiring the disease increased threefold (Hunter, 2009b; Quellette & Makowski, 2006).

B. Secondary OA

1. Definition, overview, prevalence, and incidence: Any osteoarthritic conditions that evolve from a known cause are characterized as secondary OA. The risk factors or causes of secondary OA can result from a singular instance of trauma or a confluence of biomechanical and physiologic insults, which cumulatively cause disease progression of a joint.

   Obesity significantly increases the likelihood of developing OA. This is especially true for large weight-bearing joints including the hips, knees, ankles, and feet (Felson, 2007; Schelbert, 2009). Weight excess always accounts for increased mechanical stress on all articular joint surfaces. Specifically, the risk of developing knee OA accelerates from 0.1 with a body mass index (BMI) of less than 20 kg/ml to 13.6 for a BMI of 36 kg/ml (Clark, 2007). Additionally, there is evidence that an overproduction of inflammatory compounds is produced in overweight persons, which may increase levels of pain (Clark, 2007; Schelbert, 2009).

   Congenital abnormalities, such as hip dysplasia, can produce misaligned and unstable joints, which eventually result in secondary OA (Brandt, Dieppe, & Radin, 2008; Clark, 2007). The associated malalignment, which can include either a varus ("bow-legged") or valgus ("knock-kneed") presentation, contributes to early onset arthritic changes in the knees, hips, or spine (Wilson, McWalker, & Johnston, 2008). These increased stressors are exacted by the loading forces across abnormal articular surfaces (Hunter, 2009).

   The relationship between mechanical trauma and the subsequent onset of OA has been established (Clark, 2007; Hunter, McDougall, & Keefe, 2008; Lozada & Steigelfest, 2009; Wilson et al., 2008). The specific trauma can result from a "prescribed" injury, such as surgery on a particular joint, and from deliberate and accidental insults (Fuller-Thompson & Brennenstuhl, 2009; Markenson, 2009). There is also evidence that excessive weight lifting, over time, is associated with earlier-onset OA in the shoulders, the lower spine, and knees (Kujala et al., 1995; Schumann et al., 2010).

   The preexistence of inflammatory arthropathies compounds the risk of developing OA (Harrington & Schneider, 2006; Lozada & Steigelfest, 2009). These conditions include chondrocalcinosis (also known as calcium phosphate deposition disease); RA; gout; and pseudo-gout. The inflammatory substances produced within the joints accelerate bony erosions, degeneration of cartilage, and the degradation of other soft tissue structures.

Fairly recent research implied a possible association of high bone mineral density to hip OA (Nevitt et al., 1995; Sowers et al., 1999; Zhang et al., 2000). However, later studies have indicated that the relationship between bone mineral density and OA is more complex than this association (Amin, 2002). The presence of osteoporosis in women who present with OA in the hand, for example, is statistically significant (Quellette & Makowski, 2006). The precise implications of the degree of bone mineral density and the relationship to OA remains speculative at best.

Persons with certain metabolic and pituitary diseases, such as acromegaly, Paget's disease, and hemochromatosis, have a greater likelihood of developing OA (Markenson, 2009) than individuals who do not have these conditions. Furthermore, limb immobilization and other conditions resulting in physical incapacity decrease joint stability, and the ability to absorb joint loading. When osteoarthritic pain (particularly seen with hip and knee OA) is inadequately controlled, the resultant disuse atrophy occurs approximately 40% more often than in healthy individuals (Bennell, Hunt, Wrigley, Boon-Whatt, & Hinman, 2009).

The incidence of hand OA is increased in persons with occupations that require the forceful and repetitive use of the thumb and fingers (Dillon, Peterson, & Tanaka, 2002). Additionally, nutrient and vitamin deficiencies during early childhood are risk factors for OA. Nutrients that are required for normal development and maintenance of healthy joints include calcium, vitamin D, phosphorus, protein, and zinc (Clark, 2007; Ilich & Kerstetter, 2000; O'Connor et al., 2008). An individual with a remote history of a joint infection is also at risk of acquiring OA in the respective joint (Lozada & Steigelfest, 2009).

II. Database (may include but is not limited to)

A. Subjective

1. Primary OA

   a. Past health history: unremarkable for trauma, surgery, infection, and other specific joint arthropathies.

   b. Family history: at least one sibling or a parent with a history of OA

   c. Occupational and environmental history: noncontributory

d. Personal and social history: noncontributory

e. Review of systems: Musculoskeletal (with the exception of musculoskeletal complaints, the symptoms review is usually unremarkable.)

   i. Joint pain dominates the symptom picture of OA and is the primary incentive for seeking treatment.

   ii. Exacerbated by activity, by prolonged standing, by walking up and down stairs and hills, by getting up out of a chair, and during cold and damp weather; relieved by rest. In advanced stages of the disease, particularly in large joints, joint pain interferes with sleep.

   iii. Described as not well localized, deep, aching, insidious onset. Pain characteristic of hip OA is located in the groin area and often radiating down the anterior aspect of the thigh.

   iv. Joint stiffness: generally occurs in the morning, evening, and after prolonged periods of sedentary activity; most often subsides after 10 minutes of activity.

   v. Decreased joint function inevitably takes a devastating toll on the individual's overall functional limitations, and results from decreased range of motion of the joint secondary to diminishing joint space.

   vi. Crackling in the joints that may or may not be painful, and occurs with movement of the joints, particularly in the shoulders, base of the thumbs, knees, and ankles.

   vii. Joint swelling that is typically worse in the evening.

   viii. Joint instability often described by the patient as "buckling" or "giving way" is a routine complaint of persons with knee OA. This is likely caused by a weak quadriceps femoris muscle.

   ix. Painful nodules on the dorsum of the proximal and distal interphalangeal joints of the fingers with OA of the hands.

2. Secondary OA

a. Past health history

   i. Medical illnesses

      a. RA

      b. Gout

      c. Pseudo-gout

      d. Congenital deformities

      e. Obesity

      f. Acromegaly

      g. Paget's disease

      h. Hemochromatosis

      i. Hypothyroidism

      j. Ehlers-Danlos syndrome

   ii. Surgical history on the affected joint

   iii. Obstetric and gynecological history: perimenopausal or postmenopausal

   iv. Exposure history: continuous exposure to oxidants (Felson, 2007).

   v. Medication history: systemic glucocorticoid use in the treatment of acute and chronic medical conditions. The deleterious effects of steroids on the skeletal system have been well-documented (Aaron & Ciomber, 2006). The most potentially devastating of these conditions is avascular necrosis (AVN), particularly of the femoral head.

   vi. Previous trauma to particular joints

      a. Isolated accidental

      b. History of domestic violence

      c. Repetitive trauma related to sports activities; occupational requirements; and certain religious practices, such as kneeling.

   vii. History of joint infection

   viii. Family history: noncontributory

   ix. Personal and social history

      a. Dietary

         i. Overconsumption of calories leading to obesity

         ii. Nutritional deficits necessary for optimal bone formation during infancy and early childhood

      b. Substance abuse: use of alcohol or recreational drugs increases the incidence of AVN in large joints, and subsequent advanced OA

   x. Occupational: jobs that require repetitive heavy lifting, kneeling, and deep squatting (Maly, 2008; Markenson, 2009).

   xi. Recreational: vigorous high-risk and contact sports that predispose one to frequent injury, involve running or cutting movements, and require heavy lifting.

   xii. Review of systems: systems to emphasize include

      a. Constitutional signs and symptoms: fever; chills; decreased when associated with other joint arthropathies, such as gout and RA

      b. Skin: complaints of erythema over joints when associated with other joint arthropathies or trauma

c. Musculoskeletal: see primary OA

d. Psychiatric: depression associated with increased functional limitations, chronic pain, or sleep disturbances

B. Objective

1. Physical examination

   a. General: body weight and BMI

   b. Musculoskeletal examination

      i. Inspection

         a. Mild to moderate erythema associated with recent trauma and inflammatory joint arthropathies

         b. Mild to severe effusions in any affected joints

         c. Bony deformities in the hands

            i. Heberden nodes over the dorsum of the distal interphalangeal joints

            ii. Bouchard nodes or bony enlargement of the metacarpal phalangeal joints, more often associated with mucinous cysts on the dorsum of the distal interphalangeal joints, proximal to the cuticles

            iii. Subluxation of the distal interphalangeal joints and metacarpal phalangeal joints. A positive shoulder sign can be noted in OA of the first carpometacarpal joint or the basilar joint of the thumb (Young, 2004).

            iv. Flexion contractures may occur in the elbows, fingers, hips, and knees.

            v. Muscle atrophy can be noted in association with any arthritic joint: deltoid, triceps, and biceps atrophy in shoulder OA; quadriceps and hamstring atrophy in hip and knee OA; calf atrophy in ankle OA.

      ii. Gait deformities

         a. Varus or bow-legged gait

         b. Valgus or knock-kneed gait

         c. Antalgic, characterized by a limp resulting from a shortened phase of a step on the affected side of a weight-bearing joint.

         d. Positive Trendelenburg occurs when the standing patient is asked to place all their weight on the affected side at which point their hip buckles. This finding is associated with hip OA.

      iii. Range of motion: can be decreased in any arthritic joint. Routine documentation of the affected joint range of motion is an objective measure of the patient's progress, or lack thereof.

         a. Specific joint measurements are made with an instrument called a goniometer. When measuring hinge joints, note degree of flexion and extension; for ball and socket joints, note degree of internal and external rotation.

         b. The range of motion measurements should be specified as either active (demonstrates the patient's own limits), or passive (the examiner forces the joint past the patient's self-designated limits).

      iv. Palpation

         a. Joint line tenderness

         b. Crepitus noted with passive range of motion and palpation of affected joints

         c. Instability can be noted when applying a lateral or medial force to the joint

2. Supporting data from relevant diagnostic tests

   a. Laboratory studies: there are no abnormal laboratory tests in either blood or synovial fluid that are typically associated with OA. However, there are certain laboratory tests that can be ordered to exclude the existence of other pathology in the osteoarthritic joint.

      i. Blood tests may include: complete blood count with differential to assess for infection or anemia of chronic disease, uric acid level to determine the probability of gout, rheumatoid factor to rule out RA, antinuclear antibody to aid in the determination of systemic lupus erythematosus, and erythrocyte sedimentation rate or C-reactive protein to confirm the presence of systemic inflammation.

      ii. Joint aspiration may be performed by the clinician to obtain synovial fluid for analysis. The synovial fluid analysis is requested to detect the presence of crystals and glucose. A cell count is typically ordered, in addition to a culture and sensitivity, and a Gram stain.

   b. Imaging studies

      i. Radiographs continue to be the standard measure used to confirm the presence of osteoarthritic changes in a particular joint. Radiographs are relatively inexpensive and universally available as a diagnostic tool. The specific quantities and type of radiograph views obtained are indicated by the particular joints involved. The compendium of degenerative changes used to confirm the diagnosis of OA, including subchondral sclerosis, cysts, osteophytes, loose bodies, and joint space narrowing, are almost always clearly visible on radiographs. In addition, radiographs are often sufficient to exclude the presence of other bony lesions, such as osteochondritis dessicans, osteonecrosis or AVN, fractures, and even certain bone tumors.

a. Osteophyte formation or the presence of bony growths along the joint space margins

b. Subchondral sclerosis: increased density at the ends of the bones, which is demonstrated by a bright white appearance on radiographs.

c. Degenerative cysts: small, translucent-appearing, areas of fluid-filled bone along the joint margins.

d. Joint space narrowing is a measure of the degree to which the intra-articular cartilage has degenerated. This is the radiographic finding most associated with pain. Joint space narrowing, when present, can range from mild to bone-on-bone in the most advanced cases.

e. Subluxation or malalignment of the joint is a typical finding in advanced OA.

f. Loose bodies are calcified pieces of cartilage or free-floating osteophytes that are sometimes identified either in or around synovial joints. Sometimes these can cause mechanical symptoms referred to as "locking" or "buckling," especially in the knee. Otherwise, their mere presence is without clinical significance.

g. Chondrocalcinosis can be visualized within the joint spaces as white lines that vary from faint to quite thick and chalk-like in appearance.

ii. Magnetic resonance imaging (MRI) has limited use for the actual diagnosis and therapeutic management of OA. An MRI may be indicated in the following situations

a. The radiographs are within normal limits, the diagnosis is uncertain, and the indicated therapeutic management of the condition would be affected.

b. To exclude the presence of a potentially ominous systemic abnormality.

c. The appearance of a suspicious bone lesion, which requires further study.

c. The use of computerized tomography is not routine in the diagnostic work-up of OA. Computerized tomography is considered to be superior to an MRI to assess bony alignment or the extent to which a fracture may be displaced.

d. Bone scans are occasionally used to rule out the presence, location, and extent of disease in a particular joint when not observable on radiographs.

e. Ultrasonography is sometimes ordered by primary care providers to evaluate soft tissue masses in and around joints. It is not unusual for a person with OA in the knee to complain of a "lump" in the back of their knee, which can be associated with posterior calf pain. The ultrasound confirms the diagnosis of a popliteal cyst, a benign fluid collection in the back of the knee, often associated with OA or meniscal pathology, and excludes the presence of a deep vein thrombosis, which requires urgent treatment.

III. Assessment

A. Determine the diagnosis

1. Primary OA

   The American College of Rheumatology has formulated criteria for the diagnosis of primary OA in the hands, hips, and knees only (see arc@rheumatology.org)

2. Secondary OA

3. Rule out the following conditions

   a. RA

   b. Gout

   c. Meniscal injury

   d. AVN

   e. Osteochondritis dissecans

   f. Calcium phosphate deposition disease

4. Ultimately, the diagnosis of OA is based on
   a. Patient history
   b. Physical examination
   c. Radiographs in concert with the previously mentioned details.

B. *Severity of OA is determined by the patient's overall level of functional disability*

C. *Significance of the patient's symptoms can best be determined by inquiring as to the following*

1. The limitations imposed on ability to function at home, at work, and in pursuit of satisfying recreational activities.

2. The measures, if any, the patient has taken to control or avoid pain.

D. *Overall functional capacity and motivation to follow the treatment plan must be determined with consideration given to the following*

1. Involvement of family and significant others and a social support system

2. The ease to which the patient can establish and maintain access to the resources (e.g., financial support and transportation) required to pursue adequate treatment.

3. Emotional status

IV. Goals of clinical management

A. *Screening and diagnosing OA*

1. There are presently no clinical indications to screen for OA. However, there is a case to be made for screening in childhood for the identification of risk factors, such as obesity and certain gait deformities, which may predispose one to the development of OA.

2. Plain radiographs continue to be the preferred and cost-effective diagnostic test for confirming the presence of OA, but are not universally necessary to make the diagnosis.

B. *Treatment: the goals of treatment are*

1. Pain control

2. Control of the factors that can inhibit disease progression

3. Advancement of the patient's tolerance for functional activities to their maximal level.

C. *Patient compliance*
The patient's ability to adhere to their treatment must be assessed on a continual basis.

V. Plan

A. *Diagnostic tests*

1. Imaging studies: radiographs. See Table 63-1 for recommended views of the specific affected joints

2. An MRI should be considered for further examination of
   a. Suspicious bony lesions
   b. Normal radiographs with a history and physical examination suspicious for meniscal injury
   c. Severe unexplained pain, normal radiographs, inconsistent or unremarkable examination findings

3. Synovial fluid examination is indicated when the patient has a joint effusion that is suspicious for infection. Joint aspiration and synovial fluid analysis should also be performed when the patient has sudden onset, severe, unexplained joint pain, absence of an effusion, and risk factors for infection, including diabetes. Tests may include cell count, glucose, crystals, Gram stain, and culture and sensitivity.

4. Serology tests should be obtained when there is polyarticular involvement or the presentation of a joint effusion that is suspicious for
   a. Infection.
      i. Complete blood count with differential, erythrocyte sedimentation rate, and C-reactive protein
   b. Inflammatory arthropathies
      i. Gout: uric acid level
      ii. RA: rheumatoid factor
      iii. Systemic lupus erythematosis: antinuclear antibody and erythrocyte sedimentation rate
      iv. Polymyalgia rheumatica: erythrocyte sedimentation rate
   c. Thyroid-stimulating hormone should be considered when the patient presents with multiple joint effusions and normal radiographs

B. *Management (includes treatment, consultation, indications for referral, and follow-up care)*

1. Pain management: medications and supplements
   a. Acetaminophen (Tylenol®) remains the American College of Rheumatology's (2000)

TABLE 63-1 Standard Radiograph Views and Special Views

Location	Standard Radiograph Views	Special Views*
Cervical spine	Anterior/posterior, lateral	Flexion/extension
Shoulder	Anterior/posterior, transcapular/lateral, axillary view	Anterior/posterior of the glenohumeral joint, scapular view, acromio-clavicular joint, sternoclavicular joint
Elbow	Anterior/posterior, lateral, oblique	Axial view
Wrist	Anterior/posterior, lateral, oblique, scaphoid	"Clenched fist" views
Hand	Anterior/posterior, lateral, oblique	Stress views of the first carpalmetacarpal joint
Lumbar spine	Anterior/posterior, lateral	Oblique, flexion/extension views
Hip	Anterior/posterior pelvis, lateral	Oblique or judet view
Knee	Bilateral anterior/posterior weight-bearing, lateral, bilateral merchant's views	Notch view
Ankle	Anterior/posterior, lateral, mortise view	Stress views
Foot	Anterior/posterior, lateral, oblique	Anterior/posterior weight-bearing, sesamoid view, calcaneal view

* Ordered in consultation with an orthopedic surgeon.

recommended first-line medication for OA. Dose: up to 650–1,000 mg four times a day, not to exceed 4 g in 24 hours.

b. Nonsteroidal anti-inflammatory drugs (NSAIDs), nonselective
   i. Considered to be the mainstay of systemic treatment for OA.
   ii. In general, the use of NSAIDs to alleviate the pain of OA results in an average of 30% pain relief with a 15% improvement in function.
   iii. Contraindicated in persons taking anticoagulant medication, sensitivity or allergy to NSAIDs, and history of bariatric surgery.
   iv. Should be prescribed with caution in persons with hypertension, a history of stroke, and myocardial infarction. Arterial blood pressure begins to increase within several weeks of beginning treatment with NSAIDs because of prostaglandin inhibition. It is the increase in systolic blood pressure that precipitates cardiovascular events associated with NSAIDs (Antman et al., 2007; Friedewald, Bennet, Packer, Roberts, & Williams, 2008; Risser, Donavan, Heintzman, & Page, 2009).
   v. Naproxen (Naprosyn®) presents the lowest risk of cardiovascular events among the NSAIDs (Chan, Abraham, Scheiman, & Laine, 2008).

c. Cyclooxygenase (COX)-2 selective inhibitors
   i. The use of COX-2 has decreased dramatically since 2004 when their significant association with increased cardiovascular events was widely reported.
   ii. Celecoxib (Celebrex®) is currently the only COX-2 available for use to control OA pain.
   iii. Studies to date have demonstrated that selective COX-2 may have cartilage-protective effects (Ding, Cituttini, & Jones, 2009).
   iv. The indications for prescribing Celebrex® include
      a. Treatment failures with other medications
      b. The patient has no known cardiovascular disease
      c. The patient is on anticoagulant therapy
   v. The appeal of these medications, despite the cardiovascular risks, is that COX-2 are less likely to cause gastrointestinal bleeding than other NSAIDs.

d. Opioids
   i. The use of opioids for moderate to severe pain control from chronic degenerative conditions, such as OA, has increased substantially over the past three decades. Overall, patients who take opioids for OA report an improvement of less than 35%

in pain control and only a 29% increase in their ability to function (Nuesch, Rutjes, Husni, Welch, & Juni, 2009).

   ii. The indications for opioid use for the control of chronic, nonmalignant pain may include

      a. Advanced stages of OA when pain interferes with sleep.

      b. When acetaminophen, NSAIDs, corticosteroids, and all other reasonable nonoperative treatments have failed to adequately control pain and the patient is not a candidate for surgery.

   iii. The analgesic effects of opioids result from a combination of

      a. Decreasing the perception of pain

      b. Minimizing the reaction to pain

      c. Increasing pain tolerance

   iv. The most common adverse effects of opioids include nausea and vomiting, constipation, and drowsiness

   v. Tolerance, dependence, and addiction are considerations when prescribing opioids for chronic pain. The prevailing expert opinion is that opiate addiction is not significantly higher among patients with chronic, nonmalignant pain. However, a review of the literature reveals these opinions are not generally based on rigorous study (Littlejohn, Baldacchino, & Bannister, 2004).

   vi. The most frequently prescribed opioids for control of arthritic pain are Vicodin® (hydrocodone); acetaminophen with codeine #3 or #4; and oxycodone.

   vii. Dosing needs to be titrated based on the patient's response to the medication (see Chapter 48, Chronic Pain Management)

  e. Topical treatments

   i. Nonprescription

      a. Capsaicin cream when applied to the skin overlying a painful arthritic joint decreases the amounts of "substance P," which exacerbates inflammation. Pain relief begins within a week of beginning treatment.

      b. Bengay® and Tiger Balm® are heating rubs containing camphor and menthol. Heating rubs, to the extent to which they are effective in alleviating arthritic pain, work by "camouflaging" the pain sensation in the peripheral nerve endings.

      c. The most effective nonpharmacologic topical treatment continues to be either ice packs for a total of 25 minutes or a 10-minute application of moist heat immediately followed by an ice pack for 25 minutes.

   ii. Prescription

      a. Diclofenac gel 1% is the only topical NSAID to receive Federal Drug Administration approval (as of 2007). It has been found to be effective in OA of the hands and knees. Typical dosing is between 2 and 4 g to the affected joint, to a maximum of four times a day (Altman, 2009).

      b. Lidocaine patches 5% have been used with some limited success for the relief of OA pain. Typical dosing is one to three patches over the affected joint, one time within a 24-hour period, for up to 12 hours.

      c. Phonophoresis is a treatment in which a steroid gel, typically flucinonide (Lidex®), is administered topically directly over the affected joint by a physical or occupational therapist. The treatments are typically administered every other day, for a 5- to 8-minute duration, over a 3- to 4-week period.

  f. Corticosteroids

   i. The periodic and regular use of intra-articular steroid injections has remained a very effective treatment for OA over the past 60 years.

   ii. Steroid injections can be safely administered by trained clinicians approximately every 3–4 months, as needed, for pain.

   iii. Although the potential atrophy of soft tissue structures can occur after the administration of nonarticular steroid injections, there is no evidence that corticosteroids hasten joint degradation.

   iv. The dose of the steroid depends on the size of the joint and can range from 3–5 mg of Kenalog® in certain finger joints, to 40 mg in the knee or hip.

   v. The most common reported side effects of a steroid injection include

      a. Postinjection soreness lasting from several hours to 1 week

      b. Occasional facial flushing, which subsides within 24 hours

      c. Temporary blood glucose elevation in the patient with diabetes for up to a week following the injection

g. Viscosupplementation

i. Synthetic versions comprising synovial fluid injected into an arthritic joint have become an armament in conventional OA treatment in the United States.

ii. The use of viscosupplements is approved by the Food and Drug Administration for use in the treatment of knee OA. Trials in the glenohumeral joint, hip, ankle, wrist, and finger joints have been less promising.

iii. Criteria for treatment includes

a. Moderate to severe knee pain

b. The patient has failed to benefit from other reasonable treatment, including steroid injections

c. The patient is not an appropriate candidate for knee arthroplasty

d. The patient has no known sensitivity to hyaluronans, poultry, and egg products

iv. There are approximately 10 different preparations of injectable viscosupplements on the market, two of which are predominately used in the United States: sodium hyaluronate (Supartz®) and hylan G-F 20 (Synvisc®)

v. Important considerations when prescribing treatment with viscosupplementation include

a. It is expensive, with wholesale price of approximately $500 for one series of the necessary three to five injections.

b. Treatment usually requires a referral to the orthopedic or rheumatology department.

c. It takes an average of 2–10 weeks for treatments to become effective in ameliorating pain.

d. The extent to which viscosupplementation is effective in decreasing the pain associated with knee OA has become a subject of intense debate between orthopedic surgeons and nonoperative providers. In general, it is agreed that viscosupplementation is more effective than placebo, and can result in approximately 6 months of satisfactory relief (Das & Neher, 2009).

e. The most common side effect following the administration of hyaluronate acid preparations is occasional postinjection soreness, which although severe, is not injurious, and is likely to subside within several days.

f. When effective, Supartz® or Synvisc® can be administered every 6 months, as indicated.

g. Oral supplements used for controlling OA-related pain: oral supplements do not require a prescription and are easily obtained by the consumer. The considerable cost of these supplements, in addition to the lack of oversight by the FDA, are factors to be considered by the provider when counseling the OA patient regarding alternative treatments (see Table 63-2). For additional information related to herbal and dietary supplements, visit the University of Maryland Medical Center (2009) website at http ://www.umm.edu/altmed/articles /osteoarthritis-000118.htm

h. Acupuncture: there are some studies that have demonstrated the benefits of treating chronic pain from OA with acupuncture (Markenson, 2009; Martin, 2006). It is frequently requested by patients with varying degrees of pain.

i. Transcutaneous nerve stimulation: it is usually the physical therapist who instructs the patient with chronic pain on the use of a transcutaneous nerve stimulation unit. There is some evidence that this treatment reduces arthritic pain occurring at rest.

2. Weight management

The deleterious effects of excess weight on weight-bearing joints and subsequent enhanced risk of developing knee and hip OA cannot be overstated. The risk of acquiring knee OA in persons with a BMI of 36 kg/m compared to those with a BMI of 20 kg/m or less are 14-fold. There are convincing data that demonstrate that the need for total knee arthroplasty would be reduced by 25% if the obese individual reduces their BMI to within normal range (18.5–25 kg/m) (Clark, 2007). Maintaining a nutritionally balanced diet with a prescribed caloric regimen results in decreasing inflammation in the joints and the body fat, which significantly compounds the mechanical stress on joints. A daily exercise program is an essential component of weight management.

a. Non–weight-bearing aerobic exercise, such as swimming, biking, and rowing, is generally

TABLE 63-2 Oral Supplements Used for Controlling OA-Related Pain*

Oral Supplement	Recommended Dosage	Side Effects	Comments
Glucosamine sulfate	1,500 mg/day	Mild, transient side effects, such as nausea and skin irritations, have been reported	Widely used. A study published in the *New England Journal of Medicine* in 2006 reported this preparation seemed to benefit a subgroup of persons with moderate to severe OA pain. However, the same study concluded it did not decrease OA pain, overall (Martin, 2006).
Chondroitin sulfate	1,200 mg/day		
Methylsulfonylmethane (MSM)	3 g twice a day		Odorless, tasteless sulfur compound that may reduce inflammation associated with arthritic joints. This supplement has not been studied as rigorously as glucosamine and chondroitin (Kim et al., 2005).
S-Adenosyl-l-methionine (SAMe)	800–1,200 mg/day		Reportedly has been useful in reducing OA pain by prostoeglycan synthesis and reducing inflammation (Nierenberg, 2009).
Omega-3 fatty acids	1 tbsp or 444 mg daily		Provides an anti-inflammatory effect in the treatment of OA (Leong, 2009).
Avocado soybean unsaponifiables (ASUs)	300 mg/day		In the form of natural vegetable extracts, has been used in the treatment of OA since the 1980s and has been shown to reduce inflammation, and according to at least one study actually inhibit the progression of joint degeneration (Capoor, 2005; Wei, 2004).
Hyaluronic acid	80 mg/day		Persons with an allergy to poultry products should be allergy-tested for sensitivity to hyalurons before initiating this treatment (Kallen, 2008).
Vitamin D	400–2,000 IU/day		Has preventative benefits with respect to OA. Chronic vitamin D deficiency is known to be a risk factor in the onset OA (Nierenberg, 2009).
Bromelain	250 mg twice a day		An enzyme found in pineapples, has anti-inflammatory properties. There is some indication that bromelain increases bleeding time. Patients on anticoagulant medication should consult with their primary care provider before beginning treatment. Patients with a history of peptic ulcer disease should also avoid bromelain (Meschino, 2001).
Collagen hydrolysate	5–7 g/day		A protein supplement that contains high levels glycene and praline, two amino acids essential for cartilage regeneration. This product decreases OA pain in about 70% of persons in trials within 6 months of beginning treatment (McAlindon, 2007).

* Despite the abundance of research cited in the literature on alternative treatments for OA, not one of these supplements has been proved to unequivocally alleviate pain or hinder the progression of disease as noted on a radiograph.

better tolerated by persons with OA in weight-bearing joints.

b. Walking is a low-impact form of exercise when done on level ground. Softer surfaces, such as dirt, sand, and grass, are more joint friendly than concrete and gravel.

c. The recommendation for achieving and maintaining weight loss consistent with a normal BMI is 60 minutes of sustained aerobic activity a day.

3. Nutrition and dietary considerations for the person with OA

    a. Consensus in the medical community with respect to specific dietary recommendations for the prevention and treatment of OA is confined to the inclusion of foods that contain the following

        i. Calcium: sardines and sesame seeds

        ii. Vitamin D: breakfast cereals, eggs, and legumes

        iii. Phosphorus: citrus fruits; dark yellow, green, and red fruits and vegetables

        iv. Protein: meat, fish, legumes, nuts, seeds, and eggs

        v. Zinc: lean red meat, pork, dark poultry meat, and whole grains (Clark, 2007).

    b. In general, medical experts in the area of the nutritional impact on bone and joint health admit there is not one particular diet to which all affected persons must conform (Parker-Pope, 2005). Rather, people are encouraged to simply make note of a particular food substance that exacerbated their symptoms.

    c. Dietary recommendations among contemporary researchers and healthcare practitioners advocate the importance of foods that reduce inflammation by promoting prostaglandins in the body. The typical list of these foods includes

        i. Foods containing omega-3 fatty acids, such as fish, flax seed, walnuts, and olive oil.

        ii. Fresh fruits and vegetables and whole grains that contain omega-6 fatty acids prevalent in plant oils.

        iii. Foods enriched with vitamin K contained in blackstrap molasses, alfalfa, and spinach (Balch, 2002)

    d. Foods that are considered to be inflammatory are

        i. Red meat (lean red meat contains high levels of zinc, which promotes bone health)

        ii. Dairy products

        iii. Polyunsaturated vegetable oils, such as safflower, sunflower, soy, peanut, and corn (Nierenberg, 2009)

        iv. Refined and processed foods containing white flour and white sugar

        v. Alcohol

        vi. Caffeine (Clark, 2007; Hsu-LeBlanc, 2010; Nierenberg, 2009).

4. Maintenance of maximum functioning and appropriate activity levels.

    a. Physical therapy

        i. Physical therapy is considered an essential first-line treatment for OA. Maintaining adherence to a physical therapy program for patients with significant pain can be very challenging. Adequate pain control is an important factor in adherence. In this regard, it is important to note that the type of strengthening exercise (i.e., whether isometric [when the joint or muscle is worked against resistance while static], isotonic [consistent tension during muscle-lengthening movements], or isokinetic [uses an apparatus to provide resistance during a consistent speed]), does not affect the clinical outcomes (Bennell et al., 2009).

        ii. The goals of physical therapy for the OA patient include

            a. Increasing range of motion and joint flexibility

            b. Improving the strength of major muscle groups with the desired result based on

                i. Training intensity, a byproduct of the degree of resistance and frequency

                ii. Patient compliance

                iii. Training specificity

        iii. Enhancing proprioceptive activity. The achieved benefits of physical therapy do not persist after the cessation of the regimen and have completely resolved after a period of between 3 and 6 months.

            a. Yoga has been embraced by the orthopedic community as a treatment alternative that is known to improve joint range of motion, increase large muscle mass strength, and result in significant pain reduction in the OA patient.

            b. Tai Chi, which has long been practiced in China, is recommended for patients with OA in weight-bearing joints. Data from recent studies have revealed that the benefits, similar to those seen with Yoga, have been significant for patients with hip and knee OA after 3 months of practice (Stanos, McLean, & Rader, 2007; Wang et al., 2009).

c. Assistive devices: the purpose of this aspect of treatment in OA is to alter joint biomechanics to the extent that they limit exposure to painful mechanical stresses (Wilson, McWalker, & Johnston, 2008). However, a note of caution is warranted when prescribing immobilizing splints for painful arthritic joints. When a joint is continuously immobilized, there is the inevitable soft tissue atrophy, and the onset of osteoporosis. Therefore, immobilizing splints should only be worn at night and not to avoid pain with activity during waking hours.

  i. Splints can be prescribed to stabilize or immobilize a particular joint, which is generally not indicated for OA. The exception is OA of the basilar joint of the thumb where hypermobility or instability of the joint is the primary cause of the pain. Carpometacarpal splints can be prescribed for the patient in the over-the-counter form. The splints can also be custom-made by a certified hand therapist.

  ii. Braces are often self-prescribed by the patient with knee OA and are made in a variety of styles.

   a. Elastic knee sleeves have no medical basis for use, other than most patients who wear them insist their knees "feel better" as a result. This benefit may be related to increased proprioception from the device, which is otherwise harmless.

   b. Unloader braces are mechanical devices for the severely arthritic, unstable knee that are designed to shift the load on the joint from the more severely affected side (as determined by the extent of either medial or lateral joint space narrowing) to the less affected side. These devices can be somewhat heavy and cumbersome for the patient. The amount of loading force required to shift the body weight is sometimes difficult for the patient to tolerate. These braces can be obtained "off the shelf" or may be custom-fit by an orthotist.

   c. Patients with ankle OA can benefit from relatively inexpensive devices, which include the use of an air cast or a Swedo® ankle support. Over-the-counter orthotics or arch supports benefit patients with back, hip, knee, ankle, and foot OA. Arch supports help relieve pain and improve posture by more adaptively redistributing body weight across otherwise malaligned weight-bearing joints.

  iii. Lateral or medial heel wedges can be prescribed for patients with knee OA resulting in a valgus or varus gait, respectively.

  iv. The use of a cane for someone with either hip or knee OA can reduce the loading force on the affected limb by up to 75%.

5. Indications for referral to

  a. An orthopedic surgeon are when

   i. The patient has at least moderate to advanced degenerative changes in the symptomatic joint from which the patient suffers pain and disability that interferes with the quality of their life.

   ii. The patient has tried and no longer benefits from all reasonable nonoperative treatment and is a candidate for either joint fusion or arthroplasty.

   iii. The patient meets the first two criteria and is medically stable enough to undergo joint replacement surgery.

iv. The patient has mild to moderate degenerative changes; does not meet the criteria for arthroplasty, joint fusion, or osteotomy; but has failed all reasonable nonoperative treatment to date.

b. A rheumatologist when there is
   i. Polyarticular involvement.
   ii. A reasonable index of suspicion for RA or Polymyalgia rheumatica
   iii. A questionable diagnosis.
   iv. A need for more expert evaluation and management of complex medication regimens arise (Markenson, 2009).

c. A bariatric surgeon when the patient meets the criteria for a hip or knee arthroplasty but is morbidly obese and has been unable to achieve weight loss with conventional weight-management programs.

d. A nutritionist when the patient has OA in weight-bearing joints and obesity and would benefit from dietary counseling.

e. A chronic pain program when the patient is not an appropriate candidate for surgery, has tried and failed to obtain adequately sustained relief from all reasonable nonoperative treatment, and is requiring increasing levels of opioids to manage their pain.

f. A mental health professional when the patient presents with signs and symptoms of depression, which is interfering with their ability to cope with the physical limitations of their disease.

C. Patient education

1. Determine the client's expectations with respect to their disease process and treatment options as a focal point for providing relevant information.

2. Review the patient's radiographs with the patient while explaining the course of the disease. The patient's opportunity to view their own images of the affected joint with their provider is a powerful opportunity for the patient to cultivate a fundamental understanding of the implications of the disease with respect to recommended treatment.

3. Reinforce what you have discussed with the patient with concise, printed materials, which includes illustrations of the affected joints.

4. Provide the patient with a logical, progressive treatment plan for the problems at hand. This assists the patient in maintaining reasonable expectations regarding available treatment for OA, and maintaining a perspective about the vicissitudes of chronic disease. It is an important aspect of reinforcing the patient's coping skills when they can anticipate another treatment option of their return visit, if they have failed to respond to the current interventions.

5. The patient is entitled to explanations about the indications, or lack thereof, for ordering diagnostic tests. The provider may spend considerable time reassuring the patient that there is no need to obtain an MRI of their arthritic knee to satisfy their desire to "find out what is really going on," when the purpose of these tests is elucidated.

6. The provider should make a point of acknowledging the patient's progress in achieving short-term treatment goals, in addition to reemphasizing the untoward consequences of nonadherence with treatment to which the patient agreed.

7. Before arranging consultation with an orthopedic surgeon, it is essential to educate the patient about the surgery for which they are to be considered. The patient should be given as much specific and practical information as they can assimilate. Advise the patient to bring interested significant others to the consultation.

VI. Self-management resources and tools

A. Weight-management websites

1. Weight Control Information Network, http://www.win.niddk.nih.gov/

2. Nutrition.gov

3. WeightWatchers.com

4. Weight Management: Consumers: Food & Nutrition Information center, http://fnic.nal.usda.gov/nal_display/index.php?info_center=4&tax_level=1

5. Partners In Weight Management, http://www.partnersinweightmanagement.com/

B. General information on OA

1. Rheumatology.org

2. Osteoarthritis.about.com

3. Arthritis.org

4. Healthlinkusa.com/Osteoarthritis.html

5. Preventarthritis.org

6. Arthritis Foundation@arthritis.org

7. American Academy of Orthopedic Surgeons: AAOS .org

8. The National Institute of Arthritis & Musculo-skeletal & Skin Diseases: niammsinfo@mail.nih .gov

C. Tips for accessing community resources for persons with OA

1. A number of community hospitals and recreational centers offer therapeutic aquatic exercise programs for persons with physical disabilities that are relatively inexpensive. The instructors are typically physical therapists. Certification from the primary provider that the person is medically stable and would benefit from such a program is a prerequisite for participation in these programs.

2. Community colleges frequently offer adaptive physical education classes for persons with physical limitations. These classes provide a therapeutic, nonthreatening learning environment for the person with OA to push the perceived boundaries of the physical limitations imposed by their disease.

3. Disability.gov directs the patient to a compendium of community resources pertaining to transportation issues for persons with physical limitations and disabilities.

VII. Acknowledgments

N. P. Putney extends a special thanks to James Johnson, MD, Michael MacAvoy, MD, Elizabeth Watson, MD, Lawrance Wells, MD, George Janku, MD, Christopher Lehman, MD, and Sandy Jones, PNP, for mentoring her throughout her career in orthopedic surgery.

REFERENCES

Aaron, R. K., & Ciomber, D. M. (2006). Orthopedic complications of solid organ transplantation. *Surgical Clinics of North America, 86*(5), 1237–1255.

Altman, D. (2009). Practical consideration for the pharmacologic management of osteoarthritis. *American Journal of Managed Care, 15*(8), 236–241.

American College of Rheumatology Subcommittee on Osteoarthritis Guidelines. (2000). *Recommendations for the medical management of osteoarthritis of the hip and knee.* Retrieved from http://www.rheumatology.org/practice/clinical/guidelines/oa-mgmt.asp

Amin, S. (2002). Osteoarthritis and bone mineral density. *The Journal of Rheumatology, 29*(7), 1348–1349.

Antman, E., Bennet, J., Daugherty, A., Furburg, C., Roberts, H., & Taubert, K. (2007). *Use of nonsteroidal anti-inflammatory drugs: An update for clinicians.* A Scientific statement from the American Heart Association. Retrieved from http://www.circulationaha.org

Balch, P. (2002). *Prescription for herbal healing.* New York, NY: Penguin Putnam, Inc.

Bennell, K. L., Hunt, M. A., Wrigley, T. V., Boon-Whatt, L., & Hinman, R. S. (2009). Muscle and exercise in the prevention and management of knee osteoarthritis: An internal medicine specialist's guide. *Medical Clinics of North America, 93*(1), 161–177.

Brandt, K. D., Dieppe, P., & Radin, E. L. (2008). Etiopathogenesis of osteoarthritis. *Rheumatic Disease Clinics of North America, 34*(3), 1–24.

Capoor, M. (2005). Avocado-soybean unsaponifiables (ASU). *Arthritis MD.* Retrieved from http://www.arthritismd.com/avocado-soybean-unsaponifiables.html

Chambers, A. (2005). The role of sports activity in osteoarthritis. *Arthritis MD.* Retrieved from http://www.arthritismd.com/osteoarthritis-sports-activity-html

Chan, F., Abraham, N., Scheiman, J., & Laine, L. (2008). Management of patients on nonsteroidal anti-inflammatory drugs: Clinical practice recommendation from the first international working party on gastrointestinal and cardiovascular effects of nonsteroidal anti-inflammatory drugs and anti-platelet agents. *American Journal of Gastroenterology, 103,* 2908–2918.

Clark, K. L. (2007). Nutritional considerations in joint health. *Clinics in Sports Medicine, 26*(1), 101–118.

Das, A., & Neher, J. (2009). Do hyaluronic acid injections relieve OA knee pain? *The Journal of Family Practice, 58*(5), 281c,d,e.

Dillon, C., Peterson, M., & Tanaka, S. (2002). Self-reported hand and wrist arthritis and occupation. *American Journal of Industrial Medicine, 42*(4), 318–327.

Ding, C., Cituttini, F., & Jones, G. (2009). Do NSAIDs affect longitudinal changes in knee cartilage volume and knee cartilage defects in older adults? *The American Journal of Medicine, 122*(9), 836–842. Retrieved from https://ive-wdc.kp.org/das/article/body

Doherty, M. (2004). How important are genetic factors in osteoarthritis? *The Journal of Rheumatology, 31*(4), 22–27.

Felson, D. T. (2007). Chapter 44. Osteoarthritis. In J. B. Imboden, D. B. Hellmann, & J. H. Stone (Eds.), Current rheumatology Diagnosis & Treatment (2nd ed). Retrieved from http://www.accessmedicine.com/content.aspx?aID=2727784

Friedewald, V. E., Bennet, J. S., Packer, M., Roberts, W. C., & Williams, G. W. (2008). The editor's roundtable: Nonsteroidal anti-inflammatory drugs and cardiovascular risk. *The American Journal of Cardiology, 102*(8), 1046–1055.

Fuller-Thompson, E., & Brennenstuhl, S. M. (2009). The robust association between childhood physical abuse and osteoarthritis in adulthood: Findings from a representative community sample. *Arthritis & Rheumatism, 61*(11), 1554–1562.

Guermazi, A. (2009). Preface: Osteoarthritis. From simple x-rays to compositional MRI: What have we learned? *Rheumatic Disease Clinics of North America, 35*(3), 13–14.

Harrington, L., & Schneider, J. I. (2006). Atraumatic joint and limb pain in the elderly. *Emergency Medicine Clinics of North America, 24*(2), 389–412.

Hsu-LeBlanc, E. (2010). Keep joints healthy: Diet, lifestyle, and supplements make a difference. *Taste for Life,* 30–32.

Hunter, D. J. (2009a). Preface. *Medical Clinics of North America, 1*(93), 0–3.

Hunter, D. J. (2009b). Imaging insights on the epidemiology and pathophysiology of osteoarthritis. *Rheumatic Clinics of North America, 35*(3), 447–463.

Hunter, D. J., McDougall, J. J., & Keefe, F. J. (2008). The symptoms of osteoarthritis and the genesis of pain. *Rheumatic Disease Clinics of North America, 34*(3), 515–832.

Ilich, J. Z., & Kerstetter, J. (2000). Nutrition and bone health revisited: A story beyond calcium. *Journal of American College of Nutrition, 19*(6), 715–737.

Iowa State University. (2010, August 2). High heels may lead to joint degeneration and knee osteoarthritis, study finds. *Science Daily.* Retrieved from http://www.sciencedaily.com/releases/2010/08/100802141901.htm

Kallen, B. (2008). Ease aching joints. *Natural Health,* 92–94.

Kim, L. S., Axelrod, L. J., Howard, P., Buratovich, N., & Waters, R. F. (2006.) Efficacy of methylsulfonylmethane (MSM) in osteoarthritis clinical trial. *Osteoarthritis Cartilage, 14*(3), 286–294.

Kim, L. S., Axelrod, L. J., Howard, P., Buratovich, N., Waters, R. F. (2005). Efficacy of methylsulfonylmethane (MSM) in osteoarthritis pain of the knee: A pilot clinical trial. *Osteoarthritis and Cartilage, 14*(3), doi:10.1016/j.joca.2005.10.003

Kujala U. M, Kettunen, J., Paananen, H., Aalto, T., Battié, M. C., Impivaara O., . . . Sarna, S. (1995). Knee osteoarthritis in former runners, soccer players, weight lifters, and shooters. *Arthritis & Rheumatism, 38*(4), 539–546.

Leong, K. (2009). A new natural treatment for painful osteoarthritis? *Health & Wellness.* Retrieved from http://www.associatedcontent.com/article/2443560/a_New_natural_treatment_for_painful

Littlejohn, C., Baldacchino, A., & Bannister, J. (2004). Chronic non-cancer pain and opioid dependence. *Journal of the Royal Society of Medicine, 97*(2), 62–65.

Lozada, C. J., & Steigelfest, E. (2009). Osteoarthritis. *eMedicine.* Retrieved from http://emedicine.medscape.com/article/330487

Mahajan, A., Tandon, V., Verma, S., & Sharma, S. (2005). Osteoarthritis and menopause. *Journal of the Indian Rheumatological Association, 13,* 21–25.

Maly, M. (2008). Abnormal and cumulative loading in knee osteoarthritis. *Current Opinion in Rheumatology, 20*(5), 547–552.

Markenson, J. (2009). *An in-depth overview of osteoarthritis for physicians: Hospital for special surgery.* Retrieved from http://www.hss.edu/professional-conditions_13646

Martin, S. D. (2006). *Knees & hips: A troubleshooting guide to knee & hip pain. A special report from Harvard Medical School.* Stamford, CT: StayWell Consumer Health Publishing.

McAlindon, T. E. (2007). A placebo-controlled study of collagen hydrolysate in subjects with knee osteoarthritis. *ClinicalTrialsFeeds.org.* Retrieved from http://clinicaltrialsfeeds.org/clinical-trials/show/NCT00536302

Meschino, J. P. (2001). Natural anti-inflammatory supplements: Research status and Clinical application. *Massage Today, 1,* 12.

Nevitt, M. C., Lane, N. E., Scott, J. C., Hochberg, M. C., Pressman, A. R., & Cummings, S. R. (1995). Radiographic osteoarthritis of the hip and bone mineral density. The study of osteoporotic fractures research group. *Arthritis & Rheumatology, 36,* 1671–1680.

Nierenberg, C. (2009). The ultimate guide to healthy joints. *Natural Health,* 51–56.

Nuesch, E., Rutjes, A. W. S., Husni, E., Welch, V., & Juni, P. (2009). Oral or transdermal opioids for osteoarthritis of the knee or hip. *Cochrane Database of Systematic Reviews, 4:* CD3115.

O'Connor, D. L., Khan, S., Weishuhn, K., Vaughn, J., Jefferies, A., Campbell, D. M., . . . Post Discharge Feeding Study Group. (2008). Growth and nutrient intakes of human milk fed preterm infants provided with extra energy and nutrients after hospital discharge. *Pediatrics, 12*(4)1, 766–776.

Parker-Pope, T. (2005, September 26). Need relief from arthritis? There's growing focus on food. *The Wall Street Journal.* Retrieved from http://vijayvad.com/published.html

Quellette, E. A., & Makowski, A. (2006). How men and women are affected by osteoarthritis of the hand. *Orthopedic Clinics of North America, 37*(4), 541–548.

Risser, A., Donavan, D., Heintzman, J., & Page, T. (2009). NSAID prescribing precautions. *American Family Physician, 12*(80), 1371–1378.

Rutgers, M., Saris, D., Dhert, W., & Creemers, L. B. (2010). Cytokine profile of autologous conditioned serum for treatment of osteoarthritis, in vitro effects on cartilage metabolism and intra-articular levels after injection. *Arthritis Research and Therapy, 12-R114,* 1–11.

Schelbert, K. B. (2009). Comorbidities of obesity. *Primary care: Clinics of office practice, 36*(2), 271–285.

Schumann, B., Bolm-Audorff, U., Bergmann, A., Ellegast, R., Elsner, G., Grifka, J., . . . Seidler, A. (2010). Lifestyle factors and lumbar disc disease: results of a German multi-center case-control study (EPILIFT). *Arthritis Research & Therapy, 12*(5). Retrieved from http://arthritis-research.com/content/12/5/R193

Sowers, M., Lachance, L., Jamadar, D., Hochberg, M. C., Hollis, B., Crutchfield, M., . . . Jannausch, M. L. (1999). The associations of bone mineral density and bone turnover markers with osteoarthritis of the hand and knee in pre-and perimenopausal women. *Arthritis & Rheumatism, 4*(3)2, 483–489.

Spector, T., Reneland, R. H., Mah, S., Valdes, A. M., Hart, D. J., Kammerer, S., . . . Braun, A. (2006). Association between a variation in LRCH1 and knee osteoarthritis: A genome-wide single-nucleotide polymorphism association study using DNA pooling. *Arthritis & Rheumatism, 54*(2), 524–532.

Stanos, S. P., McLean, J., & Rader, L. (2007). Physical medicine rehabilitation approach to pain. *Medical Clinics of North America, 25*(4), 721–759.

Suszynski, M. (2009). Understanding primary and secondary osteoarthritis. *Everyday Health.* Retrieved from http://www.everydayhealth.com/osteoarthritis/primary-and-secondary-osteoarthritis.aspx

University of Maryland Medical Center. (2009). *Osteoarthritis.* Retrieved from http://www.umm.edu/altmed/articles/osteoarthritis-000118.htm

Wang, L., Schmid, C. H., Hibberd, P. L., Kalish, R., Roubenoff, R., & McAlinson, T. (2009). Tai chi is effective in treating knee osteoarthritis: A randomized controlled trial. *Arthritis & Rheumatology, 61*(11), 1545–1553.

Wei, N. (2004). ASU and osteoarthritis. *Clinical Rheumatology, 23*(3), 274.

Wilson, D. R., McWalker, E. J., & Johnston, J. D. (2008). The measurement of joint mechanics and their role in osteoarthritis genesis and progression. *Medical Clinics of North America, 93*(1), 67–82.

Young, S. (2004). Thumb carpometacarpal arthrosis. *Journal of Hand Surgery, 4*(2), 73–93.

Zhang, Y., Hannan, M. T., Chaisson, C. E., McAlindon, T. E., Evans, S. R., Aliabadi, P., . . . Felson, D. T. (2000). Bone mineral density and risk of incident and progressive radiographic knee osteoarthritis in women: the Framingham Study. *The Journal of Rheumatology, 27*(4), 1032–1037.

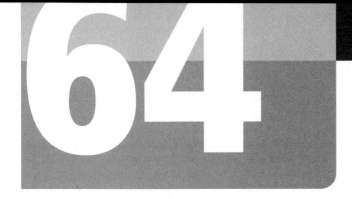

PRIMARY CARE OF HIV-INFECTED ADULTS

Suzan Stringari-Murray

I. Introduction

Since the first cases of AIDS were diagnosed in 1981, there have been significant scientific advances in the understanding of the biology, natural history, and clinical management of HIV infection. The United States Public Health Service, Department of Health and Human Services (DHHS), publishes HIV evidence-based guidelines that are continually updated (DHHS, 2011) and the Infectious Disease Society of America publishes guidelines identifying best practices in the clinical management of HIV/AIDS (Aberg et al., 2009). This chapter reviews and summarizes current DHHS and Infectious Disease Society of America guidelines for those advanced practice nurses who do not have expertise in HIV/AIDS, but who may be providing primary care for HIV-infected adolescents and adults. Clinicians who are generalists can, with expert HIV consultation and support, provide HIV-infected patients with primary care, HIV-specific healthcare maintenance and disease prevention, and follow antiretroviral therapy (ART) in consultation with HIV experts.

A. General background: HIV/AIDS updates 1998 to 2009

1. Epidemiology

   HIV is the virus that causes AIDS. AIDS represents the advanced stages of HIV and is characterized by the destruction of T-helper CD4 lymphocytes, resulting in life-threatening HIV-related opportunistic infections (OIs) and cancer. In 1993, the case definition of AIDS was expanded to include all patients with CD4 counts less than or equal to 200 mm^3, or a diagnosis of recurrent bacterial pneumonia, mycobacterium tuberculosis (TB), or cervical cancer.

The Centers for Disease Control and Prevention (CDC) has been tracking AIDS since 1981 when the first cases of a fatal pneumonia, diagnosed as *Pneumocystis carinii* (later renamed *P. jiroveci*), appeared in young otherwise healthy gay men. Now, in addition to surveillance of AIDS cases, the CDC has established an HIV incidence surveillance system to more effectively track trends in new HIV infections. A confidential names-based reporting system has been implemented in 39 states, the District of Columbia, and five United States dependent areas. As of 2009, there are an estimated cumulative total of over 1 million cases of AIDS in the United States with 583,298 deaths, and an annual incidence of 56,300 new HIV infections (CDC, 2009; Hall, Song, Rhodes, Prejean, & Qian An, 2009).

In the United States, HIV is seen predominantly in men who have sex with men, who comprise more than half of all diagnosed HIV/AIDS cases. The term "men who have sex with men" refers to all men who have sex with other men regardless of how they identify themselves (gay, bisexual, or heterosexual; http://www.cdc.gov/hiv/topics/msm/index.htm).

Women represent one quarter of all cases of HIV/AIDS in the United States, with most infections transmitted through heterosexual activity (http://www.cdc.gov/hiv/topics/women/index.htm). Globally, UNAIDS estimates a total of 33.4 million people living with HIV, with 22.4 million cases in Sub-Saharan Africa. Heterosexual transmission of HIV is the main mode of transmission in this region and women age 15 or older comprise over 60% of all living HIV/AIDS cases (UNAIDS, 2009).

In the United States, there are significant racial and ethnic disparities in reported cases of HIV/AIDS and survival following diagnosis. In 2009, African Americans accounted for 52% of all diagnoses of HIV infection (http://www.cdc.gov/hiv/topics/aa/index.htm). Historically, most HIV-positive individuals have been clustered in major metropolitan areas in three states: California, New York, and Florida. Several emerging areas of new HIV infections have been reported in rural and urban areas of the South, the Southeast, and the District of Columbia. The District of Columbia has one of the highest rates of new AIDS cases nationally at 128.4 per 100,000 cases compared to 14 per 100,000 cases in the United States overall, with most cases in the District of Columbia occurring in African American men (District of Columbia HAHSTA, 2008).

2. HIV pathophysiology and ART (Table 64-1)

HIV acquisition is followed within days to weeks by a non-specific viral syndrome or seroconversion illness, which is characterized by flu-like symptoms in most infected individuals. The period of primary HIV infection, between the acquisition of the virus and the development of a positive HIV antibody test, is accompanied by rapid depletion of CD4 lymphocytes and high levels of HIV in the plasma. Primary HIV infection is a period of high infectivity with an increased risk of transmission. Significant impairment of the immune system occurs rapidly after primary HIV infection.

Research on the immunopathogenesis of HIV has led to an improved understanding of how HIV causes AIDS. An active site of HIV replication is the lamina propria of the gut wall, which is rich in lymphoid tissue and contains large numbers of CD4 T-helper cells, the main target cell for the virus. Gut CD4 cells are rapidly infected and destroyed, leading to local inflammation and increased gut permeability. It is hypothesized that leakage of microbes or "microbial translocation" from the gut results in a state of chronic immune system activation (Douek, Picker, & Koup, 2003). Chronic immune system activation helps to sustain HIV replication through the continuous production of activated CD4 cells, which are fresh targets for the virus. In the absence of treatment, over several months to years, on average 7–11 years, progressive depletion of CD4 T-helper lymphocytes leads to immune system failure and death from HIV-related OIs. Currently approved antiretroviral drugs (ARV) control HIV replication but do not eradicate HIV from host cells. For this reason HIV treatment must be continued for the duration of the individual's life.

The primary goal of HIV treatment is to prevent HIV-related morbidity and mortality by reducing the level of HIV virus in the plasma. Recommended first-line ART regimens are durable and potent. There are now five classes of HIV drugs, with different mechanisms of action and a variety of coformulations (DHHS, 2011, p. 43). The selection of ART is complex and requires expertise in the clinical management of HIV. Potent ART,

TABLE 64-1 Indications for Antiretroviral Therapy in Adults and Adolescents

Criteria	Recommendation	Rationale
History of AIDS-defining illness	Treat	Evidence supports treatment
CD4 350 cells/mm³	Treat	Evidence supports treatment
CD4 of 350–500 cells/mm³		Observational data and nonrandomized trials support treating at CD4 counts > 350–500 cells/mm³
CD4 > 500 cells/mm³	Panel members evenly divided. 50% favor starting antiretroviral therapy at this stage of HIV disease; 50% view initiating therapy at this stage as optional	Evidence for treating at CD4 counts > 500 cells/mm³ not yet available and initiation of treatment based on expert opinion
Pregnant women	Treat regardless of CD4 count	Prevention of mother-to-chlid transmission
If treatment of HBV is indicated in HIV/HBV coinfected	Treat regardless of CD4 count	Treatment of HBV only, in coinfected patients, results in HIV drug resistance and limits future options for HIV treatment.
HIV-associated nephropathy	Treat regardless of CD4 count	Only effective treatment is antiretroviral therapy

For a complete discussion of the supporting evidence for initiating antiretroviral therapy in HIV-infected individuals see recommendations Panel on Antiretroviral Guidelines for Adults and Adolescents. Guidelines for the use of antiretroviral agents in HIV-1-infected adults and adolescents. Department of Health and Human Services. January 10, 2011; 1–166. Retrieved from http://www.aidsinfo.nih.gov/ContentFiles/AdultandAdolescentGL.pdf.

which typically consists of combinations of three or more drugs, is effective and results in durable suppression of HIV to below the limits of detection of most assays (< 40–75 copies per milliliter), if patients are engaged in care, adherent with their ARV regimens, and supported in self-managing their HIV. The January 10, 2011, ART guidelines now recommend preferred regimens for asymptomatic patients to be initiated at CD4 counts of 350 cells/mm³ to 500 cells/mm³. For patients with symptomatic HIV disease, including OIs, pregnant women, persons with HIV-associated nephropathy, and persons coinfected with hepatitis B virus (HBV), treatment of HIV is indicated regardless of CD4 cell count.

Primary care providers should be aware of the most common drug interactions that occur with ART and drugs commonly prescribed for other chronic diseases. Consultation with a pharmacist or clinician with HIV expertise is recommended before initiating new medications in patients on an ART regimen. In addition to tables in the guidelines that list significant drug interactions by class of ARV (DHHS Guidelines 2011, pp. 133–149), several Internet-based drug interaction tools are available (HIVInSite http://hivinsite .ucsf.edu/insite?page=ar-00-02). Significant drug interactions occur with rifampin; clarithromycin; statins (specifically, simvastatin and lovastatin are contraindicated in patients on protease inhibitors); oral contraceptives; anticonvulsants; erectile dysfunction drugs; proton pump inhibitors; calcium channel blockers; St. John's wort; azoles; clarithromycin; and some benzodiazepines.

3. HIV prevention: HIV testing and linkage to care

In early 2000, the CDC conducted multisite studies of standard HIV testing practices that included confidential or anonymous testing. In populations studied, close to half of all individuals who were tested in state and local health departments between May 2000 and February 2003 were late testers (HIV testing within 6–12 months of an AIDS diagnosis [CDC, 2003a]). Additional review of HIV testing practices showed that many individuals identified as HIV-infected did not return for their test results and were lost to follow-up.

The first rapid HIV antibody test was approved for use in 2002. Current whole-blood (finger stick) HIV test assays are both sensitive and specific, and the use of these assays has significantly changed the approach to screening and diagnosing HIV. The CDC now recommends HIV testing in all healthcare settings for individuals between the ages of 13 and 64, after the patient is notified that testing will be performed, unless the patient declines testing or "opts out." General consent for medical care is sufficient to cover HIV testing, and separate consent forms are not required (CDC, 2003b & 2006). Individuals at higher risk for acquisition of HIV should be tested at least once each year.

Implementation of routine HIV testing has not been widely adopted. Evidence supports the routine use of rapid HIV tests for patients in community health centers as an effective strategy for increasing the number of patients screened for HIV (Myers, Modica, Dufour, Bernstein, & McNamara, 2009). The Veterans Health Administration System, one of the largest providers of HIV care in the country, has implemented a clinical reminder system for HIV testing and found this to be an acceptable and sustainable method for adopting CDC recommendations for routine HIV testing (Goetz et al., 2009).

A critical role for the primary care clinician in controlling the HIV pandemic includes the detection of new HIV infections through routine HIV screening and the prevention of secondary transmission of HIV by those individuals who are known to be HIV-infected. Primary care providers see patients who are at risk of or infected with HIV before these individuals see an HIV expert. Clinician comfort in conducting a risk assessment of factors that increase risk of HIV transmission is essential. Recommendations have been developed to guide clinicians in providing screening and counseling to prevent HIV transmission. These recommendations contain excellent examples of prevention messages and strategies for brief behavioral interventions to reduce HIV transmission (CDC, 2003b).

4. Chronic HIV infection

As a consequence of improved survival on ART, there is an increased prevalence of persons in the United States, age 50 years or older, who are living with HIV/AIDS. It is estimated that this age group will represent approximately half of all HIV/AIDS cases by 2015 (CDC, 2009). Research in HIV and aging suggests that HIV-infected individuals are at risk for premature aging and the occurrence of common chronic conditions at a younger age compared to the general population. Additional areas of concern in aging HIV-infected individuals include early frailty and worsening HIV-associated neurocognitive disorders despite well-controlled HIV infection.

Overall, AIDS-defining illnesses are still the leading cause of death in the HIV-infected population despite improved survival. However, non–AIDS-defining illnesses (substance abuse, cardiovascular disease (CVD), non-AIDS cancers, liver cancer, and end-stage liver and renal disease) are increasing as a cause of morbidity and mortality in this population (Palella et al., 2006).

a. Metabolic syndrome and CVD in chronic HIV: Studies of observational cohorts demonstrate an increased risk of CVD and myocardial infarction in HIV-infected individuals compared to the general population (Friis-Møller et al., 2003). Atherosclerosis seems to have a different natural history and outcomes, likely related to the chronic inflammation associated with HIV infection; a higher prevalence of traditional risk factors, such as smoking and abnormal lipids; and metabolic changes that occur with use of ART regimens (Ho & Hsue, 2009). Abnormal lipids, insulin resistance, visceral adiposity, and dyslipidemias are commonly seen in HIV-infected populations on treatment. Specific strategies to address these abnormalities have included changing ART regimen components associated with abnormal lipids and body fat redistribution and an increased emphasis by HIV experts in health behavior counseling for traditional CVD risk factors, specifically smoking.

b. Malignancies: HIV increases the risk of death caused by both AIDS-defining (non-Hodgkin's lymphoma, cervical cancer, Kaposi's sarcoma) and non–AIDS-defining malignancies (lung, anal, and liver carcinomas) (Patel et al., 2008). At this time, recommendations for cancer screening do not differ for HIV-infected individuals but future recommendations may suggest that cancer screening occur at an earlier age in HIV-infected populations.

c. HIV and renal disease: Kidney function is abnormal in up to 30% of HIV-infected populations with most individuals showing histologic findings diagnostic of HIV/AIDS nephropathy (Gupta et al., 2005). Risks for renal disease include African American race; family history; low CD4 count; high HIV viral load; past use of nephrotoxic drugs; and comorbidities of hypertension, diabetes, and chronic hepatitis C virus (HCV). Assessment of kidney function and renal dosing adjustment of ARV should be done routinely (DHHS 2011, Appendix B, Table 7, pp. 1–3, ARV dosing recommendations in patients with renal or hepatic insufficiency).

d. HIV and Chronic Hepatitis B and C
Chronic viral hepatitis is more prevalent in HIV-infected populations because both infections are transmitted sexually or as a result of injection drug use. HIV-infected individuals who also have chronic HBV or HCV have a more rapid progression to cirrhosis and an increased risk of hepatocellular carcinoma than individuals with either chronic HBV or HCV alone. Both HBV and HCV complicate the treatment of HIV because of the hepatotoxicity associated with some ARV regimens. Referral to experts who treat both HIV and liver disease should be done soon after the patient enters care to plan for specific treatment of HBV and HCV if needed.

B. *Summary*
HIV-infected individuals are living longer because of effective ART regimens and are experiencing non–AIDS-defining comorbidities at an earlier age than the general population. Significant racial and ethnic disparities continue in HIV testing, access to care, and survival after diagnosis because of structural barriers, such as poverty, poor health literacy, and stigma. Improvements in life expectancy beyond those that can be achieved with the use of ART will depend on knowledge of HIV status, full implementation of CDC HIV testing recommendations, linkage of HIV-infected patients to HIV expert care, and optimal management of common comorbid conditions.

II. **Database** (to include, but not limited to)

A. *Subjective*

1. Age, gender or gender identity, race, and ethnicity.

2. Approximate date and documentation of first positive HIV-1 antibody test. If documentation is not available or cannot be obtained, repeat HIV antibody test with patient's consent.

3. Reason for testing (important in addressing the client's response to illness).

4. Emotional response to diagnosis and disclosure of HIV status to friends, family, and sexual partners. The psychosocial implications associated with HIV are numerous and significantly impact the patient's ability to adhere to therapy and stay in primary care. Assessment of the emotional impact of the diagnosis and the need for supportive counseling is essential and should be addressed before the initiation of specific therapies for HIV.

5. Past medical history

a. Acute retroviral syndrome: symptoms of acute retroviral syndrome can help estimate date of infection; screen for viral illness with myalgias, arthralgias, generalized macular-papular rash, fever, lymphadenopathy, sore throat, and aseptic meningitis.

b. CD4 nadir (lowest CD4 cell count) and HIV-1 viral loads.

c. HIV-associated complications: HIV OIs, AIDS-defining illnesses or malignancies; chronic comorbidities, such as type 2 diabetes mellitus, CVD, renal disease, chronic HBV or HCV, dyslipidemias, TB, varicella zoster virus, and abnormal cervical or anal Pap smears; and sexually transmitted infections, such as herpes simplex virus (HSV), gonorrhea, *Chlamydia*, and syphilis.

d. Transfusion of blood, platelets, or serum products; artificial insemination; and organ or tissue transplantation.

e. ARV medications: list ARV regimen components, start and stop dates for each regimen or component, CD4 and HIV-1 viral load response, reasons for stopping regimen, associated side effects or toxicities, difficulties with adherence and barriers to ARV adherence. Document dates and results of all HIV drug resistance studies: genotype, phenotype, and tropism assays if done and ARV regimen prescribed at time of resistance testing. Request medical records to verify information.

f. Other medications: list all regularly prescribed medications, complementary therapies, and over-the-counter products. Note drug allergies and screen for allergies to sulfa antibiotics.

g. Vaccination status: HBV, hepatitis A virus, tetanus-diphteria-pertussis, pneumococcal (Pneumovax), seasonal influenza, and pandemic H1N1 influenza vaccine. In non–varicella zoster virus immune patients with CD4 greater than 200 cells/mm^3 consider varicella zoster virus and mumps-measles-rubella (Table 64-2).

h. Purified protein derivative status or interferon-γ release assay results: If history of positive purified protein derivative (latent TB infection) or TB antigen assay, record dates of treatment and chest radiograph results at time of skin test.

i. Women: last menstrual period, abnormal Pap smears, and referral for colposcopy; genital or cervical condyloma, recurrent vaginal yeast infections; pelvic inflammatory disease, gravid and para status, oral contraception (ARV may reduce effectiveness of estrogen-based contraceptives); use of ARV during pregnancy

j. Foreign travel or residence in areas endemic for specific organisms (e.g., Southwestern United States, coccidioidomycosis; Ohio and Indiana, histoplasmosis). Cat ownership and uncooked beef consumption are risks for toxoplasmosis.

k. Psychiatric: history of depression, demoralization, bipolar disease, past psychiatric care and counseling, suicide attempts (methods and precipitating events).

6. Personal and social

a. Sexual practices: number of partners and gender, insertive or receptive anal sex; use of condoms or other barrier methods.

b. Substance use or addiction: alcohol use, injection drug use, needle sharing, use of needle exchange programs, injection technique and skin cleansing before injection. Drugs used: cocaine, methamphetamine, marijuana, heroin and how used (injected, inhaled, or smoked). Use of drugs or alcohol before sexual activity. Prescribed drugs obtained on the street with attention to benzodiazepines and long- and short-acting opiate pain medications.

c. Cigarette smoking: age at onset, packs per day and number of pack years, and motivation toward cessation.

d. History of incarceration, homelessness, domestic violence, or sexual assault.

e. As part of the initial assessment the patient should be evaluated for community support service needs, financial and insurance status, and referral for appropriate counseling or linkage to other services. Social support systems: family, significant others, spiritual practices, religious and community affiliations, and HIV status of dependent children and sexual partners.

7. Review of systems

a. General: usual body weight, fever or drenching sweats, unintentional weight loss of more than 10%, and persistent fatigue or anorexia.

b. Dermatologic: persistent skin rashes; recurrent outbreaks of HSV; easy bruising or bleeding; red- to violet-colored papular or macular lesions (Kaposi's sarcoma); abscesses; fungal infections, such as tinea; candidiasis; folliculitis; seborrheic dermatitis; onychomycosis; molluscum contagiosum; pruritic papules; and soft tissue infections.

c. Ear, nose, and throat: oral lesions or sores; bleeding gums; caries; painful or sensitive teeth (oral candidiasis, hairy leukoplakia, periodontal disease); and dysphagia (*Candida* esophagitis is a common initial OI)

TABLE 64-2 Immunizations for HIV-1 Infected Adults

Vaccine	Comments
Hepatitis B	Immunize if HBsAb-, HBsAg-, and HBcAb-negative with the three-dose HBV vaccination series, regardless of CD4 count or HIV viral load as early in HIV infection as possible. Verify adequate response within 1 month after completion of vaccine. Repeat series once for patients with levels < 10 mIU/ml. Patients with CD4 nadir ≤ 200 cells/mm³ may not respond. Vaccination should not be deferred while awaiting a rise in CD4 count to ≥ 350 cells/mm³. Some HIV-infected patients with CD4 counts ≤ 200 cells/mm³ may respond to vaccination. Most HIV-infected patients with isolated anti-HBc are not immune to HBV infection. Some experts recommend vaccination with a complete primary series of hepatitis B vaccine. Strategies to increase seroconversion after immunization: Use of a double-dose HBV vaccine (40 μg/ml [Recombivax HB®] administered on a three-dose schedule or two doses of 20 μg/ml [Engerix-B®] administered simultaneously on a four-dose schedule at 0, 1, 2) has resulted in higher seroconversion rates in some studies (CDC, 2009).
Influenza	Administer parenteral form of vaccine. Intranasal administration of live attenuated influenza vaccine (FluMist®) is not recommended.
H1N1 monovalent vaccine for 2009 H1N1	Safe in HIV-infected. Follow annual recommendations.
Polysaccharide pneumococcal (PPV 23)	At entry into care or as close to HIV diagnosis as possible (unless given in last 5 years). Repeat every 5 years and if initial vaccine given when CD4 < 200.
Tetanus, diphtheria, and acellular pertussis	Safe in HIV-infected.
Hepatitis A	Safe in HIV-infected. Immunize all nonimmune men who have sex with men (MSM) and those with increased risk of acquiring hepatitis A virus or at risk of experiencing severe illness if acutely infected with HAV (MSM, chronic HBV or HCV, IDU, hemophiliacs, and travel to high-risk areas).
Hepatitis A and hepatitis B combined	Not covered by some Medicaid programs. Vaccine contains insufficient antigen for HBV (separate HBV and hepatitis A virus vaccines recommended).
Hemophilus influenzae type B (Hib)	HIV-positive adults and their healthcare providers should discuss whether HIB immunization is needed. Not generally indicated for HIV-infected.
HPV	Do not administer during pregnancy. Both the bivalent and quadrivalent HPV vaccines can be administered to HIV-infected females through age 26. The immune response to the vaccine might be less than that in persons who are immunocompetent and efficacy of the vaccine has not been determined in HIV-infected men or women. Trials are underway in HIV-infected.
Mumps-measles-rubella live vaccine	Persons with HIV infection are at increased risk for severe complications if infected with measles. No severe or unusual adverse events have been reported after measles vaccination in HIV-infected persons who had no evidence of severe immunosuppression, defined as a CD4 ≤ 200 (MMWR, 2009) Newly diagnosed adults without acceptable evidence of measles immunity should receive mumps-measles-rubella vaccine unless they have evidence of severe immunosuppression (CD4 ≤ 200). If necessary separate components of vaccine can be given.
Meningococcal	Persons with HIV infection can elect to receive MCV4 or MPSV. MCV4 is licensed for persons aged 11–55 years, first-year college students living in dormitories, those with asplenia, military recruits, and travelers to endemic areas.
Varicella live vaccine	People born before 1980 do not need to receive this vaccine. No studies have evaluated the vaccine in HIV-infected adolescents or adults. Vaccine may be considered in varicella zoster virus seronegative persons > 8 years old with CD4 counts of > 200 mm³ (CDC, 2009). If exposure to person with varicella zoster virus, administer varicella zoster immune globulin within 96 hours of exposure. Do not administer during pregnancy.

TABLE 64-2 Immunizations for HIV-1 Infected Adults *(continued)*

Vaccine	Comments
Inactivated polio virus	As indicated for travel to high-risk areas.
Anthrax vaccine	Not recommended for HIV-infected.
Small pox live vaccine	Do not administer.
Zoster live vaccine	Do not administer.
Travel-related vaccines	CDC, 2009.

Inactivated, recombinant, subunit, polysaccharide, and conjugate vaccines and toxoids are safe and can be administered to all HIV-infected patients, although response to such vaccines in patients with CD4 less than 200 might be suboptimal. If indicated, vaccines are recommended at the usual doses and schedules. HIV-infected patients may be at increased risk for adverse reactions after administration of live-attenuated vaccines related to a reduced ability to mount an immune response. Live vaccines are generally contraindicated in HIV-infected patients with some exceptions, when benefits outweigh the risk of vaccines. Close contacts of persons with HIV should receive all age-appropriate vaccines, with the exception of live OPV and smallpox vaccine. Inactivated polio vaccine should be administered to close household contacts of HIV-infected individuals.

Sources: Centers for Disease Control and Prevention. Guidelines for Prevention and Treatment of Opportunistic Infections in HIV-Infected Adults and Adolescents. (2009) *Mprbidity and Mortality Weekly Report, 58* (No. RR-4); MMWR Quick Guide Recommended Adult Immunization Schedule—United States, January 2009–United States 2009. *Morbidity and Mortality Weekly Report, 57*, 53. Retrieved from www.cdc.gov /mmWR/PDF/wk/mm5753-Immunization.pdf; Department of Health and Human Services, Recommendxed immunizations for HIV-infected adults. Retrieved from aidsinfo.nih.gov/ContentFiles/Recommended_Immunizations_FS_en.pdf

or odynophagia (HSV or cytomegalovirus esophagitis if CD4 < 50 cells/mm^3).

d. Eyes: decreased visual acuity or loss of peripheral vision (CD4 < 100 cells/mm^3: cytomegalovirus retinitis, toxoplasmosis)

e. Nodes: lymph node swelling or a change in the size of node (lymphoma, TB, *Bartonella*)

f. Pulmonary: cough, dyspnea, sputum production (*P. carinii* pneumonia usually occurs at CD4 < 200 cells/mm^3); CD4 less than 200–300 cells/mm^3, increased risk of bacterial pneumonias and TB (look for atypical presentations and chest radiograph findings with CD4 < 200 cells/mm^3)

g. Cardiac: chest pain, murmurs, palpitations (CVD, endocarditis)

h. Gastrointestinal: change in bowel habits; nausea; emesis; bloating; diarrhea (parasites or bacterial enteric infections, such as *Shigella, Salmonella, Campylobacter, Clostridium difficile*); rectal pain; lesions or discharge; bright red blood per rectum; and results of previous anal pap smears. If the patient practices unprotected anal intercourse, obtain rectal swabs to screen for gonorrhea and chlamydia.

i. Gynecological and genitourinary: genital lesions or sores. In women, dysuria, vaginal discharge, pelvic pain, contraception, and use of barrier methods during sexual activity. In men, dysuria, penile discharge, and genital lesions.

j. Neurologic: persistent or severe headaches; depression; anxiety; weakness; numbness or tingling in hands or feet (neuropathy); memory loss; confusion; and personality changes (CD4 < 100, toxoplasmosis encephalitis, progressive multifocal leukoencephalopathy, cryptococcal meningitis). Screen for HIV/AIDS neurocognitive disorder, which can occur at any CD4 count.

8. Family history: Premature CVD in parent or relative, CVD, diabetes, renal disease, alcoholism, malignancies, substance use, HIV, depression, and emotional or physical abuse.

B. Objective

1. General appearance, grooming, and affect

2. Height, weight, blood pressure, body mass index, and baseline resting SaO$_2$ by pulse oximetry.

3. Skin: tinea, onychomychosis, folliculitis, seborrheic dermatitis, petechiae, Kaposi's sarcoma lesions (purplish macular, papular, or nodular lesions; discrete and well circumscribed; do not blanch with compression)

4. Lymph nodes: complete examination for presence of lymphadenopathy defined as greater than 1 cm in two or more noncontiguous extrainguinal sites, one of which may be cervical. Assess for asymmetry and consistency of node.

5. Eyes: visual acuity and visual field testing. Examine for lesions on lids or sclera; funduscopic examination screening for hemorrhage, exudate, or cotton wool

spots. Dilated retinal examination at baseline and annually for CD4 less than 100 cells mm³.

6. Mouth: ulceration (herpes or apthous stomatitis); oral candidiasis; fringed lesions on lateral border or dorsum of tongue (hairy leukoplakia); Kaposi's sarcoma; periodontal disease; and caries.

7. Chest and heart: complete examination.

8. Abdomen: enlargement of spleen or liver

9. Gynecologic: breast examination, external genital, and pelvic examination. Pap smear.

10. Rectal: digital rectal examination and anoscopy. Obtain rectal Pap on men and women.

11. Genitourinary: in women examine vulva for lesions, condyloma, HSV, and pelvic examination. In addition to Pap, screen for chlamydia and gonorrhea.

12. Neurologic: complete neurologic screening examination, including mental status examination. Standard Mini Mental Status examination is not sensitive for detecting HIV-associated neurocognitive disorders. Timed tests are a better measure of cognitive functioning. Use mental status examinations validated in HIV populations (Power, Selnes, Grim, & McArthur, 1995).

III. Assessment

A. Determine the diagnosis

1. HIV infection should be confirmed in all patients entering care. Standard testing for HIV uses an enzyme-linked immunosorbent assay (ELISA) that is highly sensitive in chronic HIV infection. If positive, the ELISA is repeated until two to three specimens are repeatedly reactive. A repeatedly reactive ELISA is then confirmed by using a Western blot, which is highly specific. A Western blot detects HIV-1 proteins (p) and glycoproteins (gp) from the viral core and envelope. A positive Western blot requires reactivity to gp120/160 plus either gp41 or p24. The Western blot is reported as indeterminate if criteria for either a positive or negative test are not met.

2. A false-negative ELISA can occur if the individual is newly infected and has not yet developed antibodies. The time period from infection to the development of antibodies is usually 2 weeks, with some individuals seroconverting at 3–6 weeks. If the patient reports significant risks for acquiring HIV the ELISA should be repeated (Hare, Futterman, & Thornton, 2011).

3. If an acute or primary HIV infection is suspected, a plasma HIV-1 RNA assay is performed to detect HIV viremia. HIV viral load tests are not approved by the Food and Drug Administration for diagnosis of HIV and must be followed by standard HIV antibody testing to confirm the diagnosis.

B. Severity

For the purposes of surveillance, patients are defined as having AIDS based on certain indicator diseases and a CD4 cell count less than 200 cells/mm³ or a lymphocyte count of less than 14%. In clinical care, severity of disease or staging is based on lowest CD4 cell, also known as "CD4 nadir."

C. Motivation and ability

Despite medical advances in the care of HIV-infected individuals, HIV is often believed to be a death sentence by those who are newly diagnosed. HIV infection is associated with significant stigma and discrimination. Mistrust of the healthcare system and the belief that AIDS is not caused by HIV contribute to the challenges of engaging patients in care.

Taking the time to establish a therapeutic relationship and identify the patient's priorities and preferences for care is critical. Because HIV is a chronic manageable disease, patient skills and abilities to self-manage chronic HIV and related comorbidities needs to be supported. Patients who are engaged in care and adherent with their ART experience improved healthcare outcomes.

IV. Plan

A. Diagnostic tests

1. Order initial laboratory and diagnostic studies (Table 64-3).

B. Management

1. Initiate HIV-specific and routine healthcare maintenance for age and gender (Tables 64-2 and 64-4).

2. Initiate primary prophylaxis for HIV OIs if needed (Table 64-4).

3. Provide screening and counseling for prevention of HIV transmission.

4. Identify and manage chronic comorbid conditions that are commonly seen in HIV-infected individuals.

5. Refer patients with serious or life-threatening OIs or illnesses of unclear etiology.

6. Refer patients who meet DHHS criteria for initiation of ART (Table 64-5).

TABLE 64-3 Initial Clinical Evaluation, Follow-up Laboratory and Diagnostic Studies

Test	Frequency	Comments
CD4 T-cell count, absolute and percentage	At baseline twice and every 3–6 months In patients with durable viral suppression and CD4 > 200, testing can be done every 6–12 months	Indicates stage of disease and time to initiate ART.[3] Normal values range from 800–1000 cells/mm³. Absolute CD4 can be highly variable based on time of day drawn, laboratory used, and presence of illness or recent immunizations. CD4 percentage less subject to variability between tests. Provides better indication of CD4 counts over time. A significant change from baseline for CD4 absolute is 30% and for CD4 percentage 3%.
HIV RNA	At baseline and every 3–6 months	Virologic failure is defined as confirmed viral load > 200 copies per milliliter. Viral load is used to follow treatment response and to diagnose acute HIV before development of HIV antibodies. Reported in copies per milliliter. Cutoff of ≥ 500–750,000 copies per milliliter for upper limits of detection and ≤ 40–75 copies per milliliter for lower limits of detection "not detected." A significant change is threefold change or 0.5 log 10 copies per milliliter increase or decrease from previous result.
HLA-B5701 testing	Once at baseline	Screens for genetic markers for risk for abacavir hypersensitivity reaction, a clinical syndrome seen within 6 weeks of initiating abacavir. Patients testing positive for HLA-B5701 should not initiate abacavir-containing regimens. Patient education and recording of positive test is important for patient safety and avoidance of serious drug reactions.
Genotypic resistance assays	At time of entry into HIV care and in acute HIV All pregnant women and women entering pregnancy with detectable HIV-1 RNA	Accuracy of results improved with viral load of > 1,000. Detects specific mutations in HIV genes known to confer resistance to nucleoside reverse transcriptase inhibitors, nonnucleoside reverse transcriptase inhibitors, and protease inhibitors. Assays are available for integrase strand transfer inhibitors and CCR5 inhibitors. Consultation recommended before ordering assays for integrase strand transfer inhibitors and CCR5 inhibitors. Interpretation requires HIV expertise regarding specific mutation patterns and cross-resistance within and across ART drug classes. Regardless of whether treatment is initiated or not. Assists in selection of optimal regimen.
Complete blood count with white blood cell count differential, chemistry profile	Baseline and every 3–6 months	Assesses for HIV-related anemia and thrombocytopenia. May influence decision regarding specific ART components.
Alanine transaminase, aspartate transaminase, T. Bili, albumin	Baseline and every 3–6 months	Required to assess for liver disease. May influence decision regarding specific ART components (nonnucleoside reverse transcriptase inhibitor nevirapine and protease inhibitors increase liver transaminases).
Fasting lipids and glucose	Baseline and every 6 months if on ART	Assess for CVD risks, insulin resistance, dyslipidemias. Low HDL seen commonly in HIV positive. May influence decision regarding specific ART components with choice of more lipid-friendly regimen.
Urinalysis, blood-urea-nitrogen, creatinine	Baseline and annually; repeat every 6 months if on tenofovir as part of a ART regimen	Assess for proteinuria caused by HIV-related nephropathy.
Pregnancy test		Indications are the same as for general population.

Source: Adapted from Panel on Antiretroviral Guidelines for Adults and Adolescents. Guidelines for the use of antiretroviral agents in HIV-1-infected adults and adolescents. Department of Health and Human Services. January 10, 2011; 1–166. Retrieved from http://www.aidsinfo.nih.gov/ContentFiles/AdultandAdolescentGL.pdf

TABLE 64-4 Specific Healthcare Maintenance for HIV-1 Infected

HIV Healthcare Maintenance	Frequency	Comments
Mycobacterium tuberculosis (MTB) TB skin test Interferon-γ release assay (IGRA)	Screen for latent tuberculosis infection annually and as needed based on symptoms and risks	If CD4 ≤ 200 mm³ at time of testing, retest once CD4 > 200 mm³. HIV-1 infected have ≥ 10% annual risk of active MTB. Positive skin test in HIV-1 infected is ≥ 5 mm induration at 48–72 hours. IGRA has high specificity compared to skin testing. IGRA has less cross-reactivity with nontuberculous mycobacteria exposures seen more commonly in resource-poor countries but use is prohibitive because of increased cost of IGRA compared to purified protein derivative skin testing. IGRA assays may be used instead of, or in conjunction with, skin testing. Reactive purified protein derivative skin test or IGRA indicates need for treatment regardless of age or CD4 count. Must rule out active MTB first.
Hepatitis A	At baseline	Immunize for hepatitis A virus if no evidence of immunity. Immunize all HIV-1 infected with chronic HCV.
Hepatitis B (HBV) HBsAb, HBcAb, HBsAg Chronic HBV HBeAg, antibody to HBeAg (anti-HBe), and HBV DNA	At baseline	Immunize all non-immune individuals. HIV-1 infected patients have an increased risk of chronic hepatitis if acutely infected with HBV. HBV DNA levels are usually high (> 20,000 IU/ml) in chronic infection. Refer to HIV specialist to evaluate need for specific HBV treatment or ART. Counsel on risk for acquisition of HBV; sexual, household, needle-sharing.
Hepatitis C (HCV) HCV Ab and HCV RNA HCV Genotype	At baseline	Screens for past exposure to HCV. Determines if infection is chronic. Can detect acute HCV before appearance of HCV specific antibodies. HCV genotype 2 and 3 is associated with improved HCV treatment outcome
Toxoplasma gondii Toxo IgG	At baseline	Counsel Toxo IgG negative adults on prevention of new *Toxoplasma* infections. Avoid eating raw or undercooked meat. If the patient owns a cat, change litter daily, preferably done by HIV-negative person. Wash hands thoroughly after changing litter box. Retest for Toxo IgG if CD4 fall to < 100 mm³ to determine need for primary prophylaxis.
Cytomegalovirus CMV Ab Varicella-zoster VZV Ab Herpes simplex virus-2 (HSV-2)	At baseline	Screen for cytomegalovirus Ab in patients where likelihood of cytomegalovirus seropositivity is low. Screen for varicella zoster virus if no history of chicken pox. Some experts recommend HSV-2 screening and initiation of secondary prophylaxis for HIV-1 infected who have evidence of HSV-2. Presence of HSV-2 lesions and viral shedding increases HIV viral loads in coinfected patients and increases transmission of HIV in sexual partners.
Glucose 6-phosphate dehydrogenase	At baseline	If deficiency present avoid antioxidant drugs, such as TMP/SMX and Dapsone.
Neisseria gonorrhoeae (GC), *Chlamydia trachomatis* (CT), *Trichomoniasis vaginalis*	At entry into care and as indicated by symptoms and risks	Several studies document the association of sexually transmitted infections with the transmission of HIV. Urine-based nucleic acid amplification test (NAAT) for CT and GC for urethral symptoms Collect specimens from all sexually active sites: anal GC and CT in men and women who report unprotected anal intercourse and pharyngeal specimens for GC if receptive oral sex reported.

TABLE 64-4 Specific Healthcare Maintenance for HIV-1 Infected (*continued*)

HIV Healthcare Maintenance	Frequency	Comments
Syphilis Venereal Disease Research Laboratory or rapid plasma regain	At baseline and as needed	Syphilis is associated with increased risk of acquiring and transmitting HIV. Some experts recommend screening rapid plasma regain at each routine follow-up visit for men who have sex with men with multiple partners or past history of syphilis. Responses to Venereal Disease Research Laboratory and rapid plasma regain are generally reliable in HIV-infected. Clinical evidence of central nervous system syphilis (headache, changes in vision or hearing) requires evaluation of the cerebrospinal fluid. Evaluation of cerebrospinal fluid is recommended for late latent and syphilis of unknown duration in HIV-1 infected.
Dilated retinal examination	At baseline CD4 < 100 annually	Screens for HIV-related retinopathy. Screens for clinical latent cytomegalovirus retinitis.
Chest radiograph	Baseline	If reactive purified protein derivative or IGRA. Consider for individuals with chronic pulmonary disease.
Men Serum testosterone level	Morning specimen	In males with fatigue, weight loss, and erectile dysfunction.
Human papillomavirus (HPV)		HPV recurrence and persistence is common in HIV-1 infected. Some experts recommend for men who have sex with men and women with referral for high-resolution anoscopy for any abnormal finding.
Anal cytology Bone mineral density screen	Annual	Men with evidence of abnormal bone mineral density. Age ≥ 50 years.
Women Cervical cytology		Pap at baseline and every 6 months. No recommendations exist for use of HPV DNA testing in HIV-1 infected women ≥ 30 years with normal cervical cytology. Perform annually after two normal Pap smears. Some experts recommend anal cytology in addition to cervical cytology. Refer any abnormal result, including atypical squamous cells of undetermined significance, for colposcopy.
Reproductive counseling		Women of childbearing age and men who are partnered with women who desire pregnancy.
Bone mineral density screen		Postmenopausal women age ≥ 65.

General healthcare maintenance for age and gender is the same for HIV-infected as for the general population with HIV-specific healthcare maintenance activities noted below. Commonly used risk assessment tools for coronary heart disease have not been validated in HIV-positive populations and risk may be underestimated in HIV-1 infected (National Cholesterol Education Project Risk Assessment Tool, http://hp2010.nhlbihin.net/atpiii/calculator.asp?usertype=prof)

Source: Adapted from Aberg, J. A., Kaplan, J. E., Libman, H., Emmanuel, P., Anderson, J. R., Stone, V. E., . . . HIV Medicine Association of the Infectious Diseases Society of America. (2009). Primary care guidelines for the management of persons infected with human immunodeficiency virus: 2009 update by the HIV Medicine Association of the Infectious Diseases Society of America. *Clinical Infectious Diseases: An Official Publication of the Infectious Diseases Society of America, 49*(5), 651–681; Centers for Disease Control and Prevention. Guidelines for prevention and treatment of opportunistic infections in HIV-1 infected adults and adolescents. (2009). *Morbidity and Mortality Weekly Report, 58* (No. RR-4). Retrieved from http://www.aidsinfo.nih.gov/Guidelines/GuidelineDetail.aspx?MenuItem=Guidelines&Search=Off&GuidelineID=15&ClassID=4

TABLE 64-5 Prophylaxis to Prevent First Episode of Opportunistic Infections in HIV-1 Infected Adults and Adolescents

Pathogen	Indication	Drug of Choice	Alternative
Pneumocystis pneumonia	CD4 count ≤ 200 cells/mm³ or oropharyngeal candidiasis CD4⁺ ≤ 14% or history of AIDS-defining illness	Trimethoprim-sulfamethoxazole, 1 DS po daily	Dapsone, 100 mg po daily or 50 mg po bid
Toxoplasma gondii	Toxoplasma IgG⁺ and CD4 ≤ 100 mm³	Trimethoprim-sulfamethoxazole, 1 DS po daily	Dapsone, 50 mg qd + pyrimethamine, 25 mg weekly + leucovorin, 25 mg weekly
Mycobacterium tuberculosis infection Treatment of latent TB infection All HIV-infected patients with diagnosed active TB should be treated with ART. See ART Treatment Guidelines for recommendations on initiation of ART in *Mycobacterium tuberculosis* and HIV coinfection.	Positive diagnostic test for latent TB infection, no evidence of active TB infection, and no prior history of treatment for active or latent TB (–) diagnostic test for latent TB infection, but close contact with a person with infectious pulmonary TB and no evidence of active TB A history of untreated or inadequately treated healed TB (i.e., old fibrotic lesions) regardless of diagnostic tests for latent TB infection and no evidence of active TB	Isoniazid, 300 mg po daily for 9 months plus pyridoxine, 50 mg daily	Rifabutin (dose adjusted based on concomitant ART) × 4 months
Disseminated *Mycobacterium avium*	CD4 ≤ 50 mm³ and no evidence of active disease or active TB	Azithromycin, 1,200 mg once weekly Clarithromycin, 500 mg bid Azithromycin, 600 mg twice weekly	Rifabutin, 300 mg daily (dose adjust for ARV drug interactions)

Source: Centers for Disease Control and Prevention. Guidelines for Prevention and Treatment of Opportunistic Infections in HIV-Infected Adults and Adolescents. (2009). *Morbidity and Mortality Weekly Review, 58*(No. RR-4).

7. Refer to social worker or community HIV/AIDS case management services to assess needs for housing, mental health and substance abuse treatment, health insurance, eligibility for AIDS programs, transportation to clinic appointments, and childcare and parenting needs.

C. Issues specific to HIV-infected women

1. Reproductive counseling: HIV-infected women of childbearing age who desire pregnancy require reproductive counseling. The landmark AIDS Clinical Trials Group (ACTG 076) study demonstrated the safety and efficacy of ART in pregnant women for prevention of mother-to-child transmission of HIV (Connor et al., 1994).

Avoidance of breastfeeding in addition to the use of ART has virtually eliminated perinatal transmission of HIV in countries where access to HIV care is available. Preconception counseling and referral to an HIV specialist should be provided for all women of childbearing age who are pregnant or desire pregnancy. If a woman does not desire to become pregnant, provide preconception counseling and initiate discussions regarding contraception. Several protease inhibitors and nonnucleoside reverse transcriptase inhibitors have drug interactions with oral contraceptives, causing changes in blood levels of ethinyl estradiol or norethindrone. Women on combined oral contraceptives and ART should use an alternative method of contraception. Progestin-only contraceptive methods seem to be effective and have no drug–drug interactions when used with currently approved ART regimens (DHHS Guidelines, 2011, pp. 133–149 and 14b). Intrauterine devices seem to be safe in women whose HIV is well controlled (World Health Organization, 2009).

2. ARV regimen considerations in women: Women seem to be more likely than men to develop severe reactions and symptomatic hepatic events from nevirapine, which is not recommended in treatment-naive women with CD4 greater than or equal to 250 cells mm³ unless risk outweighs benefits. Severe lactic acidosis is seen more commonly in women and risks for lactic acidosis include female gender, obesity, pregnancy, and use of the ARV component stavudine, and to a lesser extent, didanosine. Women have an increased risk of osteopenia and osteoporosis, especially after menopause, as a result of HIV and ARV therapies that affect bone metabolism.

D. Issues specific to HIV-infected transgender individuals

Transgender (TG) individuals are those persons whose gender identity (defined as a sense of being male or female), expressions, or behavior are not congruent with their birth sex. There are little data on this group of individuals and current evidence suggests that risks for HIV are high. The highest prevalence of HIV-positive TG individuals is among male-to-female sex workers both globally and domestically. Male-to-female TGs represent an important group for targeted HIV prevention messages. Stigma and discrimination towards TG individuals increases the likelihood of depression, suicide, intimate partner violence, psychologic abuse, substance use, and sexually transmitted diseases other than HIV. TGs are more likely to be ethnic minorities resulting in additional disparities in access to HIV care (http://www .cdc.gov/lgbthealth/transgender.htm). Some TGs may pursue sexual reassignment surgery, cosmetic surgery, or use hormones to enhance feminine or masculine physical characteristics (http://endo-society.org/guidelines /Current-Clinical-Practice-Guidelines.cfm). When caring for HIV-infected TG patients it is important to identify and link TGs with community agencies providing services for HIV-infected TGs and to consult with providers who have expertise in the care of TGs for the purposes of hormonal sex reassignment. Healthcare maintenance should be provided based on health risks and birth sex. In male-to-female TGs digital rectal examinations and prostate cancer screening is indicated based on age and other risks. In female-to-male TGs pelvic examination, Pap smear, and mammography based on recommended guidelines should be provided.

E. Patient education

HIV education should be conducted over several visits to provide basic information on HIV treatment, prevention of secondary transmission, and indications for ART. It is important to emphasize that HIV is a chronic manageable disease and that improved quality of life can be expected if individuals are engaged in care and motivated to take ART. There are several excellent websites that can provide resources and guidance in HIV/AIDS patient and provider education.

1. HIV/AIDS websites and resources
   a. U.S. HIV/AIDS Gateway for Federal/ Domestic AIDS: information and treatment guidelines (http://www.aids.gov).
   b. AIDS Education and Training Centers (AETC) Clinical Manual for HIV-infected Adults (http://www.aids-etc.org/aidsetc?page= cm-01-00).
   c. Centers for Disease Control and Prevention home page for HIV/AIDS (http://www.cdc.gov/hiv/).
   d. CDC National Center for HIV/AIDS, Viral Hepatitis, STD and TB Prevention (http://www.cdc.gov/tb).
   e. U.S. Department of Health and Human Services, Food and Drug Administration. ARV used in the treatment of HIV infection (http://www.fda.gov/oashi/aids/virals.html).
   f. Henry J. Kaiser Family Foundation, HIV Kaiser HIV/AIDS Daily Reports (http://www.kaisernetwork.org).
   g. Stanford University Drug Resistance Database (http://hivdb.stanford.edu/index.html).
   h. World Health Organization Reproductive Health Library (http://www.fhi.org/en/RH/Pubs /servdelivery/kenyabriefs/IUCD _Briefs_WHO_Update.htm).
   i. University of California, San Francisco Center of Excellence for Transgender HIV prevention (http://transhealth.ucsf.ed/trans).
   j. University of California, San Francisco HIV InSite (http://hivinsite.ucsf.edu/).
   k. University of California, San Francisco School of Medicine. Center for HIV Information (http://chi.ucsf.edu).
   l. CDC FDA-approved rapid HIV antibody screening tests (http://www.cdc.gov/hiv/topics/testing /rapid/rt-comparison.htm).

REFERENCES

Aberg, J. A., Kaplan, J. E., Libman, H., Emmanuel, P., Anderson, J. R., Stone, V. E., . . . HIV Medicine Association of the Infectious Diseases Society of America. (2009). Primary care guidelines for the management of persons infected with human immunodeficiency virus: 2009 update by the HIV Medicine Association of the Infectious Diseases Society of America. *Clinical Infectious Diseases: An Official Publication of the Infectious Diseases Society of America, 49*(5), 651–681.

Bartlett, J. G., Gallant, J. E., & Pham, P. A. (2009-2010). *Medical management of HIV infection.* Durham, NC: Knowledge Source Solutions, LCC.

Centers for Disease Control and Prevention. (2003a). Late versus early testing of HIV—16 sites—2000–2003. *Morbidity and Mortality Weekly Report, 52*(25), 581–586. Retrieved from http://www.cdc.gov/mmwr/preview/mmwrhtml/mm5225a2.htm

Centers for Disease Control and Prevention. (2003b). Incorporating HIV prevention into the medical care of persons living with HIV. Recommendations of CDC, Health Resources and Services Administration, the National Institutes of Health, and the HIV Medicine Association of the Infectious Diseases Society of America. *Morbidity and Mortality Weekly Review, 52*(RR-12), 1–24.

Centers for Disease Control and Prevention. (2006). Revised recommendations for HIV testing of adults, adolescents, and pregnant women in health-care settings. *Morbidity and Mortality Weekly Review, 55*(RR14), 1–17.

Centers for Disease Control and Prevention. (2009). Diagnosis of HIV Infection and AIDS in the United States and Dependent Areas. Retrieved from http://www.cdc.gov/hiv/surveillance/resources/reports/2009report/index.htm#1

Conde, D. M., Silva, E. T., Amaral, W. N., Finotti, M. F., & Feirera, R. G. (2009). HIV, reproductive aging, health implications in women: a literature review. *Menopause. The Journal of the North American Menopause Society, 16*(1), 199–221.

Connor, E. M., Sperling, R. S., Gelber, R. M. J., VanDyke, R., Bey, M., Shearer, W., & Jacobson, R. L. (1994). Reduction of maternal-infant transmission of human immunodeficiency virus type 1 with zidovudine treatment. *New England Journal of Medicine, 331*(18), 1173–1180.

Department of Health and Human Services, Panel on Antiretroviral Guidelines for Adults and Adolescents. (2011). *Guidelines for the use of antiretroviral agents in HIV-1- infected adult and adolescents.* Retrieved from http://aidsinfo.nih.gov/contentfiles/AdultandAdolescentGL.pdf

District of Columbia Department of Health, HIV/AIDS, Hepatitis, STD, and TB Administration (HAHSTA) District HIV/AIDS Epidemiology Update 2008. Retrieved from http://dchealth.dc.gov/doh/frames.asp?doc=/doh/lib/doh/pdf/dc_hiv-aids_2008_updatereport.pdf

Dolin, R., Masur, H., & Sagg, M. (2008). *AIDS therapy.* Philadelphia, PA: Churchill Livingstone Elsevier.

Douek, D., Picker, L. J., & Koup, R. A. (2003). T cell dynamics in HIV-1 infection. *Annual Review of Immunology, 21,* 265–304.

Friis-Møller, N., Weber, R., Reiss, P., Thiébaut, R., Kirk, O., d'Arminio, Monforte, A., . . . DAD study group. (2003). Cardiovascular disease risk factors in HIV patients-association with antiretroviral therapy. *AIDS, 17*(8), 1179–1193.

Giordano, T. P., Gifford, A. L., White, A. C., Jr., Suarez-Almazor, M. E., Rabeneck, L., Hartman, C., . . . Morgan, R. (2007). Retention in care: A challenge to survival with HIV infection. *Clinical Infectious Diseases: An Official Publication of the Infectious Diseases Society of America, 44*(11), 1493–1499.

Goetz, M. B., Hoang, T., Henry, S. R., Knapp, H., Anaya, H. D., Gifford, A. L., . . . the QUERI-HIV/Hepatitis Program. (2009). Evaluation of the Sustainability of an intervention to increase HIV testing. *Journal of General Internal Medicine, 24*(12), 1275–1280.

Gupta, S. K., Eustace, J. A., Winston, J. A., Boydstun, I. I., Ahuja, T. S., Rodriguez, R. A., . . . Szczech, L. A. (2005). Guidelines for the management of chronic kidney disease in HIV-infected patients: Recommendations of the HIV Medicine Association of the Infectious Diseases Society of America. *Clinical Infectious Diseases: An Official Publication of the Infectious Diseases Society of America, 40*(11), 1559–1585.

Hall, H. I., Song, R., Rhodes, P., Prejean, J., & Qian An, M. S. (2009). Estimation of HIV incidence in the United States. *New England Journal of Medicine, 300*(5), 520–529.

Hare, C. B., Futterman, D., & Thornton, A. C. (2011). Faculty responses to additional questions on routine testing for HIV infection in primary care settings. *Clinical Care Options.* Retrieved from http://www.clinicaloptions.com/HIV/Treatment%20Updates/HIV%20Routine%20Testing.aspx

Ho, J. E., & Hsue, P. Y. (2009). Cardiovascular manifestations of HIV. *Heart, 95,* 1193–1202.

Medicine Association of the Infectious Diseases Society of America. *Clinical Infectious Diseases: An Official Publication of the Infectious Diseases Society of America, 40*(11), 1559–1585.

Myers, J. J., Modica, C., Dufour, M. S., Bernstein, C., & McNamara, K. (2009). Routine rapid HIV screening in six community health centers serving populations at risk. *Journal of General Internal Medicine, 24*(12), 1269–1274.

Palella, F. J., Jr., Baker, R. K., Moorman, A. C., Chmiel, J. S., Wood, K. C., Brooks, J. T., . . . HIV Outpatient Study Investigators. (2006). Mortality in the highly active antiretroviral therapy era: Changing causes of death and disease in the HIV outpatient study. *Journal of Acquired Immune Deficiency Syndromes, 43*(1), 27–34.

Patel, P., Hanson, D. L., Sullivan, P. S., Novak, R. M., Moormann, A. C., Tong, T. C., . . . Adult and Adolescent Spectrum of Disease Project and HIV Outpatient Study Investigators. (2008). Incidence of Types of Cancer among HIV-Infected Persons Compared with the General Population in the United States, 1992–2003. *Annals of Internal Medicine, 148*(10), 728–736.

Perinatal HIV Guidelines Working Group. Public Health Service Task Force Recommendations for Use of Antiretroviral Drugs in Pregnant HIV-Infected Women for Maternal Health and Interventions to Reduce Perinatal HIV Transmission in the United States. April 29, 2009; pp. 1–90. Retrieved from http://aidsinfo.nih.gov/ContentFiles/PerinatalGL.pdf

Power, C., Selnes, O. A., Grim, J. A., & McArthur, J. C. (1995). HIV dementia scale: A rapid screening test. *Journal of Acquired Immunodeficiency Syndrome, 8,* 273–278.

Strategies for Management of Antiretroviral Therapy (SMART) Study Group, El-Sadr, W. M., Lundgren, J. D., Neaton, J. D., Gordin, F., Abrams, D., Arduino, R. C., . . . Rappoport, C. (2006). CD4+ count-guided interruption of antiretroviral treatment. *The New England Journal of Medicine, 355*(22), 2283–2296.

UNAIDS Joint Programme on HIV/AIDS. *AIDS epidemic update 2009.* Retrieved from http://www.unaids.org/en/KnowledgeCentre/HIVData/EpiUpdate/EpiUpdArchive/2009/default.asp

Valcour, V., & Paul, R. (2006). HIV infection and dementia in older adults. *Clinical Infectious Diseases, 42,* 1449–1454.

World Health Organization. (2009). *Gender, Women and Health. HIV and gender inequalities.* Retrieved from http://www.who.int/gender/hiv_aids/en/index.html

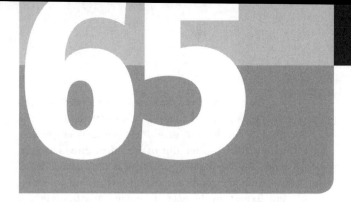

SMOKING CESSATION

Kellie McNerney
and Vicki Smith

I. Introduction and general background

A. History and politics of tobacco

American settlers adopted the ritual of smoking from Native Americans in the 1800s. In 1884, the cigarette-rolling machine was invented, allowing mass production of cigarettes. By World War I, tobacco was considered as indispensable as food and was included in ration packets distributed to Americans on the home front (Sheehan, 2004). During World War II the American military forces consumed 75% of American tobacco products. Even the journals of the American Medical Association accepted cigarette advertisements during this time (Houston, 1992).

In 1941, the insightful work of two physicians, Oschner and DeBakey, called attention to the similarity of the curve of increased sales of cigarettes to the increased prevalence of lung cancer (Wynder & Graham, 1950). Nine years later, Wynder and Graham published their results of a well-designed study linking cigarette smoking with bronchogenic carcinoma.

It was not until 1964 that the United States Surgeon General issued the first public report linking smoking with negative health consequences. Despite more than 60,000 documents proving the relationship between smoking and lung cancer, the tobacco industry continued to deny this evidence. Spending an estimated $3.5 billion a year on advertising and promotion of its products, the tobacco industry was a powerful political lobby preventing the regulation of tobacco and sale of cigarettes. It was not until June of 2009 that the Federal Drug Administration (FDA) was granted the power to regulate tobacco products, with President Obama signing HR 1256 Family Smoking Prevention and Tobacco Control Act (American Heart Association, 2009).

The three major causes of smoking-related deaths are cardiovascular disease (CVD), lung cancer, and chronic obstructive pulmonary disease (COPD). In the United States there are an estimated 443,000 premature deaths each year attributed to smoking-related diseases (Morbidity and Mortality Week Report, 2009). That is more than 1,000 deaths daily from tobacco-related disease. It is estimated that $193 billion are spent each year in direct healthcare costs and loss of productivity caused by smoking-related diseases (MMWR, 2009).

B. Prevalence and incidence

Despite the overall decline in cigarette smoking since 1965, cigarette smoking is still the leading preventable cause of death in the United States. According to data from 2007, 19.8% of the United States adult population smokes. Forty-four states show a decline in smoking since 1998. There has been no state with an increase in smoking prevalence but six states show no decrease. A state-by-state survey identified variation in prevalence of smoking rates from as high as 31% in Guam and as low as 9% in the U.S. Virgin Islands. If one looks at just the 50 states, the highest prevalence of smoking is in the states of Kentucky (28%); West Virginia (27%); and Oklahoma (26%). The lowest rates of smoking are in Utah (12%); California (14%); and Connecticut (15%) (MMWR, 2009).

Cigarette smoking causes 87% of lung cancer but is also responsible for 30% of all cancers, including cancer of the bladder, mouth, oral pharynx, larynx, esophagus, stomach, cervix, uterus, kidney, and pancreas, and myeloid leukemia (American Cancer Society, 2011; U.S. Department of Health and Human Services, 2004). It is estimated that 8.6 million people in the United States suffer from serious illness related to smoking. Chronic bronchitis and COPD comprise 59% of all serious illness attributable to smoking. Oral cancers are related to smokeless tobacco or pipe and cigar use. Clinicians in cities where immigration from Southeast Asian countries is common need to inquire about both smoking history in relation to beedi or smokeless tobacco products, such as paan or Gutkha.

C. Population-based concerns

Women who smoke have special concerns regarding reproduction and fertility. Infertility is more common in smokers as a result of the effects of nicotine on the hormonal changes responsible for menstruation. Nicotine interferes with the normal release of gonadotropins, which can result in menstrual irregularities, hirsutism, early menopause, and accelerated osteoporosis.

Other particularly high-risk groups for tobacco dependence and its related health consequences are persons with mental health or substance use disorders. Persons with mental health disorders account for 44% of the cigarettes consumed in the United States, and nationally 77–93% of persons with substance use disorders have a comorbid tobacco use disorder significantly exceeding the national prevalence for tobacco dependence (Kalman, Kim, DiGirolamo, Smelson, & Ziedonis, 2010; Schroeder & Morris, 2009). Moreover, research suggests quitting smoking cigarettes and alcohol simultaneously confers a protective factor for alcohol relapse in alcohol-dependent persons (Kalman et al., 2010). Furthermore, given the preponderance of multiple smokable drugs in substance-affected populations in addition to tobacco (e.g., marijuana, stimulants, and opiates) the risk for health consequences, particularly on the pulmonary system, may be increased (Tashkin, 2001).

D. Smoking cessation

Surveys demonstrate that 70% of smokers say they want to quit smoking and over 40% report having tried to quit in the past year (Fiore et al., 2008). Relapse rates for smokers are high. A total of 93–95% of smokers trying to quit on their own unaided relapse before 1 year is over. Most former smokers have made several attempts to quit before succeeding. The addictive nature of nicotine is the primary factor that accounts for the difficulty of quitting smoking. There are also other barriers to quitting, such as repeated behaviors and environmental circumstances that trigger the desire for a cigarette. One-year abstinent rates can be increased up to 30% with optimal therapy, usually psychosocial counseling and nicotine replacement, bupropion, or varenicline (Rennard, Rigotti, & Daughton, 2009).

Brief advice to quit smoking by the provider done routinely at each office visit increases the rates of smoking cessation. Advice to quit in addition to brief counseling strategies and follow-up improves quit rates even more (Lancaster & Stead, 2004; Rennard et al., 2009).

Three categories of pharmacotherapy have proved helpful in smoking cessation: (1) nicotine replacement therapy, (2) bupropion, and (3) varenicline. Three nicotine replacement products are sold over-the-counter: (1) nicotine patches, (2) nicotine gum, and (3) nicotine lozenges. The other nicotine replacement products (the nicotine nasal spray and the nicotine inhaler) require prescriptions. There are few studies comparing which product is more efficacious than another but several studies show all nicotine products are better compared to placebo and double cessation rates. All products also increase cessation rates when used in conjunction with a behavior modification program (Rennard et al., 2009).

To use any nicotine replacement product the smoker is counseled to pick a quit date and start the product on the quit date. Most products are recommended for 2–3 months of use. Most providers continue the nicotine replacement as long as needed if stopping the medication means returning to smoking. Experts in the field of smoking cessation say that nicotine by itself is not as harmful as tobacco smoke (Rennard et al., 2009). Combining nicotine replacement products is also considered a helpful strategy for nicotine-dependent persons trying to quit. Using a "controller" medication (patch) with a "reliever" (gum, lozenge, or inhaler) medication can be more effective to induce quitting than either medication formulation alone. The differences in pharmacology action and duration of each product make this possible. A slow-onset and long-acting product, such as the patch, can be safely combined with the use of a shorter-acting product, such as gum or lozenge.

Nicotine replacement is considered safe for use even in smokers with known CVD. Experts say the benefits of quitting smoking far outweigh any risk of the nicotine replacement product, although few studies exist (Kimmel et al., 2001; Rennard et al., 2009).

Bupropion has been used and is available in the United States as an antidepressant since 1989. Smokers who were on bupropion recognized decreased desire to smoke as an interesting side effect. A sustained-release form of bupropion was developed and marketed as a smoking cessation aid, Zyban®. Large studies demonstrate that the use of bupropion doubles the success rate of smoking cessation (Rennard et al., 2009).

Varenicline is hypothesized to both bind to nicotine receptors in the brain and block the nicotine in cigarette smoke from attaching to the receptor in the brain. It is hypothesized that this action reduces the rewarding sensation of nicotine, thus decreasing the desire to smoke. Multiple studies show efficacy. In February 2008 the FDA issued an alert that an increase in suicidal thinking and "aggressive and erratic behavior" was associated with patients being treated with varenicline (U.S. FDA, 2008). Most experts recommend taking a careful psychiatric history before starting the medication, and not using the medication for known patients with any current or past history of unstable depression or suicidality. It is important to note that neuropsychiatric side effects have been reported even in patients with no known history. It is recommended that if using this medication, use as second-line therapy, with caution and careful follow-up in 1 and 2 weeks. It is recommended that patients be told to contact the provider or the office and stop the drug if they or their family notice any unusual mood or behavior symptoms.

II. Database

A. Subjective

1. Obtain a smoking history

    a. Ask, "Do you smoke?" "For how long?" "How much do you smoke?" "Are you interested in quitting?" "Have you ever quit before?" "What made you start again?"

    b. If patient has quit, ascertain prior smoking history because recent cessation (within the year) increases the risk for relapse.

2. Past health history

    a. Medical history: illnesses specific to cardio-respiratory system, such as bronchitis, sinusitis, pneumonia, allergies, asthma, COPD, coronary artery disease, myocardial infarction, peripheral vascular disease (PVD), Reynaud's disease, hypertension, hypercholesterolemia, blood clots; cancer, such as lung, head and neck, mouth, larynx, esophagus, bladder, kidney, pancreas, brain, cervix, breast; and gastritis or peptic ulcer disease.

    b. Substance use disorders: screen with a standardized screening tool, such as CAGE-AID or other brief screening tool, and for depression using PHQ-9 or other depression screening tool (Brown & Rounds, 1995; Spitzer, Kroenke, & Williams, 1999).

    c. Psychiatric disorders: prior history of depression or other mental health diagnosis. These conditions can make cessation more difficult.

    d. Gynecological history: infertility, abnormal pap smears, low-birth-weight babies, and complications of pregnancy.

    e. Exposure history: passive smoking or asbestos.

    f. Medication history: prior use of nicotine replacement, bupropion, varenicline, or other medications related to cessation, depression, or seizures.

3. Family history: cancer, CVD, PVD, COPD, or other respiratory symptoms.

4. Personal and social history

    a. Identify social supports and living situations in terms of other smokers.

    b. Assess coexistent stressors to determine whether timing is right to introduce a major lifestyle change.

    c. Identify need for possible referrals.

    d. Use of alcohol and other substances

    e. Use of telephone-, Internet-, or office-based support groups.

5. Review of systems

    a. Constitutional for sign or symptoms as related to cancer, infection, and CVD. Generally, there are no signs or symptoms.

    b. Skin, hair, and nails: Cosmetic changes noted, such as early skin wrinkling, impaired wound healing, and finger and teeth staining.

    c. Ear, nose, and throat: allergic or irritant symptoms, postnasal drip, frequent infections, dental complaints, and dysphagia.

    d. Cardiovascular: chest pain, leg pain when walking short distances, excessively cold hands, or feet with color change. Chest pain or change in activity tolerance, paroxysmal nocturnal dyspnea, or peripheral edema.

    e. Respiratory: shortness of breath, productive or nonproductive cough, postnasal drip, wheezing, decreased exercise tolerance, frequent colds, and allergy symptoms. Cough, wheezing, mucous production, dyspnea, and paroxysmal nocturnal dyspnea.

    f. Gastrointestinal: abdominal burning or pain, acid indigestion, heartburn, constipation, diarrhea; frequent use of antacids; and food intolerance. Use of smoking to regulate bowels.

    g. Genitourinary: sexual or erectile dysfunction.

    h. Musculoskeletal: claudication or peripheral edema.

    i. Neurologic: paresthesias or depression.

B. Objective

1. Physical examination

    a. Vital signs: may include increased heart rate or blood pressure

    b. General appearance: may appear older than stated age; clothes and hair may smell of cigarette smoke

    c. Skin, hair, nails: facial wrinkles and yellow stains on teeth and fingers

    d. Head, eyes, ears, nose, and throat: assess for periodontal disease, include bimanual examination of mouth, assess for oral lesions that may be malignant or premalignant, leukoplakia, evidence of upper respiratory irritants, infection, or allergies

    e. Lymphatic: generally, there are few findings but look for lymphadenopathy in presence of any head, eyes, ears, nose, and throat symptoms

    f. Chest: generally, there are few findings unless illness is present, but assess respiratory rate, quality of cough if observed, anteroposterior diameter, presence of adventitious sounds; office spirometry or peak expiratory flow rates are usually normal

g. Cardiovascular: generally, few findings are observed but evaluate cardiac rate, rhythm, extra heart sounds, and pulses

h. Extremities: note color, temperature and pulses, note hair distribution because there is a decrease in lower extremities of those with PVD

i. Neurologic: generally, few findings but evaluation if any paresthesias; depression screen and substance abuse screen

2. Supporting data from relevant diagnostic tests

a. Complete blood count, lipid profile, and kidney functions

b. If indicated: electrocardiogram, pulmonary function tests, and chest radiograph

III. Assessment

A. *List related ICD 9 codes (e.g., 305.1 Tobacco use disorder or V15.82 History of tobacco use)*

B. *Former, current, risk of relapse*

C. *Significance of smoking history, smoking index, or pack-year in terms of disease risk*

D. *Stage of readiness to quit*

E. *Rule out concomitant physical illness*

IV. Plan

A. *Diagnostic*

1. Pulmonary function tests are usually normal unless respiratory illness is present, and is therefore not recommended.

2. Lipid panel, if elevated, may be a useful motivator for quitting and monitoring.

3. Additional testing as indicated by history and physical examination

B. *Treatment and management goals*

1. Advise patient to stop smoking. If evidence of concomitant illness or sign of abnormality on examination, use this as an indication of harmful effects of tobacco and the need to quit smoking. Provide an individualized treatment plan based on patient's readiness to quit.

a. Precontemplative: advise to quit, acknowledge lack of readiness, state availability to assist in quitting when they are ready; evaluate readiness at every visit.

b. Contemplative: advise to quit, acknowledge their consideration, provide written pamphlet or resource for review, state availability for assist in quitting when ready to set quit date.

c. Planning: help pick quit date, review behavior modification strategies, review medication available, nicotine replacement with or without bupropion or varenicline.

d. Action: follow-up and resources for relapse prevention.

C. *Behavior modification and patient education*

1. Inform patient that quitting smoking is the single most important thing he or she can do for their health.

2. Encourage patient to think of quitting smoking as "learning a foreign language." Both efforts require practice. If a relapse occurs, encourage patient not to give up and to try again. Smoking cessation may take a while to master.

3. On average, it takes three attempts before a smoker stays quit for good.

4. Encourage the smoker not to feel as if he or she has a character defect because they did not succeed in the past. Encourage them to try again.

5. Have the smoker write on a 3 × 5 file card the three most important reasons to quit, to keep this card in the same place they used to keep cigarettes, and to pull out the card and read it whenever they have an urge.

6. Have patient practice quitting a little every day, at different times of day.

a. For example, on Monday, advise patient not to smoke from 6:00 a.m. until 9:00 a.m.; on Tuesday, not to smoke from 9:00 a.m. until 12 noon; on Wednesday, not to smoke from noon until 3:00 p.m., and so on.

b. Once the week is completed, the smoker will learn which cigarettes were most important and then will know which cigarettes might prove to be harder to quit.

7. Have patient keep a smoking diary.

8. Identifying what triggers smoking (this is key to determine alternate behaviors to smoking).

9. Reward nonsmoking behaviors. Rewarded behavior is repeated.

10. Encourage patient to join a class on quitting smoking, Internet-based group, or cell phone reminder groups.

11. Ask patient to read as much as possible about the health effects of smoking, the benefits of quitting, and the tobacco industry.

12. Encourage plenty of rest, fresh air, exercise, and nutrition.

13. Ask patient to reach out to nonsmokers, to find a "buddy" in their quit smoking campaign. People with more social support have higher success rates.

14. Tell patient to expect a small weight gain.

15. Bupropion may help prevent weight gain.

16. Being overweight generally is healthier than smoking.

17. Tell patient to increase the level and frequency of exercise.

18. Advise patient to be wary of relapse. Advise patient to avoid high-risk situations initially, and to learn and practice positive imagery, meditation, or self-hypnosis techniques. Buddy up in at-risk situations.

19. Tell patient to expect success, to be confident.

20. Once patient has quit for 6 months, encourage community involvement (e.g., volunteer on "former smoker" panels, teach a quit smoking class, be a buddy for other "newly quit" smokers).

21. It is helpful to have a scheduled stop smoking visit; to establish a quit date, quit day appointment, or telephone call; and give patient homework

22. Review strategies for urge control, offer community or Internet referral sources.

23. Offer support visit at 3 months.

24. Ask at every visit about patient's efforts.

25. Praise and congratulate any quit effort, and explore what caused any relapse.

26. If quitting is recent, offer printed self-help materials and referrals to Nicotine Anonymous, American Lung Association, American Cancer Society, or Internet-based sites

D. Medications

1. Nicotine-replacement products

   a. Nicotine patch is a transdermal system absorbed through the skin over 16–24 hours depending on the brand. Patient should start use on their quit date. Apply every morning on a dry area of upper arm, stomach, or buttock. Remove at bedtime because the nicotine may interrupt sleep. However, persons who smoke immediately on waking may find it beneficial to wear the patch during sleep. Rotate sites, reusing the same site no more frequently than every 7 days. Change every day. The different brands are generally similar in dosage. Taper over 2 months (e.g., 21 mg/day for 4 weeks, 14 mg/day for 2 weeks, and 7 mg/day for 2 weeks). The 21-mg patch is equivalent to trough concentrations (i.e., lowest level of blood nicotine) in smokers averaging one pack per day. Generally well tolerated, although 50% of users experience some local skin irritation. It is acceptable to use topical steroid and continue use with rotation of sites. Can cause excessive or unusual dreams; can remove at bedtime.

   b. Nicotine gum or lozenge is an oral product containing nicotine bound to a polacrilex resin.

   c. When the gum is chewed or sucked it releases nicotine, which is absorbed through the oral mucosa. It takes 20 minutes for the nicotine level in the blood to rise. Advise the client to bite the gum slowly, not to chew like gum or the nicotine will be released faster than it can be absorbed and thus swallowed. Swallowing the nicotine causes stomach or esophageal irritation. Nicotine from the gastrointestinal tract is metabolized by the liver and essentially is ineffective. May be used with patch or after patch for "just in case." For nicotine gum, "bite and park." Bite until it tastes (radish or peppery taste) and bite again after taste disappears. It lasts approximately 20–30 minutes. Avoid coffee and carbonated drinks for up to 20 minutes before use, because this lowers the absorption of nicotine. Use 2-mg gum for most smokers; can use 4 mg for those who smoke more than 25 cigarettes per day. Use as often as an urge occurs, up to 20 pieces per day. Taper after 6 weeks; taper one to two pieces per week. Dependence on gum is not common because the delivery system essentially acts to wean the smoker, but is still considered safer than smoking (Rennard et al., 2009).

   d. For nicotine lozenges, do not chew; can be used for those with dentures or the edentulous. Place in mouth and let dissolve for 30 minutes. Use the 2-mg dose for most smokers but 4 mg is recommended for those who smoke within 30 minutes of awakening. May use one to two per hour for the first 4–6 weeks.

Taper after 6 weeks; dependence issues are not likely but see the previous discussion regarding nicotine gum.

e. Nicotine inhaler (available only by prescription): the nicotine inhaler is a plastic mouthpiece with a nicotine cartridge placed inside. When the smoker inhales through the device, nicotine vapor, not smoke is released into the mouth and throat and absorbed through the oral mucosa. The vapor mostly does not reach the lungs and is pharmacologically more similar to gum or lozenge than a cigarette. Plasma levels of nicotine are approximately one-third that of a cigarette. May be helpful in smokers to address the behavioral and sensory aspects of cigarette smoking or in those who failed gum or lozenges. Recommended dose is 6–16 cartridges per day for the first 6–12 weeks. Taper dose over the next 6–12 weeks. Avoid or use in caution in those with a history of severe reactive airway syndromes because it may cause bronchospasm.

f. Nicotine nasal spray (available only by prescription): delivers nicotine to nasal mucosa via an aqueous solution. It is more rapidly delivered with peak concentration within 10 minutes but not as rapid as a cigarette. One to two sprays per hour for the first 3 months. A high rate of nasal and throat irritation limits its use.

2. Bupropion

a. Start 1–2 weeks before quit date.

b. Start with bupropion sustained release, 150 mg once daily for 3–7 days.

c. Increase to twice a day for 7 days. If side effects occur on the 300-mg dose, continue at 150-mg daily.

d. Recommended treatment duration is 7–12 weeks, but may continue longer up to 6 months.

e. Common side effects are insomnia, dry mouth, and headache.

f. Serious side effect is seizure. Clinical trial risk of seizure is 0.1%. Contraindicated in seizure disorder or predisposition to seizure.

3. Varenicline

a. Start 0.5 mg daily for 3 days then increase to 0.5 mg twice a day for 4 days, then 1 mg twice a day for remainder of the 12-week course.

b. Advise to take with food and a full glass of water to avoid the side effect of nausea.

c. Quit smoking 1 week after start of medication.

d. Common side effects are nausea, insomnia, and abnormal dreams.

e. Because of concern regarding serious neuropsychiatric side effects, counsel patient to call office and stop medication if they or their family notice any unusual mood or behavior symptoms.

f. Use with caution with renal insufficiency and any history of depression.

4. Long-term use of nicotine replacement may increase insulin resistance, lower high-density lipoproteins, and increase risk of CVD; cancer risk is small (Dale, 2009).

5. Encourage patient enrollment in a smoking cessation class.

E. Documentation

1. Document smoking history and cessation strategies in progress notes.

2. Identify smoking status on problem list as appropriate.

V. Self-management resources and support

A. Telephone support

1. 1-800-QUIT-NOW, a national hotline for smoking cessation, or 1-800-NO-BUTTS, a California hotline for smoking cessation

VI. Consultation

A. In patients with depression or history of depression, antidepressant agents may be required. Referral for counseling is recommended.

B. In pregnant patients and patients with cerebrovascular, CVD, or seizure disorder consultation with a physician is advised before the use of pharmacologic adjuncts for smoking cessation.

C. As needed for prescriptions.

REFERENCES

American Cancer Society. (2011). *Tobacco related cancers fact sheet.* Retrieved from http://www.cancer.org/Cancer/CancerCauses/Tobacco Cancer/tobacco-related-cancer-fact-sheet

American Heart Association. (2009). *HR 1256 Family Smoking Prevention and Tobacco Control Act.* Retrieved from http://www.americanheart .org/presenter.jhtml?identifier=3010863

Brown, R. L., & Rounds, L. A. (1995). Conjoint screening questionnaires for alcohol and other drug abuse: Criterion validity in a primary care practice. *Wisconsin Medical Journal, 94*(3), 135–140.

Dale, L. C. (2009). Nicotine replacement therapy not meant for long term use. *Mayo Clinic Medical Edge Newspaper Column.* Retrieved from http://www.mayoclinic.org/medical-edge-newspaper-2009/apr-24b.html

Fiore, M. C., Jaen, C. R., Baker, T. B., Bailey, W. C., Benowitz, N. L., Curry, S. J., . . . Wewers, M. E. (2008). Treating tobacco use and dependence: 2008 update. *Clinical Practice Guidelines.* Retrieved from http://www.surgeongeneral.gov/tobacco/treating_tobacco_use08.pdf

Fiore, M. C., Bailey, W. C., Cohen, S. J., Dorfman, S. F., Goldstein, M. G., Gritz, E. R., . . .Wewers, M. E. (2000). *Treating tobacco use and dependence. Quick reference guide for clinicians.* Rockville, MD: U.S. Department of Health and Human Services.

Houston, T. P. (1992). Smoking cessation in office practice. *Primary Care, 19,* 493–507.

Kalman, D., Kim, S., DiGirolamo, G., Smelson, D., & Ziedonis, D. (2010). Addressing tobacco use disorder in smokers in early remission from alcohol dependence: The case for integrating smoking cessation services in substance use disorder treatment programs. *Clinical Psychology Revue, 30*(1), 12–24.

Kimmel, S. E., Berlin, J. A., Miles, C., Jaskowiak, J., Carson, J. L., & Strom, B. L. (2001). Risk of acute first myocardial infarction and use of nicotine patches in a general population. *Journal of the American College of Cardiology, 37*(5), 1297–1302.

Lancaster, T., & Stead, L. F. (2004). Physician advice for smoking cessation. *Cochrane Database of Systematic Reviews,* issue 4, CD000165. Update Software.

Morbidity and Mortality Weekly Report (MMWR). (2009). State-specific prevalence and trends in adult cigarette smoking—United States 1998–2007. *Morbidity and Mortality Weekly Review, 58*(09), 221–226. Retrieved from http://www.cdc.gov/mmwr/PDF/wk/mm5809.pdf

Rennard, S. I., Rigotti, N. A., & Daughton, D. M. (2009). *Management of smoking cessation.* Hardcopy received February 17, 2009, as complimentary topic downloaded from http://www.uptodate.com

Schroeder, S. A., & Morris, C. D. (2009). Confronting a neglected epidemic: Tobacco cessation for persons with mental illness and substance abuse problems. *Annual Reviews in Public Health, 31,* 297–314. . DOI:10.1146/annurev.publhealth.012809.103701

Sheehan, K. A. (2004). Smoking cessation. (2004). pp. 14-64–14-68. In W. L. Star, L. L. Lommel, & M. T. Shannon, *Women's primary health care: Protocols for practice* (2nd ed.). San Francisco: UCSF Nursing Press.

Spitzer, R. L., Kroenke, K., & Williams, J. B. W. (1999). Validation and utility of a self-report version of PRIME-MD: The PHQ primary care study. *Journal of the American Medical Association, 282*(18), 1737–1744.

Tashkin, D. P. (2001). Airway effects of marijuana, cocaine, and other inhaled illicit agents. *Current Opinion in Pulmonary Medicine, 7*(2), 43–61.

U.S. Department of Health and Human Services. (2004). *The health consequences of smoking: A report of the Surgeon General.* Atlanta, GA: U.S. Department of Health and Human Services, Centers for Disease Control and Prevention, National Center for Chronic Disease Prevention and Health Promotion, Office on Smoking and Health.

U.S. Food and Drug Administration. (2008). *Important information on Chantix (varenicline).* Retrieved from http://www.gov/drugs/drugsaffdaety/publichealthadvisories/ucm051136

Wynder, E. L., & Graham, E. A. (1950). Tobacco smoking as a possible etiological factor in bronchiogenic carcinoma. *Journal of the American Medical Association, 143,* 329–336.

THYROID DISORDERS

JoAnne M. Saxe

I. Introduction and general background

The adult thyroid gland is responsible for the production of hormones (L-thyroxine [T_4] and 3,5,3'-triiodothyronine [T_3]) that influence a variety of metabolic processes. Its structure and function are contingent on an intact axis between this gland and the hypothalamus and pituitary glands. Specifically, the hypothalamus secretes thyrotropin-releasing hormone, which stimulates the pituitary to produce and release thyroid-stimulating hormone (TSH). TSH triggers the production and secretion of T_3 and T_4 from the thyroid. Through a positive–negative feedback loop, these glands, when normally functioning, regulate T_3 and T_4 secretion so that metabolic homeostasis is ensured.

The thyroid gland is affected by a number of other extrathyroidal factors, such as the status of the immune system. Thus, alterations in the synthesis, secretion, and circulation of thyroid hormones may be caused by an array of primary or secondary thyroid disorders. The most common thyroid conditions seen in primary care settings are primary hypothyroidism, hyperthyroidism, and thyroid nodules (Saxe, 2004).

A. Primary hypothyroidism

1. Definition and overview

   This is a condition in which there is loss of thyroid function as a result of the intrinsic thyroid pathology. Primary hypothyroidism accounts for 95% of all cases of hypothyroidism (Jameson & Weetman, 2008). The most common causes of primary hypothyroidism in the United States are:

   a. Thyroid inflammatory diseases (e.g., chronic [Hashimoto's] thyroiditis, postpartum [subacute lymphocytic] thyroiditis, and subacute thyroiditis). The initial presentation of

   thyroiditis, however, often is consistent with a diagnosis of hyperthyroidism.

   b. Radioiodine-induced or surgically induced hypothyroidism.

   c. Idiopathic thyroid atrophy (Saxe, 2004).

2. Prevalence and incidence

   Data from the Whickham survey and other studies indicate that the prevalence and incidences of hypothyroidism (unsuspected overt, known overt, and subclinical) in men are extremely low (Wang & Crapo, 1997). The prevalence of primary hypothyroidism for women is less than 1% for unsuspected overt hypothyroidism, approximately 1.5% for overt hypothyroidism, and approximately 7.5% for subclinical hypothyroidism. However, the prevalence of primary hypothyroidism is higher in the geriatric female population than in women under age 40 (Wang & Crapo, 1997).

B. Hyperthyroidism

1. Definition and overview

   Hyperfunctioning of the thyroid gland can result from a variety of diseases. The most common causes of hyperthyroidism are

   a. Diffuse toxic (hyperfunctioning) goiter (Graves' disease).

   b. Toxic multinodular goiter.

   c. Toxic uninodular goiter.

   d. Thyroid inflammatory diseases (e.g., Hashimoto's thyroiditis, postpartum thyroiditis, and subacute thyroiditis, which overall cause a transient thyrotoxicosis [Saxe, 2004]).

2. Prevalence and incidence

   Data from the Whickham survey and other studies indicate that the prevalence and incidence of hyperthyroidism in men is low. In women, unsuspected and known overt hyperthyroidism is approximately 2.8 per 100 women. Like primary hypothyroidism, hyperthyroidism is more commonly seen in older women than in women before the fourth decade (Cooper, Greenspan, & Ladenson, 2007; Wang & Crapo, 1997).

C. Thyroid nodules

1. Definition and overview

   Thyroid nodules may be functional (e.g., toxic uninodular goiter) or nonfunctional (e.g., benign follicular adenomas). Most thyroid nodules are benign. However, a malignancy should be suspected particularly if an individual has the following risk profile: being relatively young (< 45 years of age); previous external head or neck irradiation; a predominant nodule or recent growth of a nodule, particularly if it does not alter thyroid functions; associated hoarseness and dysphagia; and a family history of medullary cancer of the thyroid (Cooper et al., 2007; Ward, Jemal, & Chen, 2010).

2. Prevalence and incidence

Thyroid nodules are common entities. The prevalence rates of nodules vary by detection method with rates of up to 50% of individuals who have had a thyroid ultrasound (Cooper et al., 2007). Most of the detected nodules are benign and are more commonly noted in women than in men (Cooper et al., 2007). With the exception of malignant nodules, thyroid nodules are more prevalent with increasing age as noted by incidence rates (Horner et al., 2006; Cooper et al., 2007). Since 1980, however, there has been a rising incidence of thyroid malignancies. The incidence rate was 2.4% per annum from 1980 to 1997, and 6.5% per annum from 1997 to 2006 (Horner et al., 2006).

II. Database (may include but is not limited to)

A. Subjective

1. Primary hypothyroidism
   a. Past health history
      i. Medical illnesses: assess for autoimmune thyroid disorders that can be associated with other autoimmune diseases, such as type 1 diabetes mellitus, pernicious anemia, rheumatoid arthritis, and systemic lupus erythematosus; and secondary hypothyroidism (low TSH and low FT_4) caused by pituitary or hypothalamic diseases (low TSH and low FT_4).
      ii. Surgical history: thyroid surgery or pituitary surgery
      iii. Obstetric and gynecological history: recent pregnancy or parturition
      iv. Trauma history: brain trauma
      v. Exposure history: radiation (e.g., radioiodine therapy or external neck irradiation)
      vi. Medication history: medications or supplements that influence hormone production (e.g., amiodarone, lithium, and iodine)
   b. Family history
      i. Thyroid diseases
      ii. Other endocrinopathies

   c. Occupational and environmental history: work-related exposures to radiation or radioactive iodine
   d. Personal and social history: iodine-deficient diet (uncommon because most regions have iodination programs)
   e. Review of systems: signs and symptoms vary depending on the degree of thyroid dysfunction. The individual with subclinical and mild hypothyroidism may be relatively asymptomatic. Persons with moderate dysfunction often notice constitutional and skin signs and symptoms. The individual with advanced disease often has multisystem symptoms.
      i. Constitutional signs and symptoms: fatigue, weight gain, or cold intolerance
      ii. Skin, hair, and nails: dry skin, puffy and doughy skin, and coarse hair or hair loss
      iii. Ear, nose, and throat: decreased hearing, hoarseness, dysphagia, or dysarthria
      iv. Cardiac: chest pain
      v. Abdomen: constipation
      vi. Genitourinary: oligomenorrhoea and menorrhagia
      vii. Musculoskeletal: joint stiffness or pain and myalgias
      viii. Neurologic: paresthesias, lethargy, less expressive at rest, depressed mood, or rarely ataxic gait

2. Hyperthyroidism
   a. Past health history
      i. Medical illnesses: Graves' disease, toxic uninodular or multinodular goiter, very rarely pituitary TSH-secreting tumor.
      ii. Surgical history: thyroid surgery
      iii. Obstetric and gynecological history: recent pregnancy or parturition
      iv. Exposure history: radiation (e.g., radioiodine therapy or external neck irradiation)
      v. Medication history: medications or supplements that influence hormone production (e.g., antithyroid drug use [propylthiouracil (PTU) or methimazole], amiodarone, lithium, exogenous thyroid hormone supplements, and iodine)
   b. Family history
      i. Thyroid diseases
      ii. Other endocrinopathies
      iii. Neuroendocrine disorders
   c. Personal and social history: a recent intake of an iodine-rich diet in an individual who previously had an iodine-deficient diet

(geographic regions that may not have iodination programs and that have limited access to iodine-containing foods are certain regions in South America, Africa, and Asia)

   d. Review of systems: signs and symptoms vary depending on the degree of thyroid dysfunction. The individual with subclinical and mild hyperthyroidism may be relatively asymptomatic. Persons with moderate dysfunction often notice constitutional signs and symptoms, palpitations, increased bowel motility, and neurologic signs and symptoms as depicted next. The individual with advanced disease often has multisystem symptomatology.

     i. Constitutional signs and symptoms: weakness, fatigue in the elderly, increased appetite, weight loss, insomnia, or heat intolerance

     ii. Skin: increased perspiration; pretibial myxedema in Graves' disease

     iii. Eyes: proptosis in Graves' disease

     iv. Ear, nose, and throat: hoarseness or dysphagia

     v. Pulmonary: dyspnea

     vi. Cardiac: chest pain or palpitations

     vii. Abdomen: increased bowel motility that often results in frequent bowel movements

     viii. Genitourinary: irregular menses or amenorrhea

     ix. Neurologic: tremors or nervousness and anxiety

3. Thyroid nodules

   a. Past health history

     i. Medical illnesses: thyroid disorders including thyroid cancer; and autoimmune disorders that may cause a nodular gland (e.g., Graves' disease)

     ii. Surgical history: thyroid surgery

     iii. Exposure history: radiation (e.g., radioiodine therapy or external head and neck irradiation)

     iv. Medication history: medications or supplements that influence hormone production (e.g., lithium and iodine)

   b. Family history: thyroid diseases including goitrous thyroid conditions and thyroid cancer

   c. Occupational and environmental history: work-related exposures to radiation or radioactive iodine

   d. Personal and social history

     i. Iodine-deficient diet or iodine-excessive diet (see primary hypothyroidism and hyperthyroidism for discussion)

     ii. Regular ingestion of dietary goitrogens (e.g., beets and turnips)

   e. Review of systems

The nodules may be nonfunctional, in which case the individual is clinically euthyroid. However, the nodules or nodular gland may be hypofunctioning (resulting in signs and symptoms consistent with hypothyroidism) or autonomously functioning (resulting in signs and symptoms of hyperthyroidism). See the previous discussion on "primary hypothyroidism" or "hyperthyroidism," respectively, if an altered thyroid hormone status is suspected.

It is important to inquire about symptoms, such as dysphagia, caused by an enlarged gland or hoarseness suggestive of malignant vocal cord infiltration (Cooper et al., 2007; Jameson & Weetman, 2008).

B. Objective

1. Physical examination findings (Table 66-1)

2. Supporting data from relevant diagnostic tests (Tables 66-2 and 66-3)

III. Assessment

A. *Determine the diagnosis (ready access to ICD-9 codes related to thyroid disorders is available at the American Thyroid Organization's [2008] website)*

1. Primary hypothyroidism

2. Hyperthyroidism

3. Thyroid neoplasms (benign or malignant)

4. Other conditions that may explain the patient's presentation

   a. Pituitary disease

   b. Hypothalamic disease

   c. Cardiovascular disease

   d. Extrathyroidal malignancy

   e. Psychiatric disorder

B. *Severity*
Assess the severity of the disease.

C. *Significance and motivation*

1. Assess the significance of the problem to the patient and significant others.

2. Determine the patient's willingness and ability to follow the treatment plan.

TABLE 66-1 Physical Examination Findings

Condition	Associated Findings (May or May Not Include)
Primary hypothyroidism	Assess
	1. Vital signs: hypothermia or bradycardia
	2. General appearance: flat affect or dull facial expressions
	3. Skin and hair: dry skin (early manifestation) to pasty, rough and spongy skin (advanced manifestation); coarse hair (early manifestation) to hair loss (advanced manifestation)
	4. Eyes: periorbital edema (late manifestation)
	5. Ears, nose, and throat: enlarged tongue (advanced manifestation)
	6. Thyroid: nonpalpable gland to a symmetrically enlarged and smooth gland to a multinodular enlarged gland
	7. Lungs: crackles (advanced manifestation)
	8. Cardiovascular: (+) S4, (+) S3, and jugular venous distention (advanced manifestations)
	9. Abdomen: diminished bowel sounds
	10. Neurologic: decreased tendon reflexes or enhanced relaxation phase, depressed mood, and inattentiveness or somnolence
Hyperthyroidism	Assess
	1. Vital signs: tachycardia
	2. General appearance: restless
	3. Skin and hair: moist and warm skin; pretibial myxedema (most suggestive of Graves' disease); or fine and very smooth hair
	4. Eyes: exophthalmus or proptosis caused by Graves' disease; or eye signs related to sympathetic hyperstimulation (lid lag, lid retraction, diminished blinking, inability to crease the eyebrows on upward stare)
	5. Thyroid: single nodule (toxic uninodular goiter); tender or painless, symmetrically enlarged gland (thyroiditis); or diffusely enlarged (Graves' disease) or thyroid bruit (Graves' disease)
	6. Lungs: crackles
	7. Cardiovascular: systolic murmur; or (+) S4, (+) S3, and jugular venous distention
	8. Abdomen: enhanced bowel sounds
	9. Neurologic: increased tendon reflexes or fine tremor of the hands and tongue
Thyroid nodules	The associated findings are contingent on the functional status of the thyroid
	1. Nonfunctional nodules: examination is only relevant for a thyroid gland with the palpable nodules
	2. Hypofunctioning multinodular gland (see the "Primary Hypothyroidism Associated Findings" section)
	3. Autonomously functioning nodules (see the "Hyperthyroidism Associated Findings" section)
	4. Lymph nodes: assess lymph nodes of the head and neck (may suggest a malignancy)

TABLE 66-2 Common Thyroid Tests

Test	Definition	Clinical Implications	Comments
Serum free T_4 (FT_4)	Measurement of the metabolically active T_4 (unbound to thyroid-binding globulin)	Decreased in primary hypothyroidism. Increased in thyrotoxicosis.	May be increased by various drugs or conditions in individuals who are clinically euthyroid.
Free T_4 index (FT_4I)	Indirect measurement of FT_4	Decreased in primary hypothyroidism. Increased in thyrotoxicosis. Aids with the diagnosis of conditions related to altered thyroid-binding globulins but with unaltered thyroid hormone secretion.	May be increased by various drugs or conditions in individuals who are clinically euthyroid.
Serum T_3	Measurement of bound and free serum levels of T_3	Increased in T_3 thyrotoxicosis.	May be increased by various drugs or conditions in individuals who are clinically euthyroid.
Highly sensitive thyroid-stimulating hormone (TSH)	Measurement of TSH, an anterior pituitary hormone that stimulates growth and function of thyroid cells	Sensitive and specific test for the initial assessment of thyroid dysfunction. Increased in primary hypothyroidism. Decreased in most forms of thyrotoxicosis.	Values may be altered by certain drugs (e.g., aspirin and lithium).
Serum anti-thyroid antibodies (e.g., anti-thyroid peroxidase antibodies [also known as antithyroid microsomal antibody], anti-thyroglobulin antibodies, and anti-TSH receptor antibodies)	Measurement of immunologic markers for autoimmune thyroid diseases	Increased anti-thyroid peroxidase antibodies and/or anti-thyroglobulin antibodies are seen in Hashimoto's thyroiditis and Graves' disease. Anti-TSH receptor antibodies thyroid stimulating immunoglobulin. (TSI) are commonly seen in persons with Graves' disease.	May be increased in clinically euthyroid individuals. An increase in anti-TSH receptor antibodies and thyroid stimulating immunoglobulin (TSI) are more reliably predictive of Graves' disease than the thyroidal peroxidase antibody test (Cooper, Greenspan, & Landenson, 2007).
Radioactive iodine uptake	Measurement of thyroid function via uptake of radioactive iodine (^{123}I) or technetium ^{99m}Tc pertechnetate (^{99m}TcO4)	Used to evaluate defects in thyroid hormone production. Low uptake of radioactive iodine noted with non–iodine-deficient hypothyroidism, thyroiditis and factitious thyrotoxicosis. Increased uptake is often seen with Graves' disease and toxic multinodular and uninodular goiter.	Variety of medications may interfere with uptake of the radioisotope. This test is usually not necessary for the basic evaluation of most thyroid disorders. Contraindications are iodine allergy, pregnancy, and lactation.
Thyroid scintiscan	Visualization of the thyroid gland via a scintillation camera after the administration of a radioactive isotope (e.g., ^{123}I or ^{99m}TcO4)	This test provides information about the structure and function of the thyroid gland. Increased uptake of the radioactive isotope is noted in a (hot) hyperfunctioning gland or nodules (e.g., Graves' disease and toxic uninodular goiter, respectively). Decreased uptake is seen in hypothyroidism or nonfunctioning (cold) nodule (e.g., thyroid cancer).	Variety of medications may interfere with uptake of the radioisotope. This test is usually not indicated for the evaluation of primary hypothyroidism. Contraindications are iodine allergy, pregnancy, or lactation.

Sources: Saxe, J. M. (2004). Thyroid diseases. In W. L. Star, L. L. Lommel, & M. T. Shannon (Eds.), *Women's primary health care: Protocols for practice* (2nd ed., pp. 10-33–10-39). San Francisco, CA: UCSF Nursing Press; Reassessed and adapted from Fischbach, F., & Dunning III, M. B. (2009). *A manual of laboratory and diagnostic tests* (8th ed.). Philadelphia, PA: Wolters Kluwer/Lippincott Williams & Wilkins; and Jameson, J. L., & Weetman, A. P. (2008). Disorders of the thyroid gland. In A. S. Fauci, E. Braunwald, D. L. Kasper, S. L. Hauser, D. L. Longo, J. L. Jameson, & J. Loscalzo (Eds.), *Harrison's principles of internal medicine* (17th ed., Chapter 335). Retrieved from http://www.accessmedicine.com/content.aspx?aID=2877285. Used with permission from the UCSF Nursing Press.

TABLE 66-3 Supporting Data from Other Relevant Diagnostics Studies*

Condition	Diagnostic Test	Results
Primary hypothyroidism	Serum sodium	Decreased (advanced disease)
	Serum cholesterol	Increased
	Complete blood count	Mild normocytic, normochromic anemia
	Electrocardiogram or echocardiogram	Changes secondary to a hypometabolic state or congestive heart failure
Thyrotoxicosis	Complete blood count	Elevated white blood count with some of the thyroid inflammatory conditions (e.g., subacute thyroiditis)
	Erythrocyte sedimentation rate	Elevated erythrocyte sedimentation rate with some of the thyroid inflammatory conditions (e.g., subacute thyroiditis)
	Electrocardiogram or echocardiogram	Changes secondary to a hypermetabolic state or congestive heart failure
Thyroid nodules	Hypofunctioning gland (see Primary Hypothyroidism)	Benign, malignant, or suspicious and indeterminate
	Hyperfunctioning gland (see Thyrotoxicosis)	
	Fine-needle aspiration biopsy	

* Not usually indicated for confirming the diagnosis of thyroid disease but rather for assessing target organ damage.

IV. Goals of clinical management

A. *Screening or diagnosing thyroid disease*
Choose a cost-effective approach for screening or diagnosing thyroid disease.

B. *Treatment*
Select a treatment plan that returns the patient to a euthyroid state in a safe and effective manner.

C. *Patient adherence*
Select an approach that maximizes patient adherence.

V. Plan

A. *Screening*
Some major authorities (e.g., American College of Physicians [1998] and the American Thyroid Association [Landenson et al., 2000]) recommend screening for high-risk populations (adults > 35 years of age, older women, individuals with autoimmune diseases or a strong family history of thyroid diseases) (U.S. Department of Health and Human Services, 2004). However, the U.S. Department of Health and Human Services and the American Academy of Family Physicians (2009) have noted that there is insufficient evidence to support routine screening for thyroid disease in adults. If the clinician determines that screening for thyroid disease is indicated for an individual, the initial screening test should be the highly sensitive TSH because it is more sensitive and specific than the FT_4 and the FT_4I (Jameson & Weetman, 2008). If the highly sensitive TSH is high or low, the clinician should use the suggested diagnostic approach in Table 66-4.

B. *Diagnostic tests*
See Tables 66-2 and 66-3 for the description of relevant diagnostic studies and Table 66-4 for the suggested approach for the assessment of thyroid dysfunction.

1. Common thyroid studies may include, but are not limited to: highly sensitive TSH, FT_4, FT_4I, T_3, serum antithyroid antibodies, radioactive iodine uptake, and thyroid scintigraphy.

2. Thyroid ultrasonography is indicated for an individual who has a neck mass of questionable thyroid origin.

3. Fine-needle aspiration is necessary to rule out a cancerous nodule.

4. Extrathyroidal diagnostic studies are warranted for assessing the status of other systems that may be impacted by altered thyroid functions (Table 66-3).

C. *Management (includes treatment, consultation, referral, and follow-up care)*

1. Primary hypothyroidism

a. Eliminate medications (e.g., lithium) or exposures (work-related radiation) that may negatively impact the thyroid gland.

TABLE 66-4 The Assessment of Thyroid Dysfunction

Order the Highly Sensitive Thyroid-Stimulating Hormone (TSH) Test		
↓	↓	↓
Normal TSH→ Are Secondary Causes of Hypothyroidism Suspected?	Increased TSH→ Order a Serum FT_4 or FT_4I	Decreased TSH → Order a Serum FT_4 or FT_4I
No → No further testing is indicated. The patient is clinically euthyroid.	Decreased FT_4 or FT_4I: primary hypothyroidism.	Increased FT_4 or FT_4I: Primary hyperthyroidism → order anti-TSH receptor antibodies. If the antibodies are elevated, the person has an autoimmune thyroid disease (e.g., Graves' disease). If the antibodies are normal, the patient probably has a nonimmune mediated form of thyrotoxicosis (e.g., toxic uninodular goiter). Consult with a physician to determine the need for a thyroid scintiscan.
Yes → Order a serum FT_4.	Increased FT_4 or FT_4I: pituitary (TSH-induced) thyrotoxicosis	Normal FT_4 or FT_4I: Subclinical hyperthyroidism or a rare form of primary hyperthyroidism called T_3 toxicosis → Does the patient have signs and symptoms consistent with thyrotoxicosis?
Decreased FT_4: Consult with a physician to determine the necessity for a thyrotropin-releasing hormone (TRH) stimulation test (a test for assessing the hypothalamic–pituitary function).	Normal FT_4: subclinical hypothyroidism → order thyroid peroxidase antibodies. If the antibodies are elevated, the person has compensated chronic Hashimoto's thyroiditis (subclinical hypothyroidism). If the antibodies are normal consult with a physician to determine the necessity for a TRH stimulation test.	Yes → Order FT_3 Increased FT_3–T_3 toxicosis. Consult with a physician to determine the need for a thyroid scintiscan. Normal → Consult with a physician for other diagnostic considerations.

Sources: Saxe, J. M. (2004). Thyroid diseases. In W. L. Star, L. L. Lommel, & M. T. Shannon (Eds.), *Women's primary health care: Protocols for practice* (2nd ed., pp. 10-33–10-39). San Francisco, CA: UCSF Nursing Press; reassessed and adapted from Fischbach, F., & Dunning III, M. B. (2009). *A manual of laboratory and diagnostic tests* (8th ed.). Philadelphia, PA: Wolters Kluwer/Lippincott Williams & Wilkins; and Jameson, J. L., & Weetman, A. P. (2008). Disorders of the thyroid gland. In A. S. Fauci, E. Braunwald, D. L. Kasper, S. L. Hauser, D. L. Longo, J. L. Jameson, & J. Loscalzo (Eds.), *Harrison's principles of internal medicine* (17th ed., Chapter 335). Retrieved from http://www.accessmedicine.com/content.aspx?aID=2877285. Used with permission from the UCSF Nursing Press.

b. Arrange a hospital admission for patients with severe cardiopulmonary compromise.

c. Begin oral replacement with L-thyroxine.

   i. Suggested dosing for a young adult without cardiac disorders: 50–100 mcg/day.

   ii. Suggested dosing for an elder or an individual with heart conditions: 25 mcg/day.

d. Increase dosage by 25–50 mcg every 4–6 weeks until the person's highly sensitive TSH is within normal parameters. The usual replacement dose is 1.6–1.7 mcg/kg/day for adults (Cooper et al., 2007).

e. Sustain a full replacement of L-thyroxine, which is usually 100–150 mcg daily.

f. Check the person's highly sensitive TSH every 6–12 months or as needed to assess the response to chronic therapy and to determine the need for any adjustment in daily doses (Slovik, 2009b).

2. Hyperthyroidism

a. Reduce the intake of iodine if thought to be a contributing factor.

b. Start the use of β-blocking agents (e.g., propranolol, 20 mg every 6 hours) to blunt the symptoms and signs of hyperthyroidism (e.g., palpitations, heat intolerance, nervousness, and tremor) (Slovik, 2009a).

c. Consult with a physician for the use and dosing of antithyroid agents (e.g., thionamide drugs, such as methimazole, PTU, or iodide). PTU should be given to pregnant women because methimazole can cause congenital defects. It is also recommended to give PTU to lactating women because methimazole is excreted in human milk. Although the thionamide drugs have an overall low rate of serious adverse effects, hepatotoxicity, vasculitis, and agranulocytosis are the most serious adverse sequelae. PTU is more likely to cause fulminant hepatic failure and vasculitis than methimazole. Cholestatic jaundice is more likely to occur with methimazole than PTU. An autoimmune agranulocytosis can occur with both agents. Iodide is usually reserved for individuals in thyroid storm and for those being prepared for thyroid surgery (Katz, 2010).

d. Refer the patient to a physician specialist for ablative therapy with radioactive agents (e.g., radioactive iodine) or subtotal thyroidectomy.

e. Facilitate a hospital admission for the person with severe cardiopulmonary compromise.

f. Assess TSH levels annually or as needed after the individual is in remission to determine the adequacy of treatment and the earliest evidence of overtreatment (evidence of hypothyroidism). If the values are abnormal, assess the FT_4 or FT_4I or serum T_3 levels. Antithyroid antibodies should also be obtained if the individual has Graves' disease. Consult with or refer to a physician for additional treatment if these tests are abnormal (Slovik, 2009a).

g. Screen and treat for osteoporosis in women with hyperthyroidism.

3. Thyroid nodules

a. Refer the patient with a solitary nodule or a dominant nodule within a multinodular gland to a physician for further diagnostic evaluation (fine-needle aspiration and possible thyroid scintigraphy) and for therapeutic interventions (e.g., L-thyroxine suppressive or replacement therapy or surgical therapy).

b. Stop goiter-producing medications (e.g., lithium).

c. Use the hypothyroidism treatment guidelines (see the "Management" section) for the person with a hypofunctioning multinodular goiter (e.g., chronic thyroiditis).

d. Use the hyperthyroidism treatment guidelines (see the "Management" section) for the individual with a toxic multinodular goiter.

D. Patient education

1. Information
Provide verbal and, preferably, written information regarding:

a. Risk reduction and screening (e.g., stress management and relapse prevention in autoimmune-mediated hyperthyroidism, and osteoporosis screening for women with hyperthyroidism).

b. The disease process, including signs and symptoms and underlying etiologies.

c. Diagnostic tests that include a discussion about preparation, cost, the actual procedures, and after-care.

d. Management (rationale, action, use, drug interactions, side effects, associated risks, and cost of therapeutic interventions; and the need for adhering to long-term treatment plans) (Saxe, 2004).

2. Counseling: preconception counseling as indicated.

VI. Self-management resources and tools

A. Patient and client education

1. American Thyroid Association

The American Thyroid Association's (2009) website has patient and client education brochures and frequently asked question documents in English and Spanish. The documents, albeit useful and accurate, have an average grade 10 reading level via the Flesch Kincaid assessment tool. Additionally, there are very few photographs, figures, or graphs to facilitate further understanding of challenging concepts.

2. Merck Source Resource Library

The Merck Source Resource Library (Krames, 2001) includes a consumer-friendly document entitled *The Thyroid Book*. The Flesch-Kincaid grade level is approximately grade 7. This educational resource includes colorful illustrations and culturally appropriate images.

B. Community support groups

1. Thyroid-Info

Thyroid-Info (2010) has support groups postings (e.g., How to start a thyroid support group: tips on creating a support organization in your area [Shomon, 2009]).

REFERENCES

American Academy of Family Physicians. (2009). *P-T. recommendations for clinical preventive services.* Retrieved from http://www.aafp.org/online/en/home/clinical/exam/p-t.html

American College of Physicians. (1998). Clinical guideline, part 1. Screening for thyroid disease. American College of Physicians. *Annals of Internal Medicine, 129*(2), 141–143.

American Thyroid Association. (2008). *ICD-9 Codes recommended to Medicare by the ATA.* Retrieved from http://www.thyroid.org/professionals/advocacy/icd9.html

American Thyroid Association. (2009). *Patients & the public.* Retrieved from http://www.thyroid.org/patients/index.html

Cooper, D. S., Greenspan, F. S., & Ladenson, P. W. (2007). The thyroid gland. In D. G. Gardner & D. Shoback (Eds.), *Greenspan's basic and clinical endocrinology* (8th ed.). Retrieved from http://www.accessmedicine.com/content.aspx?aID=2629192

Fischbach, F., & Dunning III, M. B. (2009). *A manual of laboratory and diagnostic tests* (8th ed.). Philadelphia, PA: Wolters Kluwer/Lippincott Williams & Wilkins.

Horner, M. J., Ries, L. A. G., Krapcho, M., Neyman, N., Aminou, R., Howlader, N., . . . Edwards, B. K . (2006). SEER cancer statistics review, 1975–2006. National Cancer Institute. Retrieved from http://seer.cancer.gov/csr/1975_2006

Jameson, J. L., & Weetman, A. P. (2008). Disorders of the thyroid gland. In A. S. Fauci, E. Braunwald, D. L. Kasper, S. L. Hauser, D. L. Longo, J. L. Jameson, & J. Loscalzo (Eds.), *Harrison's principles of internal medicine* (17th ed., Chapter 335). Retrieved from http://www.accessmedicine.com/content.aspx?aID=2877285

Katz, M. D. (2010). Thyroid disorders. In M. A. Chishom-Burns, T. L. Schwinghammer, B. G. Wells, P. M. Malone, J. M. Kolesar, & J. T. Dipiro (Eds.), *Pharmacotherapy: Principles & practice* (2nd ed., pp. 763–781). New York, NY: McGraw-Hill Medical.

Krames. (2001). *The thyroid book.* Retrieved from http://www.mercksource.com/pp/us/cns/cns_krames_template.jspzQzpgzEzzSzppdocszSzuszSzcnszSzcontentzSzkrameszSz1592_13zPzhtm

Ladenson, P. W., Singer, P. A., Ain, K. B., Bagchi, N., Bigos, S. T., Levy, E. G., . . . Cohen, H. D. (2000). American Thyroid Association guidelines for detection of thyroid dysfunction. *Archives Internal Medicine, 160*(11), 1573–1575.

Saxe, J. M. (2004). Thyroid diseases. In W. L. Star, L. L. Lommel, & M. T. Shannon (Eds.), *Women's primary health care: Protocols for practice* (2nd ed., pp. 10-33–10-39). San Francisco, CA: UCSF Nursing Press.

Shomon, M. (2009). *How to start a thyroid support group: Tips on creating a support organization in your area.* Retrieved from http://www.thyroid-info.com/articles/supportgroup.htm

Slovik, D. M. (2009a). Approach to the patient with hyperthyroidism. In A. H. Goroll & A. G. Mulley (Eds.), *Primary care medicine: Office evaluation and management of the adult patient* (8th ed., pp. 788–798). Philadelphia, PA: Wolters Kluwer/Lippincott Williams & Wilkins.

Slovik, D. M. (2009b). Approach to the patient with hypothyroidism. In A. H. Goroll & A. G. Mulley (Eds.), *Primary care medicine: Office evaluation and management of the adult patient* (8th ed., pp. 798–805). Philadelphia, PA: Wolters Kluwer/Lippincott Williams & Wilkins.

U.S. Department of Health and Human Services. (2004). Screening for thyroid disease: Recommendation statement. *Annals of Internal Medicine, 140*(2), 125–127.

Wang, C., & Crapo, L. M. (1997). The epidemiology of thyroid disease and implications for screening. *Endocrinology and Metabolism Clinics of North America, 26*(1), 189–218.

Ward, E. M., Jemal, A., & Chen, A. (2010). Increasing incidence of thyroid cancer: Is diagnostic scrutiny the sole explanation? *Future Oncology, 6*(2), 185–188. Retrieved from http://www.futuremedicine.com/doi/full/10.2217/fon.09.161

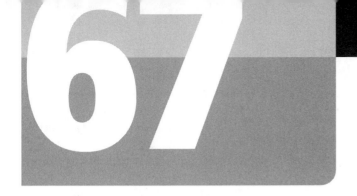

UPPER EXTREMITY TENDINOPATHY: BICIPITAL TENDINOPATHY, LATERAL EPICONDYLITIS, AND DEQUERVAIN'S TENOSYNOVITIS

Barbara J. Burgel

I. Introduction and general background

Acute and chronic injury to upper extremity tendon structures is a common health condition, often called tendinosis or tendonitis. However, the more preferred term is "tendinopathy" because the primary tendon pathology is thought to be degenerative and noninflammatory (Sharma & Maffulli, 2005). Common sites of tendinopathy in the upper extremity include the shoulder (e.g., bicipital tendinopathy); the elbow (e.g., lateral epicondylitis); and the wrist (e.g., DeQuervain's tenosynovitis).

Tendons connect muscles to bones. There are two tendon sites at risk for acute or cumulative injury. The myotendinous junction, where the muscle and tendon join, and identified as the weakest point of the muscle tendon unit (Davenport, Kulig, Matharu, & Blanco, 2005; Sharma & Maffulli, 2005); and the osteotendinous junction, the site where the tendon inserts into the bone. Strain at these sites, because of altered tendon loading from extrinsic forces or intrinsic factors, may cause inflammation to tendon sheaths and changes to the tendon cells (e.g., collagen disorganization and altered cell healing with adhesion formation) leading to tendon degeneration (Davenport et al., 2005; Sharma & Maffulli, 2005). In response to this trauma, localized pain,

warmth, swelling, and crepitus may occur in the affected region with associated functional impairment.

Mechanisms of injury include extrinsic factors, many of which are the biomechanical compressive forces, including heavy loads, repetition, overuse, awkward postures, contact stress, or cold temperature. Intrinsic factors, such as anatomy (e.g., narrowed acromium space) and excessive physical training with inadequate rest periods, also contribute to injury. Treatment with fluoroquinolones (e.g., ciprofloxacin) is associated with tendinopathy and tendon rupture, thought to be caused by inhibition of tenocyte metabolism. Tenocytes are undifferentiated fibroblasts critical to the tendon healing process (Davenport et al., 2005; Sharma & Maffulli, 2005). Psychosocial work factors, such as increased psychologic job demands, may contribute to soft tissue complaints caused by increasing speed of work, or assuming a tense posture, thereby increasing extrinsic biomechanical risks (Bongers, Ijmker, van den Heuvel, & Blatter, 2006).

A. Diagnosis: biceps tendinopathy

1. Definition and overview

   Biceps tendinopathy is defined by anterior shoulder pain, worse with overhead reaching. Tenderness is located in the bicipital groove of the humerus between the greater and lesser tuberosities, where the long head of the biceps tendon inserts at the glenoid labrum. This tendon helps to stabilize the humeral head, especially during abduction and external rotation (Durham & Chambers, 2009; van Tulder, Malmivaara, & Koes, 2007). Risk factors include

   a. Repetitive overhead motion, especially throwing sports

   b. Normal aging with degenerative changes to soft tissue and bony structures

   c. Other pathology of the rotator cuff or the labrum may contribute by placing extra force on the biceps insertion site

2. Prevalence and incidence

   In a large population-based study in the United Kingdom, the prevalence of physician-diagnosed "shoulder tendinitis" was found to be 4.5% for men and 6.1% in women, with bicipital tendinitis prevalence for both men and women documented to be 0.7% (Walker-Bone, Palmer, Reading, Coggon, & Cooper, 2004).

B. Diagnosis: lateral epicondylitis

1. Definition and overview

   Lateral epicondylitis is defined as pain in the lateral epicondyle region of the elbow, which is provoked by extension of the wrist extensors against resistance (van Tulder et al., 2007; Walker-Bone et al.,

2004). The most common risk factors for lateral epicondylitis are

    a. Repetitive and forceful movements of hands and wrists at work (Shiri, Viikari-Juntura, Varonen, & Heliovaara, 2006)

    b. High-impact sports, with force and repetition of the wrist in extension ("tennis elbow")

    c. Former or current smoking (Shiri et al., 2006)

    d. Increasing age (Shiri et al., 2006)

2. Prevalence and incidence

Physician-diagnosed lateral epicondylitis prevalence was 1.3% in a community-based sample of adults between the ages of 30 and 64 in Finland (Shiri et al., 2006). Likewise, in a large population-based study of adults in the United Kingdom, 1.3% of men and 1.1% of women were diagnosed by physical examination with lateral epicondylitis (Walker-Bone et al., 2004).

C. Diagnosis: DeQuervain's tenosynovitis

1. Definition and overview

DeQuervain's tenosynovitis is defined as pain over the radial styloid and tender swelling over the first extensor compartment, which is confirmed by pain in this location with resisted thumb extension or a positive Finkelstein's test (van Tulder et al., 2007; Walker-Bone et al., 2004). Difficulty in undoing lids on jars and bottles was reported by 28.3% of those diagnosed with DeQuervain's tenosynovitis (Walker-Bone et al., 2004). Risk factors include

    a. Repetitive, forceful, wrist or thumb motion (American College of Occupational and Environmental Medicine [ACOEM], 2004a and 2004b)

    b. Direct pressure or blunt trauma, although these are less common (ACOEM, 2004a and 2004b)

2. Prevalence and incidence

In a large population-based study in the United Kingdom, the prevalence of DeQuervain's tenosynovitis was 0.5% for men and 1.3% in women (Walker-Bone et al., 2004).

II. Database (may include but is not limited to)

A. Subjective

1. For all soft tissue complaints

    a. Past health history: any prior soft tissue complaints, any past or current workers' compensation claims

    b. Medical illnesses: inflammatory or degenerative arthritis, diabetes, or thyroid disorders

    c. Surgical history: any prior surgery to affected area

    d. Obstetric and gynecological history: current pregnancy and lactation

    e. Trauma history: acute or cumulative

    f. Medication history: nonsteroidal anti-inflammatory medication, history of cortisone injections, any allergies or sensitivity to aspirin or nonsteroidal medications

    g. Family history: arthritis, thyroid disease, or diabetes

    h. Occupational or environmental history (previous and current): work-related exposures

       i. Repetitive or awkward postures; lifting, pushing, or pulling; contact stress; vibration; or cold temperature (past and current)

       ii. Computer and telephone work: ergonomic adjustment of workstation, percent time on computer and number of keystrokes, mouse clicks, 10-key entry, and wrist rest breaks

       iii. Psychosocial work factors: psychologic demand; decision latitude; coworker or supervisor social support; rewards (esteem, respect, salary, or future job opportunities); job satisfaction; or job security

       iv. Work scheduling: number of hours worked per day and per week; overtime;

       v. Protective equipment used: splints or smart gloves, arm or wrist rests, or gloves

       vi. Coworkers with similar symptoms

       vii. Symptoms relieved on days away from work

    i. Hobbies and sports

       i. Repetitive or awkward postures; lifting, pushing, or pulling; contact stress; vibration; and cold temperature (past and current)

       ii. High-risk sports (tennis and racquetball); musical instruments; needlework (crocheting, knitting, needlepoint, or embroidery); home computer use; or motorcycling and dirt biking

    j. Personal and social history

       i. Functional impact of symptoms: assessment of activities of daily living to include dressing, bathing, shopping, housework, cooking, care-giving, and use of assistive devices

       ii. Substances: smoking and alcohol use

       iii. Sleep quality and quantity

      iv. Frequency and type of exercise (stretching and flexibility, strength, endurance conditioning, overtraining, and postural awareness)

      v. Sports: throwing or contact and racket sports, martial arts, gymnastics, or cross-training

  k. Review of systems

      i. Constitutional signs and symptoms: fatigue, fever, weight loss or gain, and night sweats

      ii. Skin, hair, and nails: erythema or warmth in affected area

      iii. Musculoskeletal: hand dominance; pain level on a 0–10 numerical or visual analogue scale; quality of pain (e.g., burning, aching, or electric shock pain); pain at rest or with activity, stiffness, limitations in motion (abrupt or chronic); presence of swelling; crepitus; locking of digits; giving way of joints; nighttime wakening with symptoms; and presence of pain in distal or proximal joints

      iv. Neurologic: paresthesias or motor weakness

B. Objective

  1. Physical examination findings

    a. Height and weight, overall conditioning

    b. General appearance, noting pain and posture

    c. Skin: erythema, bogginess, swelling, crepitus, and tenderness

    d. Musculoskeletal: bony deformity, muscle atrophy, localized tenderness and pain to palpation, anatomic distribution of pain and paresthesias, range of motion, and special maneuvers (Table 67-1)

    e. Neurologic: sensory loss mapping, motor strength, deep tendon reflexes, and special maneuvers (Table 67-1).

  2. Supporting data from relevant diagnostic tests

    a. Fasting blood sugar, hemoglobin A_{1C} (if suspect glucose impairment or diabetes)

    b. Rheumatoid factor, antinuclear antibody, erythrocyte sedimentation rate (if suspect an inflammatory rheumatologic condition)

    c. Thyroid-stimulating hormone (if suspect hypothyroidism)

    d. Radiograph (e.g., for acute trauma to rule out any underlying bony fracture)

    e. Nerve conduction studies (if suspect a peripheral nerve entrapment syndrome)

    f. Electromyogram (if suspect a cervical radiculopathy)

    g. Ultrasound (e.g., for imaging of the biceps tendon)

    h. Magnetic resonance imaging (if symptoms persist beyond 4–6 weeks of conservative treatment, and there may be a surgical intervention [e.g., a shoulder arthroscopy])

TABLE 67-1 Provocative Physical Examination Maneuvers for Selected Tendinopathy Diagnosis

Provocative Test	Diagnosis	How To
Palpation of bicipital groove	Bicipital tendinopathy	Palpate between the greater and lesser humerus tuberosities with the affected arm flexed and in 10 degrees of internal rotation
Bicipital resistance test	Bicipital tendinopathy	Shoulder flexion against resistance with elbow extended and forearm supinated produces pain for a positive test
Yergason or Speed test	Bicipital tendinopathy	Resisted supination of the wrist or with the elbow flexed at 90 degrees and the arm adducted against the body reproduces pain for a positive test
Lateral elbow palpation	Lateral epicondylitis	Palpation over the lateral epicondyle of the elbow reproduces pain for a positive test
Resisted wrist flexion	Lateral epicondylitis	Resisted extension of the wrist reproduces pain in the lateral epicondyle region for a positive test
Finkelstein's test	DeQuervain's tenosynovitis	Patient makes a fist around flexed thumb, and gently ulnar deviates the wrist. Pain is reported over the first extensor compartment (i.e., distal to the lateral aspect of radial styloid and proximal to the anatomic snuff box) for a positive test

III. Assessment

A. Determine the diagnosis based on anatomic location and mechanism of injury

1. Bicipital tendinopathy

   a. Focal tenderness over long head of biceps insertion with palpation between the greater and lesser humeral tuberosities

   b. Pain with biceps resistance test (Table 67-1)

   c. Positive Yergason or Speed test (Table 67-1)

2. Lateral epicondylitis

   a. Focal tenderness over lateral epicondyle of elbow

   b. Pain over lateral epicondyle with resisted wrist extension (Table 67-1)

3. DeQuervain's tenosynovitis

   a. Focal tenderness distal to the lateral aspect of radial styloid and proximal to the anatomic snuff box (Table 67-1)

   b. Positive Finkelstein's test (Table 67-1)

4. Other conditions that may explain the patient's presentation

   a. Referred pain from another system (e.g., Pancoast tumor in the lung with referred pain to the shoulder versus bicipital tendinopathy)

   b. Peripheral nerve entrapment (e.g., radial nerve entrapment versus lateral epicondylitis)

   c. Cervical radiculopathy (e.g., C6 radiculopathy versus DeQuervain's tenosynovitis)

   d. Other musculoskeletal conditions (e.g., acromioclavicular joint synovitis)

B. Severity

1. Assess the severity of the disease, and ability to work and do activities of daily living.

2. Assess the significance of the problem in terms of health-related quality of life and impact on productivity at work and at home.

IV. Goals of clinical management

A. Diagnosing tendinopathy

In the absence of red flags, most upper extremity soft tissue disorders can be safely diagnosed with a thorough history and physical examination. After conservative treatment for 4–6 weeks, if there is no improvement, additional diagnostic studies may be ordered or specialty referral considered.

B. Treatment

Select a treatment plan that returns the client to the preinjury functional state in a safe and timely manner.

Modify work and home activities to remove trigger events to prevent recurrence, and also protect other coworkers. Use the worksite as part of the therapeutic treatment and rehabilitation plan. Establish a plan that minimizes disability and promotes recovery.

C. Patient adherence

Emphasizes a self-care, sports medicine approach, tailoring to lifestyle and exercise patterns. Treat all work as athletic endeavors, with need for stretching and warm-up and cool-down activities.

V. Plan

A. Diagnostic tests

1. Initial laboratory and diagnostic studies

   Most initial tendinopathy work-ups do not include diagnostic studies unless there is a history of trauma.

2. Failure of conservative therapy

   After 4–6 weeks of conservative therapy, if the patient is not showing improvement, additional diagnostics are ordered.

   a. There are evidence-based imaging guidelines from the Canadian Protective Chiropractic Association for upper extremity musculoskeletal disorders (Bussieres, Peterson, & Taylor, 2008), which state that radiographs are usually not indicated when musculoskeletal pain arises from a nontraumatic origin. However, radiographs may be indicated if there has been no response to care after 4 weeks, if there is significant activity restriction beyond 4 weeks, in the presence of nonmechanical pain, or with any red flags. Red flags include

      i. History of cancer, signs or symptoms of cancer, unexplained deformity, palpable enlarging mass or swelling, or significant unexplained pain with no previous films

      ii. Red skin, fever, and systemically unwell

      iii. History of noninvestigated trauma, loss of mobility in undiagnosed condition, or loss of normal shape

      iv. Trauma, acute disabling pain, and significant weakness

      v. Unexplained significant sensory or motor deficit (Bussieres et al., 2008).

   b. See evidence-based imaging guidelines from the American College of Radiology for chronic elbow pain (Jacobson et al., 2008); for acute shoulder trauma (Steinbach et al., 2005); and for chronic wrist pain (Dalinka et al., 2005). For nontraumatic origin of pain, radiographs are the most appropriate image to order for soft tissue symptoms of more than 3 months duration.

B. Management

1. Therapeutic interventions

   For the first 4–6 weeks, if nonallergic, with normal kidney and liver function, prescribe anti-inflammatory therapeutic doses of a nonsteroidal anti-inflammatory agent, either orally or topically. Acetaminophen may additionally be added for pain control. Narcotics are rarely indicated for tendinopathy (ACOEM, 2004a and 2004b; ACOEM, 2007; van Tulder et al., 2007).

   Cortisone injections to the tendon sheath may be indicated if patient is intolerant to nonsteroidal anti-inflammatory agents, if there is one specific site of pain, or if conservative treatment is ineffective. The usual recommendation is conservative therapy for at least 3–4 weeks before cortisone injection (ACOEM, 2004a and 2004b; ACOEM, 2007; van Tulder et al., 2007). Risks of cortisone injection include not only the risk of infection, but also tendon rupture (Nichols, 2005).

2. RICE: rest, ice, compression, and elevation

   a. Relative rest: reduce or restrict any specific motion that produces symptoms by modifying work or sports activities (ACOEM, 2004a and 2004b; ACOEM, 2007; Davenport et al., 2005). There is limited evidence for rest breaks during repetitive tasks at work (e.g., 5-minute wrist rest break for every 1 hour of repetitive hand activities, or a 30-second pause for every 20 minutes of intensive work) to prevent upper extremity musculoskeletal disorders (Kennedy et al., 2010).

   b. Ice: there are consensus recommendations to use ice in the first 48 hours after initial injury to reduce inflammation and swelling, although there is currently insufficient evidence supporting this recommendation (ACOEM, 2004a and 2004b; ACOEM, 2007; van Tulder et al., 2007).

   c. Compression: compression by ace wraps, taping, splints, braces, or casting aids healing by keeping the body part in neutral position and unloading specific forces to decrease pain (Davenport et al., 2005). There are, however, risks with any compressive device, including ischemia and pressure ulcers. Likewise, prolonged immobilization may lead to muscle atrophy and joint stiffness (Boyd, Benjamin, & Asplund, 2009). Short-term splint use is recommended, with patient education to include a weaning schedule for the splint over time. Splinting during sleep prevents inappropriate wrist and thumb movements, allows for long periods of rest, and may decrease overall patient aggravation.

      i. For bicipital tendinopathy: shoulder immobilization may be indicated for 1–2 days only. Prolonged shoulder sling use could lead to a frozen shoulder (ACOEM, 2004a and 2004b; Durham & Chambers, 2009).

      ii. For lateral epicondylitis: splinting at the elbow with a dynamic extensor brace or splinting at the wrist is a consensus recommendation (although there is currently insufficient evidence) (ACOEM, 2007). In one systematic review of counterforce splinting at the elbow, there was decreased elbow pain and increased grip strength after 3 weeks of use (Burton study, as reported in Borkholder, Hill, & Fess, 2004).

      iii. For DeQuervain's tenosynovitis: a wrist and thumb splint is usually indicated during the acute treatment phase (ACOEM, 2004a and 2004b). However, in one systematic review of treatment modalities for DeQuervain's tenosynovitis, a thumb spica splint alone was the least effective treatment, with only 14% cured, whereas the most effective treatment was injection with corticosteroids (83% cure rate) (Richie & Briner, 2003).

   d. Elevation: elevation may relieve any distal swelling.

3. Referral and consultation

   a. Referral for physical or occupational therapy to aid in return to preinjury function.

      i. Ultrasound and iontophoresis are recommended as heat therapies to improve blood supply (ACOEM, 2004a and 2004b; ACOEM, 2007; van Tulder et al., 2007).

      ii. Myofascial release and soft tissue friction massage may be helpful, although there is insufficient evidence to support deep friction massage (ACOEM, 2007; Brosseau et al., 2002).

      iii. Gentle stretching during the acute treatment phase may be indicated, with introduction of a strengthening exercise program for home or work (ACOEM, 2004a and 2004b; ACOEM, 2007; Davenport et al., 2005; Kennedy et al., 2010; van Tulder et al., 2007). Postural and neuromuscular re-education is critically important to improve function and reduce pain by identifying and modifying contributing intrinsic (e.g., postural) and extrinsic (e.g., biomechanical) factors (Davenport et al., 2005).

b. Referral for ergonomic consultation to include workstation evaluation and adjustment with ergonomic training, rest breaks, new chairs, tool redesign, alternative keyboards, alternative pointing devices, and forearm and wrist supports (Kennedy et al., 2010).

c. Refer the patient to a rehabilitation or physician specialist if a more tailored rehabilitation plan or surgical intervention is needed (e.g., shoulder arthroscopy).

d. Referral for acupuncture for lateral epicondylitis may be beneficial for short-term pain relief, although there is insufficient evidence to support this recommendation (ACOEM, 2007; Green et al., 2002).

C. Client education: review

1. Self-care activities to include overall physical conditioning including stretching, core strengthening, and postural awareness. Additionally, taking intermittent rest breaks throughout any repetitive task at work and at home is important to prevent and treat tendinopathy. Reinforce that injuries of this nature generally occur over an extended period of time and that they should not expect immediate resolution of symptoms.

2. Management plan, including medication, potential side effects, and follow-up care

3. State-specific workers' compensation procedures, including any mandatory reporting, if symptoms are caused by work activities

VI. Self-management resources and tools

A. Patient and client education

1. Occupational Safety and Health Administration Ergonomics eTools

   Consumer oriented self-help tools to reduce work-related risk factors, including an eTool for baggage handling, computerized office work, and sewing

   (http://www.osha.gov/dts/osta/oshasoft/index.html#eTools)

2. Canadian Centre for Occupational Health and Safety

   (http://www.ccohs.ca/oshanswers/diseases/tendon_disorders.html)

3. Tendinopathy health education: emedicinehealth and WebMD:

   a. http://www.emedicinehealth.com/tendinitis/article_em.htm

   b. http://www.webmd.com/osteoarthritis/guide/arthritis-tendinitis

B. Community support group

There are support groups for those with repetitive strain injuries, or for those who develop chronic pain from soft tissue injuries. Contact the Alliance for Injured Workers (http://afiw.org/node/29) or the Repetitive Strain Injuries Action Group, affiliated with the Massachusetts Coalition for Occupational Safety and Health (http://www.rsiaction.org/).

REFERENCES

American College of Occupational and Environmental Medicine (ACOEM). (2004a). Shoulder complaints. In *Occupational Medicine Practice Guidelines. Evaluation and management of common health problems and functional recovery in workers* (2nd ed., Chapter 9). Elk Grove Village, IL: American College of Occupational and Environmental Medicine, 195–224.

American College of Occupational and Environmental Medicine (ACOEM). (2004b). Forearm, wrist and hand complaints. In *Occupational Medicine Practice Guidelines. Evaluation and management of common health problems and functional recovery in workers* (2nd ed., Chapter 11). Elk Grove Village, IL: American College of Occupational and Environmental Medicine, 253–285.

American College of Occupational and Environmental Medicine (ACOEM). (2007). *Elbow disorders.* Elk Grove Village, IL: American College of Occupational and Environmental Medicine. Retrieved from http://www.guideline.gov/summary/summary.aspx?doc_id=10883&nbr=005681&string=tendinopathy

Bongers, P. M., Ijmker, S., van den Heuvel, S., & Blatter, B. M. (2006). Epidemiology of work related neck and upper limb problems: Psychosocial and personal risk factors (part I) and effective interventions from a bio behavioural perspective (part II). *Journal of Occupational Rehabilitation, 16*(3), 279–302.

Borkholder, C. D., Hill, V. A., & Fess, E. E. (2004). The efficacy of splinting for lateral epicondylitis: A systematic review. *Journal of Hand Therapy, 17*(2), 181–199.

Boyd, A. S., Benjamin, H. J., & Asplund, C. (2009). Splints and casts: Indications and methods. *American Family Physician.* Retrieved from http://www.aafp.org/afp/2009/0901/p491.html

Brosseau, L., Casimiro, L., Milne, S., Welch, V., Shea, B., Tugwell, P., & Wells, G. A. (2002). Deep transverse friction massage for treating tendinitis. *Cochrane Database of Systematic Reviews, 3,* CD003528.

Bussieres, A. E., Peterson, C., & Taylor, J. A. (2008). Diagnostic imaging guideline for musculoskeletal complaints in adults—an evidence-based approach-part 2: Upper extremity disorders. *Journal of Manipulative Physiological Therapeutics, 31*(1), 2–32.

Dalinka, M. K., Daffner, R. H., DeSmet, A. A., El-Khoury, G. Y., Kneeland, J. B., Manaster, B. J., . . . Haralson, R. H. (2005). *Expert panel on musculoskeletal imaging. Chronic wrist pain.* Retrieved from http://www.guideline.gov/summary/summary.aspx?doc_id=8287&nbr=004619&string=wrist+AND+imaging

Davenport, T. E., Kulig, K., Matharu, Y., & Blanco, C. E. (2005). The EdUReP model for nonsurgical management of tendinopathy. *Physical Therapy, 85*(10), 1093–1103.

Durham, B. A., & Chambers, R. (2009). *Bicipital tendonitis.* Emedicine/Medscape. Retrieved from http://emedicine.medscape.com/article/96521-overview

Green, S., Buchbinder, R., Barnsley, L., Hall, S., White, M., Smidt, N., & Assendelft, W. (2002). Acupuncture for lateral elbow pain. *Cochrane Database of Systematic Reviews, 1,* CD003527.

Jacobson, J. A., Daffner, R. H., Weissman, B. N., Bennett, D. L., Blebea, J. S., Morrison, W. B., . . . Payne, W. K. (2008). *Expert panel on musculoskeletal imaging. ACR appropriateness criteria® chronic elbow pain.* Retrieved from http://www.guideline.gov/summary/summary.aspx?doc_id=13663

Kennedy, C. A., Amick, B. C., Dennerlein, J. T., Brewer, S., Catli, S., Williams, R., . . . Rempel, D. (2010). Systematic review of the role of occupational health and safety interventions in the prevention of upper extremity musculoskeletal symptoms, signs, disorders, injuries, claims and lost time. *Journal of Occupational Rehabilitation, 20*(2), 127–162.

Nichols, A. W. (2005). Complications associated with the use of corticosteroids in the treatment of athletic injuries. *Clinical Journal of Sports Medicine, 15*(5), 370–375.

Richie, C. A., & Briner, W. W. (2003). Corticosteroid injection for treatment of deQuervain's tenosynovitis: A pooled quantitative literature evaluation. *Journal of the American Board of Family Medicine, 16*(2), 102–106.

Sharma, P., & Maffulli, N. (2005). Tendon injury and tendinopathy: Healing and repair. *The Journal of Bone and Joint Surgery America, 87,* 187–202.

Shiri, R., Viikari-Juntura, E., Varonen, H., & Heliovaara, M. (2006). Prevalence and determinants of lateral and medical epicondylitis: A population study. *American Journal of Epidemiology, 164*(11), 1065–1074.

Steinbach, L. S., Daffner, R. H., Dalinka, M. K., DeSmet, A. A., El-Khoury, G. Y., Kneeland, J. B., . . . Haralson, R. H. (2005). *Expert panel on musculoskeletal imaging. Shoulder trauma.* Retrieved from http://www.guideline.gov/summary/summary.aspx?doc_id=8300&nbr=004632&string=shoulder+AND+imaging

Walker-Bone, K., Palmer, K. T., Reading, I., Coggon, D., & Cooper, C. (2004). Prevalence and impact of musculoskeletal disorders of the upper limb in the general population. *Arthritis and Rheumatology, 51*(4), 642–651.

van Tulder, M., Malmivaara, A., & Koes, B. (2007). Repetitive strain injury. *Lancet, 369,* 1815–1822.

WOUND CARE

Nancy A. Stotts

I. Introduction and general background

A wound is a break in the integrity of the skin. Wound healing is restoration of the functional and anatomic integrity of tissue (Lazarus et al., 1994). Wound healing occurs in all structures of the body. This chapter focuses on the skin and soft tissues. Burn wounds are not included. Healing of full-thickness wounds occurs through the processes of hemostasis, inflammation, proliferation of new tissue, and remodeling of scar tissue. Contracture also takes place when the wound is full-thickness and healing by secondary intention. Infection is the most common complication and it may occur because of contamination of the tissue with microorganisms, including tetanus. Partial-thickness wounds heal through epithelialization. Wounds are commonly divided into acute and chronic wounds.

A. Acute wounds

1. Definition and overview

   Acute wounds are those that have an abrupt onset with a short duration, recognizing that the duration is disease- or condition-specific (Lazarus et al., 1994). Surgical wounds and traumatic wounds are the most common acute wounds. Surgical wounds are deliberately made incisions. Traumatic wounds include bites, crush injuries, and lacerations. They occur abruptly, usually with significant impact and cause tissue damage. The mechanism of injury in traumatic wounds determines the extent of damage and risk of infection. The environment of the injury and the time since injury are important factors in the development of infection. A dirty environment and a significant wound that is evaluated more than 6 hours after injury is at increased risk of infection.

2. Prevalence and incidence

   In the United States, annually there are about 50 million incisions from elective surgeries and 50 million traumatic wounds (Franz et al., 2008).

B. Chronic wounds

1. Definition and overview

   Chronic wounds are those that fail to proceed through the healing process in an orderly and timely fashion to produce sustained functional and anatomic continuity (Lazarus et al., 1994). The most common types of chronic wounds are

   a. Venous ulcers: caused by chronic venous insufficiency. Most are idiopathic, although some are postthrombotic.

   b. Diabetic foot ulcers (DFU): caused by medial arteriosclerosis and neuropathy or loss of protective sensation. There are other types of neuropathic wounds (e.g., seen in persons with excess alcohol intake, spinal cord injury, and vitamin deficiency) but they are not as common as DFU. The focus here is DFU.

   c. Pressure ulcers: caused by ischemic injury as vertical pressure exceeds critical closing pressure of capillary bed or horizontal pressure results in shearing of vessels. Pressure ulcers are not addressed in this chapter because they are infrequently seen in ambulatory care.

2. Prevalence and incidence

   The prevalence of venous leg ulcers is estimated to be 1–2% of the population (Amsler, Willenberg, & Blättler, 2009). Diabetes is prevalent in approximately 7% of the United States population and the prevalence of ulcers ranges between 4 and 10% among diabetics. The incidence of ulcers is 1–4.1% and the lifetime incidence is estimated to be 25% (Wu, Driver, Wrobel, & Armstrong, 2007).

II. Database (may include but is not limited to)

A. Acute wounds

1. Subjective

   a. Past health history

      i. Medical illnesses: trauma, cardiovascular disease, or diabetes

      ii. Surgical history: recent surgery

      iii. Trauma history: recent and mechanism of injury

iv. Medication history: medications and supplements that suppress inflammation (e.g., immunosuppressive drugs and steroids, chemotherapy)

b. Family history: poor healing

c. Personal and social history: poor nutrition and such habits as tobacco, alcohol, and illicit substance use

d. Review of systems

    i. Constitutional signs and symptoms: fatigue, fever, and chills

    ii. Skin, hair, and nails: dry skin, rash, and erythema

    iii. Cardiac and circulatory: chest pain, edema, mottling, pallor, and cyanosis

    iv. Musculoskeletal: articular or nonarticular pain, swelling, and erythema

    v. Neurologic: numbness or paresthesias and gait changes

2. Objective

a. Physical examination findings (Table 68-1)

b. Supporting data from diagnostic tests (Table 68-2)

B. **Venous ulcers**

1. Subjective

a. Past medical history

    i. Medical illness: prior phlebitis; prior deep vein thrombosis or pulmonary embolus; venous disease; diabetes; end organ disease (e.g., renal failure, heart failure, or liver failure); malnutrition; pulmonary disease; prior skin ulcer; leg trauma; hypercoagulability; and varicosities

    ii. Surgical history: ligation for incompetent valves

    iii. Obstetric and gynecological history: multiple pregnancies

---

TABLE 68-1 Physical Examination Findings

Condition	Associated Findings (May or May Not Include)
Acute wounds	Assess: 1. Vital signs: increased blood pressure, increased heart rate, and signs of shock 2. Damage to underlying soft tissue, organ, bony structures, and neurovascular bundles (compartment syndromes or occult bleeding) 3. Cardiovascular and circulatory: distal mottling, pallor, coolness, cyanosis, and loss of pulses 4. Skin: tissue disrupted with open wound; note wound location, size (length, width, and depth), exudate, nature of tissue (color and consistency), odor, level of pain, uncontrolled bleeding 5. Neurologic: sensory defect caused by nerve damage from trauma, compartment syndrome, and pain
Venous ulcers	Assess: 1. Vital signs: elevated temperature 2. Skin and hair: lipodermatosclerosis, hemosiderin surrounding ulcer, stasis dermatitis, ulcer on medial lower leg (gaiter area), presence of hair and distribution 3. Cardiovascular: edema, varicosities lower extremity, and pulses (bilateral) 4. Neurologic: pain
Diabetic foot ulcer	Assess: 1. Vital signs: elevated temperature 2. General appearance: signs of poor nutrition (e.g., wasting or lethargy) 3. Skin and hair: dry fissured skin; ulcer on plantar surface of foot, dependent rubor with blanching on elevation, lack of skin hair, atrophic nails, evaluate ulcer as in acute wound calluses, and exudates* 4. Cardiovascular: presence of lower extremity pulses (dorsalis pedis and posterior tibial), presence of arterial disease in lower extremities 5. Neurologic: loss of protective sensation (use monofilament for testing), change in foot structure (Charcot), depressed mood, and inattentiveness or somnolence 6. Orthopedic: foot deformity, limited join mobility (ankles), and calluses 7. Endocrine: glycemic control

* Assess for infection with each visit and treat aggressively. Signs of infection can be subtle in the diabetic with a foot ulcer. In addition pain, as a presenting symptom, may not be present because of the loss of protective sensation. However, it may present as a change in sensation.

iv. Trauma history: leg trauma

v. Exposure history: radiation therapy

vi. Medication history: medications that influence immune function (e.g., steroids or chemotherapy)

b. Family history: maternal ulcer or varicosities

c. Occupational and environmental history: standing

d. Review of systems

i. Constitutional signs and symptoms: tired legs

ii. Musculoskeletal: neuropathy and wound-related pain (increased when dependent)

iii. Cardiac and circulatory: dependent edema

iv. Psychiatric: depressed mood

2. Objective

a. Physical examination findings (Table 68-1)

b. Supporting data from diagnostic tests (Table 68-2)

C. Diabetic ulcers

1. Subjective

a. Past health history

i. Medical illnesses: diabetes or peripheral arterial disease

ii. Surgical history: prior amputation, especially of distal lower extremity (e.g., foot or toes); alcoholism

iii. Trauma history: trauma to foot, often patient becomes aware of it with inspection because of numbness of neuropathy

iv. Medication history: medications and supplements that influence glucose control; also medications that can contribute to and precipitate nerve injury (e.g., isoniazid)

TABLE 68-2 Common Wound Care Related Tests

Test	Definition	Clinical Implications	Comments
Biopsy	Measurement of the histology and microbial invasion of the tissue.	Histology useful in differential diagnosis. Microorganisms critical to selection of appropriate antibiotic for infection.	Differential diagnosis needs to be considered in a venous ulcer that does not improve in 4 weeks of treatment. Swab culture yields false-positives and so is not useful for diagnosis.
Ankle-brachial index (ABI)	Noninvasive measure of arterial disease.	Norm = 1–1.2. ABI < 1 suggests vascular disease. Compression therapy is contraindicated with ABI < 0.7. In elderly patients, patients with diabetes mellitus, or patients with an ABI > 1.2, a toe brachial index of > 0.6 or a transcutaneous oxygen partial pressure of > 30 mm Hg near the ulcer suggests adequate arterial flow (Robson et al., 2006)	Critical to evaluate before applying compression in venous disease. If undiagnosed arterial disease is present, compression may result in ischemia and potentially result in ischemic limb and amputation.
Color duplex ultrasound scanning	Measure of vascular flow and obstruction to flow.	Used to rule out arterial disease and venous thrombosis.	
Sickle cell prep	Positive test determined by sickle appearance of red blood cells.	Can identify sickle disease or sickle cell trait	
Neuropathy testing with Semmes-Weinstein monofilament	Measurement of neuropathy using 10-g (5.07) monofilament.	Neuropathy leads to foot deformation. Lack of intact protective sensation contributes to development of ulcers in areas of high pressure, usually on plantar foot surface.	Preventive strategies include use of protective footwear to off-load high pressure areas and daily inspection of the foot for changes in temperature, color, or break in the skin. Some practitioners recommend patients wear white or light-colored socks to easily visualize drainage from foot ulcer.

b. Family history: diabetes and cardiovascular disease

c. Personal and social history: malnutrition and alcohol

d. Review of systems
   i. Skin, hair, and nails: dry or fissured skin on feet, thick nails, and calluses
   ii. Cardiac: chest pain, dyspnea, shortness of breath, and other cardiovascular symptoms
   iii. Musculoskeletal: joint stiffness or pain and myalgias
   iv. Neurologic: numbness or paresthesias, altered position sense, and depressed mood

2. Objective
   a. Physical examination findings (Table 68-1)
   b. Supporting data from diagnostic tests (Table 68-2)

III. Assessment

A. Determine the diagnosis

1. Acute wound: history of surgery or trauma

2. Chronic wound: history and underlying pathology
   a. Venous ulcers
   b. Diabetic ulcers

3. Other conditions that may explain the patient's presentation especially if failure to progress or heal with appropriate therapy or if the patient has an unusual presentation or appearance
   a. Sickle cell ulcer
   b. Arterial ulcer
   c. Pyoderma gangrenosum
   d. Cutaneous granulomatous disease
   e. Infection of bacterial or fungal origin
   f. Vasculitis
   g. Neoplasm

B. Severity

Assess the severity of the disease, especially examine for infection and limb-threatening presentation (e.g., compartment syndrome or ischemia).

C. Significance

How important is this problem to the patient and their ability to maintain their lifestyle and participate in activities of daily living (e.g., mobility or function).

D. Motivation and ability

Determine whether the patient has the ability and is willing to follow the plan that is developed by the provider with the patient.

IV. Goals of clinical management

A. Choose a cost-effective approach for diagnosing the type of wound and its severity.

B. Develop mutually acceptable goals.

C. Select a treatment plan that results in healing of the wound or palliation, if that goal is selected.

D. Develop a plan with the patient that he or she can and is willing to follow.

V. Plan

A. Screening: evaluate the wound.

B. Diagnostic tests: See Table 68-2 for common diagnostic tests

C. Management

1. Acute wounds

   a. Cleanse the wound with tap water, normal saline, or commercial cleansers. Avoid cytotoxic preparations (hydrogen peroxide, Dakin's solution, Betadine, and alcohol).

   b. Incorporate native therapies of the patient, if possible.

   c. Bite wounds and trauma wounds that are heavily contaminated should be cleansed with high-pressure irrigation (e.g., provided with #18 angiocatheter with 35-ml syringe) and monitored carefully for infection.

   d. Puncture wounds are left open to heal by secondary intention; bite wounds can be closed after cleansing with high-pressure irrigation.

   e. Close lacerations when appropriate with adhesive glue, sutures, or staples after appropriate local analgesia (see Chapter 41 for additional details) is provided. When possible avoid analgesia with epinephrine. It may result in ischemia depending on site used (i.e., ears, nose, genitalia, fingers, and toes) and slow healing.

   f. Provide an optimally moist wound bed for all wounds. The choice of dressing depends on etiology, size, location, type of tissue in wound, exudate, level of contaminations, and bioburden. Avoid wet dressings that result in maceration of tissues.

   g. Systemic prophylactic antibiotics are not a routine part of acute wound care, except for human bites, especially to the hands, and traumatic wounds, depending on the mechanism of injury.

h. Update tetanus immunization, if needed.

i. Deep traumatic wounds and those that have not improved in 2 weeks may require referral to a specialist.

2. Chronic wounds: venous ulcers

a. Compression is the mainstay of treatment for venous ulcers. Compression may be a Class 3 (most supportive) system and could be a three-layer system; four-layer system; short stretch; paste-containing bandage (Unna's boot, Duke boot); or stockings. Ulcers treated with stockings heal more effectively than with bandages (62.7% versus 46.6%) and heal faster (average time 3 weeks less with stockings). In no study did bandages perform better than compression with stockings. Pain was better controlled with stockings (Amsler et al., 2009).

b. Clean the ulcer with water, normal saline, or commercial cleanser.

c. Nonviable tissue is debrided autolytically (slowest but safest); enzymatically (e.g., Santyl® collagenase ointment); or with sharp or surgical means. Mechanical debridement is nonselective and can be painful and therefore is not recommended. Maggots may be used where other methods are contraindicated.

d. Dressings are chosen to meet goals identified during the assessment process. Goals of wound care and wound bed preparation depend on the presentation. Important parameters to assess are the presence of nonviable tissue, amount of exudate, odor, bioburden, the health of the surrounding tissue, and pain. Mitigation or control of one or all of these factors must be taken into consideration when choosing the proper dressings. Some types of dressings are transparent, foam, alginates, hydrofibers, and composite.

e. After 2 weeks of treatment, wound care is reevaluated. For ulcers that are not improving or that deteriorate, the overall plan of care is evaluated and consideration is given to adding topical antibacterial agent to the treatment. If the wound is worrisome, then weekly assessment is needed.

f. After 30 days, consideration is given to a variety of adjunctive therapies (i.e., surgical skin replacement, negative pressure therapy, electrical stimulation, radiofrequency stimulation, or ultrasound stimulation). Pharmacologic therapy is considered for those with no history of neoplasm, but generally this therapy has fallen out of favor because of the higher incidence of neoplasm reported with Regranex®.

Corrective vascular ligation or valve surgery also is considered.

g. Lifelong compression is required to prevent recurrence.

3. Chronic wounds: DFU

a. Off-loading is the mainstay of therapy in DFU. Off-loading can be accomplished with crutches, walkers, wheelchairs, custom shoes, depth shoes, shoe modifications, custom inserts, custom relief orthotics, diabetic boots, forefoot and heel relief shoes, and total contact casts. Total contact cast is the gold standard (Steed et al., 2006).

b. Nonviable tissue is debrided (see venous ulcer debridement discussion). Sharp debridement is needed for the callus that surrounds the ulcer.

c. If infection is suspected, biopsy is performed and culture is sent for aerobic and anaerobic organisms. Topical antibiotic treatment is provided if infection is confirmed with greater than or equal to 1×10^6 colony forming units per gram of tissue or any β-hemolytic streptococci. Local treatment is used because systemic antibiotics do not effectively decrease bacteria levels in granulating wounds (Steed et al., 2006).

d. Systemic antibiotics are used for infection that extends beyond the ulcer (Steed et al., 2006).

e. If osteomyelitis is suspected, differential diagnosis is made by probing the wound for bone, serial radiographs, magnetic resonance imaging, computer tomography, or radionuclide scan (Steed et al., 2006). Ideal treatment is surgical removal of the bone, followed by 2–4 weeks of antibiotics. When this is not possible, prolonged antibiotic therapy is used. Close follow-up and reevaluation of bone via the previously mentioned studies is needed.

f. Local care, including cleansing of the wound, selection of a dressing, creating and maintaining a moist environment, and use of adjunctive treatment and pharmaceutical agents, uses the same principles as for venous ulcers (see previous discussion). However, patients who fail to show improvement in the ulcer (40% or more) by 4 weeks of therapy should be reevaluated (Steed et al., 2006). It should be noted that recombinant platelet-derived growth factor (Becaplermin [Regranex®]) has been shown to be effective in treating diabetic ulcers but must be used with care in those with a history of neoplasm. Hyperbaric oxygen has been shown to be of value in reducing the amputation rate in patients with ischemic DFU.

g. In the patient with diabetes, glycemic control contributes to healing of the ulcer. All approaches that contribute to glycemic control should be considered.

h. Systemic evaluation and management of underlying diseases is pivotal to the management of the lifelong risk of diabetic ulcers (e.g., bypass to correct ischemia). The goal is to prevent loss of limb through amputation.

4. Client education

a. Patients with diabetes require lifelong management of their chronic illness and should be part of an on-going chronic illness program.

b. Referral should be made so patients and their families have information on diabetes management from experts, including ulcer management and changes in foot architecture that are part of long-term diabetes management.

VI. Self-management resources and tools

A. Patient and client education

Management of wounds and ulcers is temporal in nature. Written instruction should be provided to the patient and family specific to wound management. Management of the underlying disease in the chronic conditions of venous disease and diabetes requires patient and family education for a lifetime.

REFERENCES

Amsler, F., Willenberg, T., & Blättler, W. (2009). In search of optimal compression therapy for venous leg ulcers: a meta-analysis of studies comparing diverse [corrected] bandages with specifically designed stockings. *Journal of Vascular Surgery, 50*(3), 668–674.

Franz, M. G., Robson, M. C., Steed, D. L., Barbul, A., Brem, H., Cooper, D. M., . . . Wiersema-Bryant, L; Wound Healing Society. (2008). Guidelines to aid healing of acute wounds by decreasing impediments of healing. *Wound Repair and Regeneration, 16*(6), 723–748.

Lazarus, G. S., Cooper, D. M., Knighton, D. R., Margolis, D. J., Pecoraro, R. E., Rodeheaver, G., & Robson, M. C. (1994). Definitions and guidelines for assessment of wounds and evaluation of healing. *Archives of Dermatology, 130*(4), 489–493.

Robson, M. C., Cooper, D. M., Aslam, R., Gould, L. J., Harding, K. G., Margolis, D. J., . . . Wiersma-Bryant, L. (2006). Guidelines for the treatment of venous ulcers. *Wound Repair and Regeneration, 14*(6), 649–662.

Steed, D. L., Attinger, C., Colaizzi, T., Crossland, M., Franz, M., Harkless, L., . . . Wiersma-Bryant, L. (2006). Guidelines for the treatment of diabetic ulcers. *Wound Repair and Regeneration, 14*(6), 680–692.

Wu, S. C., Driver, V. R., Wrobel, J. S., Armstrong, D. G. (2007). Foot ulcers in the diabetic patient, prevention and treatment. *Journal of Vascular Health Risk Management, 3*(1), 65–76.

INDEX

Boxes, figures, and tables are indicated with b, f, and t following the page number.

A

AACAP. *See* American Academy of Child and Adolescent Psychiatry
AAP. *See* American Academy of Pediatrics
Abnormal cytology, 171–172, 177*f*
Abnormal uterine bleeding (AUB), 145–156
  assessment of, 146*t*, 150
  clinical management goals with, 150
  databases used for, 148–150
  diagnostic testing for, 150, 151*t*, 152
  etiologies of, 145, 146*t*
  overview of, 145, 147–148
  self-management resources and tools for, 155
  terminology of, 145, 147, 147*t*
  treatment and management of, 152–155
Abortions, spontaneous and elective, 148
Abscesses, assessment and management of, 355–359
Abuse. *See* Maltreatment of children; Physical abuse; Substance use and abuse
Acetaminophen as pain therapy, 425
Achenbach Child Behavior Checklist, 87
Acid-inhibitors
  adverse effects of, 282
  use of during pregnancy, 281–282
ACOG. *See* American College of Obstetricians and Gynecologists
Acquired Immune Deficiency Syndrome. *See* HIV-infected adults, primary care of; Postexposure prophylaxis (PEP) for HIV infection
Active vs. passive immunizations. *See* Immunizations

Acupressure wrist bands, 278
Acute bleeding, 152, 153
Acute heart failure, 448
Acute wounds, 623–624, 626–627
AD. *See* Alzheimer's disease; Atopic dermatitis
ADA. *See* American Diabetes Association
Addiction. *See* Substance use and abuse
Addiction specialists, 435
ADHD. *See* Attention-deficit/ hyperactivity disorder
Adjunctive medications, 427
Adolescence, definition of, 35
Adson test, 549*t*
Adult health maintenance and promotion, 305–351. *See also specific issues*
  developmental disabilities and, 319–335
  healthcare maintenance (HCM), 307–317
  postexposure prophylaxis for HIV infection, 343–351
  transgendered individuals and, 337–341
Adult immunizations, 45–50
Adult presentations, 353–628. *See also specific disorders*
  abscess assessment and management, 355–359
  anemia, 361–372
  anticoagulation therapy, oral, 373–385
  anxiety, 387–393
  asthma, 395–408
  benign prostatic hyperplasia (BPH), 409–416
  chronic obstructive pulmonary disease (COPD), 417–422

  congestive heart failure, 445–450
  dementia, 451–460
  depression, 461–474
  diabetes mellitus, 475–483
  epilepsy, 485–490
  gastroesophageal reflux disease (GERD), 501–507
  herpes simplex infections, 509–514
  HIV-infected adults, primary care of, 583–596
  hypertension, 515–525
  intimate partner violence (IPV), 527–535
  irritable bowel syndrome, 537–543
  low back pain (LBP), 491–500
  neck pain, 545–552
  nonmalignant pain, chronic (CNP), 423–436
  obesity, 553–565
  osteoarthritis, 567–581
  smoking cessation, 597–603
  thyroid disorders, 605–613
  upper extremity tendinopathy, 615–621
  viral hepatitis, chronic, 437–444
  wound care, 623–628
Advisory Committee on Immunization Practices, 51, 53, 54
AEDs (Antiepileptic drugs), 487, 488–489*t*
Aerobic and anaerobic wound cultures, 356
AF (Atrial fibrillation), 373, 374*t*
African Americans. *See* Ethnicity-based health issues
AGCs (Atypical glandular cells), 172, 178*f*
Ages and Stages Questionnaire (Squires & Bricker), 61

Agoraphobia, 387, 389

AIDS. *See* HIV; Postexposure prophylaxis (PEP) for HIV infection

AIDS Education and Training Centers (AETC), 595

Airway inflammation, 395

Alcohol consumption. *See also* Substance use and abuse
anxiety disorders and, 392
drug use screening and, 39
effects on INR, 375
hypertension and, 518

Allergens
asthma and, 99, 395–396, 400
atopic dermatitis and, 75–76, 81
fatigue and, 86
skin testing for, 78, 96
12–21 years, 36

Allergic rhinitis, 75, 95

Allergy & Asthma Network Mothers of Asthmatics, 102

Allergy immunotherapy, 100

Alliance for Injured Workers, 620

Alpha-hydroxy acid lotion, 81

α_2-Adrenergic agonists, 91

Alzheimer's Association, 459

Alzheimer's disease (AD), 451, 453, 456

Alzheimer's Disease Education and Referral Center, 459

AMA (American Medical Association), 41

Amenorrhea and polycystic ovary syndrome (PCOS), 157–169
assessment of, 161
clinical management goals in, 161
databases used for, 159, 161
diagnostic testing for, 161, 163–165t, 165–166
etiologies of, 159, 160–162t, 161
overview of, 157–159
physical examination findings for, 161, 162t
self-management resources and tools for, 169
treatment and management of, 166–168

American Academy of Allergy, Asthma and Immunology, 102, 403

American Academy of Child and Adolescent Psychiatry (AACAP), 88, 106, 109

American Academy of Family Physicians, 53, 267

American Academy of Orthopedic Surgeons (AAOS), 580

American Academy of Pediatrics (AAP)
Committee on Infectious Diseases, 43–44
on developmental and behavioral problems, 57–58
on healthy babies, 9
on immunizations, 43, 53
on parenting, 12
on post-NICU patients, 13, 17
on postpartum care, 255

American Academy of Rheumatology, 500

American Association for the Study of Liver Diseases, 444

American Association of Clinical Endocrinologists, 216

American Association of Diabetes Educators, 289

American Association of Family Practitioners, 12

American College of Cardiology Foundation, 445

American College of Chest Physicians, 374

American College of Nurse Midwives, 240, 267

American College of Sports Medicine, 564

American Congress of Obstetricians and Gynecologists (ACOG)
on age and genetic screening, 296
on AUB, 155
on carrier screening, 246
on cervical screening, 171–172
on hormone therapy, 212
on menopause transition, 216
on postpartum care, 255
on preeclampsia, 292
on prenatal care, 240
on sterilization, 185
on VBAC, 267

American Diabetes Association (ADA), 285, 289, 483

American Heart Association, 445, 450, 564

American Liver Foundation, 444

American Lung Association, 102, 403

American Medical Association (AMA), 41

American Pain Society, 427, 435

American Social Health Association, 514

American Society for Colposcopy and Cervical Pathology, 172

American Society for Gastrointestinal Endoscopy, 504

American Society for Reproductive Medicine, 155

American Society of Hematology, 372

American Thyroid Association, 612

American Urological Association, 411–412, 415

Ammonium lactate, 81

Amniocentesis, 295

Amphetamine salts, 89

Anaerobic and aerobic wound cultures, 356

Androgen insensitivity, 158

Anemia, 361–372
assessment of, 362t, 367–369, 369t
classification of, 361, 362t
clinical management goals with, 370, 370t
databases used for, 365–367
differentiation of, 362t
macrocytic, 364–365
microcytic, 361–363
normocytic, 363–364
overview of, 361
patient education and, 371–372
physical examination findings with, 367, 368t
pregnancy and, 263–266
screening, 27, 155
treatment of, 370–371

Anemia of chronic disease (ACD), 266, 363–364, 368–369, 371

Aneuploidy, fetal, 245–246

Anhedonia, 103

Anovulation, 148

Antepartum complications, 259

Anterior shoulder pain, 615

Anticipated early death, infants with, 15

Anticoagulation therapy. *See* Oral anticoagulant therapy (OAT)

Anticonvulsants, 427

Antidepressants, 106, 108, 390, 427, 464, 468–473t

Antiepileptic drugs (AEDs), 487, 488–489t

Antifibrinolytic agents, 154

Antihistamines, 82, 100
Antimicrobial therapy of abscesses, 356
Antiretroviral drugs (ARV) and HIV, 584–585
Antiretroviral therapy (ART) and HIV, 583–586
Anxiety, 387–393
  ADHD and, 86
  assessment of, 389
  children and adolescents and, 393
  databases used for, 388
  overview of, 387–388
  special populations and, 392–393
  treatment of, 390, 391t, 392
Anxiety Disorders Association of America, 393
Apgar scores, 10, 15, 122
Apnea
  fatigue and, 86
  in infants, 13
Apolipoprotein E4 allele, 456
Appetite suppressants, OTC, 562
Arousal disorders, 215
Arthritis. *See* Osteoarthritis (OA)
Arthritis Foundation, 580
ASC-US (Atypical squamous cells of undetermined significance), 172, 174f
Asherman syndrome, 158
Asperger syndrome, 321
Association of Asthma Educators, 403
Association of Reproductive Health Professionals, 216, 225
Asthma in adolescents and adults, 395–408
  assessment of, 397, 399
  clinical management, goals of, 399
  databases used for, 396
  diagnostic screening and testing of, 399–400, 399f
  management of, 400, 401t
  overview of, 395–396
  patient education and training in, 402–403, 402–403b
  severity and control of, 396, 397–398t
  written action plan for, 403, 404–408f
Asthma in children
  assessment of, 96
  atopic dermatitis and, 75
  classifying severity or control of, 96, 97–98t

clinical management goals in, 96
databases used for, 95–96
medication for, 99, 99t
overview of, 95
treatment and management of, 96, 99–102
Asymptomatic bacteriuria, 301–302
Atlantoaxial joints, 545
Atlanto-occipital joints, 545
Atomoxetine, 91
Atopic dermatitis (AD), 75–84
  assessment of, 79
  asthma in children and, 95
  clinical management goals in, 79–80
  conditions associated with, 78, 78f
  databases used for, 75–79
  diagnostic tests for, 78, 79t
  differential diagnoses, 79, 80f
  overview of, 75
  phases of, 76, 77f
  psychosocial and emotional support and, 83–84
  secondary opportunistic infection and, 78, 79f
  self-management of, 83
  treatment and management of, 80–83
  triggering factors for, 76, 76f
Atopic eczema. *See* Atopic dermatitis (AD)
Atrial fibrillation (AF), 373, 374t
Attention-deficit/hyperactivity disorder (ADHD), 85–94
  assessment of, 88–89
  databases used for, 86–89
  long-term issues and transition to adulthood, 93
  medications for, 89, 90t, 91–92
  overview of, 85–86
  screening tools for, 87, 87t
  treatment and management of, 89, 91–92
Attorney General opinions, 3
Atypical glandular cells (AGCs), 172, 178f
Atypical squamous cells, 172
  ASC-H, 177f
  ASC-US, 174f
AUB. *See* Abnormal uterine bleeding
Autism. *See also* Developmental delay and autism, screening for
  screening for, 57–71
  thimerosal and, 44
Autism spectrum disorders (ASD), 321

B

Babies, healthy, 9–12
Back pain. *See also* Low back pain (LBP)
  in pregnancy, management of, 274t
Back Pain Support Group, 552
Balloon distention, 573
Bariatric surgery, 563–564
Barrett's esophagus, 501
Barrier methods of contraception, 219–221, 223–224
Battering. *See* Intimate partner violence (IPV)
Beck Depression Inventory–Primary Care Version (U.S. Preventive Services Task Force), 39
Bedwetting Store, 140
Behavior Assessment System for Children (Reynolds & Kamphaus), 61
Behavior changes in adults. *See* Lifestyle changes
Benign prostatic hyperplasia (BPH), 409–416
  assessment of, 411
  clinical management, goals of, 411
  databases used for, 410–411, 415–416
  definition and overview of, 409–410
  diagnostic screening and tests for, 411, 412b, 413f
  impact index, 416
  management and treatment of, 411–413
  patient and family education on, 413–414
  symptom index, 415
Benzodiazepines, 390, 392
β_2-agonists, 400, 419–420
Beyond Blue (organization), 473
Bicipital tendinopathy, 615, 618
Bioidentical hormone therapy, 213
Biomechanical stressors, 567
Bipolar affective disorder, 103–104
Birth control. *See* Hormonal contraception; Nonhormonal contraception
Birth weight, 16, 17t
"Black box" labeling, 106
Bladder disorders. *See* Urinary incontinence (UI)
Bladder training, 230
Bladder wall muscle, 127
Bleeding
  abnormal uterine bleeding (AUB), 145–156
  acute bleeding, 152, 153

chronic anovulatory bleeding, 153
intermenstrual bleeding, 210
in postmenopause, 154–155
withdrawal bleeding, 191
Blood pressure (BP), 515, 515*t. See also*
Hypertension (HTN)
Blood thinner. *See* Oral anticoagulant
therapy (OAT)
Body mass index (BMI), 38, 553, 568
BPH. *See* Benign prostatic hyperplasia
Brain imaging, 454
Breastfeeding
bottle feeding vs., 10–11, 14,
123–124
HIV and, 594
*Brief Infant/Toddler Social Emotional
Assessment* (Briggs-Gowan), 61
Brigance Screens II (Glascoe), 61
Bronchitis, chronic. *See* Chronic
obstructive pulmonary disease
Bronchospasms, 395
Bruises on children, 114
Bupropion, 91, 598, 602
Burns on children, 114

C

Cage-Aid screening tool, 424
Calcineurin inhibitors, topical, 82
California Department of Health
Services, 44
California Developmental Disabilities
Division, 334
California Pregnancy Weight Graph,
288, 288*f*
Caloric intake and absorption,
121–122
Canadian Centre for Occupational
Health and Safety, 620
Cancer screening (all types)
recommendations, 309–310*t*
Cancer screening for cervical, vaginal,
and vulvar cancers, 171–181
abnormal cytology, management of,
172, 173–179*f*
assessment of, 179–180
Bethesda System Pap smear
classification, 172, 173*t*
cervical cancer in adolescents, 39
clinical management goals in, 180
databases used for, 179
overview of, 171–172

screening test recommendations,
309–310*t*
treatment and management of, 180
Cardiac death, sudden, 445
Cardiovascular disease (CVD). *See also*
Congestive heart failure
in children, 88
HIV and, 586
hypertension and, 520
Caregivers, 457, 459
Caregiver Strain Index, 459
Carrier screening for recessive
conditions, 246, 246*t*
Cataracts, 410
Catch-up growth, 124. *See also*
Growth trends
CBT (Cognitive behavioral therapy),
108–109, 392
CDC. *See* Centers for Disease Control
and Prevention
CDC National Center for HIV/AIDS,
Viral Hepatitis, STD and TB
Prevention, 595
Center for the Health Professions, 3
CenteringPregnancy (prenatal care
model), 249, 250*t*
Centers for Disease Control and
Prevention (CDC)
on anemia in pregnancy, 263
on asthma in children, 102
on childhood and adolescent
immunizations, 43–44
Division of Diabetes Translation, 289
on HIV/AIDS, 583, 595
on HSV infections, 514
on obesity, 553
on postexposure prophylaxis
for HIV, 343
on 12–21 years health maintenance, 41
Centers for Medicare and Medicaid
Services, 373
Cephalosporins, 83
Cerebral palsy (CP), 320–321
Cervical cancer. *See* Cancer screening for
cervical, vaginal, and vulvar cancers
Cervical spine diseases, 545–546. *See also*
Neck pain
Cesarean deliveries, 9, 267. *See also*
Vaginal birth after cesarean
(VBAC)
CHADS2 score, 373, 374*t*, 379

Chart reviews, 4
CHCs. *See* Combined hormonal
contraceptives
Chest radiographs, 96
Child abuse and neglect. *See*
Maltreatment of children
Child Abuse Prevention and Treatment
Act (PL 93-247), 111
Childbearing years, 145, 147–148
Childhood and adolescent
immunizations, 43–44
Child protective services, 111
Children. *See* Pediatric health
maintenance and promotion
Children's National Medical Center, 125
Chlamydia screening, 39
Cholesterol screening, 309–310*t*
Chorionic villus sampling, 295
Chronic anovulatory bleeding, 153
Chronic lung disease (CLD)
in infants, 13
Chronic neuropsychiatric conditions, 85
Chronic nonmalignant pain (CNP),
423–436
databases used for, 424–425,
425–426*f*
definitions and overview of,
423–424, 424*f*
diagnostic screening and tests, 425
management and treatment of, 425,
427, 430*f*, 431–435, 432–433*t*
patient education and resources on,
435
Chronic obstructive pulmonary disease
(COPD), 417–422
databases used for, 417–418
management and treatment of,
418–420, 419*t*, 421*t*, 422
overview of, 417
physical examination findings in,
418, 418*t*
spirometric testing for, 418, 418*t*
Chronic pain syndrome, 423
Chronic viral hepatitis, 437–444
assessment of, 441
databases used for, 438
diagnostic tests for, 438,
439–441*t*, 442
management and treatment of,
441–444, 441*t*
overview of, 437–438

patient education and resources on, 442t, 444

physical examination findings for, 438, 439t

Chronic wounds, 623

Cirrhosis, 437

Client education. *See* Patient and family education and resources

Clinical depression, 104

Clot risks, 373–374

CNP. *See* Chronic nonmalignant pain

Cobalamin (B₁₂ deficiency), 366–367, 369, 371

COC pills. *See* Combined oral contraceptive pills

Cognitive behavioral therapy (CBT), 108–109, 392

Cold sores. *See* Herpes simplex virus (HSV) infections

Collaborative practices, 4–5, 259–260

Colposcopic evaluation, 172

Combined hormonal contraceptives (CHCs)

assessment for, 196

COC pills, 153, 187, 190–191

contraindications to starting, 187, 188t

definition of, 187

monitoring required for, 189t

oral contraceptives, comparison of, 200–204t

transdermal patches, 191

vaginal contraceptive rings, 192

Combined oral contraceptive (COC) pills, 153–154, 187, 190–191, 196–197

Common adult presentations. *See* Adult presentations

Common obstetric presentations. *See* Obstetric presentations

Common pediatric presentations. *See* Pediatric presentations

Communication with developmentally disabled adults, 322, 324, 325–326f, 334f

Comorbidities effect on warfarin stability, 375

Complementary and alternative medicine methods, 392

Conduct disorder, 86

Congenital abnormalities and osteoarthritis, 568

Congenital hypothyroid screening of infants, 10–11

Congestive heart failure, 445–450

Conners Forms, 87

Consent, patient

adolescents and, 35

adults with developmental disabilities and, 325

for birth choice, 269, 270–271f

for HIV testing, 585

for sterilization, 185

Constipation, 541–542

Contraception. *See* Hormonal contraception; Nonhormonal contraception

Contraceptive sponges, 220

Contract breaks in opiate therapy, 434

Contraindications for stimulants, 91

Controlled substances. *See* Opiates

Controller medications, 99–100, 400

COPD. *See* Chronic obstructive pulmonary disease

Copper T 380-A intrauterine contraceptive, 221, 223–225

Cordocentesis, 295

Cortical inhibitory pathway, 127

Corticosteroids, 81–82, 574

Coumadin. *See* Oral anticoagulant therapy (OAT)

Counseling. *See* Patient and family education and resources

CP (Cerebral palsy), 320–321

CRAFFT (mnemonic), 39

Cushing syndrome, 166

Cyclooxygenase (COX)–2 selective inhibitors, 573

Cyclothymia, 103–104

Cystitis, 301–302

Cytology. *See* Abnormal cytology

D

Danazol, 154

D&C (dilation and curettage), 152, 154

Dating violence. *See* Intimate partner violence (IPV)

Defeat Diabetes Foundation, Inc., 483

Degenerative joint disease, 546

Dementia, 451–460

assessment of, 456

caregiver support and resources, 459

causes of, 451, 452t

databases used for, 452–454, 455t, 456

diagnostic tests for, 454, 456, 456t

management and treatment of, 456–458, 457t

overview of, 451–452, 452t

patient and family education, 458–459

Dementia with Lewy bodies (DLB), 452–453, 456

Denver II Developmental Screening Test (Frankenburg, Camp, & Van Natta), 61

Depression, adult, 461–474

antidepressants and, 468–471t, 472–473t

assessment of, 464–465

databases used for, 463–464, 463t

definition and overview of, 461, 463

diagnostic screening and tests, 462f, 463, 463t, 465–466

management and treatment of, 465–466, 467t

medications that may cause, 464, 465t

patient and family education on, 466, 473

in pregnancy, 273

screening test recommendations, 309–310t

Depression, childhood, 103–110

ADHD and, 86

adolescent, 39

assessment of, 105–106

databases used for, 104–105

medication for, 106, 107–108t, 108

overview of, 103–104

self-management resources in, 109

treatment and management of, 106, 108–109

Depression and Bipolar Support Alliance, 473

Depression Resource Center (AACAP), 109

DeQuervain's tenosynovitis, 616, 618

Dermatitis. *See* Atopic dermatitis (AD)

Detrusor muscle, 127

Developmental delay and autism, screening for, 57–71. *See also* Autism; Development and behavior appraisal

clinician resources for, 69–70

overview of, 57–58, 69

psychometrics, 61, 69

screening tests and tools for, 61, 62–68t

surveillance and screening algorithm for, 58–59, 59–60f, 61

Developmental Disabilities Assistance and Civil Rights Act (PL 106-402), 320

Developmental Disability Nurses Association, 334

Developmentally disabled adults, health maintenance for, 319–335

communication considerations and, 334, 334f

databases used for, 322–324

diagnostic screening and treatment, 325–326

interdisciplinary healthcare teams and, 323–324, 324f

overview and definitions of, 319–322

patient and family education and, 327–333t, 334–335

physical examination considerations and, 324, 325–326f

Developmental surveillance and screening algorithm, 58–59, 59–60f, 61

Development and behavior appraisal. *See also* Developmental delay and autism, screening for

0–3 years and, 20

3–6 years, 25–26

6–11 years, 29

infants and, 14

screening tests and tools, 57–59, 61, 62–68t, 69

Devereux Early Childhood Assessment (LeBuffe & Naglieri), 61

Dextroamphetamine, 89

DFUs (Diabetic foot ulcers), 623, 625–628

Diabetes mellitus, 475–483. *See also* Gestational diabetes mellitus

assessment of, 476–477

databases used for, 475–476

diagnosis screening and tests for, 476t, 477, 478t

foot ulcers and, 623

management and treatment of, 478–479, 478t, 479f, 480–481t, 482

overview of, 475

patient and family education on, 482–483

screening test recommendations, 309–310t

Diabetic foot ulcers (DFUs), 623, 625–628

Diagnostic and Statistical Manual for Mental Disorders (DSM-IV-TR)

on anxiety, 389

on autism spectrum disorders, 321

on childhood depression, 103–104

on dementia, 456

on depression, 461

on transgendered individuals, 337

Diagnostic screening and tests

for 0–3 years, 21, 23

for 3–6 years, 27

for 6–11 years, 31

for 12–21 years, 39

for abscesses, 356

for ADHD, 87–88

for adults, 309–310t

for amenorrhea and PCOS, 161, 163–165t, 165–166

for anemia in adults, 367–369, 368t, 370t

for anemia in children, 265f

for asthma in children, 96, 99

for atopic dermatitis, 78, 79t

for AUB, 150, 151–152t, 152–155

for benign prostatic hyperplasia, 411, 412b, 413f

for cancer, 179–180

for chronic viral hepatitis, 438, 439–441t, 442

for CNP, 425, 426f

for congestive heart failure, 447–448

for dementia, 454, 456, 456t

for depression, 61, 464–465

for developmental delay and autism, 61, 62–68t, 69

for developmentally disabled adults, 235–326, 327–333t

for diabetes in pregnancy, 286, 286f

for diabetes mellitus, 476–477, 476t

for epilepsy, 486–487

for FTT in infancy, 124

for GERD, 503–504

for HIV, 590, 591t

for hormonal contraception, 196

for HSV infections, 512

for hyperglycemia in pregnancy, 287, 287f

for hypertension, 517–518

infants and, 10–11

for intimate partner violence, 528, 530–531t, 532

for irritable bowel syndrome, 538–539, 540–541t

for low back pain, 495–496

for maltreatment in children, 118

for menopause transition, 212

for neck pain, 548–550t

for nonhormonal contraception, 224

for obesity, 556

for osteoarthritis, 570–572, 573t

for PEP and nPEP, 348, 348t

for post-NICU patients, 17

postpartum, 256–257

for preeclampsia, 292–293

pregnancy and, 239, 239b, 249, 250t

prenatal genetic, 245–247

for smoking, 600

for tendinopathy, 617t, 618

for thyroid disorders, 608–611t, 610

for transgendered individuals, 338–339

for urinary incontinence in children, 132–133t, 134, 135t, 136f

for urinary incontinence in women, 228–230, 228t

for wound care, 624–625t, 626

Diaphragm contraceptives, 220–221

Diarrhea, 539, 541–542

Diastolic dysfunction, 445

Diastolic HTN vs. elevated systolic BP (SBP), 515

Diet

diaries, 539

history and obesity, 555

interventions and patient motivation, 557, 558–560f

Differential diagnoses

for abscesses, 356

for anemia in adults, 367–369, 369t

for asthma, 96, 397

for atopic dermatitis, 79, 80f

for AUB, 145

during pregnancy, 275, 277, 278, 292

for urinary incontinence in women, 227, 228t

Dilation and curettage (D&C), 152

Diphtheria and tetanus toxoids and acellular pertussis vaccine (DTaP), 52

Disc herniation, acute, 546

Distraction test, 549*t*

DLB (Dementia with Lewy bodies), 452–453, 456

Documentation, importance of, 1, 4–5

Domestic violence. *See* Intimate partner violence (IPV)

Dopamine
    agonists, 166–167
    antagonists, 278

Down syndrome, 245–246, 321

DREAMS mnemonic (PTSD), 388

Drugs and alcohol use. *See* Substance use and abuse

DSM-IV-TR. *See Diagnostic and Statistical Manual for Mental Disorders*

DTaP vaccine, 52

Dysfunctional uterine bleeding (DUB). *See* Abnormal uterine bleeding

Dysfunctional voiding, 128

Dyslipidemia screening, 27, 31, 39

Dysmorphic features, 123

Dysthymia (minor depression), 103–104, 461

E

Eclampsia seizures, 291

ECP (Emergency contraception pill), 194–195, 198

Eczema. *See* Atopic dermatitis (AD)

Education. *See* Patient and family education and resources

eHealth Forum, 552

Elderly. *See* Older adults

Elevated systolic BP (SBP) vs. diastolic HTN, 515

EMB (endometrial biopsy), 152, 154–155

Emergency contraception pill (ECP), 194–196, 198. *See also* Hormonal contraception

Emotional or psychologic abuse, 112. *See also* Maltreatment of children

Emphysema. *See* Chronic obstructive pulmonary disease

Endocervical sampling, 172

End of life and palliative care, 448, 458–459

Endometrial biopsy (EMB), 152, 154–155

Endometrial cancer, 148

Endometrial sampling, 172

End-organ abnormalities, 158

Enuresis risoria, 128

Environmental exposures and toxins, 417

Environmental history. *See* Family and social histories

Epilepsy, 322, 485–490, 487*t*

Epilepsy Foundation, 490

Epilepsy Therapy Project, 490

Equianalgesic tables, 434

Erythropoiesis, 361

Escitalopram, 108

Esophageal carcinoma, 501

Estrogen, 145, 148, 187, 190, 212

Ethical concerns, 1, 111, 117

Ethinyl estradiol, 153

Ethnicity-based health issues
    anemia and, 363
    carrier screening and, 246, 246*t*
    cerebral palsy (CP) and, 320
    chronic viral hepatitis and, 437, 442
    congestive heart failure and, 446
    COPD and, 417
    diabetes mellitus and, 477
    HIV and, 583–584
    hypertension and, 516, 520
    intimate partner violence and, 527
    obesity and, 554
    osteoarthritis and, 567
    PCOS and, 159
    preeclampsia–eclampsia and, 291
    smoking and, 597

Exacerbations of COPD, 420, 422

Exercise. *See* Physical activity

External sphincter, 127

Eyberg Child Behavior Inventory (Eyberg & Pincus), 61

F

Failure to thrive (FTT), 116, 121–125

Fallopian tubal patency, 183

Familial transmission of depression, 103

Family and social histories
    0–3 years, 19
    3–6 years, 25
    6–11 years, 29
    12–21 years, 36–37
    abscesses and, 355
    ADHD and, 85–86, 89

    of adults, 307
    amenorrhea and PCOS, 159, 161
    of anemia in adults, 365–367
    asthma and, 95, 396
    atopic dermatitis and, 76
    AUB and, 149
    benign prostatic hyperplasia and, 410
    cancer screening and, 179
    chronic viral hepatitis and, 438
    CNP and, 424
    congestive heart failure and, 446
    COPD and, 417–418
    depression and, 103–105, 463
    of developmentally disabled, 323
    diabetes mellitus and, 286, 475–476
    epilepsy and, 486
    FTT in children and, 122
    GERD and, 502
    HIV and, 587, 589
    hormonal contraception and, 195
    HSV and, 511
    hypertension and, 516
    of infants, 10
    irritable bowel syndrome and, 538
    low back pain and, 494
    maltreatment in children and, 111, 113–114, 118
    menopause transition and, 211
    neck pain and, 547
    nonhormonal contraceptives and, 223–224
    osteoarthritis and, 568–569
    PCOS and, 159, 161
    of post-NICU patients, 15–16
    postpartum care and, 255
    pregnancy and, 238, 264
    smoking and, 599
    thyroid disorders and, 606–607
    of transgendered individuals, 338
    upper extremity tendinopathy and, 616–617
    urinary incontinence in children and, 129
    wound care and, 624–626

Family education. *See* Patient and family education and resources

Family Smoking Prevention and Tobacco Control Act (PL 111-31), 597

Family Violence Prevention Fund, 249

Fatigue. *See* Sleep

FDA. *See* U.S. Food and Drug Administration

Female condoms, 220
Female-to-male (FTM) identities, 337
FemCap contraceptives, 221
Feminization procedures, 337
Ferrous fumarate, 265
Ferrous sulfate therapy, 265
Fertility awareness methods (FAMs), 219, 222–223
Fetal fibronectin (fFN), 298
Fetal surveillance and management, 293
Fever blisters. *See* Herpes simplex virus (HSV) infections
First-trimester screening, 245
First well baby visits, 9–12
Floridex Liquid Iron Supplement, 265
Fluoxetine hydrochloride, 108
Folate (folic acid) deficiency, 263, 266, 365, 367, 369, 371
Food and Drug Administration. *See* U.S. Food and Drug Administration
Forced expiratory volume (FEV), 399, 418
Forced vital capacity (FVC), 399, 418
Formal developmental assessments, infant, 14
Fractures in children, 114
Frontotemporal dementia (FTD), 452–454, 456
FTT. *See* Failure to thrive
Functional Activities Questionnaire, 454
Functional bowel disorder. *See* Irritable bowel syndrome
Functional hypothalamic amenorrhea (FHA), 157
Functional incontinence, 227

G

Gait deformities, 570
Gallbladder disease, 276, 278–279
Gastroesophageal reflux disease (GERD), 501–507
  assessment of, 503
  clinical management goals, 503
  databases used for, 502–503
  definition and overview of, 501, 502t
  diagnostic screening and tests for, 503–504
  in infants, 14
  management and treatment of, 504, 505t, 506

patient education and resources on, 506
  pregnancy and, 278–279, 281–283
Gastrointestinal (GI) diagnosis, 501
Gastrointestinal tract during pregnancy, 276–278, 277t, 279t, 280f
GDMA1, 288–289
GDM (Gestational diabetes mellitus) in pregnancy, 285–290
Gender identity disorder. *See* Transgendered individuals, health maintenance for
General Anxiety Disorder-7 screening tool (GAD-7), 388
Generalized anxiety disorder, 387, 389
Genetics
  disorders, 321
  screening and diagnostic testing of, 245–247, 456
  transmission of depression, 103
Genital herpes, recurrent, 509, 510f
GERD. *See* Gastroesophageal reflux disease
Geriatric Depression Scale, 454, 463
Geriatrics. *See* Older adults
Gestational diabetes mellitus (GDM). *See also* Diabetes mellitus
  definition of, 475
  in pregnancy, 285–290
Giggle incontinence (enuresis risoria), 128
Glandular cells. *See* Atypical glandular cells
Glide Health Services, 427
Global Initiative for Chronic Obstructive Lung Disease (GOLD), 417, 420
Glucose challenge test (GCT), 286
Glucose intolerance, 285
Glucose tolerance test, oral (OGTT), 285–289
Goiter. *See* Thyroid disorders
Gomez criteria, 123
Gonadal dysgenesis, 158
Gonadotropin-releasing hormone agonists, 154
Gonorrhea screening, 39
Group and family therapies, 392
Growth trends
  catch-up growth, 124
  fetal, 285, 293
  FTT and, 123

infants and, 10
  placental, 276
  post-NICU patients and, 16
Gynecology. *See also specific issues*
  abnormal uterine bleeding (AUB), 145–156
  amenorrhea and polycystic ovary syndrome, 157–169
  cervical, vaginal, and vulvar cancer screening, 171–181
  hormonal contraception, 187–199
  menopause transition, 209–217
  nonhormonal contraception, 219–225
  oral contraceptives, comparison of, 200–207
  sterilization, 183–185
  urinary incontinence, 227–233

H

Haemophilus influenzae type b (Hib) vaccine, 50, 52, 314
HBV (Hepatitis B virus). *See* Chronic viral hepatitis
HCV (Hepatitis C virus). *See* Chronic viral hepatitis
Head trauma in children, 115
Healia Health Communities and Support Groups, 552
Health assessment forms, 322
Healthcare disparity, 319
Healthcare maintenance (HCM), adult, 307–317
  assessment of, 308, 308f
  databases used in, 307–308
  immunizations, 309, 311f, 312–314
  overview of, 307
  patient and family education, 314, 315–316t
  screening and secondary prevention tests, 309–310t
Health education. *See* Patient and family education and resources
Health histories
  0–3 years, 19
  3–6 years, 25
  6–11 years, 29
  12–21 years, 36
  abscesses and, 355
  ADHD in children and, 88–89
  of adults, 307

of adults with developmental disabilities, 322–323
amenorrhea and PCOS, 159
anemia and, 365–367
asthma and, 95, 396
atopic dermatitis and, 75–76
AUB and, 148–149
benign prostatic hyperplasia and, 410
cancer screening and, 179
chronic viral hepatitis and, 438
CNP and, 424
congestive heart failure and, 446
COPD and, 417
depression and, 104, 463
diabetes mellitus and, 475
epilepsy and, 486
FTT in children and, 122
GERD and, 402
HIV and, 586–587
HIV infection and, 346
hormonal contraception and, 195
HSV and, 510
hypertension and, 516
of infants, 9–10
irritable bowel syndrome and, 538
low back pain and, 491–492, 493t, 496
menopause transition and, 210–211
neck pain and, 547
obesity and, 555
osteoarthritis and, 568–569
PCOS and, 159
of post-NICU patients, 15–16
preeclampsia–eclampsia and, 291
PTB risk and, 297–298
smoking and, 599
sterilization and, 184
thyroid disorders and, 606–607
of transgendered individuals, 337–338
upper extremity tendinopathy and, 616
urinary incontinence in children and, 129
urinary tract infection and, 301–302
wound care and, 623–625
Health maintenance and promotion
in adults. *See* Adult health maintenance and promotion
in children. *See* Pediatric health maintenance and promotion
obstetric. *See* Obstetric health maintenance and promotion

Healthy People 2010 (U.S. Department of Health & Human Services), 36, 297, 553
Healthy People 2020 (U.S. Department of Health & Human Services), 553
Hearing screening
0–3 years, 11, 14, 21
3–6 years, 27
6–11 years, 31
Heartburn. *See* Gastroesophageal reflux disease (GERD)
Heart failure, 445–450
HEEADSSS (mnemonic), 37
HELLP (hemolysis, elevated liver enzymes, and low platelets) syndrome, 276–279
Hemiplegic cerebral palsy, 320
Hemoglobin
electrophoresis test, 363
and hematocrit screening, 39
Hemoglobinopathies, 263
Hemolytic anemias, 364, 369, 371
Henry J. Kaiser Family Foundation, 595
Hepatitis A (HepA) vaccine, 44, 49, 53, 55, 313–314
Hepatitis B (HepB) vaccine, 49, 52, 55, 314
Hepatitis B virus (HBV). *See* Chronic viral hepatitis
Hepatitis C virus (HCV). *See* Chronic viral hepatitis
Hepatocytes, 437
Hepcidin, 364
Herbal alternatives for menopause transition, 215
Herniated discs, 545–546
Herniated nucleus pulposus (HNP), 545
Herpes Resource Center, 514
Herpes simplex virus (HSV) infections, 83, 509–514
Herpes zoster vaccine, 48, 313
Heterosexual transmission of HIV in Africa, 583
HG (Hyperemesis gravidarum), 276
Hib vaccine, 50, 52, 314
High-fiber diets, 539, 541–542
High-grade squamous intraepithelial lesions (HSIL), 172, 176f
HIV (Human immunodeficiency virus), 583–596. *See also* Postexposure

prophylaxis (PEP) for HIV infection
assessment of, 590
databases used for, 586–587, 589–590
diagnostic screening and tests for, 590, 591t
immunizations and, 587, 588–589t
infectious fluids and, 343, 344t
management and treatment of, 588–589t, 590, 592–594t, 595
overview of, 583–586, 584t
patient and family education and resources on, 595
routes of exposure to, 343, 344t, 346
screening for, 39, 309–310t
signs and symptoms of, 349t
Hoffmann test, 549t
Hormonal contraception, 187–207
absolute and relative contraindications to, 188–190t
alternatives to oral contraception, 205–206t
assessment of, 196
clinical management goals for, 196
combined hormonal contraception (COC), 187, 189t, 190–192
contraindications to, 187
databases used for, 195–196
emergency contraception pills (ECPs), 194–195
oral contraceptives, comparison of, 187, 200–204t
overview of, 187
patient adherence, 196–198
progestin-only contraception (POP), 192, 193t, 194
treatment and management of, 196–198
Hormonal gender reassignment therapy, 338–339, 340t
Hormone therapy (HT), 210, 212
Hospital for Sick Children, 276
HPV DNA testing, 172, 179f
HPV vaccine. *See* Human papillomavirus vaccine
HSIL (High-grade squamous intraepithelial lesions), 172, 176f
HSV infections, 83, 509–514
Human immunodeficiency virus. *See* HIV
Human papillomavirus (HPV), 47, 55, 171, 312–313

Hydration and nutrition during pregnancy, 277
Hyperemesis gravidarum (HG), 276
Hyperextension and hyperflexion, 545
Hyperglycemia, 475. *See also* Diabetes mellitus
Hyperinsulinemia, fetal, 285
Hypermenorrhea, 147
Hyperprolactinemia, 157–158, 167
Hypertension (HTN), 515–525
  assessment of, 518
  classification of, 515, 515*t*
  clinical management goals for, 518
  databases used for, 515–518
  definition and overview of, 515
  diagnostic screening and tests for, 517–518, 517–518*t*
  gestational, 291–294
  management and treatment of, 518–520, 519*f*, 520–523*t*
  patient education on, 520, 524
  screening test recommendations, 309–310*t*
  substances associated with, 516, 517*t*
Hyperthyroidism, 605–607, 611–612
Hypomenorrhea, 147
Hypothalamic amenorrhea, 157, 166. *See also* Amenorrhea and polycystic ovary syndrome (PCOS)
Hypothalamic-pituitary-ovarian (HPO) axis, 145, 157
Hypothyroidism, 157
Hysterectomy, 154, 183
Hysterosalpingography, 152, 183–184
Hysteroscopy, 152, 183–184

I

IADPSGCP (International Association of Diabetes and Pregnancy Study Groups Consensus Panel), 285
IBS. *See* Irritable bowel syndrome
ICD 9 codes, 600
IFIS (Intraoperative floppy iris syndrome), 410
IgE sensitization, 75, 79, 96, 99, 395, 400
Immunizations
  0–3 years, 23
  0–6 years, 51–53, 51*f*
  3–6 years, 27
  6–11 years, 31
  7–18 years, 54–56, 54*f*

12–21 years, 36, 39
  active vs. passive, 43
  adult, 45–46*f*, 45–50, 309, 311*f*, 312–314
  childhood and adolescent, 43–44
  HIV and, 587, 588–589*t*
  infant, 11
  lag in, 39–40
  rates in the U.S., 43–44
  risks vs. benefits, 44
Immunocompromising conditions, 50, 314
Implants, contraceptive, 194, 198
IN (Intraepithelial neoplasia), 171
Inactivated poliovirus vaccine (IPV), 52, 55
Incision and drainage procedure, 357–358
Independent practices, 4
Independent reports on maltreatment of children, 117–118, 117*t*
Individuals with Disabilities Education Improvement Act, 57
Infants, healthy, 9–12
Infectious Disease Society of America, 583
Infertility, smoking and, 597
Inflammatory arthropathies, 568
Influenza vaccine, seasonal, 48, 52, 55, 100, 312
Inhaled corticosteroids (ICS), 100
Inhalers, 402, 402*b*, 419–420
Injectable progestin, 192, 197–198
Injuries, 113
INR. *See* International Normalized Ratio
Institute of Medicine, 44
Instrumental Activities of Daily Living Scale, 454
Insulin, 475, 478, 481*t*
Intellectual disability (ID), 320
Interdisciplinary healthcare teams, 323–324, 324*f*, 388
Intermenstrual bleeding, 210
International Association for the Study of Pain (IASP), 423, 435
International Association of Diabetes and Pregnancy Study Groups Consensus Panel (IADPSGCP), 285
International Children's Continence Society, 140
International Classification of Diseases–9 codes, 411, 425, 476

International Normalized Ratio (INR)
  managing variations in, 377–378, 378*t*
  variables in warfarin response, 374–376, 375–376*t*
  warfarin therapy, monitoring of, 373
International Premature Ovarian Failure Support Group, 169
Interprofessional practices, 259–260
Intimate partner violence (IPV), 527–535
  assessment of, 531, 532*t*
  clinical management goals for, 531–532
  databases used for, 528, 531, 531*t*
  diagnostic screening and tests for, 528, 530–531*t*, 532
  overview of, 527–528
  patient education and resources for, 532–533
  special risk populations for, 528, 529*t*
Intraepithelial neoplasia (IN), 171
Intraoperative floppy iris syndrome (IFIS), 410
Intrauterine contraceptives (IUCs), 219, 221–222
Intrauterine devices (IUDs), 152
Intravenous fluid therapy, 278
IPV. *See* Intimate partner violence
IPV (inactivated poliovirus) vaccine, 52, 55
Iron deficiency, 21, 367–368, 370–371
Iron deficiency anemia, 263, 264–266, 361–362, 365
Irritable bowel syndrome (IBS), 537–543
  assessment of, 538–539
  clinical management goals for, 539
  databases used for, 538
  diagnostic screening and tests for, 539, 540–541*t*
  management and treatment of, 539, 541–543, 542*t*
  overview of, 537–538
  patient and family education on, 543
Irritable Bowel Syndrome Association, 543
Irritants, asthma and, 99, 395
IUDs (Intrauterine devices), 152

J

Johns Hopkins Medical School, 414
Joint National Committee on Prevention, Detection, Evaluation, and Treatment of High Blood Pressure (JNC 7), 515

Joslin Diabetes Center, 483
Juvenile Diabetes Research Foundation International, 483

K

Kaiser Family Foundation, 41
Kaiser Permanente Chronic Pain Program and Support Group, 435

L

Labor management, preterm, 297–299
Lactational amenorrhea method (LAM), 219, 223
Lateral epicondylitis, 615–616, 618
Laughter Yoga International, 435
Laugh therapy, 425
LBP. *See* Low back pain
Lead screening
    0–3 years, 21, 22*f*
    3–6 years, 27
    6–11 years, 31
    in pregnancy, 266
Learning disabilities, screening for, 88
Left-sided heart failure, 445
Legal issues
    implications of reporting child maltreatment, 117*t*
    scope of practice, 1–5
Legislative updates, 3
Leiomyomas, 155
Levonorgestrel intrauterine system (LNG-IUS), 194, 198
Lewy bodies, dementia with (DLB), 452–453, 456
Life expectancy of adults with developmental disabilities, 319
Lifestyle changes
    for health-damaging behaviors, 308, 309*f*
    for hypertension, 518–519, 520*t*
    for menopause transition, 214
    for obesity and weight loss, 557, 561–562*t*, 562–564
    for smoking cessation, 598, 600–601
Lipid profile, 0–3 years, 21, 23
Liver diseases, 437
LNG-IUS (Levonorgestrel intrauterine system), 194, 198
Long-acting reversible contraceptives (LARC), 221

Low back pain (LBP)
    assessment of, 497
    causes of, 491, 492*t*
    databases used for, 491–492, 493*t*, 494–495, 495*t*
    diagnostic screening and tests for, 495–496
    management and treatment of, 496–498, 500
    overview of, 491, 492*t*
    patient education on, 497–498, 498–500*f*, 500
    pregnancy and, 273–276
Lower esophageal sphincter (LES), 501
Lower urinary tract symptoms (LUTS), 409
Low-grade squamous intraepithelial lesions (LSIL), 172, 175*f*
Low transverse cesarean sections (LTCS), 267
LSIL (Low-grade squamous intraepithelial lesions), 175*f*
Lucile Packard Children's Hospital, 125
Lumbopelvic pain, 273
Lung cancer, 597
Lung disease. *See* Asthma; Chronic obstructive pulmonary disease (COPD)
LUTS (Lower urinary tract symptoms), 409
Lymphadenopathy, 77

M

MacArthur Initiative on Depression and Primary Care, 473
Macrocytic anemias, 364–365, 366–367, 369
Magnetic resonance imaging (MRI), 152, 275
    for osteoarthritis, 571–572
Major depressive disorders (MDD), 103–104, 461
Male condoms, 219–220
Male-to-female (MTF) identities, 337
Maltreatment of children, 111–120. *See also specific types of abuse*
    assessment of, 117–118
    databases used for, 113–117
    independent report triggers for, 117, 117*t*
    overview of, 111–112

physical examination findings in, 114–116, 115*t*
    special considerations by age group, 114
    treatment and management of, 118–119
Mandatory reporting
    on intimate partner violence, 531
    on maltreatment of children, 117–118, 117*t*
March of Dimes, 17, 240
Masculinization procedures, 337
Maternal surveillance and management, 293
Mayo Clinic, 506
MDD (Major depressive disorder), 103–104
Mean cell volume (MCV), 362*t*, 363, 367
Measles, mumps, rubella (MMR) vaccine, 48, 52, 55, 313
Mechanical spine diseases, 545–546
Medical history. *See* Health histories
Medications. *See also* Pharmacotherapy and psychotherapy; *specific medications*
    12–21 years, 36
    as cause of depression, 464, 465*t*
    controlled substances, policies and protocols for, 427, 428–429*f*
    monitoring of, 108
    prescribing, supervision for, 4
    risks of, 106, 107*t*
    weight gain and, 555
Medroxyprogesterone acetate (MPA), 153, 155, 192
Megaloblastic anemias, 366–367, 369, 371
Menarche, 148
Mended Hearts, 450
Meningococcal vaccine, 49–50, 53, 55, 313
Menometrorrhagia, 210
Menopause transition, 209–217
    assessment of, 211–212
    clinical management goals for, 212
    clinical practice guidelines for, 216
    databases used for, 210–211
    overview of, 209–210
    self-management resources and tools for, 216
    treatment and management of, 212–216

Menorrhagia, 145, 154, 210

Menses, 145

Menstrual cycle. *See also* Amenorrhea and polycystic ovary syndrome (PCOS)

changes in, 145

disturbances in, 209, 211–212

normal, 145

regularity of, 187

Mental retardation, 320

Mental status examination (MSE), 105, 464

Metabolic syndrome, 159, 554

Methicillin-resistant Staphylococcus aureus (MRSA), 355

Methicillin-susceptible Staphylococcus aureus, 355

Metrorrhagia, 153–154

Microcytic anemias, 361–363, 365–368, 370–371

Mild cognitive impairment, 456

Mini-Mental Status Examination, 454

Minor depression (dysthymia), 103–104, 461

Mixed dementia, 451

Mixed incontinence, 227

MMR vaccine. *See* Measles, mumps, rubella vaccine

Modified Caregiver Strain Index, 459

Monophasic COCs, 153

Montreal Cognitive Assessment, 454

Mood and cognition, menopause transition and, 210, 212, 214

Morbidity and mortality

HIV and, 584

obesity and, 557

perinatal, 268–269, 291, 301, 509

Motor vehicle accidents and spine injuries, 545–546

MPA (Medroxyprogesterone acetate), 153, 155

MRI (Magnetic resonance imaging), 152

MRSA (Methicillin-resistant Staphylococcus aureus), 355

MSE (Mental status examination), 105

Müllerian abnormalities, 158

Multidisciplinary treatment teams. *See* Interdisciplinary healthcare teams

Multi-infarct dementia, 451

Musculoskeletal neck pain, acute, 545

Musculoskeletal pain in pregnancy, 273–276

differential diagnosis and management of, 273, 274*t*

"red flag" symptoms of, 273–274, 275*t*

types of, 273

Myofascial pain syndrome, 546

Myotendinous junction, 615

N

NAMS (North American Menopause Society), 212, 216

National Alliance on Mental Illness (NAMI), 393, 473

National Association for Continence (NAFC), 233

National Association of Pediatric Nurse Practitioners, 28

National Center for Health Care Technology, 267

National Center for PTSD, 393

National Diabetes Education Program, 482

National Eczema Association Support Network, 84

National Eczema Society (UK), 84

National Heart, Lung, and Blood Institute, 102, 362, 403, 450

National Institute for Diabetes, Digestive and Kidney Diseases (NIDDK), 233

National Institute for Health and Clinical Excellence (NICE), 84

National Institute of Allergy and Infectious Disease, 514

National Institute of Arthritis & Musculoskeletal & Skin Diseases, 580

National Institute of Child and Human Development, 267

National Institute of Diabetes and Digestive Kidney Diseases, 444

National Institute of Mental Health, 108

National Institutes of Health (NIH)

on anemia, 372

on BPH, 414

on dementia, 458–459

on GERD, 506

on IBS, 543

on VBAC, 267

National Jewish Medical and Research Center, 82, 84, 102

National Women's Health Information Center, 240, 334

Natural family planning (NFP), 219, 222–225

Natural remedies for gastric reflux of pregnancy, 281

Nausea and vomiting of pregnancy (NVP), 276–278

pharmacotherapy for, 279*t*

protocol for assessing and treating, 280*f*

PUQE index, 277*t*

Neck pain, 545–552

databases used for, 547–548, 547–548*t*

diagnostic screening and tests for, 549–550*t*

management and treatment of, 550–551*t*

overview of, 545–547

patient education and resources on, 549, 552

Neglect, child, 112. *See also* Maltreatment of children

Nemours Center for Child Health Media, 28

Neonatal intensive care unit (NICU), 13–18

Nerve impingement, 495*t*, 496

Neural tube defects, fetal, 263

Neurobehavioral and sensory deficits, 14

Neurogenic bladder, 227

Neurologic examinations, 494–495

Neuropsychiatric conditions and ADHD, 88

Newborn infants, 9–12

New York Health Department (NYHD), 343

New York Heart Association Functional Classification, 445

NICE (National Institute for Health and Clinical Excellence), 84

Nicotine

addictive nature of, 598

replacement products, 601–602

NICU patients, 13–18

Nocturnal enuresis, 128–129

Nonhormonal contraception, 219–225

assessment of, 224

clinical management goals for, 224

databases used for, 223–224
overview of, 219–223
treatment and management of, 224–225
Nonhormonal drugs and menopause
transition, 213
Nonmalignant pain, chronic (CNP).
See Chronic nonmalignant pain
(CNP)
Nonmechanical spine diseases, 546
Nonoccupational exposures (nPEP).
See Postexposure prophylaxis
(PEP) for HIV infection
Nonpharmacologic management of
urinary incontinence, 231t, 232t
nonpharmacologic management of
urinary incontinence, 230–231
Nonsteroidal anti-inflammatory
medications (NSAIDs),
425–426, 573
Nonstimulant medications and ADHD, 91
Normocytic anemias, 363–364, 366,
368–369, 371
Normoglycemia, 285, 288
North American Menopause Society
(NAMS), 212, 216
Novel antipsychotic medications and
weight gain, 555
Nuchal line, 545
Nuchal translucency (NT), fetal,
245–246
Nutrition
0–3 years and, 20
3–6 years, 25, 27
6–11 years, 29–30
FTT and, 121–125
infants and, 10–11, 14
menopause transition and, 216
osteoarthritis and, 577
post NICU infants and, 15–16
postpartum, 257
pregnancy and, 238–239, 251, 251t, 277
preterm labor risk and, 298
supplements use, 376
NVP. *See* Nausea and vomiting
of pregnancy

O

OAT. *See* Oral anticoagulant therapy
Obesity, 553–565
in adolescents, 38, 40
assessment of, 556–557

in children, 554
clinical management goals for, 557
databases used for, 555–556
diet interventions and, 557, 558–560f
management and treatment of, 557,
561–562f, 562–564
mental illness and, 554–555
osteoarthritis and, 568
overview of, 553–555
patient and family education and
resources on, 564
in women, 158–159
Obstetric health maintenance and
promotion, 235–260. *See also*
specific issues
genetic screening, prenatal, 245–247
medical consultation and referral
during pregnancy, 240, 247,
259–260, 260f
postpartum visits, 255–258
prenatal visits, initial, 237–243
prenatal visits, return, 249–254
Obstetric presentations. *See also*
specific issues
anemia in pregnancy, 263–266
discomforts of pregnancy, common,
273–284
genetic diagnosis, prenatal, 295–296
gestational diabetes mellitus in
pregnancy, 285–290
preeclampsia, 291–294
preterm labor management,
297–299
trial of labor vs. Vaginal birth after
cesarean, 267–272
urinary tract infection in pregnancy,
301–303
Obstructive pulmonary disease,
chronic. *See* Chronic obstructive
pulmonary disease (COPD)
Occupational exposures (PEP). *See*
Postexposure prophylaxis (PEP)
for HIV infection
Occupational Safety and Health
Administration Ergonomics
eTools, 620
OGTT (oral glucose tolerance test),
285–289
Older adults. *See also* Dementia
anxiety disorders and, 393
congestive heart failure and, 445

osteoarthritis and, 567
thyroid disorders and, 605
Oligo-ovulation, 148
Omalizumab (Xolair), 100
Open neural tube defect, fetal, 245–246
Opiates
long-acting, 433, 433t
for osteoarthritis, 573–574
policies and protocols for,
427, 428–429f
risk behaviors and, 423
short-acting, 432, 432t
Oppositional defiant disorder, 86
Oral anticoagulant therapy (OAT),
373–385
associated risks of, 373–374, 374t
dosing and follow-up in, 376, 377t
managing variations in INR,
377–378, 378t
overview of, 373
patient education and safety, 378–379,
379t, 380–384t, 384
target population for, 373, 374t
treatment duration, 374, 374t
variables in warfarin response,
374–376, 375–376t
warfarin therapy, monitoring of, 373
Oral contraceptives
comparison of, 187, 200–204t
hormonal alternatives to, 205–206t
Oral glucose tolerance test (OGTT),
285–289
Oral health
0–3 years, 20, 21
3–6 years, 27
6–11 years, 31
12–21 years, 36
developmentally disabled adults,
324, 335
Oral procedures, management of
anticoagulation during,
379, 383–384t
Oral systemic corticosteroids, 100
Osteoarthritis (OA), 567–581
assessment of, 571–572
clinical management goals for, 572
databases used for, 568–571
diagnostic screening and tests for,
572, 573t
management and treatment of,
572–575, 576t, 577–579

overview of, 567–568

patient education and resources on, 579–580

Osteophyte (bone spur) formation, 567

Osteotendinous junction, 615

Outflow tract disorders, 167–168

Ovarian disorders, 167. *See also* Amenorrhea and polycystic ovary syndrome (PCOS)

Overactive bladder, 128, 227

Overflow incontinence, 227

Overweight. *See* Obesity

P

Palliative care, 448, 458–459

Panic disorders, 387, 389

Pap smears

Bethesda System, 172, 173*t*

classifications of, 172

evaluation techniques for, 172, 174–179*f*

screening guidelines for, 171–172

Parent-child interactions

0–3 years, 19, 23

3–6 years, 25

6–11 years, 29

12–21 years, 35, 40

infants, 9–10

post-NICU patients, 16

Parent education. *See* Patient and family education and resources

Passive vs. active immunizations, 43. *See also* Immunizations

Pathologic reflux, 14

Pathophysiology, theories of for ADHD, 86

Patient and family education and resources

0–3 years, 23

3–6 years, 27

6–11 years, 31, 32*f*, 33

12–21 years, 40–41

on abscess infections, 358

on ADHD, 89, 92, 92*b*

on adult healthcare maintenance (HCM), 314, 315–316*t*

on amenorrhea and PCOS, 168–169

on anticoagulation therapy (oral), 378–379

on asthma, 100–101

on atopic dermatitis in children, 83–84

on AUB, 155

on benign prostatic hyperplasia, 413–414

on cancer, 180

on chronic viral hepatitis, 442*t*, 444

on CNP, 435

on congestive heart failure, 449

on COPD, 422

on dementia, 458–459

on depression in children, 109

on developmentally disabled adults, 334–335

on diabetes, 482–483

on epilepsy, 490

on FTT, 124–125

on GERD, 506

on HIV and PEP, 349, 595

on hormonal contraception, 196–198

on HSV infections, 512, 514

on hypertension, 520, 524

on infants, 11–12

on intimate partner violence, 532–533

on irritable bowel syndrome, 543

on low back pain, 497–498, 498*f*, 499–500*f*, 500

on maltreatment in children, 119

on menopause transition, 216

on neck pain, 549, 552

on nonhormonal contraception, 225

on obesity, 564

on osteoarthritis, 579–580

on post-NICU patients, 17

on postpartum care, 257

on pregnancy, 240, 241–242*f*, 251, 252–253*f*, 275–276, 293–294

on prenatal genetic diagnosis, 296

on smoking cessation, 600–601

on sterilization, 184–185

on tendinopathy, 620

on thyroid disorders, 612

on transgendered individuals, 339

on urinary incontinence in children, 134, 140

on urinary incontinence in women, 233

on urinary tract infection, 140

on wound care, 628

Patient consent. *See* Consent, patient

Patient Health Questionnaire–2 (PHQ-2), 461

Patient Health Questionnaire–9 (PHQ-9), 425, 462*f*, 463

Patient Health Questionnaire for Adolescents, 39

PCOS. *See* Amenorrhea and polycystic ovary syndrome

Peak Expiratory Flow Rate Monitoring, 402, 403*b*

Pediatric health maintenance and promotion. *See also specific age groups*

0–3 years, 19–23

0–6 years immunizations, 51–53

3–6 years, 25–28

6–11 years, 29–33

7–18 years immunizations, 54–56

12–21 years, 35–42

adult immunizations, 45–50

childhood and adolescent immunizations, 43–44

developmental delay and autism, screening for, 57–71

first well baby visits, 9–12

post-neonatal intensive care unit (NICU) patients, 13–18

Pediatric presentations. *See also specific disorders*

asthma, 95–102

atopic dermatitis, 85–94

attention-deficit/hyperactivity disorder (ADHD), 85–94

depression, 103–110

failure to thrive (FTT), 121–125

maltreatment, 111–120

urinary incontinence, 127–141

Pediatric psychiatric specialists, 109

Pelvic girdle pain (PGP), 273–276

Pelvic inflammatory disease (PID), 187

PEP. *See* Postexposure prophylaxis (PEP) for HIV infection

Percutaneous umbilical blood sampling, 295

Perimenopause transition, 153, 209–210

Perioperative management of anticoagulation therapy, 380–382*t*, 380*t*

Personal habits

0–3 years, 20

3–6 years, 27

6–11 years, 29–30

12–21 years, 37

adults with developmental disabilities, 323

Pertussis epidemic (2010), 44
Pervasive Developmental Disorders
    Screening Test, 61
Pessaries, 231
Petaluma Health Center, 427
Pharmacotherapy and psychotherapy
    for anxiety disorders, 390, 391t, 392
    for congestive heart failure, 448, 449t
    for dementia, 457–458
    for depression, 108–109
    for hypertension, 520, 521–523t
    for obesity, 562–563
    for PEP, 348–349, 349–351t
    for smoking cessation, 598
    for urinary incontinence, 230t, 231
Phenylketonuria (PKU) screening, 10–11
Phototherapy, 82
Physical abuse, 111–112, 114–117, 115t.
    See also Intimate partner violence
    (IPV); Maltreatment of children
Physical activity
    3–6 years, 27
    6–11 years, 31, 32f
    12–21 years, 40
    asthma and, 100
    dementia and, 458
    diabetes in pregnancy and, 288
    hypertension and, 519
    menopause transition and, 216
    obesity and, 555
    precautions for diabetes and, 478
    pregnancy and, 273, 275–276
Physical examinations
    0-3 years, 19–21
    3–6 years, 26
    6–11 years, 30
    12–21 years, 38
    for abscess assessment, 355–356
    for ADHD, 88
    for adult healthcare maintenance,
        308
    for amenorrhea and PCOS, 161, 162t
    for anemia, 264, 365–367
    for anxiety, 388
    for asthma, 95–96, 396
    for atopic dermatitis, 78
    for AUB, 149–150
    for benign prostatic hyperplasia, 411
    for bicipital tendinopathy, 617
    for cancer screening, 179
    for chronic nonmalignant pain, 425

for chronic obstructive pulmonary
        disease, 418
    for chronic viral hepatitis, 439t
    for congestive heart failure, 446–447
    for depression, 105, 463–464
    for depression in children, 105
    for developmentally disabled, 324,
        325–326f
    for diabetes mellitus, 476
    for epilepsy, 486
    for FTT in children, 123
    for GERD, 503
    for herpes simplex infections, 511
    for HIV, 589–590
    for hormonal contraception, 195–196
    for hypertension, 516–517
    infants and, 10
    for intimate partner violence,
        531, 531t
    for irritable bowel syndrome, 538
    for low back pain, 494–495
    for maltreatment in children, 114–117
    for menopause transition, 211
    for neck pain, 548t
    for nonhormonal contraception, 224
    for obesity, 556
    for osteoarthritis, 570
    for postexposure prophylaxis for HIV
        infection, 346–347
    for post-NICU patients, 16
    for postpartum visits, 256
    for preeclampsia, 292
    for pregnancy discomforts, 274–275
    for prenatal visits, 238–239, 246
    for preterm labor management, 298
    for smoking cessation, 599–600
    for thyroid disorders, 608t
    for transgendered individuals, 338
    for urinary incontinence in children,
        129, 131t
    for urinary tract infection, 302
    for wound care, 624t
Physical therapy for osteoarthritis,
    577–578
Physiologic anemia, 263
Physiologic reflux, 14
PID (Pelvic inflammatory disease), 187
Pituitary amenorrhea, 157–158, 166. See
    also Amenorrhea and polycystic
    ovary syndrome (PCOS)
Placenta accreta and previa, 268

Placental growth, 276
Planned Parenthood Federation of
    America, 185, 225
Pneumococcal polysaccharide (PPSV)
    vaccine, 48–49, 55, 313
Pneumococcal vaccine, 44, 52
Polycystic ovary syndrome (PCOS).
    See Amenorrhea and polycystic
    ovary syndrome
Polymenorrhea, 145
Polyuria, nighttime, 128
POP (progestin-only pill), 192, 197
Positive predictive value (PPV) of
    screening tests, 69
Posterior pelvic pain provocation test,
    274
Postexposure prophylaxis (PEP) for HIV
    infection, 343–351. See also HIV
    assessment of, 348
    databases used for, 343, 346
    definition and overview of, 343
    diagnostic tests for, 348, 348t
    management of, 348–349, 349–351t
    patient and family education on, 349
    risks and PEP recommendations, 343,
        344–347t
Postmenopause
    bleeding in, 154–155
    women and, 145
Postnatal growth restriction, 14
Postnatal infection, 15
Post-neonatal intensive care unit (NICU)
    patients, 13–18
Postpartum care, 255–258
Postprandial hyperglycemia, 285
Posttraumatic stress disorder (PTSD), 15,
    387, 388, 389–390, 391t
PPSV vaccine. See Pneumococcal
    polysaccharide vaccine
PPV (Positive predictive value) of
    screening tests, 69
Preeclampsia, 291–294
Pregnancy
    abuse during, 249, 250t
    anemia in, 263–266
    anxiety disorders and, 392
    AUB and, 145, 146t, 147–148,
        152–153
    consultation and referral during, 240,
        247, 259–260, 260f
    dating of, 237, 238b

depression during, 273
diagnostic testing during, 249, 250t
discomforts, 273–284
fetal evaluation, 251, 254t
gestational diabetes mellitus in, 285–290
healthcare visits, 237–243, 249–254
HIV and, 594
nutrition and, 251, 251t
patient education and counseling, 251, 252–253t
postdates, 251, 254t
smoking and, 602
urinary tract infection in, 301–303
Premature and late premature infants, 9, 13–14, 297–299
Premature ovarian failure (POF), 158
Premature Ovarian Failure Support Group, 169
Premenstrual molimina, 145
Prenatal genetic diagnosis, 295–296
Prenatal genetic screening, 245–247
Prenatal health care visits, 237–243, 249–254
Prenatal risk factors, 259–260
Preschoolers. See Pediatric health maintenance and promotion
Prescribing medications, supervision for, 4
Presenile dementia, 452–454
President's New Freedom Commission on Mental Health, 57
Pressure ulcers, 623
Preterm labor management, 297–299
Preventive services, 307, 319
Primary care, anxiety disorders and, 387
Primary hypothyroidism, 605–606, 610–611
Primary osteoarthritis, 567
Professional and ethical responsibilities, 1, 111, 117
Professional organizations, 3
Progesterone during pregnancy, 276
Progestin, 187, 190
Progestin-only contraception, 192, 194. See also Hormonal contraception
assessment for, 196
contraindications to starting, 189–190t
implants, 194
injectable, 192
levonorgestrel intrauterine system (LNG-IUS), 194

monitoring required for, 193t
POP pills, 192, 197
Progestogen therapy, 212–213
Prostate, 409. See also Benign prostatic hyperplasia (BPH)
Prostate-specific antigen (PSA), 411
Prostatic hyperplasia, benign. See Benign prostatic hyperplasia
Proteinuria, 291–292
Proton-pump inhibitors (PPIs), 282, 504
Pruritus, 76, 82
Psychoeducation and ADHD, 89
Psychological or emotional abuse. See Intimate partner violence (IPV); Maltreatment of children
Psychometrics, 61, 69
Psychosocial and emotional support
atopic dermatitis (AD) and, 83–84
postpartum care and, 255
Psychosocial assessment and support
12–21 years, 35–37, 39
atopic dermatitis in children and, 83–84
interventions, 392
Psychotherapy. See Pharmacotherapy and psychotherapy
Psychotropic medications, 104
PTB (Premature births), 297–299
PTSD. See Posttraumatic stress disorder
Puberty, 29, 31, 395
PUQE (pregnancy-unique quantification of emesis/nausea) index, 277, 277t
Purulent exudate, 355
Pyelonephritis, 274, 301–302

Q

Quad marker serum examinations, 245
Questionnaires, written, 113

R

Race. See Ethnicity-based health issues
RADAR (intimate partner violence), 531–532
Recurrent or chronic LBP, 500. See also Low back pain
Red blood cell (RBC) number, 361
Refeeding syndrome, 124
Referrals
for anxiety disorders, 392
for chronic viral hepatitis, 443

for dementia, 456
for diabetes, 482
for epilepsy, 490
for mental health and substance abuse services, 435
osteoarthritis and, 578–579
for pregnancy, 240, 247, 259–260, 260f
for tendinopathy, 619–620
Referred neck pain, 546–547
Reflex incontinence, 227
Regulations and statutes, 1–3
Regulatory agencies, 3
Reliability of screening tests, 69
Repetitive movements ("stims"), 321
Repetitive Strain Injuries Action Group, 620
Reporting, mandatory
on intimate partner violence, 531
on maltreatment of children, 117–118, 117t
Representative samples of screening tests, 69
Rescue medications, 99, 400
Respiratory diseases. See Asthma; Chronic obstructive pulmonary disease (COPD)
Respiratory syncytial virus (RSV), 15
RICE (rest, ice, compression, elevation), 619
Right-sided heart failure, 445
Rome Criteria, 537
Rotavirus vaccine (RV), 52
Rotterdam PCOS Consensus Workshop Group (2004), 159
RSV (Respiratory syncytial virus), 15
RV vaccine, 52

S

SAD PERSONS (mnemonic), 163t, 461
Safe Return program, 457
Safety
0–3 years, 23
3–6 years, 27
6–11 years, 29–31, 32f, 33
12–21 years, 37, 40
infants, 11
intimate partner violence and, 532
maltreatment of children and, 117–118
San Francisco Community Clinic Consortium Pain Clinic, 427
School-aged children, definition of, 29

Schools
    3–6 years, 27
    6–11 years, 30
    12–21 years, 37
    asthma medications and, 101–102
    outcomes for FTT children, 125
Sciatica, 494–496
Screening tests. *See also specific type*
    accuracy characteristics of, 61, 69
    standardized, 51–58
Secondary osteoarthritis, 568
Second-trimester screening, 245
Seizures. *See* Epilepsy
Seizure Tracker (website), 490
Selective serotonin reuptake inhibitors
    (SSRIs), 106, 108, 108*t*
Self-injurious behavior, 105
Self-management resources, 40–41
Senior citizens. *See* Older adults
Sensitivity of screening tests, 61
Serology tests for osteoarthritis, 572
Serotonin and serotonin-norepinephrine
    reuptake inhibitors, 390
Serum integrated screening, 245–246
Sexual abuse, 112. *See also* Maltreatment
    of children
Sexual acting out, 113
Sexual debut, 105
Sexual dysfunction, 212, 215
Sexual functioning, 210
Sexually transmitted infections (STIs),
    219, 309–310*t*
Sexual pain disorder, 215
Sexual reassignment surgeries, 337. *See
    also* Transgendered individuals,
    health maintenance for
Shingles, 44
Short-acting β-agonists (SABA), 99
Sickle cell screening, 10–11, 266
Side effects of stimulant medications, 89
Sideroblastic anemia, 363, 365, 368, 371
Simon Foundation, 233
Skin disorders. *See* Atopic dermatitis (AD)
Sleep
    0–3 years and, 20
    6–11 years, 30
    asthma and, 95, 101
    depression and, 108
    fatigue and, 86–87
    FTT and, 123
    medications and, 89

pregnancy and, 273
    urinary incontinence in children
        and, 128
Smoking. *See also* Tobacco
    asthma and, 396
    cessation of, 597–603
    COPD and, 417, 419, 422
Social and environmental risks
    0–3 years, 21
    6–11 years, 30–31
    12–21 years, 35–36, 37–38
    for asthma in children, 100
    for childhood maltreatment,
        111, 113–114
    for FTT, 121
    for major depressive disorder
        (MDD), 103
    for post-NICU patients, 15
    for suicide and self-injurious behaviors,
        105–106
    for urinary incontinence in children,
        127
Social anxiety disorder, 387, 389
Social history. *See* Family and
    social histories
Society for the Study of Behavioural
    Phenotypes, 334
Socioemotional screening tools, 61
Spastic diplegia, 320
Specific IgE immunoassay (in vitro),
    96, 99
Specificity of screening tests, 69
Spermicides, 221, 223–224
Sphincter, external, 127
Spinal disorders. *See* Low back pain
Spiritual life and menopause transition,
    216
Spirometry, 96, 399–400, 399*f*,
    418, 418*t*
Spondylosis and spondylolisthesis, 546
Spurling test, 549*t*
Squamous cells. *See* Atypical
    squamous cells
SSHADESS (mnemonic), 37
SSRIs. *See* Selective serotonin
    reuptake inhibitors
Standardized Procedures for Controlled
    Substances, 427, 428–429*t*
Standardized screening tests, 57–58
Stanford University Drug Resistance
    Database, 595

State of California Regional Center
    System, 335
State regulation of professional practice,
    1–3
Statutes and regulations, 1–3
Sterilization, 183–185
"Stims" (repetitive movements), 321
Stimulant medications and ADHD,
    89, 90*t*, 91
Stool retention and motility, 127
Stool samples, 540–541*t*
Stress
    hypertension and, 519
    urinary incontinence and, 227
Strokes
    risk factors, 373–374, 374*t*
    vascular dementia and, 451
Subacute LBP, 498. *See also*
    Low back pain
Substance use and abuse, 37, 105,
    423, 424*f*
Sudden cardiac death, 445
Sudden changes in behavior, 113
Sudden death and stimulants, 88
Suicide
    12–21 years, 37
    depression and, 105–106, 109,
        461, 463*t*
Supervision requirements, physician, 4–5
Supine active straight leg raise
    (SLR) text, 275
Surgical wounds, 623
Synovial fluid examination for
    osteoarthritis, 572
Synovial joints, 567
Syphilis screening, 39
Systolic dysfunction, 445

T

Td/Tdap vaccine. *See* Tetanus, diphtheria,
    and acellular pertussis vaccine
TE (Thromboembolism), 373–374, 379*t*
Teenagers. *See* Pediatric health
    maintenance and promotion
Tendinopathy. *See* Upper extremity
    tendinopathy
Tendinosis, 615
Tendonitis, 615
Tetanus, diphtheria, and acellular
    pertussis (Td/Tdap) vaccine,
    47, 55, 312

Tetanus prophylaxis, 356

Texas Children's Hospital, 44

Thalassemia, 266, 362–363, 363t, 365, 368, 371

T–helper CD4 lymphocytes, 583–586

Thimerosal, 44

Th1 and Th2 cytokines, 395

Thoracoabdominal trauma in children, 116

Thromboembolism (TE), 373–374

Thyroid disorders, 605–613

   assessment of, 607, 611t

   clinical management goals for, 610

   databases used for, 606–607, 608t

   diagnostic screening and tests for, 607, 609–611t, 610–612

   management and treatment of, 610–612

   overview of, 605–606

   patient and family education and resources on, 612

Thyroid nodules, 607, 612

Tic disorders, 88–89

Title V, Social Security Act, 57

Tobacco. See also Smoking

   history and politics of, 597

   mental health disorders and, 598

   smoke and asthma, 95

   smokeless and oral cancers, 597

   substance use disorders and, 598

Toddlers. See Pediatric health maintenance and promotion

TOL (trial of labor). See Vaginal birth after cesarean

Topical analgesic creams and patches, 427, 574

Toxic shock syndrome, 220

Tracheal shaving, 337

Tracking medication effects, 91–92

Transcervical tubal occlusion, 183

Transcutaneous electrical nerve stimulation, 425

Transdermal patches, 191, 197

Transgendered individuals, health maintenance for, 337–341

   gender-variant identities and, 337

   HIV and, 595

Transition from child to adult healthcare, 319–320

Transsexual individuals. See Transgendered individuals, health maintenance for

Transvaginal ultrasound (TVUS), 155

Transvestites. See Transgendered individuals, health maintenance for

Traumatic wounds, 623

Trial of labor (TOL). See Vaginal birth after cesarean

Tricyclic antidepressants, 91

Trisomies, 245–246

Tubal ligation, 183

Tuberculosis screening

   0–3 years, 21

   3–6 years, 27

   6–11 years, 31

   12–21 years, 39

TVUS (Transvaginal ultrasound), 155

Type 1 diabetes, 475. See also Diabetes mellitus

Type 2 diabetes mellitus, 286, 475, 477, 479f, 555. See also Diabetes mellitus

U

UCSF Women's Continence Center, 233

Ulcers. See Wound care

UNAIDS, 583

Underactive bladder, 128

United States Preventive Services Task Force, 263

University of California, San Francisco, 125, 595

University of Pittsburgh Medical Center, 125

Upper extremity tendinopathy, 615–621

Upper gastrointestinal tract, 501

Urge incontinence and overactive bladder, 230, 232t

Urinary diary, 228, 229t

Urinary frequency, 214. See also Urinary incontinence (UI) in women

Urinary incontinence (UI) in children, 127–141

   assessment of, 131

   clinical management goals for, 134

   databases used in, 129

   diagnostic tests for, 132–133t, 134

   medication for, 139–140t

   overview of, 127–129

   physical examination findings and, 129, 131t

   self-management resources for, 140

   treatment and management of, 134, 135t, 136f, 137–138t, 140

   voiding and elimination history and, 129

Urinary incontinence (UI) in women, 227–233

   assessment of, 229

   clinical management goals for, 229–230

   initial evaluation of, 228, 228t, 230

   nonpharmacologic treatment for, 230–231, 231–232t

   overview of, 227

   pharmacologic treatment for, 230t, 231

   self-management resources and tools for, 233

   treatment and management of, 230–233

   types of, 227, 228t

   urinary diaries and, 228, 228t, 230

Urinary tract infections (UTIs), 127, 301–303

Urogenital atrophy, 209, 211, 214

U.S. Department of Agriculture on obesity, 564

U.S. Department of Health and Human Services, 240, 583

U.S. Environmental Protection Agency, 403

U.S. Food and Drug Administration (FDA), 106, 109, 183, 365, 597

U.S. HIV/AIDS Gateway for Federal/ Domestic AIDS, 595

U.S. Preventive Services Task Force (USPSTF), 307, 461, 465, 528

U.S. Public Health Service, 43–44, 343

U.S. Surgeon General, 57, 597

Uterine bleeding. See Abnormal uterine bleeding (AUB)

Uterine ruptures, 267–268

UTIs (Urinary tract infections), 127, 301–303

V

Vaccinations. See Immunizations

Vaccine Adverse Event Reporting System (VAERS), 44–45, 54

Vaccine Injury Compensation Program, 45

Vaccine-preventable diseases, 43

Vaginal birth after cesarean (VBAC), 267–272
  patient information and consent, 269, 270–271*f*
  relative contraindications for, 268*t*
  success factors in, 269, 269*t*
  success rates of, 267, 268*t*
Vaginal cancer. *See* Cancer screening for cervical, vaginal, and vulvar cancers
Vaginal contraceptive rings, 192, 197
Vaginal deliveries, 9
Vaginal reflux and postvoid dribbling, 128
Vaginal trauma in children, 116
Vancouver Coastal Health Clinic, 339
Varenicline, 598, 602
Varicella vaccine, 47–48, 52–53, 55, 312
Vascular dementia, 451, 453, 456
Vasectomy, 184
Vasomotor symptoms, 209, 211, 212
VBAC. *See* Vaginal birth after cesarean
Venous ulcers, 623–624, 627
Vertebral compression fractures, 546
Veterans Health Administration System, 585
Viral hepatitis, chronic. *See* Chronic viral hepatitis
Viscosupplementation, 575, 576*t*
Vision screening
  0–3 years, 21
  3–6 years, 27

6–11 years, 31
  infants and, 14
Vitamin B$_{12}$ deficiency, 364–365, 366–367, 369, 371
Vitamin K antagonists, 373–375, 375*t*. *See also* Oral anticoagulant therapy (OAT)
Voiding
  elimination history and, 129, 130*t*
  postponement of, 128
  process of, 127
Vulnerable child syndrome, 15
Vulvar cancer. *See* Cancer screening for cervical, vaginal, and vulvar cancers

W

Warfarin therapy. *See also* Oral anticoagulant therapy (OAT)
  drug and nutritional supplement interactions with, 375–376, 375–376*t*
  management of, 376, 377*t*
  patient education and safety with, 378–379
  variables affecting stability of, 377
Waterlow criteria, 123
Weight changes, unintentional, 104, 108
Weight Control Information Network, 579

Weight loss
  congestive heart failure and, 448
  dieting history and, 555
  hypertension and, 518
  management programs for, 563
  osteoarthritis and, 575, 577
  urinary incontinence in women and, 230
Weight-to-age ratio, 123
WeightWatchers, 579
Well babies visits, 9–12
Wernicke encephalopathy, 278
Wet-wrap dressings, 82
Whickham survey, 605
Whiplash, 545
Withdrawal bleeding, 191
Women. *See also* Pregnancy
  HIV and, 594–595
  obesity in, 158–159
  urinary incontinence. *See* Urinary incontinence (UI) in women
Women's Health Initiative, 212
Workplace modification during pregnancy, 273, 275
World College of Gastroenterology, 537
World Health Organization (WHO), 187, 361, 461, 515
  Reproductive Health Library, 595
Wound care, 623–628

Z

Zoster vaccine, 44